Breast Surgery

Juarez M. Avelar
Editor

Breast Surgery

Aesthetic Approaches

Springer

Editor
Juarez M. Avelar
São Paulo, SP
Brazil

ISBN 978-3-030-09610-6 ISBN 978-3-319-54115-0 (eBook)
https://doi.org/10.1007/978-3-319-54115-0

Softcover re-print of the Hardcover 1st edition 2018

Printed on acid-free paper

This Springer imprint is published by Springer Nature
The registered company is Springer International Publishing AG
The registered company address is: Gewerbestrasse 11, 6330 Cham, Switzerland

Tribute to Prof. Ivo Pitanguy

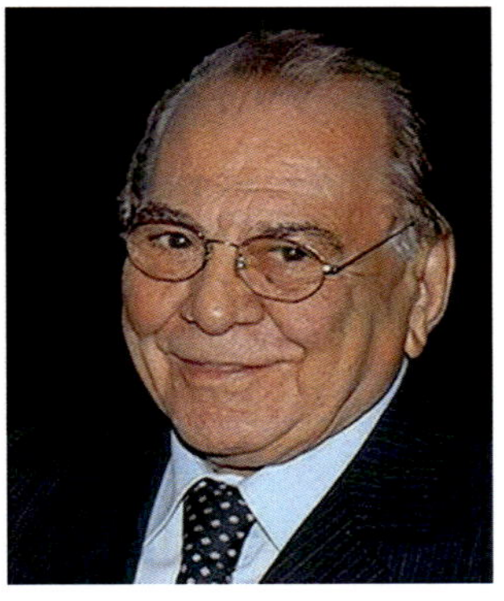

I dedicate this book to Prof. Ivo Pitanguy for his superb work over the course of 56 years devoted to the improvement of plastic surgery. Besides being an outstanding and talented surgeon, he promoted the specialization of more than 500 new plastic surgeons from all over the world, at a high level of qualification. His remarkable scientific contributions undoubtedly provide important support in every field of plastic surgery. In particular, Prof. Pitanguy developed a new technique for mastoplasty without cutaneous undermining, through kill resection of the mammary gland without dead space, with a minimal rate of complications during and after surgery. Because of several advantages, his technique is well known by plastic surgeons all over the world. Following the surgical principles of Prof. Pitanguy's technique, several plastic surgeons have developed new approaches that represent important advances in mastoplasty. For all these reasons, I am immensely thankful to Prof. Pitanguy, recognizing his important presence in my life. I dedicate this book to him, with the participation of 39 Brazilian plastic surgeons.

It was an honor and privilege for me to have been trained by Prof. Pitanguy, who opened a wide horizon in my life, giving me wonderful opportunities and the possibility of realizing my dream of being a doctor. As well as helping in my professional activity, Prof. Pitanguy also encouraged in my soul a fantastic motivation and inspired me in the scientific field, making me constantly search for more knowledge through dedicated research.

Juarez M. Avelar, M.D.

Foreword I

Dr. Juarez Avelar, during his specialization in our post-graduate course, showed a great curiosity for difficult problems, whether in ear deformities or other cases.

The hypertrophic breast is frequently encountered in our practice, causing an unpleasant series of functional problems that demand from the plastic surgeon an approach that can achieve satisfactory results with a minimum rate of complications. Juarez realized the benefits of the new techniques that we were developing and examines these and others in this book. However, he leans toward the technique, without undermining others, involving determination of the point "A" as a basic marking element, and other details that he shows clearly in this book.

In this book, Juarez also studies the progress of breast surgery, giving credit to the many authors who cooperated in developing different approaches, allowing accurate procedures for a variety of breast deformities. This book definitely deserves assessment by plastic surgeons engaged in body contour approaches, in particular for mastoplasty procedures. Its coverage is especially valuable for obtaining good results without many complications. I congratulate Dr. Juarez for outstanding editorial work in producing this important book.

Ivo Pitanguy, M.D.
Pontifical Catholic University of Rio de Janeiro
Rio de Janeiro, RJ, Brazil
Carlos Chagas Institute of Post-Graduate Medical Studies
Rio de Janeiro, RJ, Brazil
Brazilian Society of Plastic Surgery
São Paulo, SP, Brazil
American Society of Aesthetic Plastic Surgery
New York, NY, USA
International Society of Aesthetic Plastic Surgery
Hanover, NH, USA

Foreword II

> "This is the spirit that Beauty must ever induce: wonderment and a delicious trouble, longing and love and a trembling that is all delight" (Plotinus 23, [Ennead 1, 3]).

It is with great pleasure that I have been asked to write the foreword for Dr. Juarez Avelar's book on breast surgery. Dr. Avelar is a highly respected Brazilian plastic surgeon who pioneered (in the 1990s) the procedure of lipoabdominoplasty, which preserves the blood vessels of the upper abdominal wall flap during abdominoplasty. He is proliferative in authoring books on plastic surgery, such as *Creation of the Auricle* and *New Concepts on Abdominoplasty and Further Applications*, as well as journal articles and book chapters.

Dr. Avelar's new book entitled *Breast Surgery: Aesthetic Approaches* is innovative in subjects such as general information for breast surgery, surgical options for reduction breast surgery, aesthetic reparation of breast and chest wall deformities, mastopexy, and breast augmentation. Chapters include "Importance of Pitanguy's Technique for Evolution of Aesthetic Breast Surgery," "Reduction Mammaplasty in a Single Central Block," "Technical Systemization in Mammoplasy," "New Mastoplasty with Superior and Inferior Pedicles," "Mammoplasty Through Periareolar Approach," "Critical Analysis Concerning Mammary Prosthesis," and "Importance of Regenerative Medicine on Breast Augmentation." The contributors are expert Brazilian plastic surgeons with new knowledge and techniques.

This book is intended for plastic surgeons, cosmetic surgeons, general surgeons, and any surgeon performing aesthetic breast surgery. Young surgeons, experienced surgeons, and advanced breast surgeons can learn a variety of techniques and approaches to breast surgeries from the 60 chapters.

Tustin, CA, USA — Melvin A. Shiffman, M.D., J.D.

Preface

Publishing this book is an accomplishment of my professional desire to present the new techniques described by Brazilian plastic surgeons following the fundamental surgical principles and knowledge introduced by Prof. Pitanguy. In fact, a new era began in this field when Prof. Pitanguy described his novel concepts in reduction mastoplasty.

In 1980, when Prof. Jorge Psillakis and I organized the Brazilian Symposium on Breast Surgery in São Paulo, I wondered about printing a collection of contributions in this fascinating area, including several important new procedures created and developed by outstanding plastic surgeons. Some years later, I tried again to complete this work, but for unexpected reasons it was not possible. Therefore, this book represents the achievement of my dream of 37 years. It gives me special pleasure to offer readers a very wide collection of the new techniques presented at that scientific event, which represent the updated improvements in aesthetic breast surgery. I was still a young surgeon, but my mind was full of imagination and the determination to make a definitive register of new approaches to aesthetic procedures in breast surgery. Unfortunately, several of my colleagues who took part in the scientific program of that symposium are no longer with us, but I investigated their remarkable contributions and invited other plastic surgeons to write about their techniques. Besides Prof. Ivo Pitanguy, who passed away in August 2016, other authors of useful techniques left their contributions: Arié, Aleixo Sepulveda, Costa Lima, Peixoto, and Pigossi. Therefore, this publication describes modern methods that can improve plastic surgeons' aesthetic results after breast operations.

Basically, there are three main groups of techniques: (a) those that find a balance between the dimension of final scars and the shape and size of the breast after mastoplasty; (b) creation of glandular flaps that are sutured to model the breast during operation; and (c) a combination of both previous groups, which requires knowledge, good sense, and the ability to reshape the breasts in harmony with body contouring and with adequate symmetry between them.

Regarding the first group of techniques, the surgeon should not damage the final shape of the breasts in the quest for reduced and small surgical scars. I advocate that the size and form of the breasts are the main aspects for consideration after aesthetic mastoplasty. Usually, such criteria are similar to the patient's analysis. Reduced scars during operation must be a constant goal for every surgeon, as they do not jeopardize the final shape of the breasts.

Considering the second group of techniques, in which glandular flaps are created, it is a fundamental surgical principle to preserve adequate blood supply in order to avoid any risk of slough or even necrosis of mammary tissue. Readers should observe the technical descriptions given by the authors, particularly concerning complications after operations, each of which are mentioned.

The third group of methods, which is a combination of creation of mammary flaps and reduced surgical scars, require the surgeon to have good sense in order to avoid minor (or major) complications during and after surgery. Such aspects are achieved according to the knowledge, ability, and experience of the surgeon after performing a considerable number of breast operations.

Nevertheless, plastic surgeons should search continuously for new solutions to improve their results, always using their talent and stimulating their creativity to solve each problem as it comes up during an operation.

In conclusion, the main reason for publishing this book is to offer a unique opportunity to read meticulous descriptions of the personal techniques of 39 outstanding Brazilian plastic surgeons. It is important to emphasize that I invited several other well-known surgeons, but they did not join us in preparing this book. I take this opportunity to express my gratitude to all authors that accepted my invitation to participate with their contributions and to share their knowledge. Plastic surgeons and breast surgeons from all over the world may learn the techniques developed by very well qualified Brazilian specialists. I am sure that this book will introduce updated scientific methodology to the international medical literature.

São Paulo, SP, Brazil Juarez M. Avelar

Acknowledgments

While I was organizing the Brazilian Symposium on Breast Surgery in 1980, it was my dream to publish a book in which several Brazilian authors described their own techniques for mastoplasty. For various reasons, it was not possible to do this. Now, 37 years later, I have realized my project. Although, unfortunately, some of my colleagues who took part in that scientific program have passed away, it gives me great pleasure to include their contributions. Therefore, I am thankful to Profs. Ivo Pitanguy, Aleixo Sepulveda, Costa Lima, Gerardo Peixoto, and Nelson Pigossi. I also thank very much the 39 authors who have described their useful approaches.

To my parents, Anisio and Maria Ana. Although they are not with me in this world, I continuously feel their presence and I am thankful for their continuous enthusiasm and incentive.

To my loving son Thiago, and my wife Gloria, who have been constant sources of inspiration for this publication and permanent witnesses to my scientific activities.

To Professor Pitanguy, for all the knowledge I have acquired from him and for his constant encouragement of my work. He helped me throughout my professional practice by developing in me great motivation and an enthusiasm for the field of science.

To Dr. Edgar Bolanho, for the very high level of technical illustrations in this book, for the chapters I wrote as well as of other authors.

To the Plastic Surgery Unit at the Surgery Department of Science and Technology at Medical School of Marilia, and the Hospital das Clinicas of Marilia (both in São Paulo State). Professor Helio de Rezende Paoliello Jr. is the head of the Plastic Surgery Unit, who presented me with excellent conditions and support for organizing and publishing this book.

To the Federal University of Rio de Janeiro—UNIRIO and to Prof. Ricardo Cavalcanti Ribeiro, the head of the Plastic Surgery Department for their great assistance and incentive to elaborate and publish this book.

Juarez M. Avelar, M.D.

Contents

List of Contributors

Jose Horacio Aboudib, M.D., Ph.D. Plastic Surgery Pedro Ernesto University Hospital, Rio de Janeiro State University Estrada da Gávea, RJ, Brazil

Antonio Carlos Abramo, M.D., Ph.D. Division of Plastic Surgery at General Hospital São Luiz Morumbi, Post Graduate Course in Aesthetic and Reconstructive Plastic Surgery of ACA, Institute of Assistance in Plastic Surgery of São Paulo, Rua Afonso de Freitas, SP, Brazil

Christiane Vigné Alvarez de Abreu, M.D. Hospital of Plastics, Rio de Janeiro, RJ, Brazil

Yolotzin Mendez Aguilar, M.D. Global Plastic Surgery Department, Casa de Saúde Portugal, Universidade Santa Úrsula, Rio de Janeiro, RJ, Brazil

Ataliba Ronan Horta de Almeida, M.D. Sociedade Brasileira de Cirurgia Plástica, São Paulo, SP, Brazil

Plastic Surgery Training Center, Hospital Mater Dei, Belo Horizonte, MG, Brazil

Rafael Andrade Alves, M.D. Brazilian Society of Plastic Surgery, Hospital São Rafael, Salvador, BA, Brazil

Carlo Amaral, M.D. Member of the Plastic and Reconstructive Surgery Department, Ivo Pitanguy, Rio de Janeiro, RJ, Brazil

Plastic Surgery Department, Ivo Pitanguy, Rio de Janeiro, RJ, Brazil

Federal University of the State of Rio de Janeiro (UNIRIO), Rio de Janeiro, RJ, Brazil

Member of Brazilian Plastic Surgeons Society, Hospital Casa de Portugal, Rio de Janeiro, RJ, Brazil

Antonio Carlos Herrmann de Andrade, M.D. Rua Joaquim Floriano, São Paulo, SP, Brazil

Joel Araújo Silva, M.D. Hospital Belo Horizonte, Belo Horizonte, MG, Brazil

Juarez M. Avelar, M.D. Brazilian Scientific Institute of Plastic and Reconstructive Surgery, Alameda Gabriel Monteiro da Silva, São Paulo, SP, Brazil

Latus Sensus in Plastic Surgery, Federal University of the State of Rio de Janeiro, Rio de Janeiro, RJ, Brazil

Member of the Brazilian Society of Writers Doctors (SOBRAMES), São Paulo, SP, Brazil

Plastic Surgery Unit, Marília Medical School, Marília, SP, Brazil

Brazilian Society of Plastic Surgery (1986–87) and (1990–91), São Paulo, SP, Brazil

The International Society of Aesthetic Plastic Surgery (ISAPS), São Paulo, SP, Brazil

Priscilla Balbinot, M.D., M.Sc. Federal University of Paraná, Rua General Carneiro, 188—Hospital de Clínicas, Curitiba, PR, Brazil

Guilherme Cardinal Barreiro, M.D., Ph.D. Brazilian Society of Plastic Surgery, University of Campinas (UNICAMP), São Paulo, SP, Brazil

Roberto D. Basile, M.D. The American Society of Plastic Surgery, Arlington Heights, IL, USA

The Brazilian Society of Plastic Surgery, São Paulo, SP, Brazil

Department of Plastic Surgery, Basile Day Hospital, Ribeirão Preto, SP, Brazil

Adrian Bermudez, M.D. Condomínio Península, Avenida Das Acácias, Rio de Janeiro, RJ, Brazil

Antonio Roberto Bozola, M.D. Regent Cirurgia Plástica da Faculdade de Medicina de São José do Rio Preto, São José do Rio Preto, SP, Brazil

Ryane Schmidt Brock, M.D., M.Sc. Department of Plastic Surgery, The Brazilian Society of Plastic Surgery, Defeitos da Face Studies and Research Center, São Paulo, SP, Brazil

Alberto M.L. Caldeira, M.D., M.Sc., Ph.D., FACS, FICS Global Plastic Surgery Department, Casa de Saúde Portugal, Instituto de Pós-Graduação Médica Carlos Chagas, Universidade Santa Úrsula, Rio de Janeiro, RJ, Brazil

Plastic and Reconstructive Surgery Department, Caldeira-Roth Institute, Ipanema, RJ, Brazil

Humberto Campos, M.D. Bahia School of Medicine and Public Health, Salvador, BA, Brazil

Brazilian Society of Plastic Surgery, São Paulo, SP, Brazil

Sérgio Carreirão, M.D. Brazilian Society of Plastic Surgery (TSBCP), São Paulo, SP, Brazil

Brazilian College of Surgeons (ECBC), Rio de Janeiro, RJ, Brazil

American College of Surgeons (FACS), Chicago, IL, USA

Claudio Cardoso de Castro, M.D. Department of Plastic Surgery, University of the State of Rio de Janeiro, Rio de Janeiro, RJ, Brazil

Barbara de Castro Fonseca, M.D. Hospital of Plastics, Rio de Janeiro, RJ, Brazil

Armando Chiari Jr., M.D., Ph.D. Department of Surgery, Medical School, Federal University of Minas Gerais, Rua Herculano de Freitas, Belo Horizonte, MG, Brazil

Wanda Elizabeth Correa, M.D. Department of Ivo Pitanguy Plastic Surgery, Pontifical Catholic University, Rio de Janeiro, RJ, Brazil

Márcio Paulino Costa, M.D., Ph.D. Brazilian Society of Plastic Surgery, ISAPS, FILACAP, ASPS, Hospital das Clínicas, University of São Paulo Medical School, Santa Cecília, SP, Brazil

Pedro Felipe Suárez Cruz, M.D. Division of Plastic and Reconstructive Surgery, Carlos Chagas Institute, Rio de Janeiro, RJ, Brazil

Miluska Bromley Cueva, M.D. Instituto Ivo Pitanguy, Rio de Janeiro, RJ, Brazil

Instituto de Pós-Graduação Médica Carlos Chagas, Rio de Janeiro, RJ, Brazil

João Erfon, M.D. Department of Surgery, Walter Cantídio Hospital of the Federal University of Ceará, Fortaleza, CE, Brazil

Marco Aurélio Faria Correa, M.D. Dr. Marco Faria Correa Plastic Surgery Pte Ltd, Singapore, Singapore

Angela Maria Fausto Souza, Ph.D. Gynecology Department, Oswaldo Cruz Foundation, Rio de Janeiro, RJ, Brazil

Miriam Fialka, M.D. Plastic Surgery, Clínica Miranda, Curitiba, PR, Brazil

Isabel Vieira de Figueiredo-e-Silva, M.D. Brazilian Society of Plastic Surgery, Carlos Chagas Institute, The American Society of Plastic Surgeons, Rio de Janeiro, RJ, Brazil

Luis Bernardo Froes, M.D. Faculty of Medicine, University of São Paulo, Butantã, SP, Brazil

Giovani Araujo Godinho Filho, M.D. Serviço de Cirurgia Plástica da Santa Casa de Misericórdia de Goiânia, MEC/SBCP, Goiânia, GO, Brazil

Santos Espinal Gómez, M.D. Global Plastic Surgery Department, Casa de Saúde Portugal, Instituto de Pós-Graduação Médica Carlos Chagas, Universidade Santa Úrsula, Rio de Janeiro, RJ, Brazil

Ruth Graf, M.D., Ph.D. Pietà Centro Médico, Hospital de Clínicas—Rua General Carneiro, Curitiba, PR, Brazil

Farid Hakme, M.D. Hospital of Plastics, Rio de Janeiro, RJ, Brazil

Leandro Ramalho Chaves Isobe, M.D. SBCP, Plastic Surgery Medical Team, Hospital Mater Dei, Belo Horizonte, MG, Brazil

Bruna Jacobowski, M.D. Hospital of Plastics, Rio de Janeiro, RJ, Brazil

Carlos Alberto Jaimovich, M.D. Ivo Pitanguy Institute of Plastic Surgery/ PUC-RJ Post-graduation University, Rio de Janeiro, RJ, Brazil

Emília Silva Klein, M.D. Hospital Belo Horizonte, Belo Horizonte, MG, Brazil

Andrea Kocsis, M.D. Member of the Plastic and Reconstructive Surgery Department, Federal University of the State of Rio de Janeiro (UNIRIO), Rio de Janeiro, RJ, Brazil

Casa de Portugal, Rio de Janeiro, RJ, Brazil

Célio Ferreira Leão, M.D. Faculdade de Medicina da Universidade Federal de Goiás, Goiânia, GO, Brazil

Escola de Medicina da Pontifícia Universidade Católica de Goiás, Goiânia, GO, Brazil

Serviço de Cirurgia Plástica da Santa Casa de Misericórdia de Goiânia, MEC/ SBCP, Goiânia, GO, Brazil

Sociedade Brasileira de Cirurgia Plástica, São Paulo, SP, Brazil

Gheisa Moura Leão, M.D. Escola de Medicina da Pontifícia Universidade Católica de Goiás, Goiânia, GO, Brazil

Serviço de Cirurgia Plástica da Santa Casa de Misericórdia de Goiânia, MEC/ SBCP, Goiânia, GO, Brazil

Sociedade Brasileira de Cirurgia Plástica, São Paulo, SP, Brazil

Clínica de Cirurgia Plástica—Allure, Goiânia, GO, Brazil

Célio Coelho Neto Leão, M.D. Hospital of Plastics, Rio de Janeiro, RJ, Brazil

Luis Emilio Fuentes López, M.D. Division of Plastic and Reconstructive Surgery, Carlos Chagas Institute, Rio de Janeiro, RJ, Brazil

André Villani Correa Mafra, M.D. Sociedade Brasileira de Cirurgia Plástica, São Paulo, SP, Brazil

Plastic Surgery Training Center, Hospital Mater Dei, Belo Horizonte, MG, Brazil

SBCP, Plastic Surgery Medical Team, Hospital Mater Dei, Belo Horizonte, MG, Brazil

Walter Marrou Pautrat, M.D. Instituto Ivo Pitanguy/Instituto de Pós-Graduação Médica Carlos Chagas, Rio de Janeiro, RJ, Brazil

Lybio Martire Jr., M.D. University Department of Plastic Surgery, Surgical Technique and History of Medicine, Titular of Brazilian Society of Plastic Surgery, Titular of Federation Ibero Latinoamericana de Cirurgia Plástica y Reconstructiva, Titular of Brazilian College of Surgeons, Fellow of International College of Surgeons, Titular Founder of Brazilian Society of History of Medicine, São Paulo, SP, Brazil

Marcelo Paulo Vaccari Mazzetti, M.D., M.Sc. Department of Plastic Surgery, The Brazilian Society of Plastic Surgery, Defeitos da Face Studies and Research Center, São Paulo, SP, Brazil

Moacyr Pires de Mello Filho, M.D. Cirurgica, De Mello Cirurgia Plástica, São Paulo, SP, Brazil

Marcio Milman, M.D. Gynecology Department, Oswaldo Cruz Foundation, Rio de Janeiro, RJ, Brazil

José Carlos de Miranda, M.D. Plastic Surgery, Clínica Miranda, Curitiba, PR, Brazil

Arnaldo Miró, M.D. Clínica de Cirurgia Plástica e Reparadora Dr. Arnaldo Lobo Miró Ltda, Curitiba, PR, Brazil

Maria Gabriela Moreira Mangles, M.D. Division of Plastic and Reconstructive Surgery of Centro Policlinico Valencia, Valencia, Venezuela

Marcus Vinicius Alfano Moscozo, M.D. Brazilian Society of Plastic Surgery, Hospital São Rafael, Salvador, BA, Brazil

Ibero-Latin American Society of Plastic Surgery, Punta del Este, Uruguay

Roosevelt Santos Oliveira Jr., M.D. Sociedade Brasileira de Cirurgia Plástica, Santos, SP, Brazil

Daniele Pace, M.D., M.Sc. Pietà Centro Médico, Rua Albino Silva, Curitiba, PR, Brazil

Helio Paoliello Jr. Plastic Surgery Discipline, Faculdade de Medicina de Marília (FAMEMA), Marília, SP, Brazil

Ricardo Paoliello, M.D. Plastic Surgery Discipline, Faculdade de Medicina de Marília (FAMEMA), Marília, SP, Brazil

Marcelo Pastor, M.D. Condomínio Península, Avenida Das Acácias, Rio de Janeiro, RJ, Brazil

Vilibaldo Cabral de Paulo, M.D. Avenida Coremas, João Pessoa, PB, Brazil

Osvaldo Pereira, M.D. Clínica Jane Hospital Ilha, Deputado Antonio Edu Vieira, Florianópolis, SC, Brazil

Ivo Pitanguy, M.D. Pontifical Catholic University of Rio de Janeiro, Rio de Janeiro, RJ, Brazil

Carlos Chagas Institute of Post-Graduate Medical Studies, Rio de Janeiro, RJ, Brazil

Brazilian Society of Plastic Surgery, São Paulo, SP, Brazil

American Society of Aesthetic Plastic Surgery, New York, NY, USA

International Society of Aesthetic Plastic Surgery, Hanover, NH, USA

Paulo Roberto Botica do Rêgo Santos, M.D. Gynecology Department, Oswaldo Cruz Foundation, Rio de Janeiro, RJ, Brazil

Waldir Teixeira Renó, M.D. Cirurgia Plástica D'America Clinica, Plastic-Surgeon Santa Casa de Guaratinguetá, Membro Titular da SBCP, Guaratinguetá, SP, Brazil

Flávio Rezende, M.D. Plastic and Reconstructive Surgery, Universidad Federal del Estado de Río de Janeiro, Brazilian Society of Plastic Surgery, Rio de Janeiro, RJ, Brazil

Ricardo Cavalcanti Ribeiro, M.D., Ph.D. Division of Plastic and Reconstructive Surgery of Casa de Portugal, Brazilian Society of Plastic Surgery, Carlos Chagas Institute, Rio de Janeiro, RJ, Brazil

Plastic and Reconstructive Surgery Department, Federal University of the State of Rio de Janeiro (UNIRIO), Rio de Janeiro, RJ, Brazil

Manuel Torreira Rios, M.D. Division of Plastic and Reconstructive Surgery, Carlos Chagas Institute, Rio de Janeiro, RJ, Brazil

Ana Carolina Guimarães Rocha, M.D. Brazilian Society of Plastic Surgery, São Paulo, SP, Brazil

Claudio Mauricio M. Rodrigues, M.D. Unichristus University, Fortaleza, CE, Brazil

Sheyla Maria Carvalho Rodrigues, M.D. Department of Plastic Surgery, University of the State of Rio de Janeiro, Rio de Janeiro, RJ, Brazil

Sergio Romay, M.D. Division of Plastic and Reconstructive Surgery, Carlos Chagas Institute, Rio de Janeiro, RJ, Brazil

Ilson Abrantes Rosique, M.D. Sociedade Brasileira de Cirurgia Plástica, Santos, SP, Brazil

Alessandra Grassi Salles, M.D. Plastic Surgery, Hospital das Clínicas da Faculdade de Medicina da Universidade de São Paulo, São Paulo, SP, Brazil

Renato Saltz, M.D., FACS Member of the Plastic and Reconstructive Surgery Department, Federal University of the State of Rio de Janeiro (UNIRIO), Rio de Janeiro, RJ, Brazil

Mariangela Santiago, M.D. Brazilian Society of Plastic Surgery, São Paulo, SP, Brazil

International Society of Aesthetic Plastic Surgery, Hanover, NH, USA

Rayssa Sauaia, M.D. Department of Plastic Surgery

Defeitos da Face Studies and Research Center, São Paulo, SP, Brazil

William Seidel, M.D. VIVVA Clinica, Florianópolis, SC, Brazil

Fernando Serra-Guimarães, M.D., Ph.D. Plastic Surgery, Pedro Ernesto University Hospital, Rio de Janeiro State University, Rio de Janeiro, RJ, Brazil

Melvin A. Shiffman, M.D., J.D. Northwestern University, Tustin, CA, USA

Sérgio Levy Silva, M.D. Rua Real Grandeza, Botafogo, RJ, Brazil

Ramil Sinder, M.D. Member of the Brazilian Society of Plastic Surgery, Rio de Janeiro, RJ, Brazil

Irene Coelho de Souza, M.D. Cirurgia Plástica, Clínica Cirúrgica Drs. Irene e Carlos Souza, Belém, PA, Brazil

Vera Tatiana Coelho de Souza, M.D. Cirurgia Plástica, Clínica Cirúrgica Drs. Irene e Carlos Souza, Belém, PA, Brazil

Mário Junqueira Souza, M.D. Serviço de Cirurgia Plástica da Santa Casa de Misericórdia de Goiânia, MEC/SBCP, Goiânia, GO, Brazil

Ewaldo Bolivar de Souza Pinto, M.D. Sociedade Brasileira de Cirurgia Plástica, Santos, SP, Brazil

Priscilla Chiarello de Souza Pinto Abdalla, M.D. Sociedade Brasileira de Cirurgia Plástica, Santos, SP, Brazil

Ana Paula Pimentel Spadari, M.D. Sociedade Brasileira de Cirurgia Plástica, Santos, SP, Brazil

Nuberto H. Teixeira, M.D. Brazilian Society of Plastic Surgery, University of São Paulo Medical School, São Paulo, SP, Brazil

Guilherme Teles, M.D. Defeitos da Face Hospital and Santa Cruz Hospital, Fortaleza, CE, Brazil

Rawlson de Thuin, M.D. Brazilian Society of Plastic Surgery, Carlos Chagas Institute, International Society of Aesthetic Plastic Surgery, Rio de Janeiro, RJ, Brazil

Manuel Antonio Torreira Rios, M.D. Global Plastic Surgery Department, Casa de Saúde Portugal, Instituto de Pós-Graduação Médica Carlos Chagas, Universidade Santa Úrsula, Rio de Janeiro, RJ, Brazil

Johana Buitrago Valderrama, M.D. Division of Plastic and Reconstructive Surgery of Casa de Portugal, Rio de Janeiro, RJ, Brazil

Tiago Almeida Vale, M.D. Serviço de Cirurgia Plástica da Santa Casa de Misericórdia de Goiânia, MEC/SBCP, Goiânia, GO, Brazil

João Francisco Vale Pereira, M.D. Clínica Vale Pereira, Florianópolis, SC, Brazil

Part I

General Information for Breast Surgery

1 Importance of Pitanguy's Technique for the Evolution of Aesthetic Breast Surgery

Juarez M. Avelar

1.1 Introduction

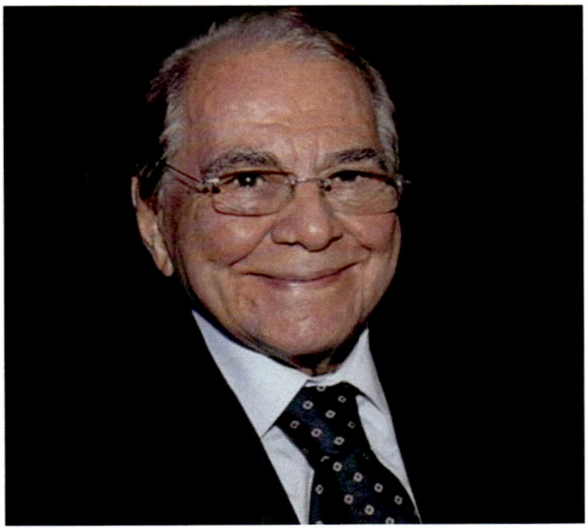

Prof. Ivo Pitanguy
1923–2016

Looking back at the history of aesthetic breast surgery, there are a few publications before the twentieth century that are the basic references on this field. According to Sinder (2003), Durston, Dieffenbach, Velpeau, Gaillard, and Thomas are the most important publications up to the eighteenth century in which mastoplasty originated. Nevertheless, during the twentieth century great improvements were achieved owing to the useful participation of several authors who introduced important knowledge on reduction mastoplasty. In the early years, Morestin and Gaudet (1905) reported an incision into the inframammary fold for the treatment of mammary hypertrophy. Later, Lexer (1912), Kausch (1916), Kraske (1923), Passot (1925), Noël (1928), and other authors introduced useful surgical steps toward improving mastopexy and reduction mastoplasty. An important reference is attributed to Biesenberger (1928), with an "S"-shaped excision of the lateral portion of the gland and rotation of the remaining glandular pedicle with the nipple attached upward. A remarkable contribution of Schwarzmann (1930) was the fashioning of a periareolar incision for the maintenance of the blood supply to the nipple, which is performed during most mastoplasty techniques. A two-stage operation was reported by Maliniac (1932), among other authors.

Gillies and McIndoe (1939) proposed a V-shaped wedge resection from the upper middle segment of the breast to reduce the incidence of avascular necrosis of the nipple, followed by mobilization of the inner and outer pedicles. Thorek (1942) reported 25 years' experience with free nipple transplantation on reduction

J.M. Avelar, M.D.
Brazilian Scientific Institute of Plastic and Reconstructive Surgery, Alameda Gabriel Monteiro da Silva, 620-Jardim Europa, Sao Paulo, SP 01442-000, Brazil
e-mail: juarezavelar@bol.com.br; institutodaorelha@uol.com.br; clinica-avelar@uol.com.br

J.M. Avelar (ed.), *Breast Surgery*, https://doi.org/10.1007/978-3-319-54115-0_1

mammaplasty. Strombeck (1960) suggested the maintenance of the lateral pedicle of the nipple–areola complex (NAC) as preservation of the principal arteriovenous and cutaneous nerve system to ensure nipple survival and using a pattern to determine the shape of the breast. Skoog (1963) described a laterally based dermal flap separated from the gland at the subcutaneous level. McKissock in (1972) described his bipedicle vertical dermal flap for nipple transposition. Dufourmentel and Mouly (1961) described a lateral wedge excision of skin, fat, and gland with a resultant lateral oblique scar.

A memorable publication by Pitanguy (1961) reported a horizontal dermal bridge and "keel"-shaped resection of the gland from the inferior and central portions of the breast, creating a "third pedicle," as he named it, to provide adequate blood supply and nerves to the NAC. As I had the privilege to be trained by Prof. Pitanguy, as a resident during my specialization in his world famous clinic, his knowledge is essential in my practice. During that useful period, I assisted with his operations and took care of his patients during postoperative recovery, which made it possible for me to confirm the excellent surgical results with minimal complications. There were a great number of patients with outstanding results, inconspicuous scars and a well-located NAC, without any sloughing or other complications.

Many plastic surgeons from all over the world used to visit Prof. Pitanguy to observe and learn from him. In fact, in every procedure he used to demonstrate his new techniques, he was always friendly with all visitors, answering questions in several languages as he was fluent in six foreign idioms. He was very kind and polite with everyone when teaching every single detail, whereby it seemed to be quite easy to learn the basic surgical principles. Also, he was happy to explain in several languages any queries presented by the plastic surgeons in the operating room and after each procedure. Undoubtedly, Prof. Pitanguy was so generous in teaching his knowledge and his own techniques. Therefore, in addition to having special opportunity to learn from him during operations, I also used to have another chance to hear his explanations about the techniques while he performed the operations. Nevertheless, during reduction mastoplasty I used to pay even more attention to learn the way in which Prof. Pitanguy demarcated the technique and how he performed glandular resection, which seemed to be very easy. All the time, he explained step-by-step all the surgical principles that are deeply embedded in my mind. For all these reasons, Pitanguy's technique for reduction mastoplasty is essential to my practice.

1.2 Method

The surgical principles presented by Pitanguy (1961, 1967, 1981) and Pitanguy and Garcia (1972) paved the way for several surgeons to perform his techniques and to introduce personal modifications for evolution of the surgical results. After his original descriptions, the number of publications in the medical literature regarding reduction mastoplasty increased enormously. In fact, Pitanguy's technique is very easy to learn and perform to treat moderate and large mammary hypertrophy.

1.2.1 Surgical Principles

Pitanguy's technique presents several surgical principles that are responsible for significant improvement in reduction mastoplasty, as he described and repeated during every operation, such as:

1. The surgical marking is done according to the surgeon's creativity with no standard pattern.
2. To determine Pitanguy's point A is the point of reference for surgical marking (Fig. 1.1). Following his technique, I introduced some modifications to his surgical marking (Avelar 1980, 1993a, b). Thus, the distance between segments AB and AC is much longer compared with his marking (Fig. 1.2). Instead of creating a classic W-shaped marking, my drawing is a long vertical area for skin

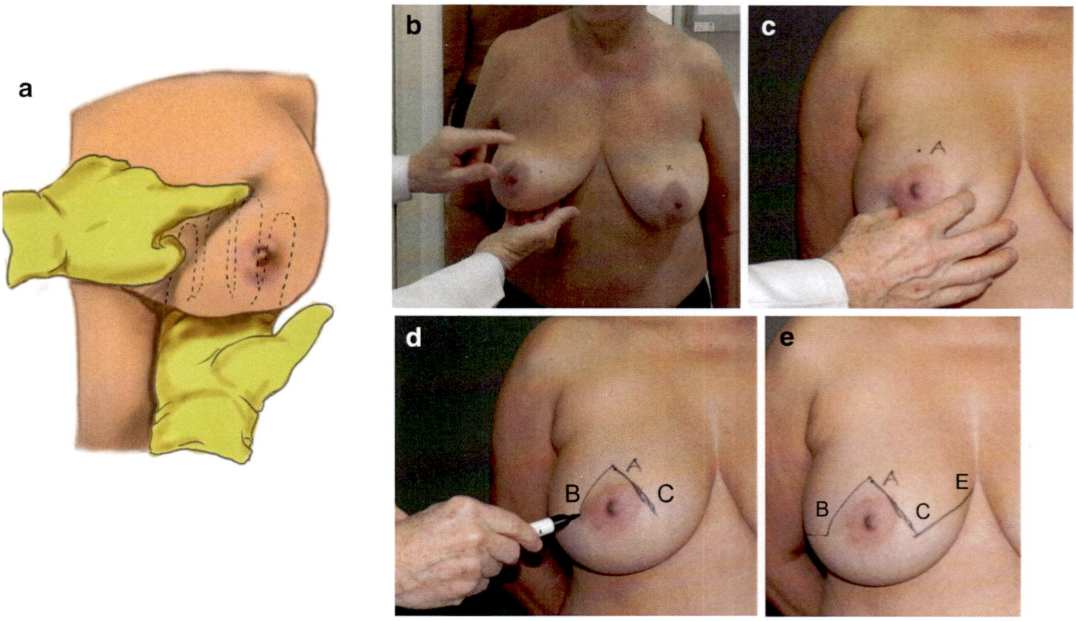

Fig. 1.1 Importance of Pitanguy's point A for surgical demarcation in mastoplasty. (**a**, **b**) Drawing and photo show the surgeon's hand to identify the point A. (**c**, **d**) Bidigital maneuver to determine the points B and C. (**e**) Two lines are marked for the W incisions

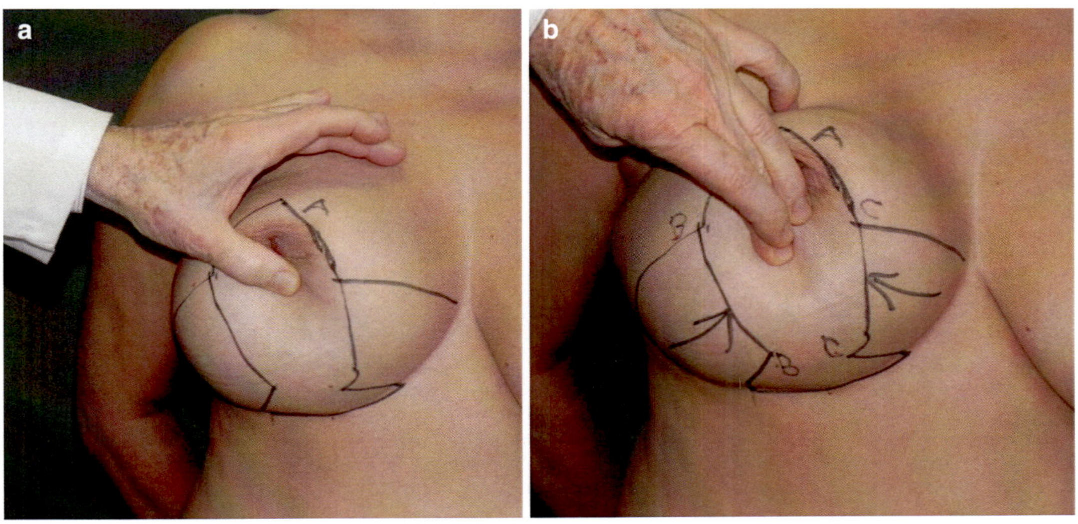

Fig. 1.2 Comparison between Pitanguy's marking and mine. (**a**) Photo of the right breast after both markings. (**b**) The same patient showing that my points B and C are very low. The arrows indicate that the excess skin of the external and internal sides of the breast will be removed in the central area of the breast

resection, as a very small area of skin is resected on the submammary fold (Fig. 1.3).

3. The resection of the mammary gland on hypertrophic breasts is performed using a "keel" shape in the medial part of the breast.
4. The creation of two mammary columns on each side of the breast, which are the essential glands after resection.
5. The creation of the "third pedicle" on the upper pole of the breast, which is an important segment

for improving vascular support to the remaining mammary gland after reduction mastoplasty.

6. The remaining mammary gland maintains anatomical communication with the galactophorous duct together with the nipple.
7. The two mammary columns are sutured together and to the muscular aponeurosis.
8. After suturing of the mammary columns, there is no "dead" space.
9. There is no cutaneous undermining.

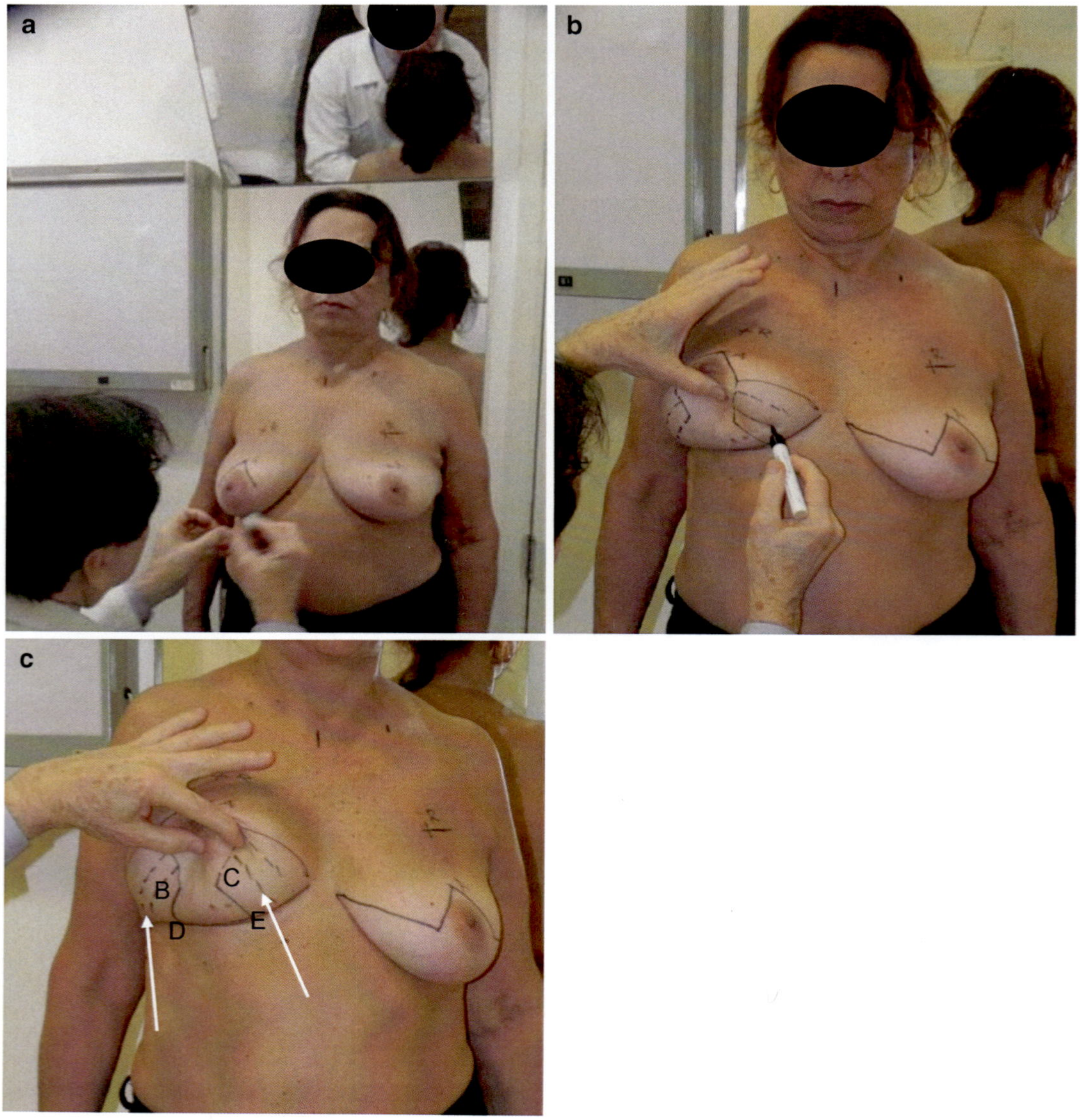

Fig. 1.3 Pre-marking with the patient in a standing position in front of two vertical mirrors. (**a**, **b**) She can observe surgical pre-marking in front of the mirrors. (**c**) Pre-marking is performed: a W drawing can be seen on the left breast and on the right one my marking shows a small area for skin resection. The lines indicated by the arrows show that the incisions CE and BD are lower so as to reduce the area for skin resection. (**d**) and (**e**) Final aspects after pre-marking

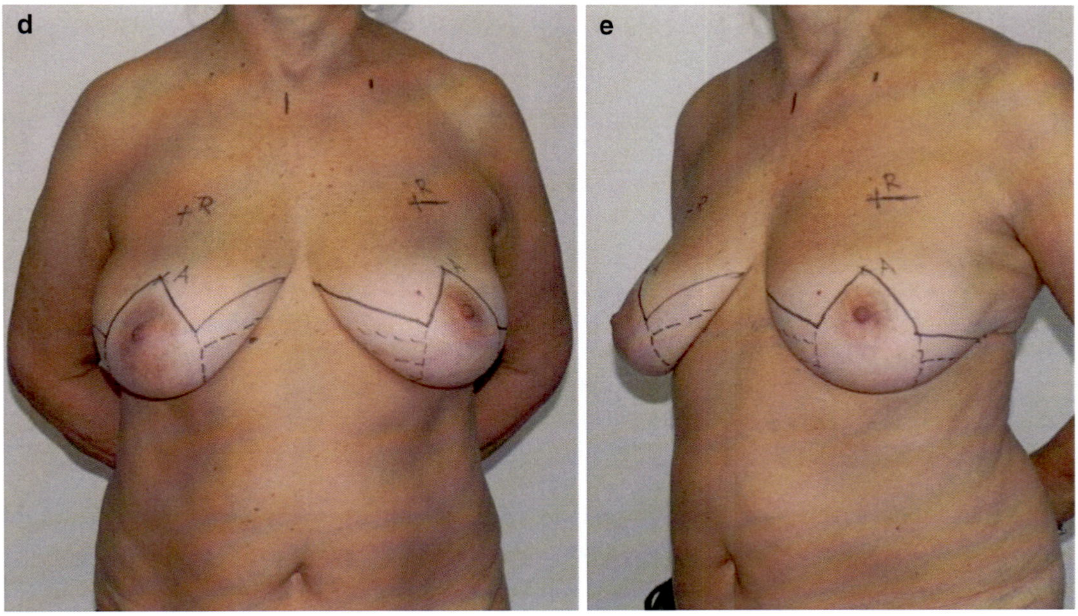

Fig. 1.3 (continued)

1.2.1.1 Surgical Marking

Surgical marking in Pitanguy's technique is done with the patient in a semi-sitting position in the operating room (Fig. 1.4). According to the history of mastoplasty, Gillies and McIndoe (1939) were the first authors to perform surgery with elevation of the patient's head on the operating table. Besides, the same authors used to measure the patient's chest for surgical marking, taking as references the sternal notch and the xyphoid process. Thus, Prof. Pitanguy introduced this routine into his practice and consequently to all surgeons who were trained by him, even those visitors who used to observe his operations. Therefore, surgical marking before reduction mastoplasty became an artistic methodology that is individual to each surgeon, who has the freedom to perform all marking according to each individual patient without any rigid points or a standard pattern. He or she may employ his or her creativity in establishing the future area for skin resection and that of the mammary gland. In this way, the measurement of the breasts and chest using a ruler or a graduated tape became a matter of routine during surgical marking. Aufricht (1949) reported a geometric method of demarcating the incisions in breast surgery. He showed the relationship between the excision of the wedge-shaped infra-areolar area and the height of the mammary cone. He also mentioned the use of long temporary stitches in the skin at the sternal notch and the level of the xyphoid process to transfer from one side to the other for symmetrical skin marking. Another important contribution was published by Fernandez (1951), in which he used a ruler placed between the breasts and thorax, to mark the new location of the NAC at the level of the inframammary crease at the hemi-mammary line.

1.2.1.2 Pitanguy's Point A

Pitanguy's point A is the point of reference for surgicalmarking. It is located on the vertical line from the midclavicular point passing by the nipple and is the projection of the submammary sulcus of the breast. The surgeon uses one hand under the breast on the submammary sulcus with his finger directed forward, and with the index finger of the other hand the surgeon touches the tip of the finger of the hand placed under the breast (Fig.1.1). Thus, this place is Pitanguy's point A. From point A, two oblique lines pass down each side of the breast to determine the points B and C and to establish the amount of skin and mammary glad that will be resected (Fig. 1.1). Nevertheless, as described above, in my marking, the lines AB and AC are drawn lower to reduce the area of skin for resection (Fig. 1.4). Therefore, during surgery a smaller area of skin is resected.

1.2.1.3 "Keel" Resection

By performing Pitanguy's resection, it is possible to remove the excess mammary gland in accordance with the surgeon's surgical planning, without causing any damage to the vascular network to the remaining parenchyma (Fig. 1.5). The main glandular resection is performed on the center of the breast, which Pitanguy named a "keel" resection. The lateral prolongations of the base of the mammary gland on each side (medial and lateral) are also resected at the same bloc (Pitanguy, 1959). Through such resection, the remaining parenchyma maintains its natural vascularization without any damage to the NAC blood supply. According to Pitanguy's publications the base of the hypertrophic breasts is the main bloc, which may be carried out without undermining any cutaneous or mammary tissue. By performing a "keel" resection, it is possible to reduce the

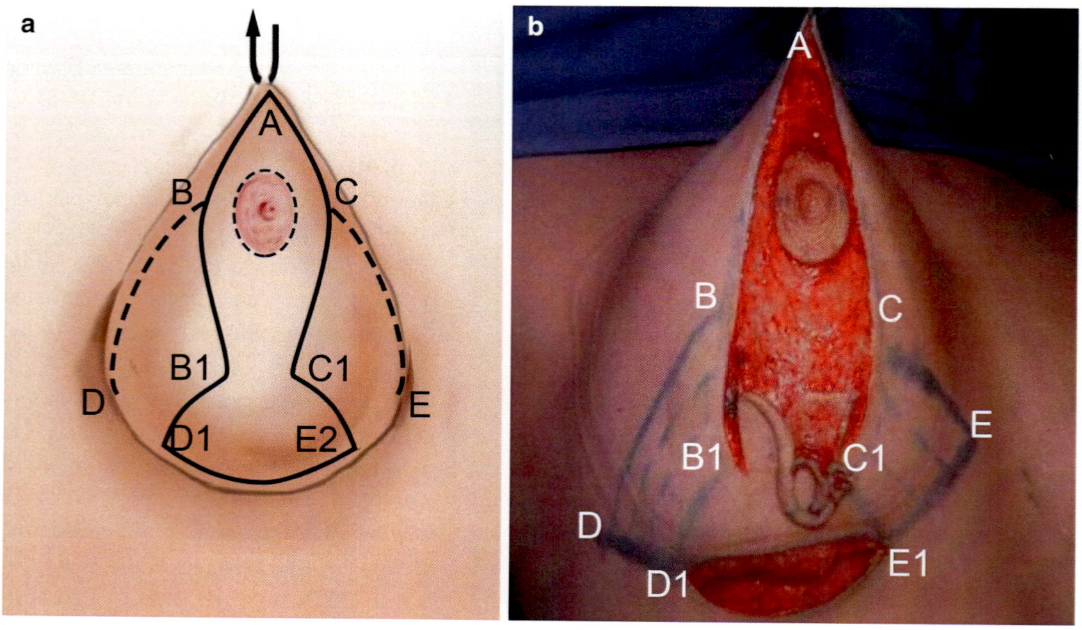

Fig. 1.4 Surgical marking during surgery. (**a**) Drawing shows a comparison between Pitanguy's marking with dotted lines (A, B, C, D, E) and mine with continuous lines (A, B1, C1, D1, E1). Between the two lines the amount of skin that is not resected during my approach can be seen, as only the rocket-shaped central area of the breast will be resected. (**b**) Photo during surgery shows that the breast is pulling up with Pitanguy's marking in comparison with my marking. The central area is already de-epithelialized and the area of skin preserved

width of the breast as much as necessary. Pitanguy also used to call his approach to the removal of excess mammary gland "gothic cathedral resection."

1.2.1.4 Creation of Two Columns

After "keel" resection, two mammary columns on each side of the breast are created, which is the essential glandular tissue after resection. Those two columns represent the natural connection with the galactophorous ducts, providing natural lactation after surgery. According to my marking, the skin that is not resected corresponds to the shape of the two columns created after glandular resection (Figs. 1.4, 1.5, and 1.6).

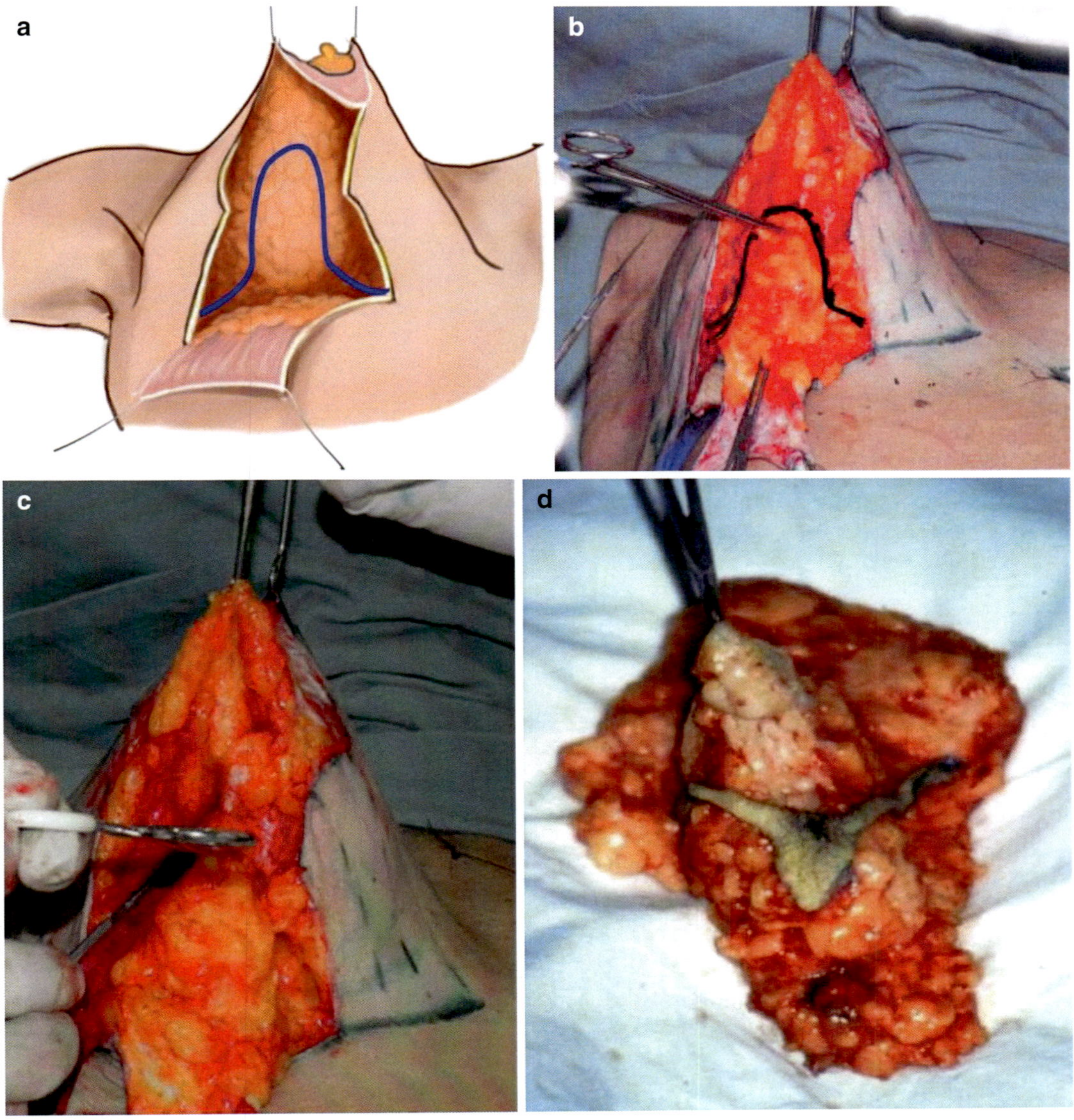

Fig. 1.5 Pitanguy's "keel" resection during mastoplasty. (**a**) Drawing shows that the central area is de-epithelialized and the "keel" resection area is marked with *blue*. (**b**) Photo during surgery shows the marking of the "keel" resection. (**c**) "Keel" resection with knife is being carried out. (**d**) A quantity of glandular tissue was removed and a small area of skin was resected

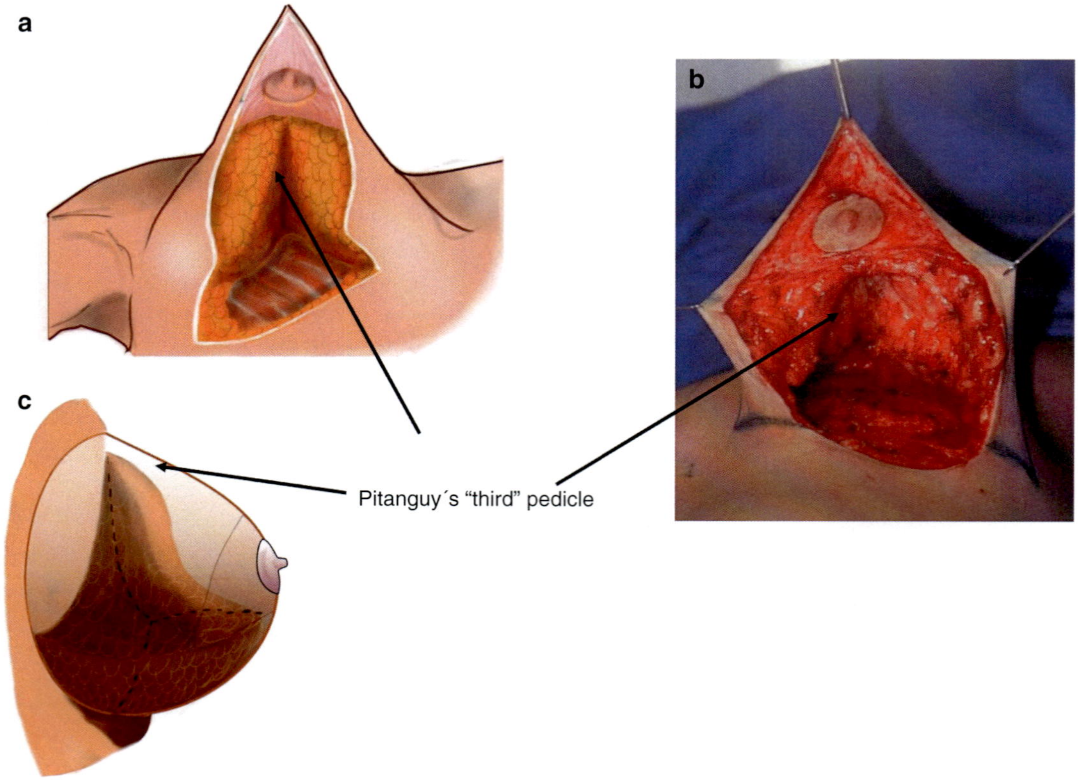

Fig. 1.6 Creation of Pitanguy's "third" pedicle. (**a**) Drawing shows remaining glandular tissue after resection; the arrows indicate the "third" pedicle. (**b**) Photo during surgery showing the "third" pedicle created after glandular resection. (**c**) Drawing in the profile view showing "keel" resection with preservation of the subcutaneous layer on top where the "third" pedicle is created

1.2.1.5 Creation of the "Third Pedicle"

Creation of the "third pedicle" on the upper pole of the breast is one of the main surgical principles of Pitanguy's technique, as the "keel" resection of the mammary gland must preserve the cutaneous and subcutaneous layers on the upper pole of the breast (Fig. 1.6). In fact, the resection of the parenchyma must be performed carefully so as not to damage the vascularization and innervation as well. The "third pedicle" provides adequate blood supply and innervation, which maintain normal sensitivity to the NAC postoperatively. If this surgical principle is not adequately followed, the final aesthetic result may cause partial or total necrosis of the NAC.

1.2.1.6 Anatomical Communication Between the Galactophorous Duct of the Mammary Tissue and the Nipple

According to Pitanguy's "keel" resection and the creation of two columns, the remaining mammary gland maintains anatomical communication between the galactophorous duct and the nipple. Therefore, patients maintain normal lactation after the operation, as the remnant mammary gland may provide regular secretion after reduction mastoplasty (Fig. 1.6).

1.2.1.7 Suturing of the Two Mammary Columns

The two mammary columns are sutured together and to the muscular aponeurosis, similar to Malbec and Quaife's (1957) suggestion to fixate breast tissue to muscle during mastoplasty. The glandular resection is performed according to each individual patient following surgical marking; particularly in asymmetrical breasts, it is possible to achieve a good balance between the two sides afterwards. In such cases, it is a fundamental step to create two similar columns on each breast to reinstate similarity after operation (Fig. 1.6).

1.2.1.8 There Is No "Dead Space"
After suture of the mammary columns there is no "dead space." After resection of the excess mammary tissue, suturing between the remaining glandular tissue and the aponeurosis of the pectoralis major. For this reason, it is not necessary to use drainage after the operation (Fig. 1.6).

1.2.1.9 No Cutaneous Undermining
This surgical principle is related to the embryological development of the breast, as it originates in dermal structures. Glandular parenchyma maintains a natural connection with the dermis, which provides a normal blood supply, avoiding bleeding and hematoma formation.

1.2.2 Surgical Marking

Before performing mastoplasty, it is a fundamental step to provide careful surgical marking. Prof. Pitanguy, with all his knowledge and experience, used to carry it out with the patient on the operating table under general anesthesia in a semi-sitting position. Although I used to assist him during my period of training, my preference is to perform a pre-marking at the office 1 day before the operation (Avelar 1993a). Some of the reference points are marked with the patient in the standing position in front of two vertical mirrors placed one in front of the other (Figs. 1.3 and 1.4). First, a point is marked at6 the center of the sternal notch. Another two points are marked laterally 7 cm away on each side in the midclavicular area. From these points, a line is pulled downwards passing the center of the nipple of both breasts. On this line a point is marked on the projection of the submammary fold (Figs. 1.1 and 1.2). This is Pitanguy's point A. The submammary folds are drawn to determine the final scars after surgery. These reference points are marked with ink and it is recommended that the patient preserves them until the next day. She can take a shower, but must be careful to maintain the references points to help the surgical marking during the operation.

I found the pre-marking very useful, as the patient is awake and observes my work by watching in the mirrors (Fig. 1.3). At that time, I am able to examine all the surgical details that were registered during the first consultation. Also, the patient signs the consent forms.

In 1949, Aufricht proposed geometric methodology as pre-surgical marking for breast operations, which has been employed by several authors. At that time, a prefabricated pattern was a very common approach. Following Aufricht's marking, Fernandez (1951) employed a ruler to measure the reference points on the chest and breast to achieve adequate projection after mastoplasty.

During the operation, surgical marking is done with the patient on the operating table under general anesthesia or local anesthesia combined with intravenous sedation under the care of an anesthesiologist. The pre-marking is very useful for performing the definitive surgical marking. A vertical line is drawn from the midclavicular point, passing through the nipple and inframammary crease (Figs. 1.2 and 1.3). The inframammary crease is also marked on each side. The nipple site (Pitanguy's point A) is identified on the midclavicular line by placing the index finger in the submammary fold and marking the point on the skin surface. The point A does not represent the exact center of the future nipple, but it is the point very near to where the nipple will be when the operation is complete. Precise nipple placement is made at the end of the operation. The amount of breast tissue to be resected is determined (Figs. 1.4 and 1.5) by grasping the breast with the thumb and index finger to establish fixed reference points B and C. These two points should not be placed higher than a transverse line passing through the nipple. According to my surgical marking, the points B and C are located much lower than in the classic Pitanguy's technique, as the skin resection is much smaller in the vertical dimension to achieve a shorter scar

(Fig. 1.4). The lengths of the distances AB and AC are not equal on both sides, even on the same breast, particularly in cases of asymmetric breasts as they are unusual in shape, thus requiring asymmetrical markings (Fig. 1.4b, c).

Points D and E represent the lateral and medial extremes respectively of the lines of resection that are marked at the ends of the inframammary incision (Figs. 1.1 and 1.2). Lines CE and BD can be straight or curved, as determined for the individual breast. Points B and C are in part determined by estimating the amount of skin and breast tissue to be removed by folding the breast (Fig. 1.7).

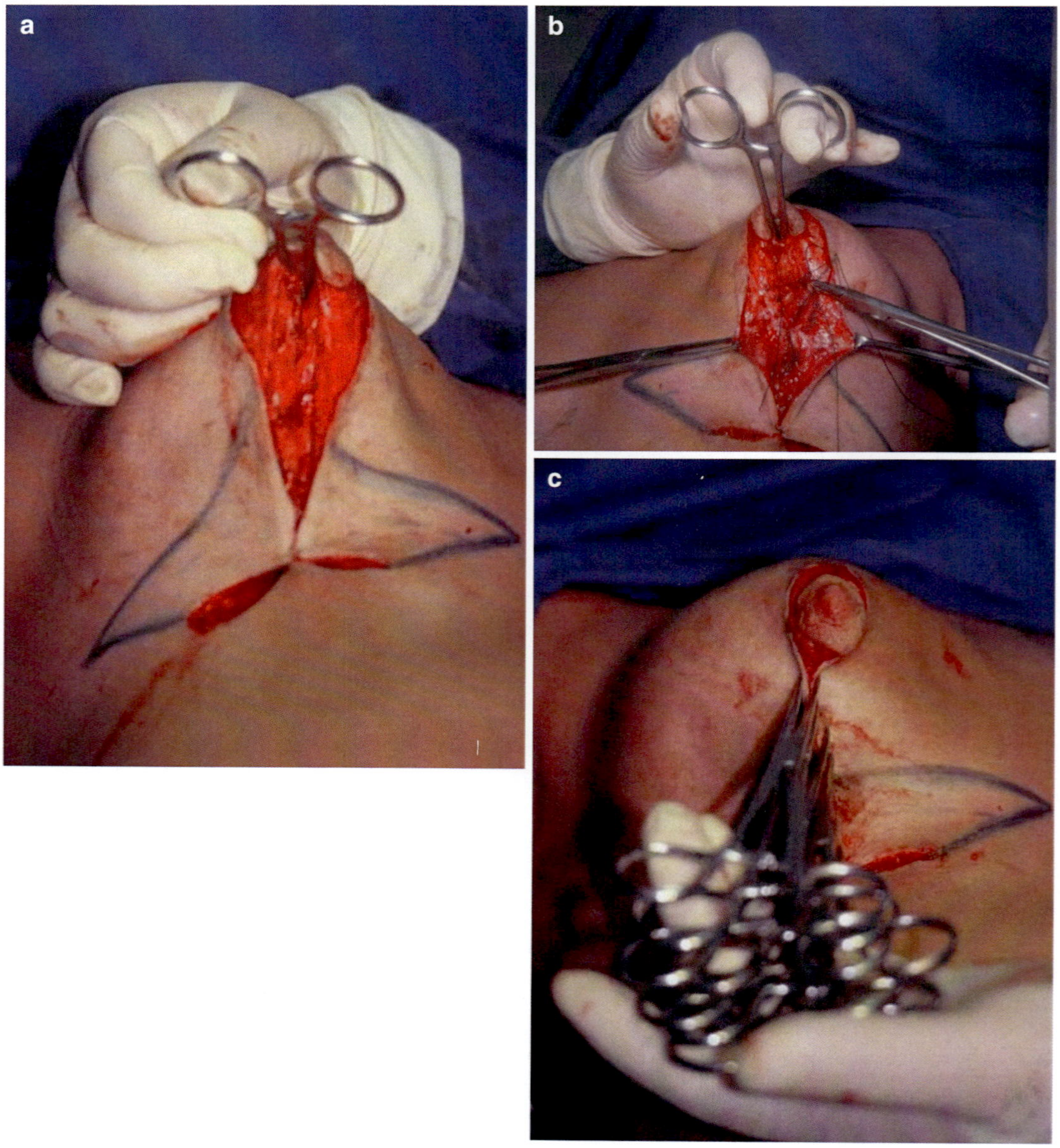

Fig. 1.7 Sequential photos during surgery showing that forceps is introduced inside the breast and lifted up where skin area preserved according to my marking can be seen. (**a**) The two columns were already sutured to the pectoralis muscle and a temporary stitch was inserted at points B and C on the medial part of the breast. (**b**) Dermal flaps were dissected on each side of the vertical incision and sutured one to another. (**c**) The excess skin was pulled forward and held by forceps at the central area of the breast

1.2.3 Glandular Resection

The operation is performed following surgical marking for the resection of mammary tissue and excess skin. With both hands, the surgeon's assistant holds the breast by its base or a strong elastic tape is wrapped around it to expose the NAC, then Schwarzmann's maneuver (1930) is performed. Afterward, using a strong hook on the point A the breast is pulled upward for skin resection (Fig. 1.5) and to remove glandular tissue following Pitanguy's technique in the shape of a "keel" in the medial part of the breast, with two wedges on each side (Fig. 1.5). After glandular resection two columns are created on each side of the breast. The skin that is not resected in my procedure corresponds to the two columns created after glandular resection (Figs. 1.2, 1.4, and 1.5b, c). The width of the "keel" and the base of the two columns constitute the amount of glandular resection that will be provided. The thickness of the columns comprises the remaining mammary tissue.

1.2.4 Creation of the "Third" Pedicle

As far as the glandular tissue is resected following Pitanguy's technique, a "third" pedicle is created on the superior segment of the breast, which is the thickness of subcutaneous tissue between the two columns (Fig. 1.6). This is an important structure for aiding the vascularization to the NAC, even though there is no cutaneous undermining.

1.2.5 Suture of Mammary Tissue to Pectoralis

Careful hemostasis is carried out so that glandular suturing can be performed. My "Z" instrument or forceps is introduced under the remaining glandular tissue between the two columns (Fig. 1.7) and the surgeon's assistant pulls it up to perform suturing of both columns to the aponeurosis of the pectoralis muscle, which avoids any "dead space." This sort of fixation was recommended by Ragnell (1946) and later by Malbec and Quaife (1957), and is a useful step during operation.

Afterward, a temporary stitch is inserted to approximate the points "B" and "C" on the midline of the submammary crease to allow evaluation of the size and shape of the future breast (Fig. 1.7).

1.2.6 Repositioning the New Nipple–Areola Complex

Determining the new position of the NAC is an important step during the mastoplasty operation. By dissection of the dermis, I introduced suturing of the dermal flaps created on both sides of the vertical segment of the breast. The dermal flaps are sutured with isolated stitches creating a dermal structure that functions as reinforcement of the vertical suture to adjust content and container (Avelar 1980, 1993a, b). Afterward, using special forceps, the skin is pulled forward to evaluate the exact amount of excess to be resected, as performed by Noël (1928), which is a useful procedure. The NAC is drawn on the vertices of the new breast using a special round marker. The NAC is pulled from the depths to the exterior and sutured on the new areolar area.

The surgical wound is then closed with a running suture and adhesive tapes are placed on it. Finally, the area is bandaged.

1.3 Discussion

Each surgeon must follow a specific technique to employ in all cases of reduction mastoplasty or mastopexy. As long as he or she follows the same surgical principles, it is possible to accumulate sufficient knowledge during each operation. This concept is a fundamental step, which is an essential guideline that gives correct orientation to perform the reduction mastoplasty.

Pitanguy's technique is easy to learn and to perform and there are no prefabricated patterns to determine the cutaneous incisions and glandular resection. Surgical marking is a fundamental step, which is done according to the surgeon's creativity and imagination for each patient. It is a versatile method, especially for medium and large hypertrophic breasts. Even in the case of asymmetry, it is a useful procedure, as the marking requires particular attention to the amount of skin and glandular tissue to be resected according to each breast. The surgical principles of the technique are very precise and must be followed during planning and when performing the operation.

Because of the versatility of the technique, it gives adequate support to several surgeons in developing new approaches as long as the essential surgical principles are preserved. My personal procedure follows Pitanguy's technique, to which I introduced some surgical detail to reduce the size of the scars; thus, the incisions on the submammary creases are very short as a great amount of cutaneous resection is carried out, pulling the skin to the medial part of the breast.

It is important to emphasize that the Pitanguy's point "A" does not represent the exact center of the future nipple after surgery, but it is a reference point very close to where the nipple will be when the operation is complete. The final marking of the precise nipple placement is performed after suturing of the two columns of the mammary gland and the skin is temporarily sutured (Fig. 1.7). It means that the nipple is placed on the vertices of the cone shape created after internal suturing of the breast tissue, and the excess skin is resected at the end of the operation. The "third pedicle" of the technique is an essential anatomical detail that is important support for adequate blood supply to the NAC. In fact, it is the superior pole of the breast located between the upper parts of the two glandular columns created during tissue resection.

During surgical marking, the surgeon may determine the amount of breast tissue to be resected by establishing fixed reference points, which are marked, even in cases of slight or severe asymmetry.

There are several advantages of Pitanguy's technique: it is easy to learn and employ, the flexibility in nipple positioning during marking and intraoperatively, the preservation of lactation in most patients, an excellent breast shape can be achieved, a very low rate of complications, and no "dead space" after suturing of the remaining mammary tissue. In summary, it is a free-handed approach to measurement and resection. The flexibility of the method is one of the most attractive features of the operation for the experienced surgeon, to create a new skin brassiere so as to achieve a good balance between the content and the continent. As I was Prof. Pitanguy's resident during my period of specialization, all surgical principles of the technique are clear in my mind. Also, I am convinced about the efficiency of the technique as I can bear testimony to the excellent results he used to achieve and the very high rate of patient satisfaction. For all those reasons, I have employed his technique since the beginning of my practice, with very small modifications, leaving nice scars located on the submammary folds (Figs. 1.8 and 1.9).

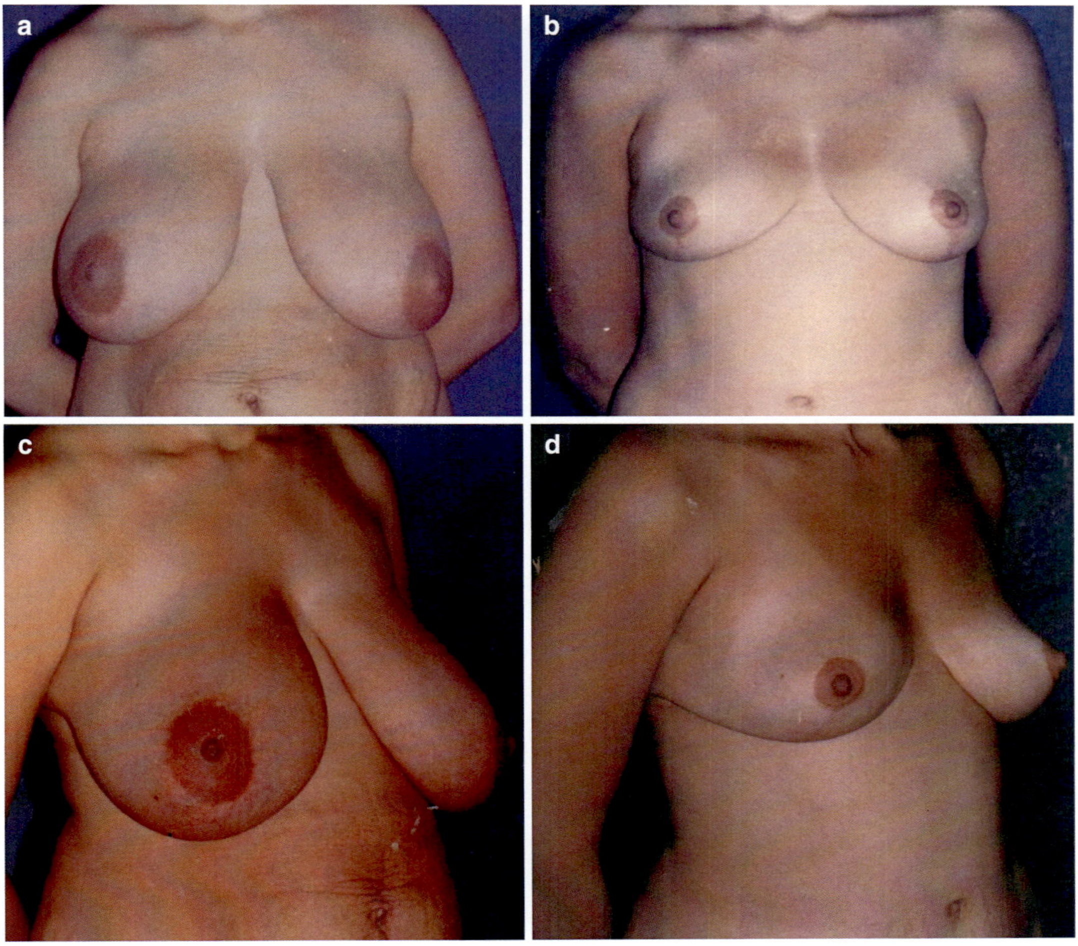

Fig. 1.8 A 35-year-old patient with large and ptotic breasts underwent reduction mastoplasty. (**a**) and (**c**) Photos before surgery. (**b**) and (**d**) Photos after the operation

If a surgeon does not have enough experience with the technique, he or she must exercise caution during all the surgical steps: marking, skin incisions, mammary tissue resection, and suturing of the columns of the remaining glandular tissue. Nevertheless, following the surgical principles of the technique, it is possible to achieve good results (Figs. 1.10 and 1.11).

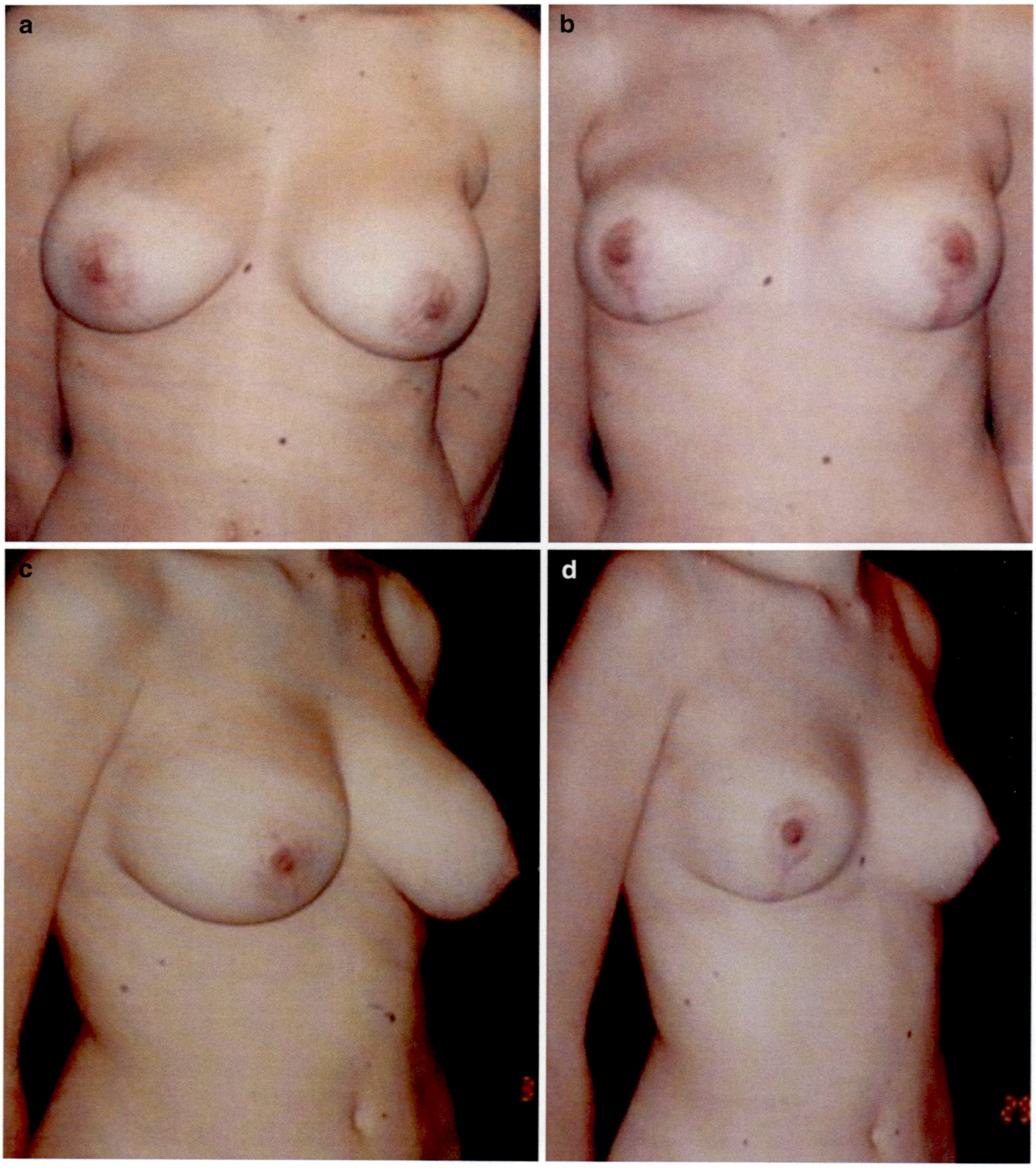

Fig. 1.9 A 28-year-old patient presenting asymmetric breasts underwent mastoplasty. (**a**) and (**c**) Photos before surgery. (**b**) and (**d**) Photos after operation

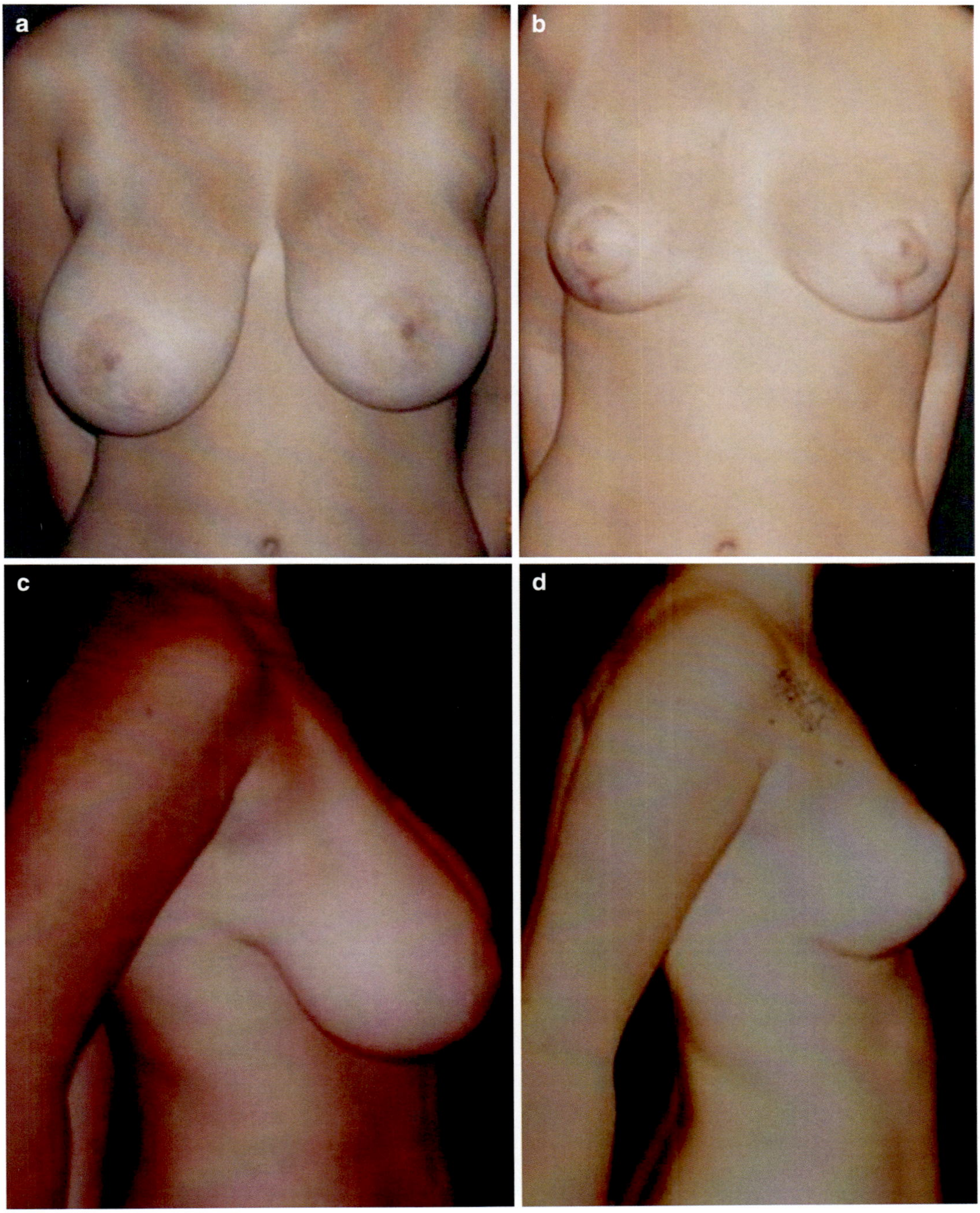

Fig. 1.10 A 25-year-old patient presenting asymmetric breasts with bilateral hypertrophy and severe ptosis with physical repercussion for her chest. (**a**, **c**, **e**) Photos before surgery. (**b**, **d**, **f**) Photos after reduction mastoplasty with resection of 950 g on the right side and 650 g from the left breast

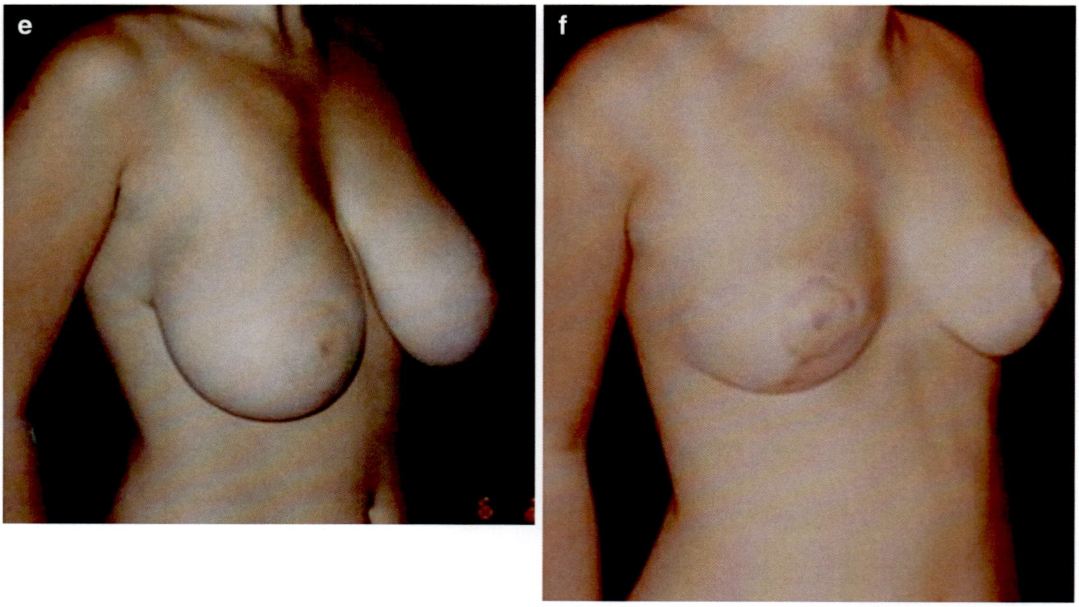

Fig. 1.10 (continued)

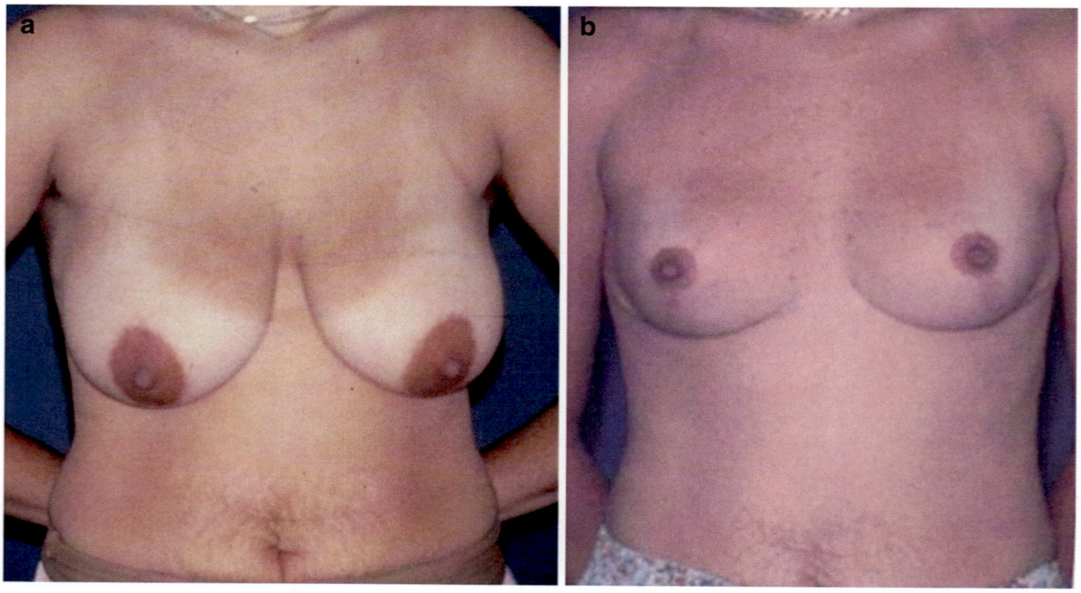

Fig. 1.11 A 28-year-old patient presenting moderate hypertrophy with ptotic and flabby breasts underwent mastoplasty. (**a**) and (**c**) Photos before surgery. (**b**) and (**d**) Photos after the operation

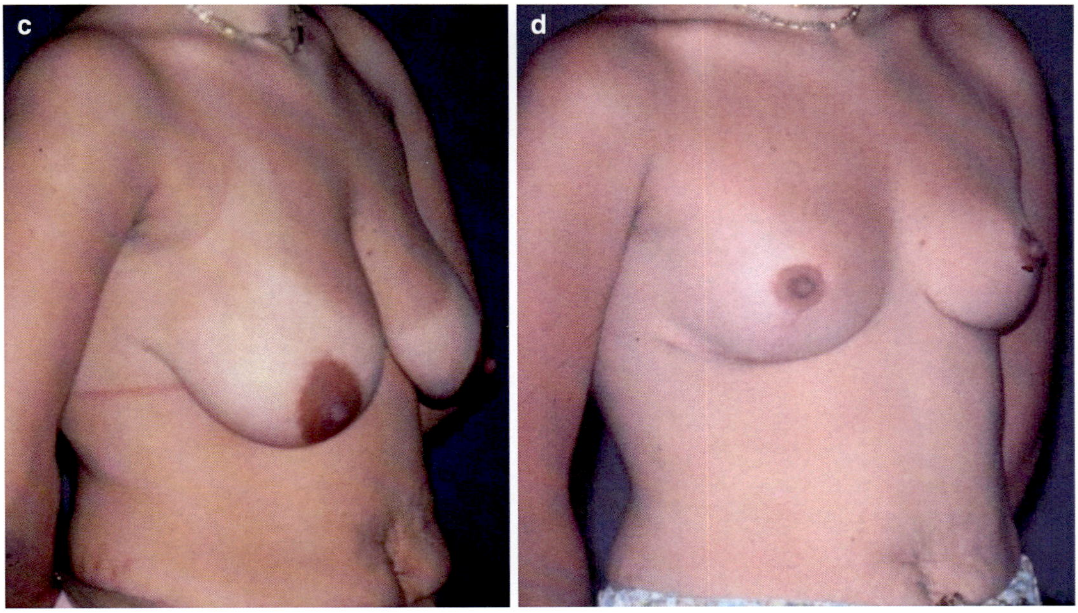

Fig. 1.11 (continued)

Conclusions

To my knowledge, there are two periods in the history of reduction mastoplasty: before and after 1960, when Pitanguy introduced his technique. Up to 1960, there were useful procedures that formed the technical platform for great development, particularly in breast reduction. I know several other techniques that were described before and after Pitanguy's publication, but I am so used to employing his technique. So far, since the beginning of my practice, I have introduced several technical modifications with regard to surgical marking with repercussions for glandular resection. As asymmetric breasts are very common, Pitanguy's technique is adequate for achieving well balanced results (Figs. 1.12 and 1.13).

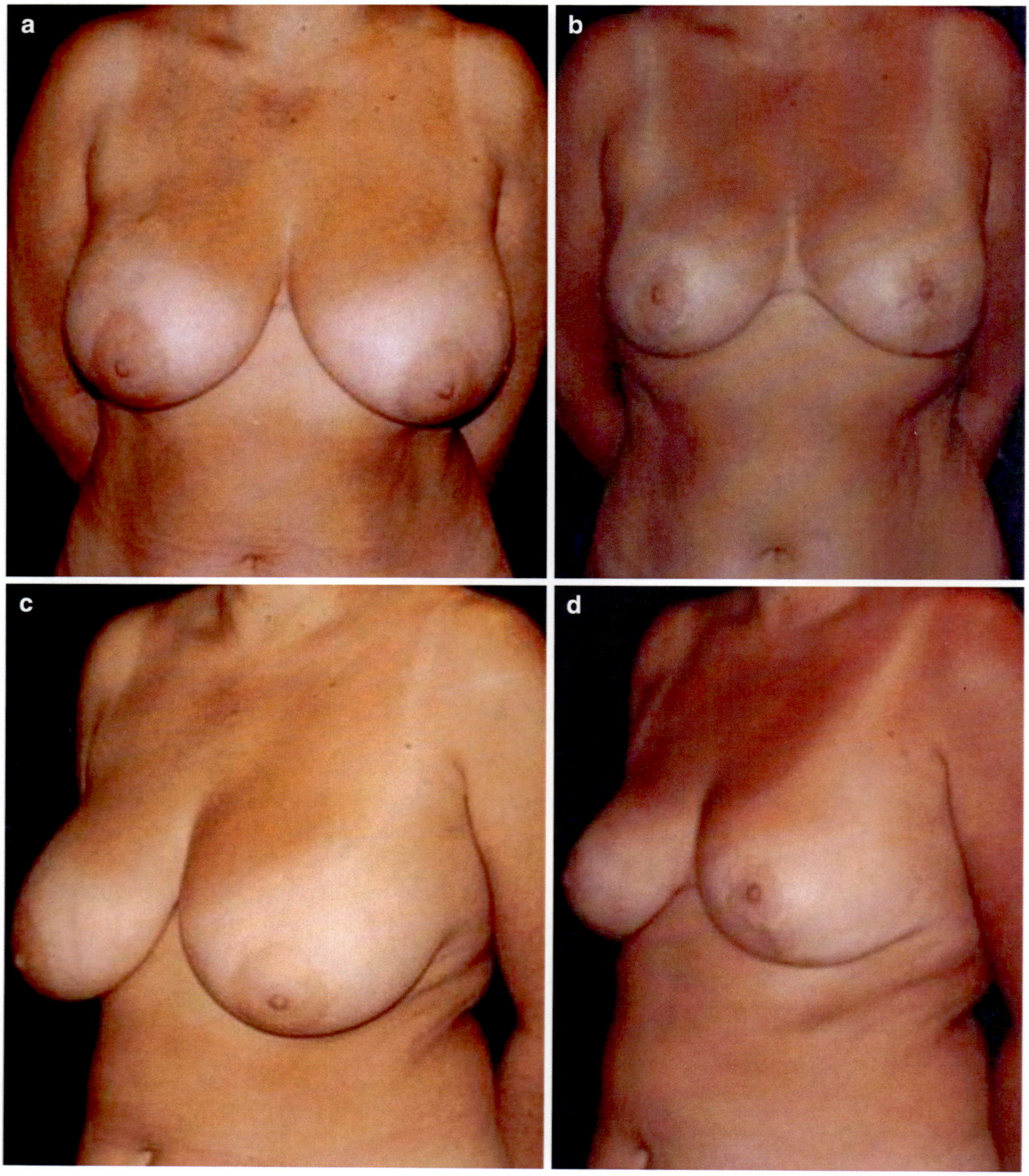

Fig. 1.12 A 51-year-old patient presenting moderate hypertrophy with asymmetrical, ptotic, and flabby breasts underwent mastoplasty. (**a**) and (**c**) Photos before surgery. (**b**) and (**d**) Photos after the operation

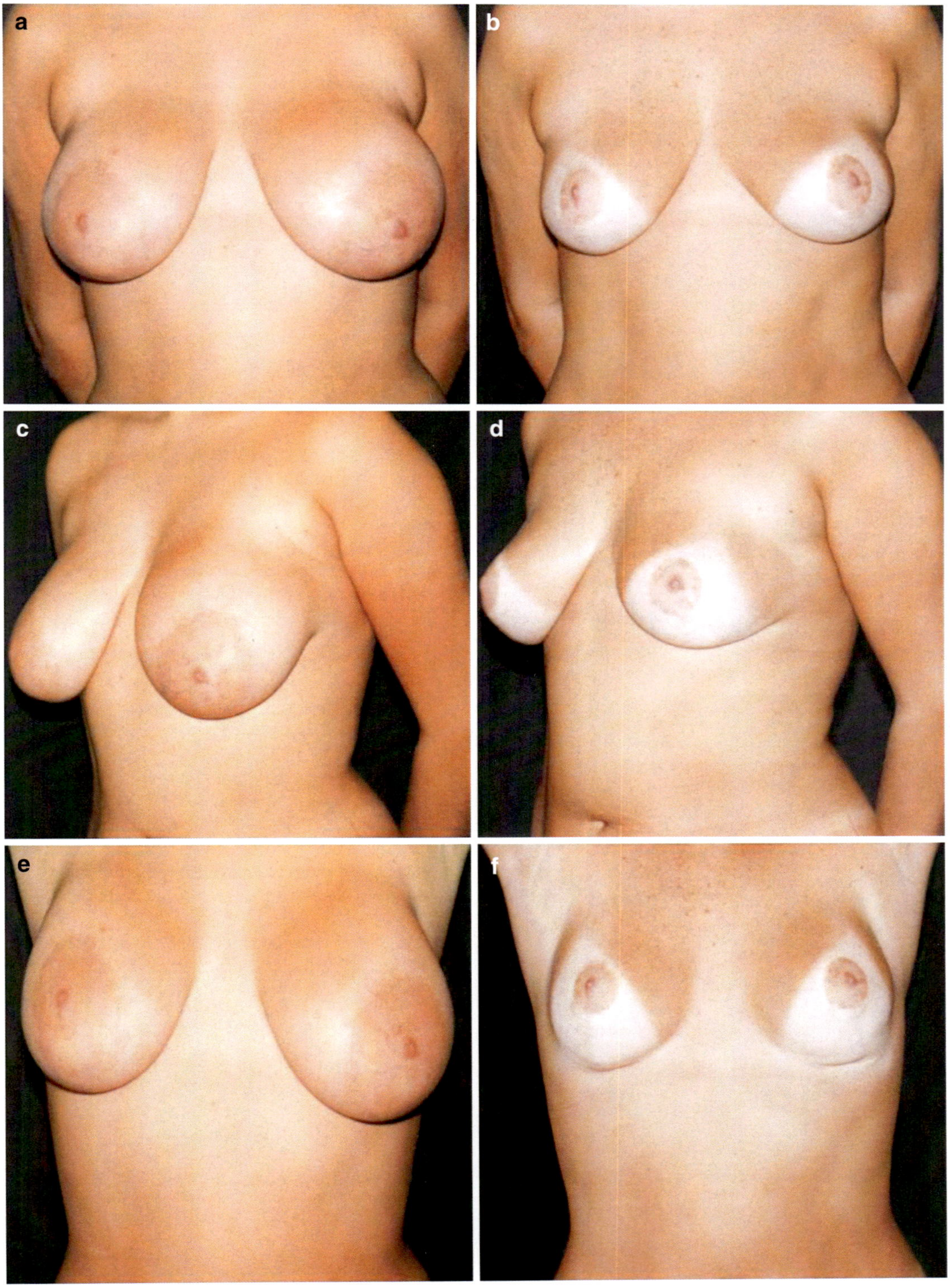

Fig. 1.13 A 19-year-old patient presenting asymmetric breasts with moderate hypertrophy and ptosis. (**a**, **c**, **e**) Photos before the operation. (**b**, **d**, **f**) Photos after reduction mastoplasty with resection of 280 g on the right side and 580 g from the left breast

References

Aufricht G (1949) Mammaplasty for pendulous breast. Empiric and geometry planning. Plast Reconstr Surg 4(1):13–29

Avelar JM (1980) Dermoadiposeglandular flap with superior pedicle on mastopexy (Retalho dermoadiposeglandular com pediculo superior nas mastopexia). Brazilian symposium on breast surgery. Brazilian Society of Plastic Surgery – Regional of São Paulo, São Paulo

Avelar J (1993a) Loco-regional anesthesia on aesthetic surgery (Anestesia Loco-Regional em Cirurgia Estética). In: Juarez M. Avelar (ed). Editora Hipócrates, São Paulo

Avelar JM (1993b) Reduction mastoplasty under local anesthesia. (Mastoplastia redutora sob anestesia local). In: Avelar JM (ed) Loco-regional anesthesia on aesthetic surgery—(Anestesia Loco-regional em cirurgia estética), vol 29. Editora Hipócrates, São Paulo, pp 244–260

Biesenberger H (1928) Blutversorsuflg und Zirkuiare Umschedung dês Warzenhofes. Zbl Chir 55:2.385

Dufourmentel C, Mouly R (1961) Plastie Mammaire par la Méthode Obliqúe. Ann Chir Plast 6:45

Fernandez J (1951) Mastoplastias, nuestra experiência editorial universitária. Buenos Aires

Gillies H, McIndoe A (1939) The technique of mammoplasty in conditions of hypertrophy of the breast. Surg Gynaecol Obstet 68:658

Kraske H (1923) Die Operation der atrophischen und hypertrophischen Hängebrust. MMW 70:672–637

Lexer E (1912) Hypertrophie bei der Mammae. Munch Med Wochenschr 59:2702

McKissock PK (1972) Reduction mammaplasty with a vertical dermal flap. Plast Reconstr Surg 49(3):245

Kausch W (1916) Die Operationen der Mammahypertrophie. Zentralbl F Chir 43:713

Malbec EF, Quaife JV (1957) Plastias mammarias. Nuestra experiências com inclusíones. Orientacián Médica 260:768

Maliniac JW (1932) Plastic repair of pendulous breasts. MJ Rec 756:312

Morestin H, Gaudet F (1905) French Congress of Surgeons, vol 82. Paris, p 125

Noël A (1928) Aesthetische Chirurgie der Weiblichen Brust. Ein neues Verfahren zur Korrektur der Hängebrust. Med Welt 2:51

Passot R (1925) La correction esthétique du prolapsus mammaire par la procede de la transposition du mamelon. Presse Méd 33:317

Pitanguy I (1959) Breast hypertrophy. In: Wallace AB (ed) Transactions of the International Society of Plastic Surgeons, Second Congress, London. Livingstone, Edinburgh, E&S, pp 509–517

Pitanguy I (1961) Estudo de 245 casos consecutivos de mamaplastia e apresentação de técnica pessoal. Rev Bras Cir:201–220

Pitanguy I (1967) Surgical treatment of breast hypertrophy. Br J Plast Surg 20(1):78–85

Pitanguy I, Garcia LC (1972) Aspectos importantes de tecnica pessoal em mammaplastia. Bol Soc Cir Plast Reconstr Cordoba 4:7

Pitanguy I (1981) Aesthetic plastic surgery of head and body. Springer, Berlin

Ragnell KGA (1946) Operative correction of hypertrophy and ptosos of the female breast: a clinical investigation of 300 cases with examination of a new method. Acta Chir Scand 1:294–296

Sinder R (2003) History of breast reduction (História da mamoplastia redutora). In: Mélega JM, Baroudi R (eds) Cirurgia plástica—fundamentos e arte. Medsi, Rio de Janeiro, pp 435–469

Skoog TA (1963) Technique of breast reduction. Transposition of the nipple on a cutaneous vascular pedicle. Acta Chir Scand 126:453

Schwarzmann E (1930) Technik der mammaplastik. Der Chirurg 2:932

Strombeck JG (1960) Mammaplasty report of a new technique based on two pedicle procedure. Br J Plast Surg 13:79–90

Thorek M (1942) Plastic surgery of the breasts and abdominal wall. Charles C. Thomas, Springfield, p 314

2 The Pitanguy Technique for the Surgical Treatment of Breast Hypertrophy

Sérgio Carreirão

2.1 Introduction

Pitanguy's technique for the surgical treatment of breast hypertrophy was introduced into the world literature in the early 1960s (Pitanguy 1978, 1960, 1961).

The procedure has been considered one of the most popular used for the treatment of breast hypertrophy. This has not occurred by chance and therefore deserves a critical evaluation.

I worked with Professor Pitanguy for 35 years without interruption, performing and teaching his technique. Thus, I had the opportunity to observe the evolution of the technique and now intend to show my point of view.

2.2 History

In 1959, Pitanguy proposed some modifications to Arié's technique for breast reduction (Pitanguy 1978). In 1960, Pitanguy published his personal technique (Pitanguy 1960).

These are the main basic principles:

- The mammary flaps of the procedure must maintain its connection to the overlying skin.
- Undermining of the flaps is consistently reduced.
- The inferior pole of the breast is removed, preserving the "adipose capsule of the superior pole of the breast"
- A keel-shaped glandular resection is performed, allowing a wide elevation of the nipple-areola complex (NAC)
- Dead spaces in the new breast are eliminated.

Since then, Pitanguy has presented important papers that have consolidated the technique (Pitanguy 1978, 1967, 1981).

2.3 The Pitanguy Technique

This technique is described in important papers published by Pitanguy (1978, 1967, 1981).

The surgical steps are as follows. Initially, a vertical line is drawn from the midpoint of the clavicular bone to the nipple (it is named the mid-clavicular line). On this line point A is marked at a level just below the projection of the inframammary fold, as shown by the finger in Fig. 2.1. This point marks the final position of the NAC, which is situated slightly above and laterall to this point, in the middle of the mammary cone.

To determine the amount of tissue to be resected, the breast is manually grasped and the points B and

S. Carreirão, M.D.
Brazilian Society of Plastic Surgery (TSBCP), Sao Paulo, SP, Brazil

Brazilian College of Surgeons (ECBC), Rio de Janeiro, RJ, Brazil

American College of Surgeons (FACS), Chicago, IL, USA
e-mail: scarreirao@hotmail.com

J.M. Avelar (ed.), *Breast Surgery*, https://doi.org/10.1007/978-3-319-54115-0_2

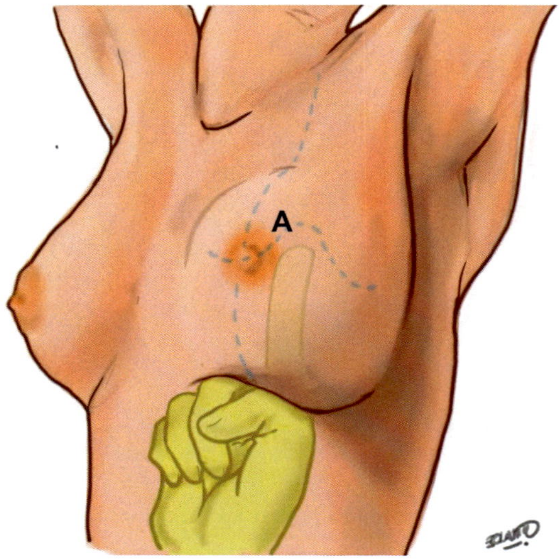

Fig. 2.1 Point A marked on the midclavicular line at the level just below the projection of the inframammary fold

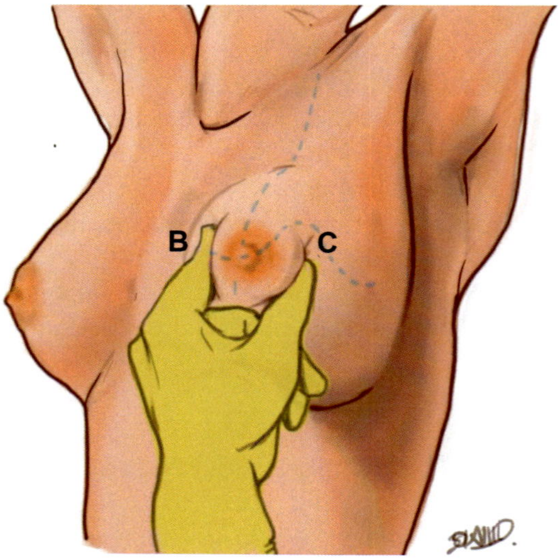

Fig. 2.2 To determine the amount of tissue to be resected, the breast is manually grasped and the points B and C are marked

C are marked (Fig. 2.2). The points can vary (range) according to the indications of each case. Pitanguy advises that the AB and AC distances should not be greater than 6–7 cm and that B and C points should not be placed higher than a transversal line passing the nipple. The distance between points B and C varies according to the amount of tissue to be removed. The lines AB and AC are drawn. Points D

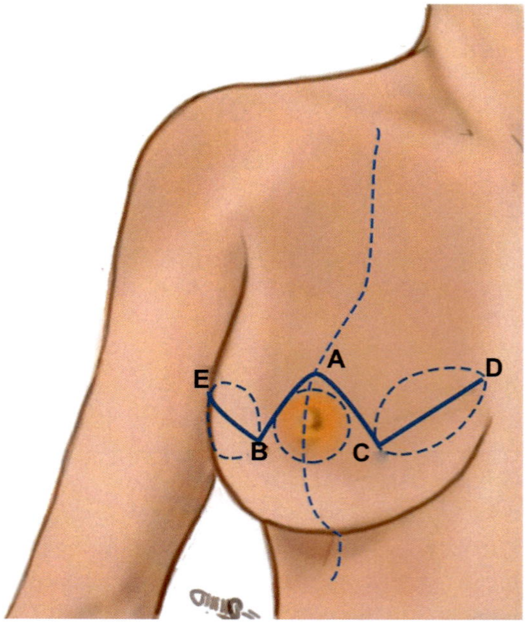

Fig. 2.3 The lines AB and AC are drawn. Points D and E are marked at the medial and lateral extremity of the inframammary fold respectively. Lines connecting points B–D, and C–E are drawn (see text)

and E are marked at the medial and lateral extremities of the inframammary fold respectively. Lines connecting B–D, and C–E are drawn. BD should not exceed the anterior axillary line. CE should not reach the median external line (Fig. 2.3). The skin area to be resected is now determined. The position and size of the NAP are evaluated using sizers that vary in diameter.

Breast distention is performed allowing Schwartzman's maneuver around the areolar skin. The skin of the ABC triangle is undermined (Fig. 2.4).

Forceps placed at point A raises the breast. CD and BE incisions are performed deep to the muscular fascia. Another incision is performed from point B to point C. Then, a keel-shaped glandular resection is performed, starting below the areola and preserving the adipose capsule, which Pitanguy considers a third pedicle (Fig. 2.5). Resection is made in one single block including skin and adipose and glandular tissues. After the desired resection, two columns or pillars (medial and lateral) are identified and put together in the middle of the breast. The breast

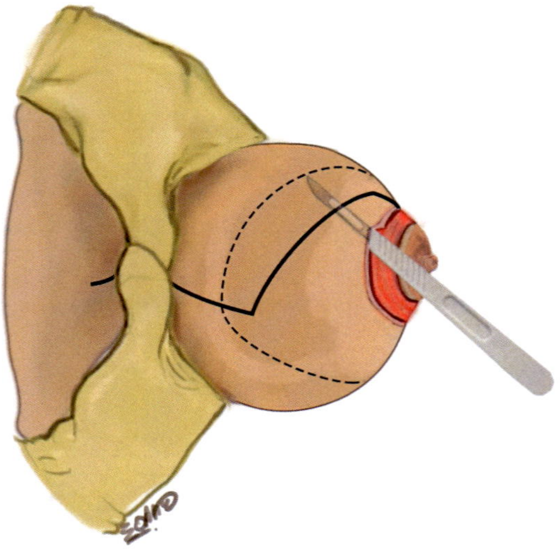

Fig. 2.4 Schwartzman's maneuver

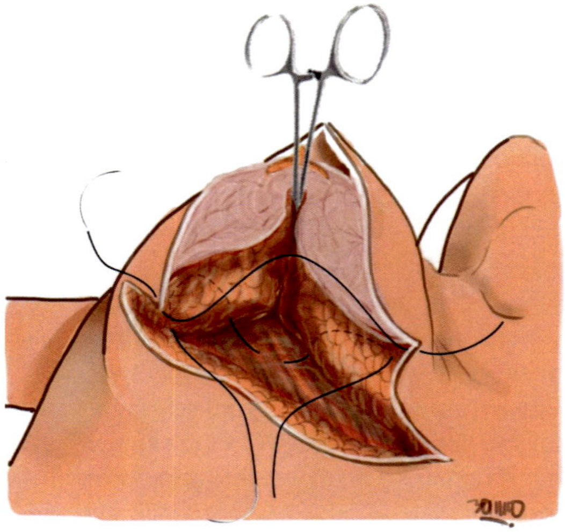

Fig. 2.6 Fixation of the columns into the chest wall

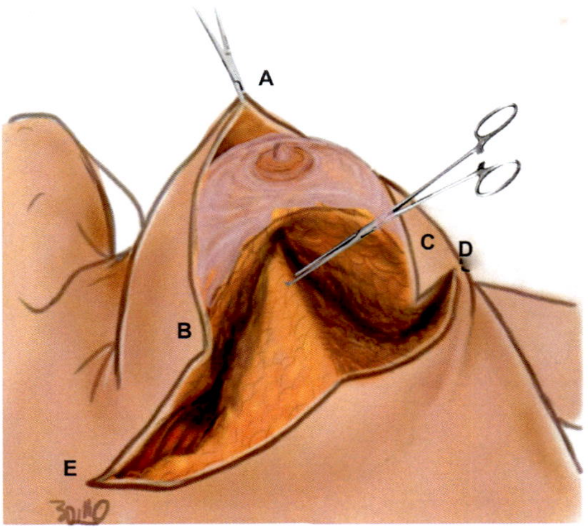

Fig. 2.5 The keel-shaped glandular resection is performed, starting below the nipple–areola complex and made in a single block

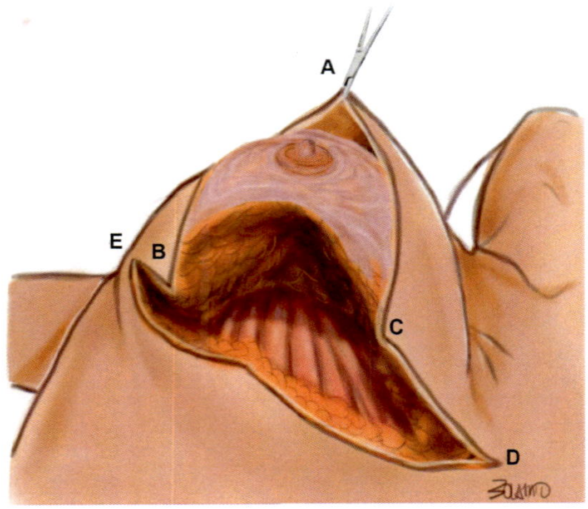

Fig. 2.7 Breast molding is completed by the union of points BC on the inframammary fold in a point that ideally corresponds to the projection of the nipple line onto this fold.

cone now formed raises the NAC to the summit of the breast. At this time, columns are fixed into the chest wall (Fig. 2.6).

Breast molding is completed by the union of points BC on the inframammary fold in a point that ideally corresponds to the projection of the nipple line on this fold (Fig. 2.7). Dead spaces inside the breast must be avoided.

When a larger resection of skin than glandular tissue is needed, the excised skin is evaluated and removed in the vertical scar (AB/AC). The final position of the NAC is then determined.

2.4 Some Considerations About the Technique

Regarding its importance in the marking of reduction mammaplasties, point A is nowadays known as Pitanguy's point by some authors.

The technique maintains skin and glandular connections in the remaining breasts, which allows normal breast feeding (lactation) and preserves nipple sensitivity. Raising the NAC flap up to the upper pole increases the fullness in this area of the breast, offering offers a better aesthetic result. The union of pillars (medial and lateral) in the middle of the breast and its fixation into the pectoral fascia gives rise to a conical and well-formed breast with an adequate position on the thoracic wall. It is Pitanguy's opinion that by preserving embryological connections between the skin and glandular tissues in the flaps, the suspension of the breast is assured. This is a very good reason for avoiding postoperative ptosis.

Pitanguy also points out the importance of drawing the points of his technique in the operating room with the patient in a semi-seated position. Before the mounting of the breasts, the resection of one side must be compared with the other to achieve better breast symmetry. In dealing with breast asymmetry, the ABC triangle should vary from one side to the other.

2.5 Author's Experience with Pitanguy Technique

My experience and results with Pitanguy's technique have been extremely favorable as I have been performing it for more than 40 years.

Keel-shaped glandular resection allowed the NAC to be raised in the most of our cases without the need for any other maneuver and providing a good shape to the upper pole (Fig. 2.8). In many cases, Letterman's maneuver (Letterman and Schurter 1981) was used to help raise the

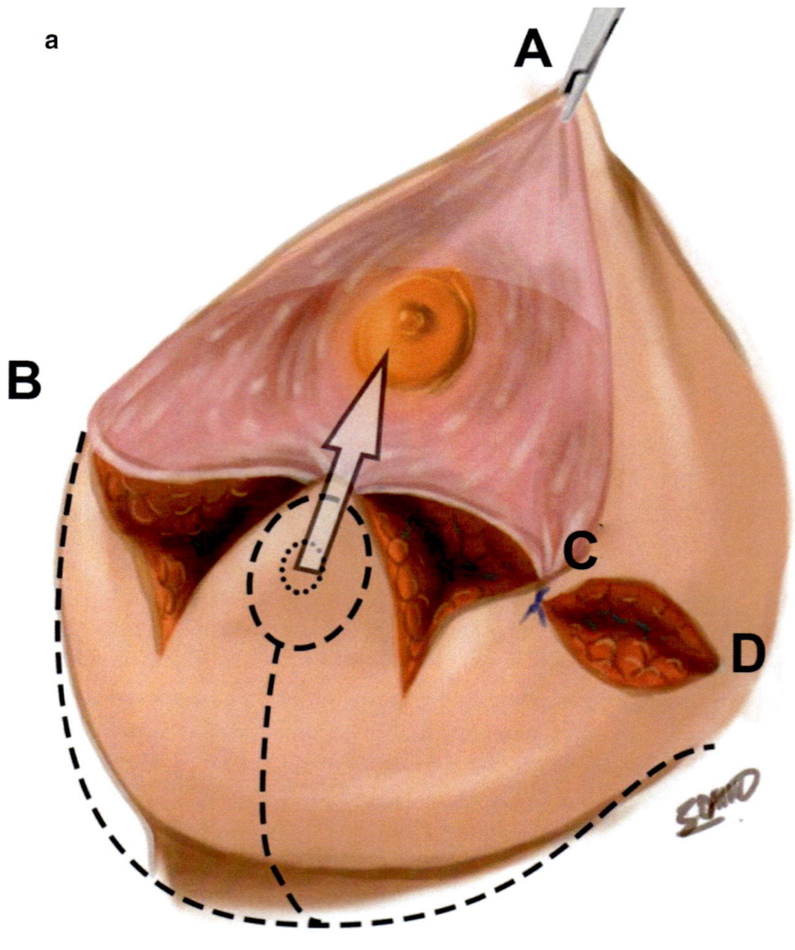

Fig. 2.8 (**a**) Nipple–areola complex elevation according to Pitanguy's technique. (**b**) Large mammary ptosis. Postoperative aspect 3 months after surgery. (**c**) Same patient, oblique view

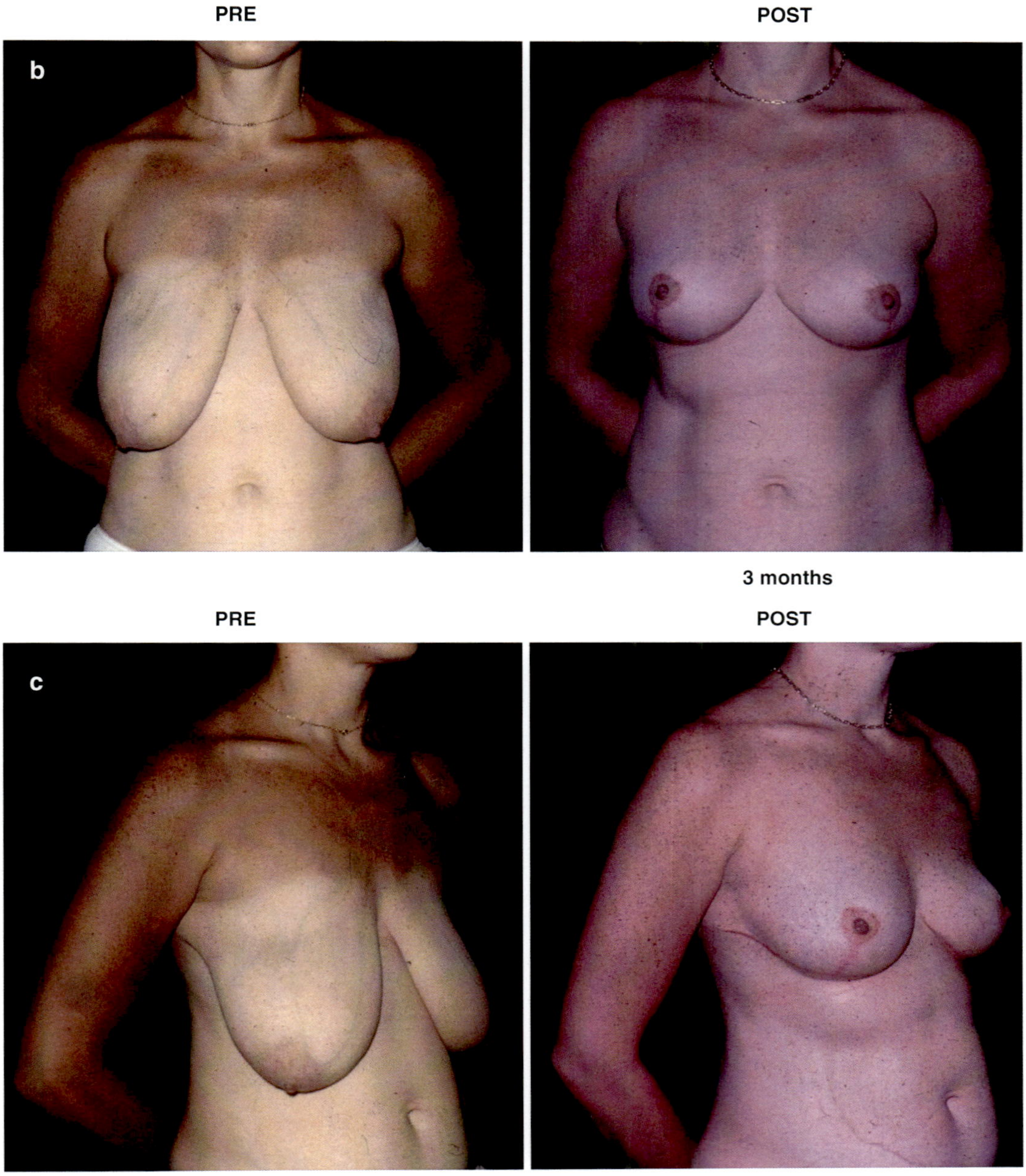

Fig. 2.8 (continued)

NAC. In a few cases of more severe ptosis we used the Silveira Neto medial flap (Silveira 1976) for providing an adequate position for the NAC.

I consider Pitanguy's technique to be a very well indicated procedure for the correction of breast asymmetry because it does not depend on a previous and rigid marking allowing different resections between one side and the other (Fig. 2.9).

Final scars, if well positioned and according to the correct principles of the technique, showed good aesthetic results in the late postoperative period (Fig. 2.10).

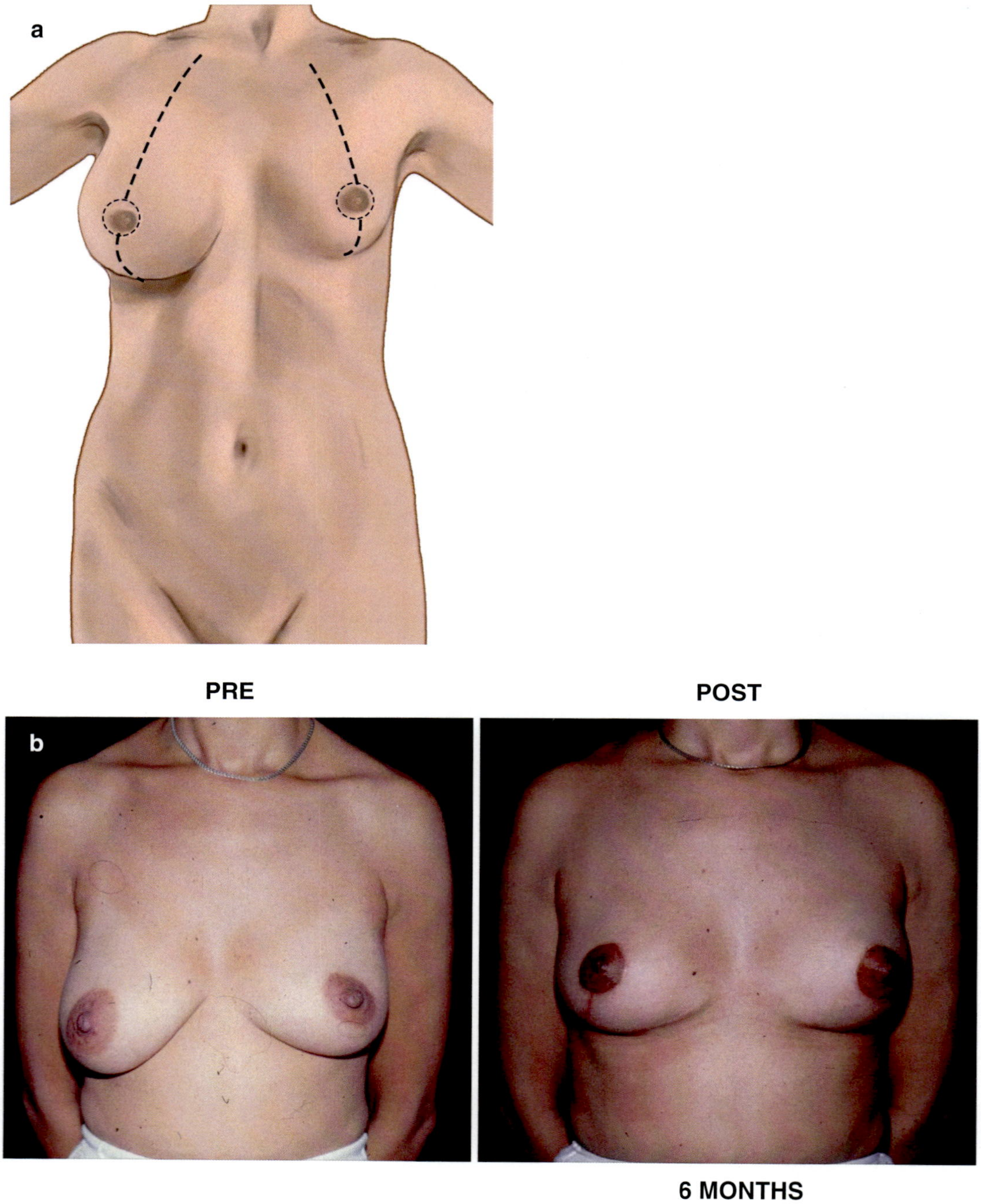

Fig. 2.9 (**a**) Drawing the Pitanguy's technique for the correction of mammary asymmetry. (**b**) Mammary asymmetry treated using Pitanguy's technique. Result 6 months after the surgery

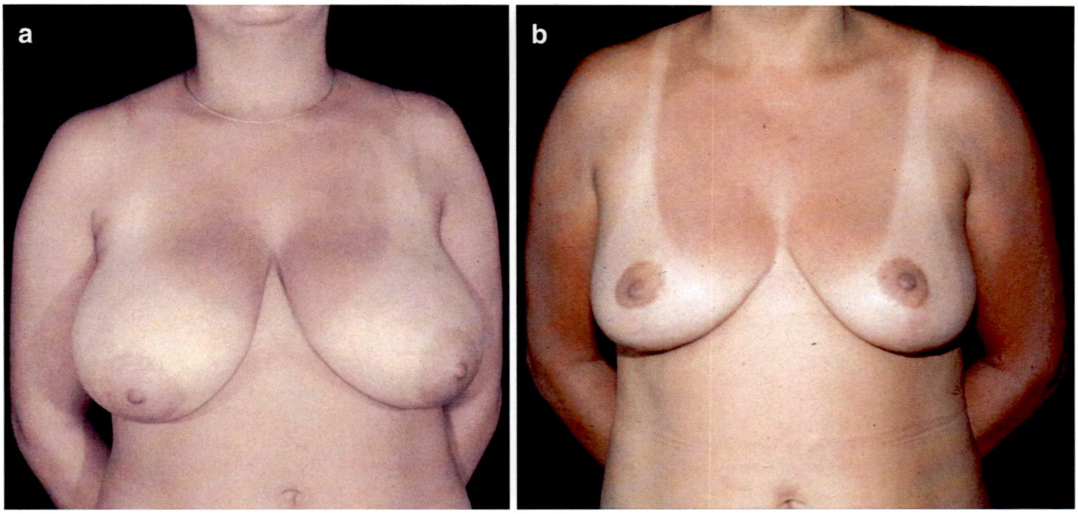

Fig. 2.10 (**a**) Preoperative aspect of a patient with massive breast hypertrophy, ptosis, and asymmetry. (**b**) Same patient. Result 18 years after the surgery was performed using Pitanguy's technique

2.6 Technical Variations

With the distribution of the procedure over a long period all around the world, many authors have adopted it and have published papers suggesting variations and contributions in the search for even better results. Some of them have proposed a greater distance between the AB and AC points of as much as 9 cm, suggesting putting the NAC in a higher position if required. Others surgeons proposed different forms of glandular resections according to the variations in breast deformities. Others proposed shorter scars on the inframammary fold. In all these proposed technical variations, and in others not mentioned here, we notice that the main principles of Pitanguy's technique have been observed (and respected).

2.7 Personal Contribution: Adjuvant Maneuver to Pitanguy's Technique

This is a procedure for patients who have large amounts of glandular tissue on the lateral quadrants of the breast that may be prolonged upward and laterally toward the axilla, forming what we call the lateral bulge of the breast. To treat these deformities, I developed a simple and efficient maneuver (Carreirão et al. 2009) (Fig. 2.11).

The glandular resection is performed according to Pitanguy's original breast reduction technique. As already described, this technique creates two pillars (medial and lateral). In these deformities, the lateral pillar is always larger than the medial one. Measurements or dimensions of the medial pillar are transposed to the larger lateral pillar. The excess inferior and lateral tissues in the lateral pillar are resected. The entire axillary extension (Spencer) is removed, leaving the two pillars of the same size. The subcutaneous tissue in the lateral border of the breast should be preserved to avoid skin retractions. The now symmetrical pillars are fixed together, into the pectoral fascia at the midline, in the way described by Pitanguy.

This maneuver, as described, allows the removal of an axillary process and the excess tissue that determined the lateral bulging of the breast. The procedure achieves a better lateral contour (Fig. 2.12).

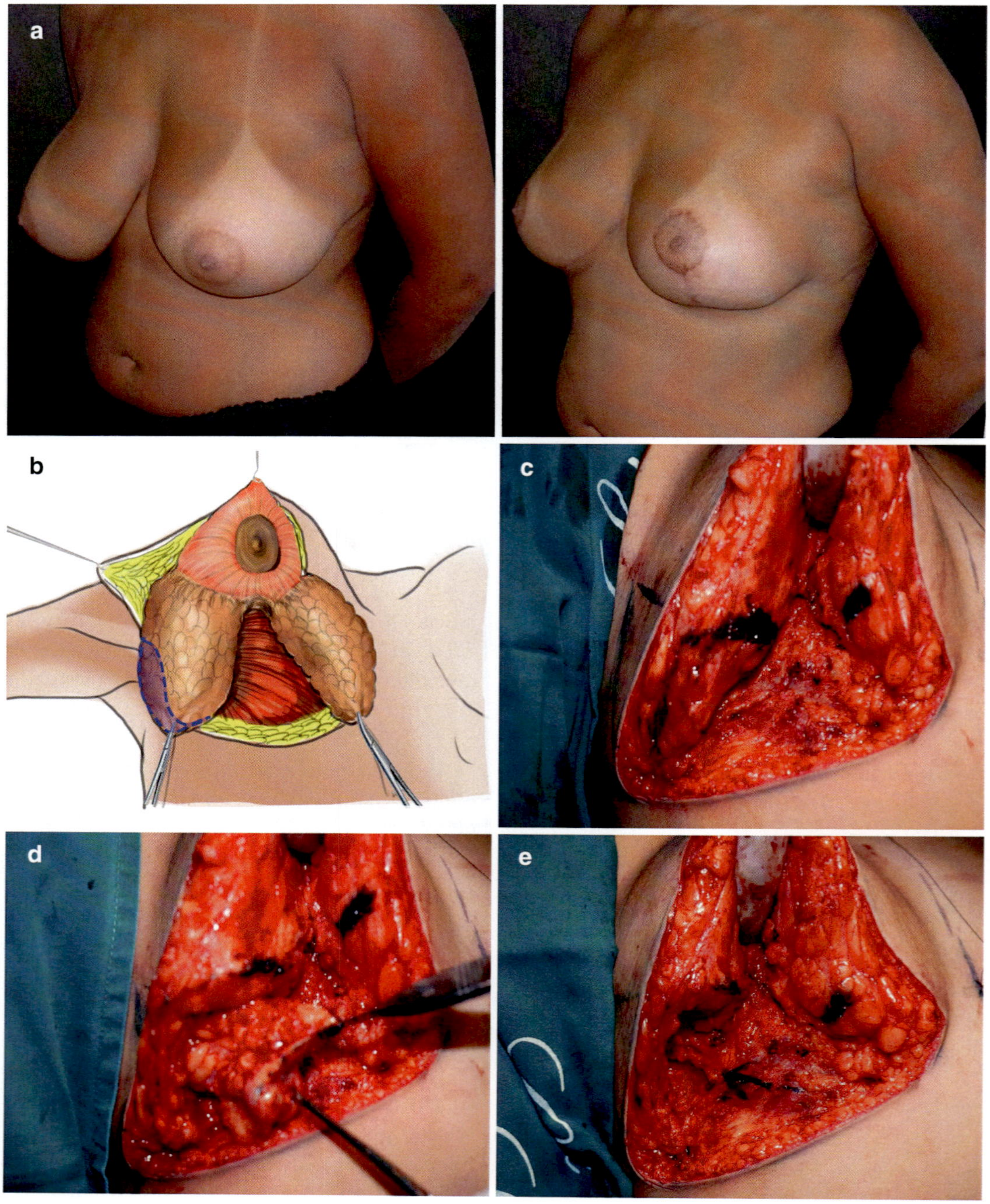

Fig. 2.11 (**a**) The deformity and the result in a patient treated with the maneuver described by the author. (**b**) The schedule of the maneuver described by the author. (**c**) Marking of tissue excess of the lateral aspect of the breast. (**d**) Resection of the demarcated area including the axillary process. (**e**) Aspect of the breast after resection of the excess lateral tissue

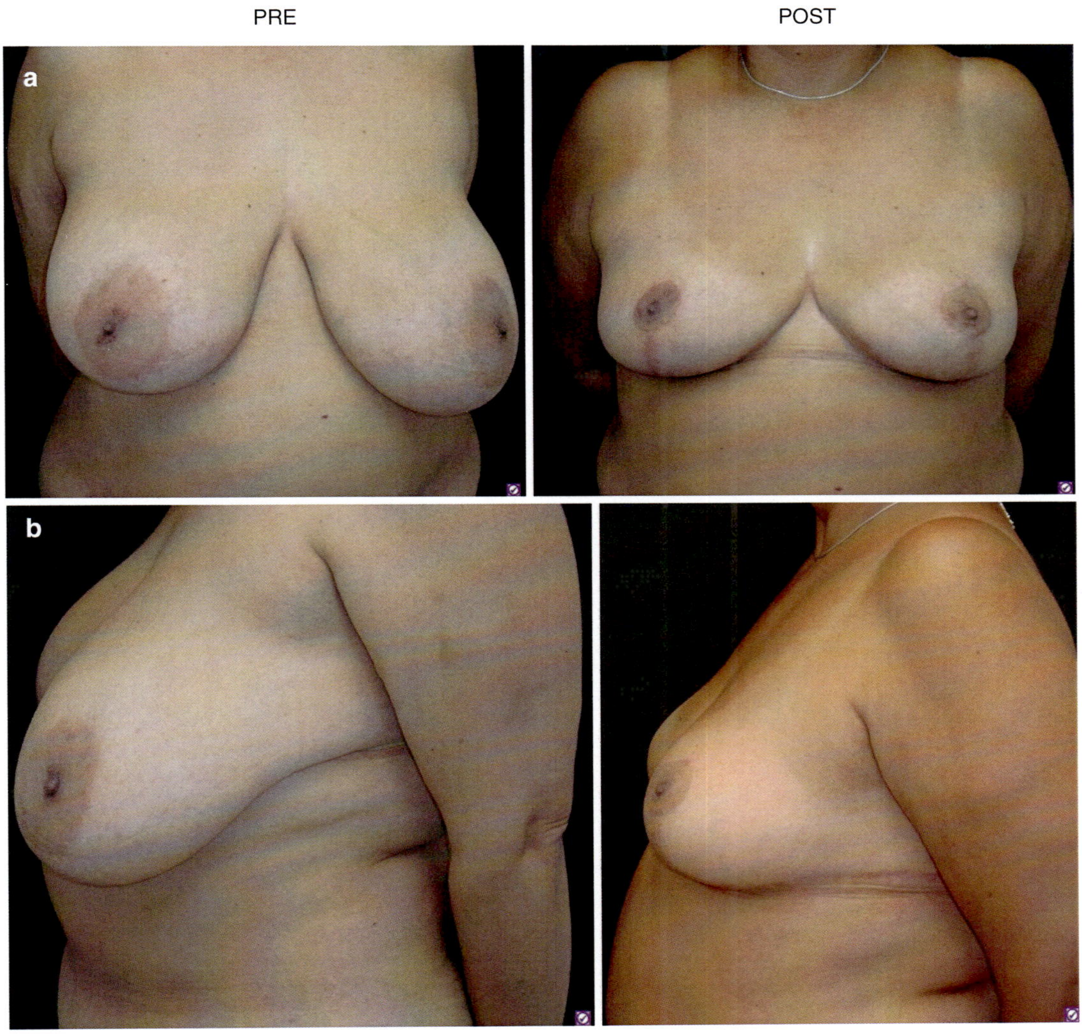

Fig. 2.12 (**a**) Patient with breast hypertrophy and lateral bulging deformity. Pre- and postoperatively (6 months). (**b**) Same patient. Notice the large deformity at the lateral aspect of the breast and the postoperative result

Conclusions

Pitanguy's technique for breast reduction is today performed all over the world. Almost all Brazilian plastic surgeons had or has had some experience with it.

It is a simple procedure, easy to learn, that has given good results for almost who used it. By following rigid anatomical criteria, it is a safe procedure with a low grade of complications. Most of the results show a breast with a natural aspect in its shape, volume, and position, and they are normally symmetrical. The final scars are well positioned and normally of good quality. Long-term results are considered to be very good (Fig. 2.12). The lack (absence) of rigid marking means that the procedure is very often used to correct asymmetries and in secondary mammaplasties. It also allows creativity on the part of the surgeons, in their search for even better results.

References

Carreirão S, Pereira L, Almeida MWR (2009) Treatment of the lateral pole: adjuvant maneuver to Pitanguy's technique. Aesthet Plast Surg 33:445–451

Letterman G, Schurter M (1981) Facilitation of the upward advancement of the nipple-areola complex in reduction mammaplasty by Kiel resection. Plast Reconstr Surg 76:793

Pitanguy I (1960) Breast hypertrophy. In: Transactions of the International Society of Plastic Surgeons. 2nd Congress, London. Livingstone, Edinburgh

Pitanguy I (1961) Aproximação eclética ao problema das mamaplastias. Rev Bras Cir 41:179–196

Pitanguy I (1967) Surgical treatment of breast hypertrophy. Br J Plast Surg 20(1):78–85

Pitanguy I (1978) Mamaplastia. Editora Guanabara Koogan, Rio de Janeiro

Pitanguy I (1981) Aesthetic plastic surgery of head and body. Springer, Berlin

Silveira Netto E (1976) Mastoplastia Redutora Setorial com Pedículo Areolar Interno. In: Transct. Anais do 13° Congresso Brasileiro de Cirurgia Plástica, Porto Alegre. Editora EMMA, Rio Grande do Sul, p 13

3 Clinical Evaluation and Surgical Planning for Aesthetic Breast Surgery

Juarez M. Avelar

3.1 Introduction

Besides its noble and divine lactation function, the female breast is an essential characteristic of identity and an important symbol of femininity on the sexual sphere. Also, it is responsible for significant expression of the harmony of the body contours. The embryological origin of the breasts is on the cutaneous integument presenting several stages from the birth until the adult life of the woman. All newborn children (female and male) present a small volume of mammary gland owing to the remaining effects of the mother's hormone. A few days after birth, that remnant volume presents total involution because of the absence of the maternal hormone. During puberty, a great physical change occurs caused by hormonal and metabolic effects on female body when the breasts start to grow, assuming enormous importance for the shape of the body. Nevertheless, abnormal development may also occur in males during puberty and in adults and is caused by a hormonal disturbance named gynecomastia, which outside the scope of this chapter.

The size, shape, and consistency of the breasts are not definitive as they may present deep alterations, secondarily to several circumstances that may happen to women throughout their lives. Initially, just after puberty, every month during the period of menstruation, the breasts present cyclical alterations with swelling due to vascular improvement followed by regression a few days later. During such natural phenomena, the breasts may feel painful. Pregnancies, obesity, massive weight loss, flabby skin, striae, and occasionally alterations of the function of the breast may have great repercussions for their appearance that requires aesthetic correction. Attention has been focused on this region of the anatomy; thus, there is a constant challenge for plastic surgeons to reinstate the shape and size of the breast itself and in the harmony with the body. Also, beauty, advertising, and fashion media affect the woman's desires, motivating her to look for aesthetic surgery.

Looking back at fashion some decades ago, it is possible to identify tremendous modifications of women's sense of aesthetic judgment. The models used to be slim with small breasts, which corresponded to the standard idea of beauty. Nowadays, the magazines and televisions show girls and women with large breasts due to implants as symbols of beauty. Therefore, there is no a pattern of beauty concerning the size and shape of the breast, as they have varied from a period to another. Several patients who underwent reduction mastoplasty during the 1970s and 1980s would certainly nowadays look for breast augmentation because of the constant advertising in the media showing the exaggerated results of too large volumes of silicone

J.M. Avelar, M.D.
Brazilian Scientific Institute of Plastic and Reconstructive Surgery, Alameda Gabriel Monteiro da Silva, 620-Jardim Europa, Sao Paulo, SP 01442-000, Brazil
e-mail: juarezavelar@bol.com.br; institutodaorelha@uol.com.br; clinica-avelar@uol.com.br

J.M. Avelar (ed.), *Breast Surgery*, https://doi.org/10.1007/978-3-319-54115-0_3

prosthesis. Our patients see themselves in the mirrors, draw conclusions about their physical changes, and indicate that they want the operation. Thus, they come to our offices with their own decisions looking for plastic surgery. On the other hand, in other specialties, the surgeons usually analyze the health problems and they indicate the need for a surgical procedure. Quite often, a patient goes to several physicians with the hope of finding clinical treatment, expecting to avoid any operation.

3.1.1 Psychological Problems of the Patients

Sometimes a plastic surgeon should not perform an operation if he or she concludes that a patient's psychological problems should be treated instead of undergoing a mastoplasty procedure (Avelar 1986, 1988). There are several circumstances regarding psychological problems of patients that demonstrate that they are not candidates for breast surgery. So far, there have been two types of patient in whom a surgeon must be careful before performing an operation: those who do not know anything about the surgery and those who know too much.

1. When a patient doesn't know anything concerning the operation she is looking for, she even believes that there will be no scars afterward, and several other circumstances during and after intervention.
2. Those patients who believe that they know so much about mastoplasty and other procedures as well, that the surgeon is obliged to do what they want. These people are so used to hearing about plastic surgery in the media, on the internet, and in conversation with friends that they think they know all the surgical details.

Each plastic surgeon should analyze his or her patient's complaints not only concerning the physical problems, but the psychological point of view as well. All members of the staff must pay attention to the reaction of the patients before consultation and to inform the plastic surgeon so that he or she is prepared and cautious about all situations (Avelar 1988, 1989).

There may be a woman with matrimonial problems not related to her breasts, who thinks that if she undergoes a mastoplasty operation the situation can be solved. Usually, it is not a matter of a conversation between the surgeon and the patient about the relationship with her family. However, sometimes someone may talk say something to the nurses or secretaries that is related to the unstable matrimonial situation. It is useful for the member of the staff to inform the plastic surgeon so that he or she can be prepared before performing the operation.

Therefore, a patient has the opportunity to choose her surgeon to perform plastic surgery following indications from friends, other patients, and through other ways. But also, each surgeon may select his or her patient by analyzing her complaints, through dialogue during consultation, according to her reactions while she is in the office. Such selection is a matter of experience during long-term practice, in addition to the surgeon's sensitivity.

Psychological problems caused by physical alterations of the body must be well identified preoperatively. If her expectations are much higher than the operation can provide she is not a good candidate for mastoplasty.

In addition, any abnormalities of the breast may be responsible for dissatisfaction of the woman, with great psychological repercussions that motivate her to request aesthetic surgery so as to improve her body contours.

3.1.1.1 Patient's Evaluation

When a patient comes to our office she should be an ideal candidate for a breast operation: she must have complaints about its size, shape, weight, asymmetry, physical effects, or bad posture. I have noticed that when breasts are too heavy, a patient's shoulders may be projected forward because of two unconscious circumstances: the weight of the breasts affects traction to the shoulders, with consequences for the vertebral column (Fig. 3.1); and owing to a psychological

Fig. 3.1 Physical deformities caused by hypertrophic breasts. (**a**), (**c**) In the frontal and oblique view asymmetry with ptotic breasts that are too heavy and near the navel can be seen. (**b**), (**d**) Postoperative photos. (**e**) In the back view the breasts projected laterally and alterations on the torso can be seen. (**f**) The same patient after reduction mastoplasty

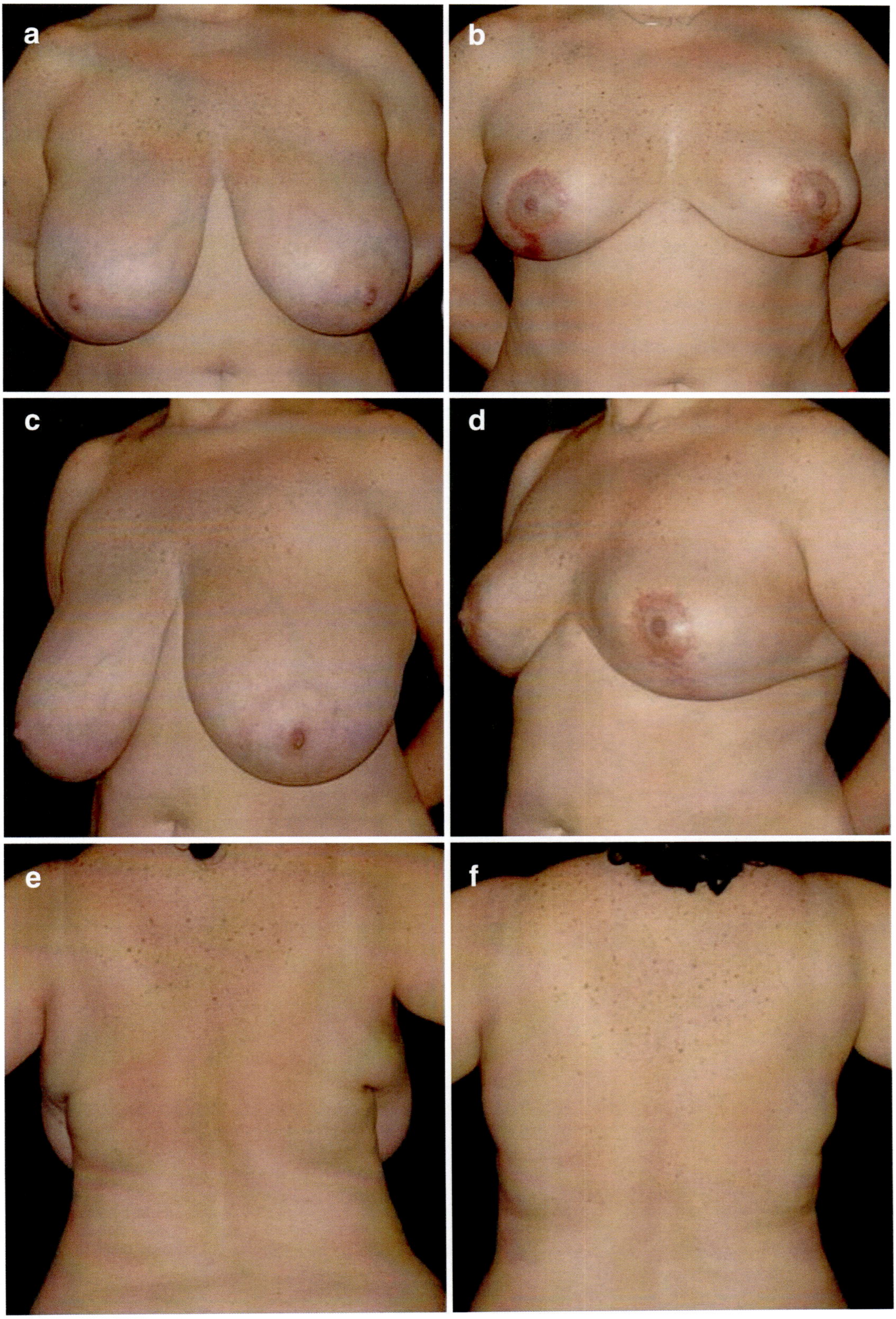
a
b
c
d
e
f

reaction, the patient tries to hide her deformity. Also, she must present well-balanced weight, stature, and height. However, some patients requesting surgery vary from slightly to significantly obese, associated with a distorted self-image. Obese patients should be required to lose excess weight preoperatively. If a woman complains about the size, shape, and weight of the breasts, she may expect to solve the abnormality of the body through reduction mastoplasty, which is incongruous, as it may well not be achieved (Avelar 1988, 1989). Young patients may complain of premenstrual pain, physical discomfort, back pain, deep striae on the skin of the sternal region caused by constant traction owing to the weight of the breasts, and even an inferiority complex, in addition to problems with her intimate relationship with her boyfriend (Fig. 3.2).

During the examination, alterations of the posture are evident. Some patients present deep grooves on the shoulders caused by straps of the brassiere (Fig. 3.3). Women with hypertrophic breasts can present cutaneous irritation on the submammary folds caused by direct contact of the skin of the breast with the cutaneous surface of the upper abdominal wall. This problem is

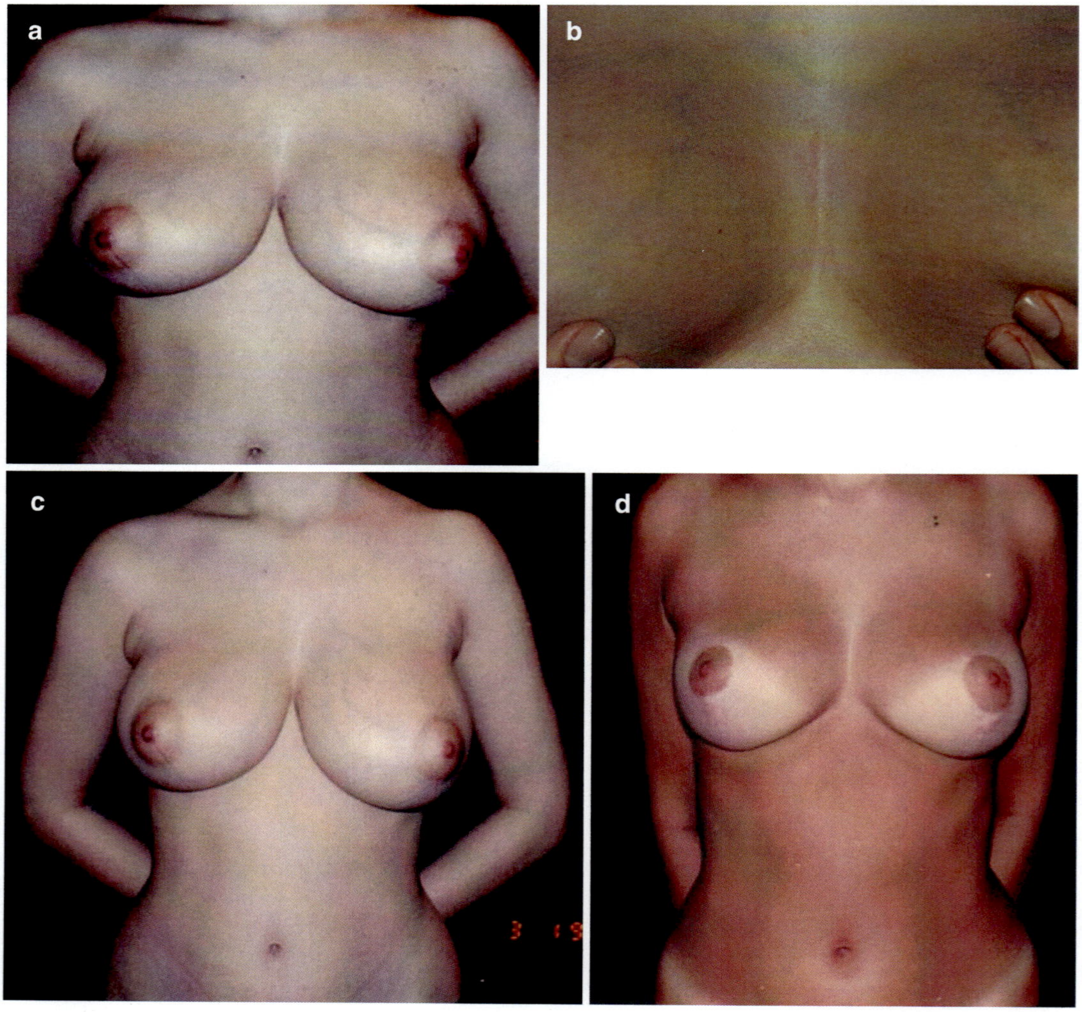

Fig. 3.2 Alterations of the skin on the external region due to traction of the heaviness of the breasts. (**a**) Photo of a 20-year-old patient showing alterations similar to a scar. (**b**) Photo in close-up of the same patient showing a deep scar on the external region. (**c**), (**e**) Photos before operation. (**d**), (**f**) Photos after reduction mastoplasty

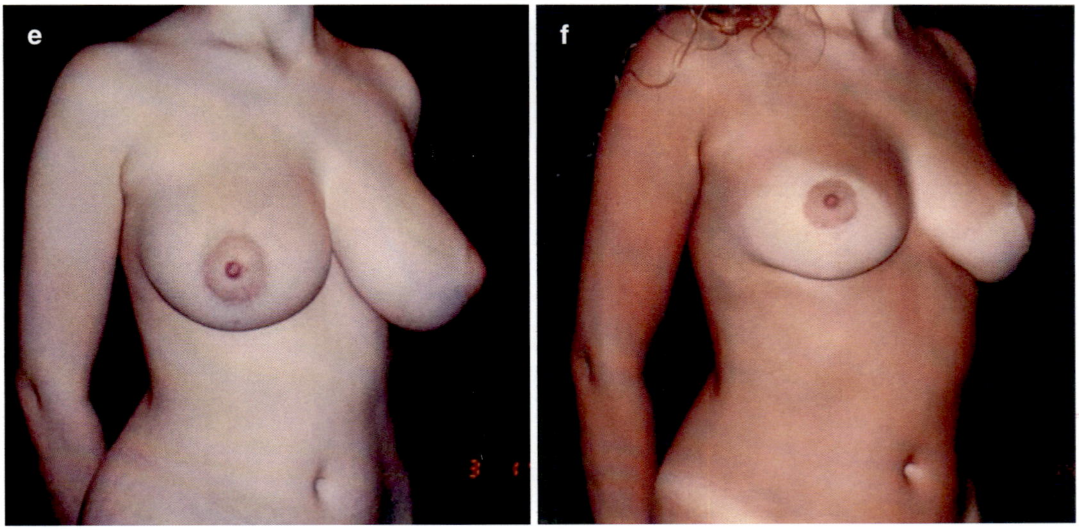

Fig. 3.2 (continued)

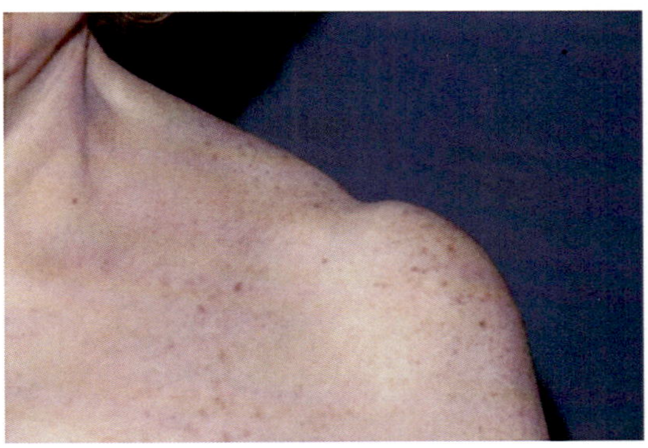

Fig. 3.3 Deformity on the shoulder caused by the brassiere strap making a deep groove

common in patients in tropical countries with warm temperatures (Fig. 3.4). If submammary intertrigo, or any other dermatological abnormalities, is present, it should be treated and eradicated before surgery. Also, edema, turgescence, and thoracic pain are seen and are caused by stretching of the skin over the breast (Figs. 3.1, 3.2, and 3.5).

Discomfort with breathing may occur because of the great effort of the muscles of the chest to elevate the large volume of glandular tissue during inspiration and expiration (Pitanguy 1960, 1961). Often multiple veins can be seen underneath the skin due to alteration of the venous circulation (Fig. 3.5). The gravity is a normal phenomenon to aid mammary venous and

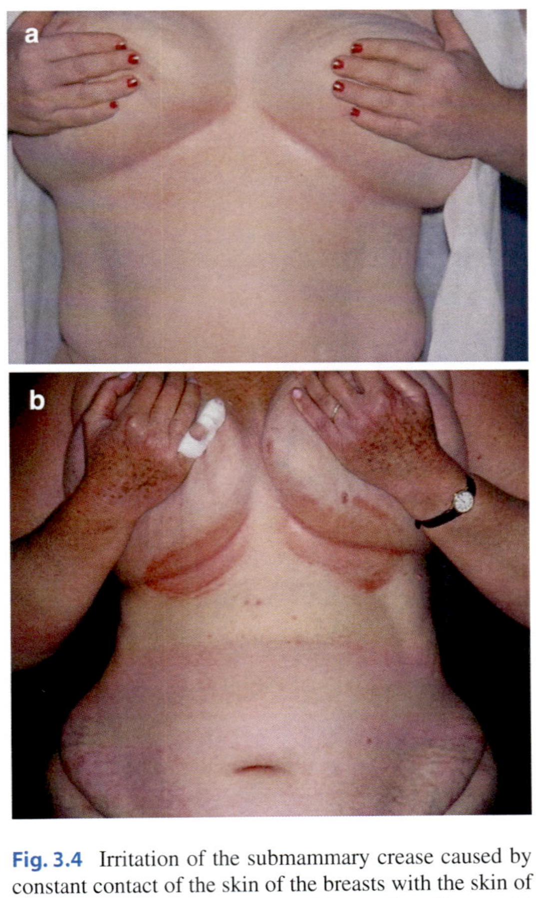

Fig. 3.4 Irritation of the submammary crease caused by constant contact of the skin of the breasts with the skin of the upper abdominal wall. (**a**) Photo of a 48-year-old patient with large breasts shows slight irritation. (**b**) Photo of a 59-year-old patient with severe dermatitis

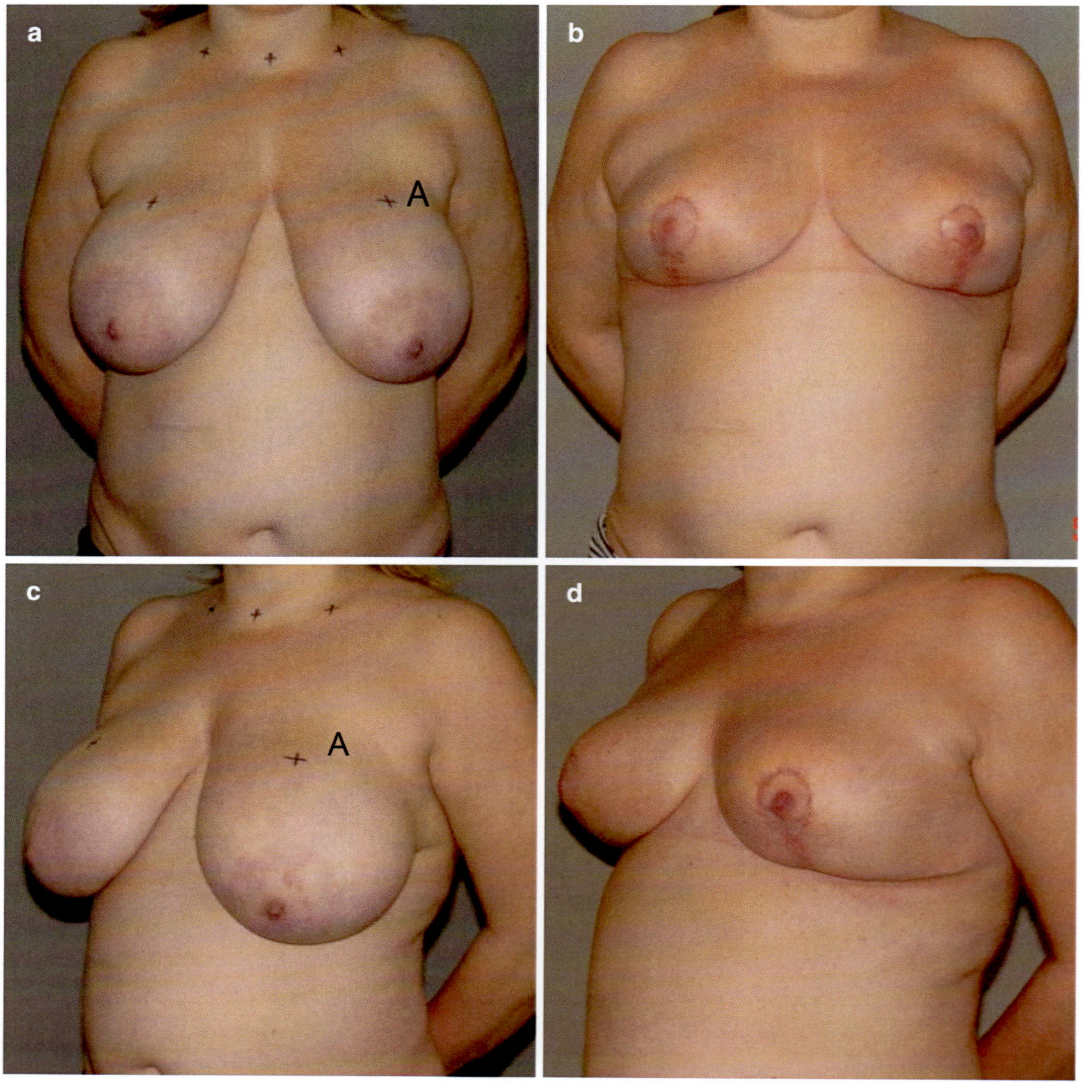

Fig. 3.5 A 44-year-old patient with large hypertrophic breasts. (**a**) and (**c**) Preoperative photos showing pre-marking with Pitanguy's point A; (**b**) and (**d**) Postoperative photos 1 year after reduction mastoplasty with resection of 850 g on the right breast and 1,080 g on the left side

lymphatic drainage, which may be jeopardized owing to ptosis with hypertrophy of the breast causing some alteration of the circulation.

3.1.1.2 Surgical Planning

During physical examination, the plastic surgeon may explain to patient how the operation may be performed. My preference is to carry out surgical planning with the patient in the standing position between two vertical mirrors placed one in front of the other with my nurse in the examination room (Figs. 3.6, 3.7, and 3.8). Thus, a patient can see her body from the front and back at the same time. Often, patients with large and heavy breasts present severe physical alterations that they had not yet noticed (Fig. 3.1). Each surgeon must be well trained in the technique he or she is performing. It is useful to show the patient the location and to estimate the extent of the scars around the areola, on the submammary folds, and the vertical distance from it to the nipple–areola complex (NAC) (Avelar 1990, 1993).

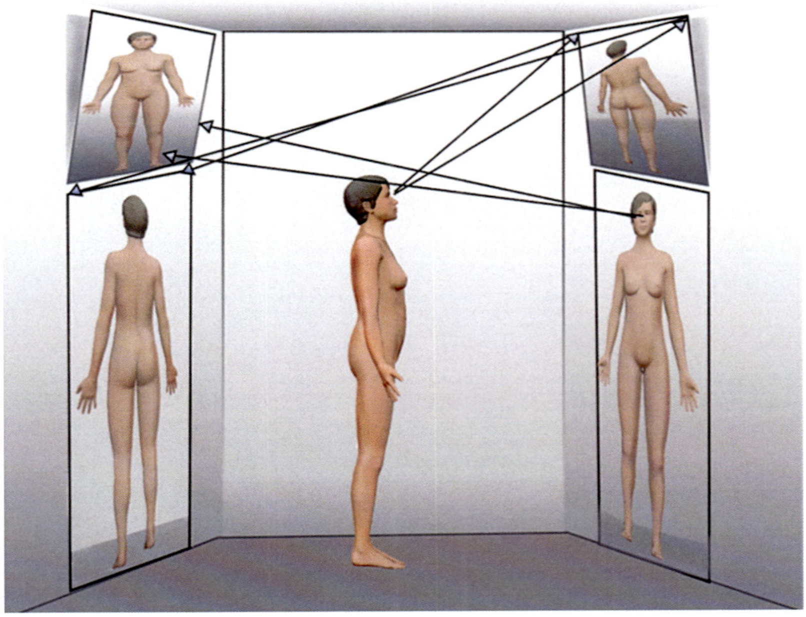

Fig. 3.6 Diagram of the examining room at my clinic. A patient in a standing position in front of two vertical mirrors placed one in front of the other combined with two small mirrors strategically located on top of the vertical ones, making a 45° inclination with the others

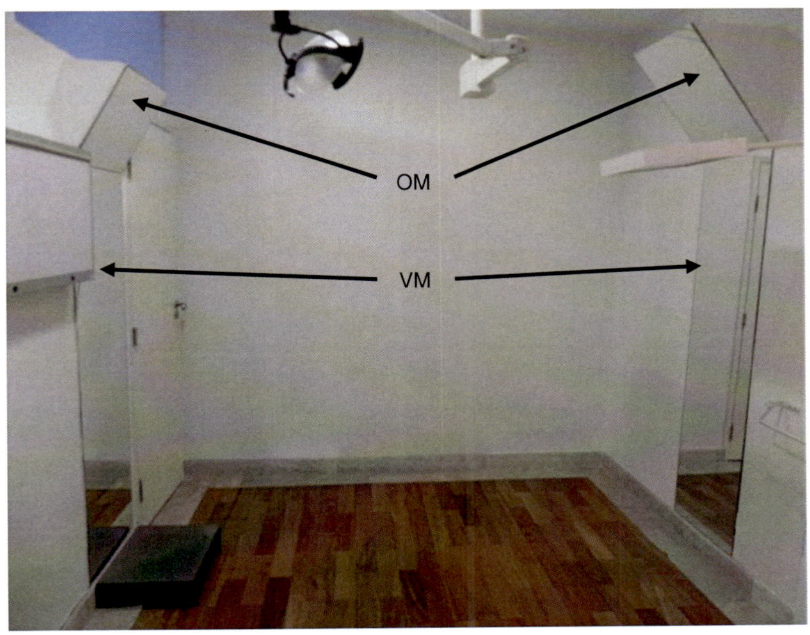

Fig. 3.7 Photo of the examining room at my clinic. Two vertical mirrors (*VM*) are placed one in front of the other combined with two oblique mirrors (*OM*) strategically located on top of the vertical ones making a 45° inclination with the others

The reference points for operation are made according to the technique employed. I usually measure the distance between both NACs and the distance to the midclavicular point. An imaginary location of the future NAC is marked. Preoperative photos are taken and blood tests, heart, and clinical evaluation must be requested according to the routine of each surgeon.

Surgical planning is a fundamental step before all operations in plastic surgery, as I have described previously for ear reconstruction and abdominoplasty (Avelar 2013, 2016).

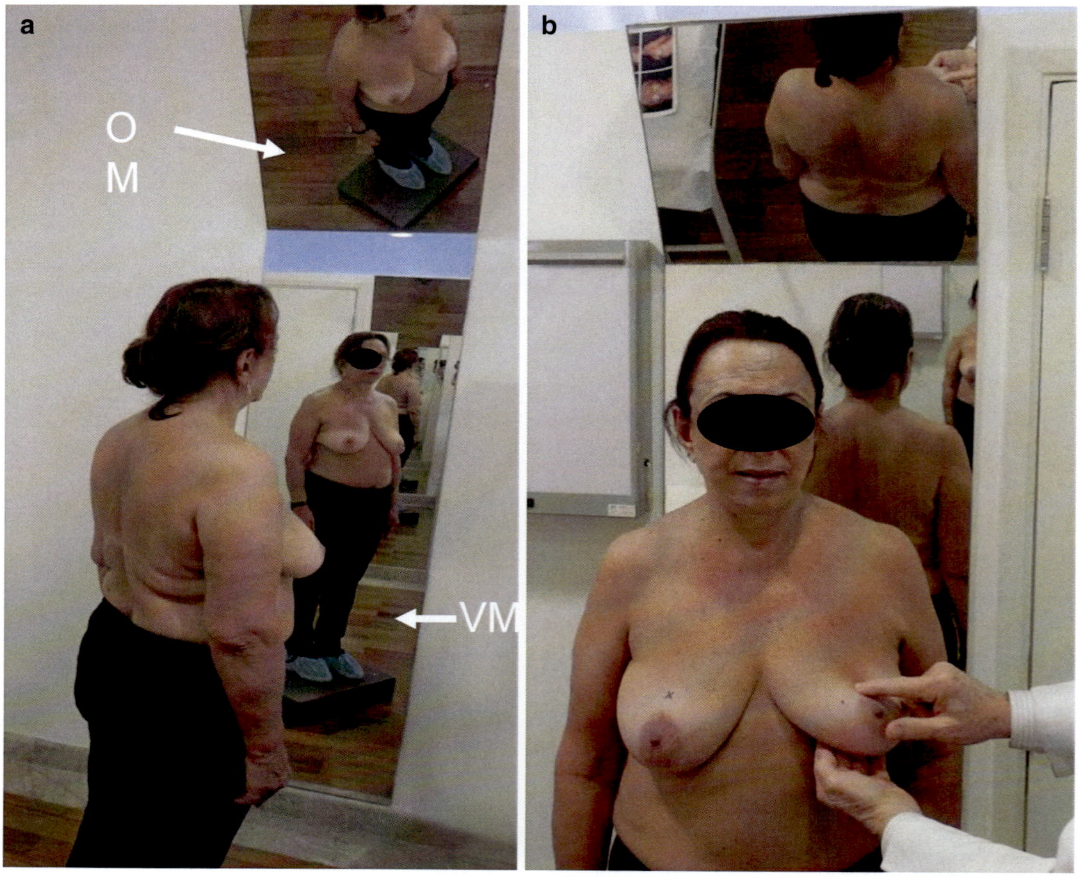

Fig. 3.8 Photo of a patient in the examining room at my clinic during examination and pre-marking. (**a**) She is in a standing position in front of two parallel VM, and sees her body in the frontal view and in the back view simultaneously through the OM. (**b**) She follows the breast examination

3.1.1.3 Pre-marking

There are some techniques that utilize prefabricated patterns for surgical marking in reduction mastoplasty. As I had the privilege to be trained by Prof. Pitanguy, he did not employ such patterns; thus, I followed his surgical guidelines for marking of the breasts before an operation (Pitanguy and Garcia 1972; Pitanguy 1981).

Once the operation is scheduled, I prefer to see my patients again at my clinic 1 day before the date. It is another opportunity to check all preoperative examinations and to re-evaluate any problems. At this time, pre-marking is carried out on the breast and chest as well. A point is marked on the suprasternal notch, and another one on each side about 7 cm from the midclavicular point. From this point, an imaginary vertical line goes downward, passing the center of the nipple. On this line, the Pitanguy's point A is drawn on the projection of the submammary fold on each side. To determine this point, the index finger of the surgeon's left hand projects the submammary fold forward onto the ptotic breast (Fig. 3.9). In conclusion, the pre-marking is done to determine two points: Pitanguy's point A and point R, as an important reference for final surgical marking during reduction mastoplasty. The patient goes home with pre-marking and the next day those reference points are very useful for performing the definitive surgical marking in the operating room (Figs. 3.10, 3.11, and 3.12).

Measurement of the chest of patients for surgical marking, taking as reference points the sternal notch and the xyphoid process, as described by

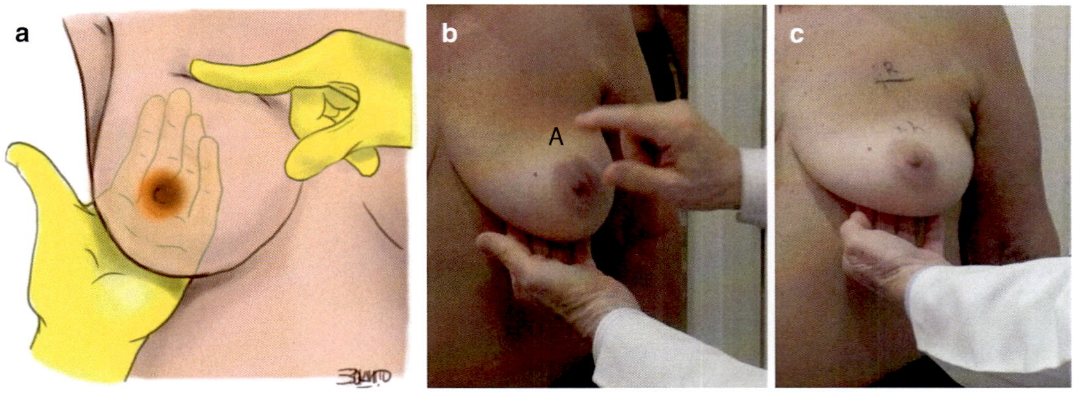

Fig. 3.9 Pre-marking of Pitanguy's point A. (**a**) Scheme to demonstrate the marking. (**b**) Photo of a patient showing the surgeon's position to determine point A. The index finger on the submammary fold shows projection of the point A, which is marked. (**c**) Point A is marked on the breast and the other point R is also marked above, as another reference

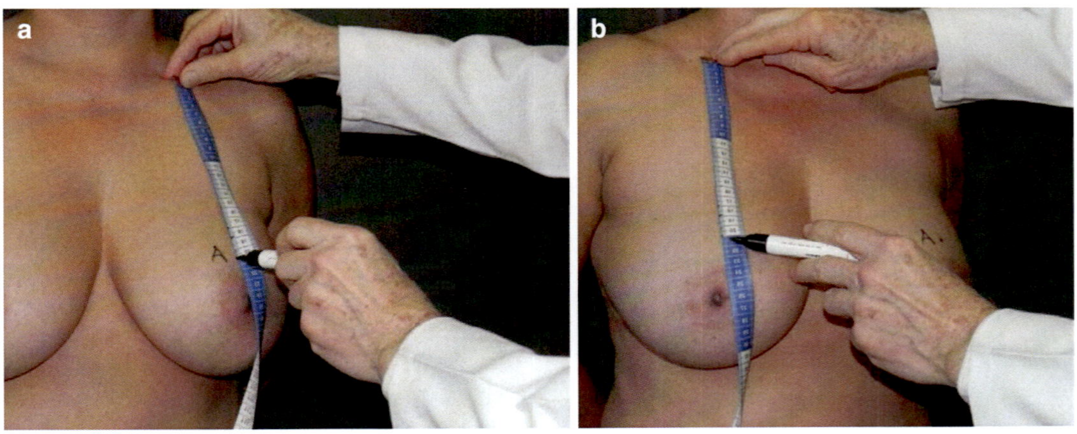

Fig. 3.10 Transposition of pre-marking on the left side to the right side. (**a**) Using a graduated tape to confirm point A and the distance from the midclavicular point. (**b**) The demarcated points are transposed to the right side

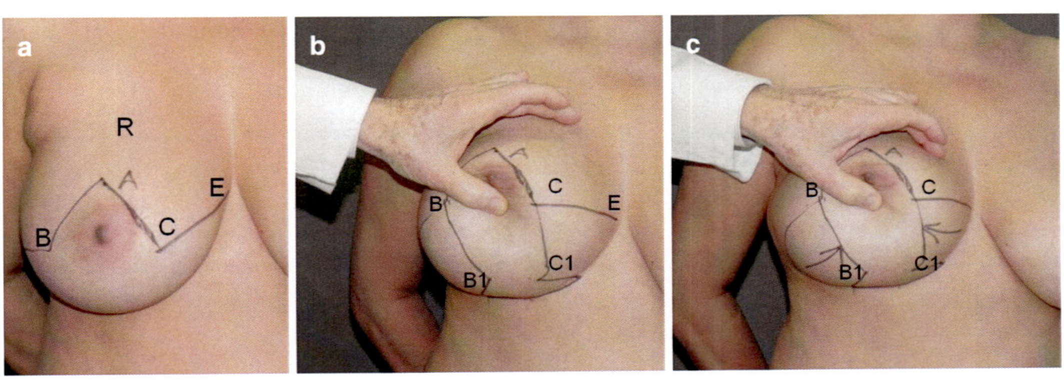

Fig. 3.11 Photos during pre-marking: Pitanguy's technique can be seen, and afterward my pre-marking was shown as an evolution of my approach. (**a**) Pitanguy's technique as a W-shaped marking (A, B, C, D, E). (**b**) After my marking, points B1 and C1 are much lower. (**c**) All pre-markings can be seen, and an arrow on each side showing the skin that will not be removed

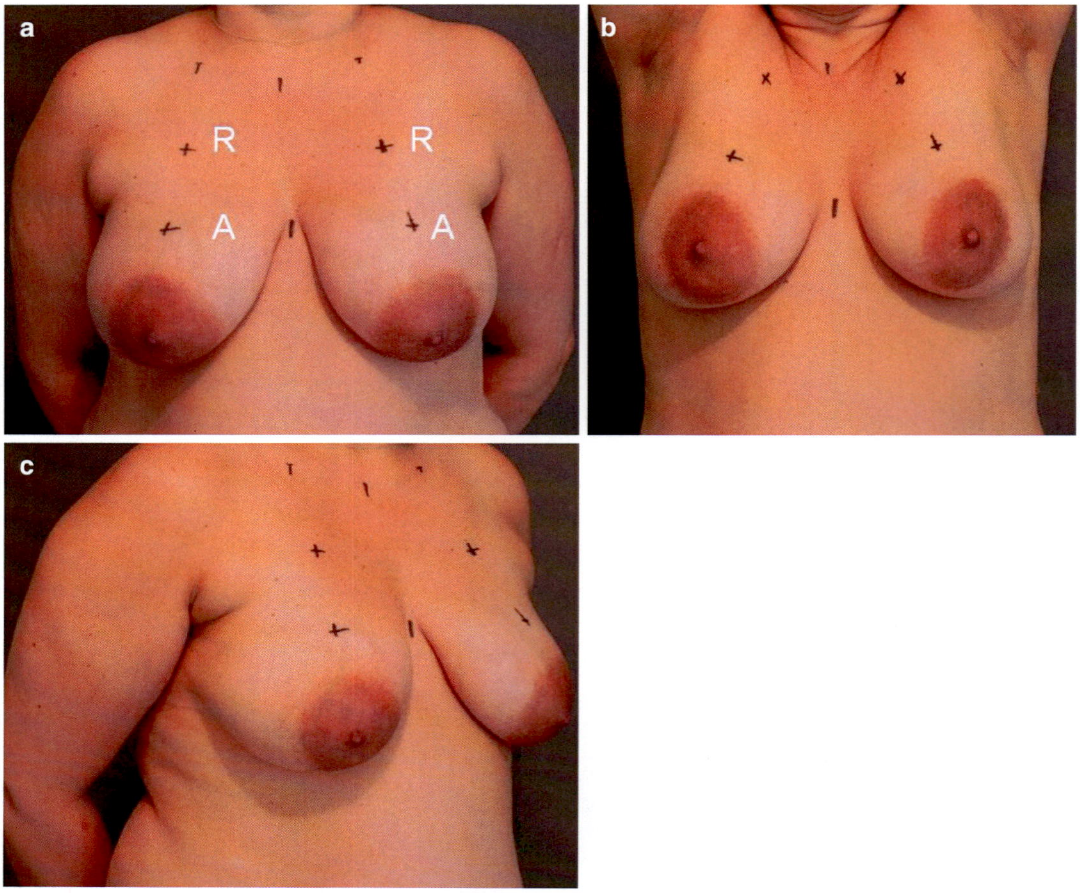

Fig. 3.12 Patient showing pre-marking. (**a**) Pitanguy's point A is on the projection of the submammary fold. The reference point R is on the midclavicular line for later orientation. (**b**) Patient with her arms up shows the alteration of the pre-marking points. (**c**) In the lateral view, the pre-marking shows the correct positions

Gillies and McIndoe (1939), and emphasized by Pitanguy (1960, 1981), and Pitanguy and Garcia (1972). Often, asymmetry of both breasts must be well identified and shown to the patient (Avelar and Anger 1989; Avelar 1989). A geometric method for surgical marking was proposed by Aufricht (1949) and has been employed by several authors, although a prefabricated pattern used to be the most frequent approach. Following similar methodology, Fernandez (1951) used to employ a ruler to measure the reference points on the chest and breast to achieve adequate projection of the breast after mastoplasty.

Once the patient is at the hospital, the premedication is carried out before she goes to the operating room, where the final surgical markings is done.

3.2 Discussion

Embryologically, the breasts originate from the cutaneous integument, presenting several modifications during female adult life. Patients with hypertrophic breasts may complaint about back pain, premenstrual pain, physical repercussions for her shoulders, which may be projected forward and put extra weight on the column (Pitanguy 1960; Pitanguy and Garcia 1972). During examination, several alterations of the posture are evident (Fig. 3.1). Some patients present deep grooves on the shoulders caused by straps of the brassiere (Fig. 3.3). I prefer to examine my patients in the examination room in front of two vertical mirrors on the wall, which allow them to see the front and back views at the same time. Also, a patient may present psychological problems caused by physical alterations of the body and her expectations may be higher than the operation can fulfil; in that case, the patient is not a good candidate for mastoplasty.

During physical examination, it is the right moment to explain to patient about surgical planning and the operation. Each surgeon must be well trained with the technique he or she is used to performing. It is useful to show to patient the location and to estimate the extent of the scars on the submammary folds and the vertical distance from the NAC. Once the operation is scheduled I prefer to carry out pre-marking on the day before the operation. A point is marked on the suprasternal notch, and another one on each side about 7 cm from the midclavicular point. From this point an imaginary vertical line goes downward passing the center of the nipple. On this line, Pitanguy's point A is drawn on the projection of the submammary fold on each side, with the surgeon's left index finger projecting the submammary fold. With the patient at the hospital, the pre-medication is given before she goes to the operating room, where the final surgical marking is done. Mastoplasty may preserve the lactation function after surgery in addition to nipple sensitivity in breast reduction, as reported by Ragnell (1957).

Mastoplasty operations must be performed with patient in a semi-sitting position to evaluate an correct position of the NAC and the final scars. This important surgical detail is described by Gillies and McIndoe (1939), who elevated the patient's head on the operating table.

Conclusions

The breasts, and indeed the whole female body start significant development during puberty due to hormonal metabolic alterations. The size and shape of the breasts present significant growth with great importance for the silhouette of female body, and breast-feeding in adult life, which I am used to confirming among my patients, may be preserved after reduction mastoplasty (Fig. 3.13), which is described by Ragnell (1957).

Often, the breasts may present several anomalies, most frequently asymmetry (Avelar 1989). Also, other deformities such as hypertrophy, hypoplasia, secondary to obesity, massive weight loss, flabby skin, striae, the consequences of pregnancies, and several other abnormalities that may require aesthetic repair (Fig. 3.1).

Usually, patients come to the plastic surgeon's office looking for a solution to their physical deformities, as they see themselves in the mirrors and realize their problems. In fact, they make the diagnosis and give indications for operation; also, they come with the decision to look for plastic surgery. However, we must evaluate the deformities, to check if the patient is really concerned about the problem. Afterward, it is essential to carry out surgical planning and finally to indicate the operation. Therefore, during physical examination, it is the right moment for the plastic surgeon to explain to patient the operation that may be performed. Surgical planning may be done with the patient in the standing position to evaluate the breasts and the relationship between them, in addition to the chest and the torso. Often, patients with large and heavy breasts present severe physical alterations that sometimes they had not yet noticed (Figs. 3.6, 3.7, and 3.8). Finally, surgical marking must be done following the physical alterations during examination.

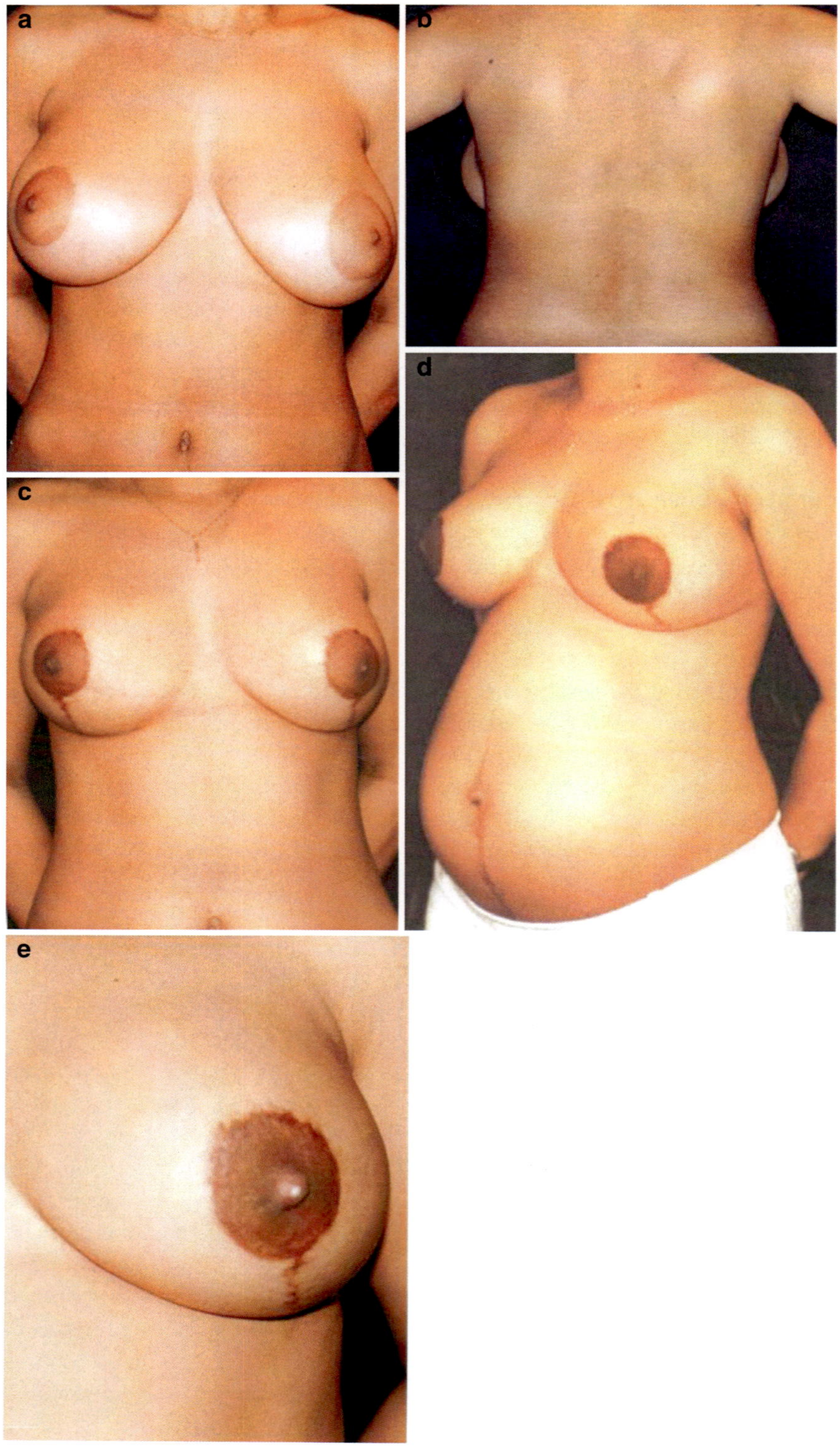

Fig. 3.13 Preservation of the lactation function after reduction mastoplasty. (**a**) A 24-year-old patient before surgery. (**b**) In the back view the breasts are projected laterally. (**c**) After reduction mastoplasty. (**d**) The same patient in the 9th month of pregnancy. (**e**) Milk on the nipple after delivery

References

Aufricht G (1949) Mammaplasty for pendulous breasts. Empiric and geometry planning. Plast Reconstr Surg 4(1):13–29

Avelar JM (1986) Perfil psicológico do paciente—Introdução ao estudo (Psychological profile of the patient—introducing to the subject). In: Avelar JM, Illouz YG (eds) Lipoaspiração (Liposuction). Editora Hipócrates, São Paulo, pp 8–18. Chapter 2

Avelar JM (1988) Abdominoplastia—reflexões e perspectiva biopsicológicas (Abdominoplasty—reflections and bio-psychological perspectives). Rev Soc Bras Cir Plast 3(2):152–154

Avelar JM (1989) Assimetria mamária (Breast asymmetry). In: Avelar JM (ed) Cirurgia Plástica na Infância (Plastic surgery in infancy). Editora Hipocrates, São Paulo, pp 413–418. Chapter 2

Avelar JM (1990) Princípios fundamentales en las mastoplastias (Fundamental principles in mastoplasty). In: Avelar JM, Malbec EF (eds) Historia, Ciência y Arte en Cirugía Estética. Ed. Hipócrates, São Paulo, pp 530–549

Avelar JM (1993) Mastoplastia redutora sob anestesia local (Reduction mastoplasty under local anesthesia). In: Avelar JM (ed) Anestesia Loco-regional em cirurgia estética—(Loco-regional anesthesia on aesthetic surgery). Editora Hipócrates, São Paulo, pp 244–260

Avelar JM (2013) Surgical principles and planning for ear reconstruction. In: Avelar JM (ed) Ear reconstruction. Springer, Heidelberg, pp 15–31. Chapter 3

Avelar JM (2016) Surgical principles and classification of abdominolipoplasty or lipoabdominoplasty. In: Avelar JM (ed) New concepts on abdominoplasty and further applications. Springer, Switzerland, pp 31–43. doi:10.1007/978-3-319-27851-3_3. Chapter 3

Avelar JM, Anger A (1989) Aspectos psicológicos do paciente infantil em cirurgia (Psychological aspects of child patient in surgery). In: Avelar JM (ed) Cirurgia Plástica na Infância. Hipócrates, São Paulo, pp 3–6. Chapter 1

Fernandez J (1951) Mastoplastias, nuestra experiência editorial universitária. Buenos Aires

Gillies H, McIndoe AH (1939) The technique of mammaplasty in conditions of hypertrophy of the breast. Surg Gynecol Obstet 68:658

Pitanguy I (1960) Breast hypertrophy. In: Wallace AB (ed) Transactions of the International Society of Plastic Surgeons, Second Congress, Edinburgh. E & S, Livingstone, p 509

Pitanguy I (1961) Aproximação eclética ao problema das mamaplastias (an eclectic approach to breast problems). Rev Bras Cir 41:179–196

Pitanguy I (1981) The breast. In: Aesthetic plastic surgery of head and body. Springer, Berlin, pp 3–62. Chapter 1

Pitanguy I, Garcia LC (1972) Aspectos importantes da tecnica pessoal em mammaplastia (Important aspects of the personal technique of mammaplasty). Bol Soc Cir Plast Reconstr. Cordoba 4:7

Ragnell KGA (1957) Further experience of preservation of lactation capacity and nipple sensitivity in breast reduction. Transactions of the International Society of Plastic Surgeons. Williams & Wilkins, Baltimore, p 379

4 Technical Systematization in Mammoplasty

Carlos Alberto Jaimovich

4.1 Introduction

The presence of the breasts is a strong factor in body contours and female identity. Therefore, it is normal for every woman to desire to have beautiful breasts in harmony with her body. This notion has been true in medicine since Hippocrates (460 to 370 BC), who used to perform mammary cauterization as a method of treatment. Nowadays, it is credited to Paul of Aegina (AD 625–690) (1846), who performed the first reduction mammaplasty in a woman, but this procedure was performed for the correction of gynecomastia. Four hundred years later, Paré (1510–1590) gave credit to Paul of Aegina for the first reduction mammaplasty operation, which has been recognized by other authors. Durston (1669) described the first complete mastoplasty operation. There are some other historical contributions reported afterward, but during the twentieth century mastoplasty underwent great developments. The contribution credited to Biesenberger (1928) is the excision of the lateral portion of the gland with rotation of the remaining glandular pedicle. Schwarzmann (1930) introduced a periareolar incision and undermining for maintenance of the blood supply to the nipple, which is still performed in most mastoplasty techniques up to the present day Biesenberguer (1928, 1931). Another major contribution was introduced by Strömbeck (1960), extending the concept of a dermal bridge technique for preservation of the principal arteriovenous and cutaneous nerve system to ensure nipple survival. He also employed a pattern to predetermine the shape of the skin flaps.

However, the most remarkable technique for reduction mastoplasty was presented by Pitanguy (1961), with new concepts that opened a wide field for the treatment of breast hypertrophy. Even he demonstrated that each breast must be evaluated with the patient in the semi-sitting position, for surgical marking, so that the surgeon has the freedom to imagine the surgical result without employing a prefabricated model. Therefore, reduction mastoplasty became an artistic approach to achieving good results with a very low rate of complications. Pitanguy introduced several surgical principles that popularized the procedure among plastic surgeons in our country and all over the world. Because of such valuable improvements, mastoplasty is one of the most frequent procedures performed by plastic surgeons.

Although the breasts are organs with well-known anatomy, histology, and physiology with updated surgical techniques, each surgeon must be aware of the possibility of unexpected situations and some complications. For these reasons, a meticulous and careful technical systematization before operation is fundamental.

C.A. Jaimovich, M.D.
Ivo Pitanguy Institute of Plastic Surgery/PUC-RJ
Post-graduation University, Av N S Copacabana, 680/501, Rio de Janeiro, RJ 22050-001, Brazil
e-mail: jaimail@iis.com.br

J.M. Avelar (ed.), *Breast Surgery*, https://doi.org/10.1007/978-3-319-54115-0_4

4.2 Method

Before Pitanguy's technique it was quite frequent to employ prefabricated pattern, which used to be a useful approach to simplifying marking. Since that time with the use of pattern positioning of the future nipple-areola location, it has been the key to achieving good surgical results. However, the pattern provides only the basic outline, as the drawings must be modified so as to obtain the desired result in each patient. Ever since Pitanguy (1961a, b) developed his new technique, use of a pattern became an unnecessary procedure. Therefore, owing to new concepts for surgical marking before mastoplasty, it became an important preoperative step. Consequently, surgical planning is a mandatory approach before marking, as the surgeon and the patient may achieve a good understanding.

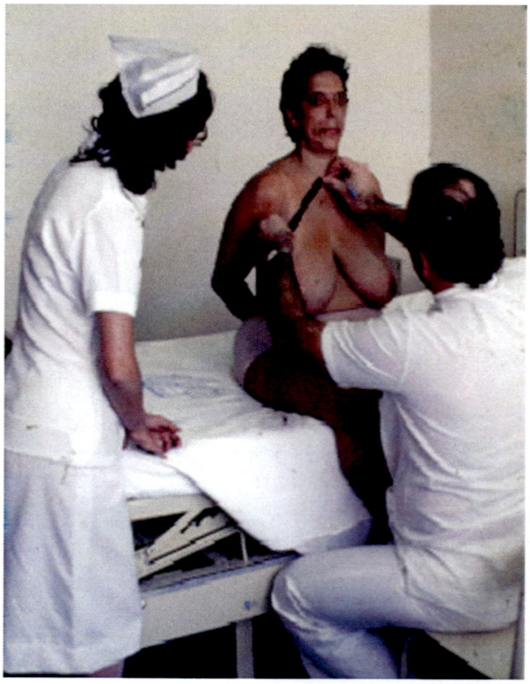

Fig. 4.1 Surgical marking. Patient is awake in a sitting position. The surgeon carries out pre-marking to give adequate support during the surgery

4.2.1 Surgical Marking: Pre-marking

Following surgical principles introduced by Pitanguy surgical marking must be carried out with the patient in a semi-sitting position. However, my preference is to perform pre-marking before she goes to the operating room, while she is awake, in a standing position (Fig. 4.1). The main topic is to determine the future nipple–areola region as in most cases of hypertrophic breasts, they are in an ectopic position. The pre-marking starts by marking the medial line from the suprasternal notch to the projection of the xyphoid process. Afterward, the midclavicular point is marked laterally about 10 cm away from the suprasternal notch (Fig. 4.2). From this point, a vertical and oblique line goes downward passing by the nipple–areola region. The key to the marking is to find Pitanguy's point A (Fig. 4.3). The submammary sulcus is drawn to orientate the future scar after reduction mastoplasty.

With one hand on the submammary fold under the breast the surgeon projects his finger forward onto the vertical line (Fig. 4.3), whereby it becomes possible to determine a point on the vertical line. Using a ruler or his hand, it is possible to measure the distances to determine Pitanguy's point A, which is key for mastoplasty marking (Fig. 4.3). From this important reference point, two oblique lines are marked on internal and external segments of the breast to determine points B and C (Fig. 4.4). From these points, a line is drawn on the internal and external sides of the breast until the submammary line previously marked is reached (Fig. 4.5).

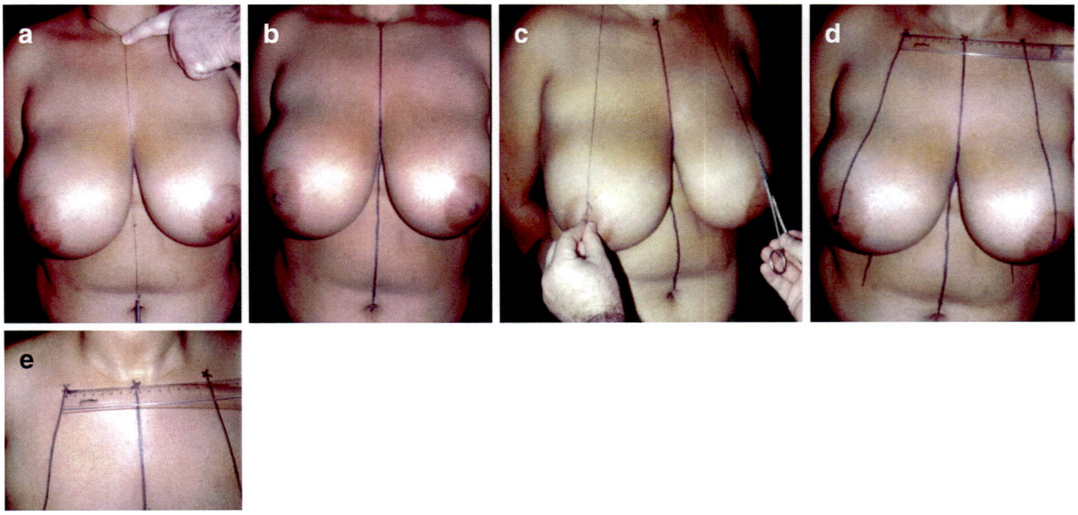

Fig. 4.2 (**a**, **b**) A midline is drawn. (**c**, **d**) A midclavicular line is drawn on each side up to the nipple. (**e**) The distances are adequately demarcated using a ruler

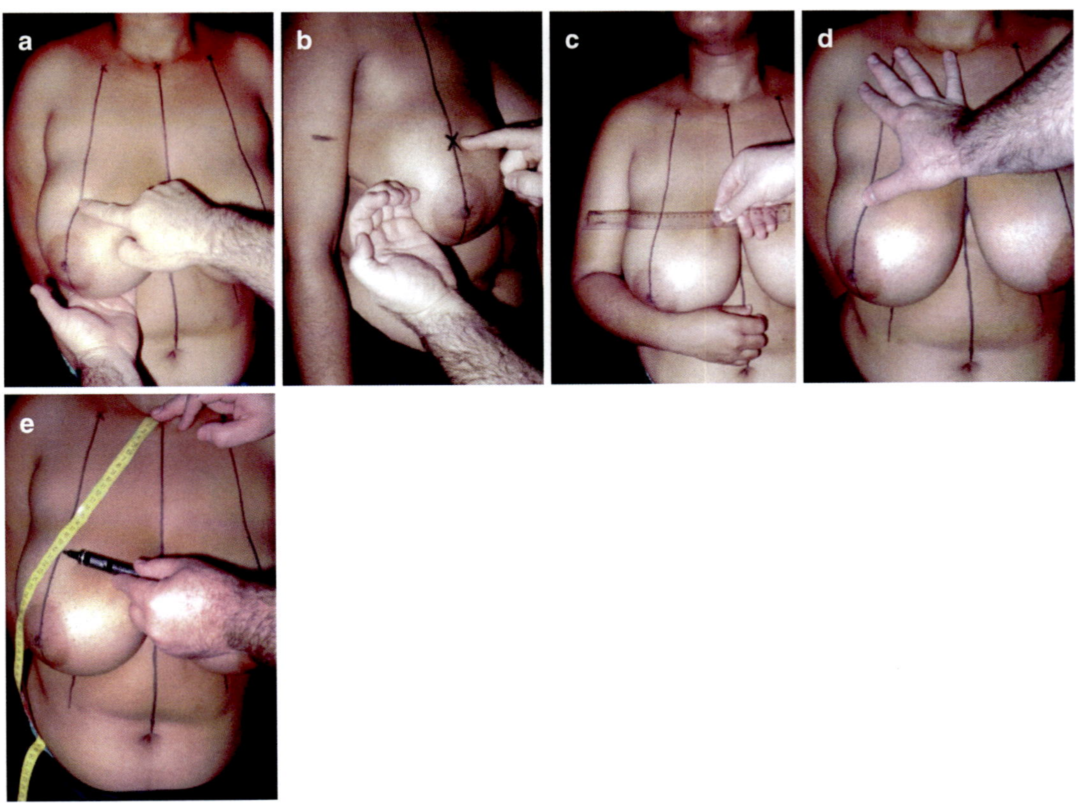

Fig. 4.3 Marking of Pitanguy's point A. (**a**, **b**) With the left hand placed under the breast, the surgeon projects the submammary sulcus on the breast and with his right index finger, point A is located. (**c–e**) Using a ruler and the hand to measure the medial part of the arm as a reference

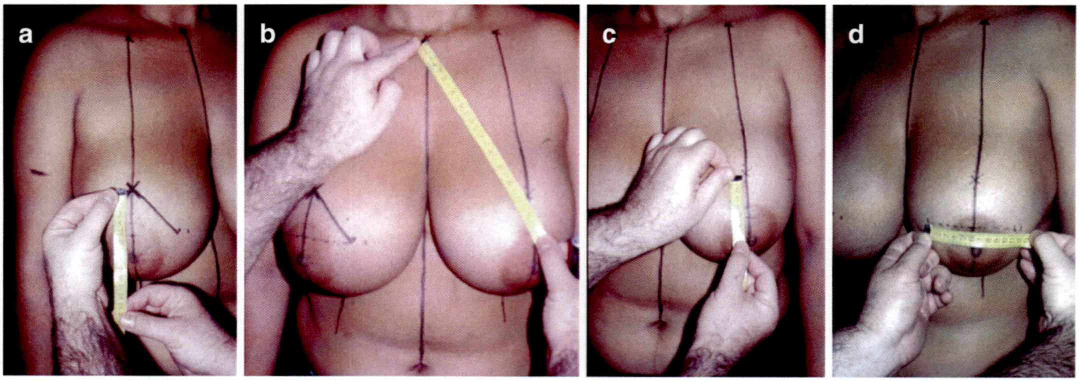

Fig. 4.4 Marking of points B and C taking point A as a reference. (**a**) An oblique line from point A to each side of the breast. (**b–d**) The measurement is made as an artistic apraoch with use of a ruler

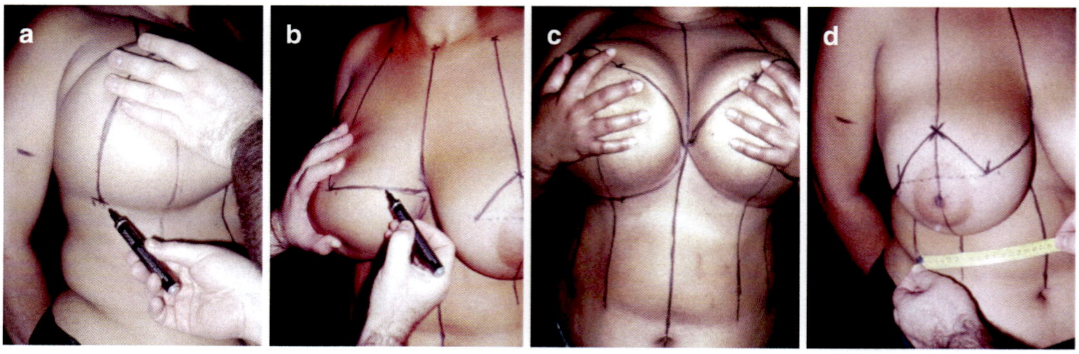

Fig. 4.5 Marking of lateral incisions of the breast. (**a**, **b**) From points B and C, two lines are demarcated laterally until they join the submammary sulcus. (**c**, **d**) The final marking can be seen

4.3 Surgical Technique

4.3.1 Anesthesia

The anesthesia for reduction mastoplasty is a matter of a good understanding among the patient, surgeon, and anesthesiologist, and should be considered according to each case and each patient. There are four options: general anesthesia, epidural anesthesia, local anesthesia combined with intravenous sedation, and local anesthesia. Local infiltration with epinephrine solution is a useful procedure for avoiding bleeding during surgery.

4.3.2 Anesthetic Infiltration

In all anesthesia options, it is useful to perform local infiltration on both breasts before operation. Usually 200 mL of a solution is enough for infiltration of both breasts. The solution is: 500 mL of serum + 20 mL of lidocaine (2%) + Naropin® (20 mL) + 1 mL of epinephrine (1/1000).

4.3.3 Glandular Resection

Once the anesthesia is done and surgical marking is again performed, the surgeon's assistant holds the base of the breast to facilitate the start of the operation by making a circular incision around the areola. Also, it is possible to use an elastic tape to hold the base of the breast to expose the nipple–areola region (Fig. 4.6). This maneuver was introduced by Schwarzmann (1930) and is employed in most mastoplasty techniques. Because of that maneuver, it is possible to perform a superficial incision all around the areola to maintain and preserve good vascularization to the nipple–areola region, avoiding sloughing or even necrosis. It may occur, but it is rare, as enough blood supply is provided to the nipple–areo-

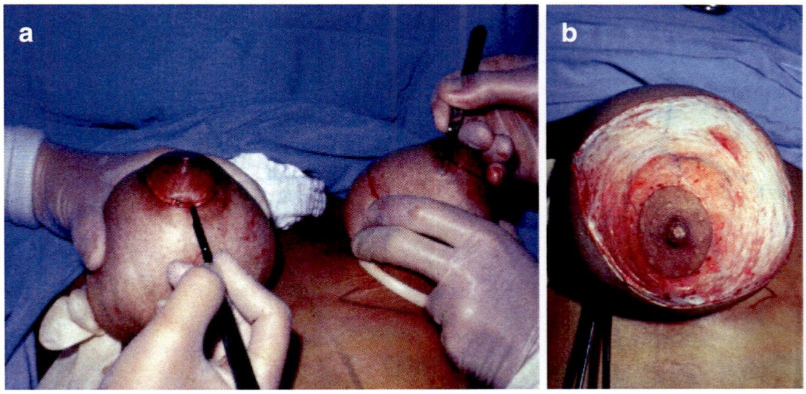

Fig. 4.6 Schwarzmann's maneuver. (**a**) Peroperative photo shows periareolar incisions being made simultaneously on both breasts by two surgeons. (**b**) Photo shows one breast after periareolar deepitheliazation

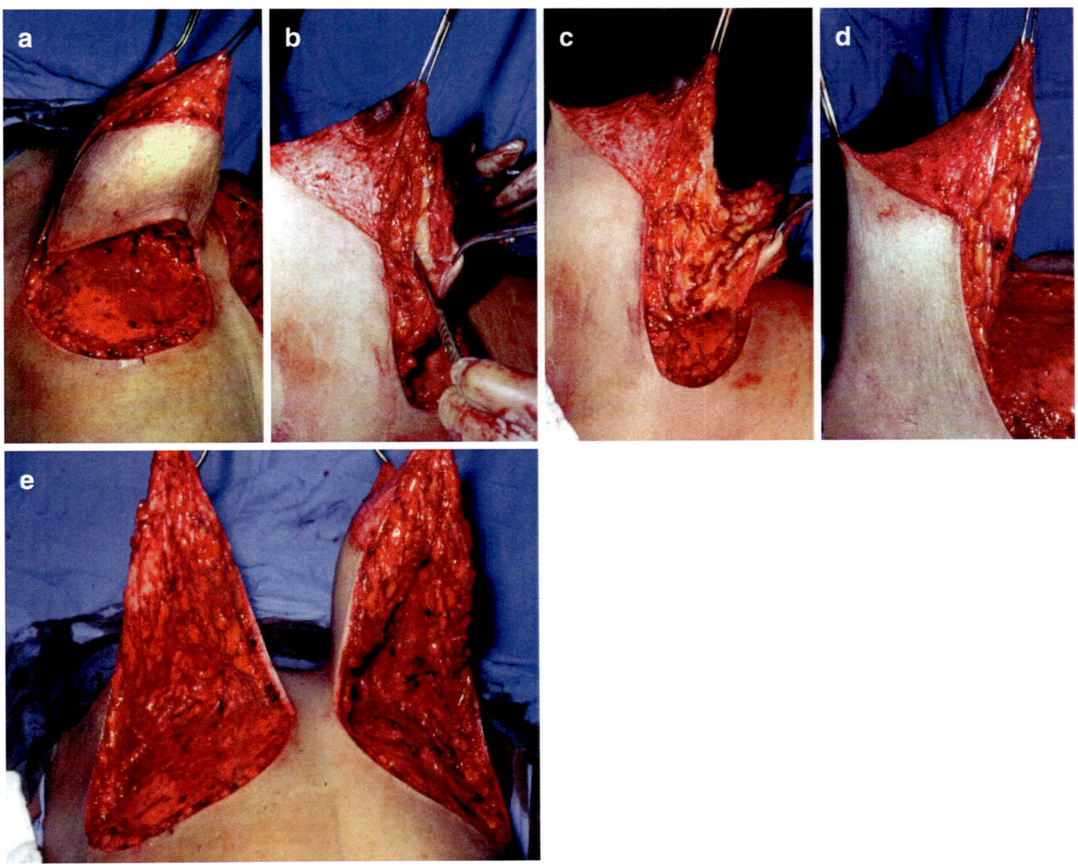

Fig. 4.7 Sequential photos to show glandular resection according to Pitanguy's "keel" resection. (**a**) An incision was made in the submammary sulcus. (**b, c**) A lateral incision is made to create Pitanguy's glandular columns and "keel" resection. (**d**) Profile view after resection. (**e**) Frontal view after glandular resection on both sides showing that "keel" resction was done and Pitanguy's "third pedicle" was preserved in the medial part

lar region during surgery (Fig. 4.6). Afterward, the breast is pulled upward to expose the mammary tissue to be resected. At this point, Pitanguy (1961a, b) again made a valuable contribution, with the term "keel" resection during reduction mastoplasty (Fig. 4.7). In fact, "keel" resection is an important approach to removing excess breast tissue without any cutaneous undermining. As a consequence of "keel" resection, two columns of remaining mammary tissue are created on each side of the breast (Fig. 4.7). Careful cauterization is carried out all over the raw area after glandular resection.

4.3.4 Suture of Glandular Tissue

The next step of the operation is the suturing of remaining glandular tissue. To facilitate this procedure, the surgeon's assistant maintains the remaining breast tissue using forceps to suture the two columns of mammary tissue created during resection, as described above (Fig. 4.8). It is important to emphasize that reduction mastoplasty using Pitanguy's technique does not leave any "dead" space post-surgery, after suturing of the two mammary columns (Fig. 4.8). Simultaneously, the same procedure is performed on the opposite breast. The mammary gland resected from each breast must be analyzed by the anatomopathologist, even when patient does not present any problems during clinical evaluation.

4.3.5 Repositioning the Nipple–Areola Regions

Afterward, the new nipple–areola regions are drawn on the vertices of the breasts. With the patient in a lying down position, the surgeon may project the new regions according to his or her sense of aesthetic (Fig. 4.8). When a patient presents with very fatty breasts, repositioning the nipple–areola region may be difficult so as to achieve a satisfactory position as the glandular flaps are quite thick. To solve such a situation, Silveira Neto's maneuver is employed to elevate the nipple–areola region to the correct position (Fig. 4.9).

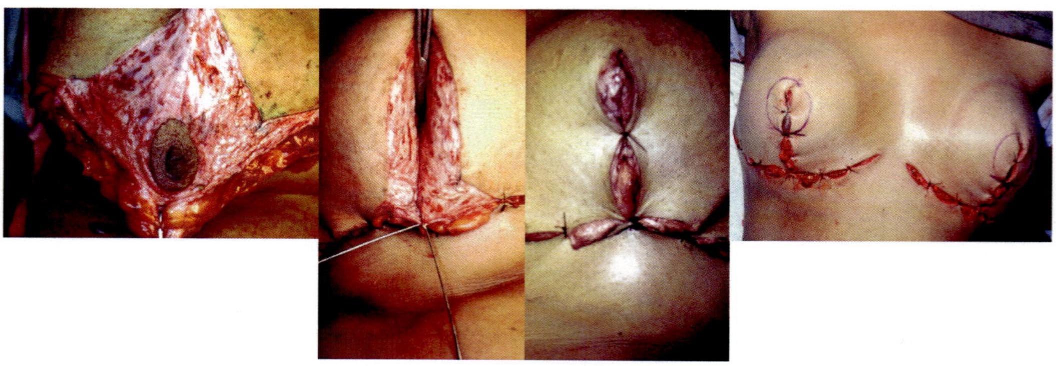

Fig. 4.8 Suturing of Pitanguy's columns and marking of the future nipple–areola regions. (**a**) The nipple–areola region in the center. (**b**, **c**) Temporary stitches were inserted laterally and medially. (**d**) The new nipple–areola regions are demarcated on the vertices of the breasts

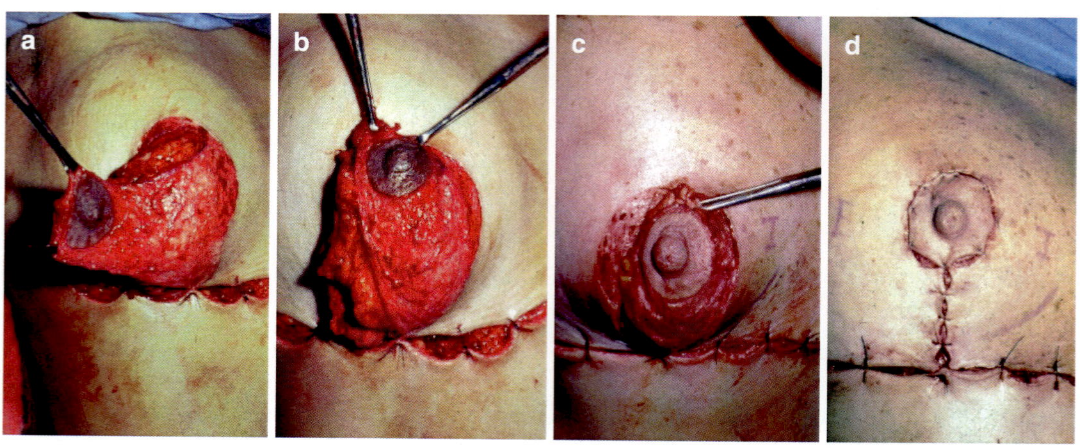

Fig. 4.9 Silveira Neto's (1990) maneuver for elevation of the nipple–areola region in very large and fatty breasts. (**a**) A lateral incision was made. (**b**) The nipple–areola region is rotated and elevated. (**c**, **d**) The nipple–areola region is placed and sutured on natural vertices of the breast after mastoplasty

4.3.6 Suturing of the Skin

Finally, the borders of the wound are sutured using a running internal suture. Adhesive tapes are then applied to the surgical wound. At the end the new breast undergoes bandaging.

4.4 Discussion

Reduction mastoplasty is one of the most frequently performed procedures in plastic surgery in our country and around the world. When young girls present with hypertrophic breasts they may have several secondary signs and symptoms. Often, they complaint of back pain, heavy breasts, alteration of the posture, pre-menstrual pain causing physical discomfort, which may all be solved by reduction mastoplasty (Fig. 4.10).

After pregnancy, the breasts may undergo severe changes, leaving unaesthetic alterations that may bother the woman. Striae and flabby skin may also cause problems, inducing severe physical and psychological disturbances that may be adequately treated by reduction mastoplasty (Figs. 4.11 and 4.12).

Reduction mastoplasty may be performed in patients of any age, if they have adequate reason to complain about their breasts. As the use of Pitanguy's technique of reduction mastoplasty preserves the function of the breast, the operation may be performed in young patients (Figs. 4.13 and 4.14). Even combined procedures with abdominoplasty or any other aesthetic approach may be carried out with gratifying results. It is important to emphasize that the systematization described above may be employed in other circumstances of mastoplasty combined with silicone prosthesis implants.

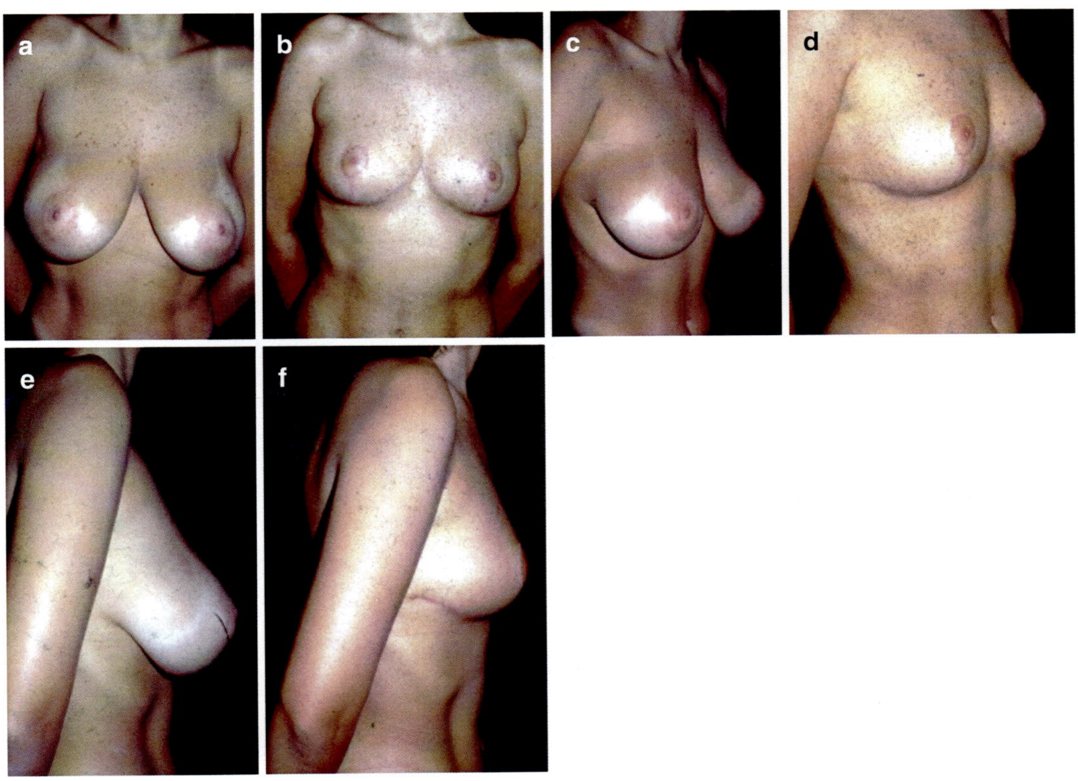

Fig. 4.10 Surgical results in hypertrophic, ptotic, and asymmetric breasts. (**a**, **c**, **e**) Preoperative photos. (**b**, **d**, **f**) Final results after reduction mastoplasty

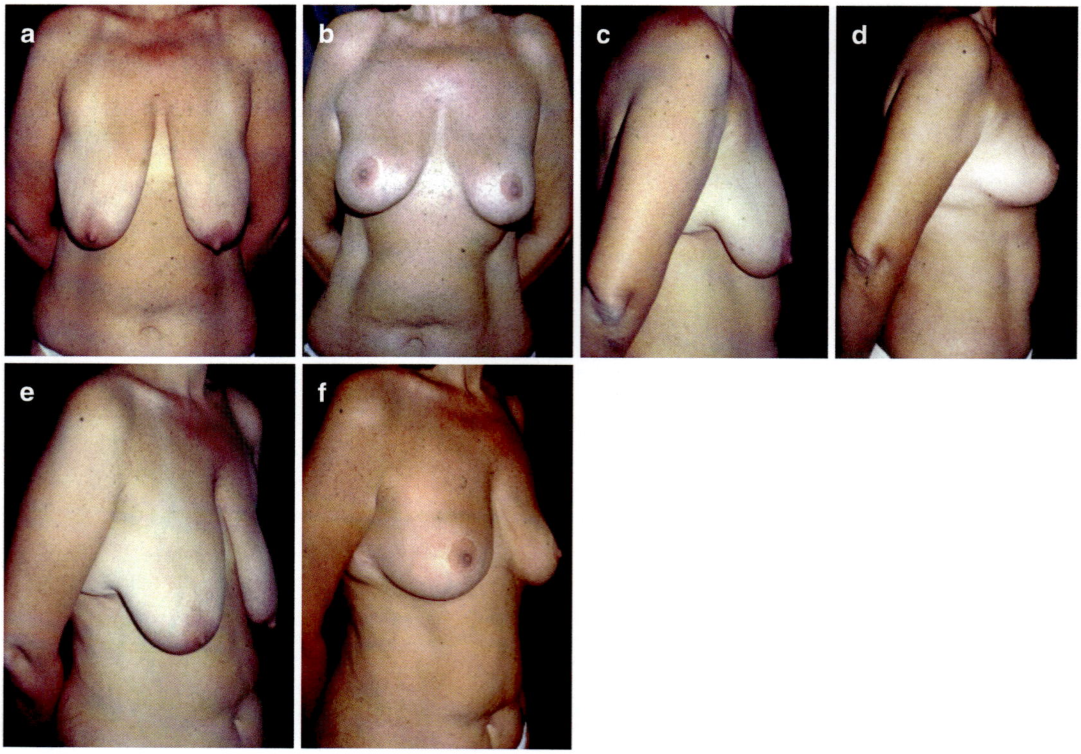

Fig. 4.11 Surgical results of severe ptotic and flabby breasts. (**a**, **c**, **e**) Preoperative views. (**b**, **d**, **f**) Final results after reduction mastoplasty

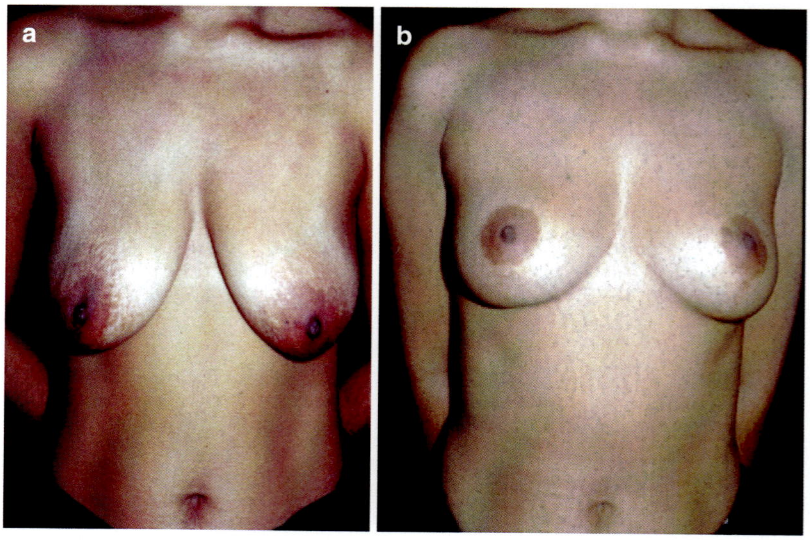

Fig. 4.12 Surgical results in hypertrophic, ptotic, flabby, and asymmetrical breasts. (**a**, **c**) Photos before surgery. (**b**, **d**) Final results after reduction mastoplasty

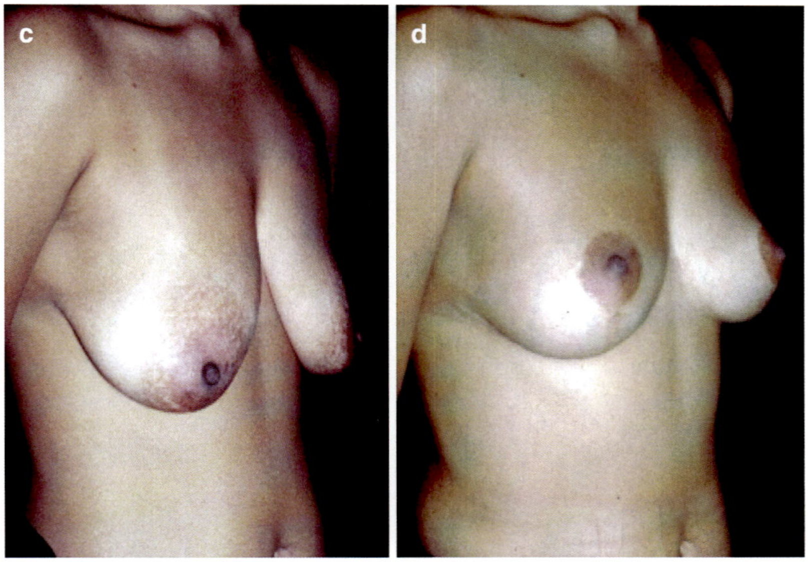

Fig. 4.12 (continued)

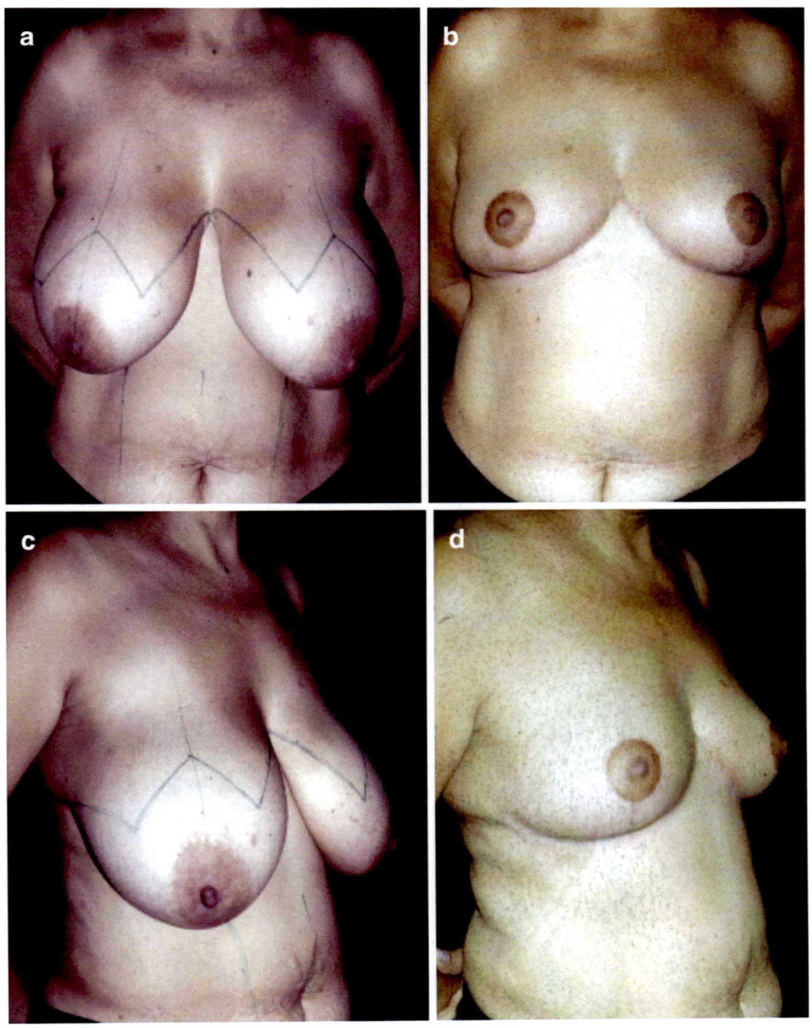

Fig. 4.13 Surgical results in large hypertrophic and ptotic breasts. (**a**, **c**) Preoperative photos showing surgical marking. (**b**, **d**) Final results after reduction mastoplasty

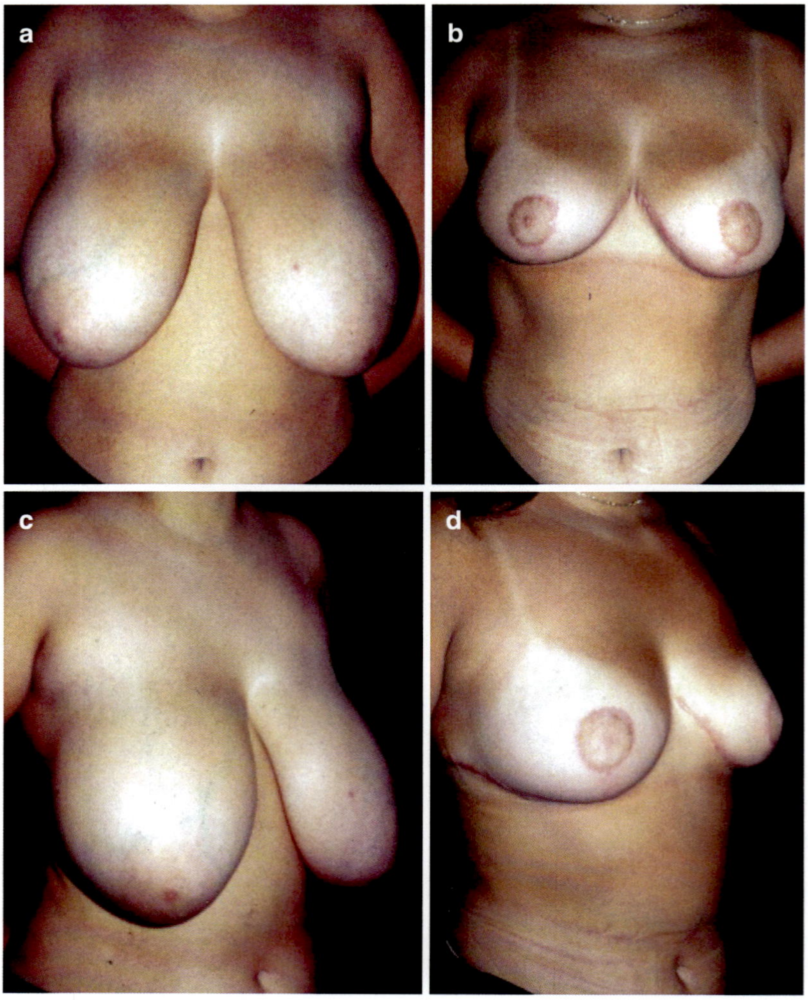

Fig. 4.14 Surgical results in large hypertrophic and ptotic breasts. (**a**, **c**) Preoperative photos. (**b**, **d**) Final results after reduction mastoplasty

Surgical planning is a fundamental step before surgery, as the decision regarding operation is a matter of good understanding between the patient and surgeon. Once the operation is adequately planned surgical marking is a mandatory step before the procedure. Owing to Pitanguy's technique, mastoplasty has become popular, with minimal complications and outstanding aesthetic results. Even in the treatment of asymmetry, it is possible to achieve good surgical correction. The use of a prefabricated pattern is no longer necessary, as surgical marking is a matter of artistic approach.

4.5 Complications

Nowadays, there is a minimal rate of complications in the use of Pitanguy's technique, as there is no cutaneous undermining. Hematoma formation is rare because of the absence of "dead space" after surgery. As long as the surgical marking is well done, the final scars will be well located on the submammary sulcus, which presents good anatomical and histological characteristics for healing. The vertical scar usually also has an agreeable appearance. It is rare, but some sloughing of the areolar regions may occur or even a small area of necrosis, which should heal well.

Conclusions

Because of the great developments in reduction mastoplasty techniques, patients have enough motivation to undergo the operation, as the breasts can cause physical and psychological discomfort. The decision to undergo operation must entail a good understanding between the patient and surgeon. Surgical marking is the key to the surgeon achieving adequate results, because each patient requires an individual approach, but using the same basic surgical principles. The operation may be performed under epidural anesthesia, general anesthesia or local anesthesia combined with intravenous sedation, always under the care of an anesthesiologist.

References

Aegina P (1846) Book II. Adams Francis (Trans). London, England: Sydenham Society; 334–335

Biesenberger H (1928) Eine neue Methode der Mammaplastik. Zentralbl Chir 55:2382

Biesenberguer H (1931) Deformitaten und Kosmetische Operationen der Weiblichen Brust . Wilhem Maudich, Wien

Cunha RJC, Jaimovich CA, Nogueira AJS, Lins DSMR, Nogueira CF (1990) Reduced mastoplasty: modified Silveira Neto's tactical maneuver for ascension of the nipple-areola complex. Arq Bras Med Nav 52(3);65

Durston W (1669) Concerning a very sudden and excessive swelling of a womans breasts. Phil Trans 4:1047–1049. Royal Society, London, 1670

Letterman G, Schurter M (1974) Will Durston's mammaplasty. Plast Reconstr Surg 53(1):48

Paré A (1510–1590) According to Letterman G, Scharter M (1974) Inframammary based dermofat flaps in mammary reconstruction following a subcutaneous mastectomy. Plast Reconstr Surg 55:156–159

Passot R (1925) La correction esthétique du prolapsus mammaire par la procede de la transposition du mamelon. Presse Méd 33:317–318

Paulus A (625–690 d. C.) Referred by Sinder R (2003) History of reduction mastoplasty (História da mamoplastia redutora). In: Mélega JM, Baroudi R (eds) Cirurgia plástica: fundamentos e arte, vol. 31. Medsi, Rio de Janeiro, pp 435–469

Pitanguy I (1961a) Aproximação eclética ao problema das mammaplastias. Rev Bras Cir 41:179–196

Pitanguy I (1961b) Mammaplastic—Estudo de 245 casos consecutivos de mamaplastia e apresentação de técnica pessoal. Rev Bras Cir Out 42:201–220

Schwarzmann E (1930) Die Technik der Mammaplastik. Chirurg 2:932

Strömbeck JO (1960) Mammaplasty. Report of a new technique based on the two pedicle procedure. Br J Plast Surg 13(1):79

5 Anesthesia for Aesthetic Breast Surgery

Juarez M. Avelar

5.1 Introduction

Anesthesia is an important specialty in medicine with great developments since the first decade of the twentieth century, which provides fantastic support to the progress in all surgical fields, particularly plastic surgery. The first anesthesia is credited to Crawford Williamson Long in 1846 (Reis Junior 2006) using sulfuric ether for surgical procedures, which opened up a wide field. Later, Long was serving in the Army during the North American Civil War (1861–1865) when he had opportunity to do a great deal of work using his knowledge. Afterward, chloroform was also employed for surgical amputations. During the World War I in Europe, as there were many people requiring surgical repairs, Long's knowledge was useful (Reis Junior 2006). Several other types of anesthesia emerged for performing operations without pain during World War II in several fields of medicine, especially disfigurement of the human body, as described by Gillies and Millard (1957). Unfortunately, during those periods of great bloodshed, some specialties showed remarkable improvements and evolution because of the emergency procedures for repairs of physical deformities.

Ever since I made the decision to publish a book concerning aesthetic surgery of the breast, it was clear in my mind that it was necessary to include a chapter dedicated to anesthesia, that could be written by a well-qualified anesthesiologist. However, the purpose of this chapter is not to teach how to perform anesthesia, or even to inform the reader about particular details concerning drugs and some technical topics. This knowledge may be very well described in books and in the *Journal of Anesthesia* along with all the technical information. As I have always been interested in this subject, I edited a book called *Local and Regional Anesthesia in Aesthetic Plastic Surgery* (Avelar 1993a, b) focusing on information for plastic surgeons. The main purpose of that book was not to encourage other plastic surgeons to perform operations by themselves alone without the active presence of an anesthesiologist. There are 45 outstanding Brazilian authors who wrote other chapters about their methodology for performing aesthetic plastic surgery under local or regional anesthesia. All authors described updated topics along the lines of not encouraging our colleagues to perform aesthetic procedures without the participation of anesthesiologists. In mean time, aesthetic breast surgeons were fascinated to perform surgery under local anesthesia combined with intravenous sedation under the care of an anesthesiologist (Avelar 1980, 1993b; Avelar and Catunda 1985).

J.M. Avelar, M.D.
Brazilian Scientific Institute of Plastic and Reconstructive Surgery,
Alameda Gabriel Monteiro da Silva, 620-Jardim Europa, Sao Paulo, SP 01442-000, Brazil
e-mail: juarezavelar@bol.com.br; institutodaorelha@uol.com.br; clinica-avelar@uol.com.br

J.M. Avelar (ed.), *Breast Surgery*, https://doi.org/10.1007/978-3-319-54115-0_5

Performing an aesthetic breast operation requires a surgeon's ability, creativity, knowledge, mental concentration, and adequate ambiance in the operating room. Thus, on top of all those surgical steps, it is not appropriate for he or she to take care of the patient's condition as well, i.e., fluctuations in blood pressure, pulse, irregularity of respiratory depth and rate, bucking and coughing, increased bleeding in the wound, straining and moving during application of the surgical dressing, all signs and symptoms that require special attention and immediate treatment. For all these reasons, the presence of an anesthesiologist during surgery in the operating room may deal with any problems, providing adequate support for the surgeon in performing the operation (Avelar 1993b). As I had the privilege to be Prof. Pitanguy's resident, I learned from him, as he always used to perform his operations with an anesthesiologist, and this is mentioned in some of his publications (Pitanguy 1961; Pitanguy et al. 1971, 1977; Pitanguy and Garcia 1972). Problems that are considered to be of little consequence in other specialties are of major importance to the patients undergoing breast aesthetic surgery, during the operation as well as postoperatively regarding pain, which should be minimal (Avelar 1993a).

5.2 Method

5.2.1 Preoperative Evaluation

Before a patient goes to the hospital to undergo a breast operation, his or her surgeon has already examined her during previous consultations for surgical indications and planning in addition to surgical pre-marking, according to the routine of each surgeon.

My preference is to demarcate some reference points 1 day before surgery and once more to examine the breasts and take other photos. It is useful to do pre-marking at my clinic to provide essential orientation, as the patient is awake and follows my work, which is done in front of two parallel vertical mirrors strategically placed on the walls of examination room (Fig. 5.1). Under this system, each patient sees my pre-marking and she can confirm all the information about location and size of the scars as well. She can even observe again her asymmetric breasts and the posterior aspect of the torso and chest deformities secondary to the hypertrophic breasts. After pre-marking, my patients sign informed consent.

Routine blood test, heart examination and other specific examinations according to the surgical planning are always carried out, which are carefully observed.

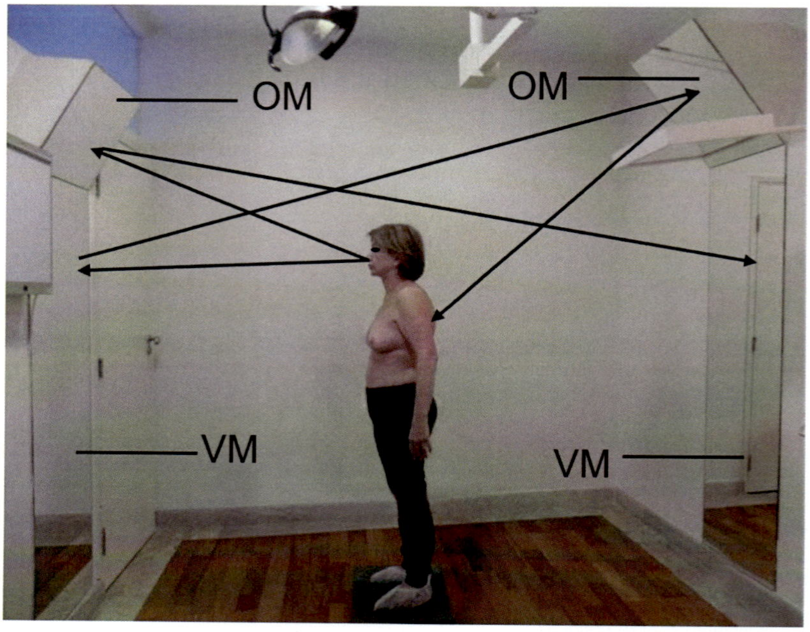

Fig. 5.1 Photo of a patient in the examination room at my clinic. She is in a standing position in front of one vertical mirror (VM), she sees her body from the frontal view and from the back view simultaneously through the oblique mirrors (OM), as indicated by the *arrows*

5.2.1.1 At the Hospital

When a patient goes to the hospital it is essential that the anesthesiologist visits and examine her before aesthetic breast surgery to gain the confidence of the patient and to relieve any fears and anxieties. In fact, this is the first time they meet each other. That brief moment is adequate opportunity for a good understanding between them. Also, a patient with a history of heart, lung, chronic kidney disease, unstable blood pressure, and other circumstances that raise concerns regarding anesthesia for the operation, is given careful consideration. Because of the increased risk involved, elective surgery should not be attempted following any previous disease. A patient who is accustomed to a daily alcohol intake, or who routinely takes sedatives for insomnia should be well evaluated before premedication, and, most likely, given higher concentrations of anesthetic agents to produce a satisfactory state of unconsciousness. A detailed oral examination is mandatory because of the many delicate dental restorations commonly observed today. Most potential errors in the management of anesthesia can be avoided by careful preoperative evaluation and planning. Finally, the patient should have confidence in the anesthesiologist before undergoing breast surgery (Avelar 1993b).

Gentleness is an art when inducing and sustaining a pain-free unconscious state. Administering an anesthetic means applying a measured physiological insult to a patient under precise pharmacological control. The choice of premedication and anesthetic agents is made at this time, according to anesthesiologist's decision.

5.2.2 Premedication

The patient who has undergone proper administration of premedication usually arrives in the operating room in a drowsy, amnesic, and cooperative estate, with no circulatory or respiratory depression. This optimal condition may be achieved by a combination of drugs, which is given by anesthesiologist. Because of its pharmacological activity, each drug plays an important role in the final result. Drugs used for premedication include barbiturates, belladonna alkaloids, tranquilizers, and narcotics. All these decisions and drug administration are under the anesthesiologist's control. Even if he or she takes the decision not to administer any drugs as premedication, it means that it is an appropriate condition for the patient undergoing the operation. Such a circumstance sometimes occurred with my patients, that I did not take part in the decisions, as long as the operation is carried out under good conditions.

5.2.2.1 Breast Surgery

The choice of the anesthesia technique is a matter of a good understanding between the plastic surgeon and the anesthesiologist. I do not feel comfortable decide which method must be followed. In fact, each surgeon may take his or her decision in accordance with the anesthesiologist so that they are both comfortable bearing in mind that the patient's life is in their hands. Sometimes, a patient says that her preference for one or other type of anesthesia, which should have been previously well-evaluated during consultation at the office and during premedication. As long as the patient's suggestion is well understood and accepted by the surgeon and the anesthesiologist it is a matter of good sense and reasonable to do that.

5.2.3 The Choice of Anesthesia

There are five types of anesthesia used for performing breast surgery:

(1) General anesthesia (Fig. 5.2)
(2) Local anesthesia combined with intravenous sedation (Fig. 5.3)
(3) Epidural anesthesia combined with intravenous sedation (Fig. 5.4)
(4) Intercostal block infiltration combined with intravenous sedation
(5) Local anesthesia without participation of an anesthesiologist

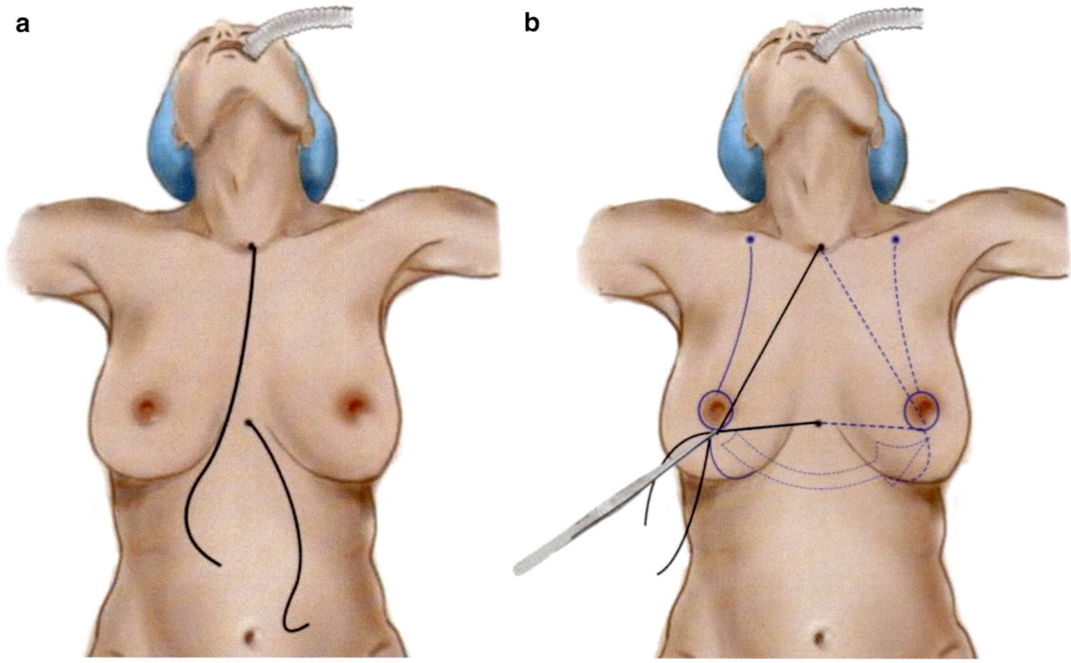

Fig. 5.2 Drawings to demonstrate surgical marking during the operation under general anesthesia with endotracheal intubation. (**a**)—A long line is stitched on the sternal notch and another on the xyphoid process. (**b**) Using forceps, the two lines are held for comparison of the two breasts after surgical marking and during surgery

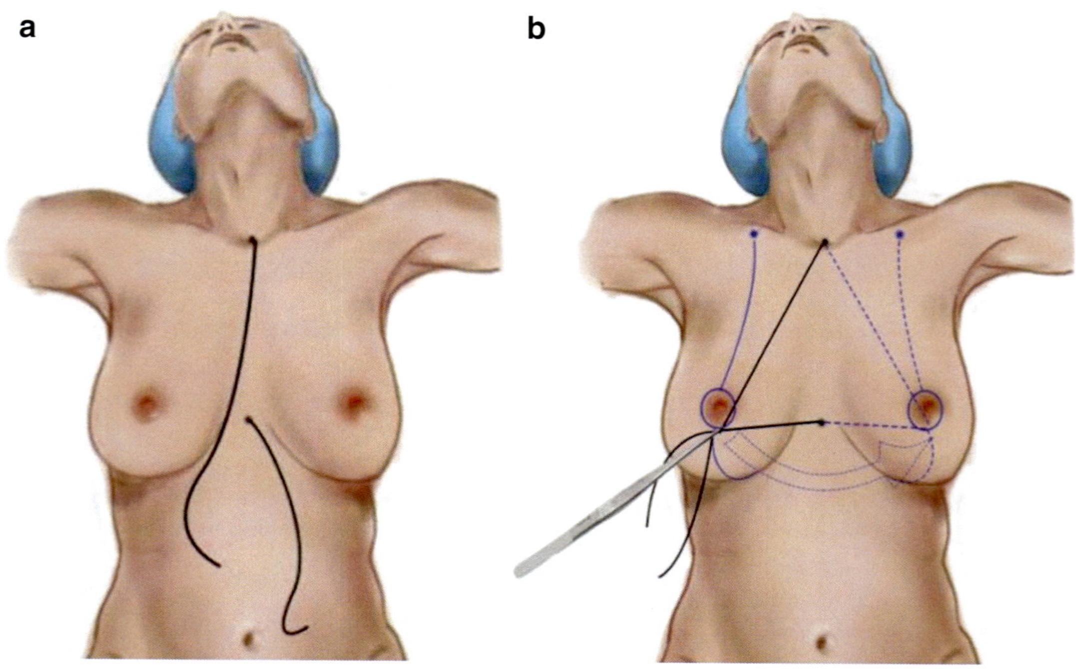

Fig. 5.3 Two drawings show surgical marking during the operation under local anesthesia combined with intravenous sedation. (**a**) A long line is stitched on the sternal notch and another on the xyphoid process. (**b**) Using forceps, the two lines are held for comparison of the two breasts after surgical marking

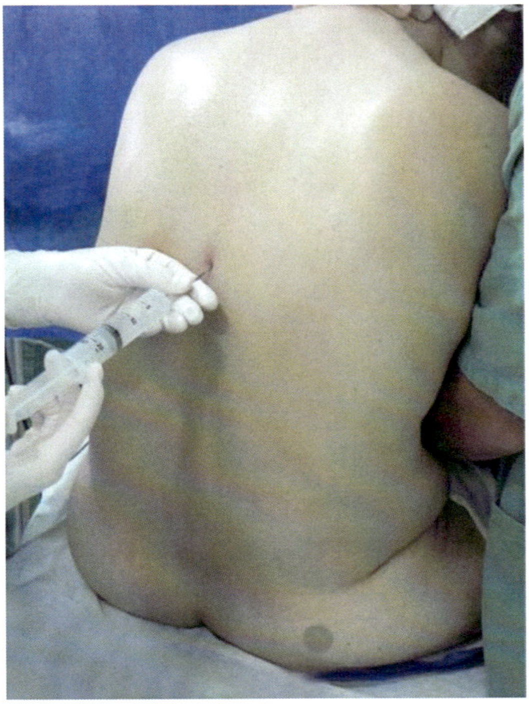

Fig. 5.4 Epidural anesthesia for aesthetic breast surgery. Photo shows the epidural being performed by the anesthesiologist with the patient sitting on the operating table

5.2.3.1 General Anesthesia

Performing breast surgery under general anesthesia is the most frequent procedure, as the patient's condition is under the control of the anesthesiologist and the surgeon may work comfortably. Even when associated surgical procedures are scheduled, general anesthesia provides adequate and safe conditions. Nevertheless, local infiltration can be performed to avoid too much bleeding during the operation. The patient's breathing (through the endotracheal tube), heart control, drug administration, and all other aspects during surgery are under the rigid control of the anesthesiologist, who should provide the surgeon with peaceful conditions under which to work (Fig. 5.2).

My preference is to perform breast surgery with the patient in a semi-sitting position with the arms at a 45° angle from the body laterally on each side of the torso (Fig. 5.3) (Pitanguy 1961; Gillies and McIndoe 1939). When I perform a combined procedure of mastoplasty with rhytidoplasty, or rhinoplasty, or with abdominoplasty, or any procedure on the lower extremities, I always start the operation by first performing the mastoplasty because of the semi-sitting position of the patient on the operating table. I consider this safer than vice versa (Pitanguy 1981). It is important to emphasize that I perform only one procedure associated with the breast operation on a patient if she is in good health and the anesthesiologist is in agreement to performing the two procedures.

After endotracheal intubation and all the activities concerning the anesthesiologist's medications providing good conditions for anesthesia, the patient is then prepared for the operation according to the routine of each surgeon. I prefer to raise the table to about 45° to elevate the head and torso of the patient so that the breasts show the natural degree of ptosis. I had the privilege of being trained by Prof. Pitanguy, who used to perform combined procedures and mastoplasty with the patient in the semi-sitting position (Pitanguy 1975; Pitanguy and Garcia 1972; Pitanguy et al. 1977).

In addition to the patient being under general anesthesia, local infiltration may be done with the use of vasoconstrictor agents to reduce bleeding during surgery. These agents, by causing local vasoconstriction (a chemical tourniquet effect), reduce the rate of absorption of the local anesthetic agent, if it is added to the solution in accordance with the anesthesiologist and thus reduces the incidence of adverse reactions. They also prolong the duration of the anesthetic. The dangers of these agents, particularly epinephrine (which is the best), lie in the use of unnecessarily high concentrations. The solution I am used to employing is 1:200,000 (1 mL of epinephrine (1:1000) and 200 mL of serum) produces a proper degree of vasoconstriction (Pitanguy et al. 1971). Stronger solutions increase the vasoconstrictor effect and may induce complications of epinephrine intoxication, which are nervousness, cold sweats, hypertension, and tachycardia, in addition to severe arrhythmias. Errors in the preparation of local analgesic agents containing epinephrine should be avoided.

Usually, a volume of 200 mL of solution is enough to perform local infiltration for both breasts, even in large hypertrophic breasts, as it is not necessary to infiltrate the mammary gland (Avelar 1993a, b).

Infiltration of the solution with epinephrine is done on three levels (Fig. 5.5a):

(a) Below the mammary gland. Using a long needle, infiltration is carried out all over the area below the mammary gland. With left hand, the surgeon holds the breast and pulls it forward to create a natural space between the mammary gland and the aponeurosis of the pectoralis major (Fig. 5.5b–d). Caution is necessary to avoid infiltration inside the muscle, which leads to massive absorption of the solution with undesirable consequences. With the left

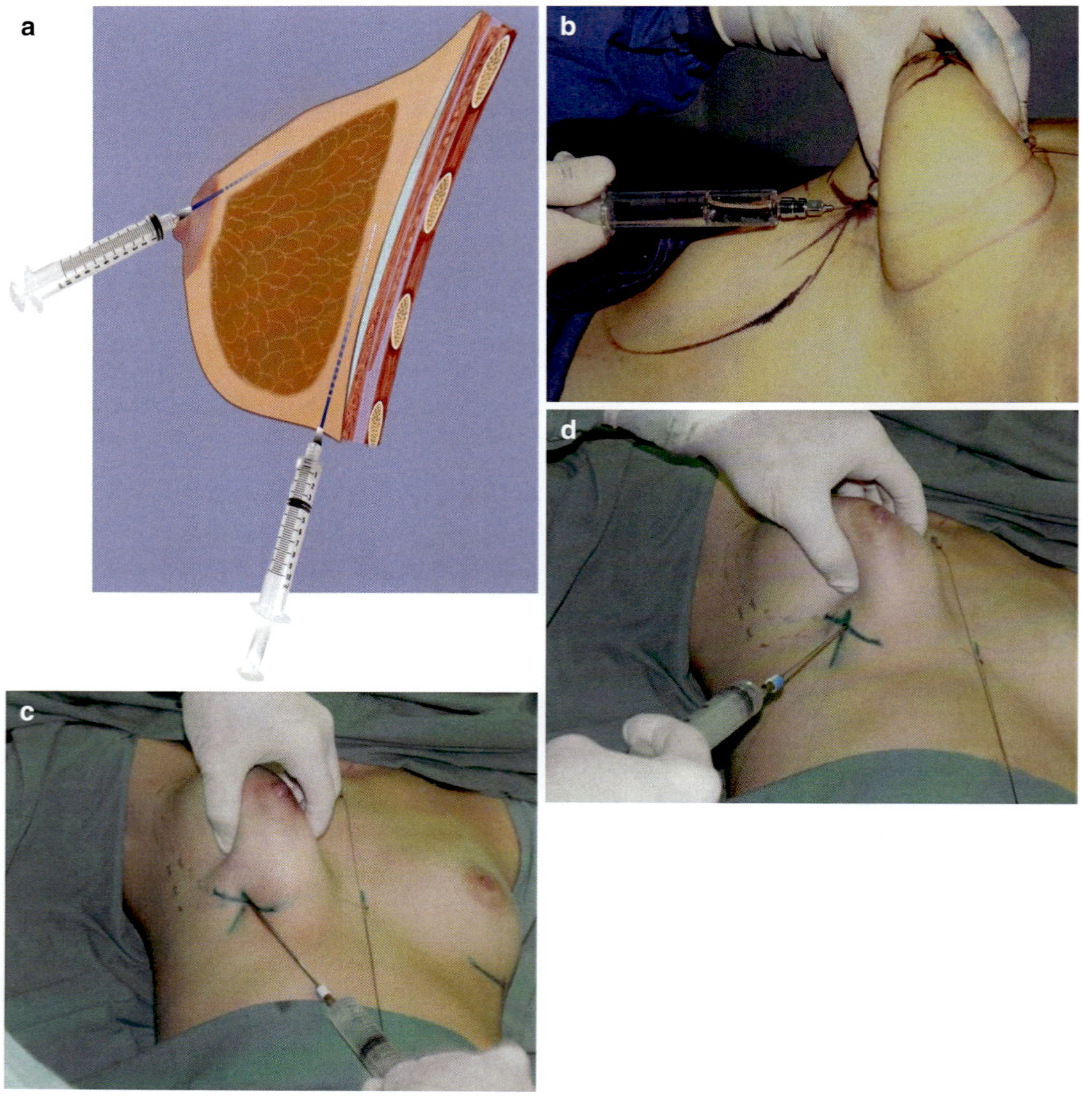

Fig. 5.5 Local infiltration is performed by the surgeon at two levels: on the subcutaneous plane and between the mammary gland and the fascia of the pectoralis major muscle. (**a**) The drawing demonstrates the two levels of infiltration. (**b**) Photo during infiltration shows the surgeon holding the left breast with one hand and using a long needle that is being introduced below the mammary gland. (**c**) Photo shows the surgeon holding the right breast and using a long needle to infiltrate below the mammary gland and above the fascia of the pectoralis major muscle. (**d**) Photo showing the infiltration in a different direction below the mammary gland

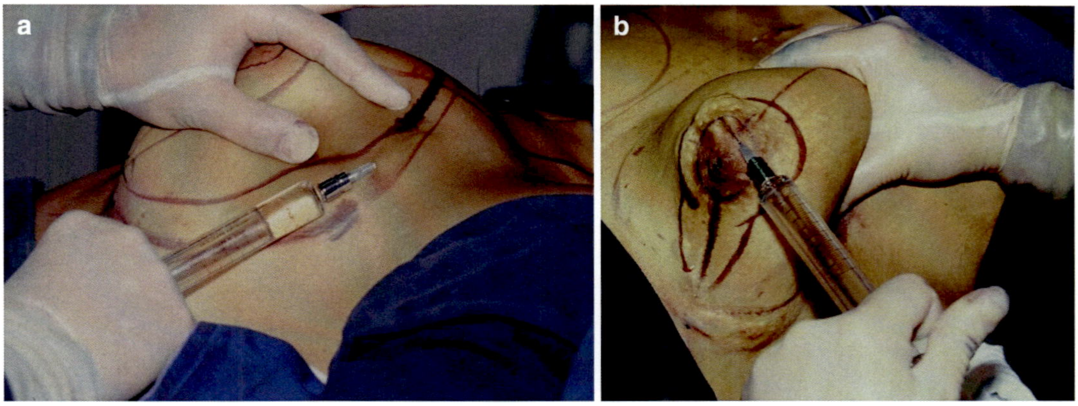

Fig. 5.6 Local infiltration is being performed by the surgeon on a subcutaneous level. (**a**) Photo shows the surgeon holding the left breast to infiltrate the external border on the pre-axillary line to block the innervation of the ending of the intercostobrachial nerve in the subcutaneous plane. (**b**) Photo during infiltration shows the surgeon holding the left breast with one hand and using a regular needle to infiltrate the demarcated lines of the mastoplasty

hand holding the breast, the surgeon can be sure that the needle is passing just below the tip of his fingers and above the muscular level. Under this maneuver, the needle passes on "dead" space between the mammary gland and the pectoralis major. This infiltration provides good conditions for surgery, as there is minimal absorption of the solution.

(b) On a subcutaneous level on the pre-axillary line at the external border of the breast. Through this infiltration good anesthesia is achieved during and after the operation, as branches of the intercostobrachial nerve and the ends of the intercostal nerves are adequately infiltrated (Fig. 5.6a).

(c) On a subcutaneous level, all around the areola and the demarcated lines on the anterior surface of the breasts (Fig. 5.6b). Once again, it is important to emphasize that it should not infiltrate the mammary gland.

Afterward, reduction mastoplasty or mastopexy is performed following surgical demarcations.

5.2.3.2 Local Anesthesia Combined with Intravenous Sedation

This is my favorite choice, as long as the anesthesiologist can induce good sedation to provide comfortable conditions. Once again, pre-marking and premedication follow the same methods described above. Pre-marking is done at my clinic on the day before the operation.

In the operating room, the anesthesiologist administers proper intravenous sedation according to his criteria and decision. Afterward, the patient is prepared for surgery, as described for general anesthesia (Figs. 5.5 and 5.6).

Local infiltration is carried out according to the previous description. In this type of local anesthesia combined with intravenous sedation, it is mandatory to add anesthesia (my preference is lidocaine) to the solution, which I call 201 (Avelar 1993a, b), as it is easily prepared by this method: 160 mL of serum + 40 mL of lidocaine (2%) + 1 mL of epinephrine (1/1000).

The technique of infiltration is similar to that previously described, that is it: below the mammary gland, on the lateral and external borders of the breast, underneath of the areola and subcutaneously on the demarcated area for mastoplasty (Figs. 5.3, 5.5 and 5.6). Once again, it is important to emphasize that it is not necessary to infiltrate the mammary gland.

5.2.3.3 Epidural Anesthesia Combined with Intravenous Sedation

This type of anesthesia is not at all my preferred option, but it may be the anesthesiologist's preference. If the surgeon has enough confidence in the anesthesiologist, it is possible to perform breast surgery (Fig. 5.4). I used to perform operations at a hospital where the anesthesiologists are very well trained and they perform outstanding epidural anesthesia, which provides excellent conditions for performing breast operations. In addition to the epidural anesthesia, I do carry out local infiltration in all patients without anesthetic drugs, but only with epinephrine to avoid bleeding during the operation (Figs. 5.3 and 5.4). It is important to emphasize that the patient chooses her surgeon to perform breast surgery; therefore, he takes all responsibility for the operation.

When this type of anesthesia is administered, all conditions for the operation may be organized according to the surgeon's necessities: the position of the patient on the operating table, the position of the table, local infiltration to avoid too much bleeding, etc. (Fig. 5.7).

There is no relationship between the type of anesthesia and the surgical results, as long as the patient feels very comfortable after surgery (Figs. 5.8 and 5.9). Such a procedure may also be employed for breast augmentation with silicone prosthesis (Fig. 5.10), even when mastoplasty is performed for removal of the breast implant combined with mastopexy (Fig. 5.11).

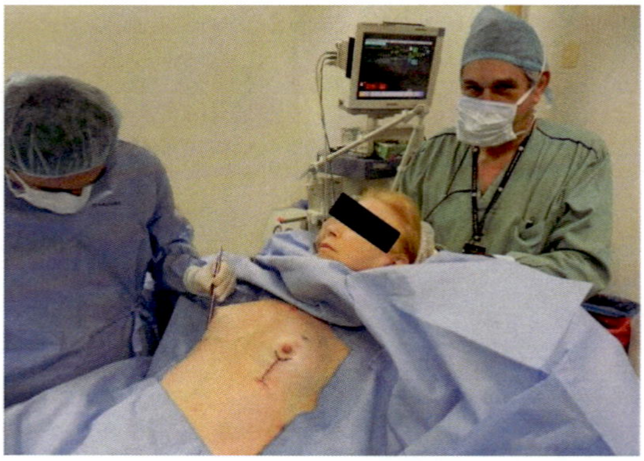

Fig. 5.7 Epidural anesthesia for aesthetic breast surgery. Photo during surgery shows a patient under local anesthesia combined with intravenous sedation under the care of an anesthesiologist behind the patient with all equipment in the operating room

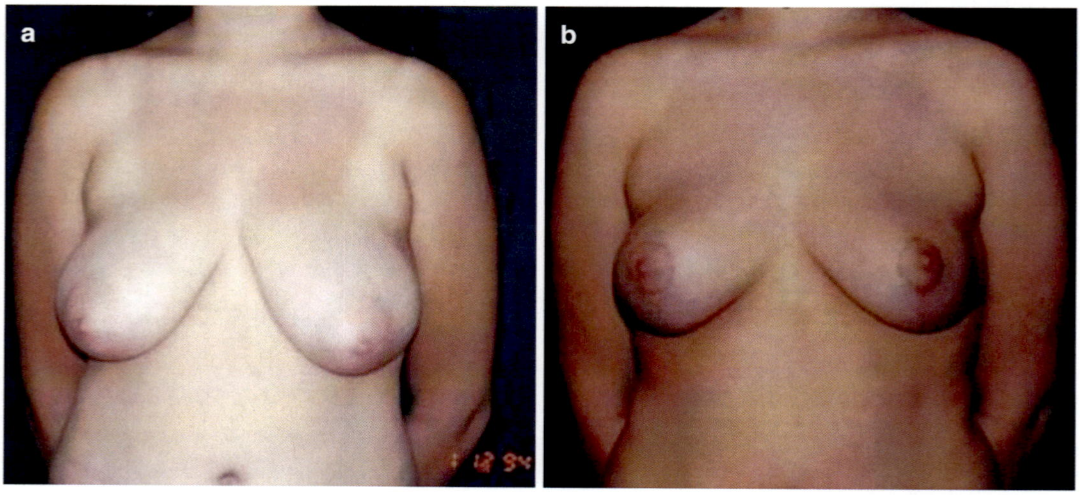

Fig. 5.8 A 49-year-old patient with hypertrophic, asymmetrical, and ptotic breasts underwent reduction mastoplasty. (**a**, **c**, **e**, **g**) Photos before surgery. (**b**, **d**, **f**, **h**) Photos after reduction mastoplasty under local anesthesia combined with intravenous sedation

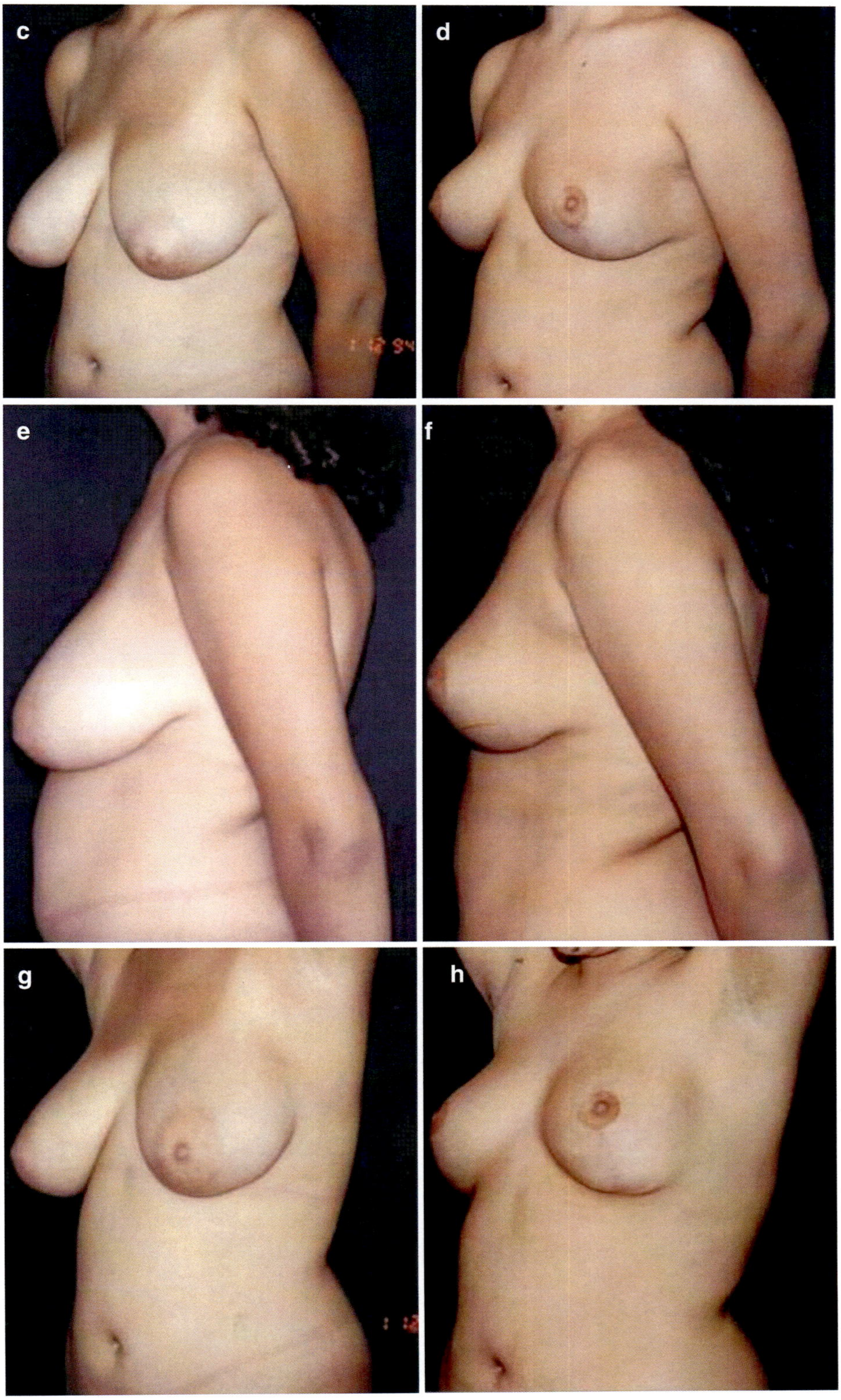

Fig. 5.8 (continued)

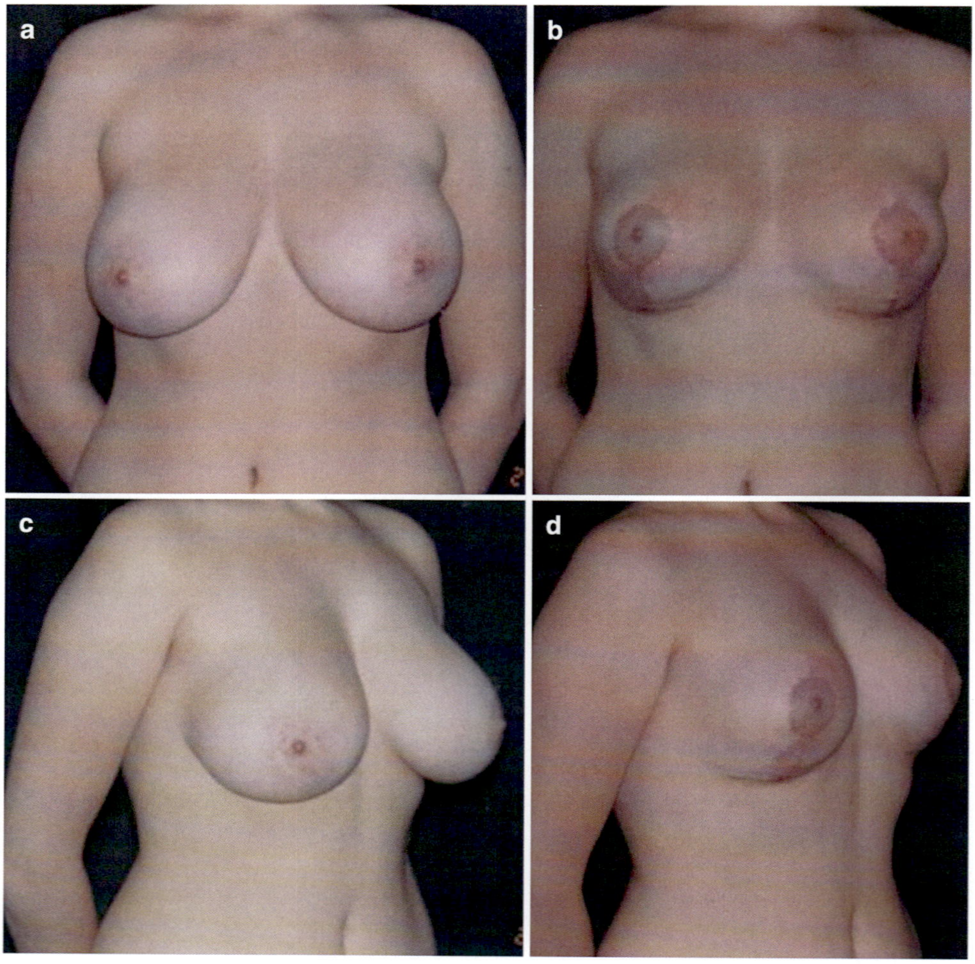

Fig. 5.9 A 38-year-old patient with hypertrophic breasts underwent reduction mastoplasty. (**a**, **c**) Photos before surgery. (**b**, **d**) Photos after reduction mastoplasty under local anesthesia combined with intravenous sedation

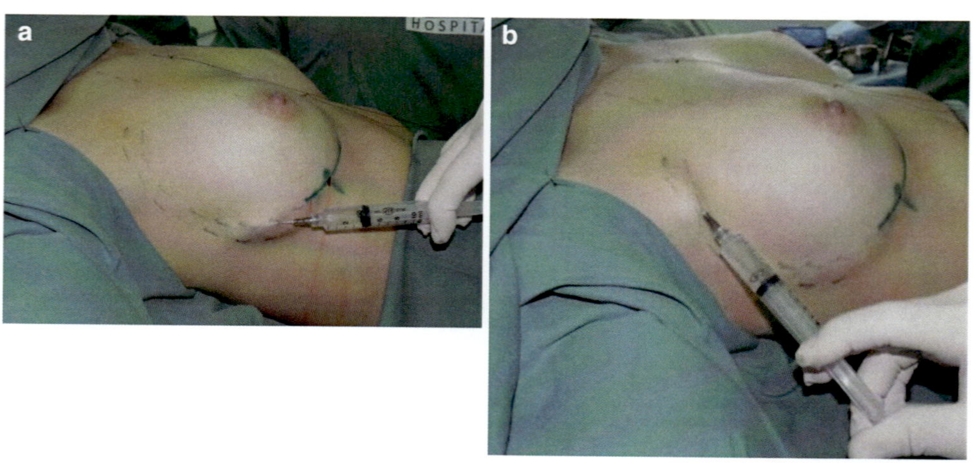

Fig. 5.10 Local infiltration for augmentation mastoplasty with a silicone prosthesis implant. (**a**) Photo shows the surgeon infiltrating the external border of the right breast on the pre-axillary line to block the innervation of the ending of the intercostobrachial nerve in the subcutaneous plane using a regular needle. (**b**) The infiltration is done all way to the external border of the breast

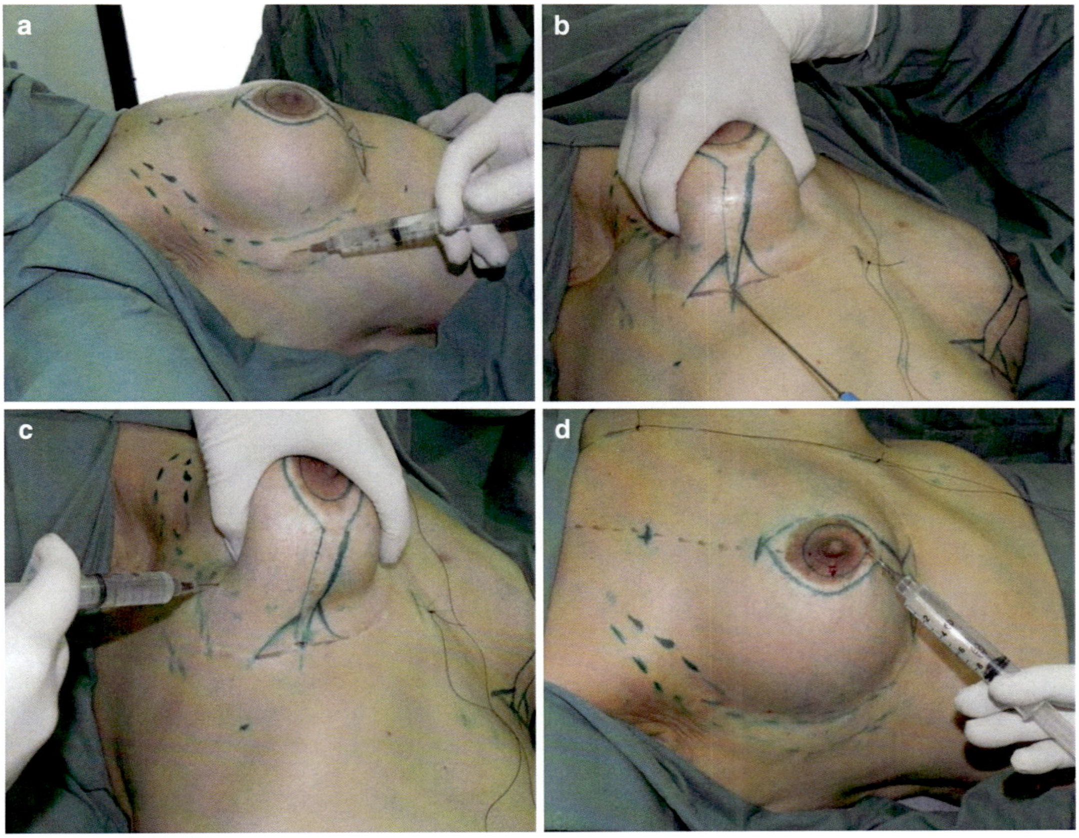

Fig. 5.11 Local infiltration for removing of a mammary implant followed by mastopexy. (**a**) Photo shows the surgeon infiltrating the external border of the right breast on the pre-axillary line to block the innervation of the ending of the intercostobrachial nerve in the subcutaneous plan using a regular needle. (**b**) Photo during infiltration shows the surgeon holding the right breast with one hand and using a long needle to infiltrate below the mammary implant and above the pectoralis major muscle. (**c**) Photo shows the surgeon holding the right breast and using a long needle to infiltrate below the mammary implant and above the fascia of the pectoralis major muscle. (**d**) Photo showing the infiltration of the demarcated lines of the mastoplasty using a regular needle

5.2.3.4 Intercostal Block Infiltration Combined with Intravenous Sedation

5.2.3.5 Local Anesthesia Without Participation of an Anesthesiologist

I consider both types of anesthesia the worst for breast operations, no matter whether intercostal block infiltration is carried out by the anesthesiologist or by the surgeon, as reported by Huang et al. (1979). There has already been some sort of complications during such anesthesia with severe problems for patients and surgeons alike. It is mentioned here only to demonstrate the possibility, but I do not at all recommend it. I have heard about perforation of the chest wall with tearing of the pleura with the needle due to intercostal block infiltration. Infiltration may not be regular throughout the intercostal spaces if some of the injections do not reach the nerves. Therefore, the effect of the anesthesia will not be satisfactory. If other injections have to be administered during surgery, this may spoil the ambience of the operation.

5.3 Discussion

Local anesthesia for breast surgery associated with general anesthesia or with intravenous sedation under the care of an anesthesiologist is a useful procedure. Safe administration depends on certain conditions, such as.

1. Proper dose of premedication.

It is my personal preference that it is not wise for a surgeon to perform breast operations by himself or herself with only his or her staff, without the participation of an anesthesiologist. The desire to avoid patient discomfort during local anesthesia leads the surgeon to attempt to produce the state of general anesthesia by ordering heavy premedication. The presence of an anesthesiologist who has enough knowledge provides adequate support for the surgeon to perform aesthetic surgery on the breast in addition to other types of surgery. Premedication is designed merely to produce a state of calm relaxation, while unusual or uncomfortable situations may occur before the operation. The patient should sustain all vital functions, including responsiveness. It is much safer for the surgeon to perform his or her operations under adequate medication than to run the risk of any iatrogenic complications.

2. The application or injection of the adequate concentration of the selected agent.

The surgeon must remember that it is almost impossible to predetermine the exact amount of premedication that will be effective for each patient. Continuous injection of small doses intravenously may not produce an adequate degree of control.

3. Avoidance of intravenous injections of solutions.

This circumstance may occur accidentally during surgery with an unexpected patient's reaction. For this reason, I consider that it is not safe for a surgeon to perform any operation without the participation of an anesthesiologist.

4. Well-balanced vasoconstrictor drugs.

Each surgeon must have as a matter of routine the adequate solution to use during surgery to avoid bleeding. In my practice, I am used to employing local infiltration during breast surgery under general anesthesia under the care of an anesthesiologist. My preferred solution is: 1:200,000 (1 mL of epinephrine (1:1000) and 200 mL of serum), which produces the proper degree of vasoconstriction.

Nevertheless, when mastoplasty is performed under local anesthesia combined with intravenous sedation under the care of an anesthesiologist my solution is: 160 mL of serum + 40 mL of lidocaine (2%) + 1 mL of epinephrine (1/1000). With the use of this volume, it is possible to infiltrate both breasts for mastopexy or even reduction mastoplasty.

5. Constant vigilance to treat adverse reactions.

This is the main reason why a surgeon should work with an anesthesiologist during an operation. If some unexpected reaction is caused by injection of the solution, the surgeon is not adequately prepared for immediate treatment, as he or she is concentrating on the operation.

The use of vasoconstrictors is useful to avoid bleeding during the operation and to prolong the duration of the anesthetic. The dangers of these agents, particularly epinephrine, lies in the use of unnecessarily high concentrations. Each surgeon may have a routine solution that all members of staff are used to so as to observe the preparation and the volume during administration (Figs. 5.13 and 5.14).

After the operation, the patient can usually sit on the operating table, which is useful for performing the bandaging (Fig. 5.12).

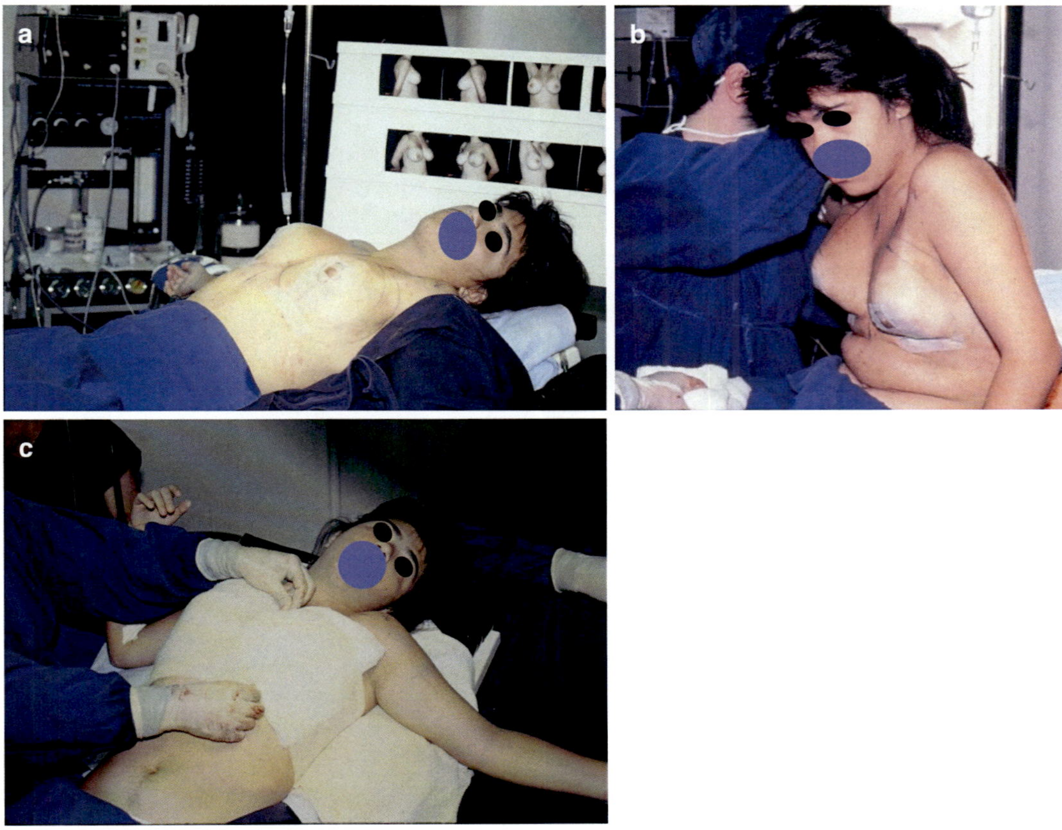

Fig. 5.12 After reduction mastoplasty the patient is awake and in a good enough condition to sit on the operating table for application of the dressing. (**a**) The patient can be seen on the operating table with adhesive tapes on her breasts; her preoperative photos and the anesthesiologist's equipment can also be seen. (**b**) She is sitting in a good enough condition undergo bandaging around the chest. (**c**) The bandaging is done

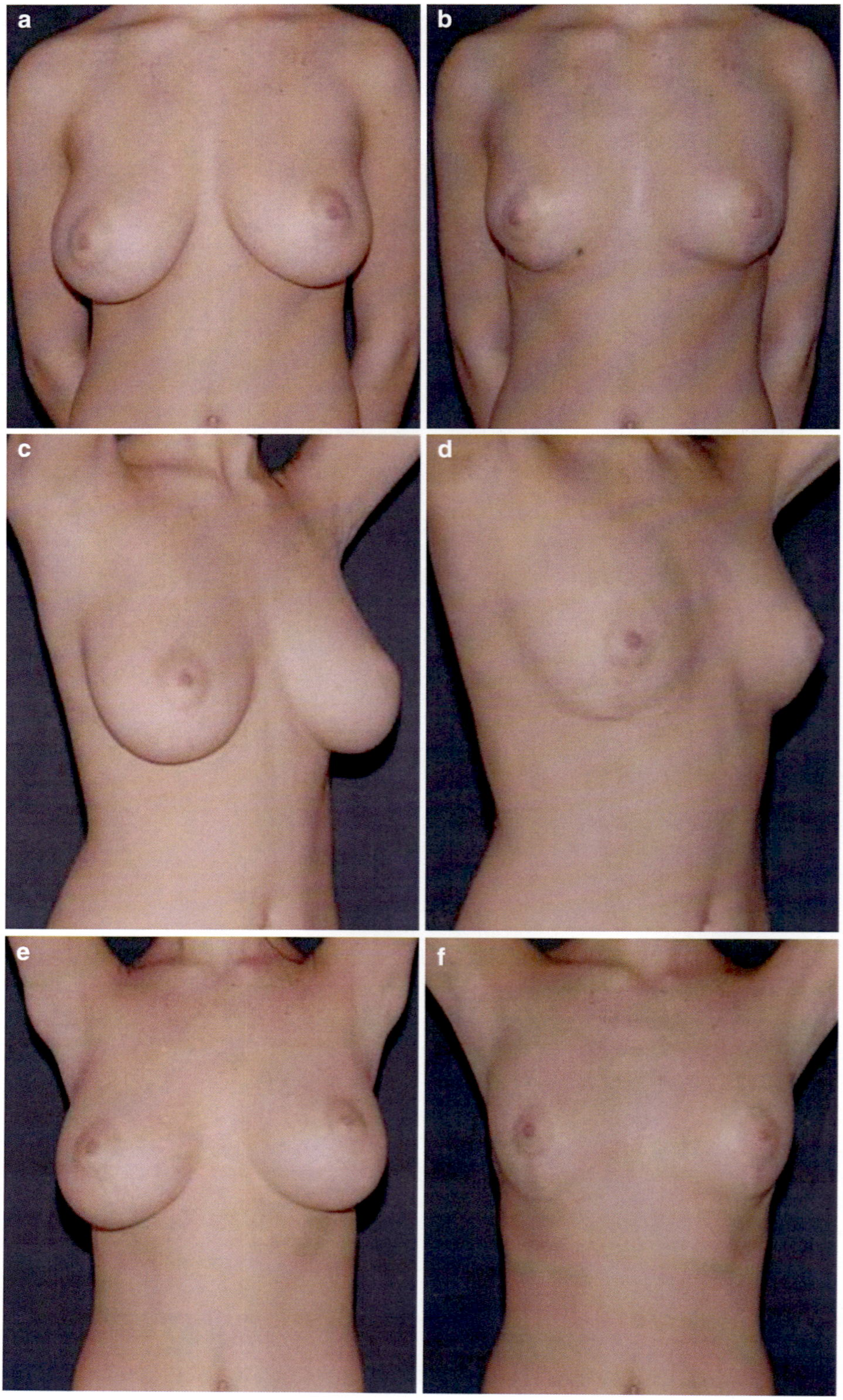

Fig. 5.13 A 26-year-old patient with hypertrophic, asymmetrical, and ptotic breasts underwent reduction mastoplasty. (**a**, **c**, **e**) Photos before surgery. (**b**, **d**, **f**) Photos after reduction mastoplasty under epidural anesthesia combined with intravenous sedation

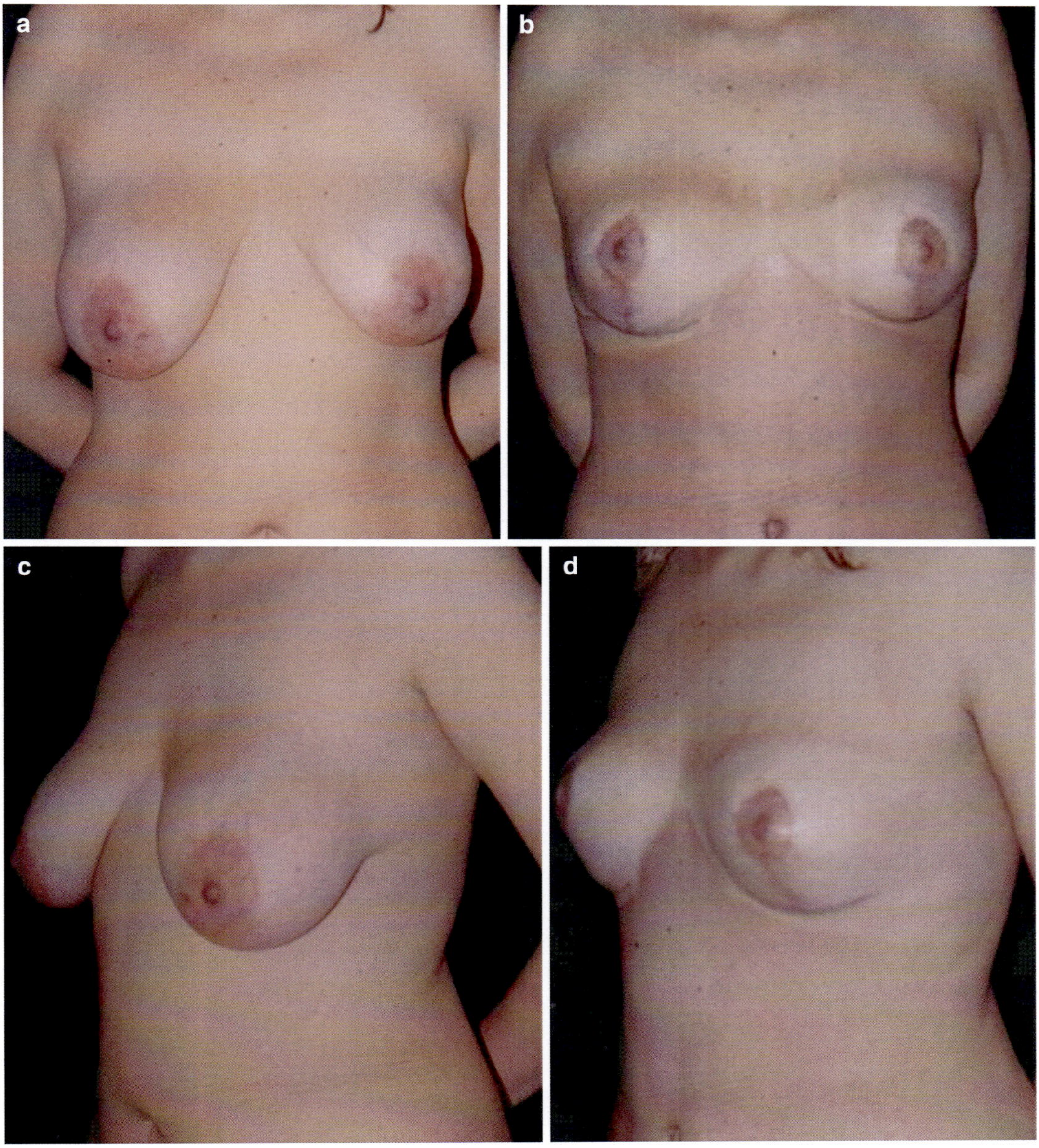

Fig. 5.14 A 31-year-old patient with hypertrophic, asymmetrical, and ptotic breasts underwent reduction mastoplasty. (**a**, **c**, **e**) Photos before surgery. (**b**, **d**, **f**) Photos after reduction mastoplasty under epidural anesthesia combined with intravenous sedation

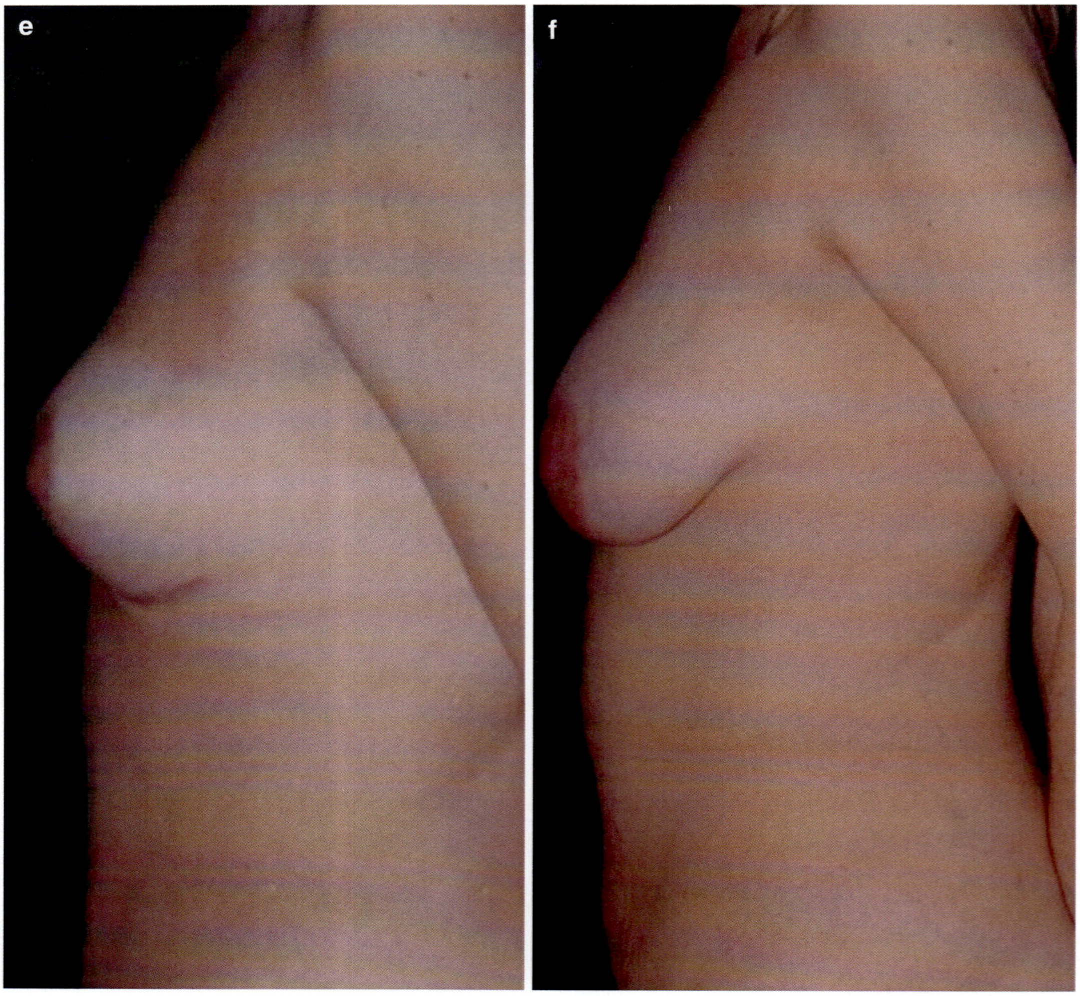

Fig. 5.14 (continued)

5.4 Complications

Complications related to anesthesia during aesthetic breast surgery may occur because of:

(1) The dose of drug administration
(2) Unexpected metabolic reactions
(3) Allergic reactions
(4) Postural imbalance
(5) Respiratory depression
(6) Cardiac arrhythmias

As long as an anesthesiologist is in charge of the anesthesia he or she must take care of the patient all the time, from the premedication until after the operation while she stays in the recovery room.

In the case of circulatory depression, as indicated by hypotension, the anesthesiologist should immediately check the respiration, pulse, and blood pressure, as tachycardia, tachypnea, and hypotension are the adverse signs most frequently encountered.

The anesthesiologist must check if inadvertent intravenous injection was administered or an incorrect dose of the drug concentration, or the toxic dose of an agent was exceeded, which are some common errors.

A patient should never be left unattended: a means of monitoring the patient's vital signs must be used at all times. This essential monitoring must be carried out by efficient electronic devices throughout the operation.

No matter whether the operation was performed under general anesthesia, local anesthesia combined with intravenous sedation, or epidural anesthesia, the final step for the anesthesiologist is when the patient goes out of the postoperative recovery room.

Conclusions

Any breast operation must be well evaluated preoperatively by the surgeon from the point of view of the patient's complaints. The operation must be well planned to be performed at the hospital under the care of an anesthesiologist. Blood tests, heart examination, and others must be carried out preoperatively according to the routine of each surgeon. Premedication is an important step before surgery as it is the first time that the patient speaks to the anesthesiologist. The choice of anesthesia is a matter of a good understanding between the surgeon and the anesthesiologist, and may be general anesthesia; local anesthesia combined with intravenous sedation; or epidural anesthesia combined with intravenous sedation. There are other possibilities for performing mastoplasty, but they are not safe.

References

Avelar JM (1980) Retalho dermo-adiposo-glandular de pedículo superior nas ptoses mamárias (Dermal-adipose-glandular flap with superior pedicle in ptotic breasts). Simpósio Brasileiro de Cirurgia da Mama, São Paulo, August

Avelar J (1993a) In: Avelar JM (ed) Anestesia Loco-Regional em Cirurgia Estética (Loco-regional anesthesia on aesthetic surgery). Editora Hipócrates—Brazil, São Paulo

Avelar JM (1993b) Mastoplastia redutora sob anestesia local (Reduction mastoplasty under local anesthesia). In: Avelar JM (ed) Anestesia Loco-regional em cirurgia estética—(Loco-regional anesthesia on aesthetic surgery). Editora Hipócrates, São Paulo, pp 244–260

Avelar JM, Catunda MM (1985) Anestesia local na cirurgia do contorno corporal (Local anesthesia on body contour surgery). Anais do XII Congresso Brasileiro de Cirurgia Plástica (Annals of the XII Brazilian Congress of Plastic Surgery)—Gramado, RS—Brazil—Novembro, pp 415–416

Gillies H, McIndoe AH (1939) The technique of mammaplasty in conditions of hypertrophy of the breast. Surg Gynecol Obstet 72(68):658

Gillies H, Millard R Jr (1957) The principle and art of plastic surgery. Little Brown, Boston

Huang TT, Parks DH, Lewis SR (1979) Outpatient breast surgery under intercostal block anesthesia. Plast Reconstr Surg 63(3):299–303

Pitanguy I (1961) Aproximação eclética ao problema das mamaplastias (An eclectic approach to breast problems). Rev Bras Cir 41:179–196

Pitanguy I (1975) Abdominal lipectomy. Clin Plast Surg 3:401–410

Pitanguy I (1981) The breast. In: Aesthetic plastic surgery of head and body. Springer-Verlag, Berlin. pp 3–62

Pitanguy I, Garcia LC (1972) Aspectos importantes de técnica pessoal em mamaplastia (Important aspects of personal technique on mastoplasty). Soc Cir Plast Reconstr. sumário, Córdoba, Argentina

Pitanguy I, Cansação Á, Ramos H, Araújo M (1971) Mamaplastias. Estudo comparativo da evolução técnica em torno de 1196 casos pessoais (Mammaplasties comparative study of the technique evolution around 1196 personal cases) Rev Bras Cirurgia Nov/dez: 227–236

Pitanguy I et al (1977) Cirurgias Estéticas Combinadas (Combined aesthetic surgeries). Rev Bras Cir 67(7/8): 265–272

Reis Junior A (2006) The first to use surgical anesthesia was not a dentist, but the physician Crawford Williamson Long. Rev Bras Anestesiol 56(3):304–324

History of Breast Reduction

6

Ramil Sinder

The history of mammaplasty has been reported for several centuries , but there are few reports; therefore, it deserves careful study to understand the value of the surgeons who worked in adverse surgical conditions. Currently, breast reduction is a very frequent intervention in our country, but not in other countries. Numerous authors with their publications and papers presented at conferences and scientific meetings attest to its great importance. Surgery should be performed safely to reduce or even avoid complications that may be harmful to patients and surgeons. Mammaplasty aims to produce a breast with natural, proportional volumes and minimal scars and challenges the creative ability of the surgeons devoted to it and that seems to have no limits. There is no doubt that it is a constant challenge to the plastic surgeon and consists of a set of techniques or a combination of surgical maneuvers that enriches the medical literature. Among them, we can mention some that have become classic, such as the skin incision marked in a W shape; peri-areolar de-epithelialization or Schwarzmann's maneuver; the longitudinal fusiform infra-areolar incision, oblique and/or transverse; undermining and incisions of the adipose–glandular tissue at the base of the breast; the use of various types of areolar and de-epithelialized flaps with proximal, distal pedicle, and superomedial and superolateral to transpose the nipple–areola complex (NAC).

The purpose of this chapter is to report the contributions of a large number of highly qualified professionals who are interested in this surgery. However, just to remind us of the extensive existing literature, we reviewed numerous publications presented below in chronological order. It is not a complete list, because the goal is not to exhaust the subject. We apologize if equally as significant or more important works are not mentioned.

625–690 AD—**Paul of Aegina (Sinder 2003).** According to Letterman and Schurter (1974), the first description of breast reduction was written by Paul of Aegina, or Paulus Aegineta, for the surgical correction of gynecomastia with tissue resection of the excess of tissue at the level of the inframammary crease.

1556—**Paulus.** *Medicinae Totius Enchirifion Septem Libris Universam Recte Mectendi Rationem Comnpectus*.

1669—**Durston**. According to Letterman and Schurter (1974), Durston made a 7-cm length incision for the application of caustic, in a patient with hypertrophic breasts. After the death of this patient, he resected her left breast for examination, which may have generated the hypothesis that he was the first surgeon to carry out a partial amputation of the breast.

R. Sinder, M.D.
Member of the Brazilian Society of Plastic Surgery,
Av. Rui Barbosa, 532 Apto. 1501—Flamengo,
Rio de Janeiro, RJ CEP 22250-020, Brazil
e-mail: ramilsinder@hotmail.com

J.M. Avelar (ed.), *Breast Surgery*, https://doi.org/10.1007/978-3-319-54115-0_6

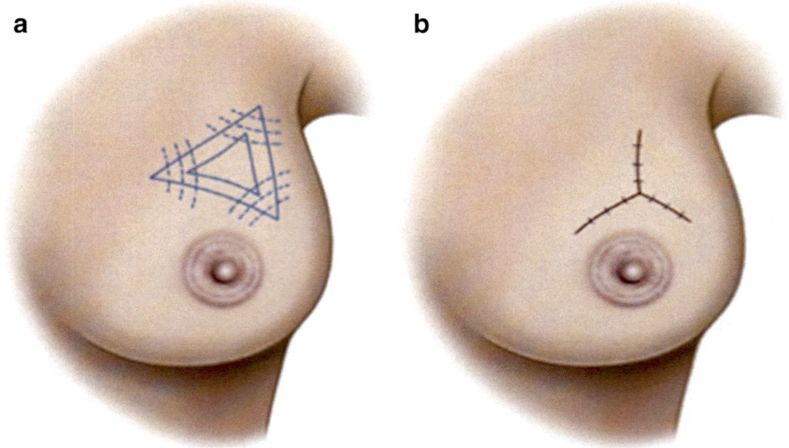

Fig. 6.1 Verchêre—1898

1669—**Durston.** Concerning a very sudden and excessive swelling of a woman's breast.

1847—**Paulus.** The seven books of Paulus A. Translated from the Greek by Francis Adams, London Sydenham Society.

1848—**Dieffenbach. R**eported that he had been performing breast reduction by making an incision in the inframammary crease.

1852—**Paul.** Total absence of the left mammary gland.

1854—**Velpeau.** Published work about breast disease in which he also addressed the problem of breast ptosis.

1882—**Gaillard and Thomas.** A surgeon from New York, who described an incision at the inframammary crease level used for excision of benign tumors and through which the breast was raised, fixing it in the cartilage of the second rib.

1886—**Hutchinson.** Congenital absence of hair and mammary glands.

1888—**Batchelor.** Absence of mammae in a woman.

1891—**Williams.** Polymastia with special reference to mammae erraticae and development of neoplasms for supernumerary mammary structures.

1893—**Basch and Thorek.** Undertook combined mammoplasty surgery with the abdominal wall.

1895—**Czerny.** Reconstituted with a lipoma removed from the thigh of a patient a breast that had undergone excision of a benign tumor.

1897—**Michel and Pousson.** Described a technique consisting in a semi-conic excision of the proximal part of the breast, through two concave incisions, from the skin to the aponeurosis, of the chest, which was fixed to the breast using catgut.

1898—**Verchêre.** Performed triangular excision on the superolateral aspect of the breast, including skin, fat layer, and mammary gland (Fig. 6.1).

1903—**Morestin.** Described removing a small benign breast tumor by making an incision at the level of the axilla. Some believe that in 1909, Morestin had already used the grafting technique between the papilla and areola.

1903—**Guinard.** Presented a technique that consisted in the conical excision of adipose and glandular tissue of the dorsum of the breast, with aponeurosis of the pectoralis major muscle, using a semicircular incision at the level of the inframammary crease.

1907a, b—**Morestin.** Reported the excision technique used since 1905 that is similar to a shaped disk of the dorsal part of the mammary gland with the aponeurosis of the pectoralis major muscle through an incision at the level of the inframammary crease. Because of its resemblance to the Guinard's technique, Joseph called this type of surgery Morestin-Guinard's technique (Fig. 6.2).

1907—**Hubert.** Published *Etude sur l'amastic. Thèse pour le doctorate médecine.*

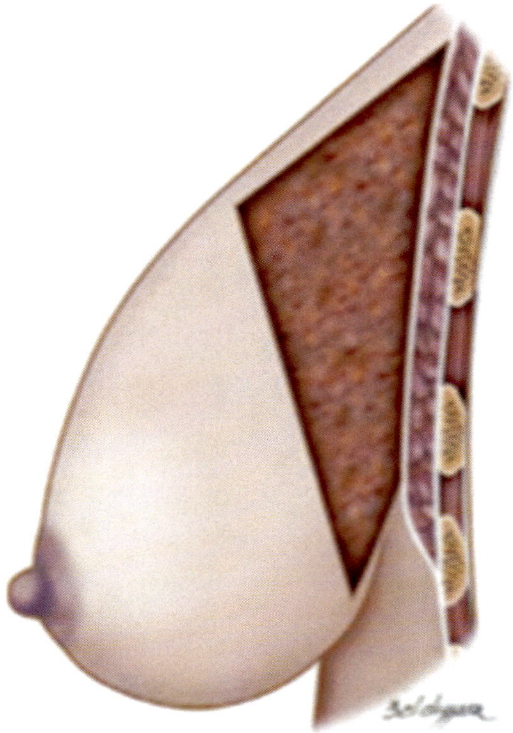

Fig. 6.2 Morestin and Guinard—1907

1907—**Warren.** Presented radial resection of the gland in relation to the papillary wedge from the chest to the aponeurosis to subcutaneous tissue, followed by fixation of the gland to the pectoralis fascia. He used this technique for excision of benign tumors with access via the inframammary crease.

1908—**Dehner.** Described the technique that consists of fusiform excision of the proximal part of the breast and its fixation on the periosteum of the third rib.

1910—**Girard.** Described surgery identical to that of Guinard, but added fixation of the breast to the cartilage of the second rib.

1911—**Villandre (Sinder 2003).** Reported mammoplasty with transposition of the nipple and areola by a cutaneous opening consisting in the original location of these elements.

1912—**Lexer.** In addition to the transposition of the nipple and areola, reduction of the breast was performed reduction, excising tissue from the distal pole, without skin undermining. He left peri- and infra-areolar scars shaped like an inverted T, with the transverse line at the level of the inframammary crease. From the historical point of view, perhaps this is the most important breast reduction technique, being the precursor of modern mammaplasties, which differ mainly by not performing Schwarzmann's maneuver. According to Maliniac and Thomas Rees, Lexer also carried out partial excision of the breast with grafting of the nipple and areola (Fig. 6.3).

1912—**Holländer.** Published a book about cosmetic surgery.

1913—**Simpson.** Published a case of amastia.

1914—**Göbell.** Described the suspension of the breast using fascia lata strips attached to the third rib.

1916—**Dufourmentel.** Described transposition of the nipple and areola similar to Villandre's technique.

1916—**Kausch.** Performed excisions similar to a ring around the areola. He reported extensive necrosis in the left breast operated on in one stage. He operated on the right breast in two stages, without necrosis.

1917—**Deaver, McFarland.** *The breast: its anomalies, its diseases, and their treatment.*

1923—**Aubert.** Performed skin incisions with resection of rings of skin around the areola to reduce its size. Incision supra-areola with small inverted V in the center and the edges on the side limits and the medial inframammary crease. Undermining and excision of skin between this incision and the inframammary crease (except the nipple and areola). Excision of the glandular tissue on the distal base and suture of the gland, giving the conical shape. Transposition of the nipple and areola and suturing of the skin. The final peri-areolar and infra-areolar scar was shaped like an inverted T.

1923—**Passot (Sinder 2003).** Performed a half-moon excision of the skin with nipple–areolar transposition similar to Villandre's technique.

1923—**Kraske.** Described and disclosed Lexer's technique, as he was trained by him, and it became known as Lexer–Kraske's technique.

1923—**Lotsch.** Made circular incisions around the areola and vertical fusiform excision

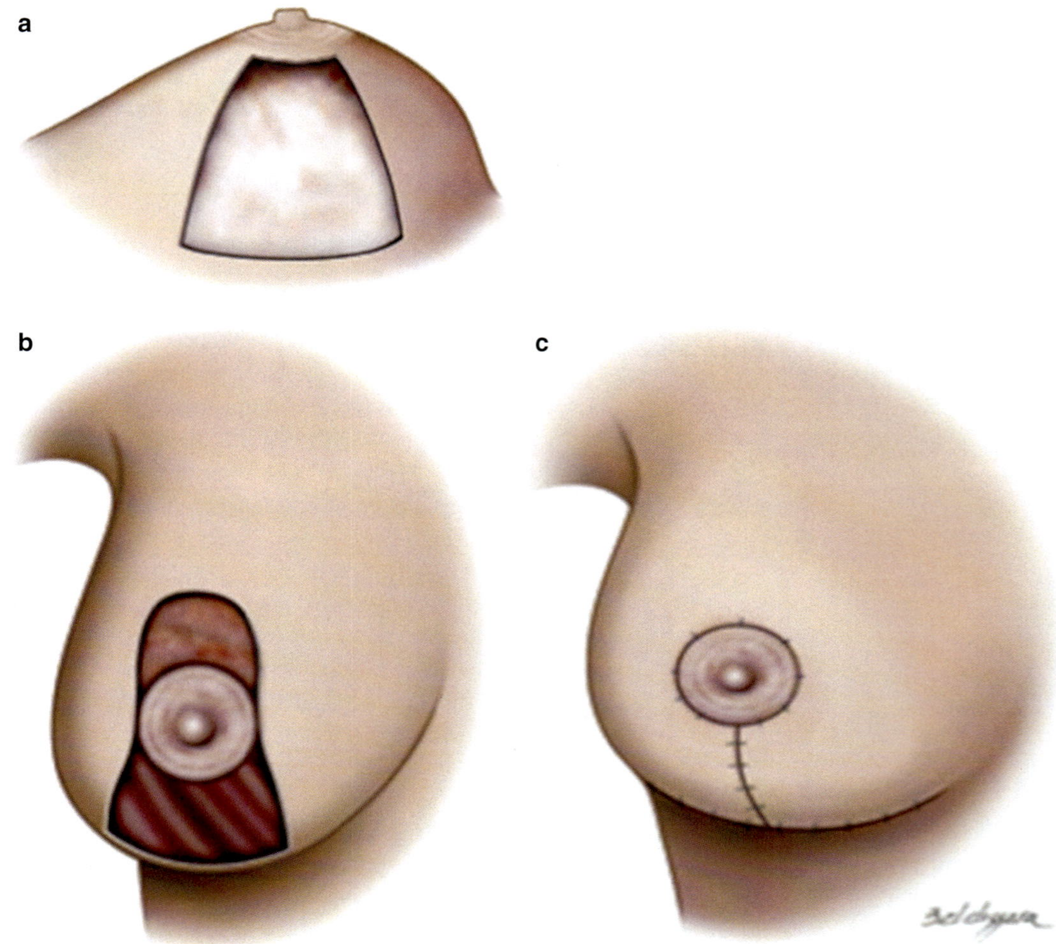

Fig. 6.3 Lexer—1912

between the areola and the inframammary crease. Also, the nipple and areola were transposed into their new positions, by making a circular skin excision. The final scars were peri-areolar and vertical infra-areolar.

1924—**Holländer.** Performed excision of the inferolateral part of the breast to the fascia of the pectoralis major and resection of the supra-areolar skin. Suturing by planes, leaving L or J-shaped scars or point with an oblique branch of the areola to the inframammary crease and another branch at the level of this inferolateral groove (Fig. 6.4).

1924—**Dartigues.** Described suspension and mastopexy techniques via the axilla.

1925—**Dufourmentel.** Performed transposition of the NAC and distal excision of excess tissue, similar to Villandre's and Passot's techniques.

1925—**Joseph.** Published his mammoplasty method in two phases, which has been used since 1922. Transplantation of the NAC through a pedicle flap with the distal level of the inframammary crease and excisions in the distal pole of the breast. In a second operation, about 1 month later, excision of the pedicle of the flap of the areola and final revision of scars.

1925—**Passot**. Performed aesthetic correction of the ptotic breast through transposition of the nipple.

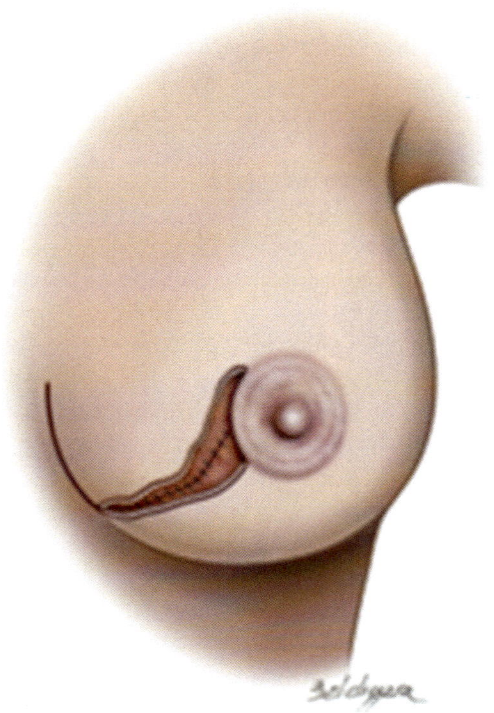

Fig. 6.4 Holländer—1924

1925—**Adair and Bagg.** Reported breast stasis to be the cause of mammary cancer.

1926—**Axhausen.** Performed peri-areolar resection of the skin through a ring and above this, made a curved incision with proximal concavity and almost complete undermining of the skin. Also, he carried out excision of the excess skin between the supra-areolar incision and the inframammary crease, and transposition of the NAC. Finally, he sutured the peri-areolar skin and inframammary crease.

1926—**Mornard.** Performed peri-areolar skin excision and on the inframammary crease, and detachment of the skin and partial excision of the gland wedge-shaped or infra-areolar "keel". He also carried out vertical and longitudinal suturing of the gland with transposition of the NAC, Followed by excision of excess skin and peri-areolar cutaneous and inframammary crease suturing.

1926—**De Quervain (Sinder 2003).** Performed skin incision just above the inframammary crease and detachment of the skin, together with excision of the peripheral gland, leaving the central part that remains attached to NAC. He also carried out gland fixation to the pectoralis fascia and cutaneous suturing on the inframammary crease.

1926—**Küster no. 1. (Sinder 2003).** Performed partial excision of the breast, with half-moon or lateral concavity.

1926—**Küster no. 2. (Sinder R. 2003).** Performed partial excision of the breast with a half-moon shaped approach with proximal concavity.

1926—**Weinhold.** Performed semicircular excisions above and below the NAC.

1927—**Cesari.** Performed breast surgery in ptotic breasts.

1928—**Joseph.** Described his mastopexy technique or suspension of the breast using the axillary method, that is, supra-areolar excision using an inverted U-shaped incision with suturing of the areola in the proximal-most position. Vertical incision was made at the level of the anterior axillary line and the breast lifted, making two "dog ears," which were excised and sutured by a "z-plasty."

1928—**Noël a.** Performed skin resection using half-moon incisions on the supra-areolar area two or three times until the desired position of the areola was achieved. Sometimes, infra-areolar excisions were also made to distribute the scar around the areola in a regular fashion.

1928—**Noël b** Circular skin excisions were made up to the NAC to achieve the desired position. Straight skin incisions were made to join the peri-areolar circular incision to another one on the inframammary crease. Skin was detached to provide resection of the distal part of the mammary gland and transposition of the NAC. Forceps were used to evaluate the amount of excess skin on the vertical segment to be removed. After the infra-areolar vertical suturing was done, the excess skin on the submammary crease was removed and the final scar was an inverted T (Fig. 6.5).

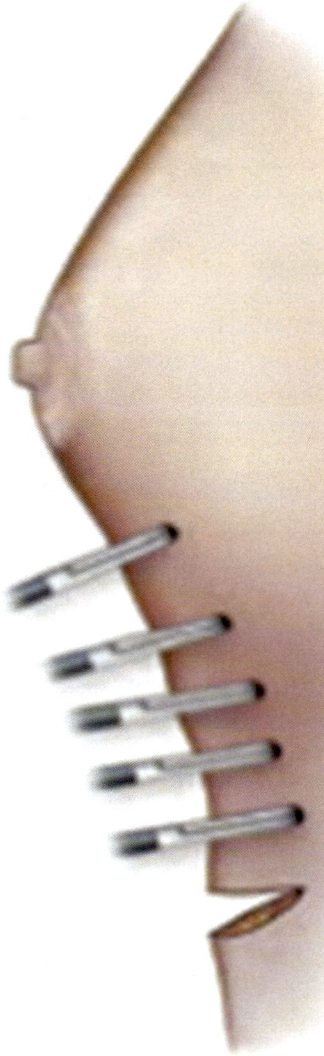

Fig. 6.5 Nöel—1928

1928—**Cesari, de Bolonha (Sinder R. 2003).** Checking the difference in length between the two half-moon incisions performed by Noël's first technique, he removed small triangles on the proximal segment of the wound to make it easy to suture.

1928—**Dartigues**. Performed vertical skin incision on the infra-areolar segment after detachment of the skin. Excision of excess fat and glandular tissues of the distal portion of the breast was carried out. With the use of a curved intestinal clamp, he demarcated the excess skin to be removed combined with fixation of the glandular tissue to the fascia of the pectoralis major muscle. He also made partial excision of the breast and nipple–areola graft using a special instrument to delimit the circular incision on the areola. In some cases, intra-areolar excisions were carried out without peri-areolar incision.

1928—**Lotsch no. 2**. Described his infra-areolar method using an anchor-shaped incision to undermine the skin to resect the excess adipose and glandular tissues and suture the skin leaving an inverted T scar.

1928—**Biesenberger**. Performed skin excision of the areola using a ring-shaped incision to reduce the diameter of the areola. Curve incision was done from the areola to the inframammary crease followed by wide detachment of the skin. Excision through an S-shaped incision of the lateral and distal portions of the gland and adipose tissue was carried out. Rotation in the lateral and cranial direction of the remaining glandular tissue (with the nipple and areola) and its fixation with simple stitches, giving the breast a conical shape. Delimitation and excision of excess skin (vertical and horizontal) with suturing of the skin leaving at the end a peri-areolar and inverted T.

1928—**Dufourmentel L.** Performed an areolar incision for breast surgery.

1929—**Virengue (Sinder 2003).** He published a book *Le Sein* (*The breast*) on cosmetic breast surgery in which he described a technique similar to Thorek's (reduction mammoplasty with graft of the nipple and areola). He used local anesthesia with adrenaline and placed drains that were removed on the third or fourth day after surgery. He used to perform surgery in one go in cases of ptosis and moderate hypertrophy, and a two-stage operation for gigantomastia that he called "localized or generalized fat degeneration."

1929—**Schreiber (Sinder 2003).** Performed mammoplasty in two stages: in the first, a skin excision was made through an inverted U-shaped incision between the areola and its future position; also, with partial resection of the supra-areolar gland and fixing to the fascia of the pectoralis major. In the second stage, he performed excision of the skin on the vertical segment between the areola and the submammary

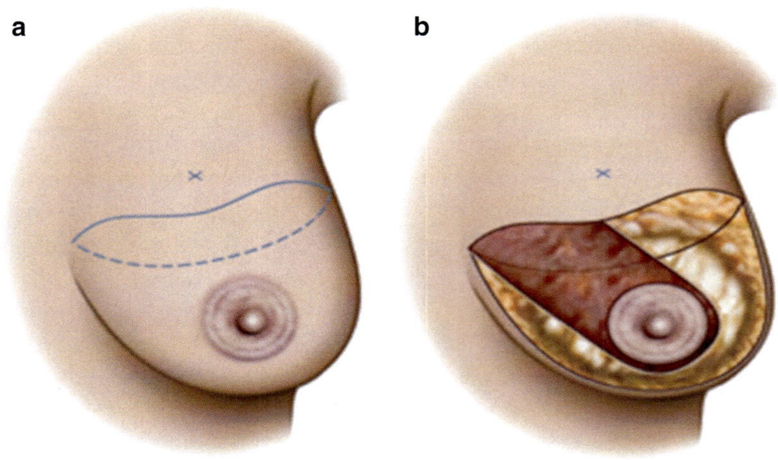

Fig. 6.6 Schwarzmann —1930

fold; glandular resection was carried out, forming a wedge below the areola with the vertical suturing of the gland and the final scar was an inverted T on the infra-areolar area.

1930—**Schwarzmann**. Resected the distal and lateral parts of the breast and the NAC was transposed by a de-epithelialized dermal–adipose–glandular flap with a superior and medial pedicle. The peri-areolar de-epithelialized procedure became a classic one and bears his name, Schwarzmann's maneuver (Fig. 6.6).

1930—**Glässmer.** Performed skin resection just above the areola and lateral transposition of the nipple and areola. The final scar was transverse, lateral, proximal and peri-areolar.

1931—**Kurtzahn.** Performed vertical mammoplasty: detachment and skin excision around and below the areola in a J-, comma- or L-shaped scar.

1931—**Passot.** Published a book: *La chirurgie esthétique pure* (*Pure cosmetic surgery*).

1931—**Lexer.** Published a book: *Die gesamte Wiederherstellung Chirurgie* (*The entire reconstructive surgery*).

1932—**Eitner.** Employed two techniques: first, to correct small breast ptosis in one go (skin excision above the areola in the inverted U-shaped incision and transposition of the nipple and areola). The second in two stages for gigantomastia correction. The first stage of the second technique consisted of a supra-areolar incision, undermining of the skin, a wedge resection of the superomedial part of the gland and fixation to the fascia of the pectoralis major muscle; supra-areolar excision of excess skin, and transposition of the papilla and areola. In the second stage, he made a wedge-shaped excision of the breast of the distal portion and vertical sub-areolar suture. It is mentioned that in 1935, he used to perform breast reduction using peri-areolar incision.

1933—**Nissen (Sinder 2003).** Mastoplasty was performed in two stages. In the first stage: a peri-areolar and transverse incision on each side of the areola; cutaneous detachment; wedge-shaped glandular excision in the superomedial area of the breast; and transposition of the nipple and areola. In the second stage (15 days later): excision of the distal part of the breast; suturing at the level of the inframammary crease.

1935. **Ehrenfeld (Sinder 2003).** Drew a line around the base of the breast with the aid of an apparatus called a "*mastômetro*": a segment directed downward to determine the radius of the circumference of the base of the breast and was used to mark the new position of the papilla. Marking the excision of the excess tissue by means of two curved lines whose lateral and medial ends joined in the submammary fold, such that the distal curved line, as in the U shaped incision, to delimit a flap with an areolar and dorsal pedicle, whose excessive skin was used to transpose the papilla and areola.

1936—**Prudente.** Published a book (*Contribution to Study of Plastic of the Breast—Aesthetic Surgery Breast*) in which he described several types of flaps to cover large wounds resulting from mastectomies and various reduction mammaplasty techniques in one and two surgical stages, with scars in the inframammary crease, on the vertical and areola, leaving an inverted T-shaped scar. He employed vertical methods based on Kurtzahn's publication in 1931, with and without circumcision of the areola. In the method with an inverted T-shaped scar, which he considered the most complete, was a supra-areolar incision in the shape of a W opened with the medial branches and horizontal side, ending the incision at the level of the inframammary crease. He used a circular device, which he called "*haloniótomo*" to make the areolar incision.

1936—**Claqué I, Bernard.** They described about mammaplasty.

1938—**Nedkoff.** Marked the skin excisions by drawing a W above the areola with the medial and lateral branches slightly curved. Excision of all skin between this route and the inframammary crease (except for the NAC); adipose–glandular excision wedge-shaped distal base with transposition of the areola. Peri-areolar scar and inverted T-shaped scar.

1938—**Burian F.** Described his experience with mammaplasties

1939—**Claoué (Sinder 2003).** Published a book: *Breast Plastic Surgery* (*Plastique Mammaire*) in which he addressed several issues of mammoplasty and described in detail his personal technique and several surgeons such as Pousson, Dartigues, Noel, Glässmer, Guinard, Morestin, Girard, Dehner, Goebell, Aubert, Mornard, Dufourmentel, Villandre, Joseph, Hollander, Biesenberger, and Schwarzmann. Claoué developed a complex technique using multiple points, lines, and angles to measure the breast and chest on the horizontal, vertical, and oblique.

1939—**Gillies and McIndoe**. Elevated the operating table so that the patient stays in a semi-sitting position. The new position of the NAC was determined by the intersection of two circles with centers respectively at the sternal notch (15–19 cm in radius) and the base of the xiphoid process (such as 1.27 cm smaller radius than the former); with an interpapillary distance of approximately 23 cm. Schwarzmann's maneuver with bimanual stretching of the skin was performed. They used two methods to incise the skin and to resect any excess:

(1) Vertical incision above and infra-areolar, resulting in a final peri-areolar and infra-areolar inverted T-shaped scar.
(2) Transverse or horizontal supra-areolar incision, resulting in a final peri-areolar scar and the level of the inframammary crease. They carried out extensive skin displacement and used two methods of adipose–glandular excision: the Biesenberger technique, preserving the vascular superomedial pedicle; and a U-shaped incision above the areola and an infra-areolar, half-moon-shaped proximal concavity maintaining the two major vascular pedicles.

1942a**, b—Thorek.** Reported his technique of excision of the distal part of the breast and free graft of the nipple and areola he had already used some years before. According to Maliniac and Thomas Rees, this technique had already been used by Lexer (1912) and by Dartigues.

1942—**Nagel.** Verified histologically the presence of smooth muscle cells in the nipple graft, which would explain its contractility.

1942—**Prudente.** Worked on glandular regeneration in patients with chronic cystic fibrous mastopathy, undertaking partial amputation of the breast.

1943—**May.** Started surgery with the patient in the semi-sitting position. Peri-areolar incisions with Schwarzmann's maneuver. Also, he performed a straight supra-areolar incision up to the new position of the areola and infra-areola up to one third of the distance from the papilla to the inframammary crease, with wide skin undermining. After excision of the wedge-shaped gland and suturing, he then placed the patient in a horizontal position. Afterward, he re-adapted the skin on the gland as a brassiere, temporarily covering the breast. He then evaluated and excised the excess skin using forceps. The final scar was peri-areolar and infra-areolar like an inverted Y-shape.

1943—**Maliniac.** Concerned with important arterial blood supply of the breast.

1944—**Adams.** First author to mention the importance of the conical shape of the breast for marking of the NAC on the top.

1945—**Gillies.** Published personal analyses after plastic surgery of the breast.

1945a, b—**Maliniac.** *La mamaplastic en deux temps en report avec la vascularization.*

1945a, b—**Maliniac.** Published two-stage mammaplasty in relation to the blood supply.

1946—**Ragnell.** In breasts with flaccidity, ptotic breasts, or those with or without moderate hypertrophy, he performed mammoplasty in one stage: superficial skin peri-areolar resection with wide cutaneous undermining and glandular resection on a supra- and infra-areolar wedge-shape with suturing of the gland to the fascia of the pectoralis major muscle. The excess skin was resected and sutured, resulting in peri-areolar and infra-areolar scarring with an inverted T shape. In large hypertrophy, he performed mammoplasty in two stages. First, he carried out a large-scale detachment of the skin, a glandular excision above the areola with a wedge-shaped resection and suturing, resulting in peri-areolar scarring and on the inframammary crease. In the second stage, he made an incision in the inframammary crease and carried out skin detachment, glandular excision through a half-moon shape on the distal part as a wedge-shaped resection, and the excess skin was excised with suturing in the inframammary crease.

1946—**Thorek.** Published important considerations about breast reconstruction with free transplantation of the nipple.

1947—**Adams.** Performed a free compound graft of the nipple in mammoplasty.

1948—**Maliniac.** Carried out a comparative study of the amputation methods with nipple–areola grafting and transposition. He used to prefer the transposition method; however, in gigantomastia, he indicated amputation with a nipple–areola graft. He presented an important anatomical study of the vascularization of the breast, especially on the plexus supplying the NAC. He gave credit to Dartigues for the pioneering amputation method with the nipple–areola graft.

1948—**Viegas.** Published a case of amastia.

1949—**Adams.** First author to perform transplantation of the genital labia as a graft for nipple correction.

1949—**Aufricht.** Presented a geometric method of tracing incisions in breast surgery. He showed the relationship between the infra-areolar excision with a wedge-shape and the height of the mammary cone. Also, he reported the use of long temporary stitches on the skin of the sternal notch and at the level of the xyphoid process to transfer from one side to another of the symmetrical points of the skin marking. He performed glandular resection excisions above the areola, and, like most of the surgeons of that time, he used to carry out extensive skin detachment.

1949—**Bames.** After extensive skin detachment, he excised the inferolateral part and sometimes also inferomedial part of the gland and excess skin, and with transposition of the NAC. In patients with gigantomastia, however, he preferred amputation with a nipple–areola graft. His final scar was peri-areolar and infra-areolar with an inverted T shape.

1949a, b—**Maliniac.** Published an article about the indication for and basic care of mammaplasties. He preferred to carry out reduction mammaplasty with transposition of the NAC in one or two stages, according to the degree of hypertrophy. In gigantomastia, he performed a nipple–areolar graft. He stressed the advantages of glandular excision at the base of the breast close to the aponeurosis of the pectoralis major muscle by incision into the inframammary crease.

1949—**Harris.** Published a description of a peri-areolar mammaplasty.

1949a, b—**Maliniac.** Published an important evaluation of the surgical principles of mammaplasty.

1950—**Harris.** Presented valuable considerations of the status of plastic surgery of the breast.

1950a, b—**Maliniac.** Published the book *Breast Deformities and Their Repairs*. He has written numerous articles related to breast plastic surgery, such as a study of arterial vascularization in 1943; a critical analysis of mammectomy and nipple and areola graft in 1944; mammoplasty in two stages and breast vascularity in 1945; he also made a comparative study of transposition and nipple–areolar graft in mammoplasty in 1943; the evolution of the main techniques of mammoplasty in 1949; and the use of a de-epithelialized dermal-adipose flap in mammoplasty in 1953. In the latter technique, he resected the mammary gland and de-epithelialized the skin infra-areolar, forming a flap with the distal pedicle in the inframammary crease, which was used as "refilling" behind of the supra-areolar flap with a NAC graft. In 1959, he presented a paper on poor results in mammoplasty.

1950—**Hanrahan.** Performed wide detachment of the skin, with adipose–glandular excision supra-areolar, similar to a wedge shape with transposition of the NAC. On excising the excess skin, he used to leave a triangular flap with a distal base to the inframammary crease to decrease the tension at the union of the vertical and horizontal sutures.

1950—**Skoog.** Published a description of a new surgical instrument to be used in mammaplasty.

1950—**Spina.** Performed neo-areoloplasty with labial transplant.

1951—**Fernandez.** With a ruler placed between the breast and thorax, to mark the new location of the NAC to the level of the inframammary crease at the hemi-mammary line. He used to carry out bidigital clamping to evaluate the excess skin to be excised, similar to a lozenge-shape between the inframammary crease and this new position, with transposition of the NAC.

1951—**Tamerin.** Performed a wedge-shaped excision with its vertex at the center of the nipple and based on the inframammary crease, including a distal triangular flap of the nipple and areola. Excision of the two "dog ear," which were formed on each side of the base, resulting in a final scar with an inverted T shape.

1951—**Thale.** Presented a paper on the complications of mastoplasty, paying special attention to nipple–areolar necrosis and reconstruction with a small genital lip graft.

1951—**Malbec.** Published an important review of mammaplasty.

1952—**Conway.** Presented his experience in 110 consecutive cases of mammaplasty, 68 of which by amputation with nipple–areolar graft, which was the method of choice. He concluded that, in most cases, there was recovery of contractility and sensitivity of the NAC graft.

1952—**Gillet.** Suspension and support of the mammary gland through a network of nylon threads anchored in the collarbone.

1953—**Maliniac.** Published his technique on subcutaneous excision of the mammary gland and use of a dermal–adipose de-epithelialized flap with a distal pedicle at the level of the inframammary crease, used to "refill" the breast, with a NAC graft (Fig. 6.7).

1953—**Malbec (Sinder 2003).** Performed mammoplasty in two stages. He carried out the second stage about 45 days afterward. In the first

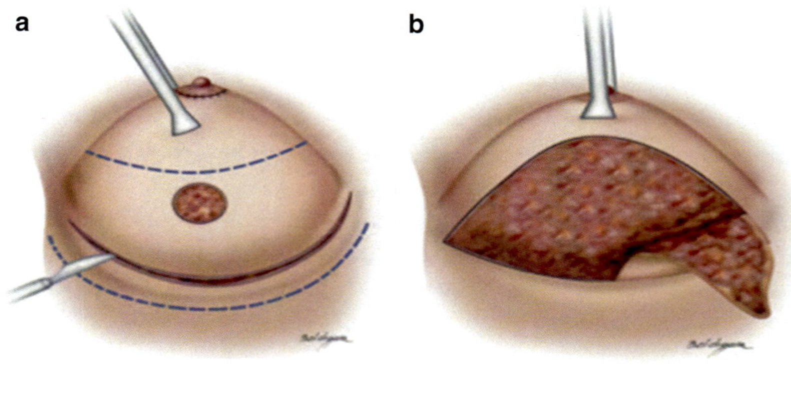

Fig. 6.7 Maliniac—1953

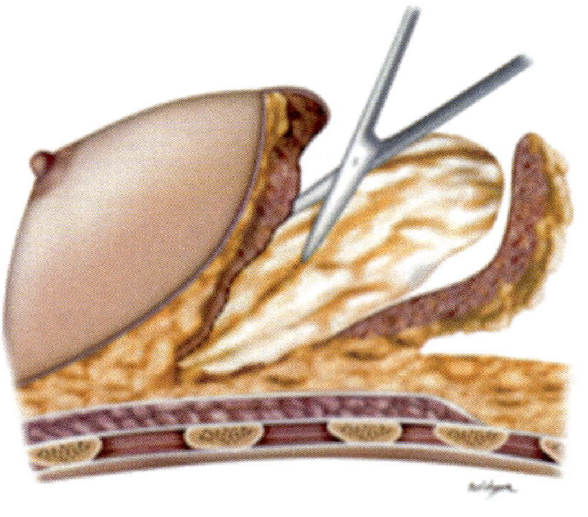

Fig. 6.8 Longacre—1954

stage, he excised a segment of the supra-areola and positioned the NAC. In the second stage, he dealt with excess of skin and modeling of the breast.

1953—**Gilliles, Marino.** Published "periwinkle shell" principles in the treatment of the small ptotic breast.

1954—**Longacre.** Presented a technique for the correction of hypoplastic breasts, utilizing a dermal-adipose de-epithelialized flap, with a half-moon shape, which was introduced under the gland to increase the volume of the breast. He carried out undermining of the dermal-adipose segment allowing a submammary skin advancement flap to close the donor area, resulting in a scar in the submammary crease (Fig. 6.8).

1955—**Erczy.** Performed mammoplasty in two stages, with a 6-week interval. In the first stage, he carried out extensive undermining of the skin with excision of the glandular tissue supra-areolar with suturing and fixation to the pectoralis major muscle, and transposition of the nipple and areola. In the second stage, he used to perform infra-areolar excision, including skin, fat, and glandular tissue, for modeling and final suturing peri-areolar and infra-areolar with an inverted T-shaped scar.

1955—**Jack Penn.** He published the technique called "Jack Penn #1": infra-areolar excision in a wedge-shape, with transposition of the nipple–areolar complex. He used to suture the infra-areolar and vertical wound to the inframammary crease, which decreased the distance from the areola to the submammary fold; the two "dog ears" were resected on the submammary fold. The final scars were peri-areolar and infra-areolar with an inverted T shape.

1955—**Ragnell.** Analyzed over a 1,000 cases operated on using the method of the proximal double vascular NAC pedicle, described in 1946: wide detachment of the skin, with adipose–glandular excision supra- and infra-areolar, modeling of the breast, with suturing of the skin. He used to carry out gigantomastia in two stages. Good lactation capacity was reported in most patients who became pregnant after surgery.

1955—**Guillera.** Published the book: *Breast Disease*.

1956—**Longacre.** Based on his technique published in 1954 for the treatment of hypoplastic breast, the author modified this, adapting it to flaccid and discoid breast correction, making a de-epithelialized dermal–adipose flap with a half-moon shape with a proximal infra-areolar pedicle. This flap was folded back and up with its lateral and medial extremities united behind and above the areola with the pectoralis major, projecting the NAC and improving the conical shape of the breast.

1956—**O'Connor and Watron (Sinder 2003).** Published a wide review of the mastoplasty techniques most frequently used in the previous 10 years and a summary of the care that was considered fundamental in these surgeries.

1956—**May.** He performed a wide detachment of the skin, adipose–glandular excision in the superolateral quadrant, skin rehabilitation with the help of a brassiere temporarily covering the papilla and areola, excision of the excess skin with the aid of forceps, leaving a lower triangular flap based on the inframammary crease and the top 2.5 cm from the center of the crease. In gigantomastia, he preferred amputation with a nipple and areolar graft.

1956—**Wise.** Published a mammoplasty technique employing a plastic ring to enclose the periphery of the base of the breast and latex molds to draw the skin incisions. Assessed resection with the aid of a model, also made of plastic.

The molds were based on the shape and volume of normal breasts and a good aesthetic standard.

1957—**Adams.** Performed a free transplant of the NAC in mammoplasty.

1957—**Marino, Uriburu.** Published the book: *The Breast*.

1957—**Ragnell.** Further experience of the preservation of the capacity for lactation and nipple sensitivity after breast reduction.

1957—**Arié.** Published a technique for the correction of hypertrophy and ptotic breast: Schwarzmann's maneuver, infra-areolar excision in a wedge-shape and transposition of the NAC. He did not perform any cutaneous undermining and obtained great dissemination and acceptance owing to the simplicity of the procedure. It represented an important contribution to modern mammoplasty, especially in Brazil.

1957—**Malbec.** Stressed the importance of suturing the mammary gland to the musculoaponeurotic plain because, in his view, the skin does not serve to support the breast, but merely to wrap it.

1957—**Gillies H, Millard Jr.** Published an remarkable book: *Principle and Art of Plastic Surgery*.

1957—**Malbec**. Described important aspects of mammaplasties.

1958—**Gillies and Marino.** In ptosis, small breasts underwent extensive skin detachment, rotating the side portion of the gland on the proximal portion so as to increase the volume of the cranial pole and readaptation of the skin. This technique, based on Biesenberger's method was called the periwinkle shell principle or the snail technique.

1958—**Marino.** Described important considerations regarding mammaplasties.

1958—**Conway, Smith.** Analyzed 245 cases for: reduction mammaplasty, mastopexy, augmentation mammaplasty, and mammary construction.

1958a, b—**Bames.** Described reduction mammaplasty performed in two operative stages.

1958a, b—**Bames.** Described breast reduction in major hypertrophy.

1958—**McIndoe and Rees.** Also used the technique that Biesenberger modified.

1958—**Malbec.** Reported on postoperative complications after mammaplasties.

1959—**Maliniac.** Presented important considerations: harmful fallacies in mammoplasty.

1959—**Pitanguy.** Presented an analysis of 120 cases of breast lift operated by several techniques, depending on the type of breast, giving preference to nipple–areola transposition methods. Underlines the good results obtained with Arié's technique, especially in small ptosis and hypertrophy, adding significant changes in surgical principles that gave a huge boost to reduction mammaplasty.

1960—**Strömbeck.** Planned the incisions on the skin with the aid of a mold similar to that described by Wise; Schwarzmann's maneuver; dermal–adipose–glandular excision infra-areolar and a supra-areolar cylinder to facilitate the transposition of the NAC, which has two pedicles: one superomedial and the other superolateral. The skin was not detached.

1960—**Penn.** Published breast reduction II.

1960—**Fomon**. Published: *Cosmetic Surgery. Principles and Practice*.

1961a, b—**Pitanguy.** Described his personal technique and important aspects of a study of 245 consecutives cases of mammaplasty (Fig. 6.9).

1961a, b—**Pitanguy.** Described an eclectic approach to the problems of mammaplasties.

1961—**Dufourmentel and Mouly**. Schwarzmann's maneuver; skin and fat–glandular excision in the laterodistal portion of the breast, resulting in peri-areolar and infra-areolar scarring, the latter angled, from the distal-most part of the areola to the lateral end of the inframammary crease.

1961a, b—**Pitanguy.** Presented a mammoplasty technique with dermal–adipose–glandular excision infra-areolar after Schwarzmann's maneuver, without undermining of the skin. The evaluation and marking of the portion to be excised were made individually on each breast of each patient and depended on several factors, such as volume, skin elasticity, and consistency

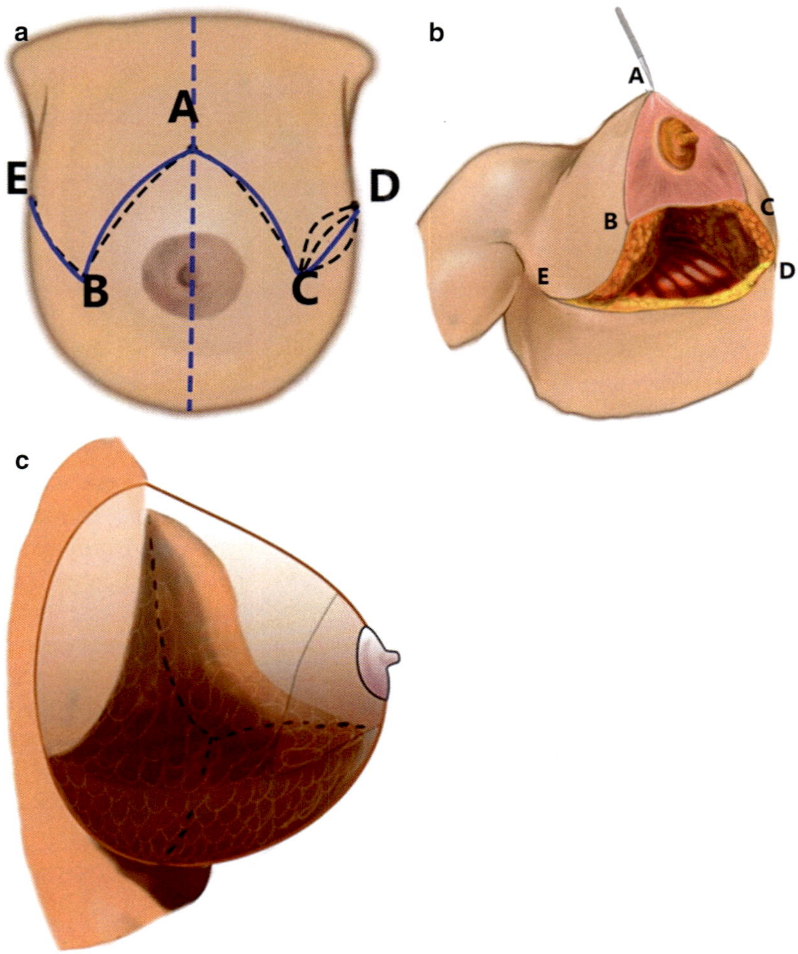

Fig. 6.9 Pitanguy—1961a, b

of the gland. The NAC was positioned in the apex of the cone obtained after mastopexy of the breast tissue. It had indications for various types of breast ptosis and hypertrophy and is one of the most frequently used techniques in recent years by many surgeons. Pitanguy was author of a book and several publications on mammaplasty. The details of his technique, with or without modification, have been the basis for numerous current methods of mammaplasty, in the endless pursuit of surgical improvement.

1962a, b—**Pitanguy.** Published a new technique for mammaplasty.

1962a, b—**Pitanguy.** Carried out an extensive histopathological study of the breast tissue removed during mammaplasties.

1963—**Cronin and Gerow.** Published augmentation mammaplasty: a new "natural feel" prosthesis.

1963—**Da Silva.** Presented a geometric method to make the planning of the incisions, using as a basic measure the distance from the papilla to the inframammary crease of a woman with normal breasts (8 cm). His method can be used with transposition of the nipple and areola or even for a nipple–areola graft.

1963—**Marino.** Made interesting comments on the new trends in breast reduction. He gave preference to techniques that respect the early embryological relationship between the coating skin and the glandular tissue, to avoid or reduce to a minimum of detachment of the skin and moreover, maintaining full vascularization of the NAC. Within these principles, he made special reference to Jack Penn's technique #1, in addition to Arié's, Strömbeck's, and Pitanguy's techniques, which resembled Lexer's technique, considering them safer. Also, Dufourmentel and Mouly's method, in which an inferolateral excision, reminiscent of Hollander's technique, was executed, made a great impression upon him.

1963—**Robertson.** Described mammoplasty by a dermal–adipose–glandular excision between two incisions: one above and one below the areola, both curves. The NAC was grafted. The skin suture was made around the areola and a horizontal line on each of its sides.

1963—**Skoog.** Presented a mammoplasty technique with transposition of the nipple and areola, through a de-epithelialized flap with a superolateral pedicle (Fig. 6.10).

1963—**Tamerin.** Stressed the importance of the technique used by Lexer in 1912 and published by Kraske in 1923—"Lexer—Kraske technique"—and he considers one of the best. Made suggestions and personal technical details for their implementation.

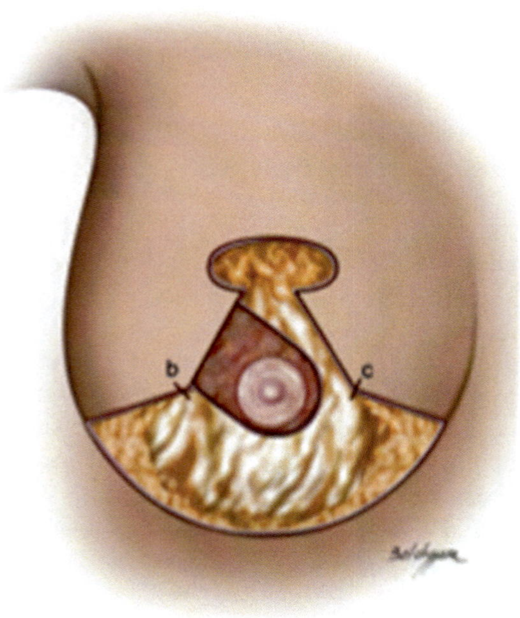

Fig. 6.10 Skoog—1963

1963a, b—**Pitanguy.** Contributed to the free graft technique for the correction of large breast hypertrophy.

1963a, b—**Pitanguy.** Contributed to the technique of mammaplasties.

1963—**Wise, Gannon, and Hill.** Reported good results with the technique presented by the senior author in 1956, performing transposition of the NAC. Basically, using the same technique, a pattern to trace the skin incisions, plastic rings to enclose the periphery of the base of the breast, which may also the graft NAC in gigantomastia, and studies related to the use of same technique in two stages in young patients.

1963—**Dufourmentel.** Performed mammaplasty using a lateral method.

1963—**Elbaz.** Published a useful thesis about the treatment of hypertrophic breast with or without ptosis using the "external oblique" method.

1964a, b—**Da Silva.** Presented mammoplasty technique of mastopexy: de- epithelialized skin to be spliced, which, in the form of a dermal tape, was used to lift the breast, fixing it to the pectoralis major muscle.

1964a, b—**Strömbeck.** Performed mammaplasty in hypertrophy of the female breast.

1964a, b—**Strömbeck.** Performed reduction mammaplasty. *Modern Trends in Plastic Surgery*.

1964—**Crickelair, Richey, Symonds.** Carried out histological studies of the female breast before and after nipple transplant.

1965—**Farina.** Published an article: *Plastic and Reconstructive Surgery*.

1965—**Dufourmentel, Mouly.** Developed the latero-oblique method.

1966—**Zilbsky.** Published a mammoplasty technique for cases of benign disorders such as cystic mastitis and fibroadenomas. In a first stage, a gland excision was carried out using the modified Strömbeck technique, leaving a supra-areolar vertical pedicle of denuded skin, so that the NAC had three pedicles, one at the top and two on the sides; infra-areolar skin was denuded, also forming a bifurcated flap based on the infra-mammary crease, as in the Longacre technique for discoid breast, in that the ends were sutured behind the NAC to serve as fullness. In a second stage, silicone inclusion was performed.

1966a, b, c—**Pitanguy.** Published a new approach: transareolar incision for gynecomastia.

1966a, b, c—**Pitanguy.** Made a critical study of his personal technique for breast hypertrophy.

1966—**Pitanguy, Franco.** Published on the agenesis of the pectoral muscle associated with deformity of the hand (syndactyly and ectrodactyly).

1966—**Dufourmentel, Mouly.** Performed mammaplasty using the lateral method: reconstructive surgery of thermal injuries and other subjects.

1967—**Clarkson and Jeffs.** Carried out a study on various methods of mammoplasty, stressing the mainly good results obtained with use of the Strömbeck technique, which was considered to be among the best for correction of breast hypertrophy. In cases of gigantomastia he prefers amputation with a graft of the NAC.

1967—**Beare.** Performed reduction mammaplasty.

1967—**Pitanguy, Franco.** Reported on hypomastia and its surgical treatment.

1967—**Pitanguy.** Reported on surgical treatment of breast hypertrophy.

1967—**Kohn.** Performed cross-excision of the skin and adipose tissue in the glandular form of two trapezoids, one on each side of the areola, with the smaller base adjacent to it. The skin of the distal part of the breast was completely denuded, forming a dermal–adipose–glandular flap composed of a posterodistal pedicle with the NAC at its proximal end. The de-epithelialized flap was covered by the above-mentioned areolar flap, which was a circular opening to receive the NAC. The surgery results in a peri-areolar and submammary scar, as in Passot's technique.

1967—**Burian.** Performed a de-epithelialized dermal–adipose flap in a half-moon proximal concavity whose cranial margin corresponded to the inframammary crease; its central part, not removed, was the posterosuperior pedicle. He raised the medial and lateral parts and fixed them to the fascia of the pectoralis major muscle behind the gland, increasing the volume of the breast. Skin and subcutaneous adipose tissue distal to this flap were hipsters and advanced by sliding to close the donor area, which created fullness for the retro-areolar defect, improving or restoring the conical shape of the breast and designing the NAC. Some believe that Burian had used this technique since 1931.

1967—**Mathews.** Published a technique in which the planning of skin incisions and the volume to be excised was based on a path that takes into account not only fixed points, such as the sternal notch, xiphoid process, and midclavicular line, but also skin elasticity, the volume and the consistency of the breast. Excision was made after extensive skin detachment, achieving a NAC with two proximal pedicles, as in techniques already published by Gilles and Mclndoe in 1939 Maliniac in 1945 and Ragnell in 1946.

1967—**Pesková.** Presented a technique in which a NAC graft was made after gland excision of the skin and fat; scarification of the ends of two sub-areal flaps with a proximal pedicle and a circle in the new position of the areola to receive the NAC graft. The denuded portion of the sub-areal flaps was used as the "stuffing" of the breast.

1967—**Robertson.** Performed the inferior flap mammaplasty technique.

1968—**Dufourmentel and Mouly.** Used a breast ptosis correction technique based on the method proposed by Barnes in 1950: spin the inferolateral part of the gland upward and inward, also called *operation colimaçon* in French and in English periwinkle shell based on Biesenberger's technique. Among other changes, minimal detachment of the skin was made, the inferolateral part of the gland was introduced behind its proximal part, and the lower skin of the breast inferolateral was excised, so that the resulting scar directed the areola downward and out, like an L, a J, or a comma.

1968—**Berry.** Carried out geometric planning in reduction mammaplasty.

1968—**Rees, Dupeurs.** Treated unilateral mammary hypoplasia.

1968—**Myr y Myr.** Presented a study on breast lift, stressing the causes of poor results in the late postoperative period. Complaints, in most cases, were caused by the rise of the NAC with an increase in the distal pole of the breast as if it executed one folding movement; loss of the single cone shape of the breast, and asymmetries and extended medial or hypertrophic scars. He usually used Biesenberger's technique modified by McIndoe; however, instead of the infra-areolar inverted T-shaped scar, a side concave curve leaves scarring in a U or J shape.

1968—**Pastoriza.** Made an extensive comparative study of various mammoplasty techniques, taking into account the innervation and vascularization of the NAC, the shape and volume obtained after breast reduction, the resultant scars, and other factors. It was concluded that the maintenance of the results was conditioned by an appropriate reduction in the volume and sufficient excision of the skin, which should be sutured without undue stress; decreasing the function of the skin as breast support was advised, preferably using de-epithelialized skin flaps.

1969—**Mendes Filho and Lodovici.** In breast hypertrophy, removal of the gland as completely as possible was considered important. To create fullness in place of the gland, de-epithelialized skin flaps from the distal part of the breast were used, as in the technique published by Maliniac, 1953.

1969—**Goulian Jr, Gonway.** Reported correction of the moderate ptotic breast.

1969—**Lassus.** Mentioned the possibilities and limitations of plastic surgery on female silhouette.

1969—**Hoopes, Jabaley.** Made a comparison between reduction mammaplasty: amputation and augmentation.

1969 **and** 1972—**Hinderer.** Proposed in small ptotic and tubular breasts to excise one peri-areolar skin ring off the pectoral fascia in the distal part of the gland and make plication of the dermis and the gland below the areola.

1970—**Ramil Sinder.** Presented at the former National School of Medicine, at the current Federal University of Rio de Janeiro (UFRJ), a thesis on mammoplasty in which, in addition to a comprehensive literature review, he described how they treated medium and large hypertrophy. Usually, he used Pitanguy's modified technique. In large hypertrophies or gigantomastia, he carried out a true "emptying" of the fatty glandular breast, leaving the NAC at the distal end of a broad and thin de-epithelialized skin–fat flap of the proximal pedicle, in which a vertical supero-areolar incision was then made to transpose the NAC, in which it doubles over itself twice, first back and up and then back and down. Also, he made the flap behind and above the areola, with aponeurosis of the pectoralis major muscle, to provide more projection to the NAC. To join the vertical suture with the horizontal he used a triangular flap with a pedicle in the inframammary crease, resulting in a Y-shaped scar on the infra-areolar segment.

From 1972, he began to use a trapezoidal de-epithelialized flap based on the inframammary crease, whose height was identical to that from the groove to the areola after removal of excess tissue. Also, during the suturing of mammary tissue this flap was placed under the skin between the areola and the submammary groove. He inserted some stitches into the vertical infra-areolar skin and on the distal peri-areolar transfixing the dermal side and the proximal end of the flap respectively, leaving the distal pole of the breast supported by a subcutaneous dermal enhancement at the level of the anchor-shaped scar or inverted T-shaped scar. He performed that maneuver to decrease or to avoid flattening of the proximal segment and the distal pole bulging or folding movement, which may occur in the post-operative period. This flap was identical to the suprapubic one used in abdominoplasty described by the author, in which the surgery begins with an incision and undermining of the supraumbilical flap, followed by distal traction to assess the extent of infra-umbilical resection. From 1980, he began to use a similar flap in breast reconstruction with a myocutaneous transverse rectus abdominalis (TRAM) flap. From that year, when there was some difficulty in performing transposition of the NAC, the lateral portion of the supra-areolar flap became separated from the areola, as in the disclosure by Schwarzmann's maneuver (1930). A similar approach has been reported by Orlando and Guthrie (1975); Silveira Neto (1976), and Haben (1984), making it easier and safer to position the NAC by rotation of the superomedial flap. It was also possible to use the superolateral flap similar to that described by Skoog. If, despite the above-mentioned maneuvers, ischemia and/or cyanosis of the NAC were found, this was carefully excised and used as a graft.

1970—**Craig, Skyes.** Investigated nipple sensitivity following reduction mammaplasty.

1970—**Sinder.** Thesis on mammaplasty presented and approved for Associate Professor at the former National Medical School (Faculdade Nacional de Medicina), the current Federal University of Rio de Janeiro (UFRJ).

1970—**Felix, Sethi, Ransdel, and Lissner.** Published a modification of Strömbeck's technique in which, instead of making transposing the NAC, they grafted it.

1970—**Arufe and Juri.** Presented modification of Strömbeck's technique. Instead of excising a cylinder or a cone of dermal–adipose–glandular supra-areolar tissue, they leave it fixed by its pedicle on depth. When they performed transposition of the NAC, the cylinder or cone was positioned behind the nipple and areola, to improve its projection and the conical shape of the breast. At the end of surgery, the distance from the areola to the inframammary crease should be about 4 cm. If it was greater, it was necessary to carry out deepithelialization of the distal end of the flap, so that, when approximated in the areola, the vertical scar between them was 4 cm in length.

1970—**Souza.** Performed a wide review of techniques that employ supra-areolar incisions. He advised this type of approach in cases of ptosis in small breasts.

1971—**Pitanguy.** Described his personal technique for hypertrophic breast in a clinical study.

1971—**Goulian.** Published a technique for the correction of ptotic breasts.

1971—**Ress.** Reported an historical review of reduction mammaplasty.

1971—**Fisher, Smith.** Presented work on macromastia during puberty.

1971a, b—**Franco.** Published work on the heterotopic conservation of the nipple–areola segment for later implantation.

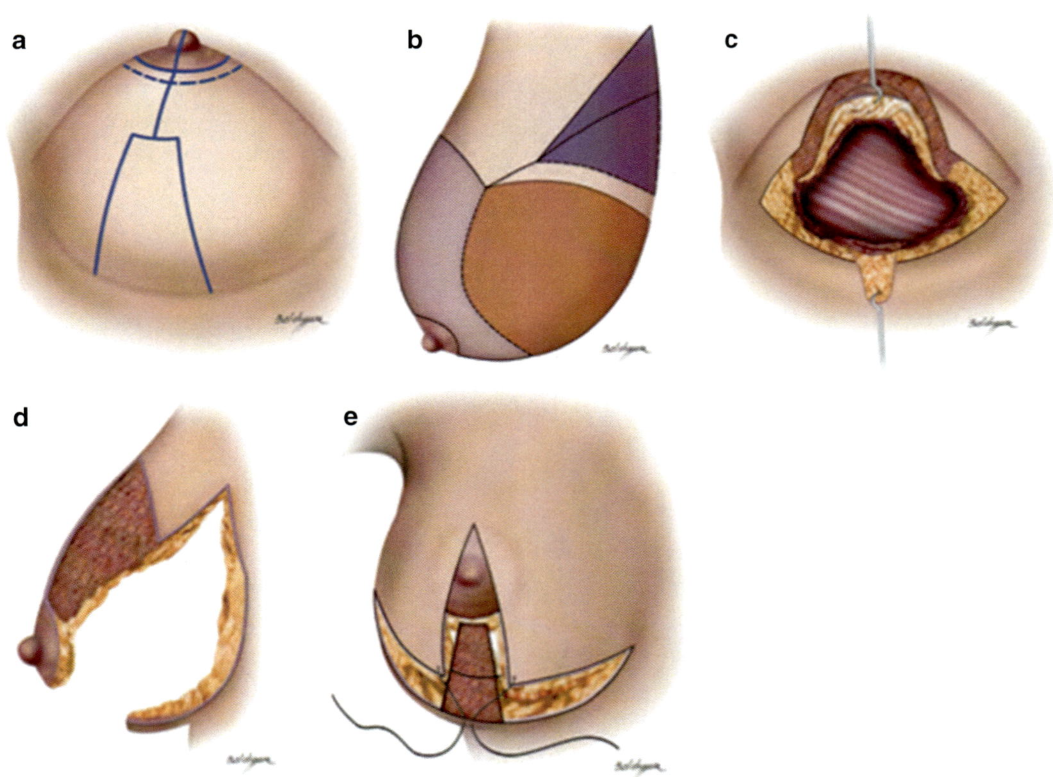

Fig. 6.11 Sinder—1972

1971—**Ship.** Described virginal and gravid mammary gigantism.

1972—**Ramil Sinder.** Presented a technique for treatment of gynecomastia using as access a Z-shaped incision within the limits of the areola. He also used this excision for access in benign tumor resections and to insert silicone into women's breasts. This technique extended the surgical field, facilitating hemostasis and avoiding scars outside of the areolar region (Fig. 6.11).

1972—**Lemos.** Presented personal communication for the improvement of breast surgery. Comunicação pessoal. I Congresso da ISAPS—Rio de Janeiro 1972. First Congress of the International Society for Aesthetic Plastic Surgery. Rio de Janeiro—January, 1972.

1972—**McKissock.** Published a breast reduction technique in which the NAC was in a de-epithelialized, bipedicled vertical flap. When nipple–areola transposition was carried out the flap folds in on itself, helping to increase the projection of the proximal pole, or supra-areola, when the mammary gland was sutured and afterward the skin.

1972—**Franco, Luz, Rebello.** Described mammaplasty by an incision into the upper pole of the breast.

1973—**Pontes.** Presented a personal technique in which surgical marking of the skin incisions was shaped like a W. After Schwarzmann's maneuver and skin incisions, he made a horizontal incision into the mammary gland 2 cm below the areola.

1973—**Weiner.** Published on transposing the NAC through a de-epithelialized flap with a proximal pedicle.

1973—**Pitanguy, Carreirão, Garcia.** Published on a transareolar incision for augmentation mammaplasty.

1973—**Farina.** Described breast hypertrophy treated by a mammoplasty with a free areola transplant.

1973—**Wexler, O'Neil.** Reported areolar sharing to reconstruct the absent nipple.

1974—**Letterman and Schurter.** Wrote an interesting article based on historical documents. They concluded that, contrary to what was found in many books, the first mammoplasty was not performed by Durston in 1669, but by Paulus Aegineta , a Byzantine physician who in the sixth century BC, described a technique for the surgical treatment of gynecomastia.

1974—**Gsell.** Published a technique of mastoplasty with transposition of the NAC for cases of gigantomastia. As in Strömbeck's technique, he made surgical marking for the skin incisions with the use of a modified Wise's mold.

1974—**Regnault.** Published a method called the b technique of breast reduction, because of the original layout of similar incisions to that letter of the alphabet. She did not perform cutaneous undermining, and the resulting scar was relatively small.

1974—**Meijer.** He presented a procedure that was based on Aufricht's modified technique, not only regarding the surgical marking for the skin incisions, but also the shape of the flaps, which resembles a pyramid with a proximal apex similar to the keel-shaped excision of Pitanguy's technique.

1974—**Aíache.** Based on the mastopexy technique that was presented by Lerner and Tittiranonda, at the First Congress of ISAPS in Rio de Janeiro in 1972. The mammaplasty technique was indicated for ptotic breasts and moderate hypertrophy. The surgical marking was a circle, to determine the future position of the areola, with two descending lines at the lateral and medial margins of the breast. Below the areola the two lines converged to a point in the inframammary crease, forming a proximal triangle at the distal edge of the areola.

1974a, b—**Sinder.** Employed a dermal–adipose flap on the reduction mastoplasty and in abdominoplasty (personal techniques).

1974—**Sperli.** Described a technique of reduction mastoplasty with functional preservation of the nipple.

1974—**Townsend.** Described nipple sensation following breast reduction and free nipple transplantation.

1975—**Parsons, Burton, and Shaw.** Published a paper stressing the importance of a pre-fabricated pattern presented by Wise in 1956 to demarcate the skin incisions for mastoplasty. This model was adopted or modified by other surgeons as Strömbeck, Weiner, McKissock, and Lewis.

1975—**Meyer and Kesselring.** Preferred to make an infero-lateral excision with de-epithelialization peri- and infra-areolar and with elevation of the inframammary crease. Surgical marking was done according to the size and shape of the breast. The final scar was similar to an L or a J, reminiscent of Hollander's technique, which has been modified and improved by several authors such as Dufourmentel and Mouly, Elbaz and Verheecke.

1975—**Carlsen and Tershakowsec.** Made a circular incision of 5 cm in diameter around the NAC and Schwarzmann's maneuver followed by detachment from the skin with resection of fat and glandular tissue similar to the cone above the areola and a wedge-shape or a keel. The final scar was around the areola and it was a vertical one similar to an inverted T shape.

1975—**Andrews, Yshizuki, Martins, and Ramos.** In selected cases of small hypertrophy and breast ptosis, they exclusively used a periareolar approach through Schwarzmann's maneuver, skin undermining, glandular resection, and deep suture, modeling the gland.

1975—**Rudolph, Earle, and Fratianne.** Using the technique described by Dufourmentel and Mouly: they made an inferolateral excision with some personal modifications and refinements.

1975—**North.** Published an article about surgical correction of breasts that, after lactation, suffered a process of severe involution and ptosis. He employed Wise's model, similar to Strömbeck's technique. He did not carry out adipose-glandular resection, only de-epithelialization of the area limited by surgical marking for skin resection. The infra-areolar flap of dermal–adipose—glandular tissue was fixed between the mammary gland and the pectoralis major muscle, to improve the volume and projection of the breast.

1975—**Ribeiro.** Presented a technique of de-epithelialization of the skin between the submammary crease and a line joining the ends of the inframammary crease with the areola, which was shared with Schwarzmann's maneuver. The skin was incised with a proximal concave curved line connecting the ends of the inframammary crease and a circle around the areola above its proximal edge. Like the techniques of Passot and Kohn, only two scars were left on the skin: one peri-areolar and another in the inframammary crease.

1975—**Schatten, Hartly, and Crow.** Employed the technique published by Dufourmentel and Mouly, in 1961 and 1965, leaving an infra-areolar scar similar to an L or J shape. In some cases, it was necessary to perform wide glandular excision, de-epithelializing the NAC into a thin flap. In small and flabby breasts, instead of excising the infero-lateral portion, de-epithelialization was carried out and used as a composite dermal–adipose—glandular flap, which was introduced between the mammary gland and the pectoralis major muscle.

1975—**Herman, Hoffman, and Kahn.** Published an article about the sequelae of mastoplasty with unaesthetic scars with depigmentation, recurrence of ptosis or hypertrophy, asymmetry, changes in the shape, unaesthetic position inversion or loss of the papillae, and others. They investigated the causes and made suggestions for prophylaxis and treatment of these sequelae.

1975—**Orlando and Guthrie.** The surgical marking was done using the model described by Wise in 1956. Transposition of the NAC through a de-epithelialized flap with a supero-medial pedicle obtained by Schwarzmann's maneuver. An incision that extends from the side margin of the areola to the lateral limit of this new position was made. This flap with the areola maintains good vascularization.

1975—**Fischi, Kahn Simon.** Published on Mondor's disease: an unusual complication of mammaplasty.

1975—**Rees.** Described a useful method for reconstruction of the areola by tattooing.

1975—**Hartley JH, Schatten WE, Griffin M.** the authors described about redundancy of skin during subcutaneous mastectomy.

1976—**Rubin.** Wrote a chapter on the surgical treatment of the massive hypertrophic breast.

1976—**Silveira Neto.** Described a technique with transposition of the NAC through a de-epithelialized flap with a superomedial pedicle that was obtained by performing Schwarzmann's maneuver. A straight incision was made extending from the side edge of the areola to about 1 cm from point A. A lateral incision was made to facilitate the rotation of the areola up and out to its new position.

1976—**Jacques W, Silveira Neto J A.** they described a miomastopexy technique for mastoplasty.

1976—**Franco.** Made an incision in the small and ptotic breast, similar to a key-hole.

1976—**Horibe, Spina, and Lodovici.** Performed breast reduction with oblique lateral skin excision and infra-areolar glandular excision leaving a lateral scar.

1976—**Baroudi and Lewis.** Published an article in which they addressed surgical treatment for small and ptotic breasts. Skin excision with transposition of the areola associated with inclusion of a silastic implant, leaving the peri-areolar and infra-areolar scar as an inverted T shape.

1976—**Bartels et al.** Published a study on mammoplasty using a technique similar to that described by Andrews in 1975, excising a skin ring on the edge of the areola, leaving only a peri-areolar scar.

1976—**Goldwyn.** He published a book on mammoplasty, *Plastic and Reconstructive Surgery of the Breast*, with a large number of authors, about aesthetic and reconstructive surgery.

1976—**Jurado.** Carried out transposition of the NAC through a dermal–adipose–glandular de-epithelialized flap with the areola. The base of the flap was at the level of the inframammary crease. A peri-areolar and infra-areolar scar was an inverted T shape.

1976—**Coutriss.** Transposition of the NAC through a pyramidal and de-epithelialized flap with a pedicle on the distal base at the level of the inframammary crease. The outline of the skin incisions is shown as in Strömbeck's technique.

1977—**Dinner and Chait.** Use the technique described by McKissock, but with fixation to the aponeurosis of the pectoralis with isolated and non-absorbable stitches on infra-areolar part of the bipedicled vertical de-epithelialized flap.

1977—**Courtiss and Goldwyn.** Transposed the NAC using a de-epithelialized flap with a half-moon pedicle based on the entire length of the inframammary crease. The outline of the skin incisions were made with the aid of a key-hole-shaped mold as used in McKissock's technique.

1977—**Fígallo.** In ptosis without hypertrophy, designed an equilateral triangle around the areola with a 6- to 8-cm side and distal base, below which the outline of the recessed area was traced, as in Strömbeck's technique. The de-epithelialized skin between the areola and equilateral triangle up to the groove was delimited by the Wise's mold and the inframammary crease, as in Strömbeck's technique. The skin around the triangle was carefully undermined. Below the triangle and with the same width of the base, he created a dermal–adipose flap with a proximal pedicle and separated the gland from the aponeurosis of the pectoralis major. Introduced the distal end of this flap into the retroglandular space and sutured it to the fascia of the pectoralis major, at the level of the third intercostal space.

1977—**Arufe, Erenfryd, and Saubidet.** Carried out the transposition of the NAC through a de-epithelialized vertical flap with a proximal pedicle with the areola and nipple free at its extreme or distally. The flap was narrow; its distal and lateral margins were only 0.5 cm from the margin of the areola.

1977—**Sperli.** Treated breast ptosis using Arié and Pitanguy's technique modified using de-epithelialized flaps for fullness of the breast. Three to six months later when necessary, silicone implants were inserted.

1977—**Franco, Rebello.** Published a book entitled *Aesthetic Plastic Surgery*.

1977—**Uriburu.** Published a book entitled *The Breast*.

1978—**Kaplan.** Made a circular incision around the areola 4–5 cm in diameter, completely separate from the breast, excised the adipose–glandular tissue that had hypertrophied, leaving the NAC fixed to the part not excised from the proximal or distal quadrant with transposition of the NAC and excision of the excess skin. Cutaneous suture left peri-areolar and infra-areolar inverted T-shaped scars.

1978—**Spadafora.** Cutaneous incisions designed with the aid of Wise's mold, as in Strömbeck's technique, which was modified using similar maneuvers to Pitanguy technique.

1978—**Whidden.** In cases of ptotic breast with flaccidity, he carried out a vertical pinch maneuver from the nipple to the inframammary crease with invagination of the skin. He kept the invaginated skin and made several simple provisional points. Then, he carried out the same maneuver, pinching the skin horizontally above the inframammary crease and with simple provisional points, kept the invaginated skin. Thus, with the provisional points, a shaped breast resulted. After obtaining the desired shape and position, the position of the points was marked with transcutaneous methylene blue and removed, obtaining a design that limited the skin area to be ablated.

1978—**Pitanguy.** Published a book on mammoplasty in which the principles and technical details that were employed were analyzed and described.

1979—**Hugo and McClellan.** Marked the skin incisions as in Strömbeck's modified technique, to effect the transposition of the NAC through a narrow and thin de- epithelialized flap with the nipple and areola and the proximal pedicle. Excision proceeds as in McKissock's technique as if excising the infra-areolar pedicle.

1979—**Baroudi, Keppke, and Carvalho.** In selected cases, they carried out breast reduction associated with inverted abdominoplasty. For the mammoplasty, they used Pitanguy's technique and in the inverted abdominoplasty the technique described by Franco and Rebello.

1979—**Hoopes and Maxwell.** Marked the skin incisions with the aid of Wise's model. They carried out a large detachment of the skin to facilitate the lateral and medial gland excision, leaving much of the gland behind the NAC to give it greater projection.

1979—**Peixoto.** Made minor skin excisions, even when the gland excisions were large, giving an infra-areolar scar, resulting in an inverted T shape with the horizontal branch in a much smaller submammary groove that occurs in most of the techniques that result in this type of scar. The surgical marking for medium and large hypertrophy, differed only slightly in the dimensions of the infra-areolar lines. The author based this technique on the capacity for skin contraction and informed that, after a few months, the skin wrap to readjust the content was decreased. The glandular excision was made on the dorsal part of the gland, with the pectoralis major muscle.

1979—**Riquet.** He used Pitanguy's technique plus a triangular dermal—adipose flap technique with the lateral base of the distal part of the breast and sutured to the pectoralis major muscle. He reported that, with this flap, the transposition of the NAC was facilitated.

1979—**Castro.** Employed Pitanguy's basic technique, making the curved incisions to achieve more stable surgical results.

1979a, b—**Lima.** In patients with small hypertrophy, he did not perform nipple–areolar transposition or excision of the skin. Through an incision in the inframammary crease, glandular tissue was excised with the same shape as a silicone breast implant. He believed in the contraction of the skin, as described by Peixoto.

1979a, b—**Lima.** In large hypertrophy, he performed extensive glandular excision, emptying the breast behind the NAC, which was implemented through a wide and thin de-epithelialized flap, with a proximal pedicle, leaving the infra-areolar scar in an inverted T shape. The procedure was similar to the technique described by Ramil Sinder (1970).

1979a, b—**Goergiade et al.** Analyzed the results of reducing mammaplasties performed in 218 patients using various techniques over a period of 5 years. They gave preference to using a de-epithelialized flap with a distal pedicle with 6–7 in width for transposition of the NAC, but maintained their connection to the pectoral fascia. In some cases, they added a small de-epithelialized flap on the inframammary crease, similar to that described by Ramil Sinder (1972).

1979—**Herrera and Heredia.** Marked the incisions using Strömbeck's pattern, and de-epithelialized the area to a transverse line through points B and C, forming a flap with the distal pedicle in the center of the inframammary crease. The medial and lateral parts were undermined and its extremities were sutured together in the midclavicular line, increasing the central volume of the flap, which was introduced behind the NAC.

1979—**Cloutier.** Reported on volume reduction mammaplasty.

1979—**Huang, Parks, Stephen.** Performed outpatient breast surgery under intercostal block anesthesia.

1979—**Myr y Myr, Planes, Caragol.** Reported the value of preoperative thermography in patients undergoing reduction mammaplasty and mastopexy.

1980—**El-Sahy.** Employed McKissock's technique, but positioned the NAC after excision of the excess tissue and suturing of the glandular breast, as already advocated by Adams in 1944. He also made combined use of Wise's model, as in Strömbeck's technique, and McKissock's keyhole-shaped mold incisions to mark the new areola.

1980—**Psillakis and Avelar.** Organized the Brazilian Symposium on Breast Surgery sponsored by the Brazilian Society of Plastic Surgery—Region of Sao Paulo, with participation of a large number of Brazilian plastic surgeons. Surgical demonstrations were performed by Pitanguy and John Bostwick. During the event, several new techniques were presented by Brazilian plastic surgeons (such as Peixoto, Aleixo Sepúlveda, Costa Lima, Avelar, Pigossi, Chidid, Cardoso, Ribeiro, Pontes, Carreirão, Estima, Sperli, Silveira Neto, Souza Pinto, Andrews, and Sinder), which became important contributions to breast surgery. It was a remarkable meeting with great improvements being made in the mammaplasty field (Fig. 6.12).

1980—**Costa Lima.** Described a technique for reduction mammaplasty in large hypertrophic breasts and gigantomastia without a nipple–areola graft. He created a long de-epithelialized flap with transposition and ascension of the areola and nipple.

1980—**Erol and Spira.** In medium and moderate ptosis without hypertrophy, they made a circular incision around the areola with wide undermining of the skin and vertical plication of the gland in two or three planes between the areola and the submammary groove, and sutured the peri-areolar incision. They believed that the contraction of the skin occurred after some time; there was the same accommodation for the gland as described by Peixoto.

1980—**Mathes, Nahay, and Hester.** In patients with small hypertrophy, they carried out NAC transposition using a de-epithelialized flap with a proximal pedicle. In gigantomastia they performed a NAC graft. In both cases, they used a de-epithelialized flap, which was inserted between the gland and the pectoralis major muscle.

1980—**Avelar.** Presented a dermal–adipose–glandular flap with a superior pedicle and rotation from down to upward for correction of breast ptosis with or without inclusion of silicone implants (Fig. 6.13).

1980—**Ariyan.** Transposed the NAC using a de-epithelialized vertical flap with the nipple and areola with one distal pedicle or with two pedicles: one proximal and one distal. He mentioned that he used a monopedicle 30 cm in length and 51-cm bipedicles.

1980—**Peixoto.** Presented his new technique on mammaplasty with mention of a reduced scar with skin retraction after the operation.

1980—**Chidid.** Made dermal–adipose flaps with a proximal pedicle to create fullness in subcutaneous mastectomies.

1980—**Ashbell.** Commented on the paper: *Out Patient Breast Surgery under Intercostal Block Anesthesia.*

1980—**Farina, Newby, and Alani.** Published a very important investigation about innervation of the NAC.

1980—**Franco.** Axial flap from the inferior pole of the breast.

1980—**Pigossi.** Presented a new technique for reduction mammoplasty at the Brazilian Symposium on Breast Surgery. Sponsored by the Brazilian Society of Plastic Surgery—Region of São Paulo, August 1980, São Paulo.

1980—**Planas and Mosely.** Employed Strömbeck's modified technique. They maintained connection to the distal part of the tissues that they planned to excise to ensure that they were not missed. They did not excise the glandular cylinder's supra-areolar surface delimited by Wise's and Strömbeck's models and caused a small amount of undermining at the ends of the horizontal bipedicled flap used for NAC transposition.

1980—**Mathes, Nahai, Hester.** Published the article *Avoiding the flat breast in reduction mammaplasty.*

1980—**McKissock.** Made an interesting discussion about the article *Avoiding the flat breast in reduction mammaplasty.*

1981—**Sepúlveda.** Presented a new approach to ptotic mastoplasty, leaving a small scar around the areola and a J- or L-shaped one.

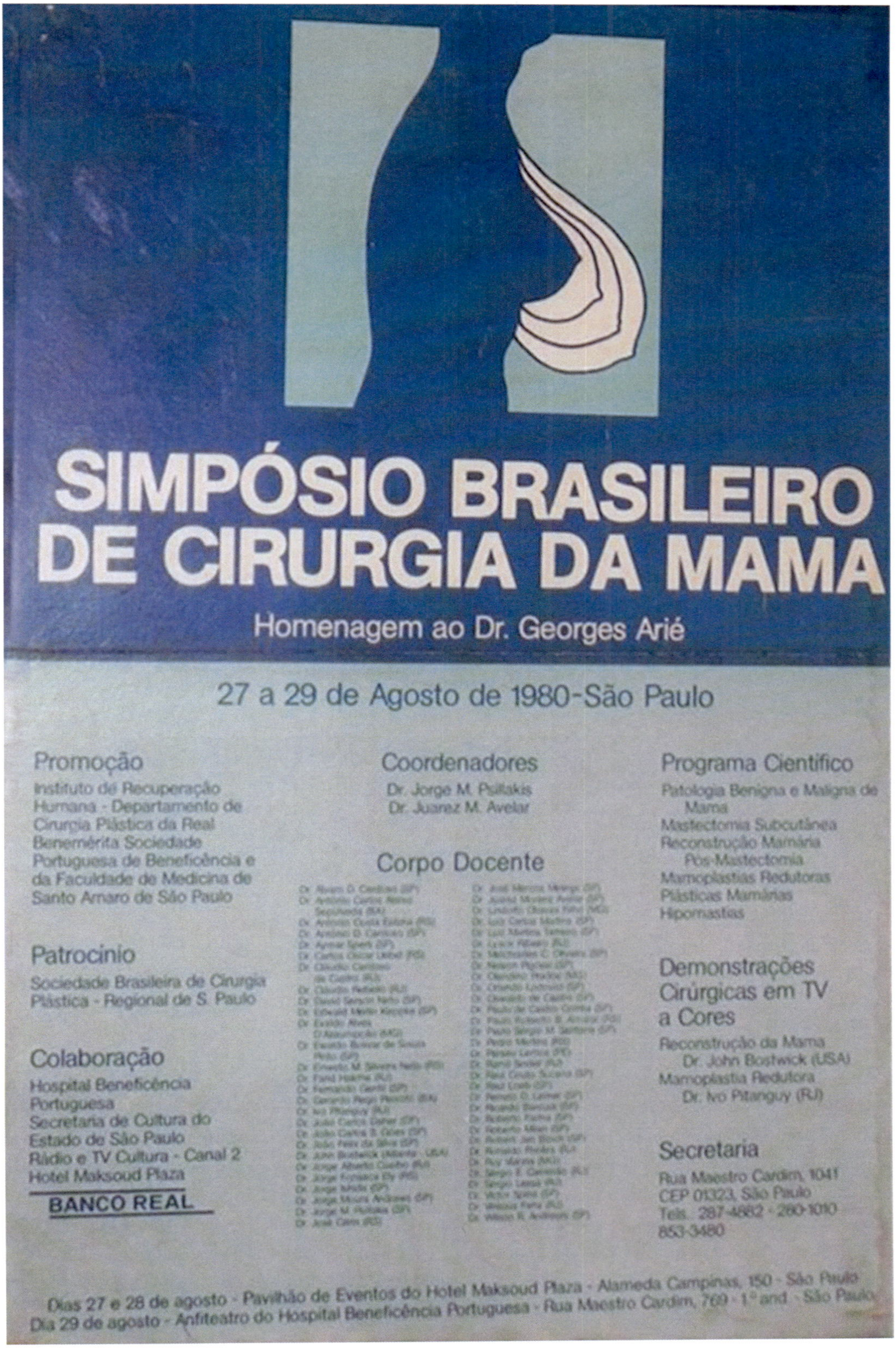

Fig. 6.12 Brazilian Symposium of Breast Surgery—August 1980

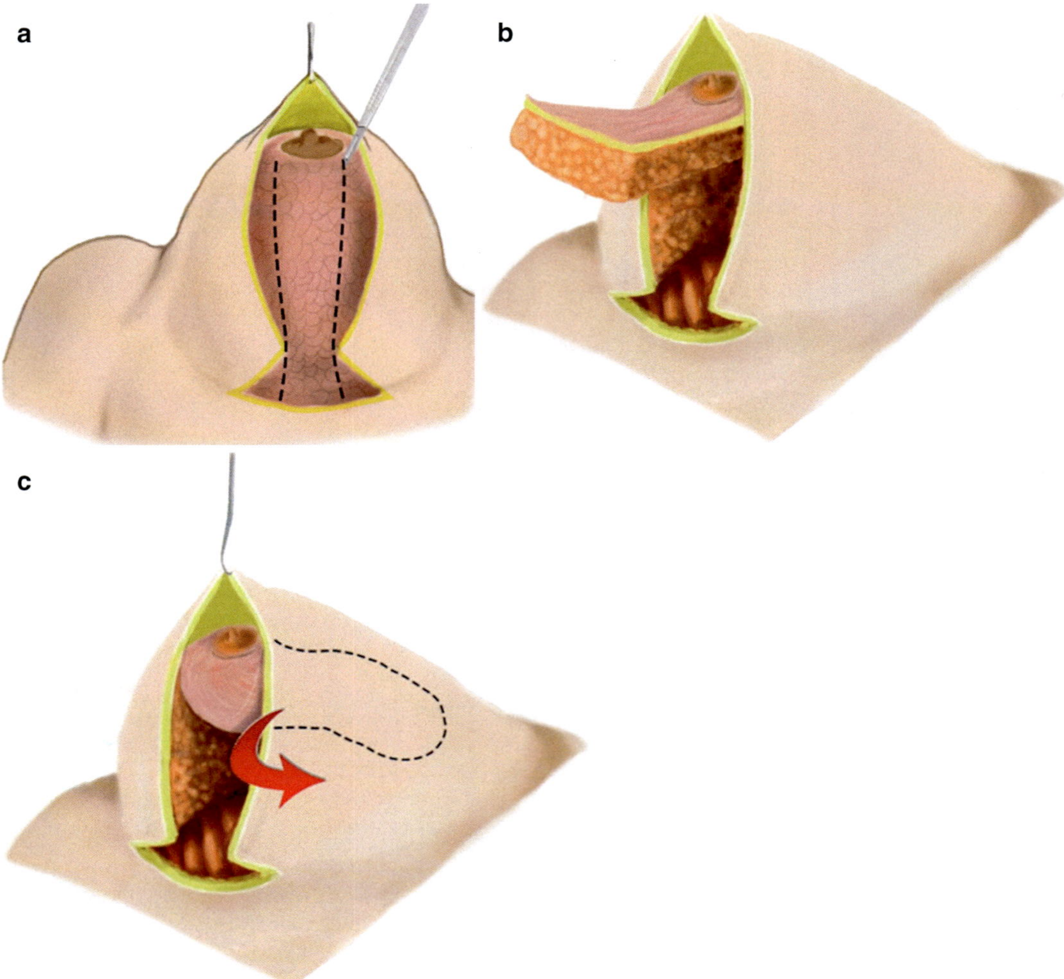

Fig. 6.13 Avelar—1980

1981—**Lassus.** Reported on vertical mammoplasty. Transposition of the NAC through a vertical flap with the areola with a proximal pedicle, an infra-areolar vertical excision, resulting in peri-areolar and vertical infra-areolar scars.

1981—**Balch.** Operated with the patient in the Trendelenburg position, with 10–15°. He de-epithelialized around the areola, an elongated vertical area in the shape of a keyhole. He performed dermal–adipose–glandular excision with infra-areola-shaped horizontal incision. The resulting scar was peri-areolar and infra-areolar in an inverted T shape.

1981—**Zelnik et al.** Studying vascularization of the NAC, they found that, in most cases, there were three intercostal perforations in each of the fourth, fifth, and sixth intercostal spaces. Based on this finding, these spaces are now included in the de-epithelialized flap base with the distal pedicle used for transposition of the NAC.

1981—**Spadafora et al.** In young patients with small hypertrophy, glandular excision was made through a small incision in the inframammary crease. The excision was carried out on the dorsal surface of the gland and not on excised skin.

1981—**Wray and Luce.** Reported the approach followed in two cases of sloughing of the nipple observed on the first day after breast reduction. They excised devitalized tissue with remodeling of the breasts and made a nipple–areola graft.

1981—**Shanoff and Tsur.** Reported a case of a complication 1 month after breast reduction in which necrosis and suppuration were observed. They excised the commitments tissues and created a NAC graft on both sides.

1981—**Schultz and Markus.** Created a NAC using a vertical de-epithelialized flap with a distal pedicle 8–10 cm in width. In the new position of the NAC, they de-epithelialized the skin, forming a circular flap with a proximal pedicle as a platform to project it.

1981—**Sepúlveda.** Carried out excision in the infero-lateral segment of the breast. The excess skin was excised and de-epithelialized partly so that the resulting scar was peri-areolar and infra-areolar with a U or J shape, without extending to the inner side of the inframammary crease.

1981—**Raventós.** Employed a modified Dufourmentel and Mouly technique. He de-epithelialized a segment of skin in the infero-lateral part of the breast and excised a radial segment of the glandular tissue.

1981—**Pontes.** Based on his work published in 1973, the author presented two variants of his mammoplasty method: variant I was used in small and medium hypertrophy after incising the gland at right angles to the chest wall and excising the distal excess glandular and fatty tissues. Variant II was employed in large hypertrophic breasts in which adipose tissue in the glandular breast base of the cone was excised and this excision was extended, removing more tissue contour around the gland, leaving the central portion intact to the papilla and areola.

1981—**Letterman and Schürter.** Performed excisions of the glandular tissue similar to a keel shape on an infra-areolar segment. To facilitate elevation of the NAC they made two incisions on the adipose–glandular tissue on each side of it at the base of the de-epithelialized triangle after Schwarzmann's maneuver.

1981—**Marchac and Clarte.** In small and moderately hypertrophic breasts they made a transverse skin incision of 6–12 cm in length about 4–5 cm above the NAC, with the center of the nipple and another vertical line about 10 cm from the medial line. To excise the excess glandular tissue, an incision was made above that line. When the vertical cutaneous suturing was performed, "dog ears" were formed on each side, which were removed. The final scar was an inverted T shape, as the horizontal or transverse segment was smaller than in other techniques.

1981—**Dargallo.** Published the paper entitled *Mammary reduction with dermopexy*.

1981—**Goldwyn.** Wrote a discussion about the paper *An Urgent Reduction Mammaplasty*.

1981—**Pitanguy.** Published the book *Aesthetic Plastic Surgery of Head and Body*.

1981—**Singer, Krant.** Carried out intravenous fluorescein for evaluation of the dusky NAC during reduction mammaplasty.

1981—**Sperli.** Published the article *Shaping surgical dressing in mammaplasty (new reusable method)*.

1982—**Avelar and Padovez.** Described mastoplasty in association with abdominoplasty with evaluation of surgical results in 40 operated patients.

1982—**Carvalho and Baroundi.** Used the technique described by Pontes in reducing mammaplasty and Arié's modified technique in cases of mastopexy. They presented technical details that were employed for best projection to the NAC. They drew a circle 4 cm in diameter at the new position of the areola.

1982—**Claredon.** Transposed the NAC through a de-epithelialized flap with a distal pedicle at the level of the inframammary crease. The mammary gland was sutured to achieve the best projection of the NAC.

1982—**Juri et al.** In small hypertrophy and ptosis, they carried out vertical mammoplasty. After excision of excess fat and glandular tissue they made a triangular skin excision with a proximal base and understanding held by the areola.

1982—**Nicolle.** Used Wise's mold placed obliquely on the inframammary crease; thus, the final scar was also obliquely papillary–areolar. The transposition of the NAC was carried out using a dermal–adipose–glandular de-epithelialized flap with s superolateral pedicle.

1982—**Bozzolla.** Performed mammoplasty through an inferolateral excision, leaving an L- or J-shaped scar. His method could be performed by surgeons who were not used to employing it.

1982—**Loya and Ryan.** Made a peri-areolar incision similar to a ring. Through this opening, they excised and sutured part of the glandular tissue. Then, they found that the external incision was larger than the internal one. They sutured the skin and resected a triangular segment and on the external margin. After suturing, they concluded that some small scars were left around the areola.

1982—**Kostionovsky.** Described the adaptability of McKissock's technique in diverse mastoplasties.

1982—**Bernadello and Bragadini.** Reported on glandular resection in reduction plasties for mammary dysplasia.

1982—**Mouffarege.** Described mammaplasty with an inferior dermal glandular pedicle.

1982—**Fará and Hrivnakova.** Carried out transposition of the NAC in patients with large hypertrophy through a long de-epithelialized flap with a proximal pedicle folded over itself. The resulting scar was around the areola and shaped like an inverted T.

1982—**Labandter, Dowden, Dinner.** Advocated the inferior segment technique for breast reduction.

1982—**Nicole.** Published on improved standards in reduction mammaplasty and mastopexy.

1983a, b—**Reich.** Left the NAC in the central and distal segments of the breast, which remains attached to the chest, forming a de-epithelialized flap with dorsal and distal pedicles consisting of derma, fat, and gland. The excision of the excessive tissue was done above and on the side of this flap. The final scar was peri-areolar and infra-areolar with an inverted T shape.

1983—**Elly.** In ptotic breasts he made a superficial skin incision in a half-moon shape with the distal edge of the areola, and de-epithelialized a vertical segment of skin in the infra-areolar region. The distal end of the flap had a proximal pedicle and was folded and positioned behind the NAC, to improve its projection.

1983—**Hurst, Evans, and Murray.** Presented modifications of Robertson's technique, which used areolated distal pedicle flaps.

1983—**Soussaline.** Presented a technique for the transposition of the NAC using a nipple–areolar flap with a proximal pedicle. The final scars were peri-areolar and infra-areolar in an inverted V shape.

1983—**Meline.** Described a procedure for the treatment of moderate ptotic breast through cutaneous excision of a vertical fusiform on the distal pole, including a sector or triangle of the areola. The final scar was infra-papillary, vertical, and an inverted T shape, avoiding the peri-areolar scar.

1983—**Ho and Pelly.** Showed technical details for optimal positioning of the NAC and the vertical and horizontal sutures, especially when resulting in scar with a U or J shape.

1982—**Hirshowitz and Moscona.** Published some modifications of McKissock's technique.

1983—**Palma.** Presented surgical details of his method that avoided medial scarring on the nipple–areolar inframammary to increase its projection. The resulting scar was vertical infra-areolar and there was distal curvature of the areola.

1983—**O'Keeffe.** Described a method of mammaplasty with absence of the medial scar.

1983—**Teimurian and Adham.** Presented treatment for the tuberous breast, performing ring de-epithelialization of the peri-areolar skin to give a conical shape to the breast, excising four wedges in the peripheral area of the NAC with inclusion of the subpectoral breast implant.

1983—**Brown, Raunsley, Lawe.** Presented on autologous blood in patients undergoing subcutaneous mastectomy or reduction mammaplasty.

1983—**Castro et al.** Described reduction mammaplasty through the technique of dermal–adipose flap with an inferior pedicle.

1983—**Castro, Araújo.** Reported on later results of mammoplasty.

1983—**Crow.** Reported on the refinements of reduction mammaplasty.

1983—**Pina.** Published technical refinements for mammaplasty.

1984—**Hauben.** Carried out NAC transposition through a flap with the areola on the superomedial pedicle that was obtained for the area after Schwarzmann's maneuver by an incision extending from point A of the midclavicular line to the lateral margin of the areola, which was rotated upward and out to its new position. He achieved greater projection of the NAC.

1984—**Cardoso.** Performed mammoplasty with transposition of the NAC in a de-epithelialized flap with three pedicles: two proximal supra-areolar and the other one distal or infra-areolar.

1984—**Chidid.** Used de-epithelialized triangular flaps at the distal part of the flap sutured below the areola to reinforce the union of the vertical scar with the horizontal scar.

1984—**Nicolle.** Used two molds (left and right) similar to those described by Wise and Strömbeck, but with the most elongated medial part of the side. He performed transposition of the NAC using a supero-lateral flap, leaving an infra-areolar scar in an inverted T shape.

1984—**Andrews.** Reduced the horizontal branch of the inverted T-shaped infra-areolar scar, excising less skin on the medial and lateral sides.

1984—**Dowden et al.** Showed surgical details of the modification of McKissock's technique for mammoplasty with a vertical de-epithelialized flap in asymmetric hypertrophy.

1984—**Spence.** Proposed designation of symmastia for cases of breasts together in the midline. He described treatment of two patients with this feature.

1985—**Bustus.** Described mammoplasty by peri-areolar incision using a tripartite flap with distal pedicles.

1985—**Felicio.** Performed a peri-areolar breast lift, leaving the NAC with a glandular pedicle and two dermal pedicles: one was medial and the other lateral.

1985—**Peled.** Proposed intradermal peri-areolar suturing as a tobacco packet shape with nylon or Dexon for the surgical treatment of gynecomastia and tuberous breast, for reduction and better distribution of the tension.

1985—**Hester et al.** Performed skin undermining with 2 cm of adipose tissue up to 2–3 cm from the chest wall; excised the periphery of the gland, leaving intact its central part with NAC and excised the excess skin. The final infra-areolar scar was an inverted T shape.

1985—**Peixoto.** Performed the infra-areolar longitudinal incision in reduction mammaplasty.

1986a, b—**Avelar.** Described liposuction associated with reduction mammaplasty as an important complement to facilitate the surgical procedure and to reduce the final scarring.

1986—**Tostes.** In moderate ptosis and hypoplasia, he used two dermal–adipose–glandular flaps with a proximal pedicle fixed behind the NAC to increase its projection. The infra-areolar scar was shaped like an inverted T.

1986a, b—**Avelar.** Described the importance of the liposuction technique for the treatment of adipose gynecomastia. It showed that only the adipose tissue was aspirated, as the mammary parenchyma must be resected after liposuction.

1986—**Lassus.** Performed transposition of the NAC in a flap with a proximal pedicle. Infra- and retro-areolar excision was carried out, leaving a vertical infra-areolar scar.

1986—**Maillard.** Performed partial adipose–glandular excision at the base of the breast. Infra-areolar Z-shaped scar.

1987—**Bozzolla et al.** Systematized mammoplasty technique with an infra-areolar L- or J-shaped scar, which had been presented in 1982.

1988—**Berrino et al.** Treated unilateral hypertrophy through vertical and infra-areolar adipose–glandular excision at the base of the breast.

1988—**Elliot.** For treatment of tuberous breasts, he employed a horizontal triangular flap along the inframammary crease transposed to the central infra-areolar part, increasing the width of the base of the breast.

1988—**Kroll.** Studied the use of a de-epithelialized flap with a distal pedicle compared with the same type of flap without the skin, concluding that there was no difference in the safety of vascularization.

1988—**Gradinger.** Preferred to use free NAC graft in cases of large hypertrophy and gigantomastia, and showed surgical details that facilitate improving the results.

1988—**Benelli.** Performed peri-areolar mammoplasty by suturing the external border of the circular wound to reduce the centrifugal tension, similar to the method employed by Isaac Peled (1985) in cases of gynecomastia and tuberous breast.

1989—**Ribeiro.** Published the book *Plastic Surgery of the Breast* published by MEDSI, in which a variety of uses of de-epithelialized infra-areolar flaps in reduction mammoplasty were shown, with transposition of the NAC.

1989—**Toledo et al.** Performed peri-areolar reduction mammoplasty in association with liposuction.

1989—**Ship et al.** Employed two de-epithelialized flaps with the same pedicle in the distal pole fixed in the aponeurosis and pectoral muscle.

1989—**Martins.** Described peri-areolar breast reduction by excising the excess adipose–glandular tissue of the proximal part of the breast.

1989—**Goes.** Described peri-areolar mammoplasty using a circular peri-areolar dermal flap as an external reinforcement.

1989—**Sinder.** Wrote the first chapter of the book *History of Breast Reduction*, edited by Liacyr Ribeiro (published by MEDSI).

1990—**Lejour.** Published on mammoplasty with an almost vertical infra-areolar scar with transposition of the NAC using a flap with a proximal pedicle. She sutured the gland to improve the shape of the breast through discreet skin detachment.

1990—**Lejour.** Described liposuction in association with vertical mammoplasty (no scar on the submammary groove).

1990—**Hinderer.** Based on Peled's publications (1985) and Benelli (1988), he added a second purse string suture to achieve better projection of the NAC.

1991—**Bozolla et al.** Presented a method for calculating preoperatively the extent of the horizontal final scar of the reduction mammoplasty as L-shaped, based on breast ptosis.

1992—**Almeida.** In moderate hypertrophy, he made a distal peripheral intra-areolar semicircular incision, similar to that published by Webster in 1946 to treat gynecomastia.

1992—**Bustos.** Presented breast reduction and peri-areolar and made a silicone blade in the skin for gland support, which developed severe complications.

1992—**Chiari.** Published mammoplasty with an L-shaped scar with geometric planning and marking for the skin incisions and glandular resection.

1992—**Robbins and Hoffman.** Performed transposition of the NAC through a supra-areolar vertical de-epithelialized flap identical to the flap published by Weiner et al. in 1973.

1992—**Erfon et al.** Carried out NAC transplantation in a thick dermal–adipose–glandular flap with a reduced final scar.

1992—**D' Assumpção.** Used a triangular cutaneo-adipose flap with a distal pedicle in the inframammary crease, achieving a final scar similar to a W.

1992—**Fuente and Yesso.** Presented peri-areolar mammoplasty with glandular excision in the shape of an infra-areola keel.

1992a, b—**Aiache.** Presented a semi-circular peri-areolar incision in reduction mammaplasty.

1992—**Yousif et al.** Preferred to avoid a vertical infra-areolar scar. They employed areolar and inframammary crease incisions.

1992a, b—**Hinderer.** Published *Mammaplasty with a periareolar scar: historical evolution and actual state.*

1993—**Auclair and Mitz.** Presented peri-areolar mammoplasty; superomedial, superolateral and infra-areolar glandular excision, including a Vicryl network as a "subcutaneous suture".

1993a, b **Avelar.** Wrote the book: *Loco-Regional Anesthesia for Aesthetic Plastic Surgery* with emphasis on mastoplasty under local anesthesia, published by Hypocrates Ed., São Paulo, Brazil.

1993a, b **Avelar.** Published a chapter with emphasis on the use of his dermal–adipose–glandular flap with superior pedicle in mastopexy.

1993a, b—**Marconi and Cavina.** They presented the three dermal flaps with proximal pedicles: one infra-areolar rectangular and two triangular, one on each side of the areola, which, after infra-areolar glandular excision, were sutured as subcutaneous reinforcement for the areola and the inframammary crease.

1993a, b—**Avelar.** Published on reduction mammoplasty using local anesthesia combined with intra-venous sedation.

1993a, b—**Avelar.** Published a chapter about augmentation mammoplasty through mastopexy using a dermal–adipose–glandular flap versus silicone prosthesis insertion. His flap had been previously described in 1980 at the Brazilian Symposium of Breast Surgery.

1993—**Courtiss.** In selected cases of breast reduction he employed liposuction only.

1993—**Daniel.** Described mastopexy with fixation of a sub-areolar de-epithelialized flap with a distal pedicle under a horizontal bipedicled flap of the pectoralis major muscle.

1994—**Born.** Presented a procedure: after infra-areolar, to close the pectoralis muscle excision of excess tissue, two flaps were made: a lateral rectangular and a medial triangular, which were imbricated, resulting in an infra-areolar horizontal V-shaped scar with a medial vertex or an L-shaped scar in a "lying position".

1994a, b—**Caldeira.** Described the use of the pectoralis major muscle flap to create important fixation of the glandular flaps during reduction mammoplasty and mastopexy.

1994—**Koger.** In gigantomastia, he made a graft of the NAC associated with an infra-areolar de-epithelialized flap with a dorso-distal pedicle to give more projection to the CAP and the proximal pole.

1994—**Daniel.** Published on mastopexy with muscular support. A dynamic and definitive approach to ptosis.

1995—**Harouche.** Used a mold similar to McKissock to mark the incisions. He de-epithelialized a triangular flap with a distal base on each side of the sub-areolar flaps to reinforce the union of the vertical suture with the horizontal suture.

1995—**Caldeira.** Described technical developments to create muscle flaps of the pectoralis major as a resource for fixing the glandular flaps in reduction mastoplasty and mastopexy.

1995—**Ferreira et al.** Separated the infra-areolar flaps of the gland with resection of the excess tissue with direct or crossed sutures.

1995—**Correa.** Through an instrument that was named a subcutaneous endoscope, he performed reduction mammoplasty or mastopexy and abdominoplasty with plication of the aponeurosis, using the same resources as endoscopic surgery.

1996—**Caldeira and Luca.** Published a method through which the breast implant was inserted and fixed inside an envelope created by the inferior segment of the pectoralis muscle. In an adipose breast, with axillary projection, a bipedicled muscular flap was created for fixation to the adipose–glandular tissue. In an adipose breast with discrete axial projection, a muscular flap was sutured to the glandular flap. They used the pectoralis major muscle to sustain the mammary gland. In glandular breasts, its central adipose–glandular pole was covered by two fatty–glandular flaps, one medial and one lateral.

1996—**Goes.** Described peri-areolar mammoplasty with dermal support using an absorbable polyglactin 910 mesh or a mixed network with polyester.

1996—**In Longir.** Presented mammoplasty with an L- or J-shaped scar with fixation of a de-epithelialized triangular flap under the infra-areolar through the pectoralis major muscle.

1996—**Sperly.** Published a book entitled *Mammaplasty. Brazilian procedures, with 49 Coauthors, featuring 62 specific procedures.*

1996—**Gulyás.** Associated peri-areolar mammaplasty with excision of infra-areolar resection to reduce the extent of a vertical scar, avoiding scarring on the submammary groove.

1996—**Saccomanno.** Presented a procedure of breast reduction for moderate and large hypertrophy, based on previous marking of the inframammary sulcus, with an equatorial line crossing below the areola from one end to the other. Dermal–adipose–glandular excision was carried out through a transverse and longitudinal incision following marking. Suturing of the skin was done with stitches similar to a tobacco packet.

1997—**Chen and Wei.** Described a method for reduction mammaplasty with a glandular flap with a proximal pedicle sutured to the periosteum of the fifth rib. The resulting scar was in an S shape, being on the peri-areolar and the other on the infra-areolar segment.

1997—**Oliveira.** Developed a quantitative preoperative evaluation for breast ptosis: except for the thumb, how many fingers found in adduction of the open hand fit between the submammary groove and the free or distal edge of the breast.

1998—**Cerqueira.** Mammoplasty with a de-epithelialized infra-areolar flap with a proximal pedicle was described. The distal part of this flap was folded back and up and introduced into the pectoralis major muscle by a horizontal opening made through the muscular fibers.

1998—**Fayman.** Vertical mammoplasty was performed: according to the type of breast, he carried out transposition of the NAC with a proximal or distal flap.

1998—**Ribeiro et al.** Correction of tuberous breasts was performed using a peri-areolar technique. They divided the mammary gland using a transverse incision, maintaining the NAC in the proximal half, which corrected the typical constriction of this deformity. The adipose–glandular distal flap was fixed behind the proximal one.

1998—**Atiyeh et al.** Treated tuberous and tubular breasts excising a ring of epidermis around the nipple, but a segment of the peripheral part of the areola was preserved. The derma was then incised to insert the breast implant at the retro-glandular level.

1998—**Würinger et al.** Carried out a breast vascularity study, showing the presence of a ligament or fibrous septum at the level of the fifth rib, containing blood vessels directed to the NAC.

1998—**Aboudib and Castro.** Presented periareolar mammaplasty with extensive skin detachment and excision of the excess glandular tissue by a wedge- or V-shaped supra-areolar resection.

1999—**Aiache.** Breast reduction with NAC transposition through a triangular flap with a pedicle in the inframammary crease, resulting in a peri-areolar scar and another infra-areolar scar as an inverted V shape.

1999—**Neuprez et al.** Associated Thorek's technique (breast reduction with NAC graft) with a de-epithelialized flap with a pedicle in the inframammary crease.

1999—**Würinger.** After Schwarzmann's maneuver, made an dermal incision on the outskirts of the skin detachment and performed extensive detachment of the skin; excised the excess proximal adipose–glandular tissue and distal to the ligament or membranous septum described by the author and colleagues in 1998; set the same pectoral aponeurosis and excised the excess skin.

1999—**Bozzolla, Cunha, and Mattisti.** Reported on L-shaped mammoplasty.

1999—**Haykal, Calteux**. Employed Thorek's technique with a dermal–glandular flap with an inferior pedicle that they had developed.

1999—**Hall-Findlay.** Described vertical breast reduction based on Lejour's technique, but with NAC transposition using a de-epithelialized flap with a medial or lateral pedicle.

2000—**Nahabedian et al.** In severe hypertrophy, they carried out NAC transposition using a supero-medial de-epithelialized flap.

2000—**Graf et al.** Used a dermal–adipose flap with a distal pedicle fixed cranially under the pectoralis major muscle to increase the projection or filling, based on the technique described by Daniel Milton.

2000—**Caldeira and Luca.** Developed three types of glandular flaps in the distal third of the pectoralis major muscle for breast support. Each one was indicated according to the anatomical and histological type of breast.

2001—**Ribeiro RC, Saltz R.** They published a book about aesthetic and reconstructive breast surgery.

2003—**Sinder.** Published a chapter called *History of Reduction Mammoplasty*.

References

Aboudib JH, Castro CC (1998) Mammaplasty utilizing the periareolar approach. Aesthet Plast Surg 22:51–57

Adair FE, Bagg HJ (1925) Breast stasis as the cause of mammary cancer. Intern Clin 4:19

Adams WM (1944) Free transplantation of the nipples and areolae. Surgery 15:186

Adams WM (1947) Free composite grafts of the nipples in mammaplasty. South Surg 12:715

Adams WM (1949) Labial transplant for correction of the loss of the nipple. Plast Reconstr Surg 4:295

Adams WM (1957) Mammaplasty with free transplantation of the nipple and areolae. Transactions of the International Society of Plastic Surgeons (1st Congress). William and Wikins, Baltimore, p 317

Aiache AE (1974) Mammplasty: a technique for the ptotic and enlarged breast. Br J Plast Surg 27:318

Aiache R (1992a) Referred by Sinder R (2003) History of reduction mastoplasty (História da mamoplastia redutora). In: Mélega JM, Baroudi R (eds) Cirurgia

plástica: fundamentos e arte, vol 31. Medsi, Rio de Janeiro, p 435–469
Aiache R (1992b) A semicircular periareolar incision for reduction mammaplasty, vol 24. III RAPS, São Paulo, March, p 119
Aiache AE (1999) Arch reduction mammaplasty. Plast Reconstr Surg 103(3):862–868
Almeida R (1992) A semicircular periareolar incion for reduction mammplasty. III RAPS 119–124, March
Andrews JM (1984) A technique for reduction mammaplasty. Aesthet Plast Surg 8:55–58
Andrews JM, Yshizuki MM, Ramos RR (1975) An areolar approach to reduction mammaplasty. Br J Plast Surg 28:166
Arié G (1957) Nova técnica em mammplastia. Rev Lat Am Cir Plast 3:28
Ariyan S (1980) Reduction mammaplasty with the nipple areola carrid on a single, narrow inferior pedicle. Ann Plast Surg 5(3):167
Arufe HN, Juri (1970) Referred by Sinder R (2003) History of Reduction Mastoplasty (História da mamoplastia redutora). In: Mélega JM, Baroudi R (eds) Cirurgia plástica: fundamentos e arte, vol 31. Medsi, Rio de Janeiro, p 435–469
Arufe HN, Erenfryd A, Saubidet M (1977) Mammaplasty with single vertical superiorly-based pedicle to support the nipple-areola. Plast Reconstr Surg 60:221
Ashbell TS (1980) Comentário sobre o traablho "out patient breast surgery under intercostal block anesthesia". Plast Reconstr Surg 65(2):239
Atiyeh et al (1998) Referred to by Sinder R (2003) History of reduction mastoplasty (História da mamoplastia redutora). In: Mélega JM, Baroudi R (eds) Cirurgia plástica: fundamentos e arte, vol 31. Medsi, Rio de Janeiro, p 435–469
Aubert V (1923) Hypertrophie mammaire de la puberté, resection partielle restauratrice. Arch Fr Belg Chir 3:287
Auclair ER, Mitz V (1993) Repair of mammary ptosis by insertion of an internal absorbable support and periareolar scar. Ann Chir Plast Esthet 38(1):107–113
Aufricht G (1949) Mammaplasty for pendulous breast. Empiric and geometry planning. Plast Reconstr Surg 4(1):13–29
Avelar JM (1980) Creation of a dermoadiposeglandular flap with superior pedicle on mastopexy with or without silicone prosthesis inclusion (Criação de retalho dermo-adiposo-glandular de pedículo superior nas mastopexia com ou sem inclusão de próteses de silicone). Brazilian Symposium on Breast Surgery. Sponsored by Brazilian Society of Plastic Surgery—Region of São Paulo, August, São Paulo
Avelar JM (1986a) Liposuction on treatment of gynecomasty. (Lipoaspiração no tratamento de Ginecomastia). In Liposuction (Lipoaspiração). Ed. by Avelar JM and Illouz YG, Editora Hipócrates, São Paulo; 26:153–156
Avelar JM (1986b) Reduction mastoplasty combined with liposuction technique (Lipoaspiração Associada a Mastoplastia Redutora). In Liposuction (Lipoaspiração). Ed. by Avelar JM and Illouz YG, Editora Hipócrates, São Paulo; 25:148–151.
Avelar JM (1993a) Augmentation mastoplasty—mastopexy versus silicone inclusion (Mastoplastia de aumento—Mastopexia X Inclusão de silicone). In: Avelar JM (ed) Loco-regional anesthesia on aesthetic surgery— (Anestesia Loco-regional em cirurgia estética), vol 33. Editora Hipócrates, São Paulo, pp 284–300
Avelar JM (1993b) Reduction mastoplasty under local anesthesia (Mastoplastia redutora sob anestesia local). In: Avelar JM (ed) Loco-regional anesthesia on aesthetic surgery— (Anestesia Loco-regional em cirurgia estética), vol 29. Editora Hipócrates, São Paulo, pp 244–260
Avelar JM, Padovez JC (1982) Mammoplasty combined with abdominoplasty—analyses about 40 consecutive cases (Mamaplastia e abdominoplastia combinadas. Análise de 40 casos consecutivos). In: Annals of Brazilian Symposium on Abdominoplasty. Ed by Brazilian Society of Plastic Surgery—Regional of São Paulo, September, São Paulo, p 141–148
Axhausen G (1926) Über Mammoplastik. Méd Klin 22:976
Balch CR (1981) The central mound techniques for reduction mammaplasty. Plast Reconstr Surg 67(3):305
Bames HO (1938) Los problemas de la cirurgia plástica y de la cirurgia de lãs glândulas mammarias em particular. El Dia Méd 10:907
Bames HO (1958a) Gigantomastia—the two-stage operation for reduction of extremely large breasts vs. the one-stage technique. Plast Reconstr Surg 3(5):560–569
Bames HO (1958b) Reduction of massive breast hypertrophy. Plast Reconstr Surg 3(5):560–569
Baroude, Keppke and Carvalho (1979) Referred to by Sinder R (2003) History of reduction mastoplasty (História da mamoplastia redutora). In: Mélega JM, Baroudi R (eds) Cirurgia plástica: fundamentos e arte, vol 31. Medsi, Rio de Janeiro, p 435–469
Bartels RH, Strickland OM, Douglas WM (1976) A new mastopexy operation for mild and moderate breast ptosis. Plast Reconstr Surg 57:687
Basch K, Thorek M (1893) Plastic surgery of the breast and abdominal wall. Charles C. Thomas, Springfield, p 1942
Batchelor HT (1888) Absence of mammal in a woman. Br Med J 2:876
Beare R (1967) Reduction mammaplasty. Presented at the Fourth International Congress of Plastic Surgery, Rome, October
Benelli L (1988) Technique de plastic mammaire: le round block. Rev Fr Chir Esth 13(50):7–11
Bernadello ET, Bragadini IA (1982) Glandular resection in reduction plasties for mammary dysplasia. Rev Argent Cir 42:45
Berrino P, Galli A, Rainero ML et al (1988) Unilateral reduction mammaplasty sculpturing the breast from the undersurface. Plast Reconstr Surg 1:88
Berry ER (1968) Geometric planning in reduction mammaplasty. Plast Reconstr Surg 42(3):232
Biesenberger H (1928) Blutversorgung und zirkulare Umscheidung des Warzenhofes. Zbl Chir 55(2): 385

Born G (1994) The "L" reduction mammaplasty. Ann Plast Surg;324:383–387.
Boroudi, Lewis (1976) Referred to by Sinder R (2003) History of reduction mastoplasty (História da mamoplastia redutora). In: Mélega JM, Baroudi R (eds) Cirurgia plástica: fundamentos e arte, vol 31. Medsi, Rio de Janeiro, p 435–469
Bozolla AR (1991) Referred to by Sinder R (2003) History of reduction mastoplasty (História da mamoplastia redutora). In: Mélega JM, Baroudi R (eds) Cirurgia plástica: fundamentos e arte, vol 31. Medsi, Rio de Janeiro, p 435–469
Bozzolla AR et al (1987) Referred to by Sinder R (2003) History of reduction mastoplasty (História da mamoplastia redutora). In: Mélega JM, Baroudi R (eds) Cirurgia plástica: fundamentos e arte, vol 31. Medsi, Rio de Janeiro, p 435–469
Bozzolla AR, Cunha MTR, Mattisti E (1999) Mamoplastia em L. Ver Bras Cir Plast 6(33):108
Bozzolla AR, Oliveira HC, Sanchez WH et al (1982) Mamoplastia em L;Contribuição pessoal. R Amriggs 26(3):207
Brown FE, Raunsley HM, Lawe JE (1983) Use of autologous blood in patients undergoing subcutaneous mastectomy or reduction mammaplasty. Ann Plast Surg 10:186
Burian F (1938) Our experience with mammaplasties. Rev Chir Struct 1:35
Burian F (1967) The plastic surgery atlas. Butterworths, London
Bustus RA (1992) Referred to by Sinder R (2003) History of reduction mastoplasty (História da mamoplastia redutora). In: Mélega JM, Baroudi R (eds) Cirurgia plástica: fundamentos e arte, vol 31. Medsi, Rio de Janeiro, p 435–469
Bustus RA, Loureiro LEK (1985) Mamoplastia Redutora de Retalho Glandular Trilobulado de Pedículo Inferior por Incisão Periareolar. Trans XXIV Cong. Cir Plast. Gramado, APLUB, p 484
Caldeira AML (1994a). New Approach de Sustentação nas Mamoplastias. Personal Tecnique. Annals 8th International Congress on Senology, Rio de Janeiro, p 1400
Caldeira AML (1994b) Nova Abordagem de Sustentação nas Mamoplastias Redutoras. Communication to the X Congreso Iberoamericano de Cir. Plást. Viña del Mar, Chile
Caldeira AML (1995) A new support approach to mammaplasties; pectoralis maior muscle flap. 11th Congress of the International Confederation of Plastic, Reconstitutive and Aesthetic Surgery, Yokojama
Caldeira AML, Lucas A (1996) Retalho do músculo grande peitoral em mamoplastia redutora e mastopexia. Rev Bras de Mastol 6:111–118
Caldeira AML, Lucas A (2000) Pectoralis major muscle flap: a new approach to mammaplasty—personal technique. Aesthet Plast Surg 24:58–70
Cardonal-Loya O, Arrillaga A, Ryan RF (1982) Toroidal breast reduction: an unsatisfactory procedure. Plast Reconstr Surg 70(1):46
Cardoso AD (1984) Three dermal pedicles for nipple-areola complex movement in reduction gigantomastia. Ann Plast Surg 12(5):419–427
Carlsen L., Tershakowec MG (1975) Variation of Biesenberg technique of reduction mammaplasty. Plast Reconstr Surg 55:653.
Carvalho CG, Baroudi R (1982) Mammplasties: surgical refinements of the nipple-areola complex. Ann Plast Surg 8(6):458
Castro CC (1979) Mamaplastia de redução. Rev Col Bras Cir 6:85
Castro CC et al (1983) Redução mamária pela técnica do retalho dermoadiposo de pedículo inferior. Rev Col Bras Cir 73:47
Castro CC, Araújo MR (1983) Mamaplastia: avaliação de resultados tardios. Rev Col Bras Cir 73:21
Cerqueira AA (1998) Mammoplasty: breast fixation with dermo glandular mono upper pedicle flap under the pectoralis muscle. Aesthet Plast Surg 22:276–283
Cesari M (1927) Spunti di chirurgia del prolasso mammario. Bull Sci Méd Bologna 5:373
Cesari M, Bolonha (1928) Referred to by Sinder R (2003) History of reduction mastoplasty (História da mamoplastia redutora). In: Mélega JM, Baroudi R (eds) Cirurgia plástica: fundamentos e arte, vol 31. Medsi, Rio de Janeiro, p 435–469
Chen TH, Wei FC (1997) Evolution of the vertical reduction mammplasty: the S approach. Aesthet Plast Surg 21:97–104
Chiari AJ (1992) The short scar mammaplasty: a new approach. Plast Reconstr Surg 90(2):233
Chidid N (1980) Comunicação pessoal. Uso de retalhos dermoadiposos com pedículos proximais nas mastectomias subcutâneas. 17° Congresso Brasileiro de Cirurgia Plástica
Chidid N (1984) Referred to by Sinder R (2003) History of reduction mastoplasty (História da mamoplastia redutora). In: Mélega JM, Baroudi R (eds) Cirurgia plástica: fundamentos e arte, vol 31. Medsi, Rio de Janeiro, p 435–469
Claoué (1939) Referred to by Sinder R (2003) History of reduction mastoplasty (História da mamoplastia redutora). In: Mélega JM, Baroudi R (eds) Cirurgia plástica: fundamentos e arte, vol 31. Medsi, Rio de Janeiro, p 435–469
Claqué I, Bernard (1936) Plastique mammaíre: considérations médico-Chirurgicales. Librarie Maloine SA—27 rue de l'Ecole-de-Medicine, Paris
Claredon CCD (1982) A breast "seat" techinique for reduction mammaplasty. Ann Plast Surg 9(4):350
Clarkson, Jeffs (1967) Referred to by Sinder R (2003) History of reduction mastoplasty (História da mamoplastia redutora). In: Mélega JM, Baroudi R (eds) Cirurgia plástica: fundamentos e arte, vol 31. Medsi, Rio de Janeiro, p 435–469
Cloutier AM (1979) Volume reduction mammaplasty. Ann Plast Surg 2(6):475
Conway H (1952) Mammaplasty: analysis of 110 consecutive cases with end results. Plast Reconstr Surg 10(5):303–315

Conway H, Smith J (1958) Breast plastic surgery: reduction mammaplasty, mastopexy, augmentation mammaplasty and mammary construction; analysis of two hundred and forty-five cases. Plast Reconstr Surg 21(1):8–19

Corrêa (1995) Referred to by Sinder R (2003) History of reduction mastoplasty (História da mamoplastia redutora). In: Mélega JM, Baroudi R (eds) Cirurgia plástica: fundamentos e arte, vol 31. Medsi, Rio de Janeiro, p 435–469

Courtiss EH (1993) Referredto by Sinder R (2003) History of reduction mastoplasty (História da mamoplastia redutora). In: Mélega JM, Baroudi R (eds) Cirurgia plástica: fundamentos e arte, vol 31. Medsi, Rio de Janeiro, p 435–469

Courtiss EH, Goldwyn RM (1977) A reduction mammaplasty by the inferior pedicle technique. An alternative to free nipple and areola grafting for severe macromastia extreme ptosis. Plast Reconstr Surg 59:500

Craig ROP, Skyes P (1970) Nipple sensibility following reduction mammaplasty. Br J Plast Surg 23:16

Crickelair GF, Richey OW, Symonds EG (1964) Histologic studies of the female breast before and after nipple transplant. Plast Reconstr Surg 34(6):590

Cronin TD, Gerow FJ (1963) Augmentation mammaplasty: a new "natural feel" prosthesis. Presented at the Third International Congress of Plastic Surgery, Washington, DC, October

Crow RW (1983) Refinements of reduction mammaplasty. Plast Reconstr Surg 71(2):205

Czerny V (1895) Plastischer Ersatz der Brustdruse durch ein Lipom. Zentralbl Chir 27:72

Daniel MJB (1993) Mamoplastia com músculo peitoral. Comunicação no 31o Congresso Brasileiro de Cirurgia Plástica, Curitiba PR

Daniel MJB (1994) Mastopexia com suporte muscular. Uma abordagem dinâmica e definitiva contra a ptose. Clin de Cir Plást. Hospital Nossa Senhora Aparecida e Hospital Cemil. Paraná, Brasil: Umuarama, 25 July

Dargallo R (1981) Mammary reduction with dermopexy. Cir Plast Iber Latin Am 107

Dartigues L (1924) Procédé de incision et mastopexie par voie axillotomique. Bull Soc Méd. Paris, February 23

Dartigues L (1928) Procedé de suspension et mastopexie par voie axilotomique. Bull Soc Méd 38:75

Dartigues L (1935) Les anomalies du sein em dehors dês hypertrophies et dês prolapsus. Bull Mém Soc Méd (Paris) 139:575

D'Assumpção EA (1992) Mamaplastia redutora com cicatriz final em "W". Rev Bras Cir 82(6):244

De Longir (1996) Referred to by Sinder R (2003) History of reduction mastoplasty (História da mamoplastia redutora). In: Mélega JM, Baroudi R (eds) Cirurgia plástica: fundamentos e arte, vol 31. Medsi, Rio de Janeiro, p 435–469

De Quervain (1926) Referred to by Sinder R (2003) History of reduction mastoplasty (História da mamoplastia redutora). In: Mélega JM, Baroudi R (eds) Cirurgia plástica: fundamentos e arte, vol 31. Medsi, Rio de Janeiro, p 435–469

Deaver JB, McFarland J (1917) The breast: its anomalies, its diseases, and their treatment. Philadelphia: P. Blakiston's Son and Company.

Dehner J (1908) Mastopexie zur Beseitgung der Hängebrust. München Med Wochenschr 36(1):878

Dieffenbach JF (1848) Die operative Chirurgie. Brockhaur FA, Leipzig

Dinner, Chait (1977) Referred to by Sinder R (2003) History of reduction mastoplasty (História da mamoplastia redutora). In: Mélega JM, Baroudi R (eds) Cirurgia plástica: fundamentos e arte, vol 31. Medsi, Rio de Janeiro, p 435–469

Dowden RV, Dinner M, Labandter HP (1984) Breast reduction for asymmetrical hypertrophy. Plast Reconstr Surg 73(6):928

Duformentel C, Mouly R (1968) Modification of "periwinkleshell" operation for small ptotic breast. Plast Reconstr Surg 41:523

Duformentel C, Mouly R (1961) Plastie mammaire par la méthode oblique. Ann Chir Plast 6:45

Duformentel C, Mouly R (1965) Dévelopments récents de la méthode oblique lateral. Ann Chir Plast 10:227

Duformentel C, Mouly R (1966) Mammaplasty by the lateral method: reconstructive surgery of thermal injuries and other subjects. Excerpta Med Int Congr Ser 414:131

Duformentel C (1963) Plastie mammaire par lê méthode laterale. Transaction of the Third Congress of Plastic Surgery

Dufourmentel L (1916) Referred to by Sinder R (2003) History of reduction mastoplasty (História da mamoplastia redutora). In: Mélega JM, Baroudi R (eds) Cirurgia plástica: fundamentos e arte, vol 31. Medsi, Rio de Janeiro, p 435–469

Dufourmentel L (1925) La mastopeixe par déplacement sous-cutané avec transposition du mamelon. Soc Chir Paris, séance du 20 mars

Dufourmentel L (1928) L'incision areolaire dans la chirurgie du sein. Bull Mem Soc Chir Paris, 209

Durston W (1669) Concerning a very sudden and excessive swelling of a woman's breast. Phil Trans IV:1047–1049. Royal Society London, (apud Leterman C, Schurter M)

Ehrenfeld (1935) Referred to by Sinder R (2003) History of reduction mastoplasty (História da mamoplastia redutora). In: Mélega JM, Baroudi R (eds) Cirurgia plástica: fundamentos e arte, vol 31. Medsi, Rio de Janeiro, p 435–469

Eitner E (1932) Kosmetische Operationen. Springer, Berlin

Elbaz J (1963) Traitmeent des hypertrophies mammaires avec ou sans ptose par la méthode dite "oblique extern". thesis, Paris

Elliot MP (1988) A musculocutaneous transposition flap mammaplasty for correction of the tuberous breast. Ann Plast Surg 20(2):153

Elly JF (1983) The Devil's incision mammaplasty. Aesthet Plast Surg 7:159–162

El-Sahy NI (1980) The modified McKissock technique for reduction mammaplasty. Egypt J Plast Reconstr 4:155

Erczy M (1955) New method of mammaplasty by double wedge shaped excision and submuscular suspension of gland. Plast Reconstr Surg 16:374

Erfon J, Barbosa V, Brasil Jr AA (1992) Reduction mammaplasty in a single block: plastic surgery. Hunderer VT: Elsevier Science 2:629–634

Erol OO, Sprira M (1980) A mastopexy technique for mild to moderate ptosis. Plast Reconstr Surg 65(5):603

Fará M, Hirivnakova J (1982) Reduction mammaplasty in gigantomastias with a single pedicle superiorly based flap. Rozhl Chir 61:803

Farina MA, Newboby BG, Alani HM (1980) Innvervation of the nipple areola complex. Plast Reconstr Surg 66(4):497

Farina R (1965) Cirurgia plástica e reparadora. Gráfica São José, São Paulo

Farina R (1973) Hipertrofia mamária: mamaplastia com transplante livre de aréola. Ars Curandi :81–87

Fayman MS (1998) Short scar mastopexy with flap transposition. Aesthet Plast Surg 22:134–141

Felicio Y (1985) Mamaplastia com uma só cicatriz areolar. Transaction XXV Congr Brás Cir Plast. Aplub, Gramado RS, p 481

Felix ER, Sethi SM, Randesdell AM, Lissner AB (1970) Strombeck mammaplasty with free nipple grafts. Plast Reconstr Surg 45:47

Fernandez J (1951) Mastoplastias, nuestra experiência editorial universitária. Buenos Aires

Ferreira et al (1995) Referred to by Sinder R (2003) History of reduction mastoplasty (História da mamoplastia redutora). In: Mélega JM, Baroudi R (eds) Cirurgia plástica: fundamentos e arte, vol 31. Medsi, Rio de Janeiro, p 435–469

Fígallo E (1977) Surgical treatment of mammary ptosis without hypertrophy. Plast Reconstr Surg 60(2):189–196.

Fischi RA, Kahn Simon BE (1975) Mondor's disease: an unusual complication of mammaplasty. Plast Reconstr Surg 56(3):319

Fisher W, Smith JW (1971) Macromastia during puberry. Plast Reconstr Surg 47:445

Fomon S (1960) Cosmetic surgery. Principles and practice. JB Lippincott, Philadelphia

Franco T (1976) Incisão "em fechadura" no tratamento cirúrgico das pequenas ptoses mamárias. Rev Bras Cir 66(1/2):43

Franco T (1980) Axial flap from the inferior pole of the breast. Ann Constr Surg 5(4):260–265

Franco T, Rebello C (1977) Cirurgia estética. Atheneu, Rio de Janeiro

Franco T (1971a) Conservação heterotópica de papila para reimplante ulterior. Rev Col Bras Cir III 4(263)

Franco T (1971b) Conservação heterotópica de papila para reimplante ulterior. Rev Col Bras Cir III 4:263

Franco T, Luz SAR, Rebello C (1972) Mamaplastia por incisão do pólo superior da mama. A Folha Méd 64(3):559

Fuente A, Yerro LM (1992) Mamaplastia periareolar com excisão glandular em forma de quilha. Plast Surg 2:579

Georgiade G, Serafin O, Reifkohi R et al (1979a) Reduction mammaplasty utilizing an inferior pedicle nipple-areolar flap. Ann Plast Surg 3(3):211

Georgiade NG, Serafin O, Reifkohl R et al (1979b) Is there is a reduction mammaplasty for "all seasons"? Plast Reconstr Surg 63(6):765

Gillet (1952) Referred to by Sinder R (2003) History of reduction mastoplasty (História da mamoplastia redutora). In: Mélega JM, Baroudi R (eds) Cirurgia plástica: fundamentos e arte, vol 31. Medsi, Rio de Janeiro, p 435–469

Gillies H (1945) Refection operatoire de la preominence mammaire. Br J Surg 32(3):477

Gillies H, Marino H (1958) The "periwinkleshell" principles in the treatment of the small ptotic breast. Plast Reconstr Surg 21(1):1–7

Gillies H, McIndoe H (1939) Technique of mammaplasty in conditions of hypertrophy of breast. Surg Gynecol Obstet 68:658

Gillies H, Millard R Jr (1957) The principle and art of plastic surgery. Little Brown company, Boston

Gilliles H, Marino H (1953) The "periwinkleshell" principles in the treatment of the small ptotic breast. Plast Reconstr Surg 21(1):1

Girard C (1910) Über Mastoptose undMmastopexie. Chir Beilage Zentbl Chir 31:70

Gläsmer E (1930) Die Formfehler und die plastischen Operationen der weiblichen Brust. Stuttgart: Ferdinand Enke.

Goes JCS (1989) Mamaplastia periareolar usando como reforço um retalho dérmico periareolar circular sob o revestimento cutâneao externo. Rev Bras Cir Plast 4(2, 3):55–67

Goes JCS (1996) Periareolar mammaplasty: double skin technique with application of polyglactine or mixed mesh. Plast Reconstr Surg 97:959–968

Goldwyn RM (1976) Plastic and reconstructive surgery of the breast. Little Brown and Co, Boston

Goldwyn RM (1981) Comentário sobre o trabalho "an urgent reduction mammaplasty". Plast Reconstr Surg 67(3):357

Golell R(1914) Mamma pendula und heftiger Mastodynie Munch Med Wochenschr. 611760.

Goulian D Jr (1971) Dermal mastopexy. Plast Reconstr Surg 47(2):105

Goulian O Jr, Gonway H (1969) Correction of the moderately ptotitc breast. Plast Reconstr Surg 43(5):478

Gradinger GP (1988) Reduction mammaplasty utilizing nipple-areola transplantation. Clin Plast Surg 15(4):641

Graf R, Biggs TM, Steel RL (2000) Breast shape: a technique for better upper pole fullness. Aesthet Plast Surg 24:348–352

Gsell F (1974) Reduction mammaplasty for extremely large breasts. Plast Reconstr Surg 53(6):643–646

Guillera G (1955) Enfermedades de la mama. Salvat editors, Barcelona

Guinard A (1903) In discussion of report by Morestin on the removal of benign tumors of the breast. Bull et mém Soc de Chir Paris Leay: 27

Gulays G (1996) Combination of the vertical and periareolar mammaplasty. Aesthet Plast Surg 20:369–375
Hall-Findlay EJ (1999) A simplified vertical reduction mammaplasty: shortening the learning curves. Plast Reconstr Surg 104(3):748
Hanrahan EM (1950) Mammaplasty: the one-stage transposition operation. Plast Reconstr Surg 6:110
Harouche EF (1995) The double dermal keyhole pattern for breast reduction. Plast Reconstr Surg 1:451
Harris HI (1949) Automammaplasty. J Int Coll Surg 12:827
Harris HI (1950) The present status of plastic surgery of the breast. Med Arts Sci 4:95
Hartley JH, Schatten WE, Griffin M (1975) Subcutancous mastectomy: the excess skin problem. Plast Reconstr Surg 56(1):5
Hauben DJ (1984) Experience and refinement with the supeonmedial dernal pedicle for nipple-areola transposition in reduction mammoplasty. Aesthet Plast Surg 8:189–184
Haykal S, Calteux N (1999) Utilisation d'um lambeau dermo glandulaire inferieur dans la technique de Thorek. Ann Chir Plast Esthet 44(3):231
Herman S, Hoffman S, Kahn S (1975) Revisional surgery after reduction mammaplasty. Plast Reconstr Surg 55(4):422–427
Herreira, Heredia (1979) Referred to by Sinder R (2003) History of reduction mastoplasty (História da mamoplastia redutora). In: Mélega JM, Baroudi R (eds) Cirurgia plástica: fundamentos e arte, vol 31. Medsi, Rio de Janeiro, p 435–469
Hester Jr TR, Bostwick J 3rd, Muller L Cunningham SJ (1985) Breast reduction utilizing the maximally vascularized central breast pedicle. Plast Reconstr Surg; 76(6):890
Hinderer UT (1969) Primera experiência com uma nueva técnica de mammaplastia para ptosis ligeras. Madrid, Espanha: VI Reunion Nac Soc Esp Cir Plast (Noticias Medicas y Tribuna Medica)
Hinderer UT (1972) Plástica mamária modelante com dermopexia superficial y retromamária. Rev Esp Cir Plast 5:65
Hinderer UT (1990) Development of concepts in reduction mammaplasty and ptosis. Philadelphia: WB Saunders Co: 575–576
Hinderer UT (1992a) Referred to by Sinder R (2003) History of reduction mastoplasty (História da mamoplastia redutora. In: Mélega JM, Baroudi R (eds) Cirurgia plástica: fundamentos e arte, vol 31. Medsi, Rio de Janeiro, p 435–469
Hinderer UT (1992b) Mammaplasty with a periareolar scar: historical evolution and actual state, vol II. In Hinderer UT (ed) Plastic Surgery. Elsevier Science. p 569–584
Hirshowitz B, Moscona AR (1982) Modification of the bipedicle vertical dermal flap technique in reduction mammaplasty. Ann Plast Surg 8(5):363
Ho, Pelly (1983) Referred to by Sinder R (2003) History of reduction mastoplasty (História da mamoplastia redutora. In: Mélega JM, Baroudi R (eds) Cirurgia plástica: fundamentos e arte, vol 31. Medsi, Rio de Janeiro, p 435–469
Holländer E (1912) Handbuch Kosmetik. Vexit, Leipzig
Holländer E (1924) Die Operation der Mammahypertrophie und der Hãngebrust. Dtsch Med Wochenschr 50(1):400
Hoopes JE, Jabaley ME (1969) Reduction mamnmaplasty: amputation and augmentation. Plast Reconstr Surg 44(5):441
Hoopes JO, Maxwell GP (1979) Reduction mammaplasty: a technique to achieve the conical breast. Ann Plast Surg 3(2):106
Horibe K, Spina V, Lodovic O (1976) Mamaplastia redutora: Nuevo abordaje Del método lateral oblíquo. Cir Plast Ibero Am 1:7
Huang TT, Parks OH, Stephen RL (1979) Outpatient breast surgery under intercostal block anesthesia. Plast Reconstr Surg 63(3):299
Hubert C (1907) Etude sur L'amastic. Thèse pour le doctorate médecine. Michalon A, Paris
Hugo, Mc Clellan (1979) Referred to by Sinder R (2003) History of reduction mastoplasty (História da mamoplastia redutora. In: Mélega JM, Baroudi R (eds) Cirurgia plástica: fundamentos e arte, vol 31. Medsi, Rio de Janeiro, p 435–469
Hurst LN, Evans HB, Murra KA (1983) Inferior flap reduction mammaplasty with pedicled nipple. Ann Plast Surg 10(6):483–485
Hutchinson J (1886) Congenital absence of hair and mammary glands. Proc R Med Chir Soc London 69:173
Jacques W, Silveira Neto J (1976) A mastomiopexia nas mamaplastias. Anais do 13° Congresso Bras Cir Plást. Meridional, Porto Alegre
Joseph J (1925) Zur Operationen der hypertrophischen Hängebrust. Deutsche Med Wochenschr 51(1):103
Joseph J (1928) Nasenplastik und sonstige Gesichtsplastik nebst einem Anhang über Mammaplastik. Curt Kabitzch, Leipzig
Jurado J (1976) Anais do XIII Congresso Brasileiro de Cirurgia Plática e I Congresso Brasileiro de Cirurgia Estética. Emma, Porto Alegre, pp 29–30
Júri J, Jarí C, Cutini J et al (1982) Vertical mammaplasty. Ann Plast Surg 9(4):298
Kaplan I (1978) Reduction mammaplasty. Nipple-areola survival on a single breast quadrant. Plast Reconstr Surg 61(1):27–31
Kausch W (1916) Die Operationen der Mammahypertrophie. Zentralbl F Chir 43:713
Koger (1994) Referred to by Sinder R (2003) History of reduction mastoplasty (História da mamoplastia redutora). In: Mélega JM, Baroudi R (eds) Cirurgia plástica: fundamentos e arte, vol 31. Medsi, Rio de Janeiro, p 435–469
Kohn (1967) Referred to by Sinder R (2003) History of reduction mastoplasty (História da mamoplastia redutora). In: Mélega JM, Baroudi R (eds) Cirurgia plástica: fundamentos e arte, vol 31. Medsi, Rio de Janeiro, p 435–469
Kostionovsky AS (1982) Adaptability of McKissock's technique in diverse mastoplasties. Cir Plast Argent 6:17

Kraske H (1923) Die Operation der atrophischen und hypertrophischen Hängebrust. Munchen Med Wochenschr 70:672

Kroll (1988) Referred to by Sinder R (2003) History of reduction mastoplasty (História da mamoplastia redutora). In: Mélega JM, Baroudi R (eds) Cirurgia plástica: fundamentos e arte, vol 31. Medsi, Rio de Janeiro, p 435–469

Kurtzahn (1931) Zur Beseitigung der Formfehler der weiblichen Brust. Der Chirurg p 20

Küster no 2 (1926a) Referred to by Sinder R (2003) History of reduction mastoplasty (História da mamoplastia redutora). In: Mélega JM, Baroudi R (eds) Cirurgia plástica: fundamentos e arte, vol 31. Medsi, Rio de Janeiro, p 435–469

Küster n°1 (1926b) Referred to by Sinder R (2003) History of reduction mastoplasty (História da mamoplastia redutora). In: Mélega JM, Baroudi R (eds) Cirurgia plástica: fundamentos e arte, vol 31. Medsi, Rio de Janeiro, p 435–469

Küster H (1926) Operation bei Hängebrust and Hängeleib. Monatsschr Geburtshilfe Gynäkol 73:316

Labandter HP, Dowden RV, Dinner M (1982) The inferior segment technique for breast reduction. Ann Plast Surg 8:493–503

Lassus C (1969) Possibilities et limites de la chirurgie plastique de la silhouette feminine. L'Hospital 801:575

Lassus C (1981) Referred to by Sinder R (2003) History of reduction mastoplasty (História da mamoplastia redutora). In: Mélega JM, Baroudi R (eds) Cirurgia plástica: fundamentos e arte, vol 31. Medsi, Rio de Janeiro, p 435–469

Lassus C (1986) Referred to by Sinder R (2003) History of reduction mastoplasty (História da mamoplastia redutora). In: Mélega JM, Baroudi R (eds) Cirurgia plástica: fundamentos e arte, vol 31. Medsi, Rio de Janeiro, p 435–469

Lejour M (1999) Vertical mammaplasty: early complications after 250 personal consecutive cases. Plast Reconstr Surg 104(3):764–770

Lejour M, Abboud M, Declety A et al (1990) Reduction dês cicatrices de plastie mammaire: de l'ancre courte à la verticale. Ann Chir Plast Esthet 35:369

Lemos P (1972) Comunicação pessoal—1° Congresso ISAPS. Rio de Janeiro. I Congress of the International Society for Aesthetic Plastic Surgery. Rio de Janeiro—January, 1972

Letterman G, Schurter M (1981) Facilitation of the upward advancement of the nipple-areola complex in reduction mammaplasty by Kiel resection. Plast Reconstr Surg 67(6):793

Letterman G, Schurter M (1974) Will Durston's mammaplasty. Plast Reconstr Surg 53(1):48

Lexer E. (1912) Hypertrophie bei der mammae. Munch Med Wochenschr. 59:2702.

Lexer E (1931) Die gesamte Wiederherstellung Chirurgie. Johann a. Barth, Leipzig, p 555

Lima JC (1979a) Referred to by Sinder R (2003) History of reduction mastoplasty (História da mamoplastia redutora). In: Mélega JM, Baroudi R (eds) Cirurgia plástica: fundamentos e arte, vol 31. Medsi, Rio de Janeiro, p 435–469

Lima JC (1979b) Breast reduction: new methods and refinements. Transaction of the International Congress of Plastic Rec Surg Cartgraf, São Paulo

Lima JC (1980) Reduction mastoplasty on large hypertrophic breast—new technique. (Mamoplastia redutora nas grandes hipertrofias—Nova técnica). Brazilian Symposium on Breast Surgery. Brazilian Society of Plastic Surgery—Region of São Paulo, September, São Paulo (_impósio Brasileiro de Cirurgia da Mama. Sociedade Brasileira de Cirurgia Plástica—Regional São Paulo—setembro, São Paulo)

Longacre JJ (1954) Correction of the hypoplastic breast with special reference to reconstruction of the "nipple type breast" with local dermofat pedicle flaps. Plast Reconstr Surg 14(6):431

Longacre JJ (1956) Surgical reconstruction of the flat discoid breast. Plast Reconstr Surg 17(5):358–366

Lotsch F (1923) Über Hängebrustplastik. Zentralbl F Chir 50:1241

Lotsche, F (1928) Über Hängebrustplastitik Klin Wochenschr; 7:603.

Maillard (1986) Referred to by Sinder R (2003) History of reduction mastoplasty (História da mamoplastia redutora). In: Mélega JM, Baroudi R (eds) Cirurgia plástica: fundamentos e arte, vol 31. Medsi, Rio de Janeiro, p 435–469

Malbec EF (1951) Plastias mamárias. Comentários operatórios. El Dia Méd 23:2956

Malbec EF (1953) Referred to by Sinder R (2003) History of reduction mastoplasty (História da mamoplastia redutora). In: Mélega JM, Baroudi R (eds) Cirurgia plástica: fundamentos e arte, vol 31. Medsi, Rio de Janeiro, p 435–469

Malbec EF (1957) Plastias mammarias. El Dia Méd 93(3):593

Malbec EF (1958) Plastias mammarias. Complicationes pós-operatórias. El Dia Méd 30(32):1.097

Maliniac JW (1943) Arterial blood supply of the breast. Arch Surg 47:329

Maliniac JW (1945a) La mamaplastic en deux temps en report avec la vascularization. Am J Surg 67(1):55

Maliniac JW (1945b) Two-stage mammaplasty in relation to blood supply. Am J Surg 68:55

Maliniac JW (1948) L'Amputatíons opposée a la transposition de la glande et du mamelon dans la plastie mammaire. Plast Reconstr Surg 3:37

Maliniac JW (1949a) A mammaplastic substitute for amputation in hypertrophies. Surgery 26:573

Maliniac JW (1949b) Evaluation of principal mammaplastic procedures. Plast Reconstr Surg 4(4):359–373

Maliniac JW (1950a) Asymmetrical breast deformities. Am Surg 1934:734

Maliniac JW (1953) Use of pedicle dermo-fat flap in mammaplasty. Plast Reconstr Surg 12:110

Maliniac JW (1959) Harmful fallacies in mammoplasty. Personal Communícation. Abstract, International Congress of Plast Surgery, London

Maliniac JW (1950b) Breast deformities and their repairs. Grune & Stratton, New York
Marchac O, Clarte G (1981) Reduction mammaplasty and correction of ptosis with a short inframammary scar. Plast Reconstr Surg 69(1):45
Marconi, Cavina (1993a) Referred by to Sinder R (2003) History of reduction mastoplasty (História da mamoplastia redutora). In: Mélega JM, Baroudi R (eds) Cirurgia plástica: fundamentos e arte, vol 31. Medsi, Rio de Janeiro, p 435–469
Marconi, Cavina (1993b) Referred to by Sinder R (2003) History of reduction mastoplasty (História da mamoplastia redutora). In: Mélega JM, Baroudi R (eds) Cirurgia plástica: fundamentos e arte, vol 31. Medsi, Rio de Janeiro, p 435–469
Marino H (1958) Plásticas mamárias. Científica Argentina, Buenos Aires
Marino H (1963) A review of new trends in corrective mammaplasty. Transactions of the Third International Congress of Plastic Surgeons, vol 66, Washington, p 73
Marino H, Uriburu JV (1957) La Mama. Científica Argentina, Buenos Aires
Martins (1989) Referred to by Sinder R (2003) History of reduction mastoplasty (História da mamoplastia redutora). In: Mélega JM, Baroudi R (eds) Cirurgia plástica: fundamentos e arte, vol 31. Medsi, Rio de Janeiro, p 435–469
Mathes SJ, Nahai F, Hester R (1980) Avoiding the flat breast in reduction mammaplasty. Plast Reconstr Surg 66(1):63
Mathews (1967) Referred to by Sinder R (2003) History of reduction mastoplasty (História da mamoplastia redutora). In: Mélega JM, Baroudi R (eds) Cirurgia plástica: fundamentos e arte, vol 31. Medsi, Rio de Janeiro, p 435–469
May H (1943) Reconstruction of breast deformities. Surg Gynecol Obstet 77:523
May H (1956) Breast plasty in the female. Plast Reconstr Surg 17(5):357
McIndoe AH (1938a) Considerations in plastic repairs. Am J Surg 39:54
McIndoe AH (1938b) Review of 80 cases of mammaplasty. Rev Chir Structive 8:39
McIndoe AH, Rees O (1958) Mammaplasty: indications, technique and complications. Br J Plast Surg 10:307
McKissoc PK (1980) Discussão sobre o trabalho “avoiding the flat breast in reduction mammaplasty”. Plast Reconstr Surg 66(1):69
McKissock PK (1972) Reduction mammaplasty with a vertical dermal flap. Plast Reconstr Surg 49(3):245
Meijer R (1974) A modified Aufricht reduction mammaplasty. Plast Reconstr Surg 53(2):129
Meline (1983) Referred to by Sinder R (2003) History of reduction mastoplasty (História da mamoplastia redutora). In: Mélega JM, Baroudi R (eds) Cirurgia plástica: fundamentos e arte, vol 31. Medsi, Rio de Janeiro, p 435–469
Mendes Filho A, Lodovici O (1969) Bases fisiopatológicas para a correção da hipertrofia mamária pela adenomastectomia bilateral. Rev Lat Am Cir Plást 13(1–4):17
Meyer R, Kasselring VK (1975) Reduction mammaplasty with an L-shaped suture line. Plast Reconstr Surg 55(2):139
Michel, Pousson (1897) De la mastopexies. Bull Set Mém Soc Chir Paris 23:507 (Citado por Thorek, 1942)
Morestin H (1903) De L'ablation estpétique dês túmeurs du sein. Bull et Mém Soc Chir Paris 29:62
Morestin H (1907a) Bilateral mammary hypertrophy corrected by discoid resection. Bull Mém Soc Chir Paris 33:201
Morestin H (1907b) Bull Soc Chir Paris 29, 1903, tome 33
Mornard P (1926) Mastopéxie esthetique par transplantation du mamelon, pratique chirurgicale illustrée (Pauchet). G. Doint et Cie, Paris
Mouffarege E (1982) Mammaplasty with an inferior dermal glandular pedicle. Ann Chir Plast 27:249–254
Myr y Myr I, Planes AB, Caragol SM (1979) The value of preoperative thermography in patients undergoing reduction mammaplasty and mastopexy. Ann Plast Surg 3:505
Myr y Myr L (1968) Reduction mammaplasty. Plast Reconstr Surg 41(4):352–355
Nagel A (1942) Das elastisch-musculose System der Brustwarze und seine functionelle Bedeutung. Jahrb Morphe und Microsc Anat 87:216
Nahabedian MY, Bernard MG, Manson PM (2000) Medial pedicle reduction mammaplasty for severe mammary hypertrophy. Plast Reconstr Surg 105(3):896
Nedkoff N (1938) New corrective for method for breast hypertrophy. Zentralbl Chir 65:1503
Neuprez A, Haykal S, Calteux N (1999) Utilison d'un Lambeau Dermo Glandulaire Inferieur dans la Technique de Thorek. Ann Chir Plast Esthet 44(3):231
Nicole E (1982) Improved standards in reduction mammaplasty and mastopexy. Plast Reconstr Surg 69:453
Nicolle E (1984) Referred to by Sinder R (2003) History of reduction mastoplasty (História da mamoplastia redutora). In: Mélega JM, Baroudi R (eds) Cirurgia plástica: fundamentos e arte, vol 31. Medsi, Rio de Janeiro, p 435–469
Nissen (1933) Referred to by Sinder R (2003) History of reduction mastoplasty (História da mamoplastia redutora). In: Mélega JM, Baroudi R (eds) Cirurgia plástica: fundamentos e arte, vol 31. Medsi, Rio de Janeiro, p 435–469
Noël A (1928) Aesthetische Chirurgie der weiblichen Brust. Ein neues Verfahren zur Korrektur der Hängebrust. Med Welt 2:51
Nöel A, Lopez-Martínez M (1928) La chirurgie esthétique, nouveaux procedes chirirgicaux de correction du prolapsus mammaire. Lê Concours Méd 2:41
Noel A, Lopez-Martínez M (1928) Nouveaux procedes chirurgicaux de correction du prolapsus mammaire. Arch Franco-Belges Chir 31:138
North (1975) Referred to by Sinder R (2003) History of reduction mastoplasty (História da mamoplastia

redutora). In: Mélega JM, Baroudi R (eds) Cirurgia plástica: fundamentos e arte, vol 31. Medsi, Rio de Janeiro, p 435–469

O'Connor, Watron (1956) Referred to by Sinder R (2003) History of reduction mastoplasty (História da mamoplastia redutora). In: Mélega JM, Baroudi R (eds) Cirurgia plástica: fundamentos e arte, vol 31. Medsi, Rio de Janeiro, p 435–469

O'Keeffe PJ (1983) Draftmanship for reduction mammaplasty. Ann Plast Surg 10(6):467

Oliveira MM Jr (1997) Ptose mamária—Uma graduação prática. Rev Bras Cir 97(1):9–11

Orlando JC, Guthrie RH (1975) The supero-medial dermal pedicle for nipple transposition. Br J Plast Surg 28:42

Palma (1983) Referred to by Sinder R (2003) History of reduction mastoplasty (História da mamoplastia redutora). In: Mélega JM, Baroudi R (eds) Cirurgia plástica: fundamentos e arte, vol 31. Medsi, Rio de Janeiro, p 435–469

Parsons RW, Burton FC, Shaw RC (1975) The versatile mammaplasty pattern of Wise. Plast Reconstr Surg 55:1–4

Passot R (1923) Referred to by Sinder R (2003) History of reduction mastoplasty (História da mamoplastia redutora). In: Mélega JM, Baroudi R (eds) Cirurgia plástica: fundamentos e arte, vol 31. Medsi, Rio de Janeiro, p 435–469

Passot R (1925) La correction esthétique du prolapsus mammaire par la procede de la transposition du mamelon. Presse Méd 33:317–318

Passot R (1931) La chirurgie esthétique purê. G Doin, Paris

Pastoriza J (1968) Hypertrophies et ptoses mammaires. CM France 75(28):5.569

Paul E (1852) Total absence of the left mammary gland. Non development. Lancet 1:648

Paulus A (625–690 AD) Referred to by Sinder R (2003) History of reduction mastoplasty (História da mamoplastia redutora). In: Mélega JM, Baroudi R (eds) Cirurgia plástica: fundamentos e arte, vol 31. Medsi, Rio de Janeiro, p 435–469

Paulus A. (1556) Medicinae Totius Enchirifion Septem Libris Universam Recte Mectendi Rationem Comnpectus. Opera Basilae, lib 6:46

Paulus A. (1847) The seven books of Paulus A. Translated from the Greek by Francis Adams, vol 2. London Sydenham Society, p 334, book 5, sect 46

Peixoto GR (1979) Reduction mammaplasty: a personal method. Transactions of the 7th International Congress of Plastic Reconstructive Surgery, São Paulo

Peixoto G (1980) Reduction Mammaplasty: A Personal Technique. Plast Reconstr Surg 65(2):217–225

Peixoto GR (1985) The infra-areolar longitudinal incision in reduction mammaplasty. Aesthet Plast Surg 9(1):1–5

Peled (1985) Referred to by Sinder R (2003) History of reduction mastoplasty (História da mamoplastia redutora). In: Mélega JM, Baroudi R (eds) Cirurgia plástica: fundamentos e arte, vol 31. Medsi, Rio de Janeiro, p 435–469

Penn J (1955) Breast reductions. Br J Plast Surg 7:357

Penn J (1960) Breast reduction II. Transactions of the International Society of Plastic Surgeons. 2nd Congress, London, 1959, E S 300. Edinburgh: Livingstone, p 502

Pesková (1967) Referred to by Sinder R (2003) History of reduction mastoplasty (História da mamoplastia redutora). In: Mélega JM, Baroudi R (eds) Cirurgia plástica: fundamentos e arte, vol 31. Medsi, Rio de Janeiro, p 435–469

Pigossi N (1980) New technique for reduction mammoplasty. Presented at the Brazilian Symposium on Breast Surgery. Sponsored by the Brazilian Society of Plastic Surgery—Region of São Paulo, August, São Paulo

Pina OP (1983) Technical refinements in mammaplasty. Plast Reconstr Surg 77(1):50

Pitanguy I (1959) Breast hypertrophy. Transactions of the International Society of Plastic Surgeons. 2nd Congress, London, 1959, E. & 5. Livingstone, Edinburgh

Pitanguy I (1961a) Aproximação eclética ao problema das mammaplastias. Rev Bras Cir 41:179–196

Pitanguy I (1961b) Mammaplastic—Estudo de 245 casos consecutivos de mamaplastia e apresentação de técnica pessoal. Rev Bras Cir Out

Pitanguy I (1962a) Estudo histopatológico de tecido mamário retirado para fins de plástica. Rev Bras Cir 43(3)

Pitanguy I (1962b) Une nouvelle techinique de plastic mammaire. Ann Chir Plast 7:199

Pitanguy I (1963a) Contribuição à técnica do enxerto livre para correção das grandes hipertrofias mamárias. Rev Lat Am Cir Plast 7(2):75

Pitanguy I (1963b) Mammaplastias—Contribuição ao seu tratamento. Rev Lat Am Cir Plast 7(3):142

Pitanguy I (1966a) Ginecomastia. Rev Bras Cir 51(2):59

Pitanguy I (1966b) Hipertrofias mamárias. Estudo crítico da técnica pessoal. Rev Bras Cir 56:263–266

Pitanguy I (1966c) Transareolar incision for gynecomastia. Plast Reconstr Surg 38(5):414

Pitanguy I (1967) Surgical treatment of breast hypertrophy. Br J Plast Surg 20:78

Pitanguy I (1971) Hipertrofias mamárias. Estudo crítico de técnica pessoal. Rev Bras Cir 51:263

Pitanguy I (1978) Mamaplastia. Guanabara Koogan, Rio de Janeiro

Pitanguy I (1981) Aesthetic plastic surgery of head and body. Springer, Berlin

Pitanguy I, Carreirão E, Garcia LC (1973) Transareolar incision to augmentation mammaplasty. (Incisão transareolar para mamoplastias de aumento). Rev Bras Cir 63(9/10):301

Pitanguy I, Franco T (1966) Agenesia peitoral associada a deformidades da mão (sindactilia e ectrodactilia). A Folha Méd 53(1):1

Pitanguy I, Franco T (1967) As hipomastias e seu tratamento cirúrgico. O Hospital 72(5):13

Planas J, Mosely LH (1980) Improving breast shape and symmetry in reduction mammaplasty. Ann Plast Surg 4(4):297
Pontes R (1973) A technique of reduction mammaplasty. Br J Plast Surg 26:365–370
Pontes R (1981) Reduction mammaplasty—variations I and II. Ann Plast Surg 6(6):437
Pousson M (1897) De la mastopexies. Bull Set Mém Soc Chir Paris 23:507 (Referred to by Thorek M (1942) Plastic surgery of the breast and abdominal wall. Springfield, IL: Charles Thomas.)
Prudente A (1936) Contribuição ao estudo da plástica mamária—Cirurgia estética dos seios. Casa Editora "Publicitas", São Paulo
Prudente A (1942) Amputação plástica da mama na mastopatia fibrosa crônica cística. Regeneração glandular. Arg Cir Clin e Exper 6(2–3):67
Psillakis, Avelar (1980) They organized the Brazilian Symposium on Breast Surgery. Sponsored by Brazilian Society of Plastic Surgery—Region of Sao Paulo—August, São Paulo
Ragnell KGA (1946) Operative correction of hypertrophy and ptosis of the female breast: a clinical investigation of 300 cases with examination of a new method. Acta Chir Scand 94(1):296
Ragnell KGA (1957) Further experience of preservation capacity and nipple sensitivity in breast reduction. Transactions of the International Society of Plastic Surgeons, 1st Congress, Sweden. Williams & Wilkins, Baltimore
Ragnell A (1955) Further experience of preservation of lactation capacity and nipple sensitivity in breast reduction. Transactions of the International Society of Plastic Surgeons, 1st Congress, Sweden
Raventós (1981) Referred to by Sinder R (2003) History of reduction mastoplasty (História da mamoplastia redutora). In: Mélega JM, Baroudi R (eds) Cirurgia plástica: fundamentos e arte, vol 31. Medsi, Rio de Janeiro, p 435–469
Rees T (1975) Reconstruction of the breast areola by intradermal tattooing and transfer. Plast Reconstr Surg 55(5):620
Rees T, Dupeurs CC (1968) Unilateral mammary hypoplasia. Plast Reconstr Surg 41(4):307
Regnault P (1974) Reduction mammaplasty by the "B" technique. Plast Reconstr Surg 53(1):19
Reich n°1 (1983a) Referred to by Sinder R (2003) History of reduction mastoplasty (História da mamoplastia redutora). In: Mélega JM, Baroudi R (eds) Cirurgia plástica: fundamentos e arte, vol 31. Medsi, Rio de Janeiro, p 435–469
Reich n°2 (1983b) Referred to by Sinder R (2003) History of reduction mastoplasty (História da mamoplastia redutora). In: Mélega JM, Baroudi R (eds) Cirurgia plástica: fundamentos e arte, vol 31. Medsi, Rio de Janeiro, p 435–469
Ress T (1971) An historical review of reduction mammaplasty. Transactions of the 5th International Congress of Plastic Reconstructive Surgery. Butterworths, Melbourne
Ribeiro L (1975) A new technique for reduction mammaplasty. Plast Reconstr Surg 55(3):330
Ribeiro L, Canzi V, Accorsi A Jr (1998) Tuberous breast: a new approach. Plast Reconstr Surg 101:42
Ribeiro R (1989) Cirurgia Plástica da Mama. MEDSI, Rio de Janeiro
Ribeiro RC, Saltz R (2001) Cirurgia da mama estética e reconstrutiva. Revinter, Rio de Janeiro, pp 351–386
Riquet G (1979) Refinamentos em mamaplastia. Ceará Méd 1:58
Robbins, Hoffman (1992) Referred to by Sinder R (2003) History of reduction mastoplasty (História da mamoplastia redutora). In: Mélega JM, Baroudi R (eds) Cirurgia plástica: fundamentos e arte, vol 31. Medsi, Rio de Janeiro, p 435–469
Robertson (1963) Referred to by Sinder R (2003) History of reduction mastoplasty (História da mamoplastia redutora). In: Mélega JM, Baroudi R (eds) Cirurgia plástica: fundamentos e arte, vol 31. Medsi, Rio de Janeiro, p 435–469
Robertson O (1967) The technique of inferior flap mammaplasty. Plast Reconstr Surg 40(4):372
Rubin LR (1976) Surgical treatment of the massive hypertrophic breast. In: Georgiade NG (ed) Reconstructive breast surgery. CV Mosby, St. Louis
Rudolpf, Earle, Fratianne (1975) Referred to by Sinder R (2003) History of reduction mastoplasty (História da mamoplastia redutora). In: Mélega JM, Baroudi R (eds) Cirurgia plástica: fundamentos e arte, vol 31. Medsi, Rio de Janeiro, p 435–469
Saccomanno (1996) Referred to by Sinder R (2003) History of reduction mastoplasty (História da mamoplastia redutora). In: Mélega JM, Baroudi R (eds) Cirurgia plástica: fundamentos e arte, vol 31. Medsi, Rio de Janeiro, p 435–469
Salmon M (1939) Lês artères de la glande mammaire. Ann Anat Pathol (Paris) 16:477
Schatten WE, Hartley JH Jr, Crow RW, Griff IM (1975) Further experience with lateral wedge resection mammaplasties. Br J Plast Surg 28:37
Schreiber (1929) Referred to by Sinder R (2003) History of reduction mastoplasty (História da mamoplastia redutora). In: Mélega JM, Baroudi R (eds) Cirurgia plástica: fundamentos e arte, vol 31. Medsi, Rio de Janeiro, p 435–469
Schultz, Markus (1981) Referred to by Sinder R (2003) History of reduction mastoplasty (História da mamoplastia redutora). In: Mélega JM, Baroudi R (eds) Cirurgia plástica: fundamentos e arte, vol 31. Medsi, Rio de Janeiro, p 435–469
Schwarzmann E (1930) Technik der Mammaplastik. Chirurg 2:932
Sepúlveda A (1981) Tratamento das Assimetrias Mamárias. Ver Bras Cirurgia 71:11–18
Shanoff E, Isur H (1981) An "urgent" reduction mammaplasty. Plast Reconstr Surg 67(3):355
Ship AG (1971) Virginal and gravid mammary gigantism. Recurrence after reduction mammaplasty. Br J Plast Surg 24:396

Ship AG et al. (1989) Referred to by Sinder R (2003) History of reduction mastoplasty (História da mamoplastia redutora). In: Mélega JM, Baroudi R (eds) Cirurgia plástica: fundamentos e arte, vol 31. Medsi, Rio de Janeiro, p 435–469
da Silva G (1964a) Accurate ruler for preoperative marking in mammaplasty. Transactions Of the 3rd International Congress of Plastic Surgeons, Washington, 1963, Excerpta Med Found, p 50–59
da Silva G (1964b) Mastopexy with dermal ribbon for supporting the breast and keeping it in shape. Plast Reconstr Surg 34(4):403
Simpson G (1913) A case of mastia. Br J Surg 7:336
Sinder R (1970) Thesis presented and approved for Associated-Professor at the former National School of Medicine (Faculdade Nacional de Medicina), current Federal University of Rio de Janeiro (UFRJ), with subject on mammoplasty
Sinder R (1972) Referred by Sinder R (2003) – History of Reduction Mastoplasty (História da mamoplastia redutora). In: Mélega JM, Baroudi R, eds. Cirurgia plástica: fundamentos e arte. Rio de Janeiro: Medsi; (31):435–469
Sinder R (1974a) Referred to by Sinder R (2003) History of reduction mastoplasty (História da mamoplastia redutora). In: Mélega JM, Baroudi R (eds) Cirurgia plástica: fundamentos e arte, vol 31. Medsi, Rio de Janeiro, p 435–469
Sinder R (1974b) The use of dermo-adipose flap in abdominoplasty and mammoplasty—personal technique. (Uso de retalho dermo-adiposo em plásticas de mamas e de abdome—técnicas pessoais). XI Cong Bras Cirurgia Plástica. Belo Horizonte-MG
Sinder R (1975) Use of decorticated dermo-adipose flap in abdominoplasty and mammaplasty. VI International Congress of Plastic Surgery. 24–29 August. (page 58 of the abstracts)
Sinder R (1989) Ginecomastia – In Cirurgia Plástica na Infância. Ed. Juarez M. Avelar, Editora Hipócrates, São Paulo, p 425–436
Sinder R. (2003) History of reduction mammoplasty (História da mamoplastia redutora). In: Mélega JM, Baroudi R, editores. Cirurgia plástica—fundamentos e arte. Rio de Janeiro: Medsi; 435–469
Singer R, Krant SM (1981) Intravenous fluorescein for evaluation of the dusky nipple-areola during reduction mammaplasty. Plast Reconstr Surg 67(4):534
Skoog T (1950) A new instrument to be used in mammaplasty. Plast Reconstr Surg 5(6):507–511
Skoog TA (1963) Technique of breast reduction. Transposition of the nipple on a cutaneous vascular pedicle. Acta Chir Scand 126:453
Soussaline M (1983) Plastie mammaire: technique en "V" inverse. Ann Chir Plast Esthet 28(2)
Souza AM (1970) Mastoplastia por incisão periareolar superior. Ars Curandi:80–82
Spadafora A (1978) Hipertrofia mamaria y ptosis: Uma técnica baseada em el dibujo de Strömbeck. Cir Est Argent 3:23
Spadafora A, Viñas JM, Durand A (1981) Mammary reduction. Cloutier's operations. Prensa Méd Argent 68:895
Sepúlveda A (1981) Tratamento das Assimetrias Mamárias. Ver. Bras. Cirurgia. 71:11–18
Sperli AE (1974) Cosmetic reduction of the nipple with functional preservation. Br J Plast Surg 27(1):42
Sperli AE (1977) Mastoplastia estética nas ptosis: o limite entre o uso do silicone e a mastopexia. Cir Est Argent 2:93
Sperli AE (1981) A shaping surgical dressing in mammaplasty (new reusable method). Folha Méd 83:627
Sperly AE (1996) Mammaplasty. Brazilian procedures, with 49 coauthors, featuring 62 specific procedures, PC 486, 4Mb RAM, CD-ROM, São Paulo, Brazil
Spina V (1950) Neoareoloplasty with labial transplant. Plast Reconstr Surg 6(5):400
Strömbeck JO (1960) Mammaplasty. Report of a new technique based on the two pedicle procedure. Br J Plast Surg 13(1):79
Strömbeck JO (1964a) Mammaplasty in hypertrophy of the female breast. Transactions of the 3rd International Congress of Plastic Surgeons. Excerpta Med Found, Washington 1963, p 87–96
Strömbeck JO (1964b) Reduction mammaplasty. In: Gibson T (ed) Modern trends in plastic surgery I. Butterworth, Philadelphia, p 237
Tamerin JA (1951) A mammmaplastic procedure. Plast Reconstr Surg 7:288
Tamerin JA (1963) The Lexer-Kraske mammaplasty: a reaffirmation. Plast Reconstr Surg 31:442
Teimurian, Adham (1983) Referred to by Sinder R (2003) History of reduction mastoplasty (História da mamoplastia redutora). In: Mélega JM, Baroudi R (eds) Cirurgia plástica: fundamentos e arte, vol 31. Medsi, Rio de Janeiro, p 435–469
Thale HB (1951) Mammplasty and its complications with special reference to nipple loss and its replacement. Plast Reconstr Surg 7:296
Thomas LG (1882) On the removal of benign tumours of the mamma without mutilation of the organ. New York Med J Obstet Rev 35:337–340
Thorek M (1942a) Plastic surgery of the breast and abdominal wall. Charles C. Thomas, Springfield [Basch apud (1893] .
Thorek M (1942b) Plastic surgery of the breast and abdominal wall. Charles Thomas, Springfield, p 314
Thorek M (1946) Plastic reconstruction of the breast and free transplantation of the nipple. J Int Coll Surg 9:194
Toledo LS (1989) Syringe liposculpture for face and body. In: Annals of the International Symposium "Recent advance in plastic surgery", São Paulo, Brazil, Estado, 3–5 March, p 177
Tostes (1986) Referred to by Sinder R (2003) History of reduction mastoplasty (História da mamoplastia redutora). In: Mélega JM, Baroudi R (eds) Cirurgia plástica: fundamentos e arte, vol 31. Medsi, Rio de Janeiro, p 435–469
Townsend PLG (1974) Nipple sensation following breast reduction and free nipple transplantation. Br J Plast Surg 27:308
Uriburu JV (1977) La mama. Los Libreros Lopez, Buenos Aires

Velpeau AALM (1854) Traité de maladies du sein et de la region mammaire. Masson, Paris
Verchere F (1898) Mastopexie laterale control la mastoptose hypertrophique. Paris: Méd Mod 1989:340
Viegas AP (1948) Amastia. Referência de um caso. Bras Méd 62:201
Villandre (1911) Referred to by Sinder R (2003) History of reduction mastoplasty (História da mamoplastia redutora). In: Mélega JM, Baroudi R (eds) Cirurgia plástica: fundamentos e arte, vol 31. Medsi, Rio de Janeiro, p 435–469
Virengue (1929) Referred to by Sinder R (2003) History of reduction mastoplasty (História da mamoplastia redutora). In: Mélega JM, Baroudi R (eds) Cirurgia plástica: fundamentos e arte, vol 31. Medsi, Rio de Janeiro, p 435–469
Warren JC (1907) Plastic resection of the mammary gland. Ann Surg 45:801
Weiner OL (1973) A single dermal pedicle for nipple transposition in subcutaneous mastectomy, reduction mammaplasty or mastopexy. Plast Reconstr Surg 51:115
Weinhold E (1926) Discussion zum Vortrag Küster: operation bei Hängebrust und Hängebauch. Zentralbl Gynak 50(2):581
Wexler MR, O'Neil RM (1973) Areolar sharing to reconstruct the absent nipple. Plast Reconstr Surg 51(2):176–178
Whidden (1978) Referred to by Sinder R (2003) History of reduction mastoplasty (História da mamoplastia redutora). In: Mélega JM, Baroudi R (eds) Cirurgia plástica: fundamentos e arte, vol 31. Medsi, Rio de Janeiro, p 435–469
Williams WR (1891) Polymastism with special reference to mammae erraticae and the development of neoplasms from supernumerary mammary structures. J Anat Physiol 25:225
Wise RJ (1956) A preliminary report on a method of planning the mammaplasty. Plast Reconstr Surg 17:367
Wise RJ, Cannon JP, Hill JF (1963) Further experience with reduction mammaplasty. Plast Reconstr Surg 32:12
Wray RC, Luce EA (1981) Treatment of impending necrosis following reduction mammaplasty. Plast Reconstr Surg 68(2):242
Würinger E (1999) Refinement of the central pedicles breast reduction by application of the ligamentous suspension. Plast Reconstr Surg 103(5):1400–1410
Würinger E, Mader N, Posche E et al (1998) Nerve and vessel supplying ligamentous suspension of the mammary gland. Plast Reconstr Surg 101:1486
Yousif NJ, Larson DL, Sangers S (1992) Elimination of the vertical scar in reduction mammaplasty. Plast Reconstr Surg 89:459–567
Zelnik JN, Pearls RM, Johnson D (1981) Use of an axial flap for reduction mammaplasty. Ann Plast Surg 7:204
Zilbsky JN (1966) Adenomamectomy and breast reconstruction. Plast Reconstr Surg 37:1

Part II

Surgical Options for Reduction Mammaplasty

7 Reduction Mastoplasty with a Short Scar

Juarez M. Avelar

7.1 Introduction

Mastoplasty is an extremely popular and very common surgical procedure in Brazil compared with other countries. A highlight for the development and progress resulting from the effort, commitment, and creativity of surgeons all over the world, seeking new approaches to creating an organ with immense significance for women's personal lives. As long as a surgeon respects the anatomy, physiology, and basic surgical principles, it is possible to develop new approaches to reshaping the breasts.

Breast hypertrophy is a very common problem for physical reasons, but also for psychological conditions. Patients complaint of the unaesthetic appearance of the breasts; quite often, they refer to back pain, sulcus on the shoulders caused by the brassiere, bad posture because of the overweight of the breasts, cutaneous irritation on the submammary crease caused by constant contact of the breast with the skin of the upper abdominal wall.

Because of the progress and development of our specialty, technical improvement has taken place in mastoplasty with the significance that it is safe to perform surgery, even in young patients. In fact, the basic technical principles and anatomical knowledge allow us to perform surgery on patients with marriage prospects, and on those who are pregnant or breast-feeding children.

The resulting scars after reduction mastoplasty are extensive according to skin resection, which may bother patients because of the unaesthetic appearance. Usually, surgeons are very concerned about the final scars and several procedures have been presented to suggest how to perform the operation leaving reduced scars. As I had the privilege to be Prof. Pitanguy's resident, I learned his technique in detail, which has been of fundamental importance in my practice. Nevertheless, as soon as I started my private activities, some modifications were introduced to achieve reduced scars after mastoplasty. Thus, the area of skin on the internal and external sides of the breast have a similar shape to the glandular columns to be created after "keel" resection. In my mind, it is like two arms hugging.

7.2 Method

7.2.1 Surgical Planning

According to Pitanguy's publications (Pitanguy 1960; Pitanguy and Garcia 1972), surgical planning is the basic step before performing mastoplasty. As in any other field, surgical planning must be a fundamental stage before all surgeries, as I have already described in

J.M. Avelar, M.D.
Brazilian Institute of Surgery Plastic and Reconstructive, Alameda Gabriel Monteiro da Silva, 620 JD Europa, São Paulo, SP 01442000, Brazil
e-mail: juarezavelar@bol.com.br; institutodaorelha@uol.com.br; clinica-avelar@uol.com.br

J.M. Avelar (ed.), *Breast Surgery*, https://doi.org/10.1007/978-3-319-54115-0_7

my previous publications (Avelar 2013, 2016). The surgeon must talk peacefully with patient who comes to the office to seek a surgical solution for breast hypertrophy. In a subsequent stage, the physical examination is valuable step in analyzing the breasts and preparing the operative plan. If there is hypertrophy with or without ptosis, the recommended treatment is surgical resection, as there is no other effective therapy.

Nevertheless, there are several aspects that should not be forgotten by a surgeon when examining a patient. First, any asymmetry can be seen and the surgeon should note this and advise the patient to observe her own body. Second, the surgeon should check if there is only ptosis with sagging but without hypertrophy. and third, if there is hypertrophy combined with ptosis. The surgical technique used is different and the patient should be advised of the position, location, and size of the scars.

Although there are many techniques, the surgeon should employ the one that he or she is used to performing and over which he or she has total control. Excessive disclosure on the subject may give false information to the public causing professional problems. However, the doctor may evaluate the problem of each patient and prepare a specific operative plan for each case.

Often patients may opt for surgery that leaves one vertical scar or even a periareolar one, thinking that such a procedure is an updated one to correct her problem. In fact, she wants the best for her, but her intellectual capacity cannot exceed that of the doctor who will perform it.

If we have a patient with bilateral breast hypertrophy, the technique is aimed at reducing the volume, but she also deserves explanations about the position and other characteristics of the scars.

7.2.2 Surgical Technique

Among several techniques for the treatment of breast hypertrophy, my description basically addresses the one that I am most convinced of. My methodology is developed from Pitanguy's technique, with whom I had the privilege to be his resident during my specialization and training. Some of the improvements I added to the original technique are due to my own style, attention to detail, and surgical refinements, especially in the long-term observation of my patients.

At the beginning of my practice, I concluded that it would be possible to reduce it without any damage to the aesthetic characteristics of the operated breast. In fact, achieving small scars should not be given priority over the shape, harmony, and symmetry of the breasts. Patients are basically concerned about the shape of the breasts and their harmony with the body contour. The surgeon may be concerned about reducing the size of the scars, but should not jeopardize the shape of the breasts.

7.2.3 Surgical Marking

Surgical marking is an essential and fundamental procedure before mastoplasty to provide adequate orientation during surgery concerning skin and glandular resection. As Prof. Pitanguy had so much experience, he usually did it with the patient on the operating table under general anesthesia in a semi-sitting position. However, I prefer to do the surgical pre-marking on my patients 1 day before the operation.

7.2.3.1 Pre-Marking

Reference points are marked with the patient standing in front of two vertical mirrors placed strategically one in front of the other in my examination room at my clinic (Fig. 7.1). Initially, a point is marked on the center of sternal notch. Afterward, another two points are marked laterally 7 cm away on each side on the midclavicular point. Those vertical lines are not parallel as they diverge in a lateral direction through the nipples. The inframammary crease is marked by gently elevating the breast. Afterward, I follow Pitanguy's description, such as placing my index finger of one hand under and behind the breast up to the inframammary crease (Fig. 7.1). The opposite index finger palpates through the breast to determine the level of the tip of my finger in the inframammary crease, and the surface of the breast is marked at this point (Fig. 7.1). It is the

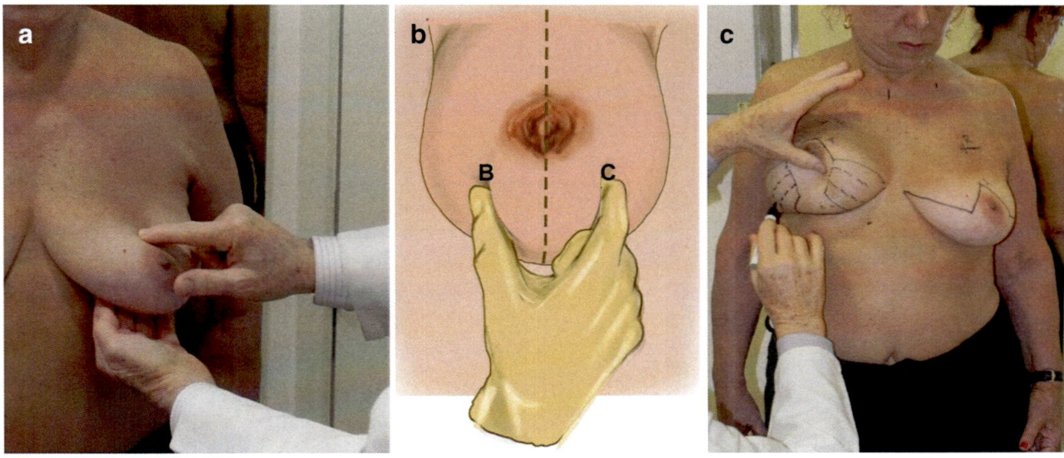

Fig. 7.1 Pre-marking 1 day before the operation at my clinic with a patient in front of two vertical mirrors. (**a**) Photo with the patient in a standing position: Pitanguy's point A is demarcated. (**b**) Drawing shows the position of fingers to mark points B and C, which are always below the nipple–areolar complex (NAC). (**c**) Photo shows the breasts already demarcated

approximate site of the new nipple, which is shown to the patient in front of the mirror. This is the Pitanguy's point A, which is marked to give adequate orientation during surgical marking in the operating room. There is no fixed position for the new nipple site, but to show that it allows for upward migration. In fact, the nipples are projected onto the vertical lines depending upon the height of the patient, the size of the breasts, and the dimensions of the thorax, in addition to the age of the patient. When the breasts are very large and the skin is stretched, the nipples may move up after the weight and stretch have been reduced. Correction of mild ptosis may only require a small amount of upward nipple movement. For this reason, I consider pre-marking a useful procedure to determine the reference points before surgery.

These reference points are marked with ink and the patient is recommended to preserve them until next day. She can take a shower, but must be careful to maintain those points to help the surgical marking during the operation.

I found those pre-markings to be very useful, as the patient is awake and observes my work in the mirrors. At this time, I have one more chance to examine all the surgical details that were registered during the first consultation. I check the blood tests, heart and clinical examination, ultrasound or mammography of patients over 30 years of age. Also, the patient signs the consent form.

The next day, when the patient is in the operating room, the references points previously marked are useful for determining the surgical marking. My preference is to perform reduction mastoplasty under local anesthesia combined with intravenous sedation under the care of an anesthesiologist. A stitch is made in the sternal notch and another one on xyphoid process for surgical marking (Fig. 7.2). With the patient placed in the supine position, the operating table is raised to about 45°, with elevation of the chest so that the breasts show the ptotic position and the inframammary creases are marked (Fig. 7.2). At this moment, Pitanguy's point A is a fundamental reference for the marking of the surgery. The submammary folds are drawn to determine the location of the final scars after surgery.

I have never employed any of the prefabricated patterns advocated a long time ago by several authors (Wise 1956; Strömbeck 1960), as Prof. Pitanguy did not use them. My marking presents some modifications of Pitanguy's original descriptions. First, I changed the position of points B and C, which were placed lower than a horizontal line with the nipple (Fig. 7.1b). As

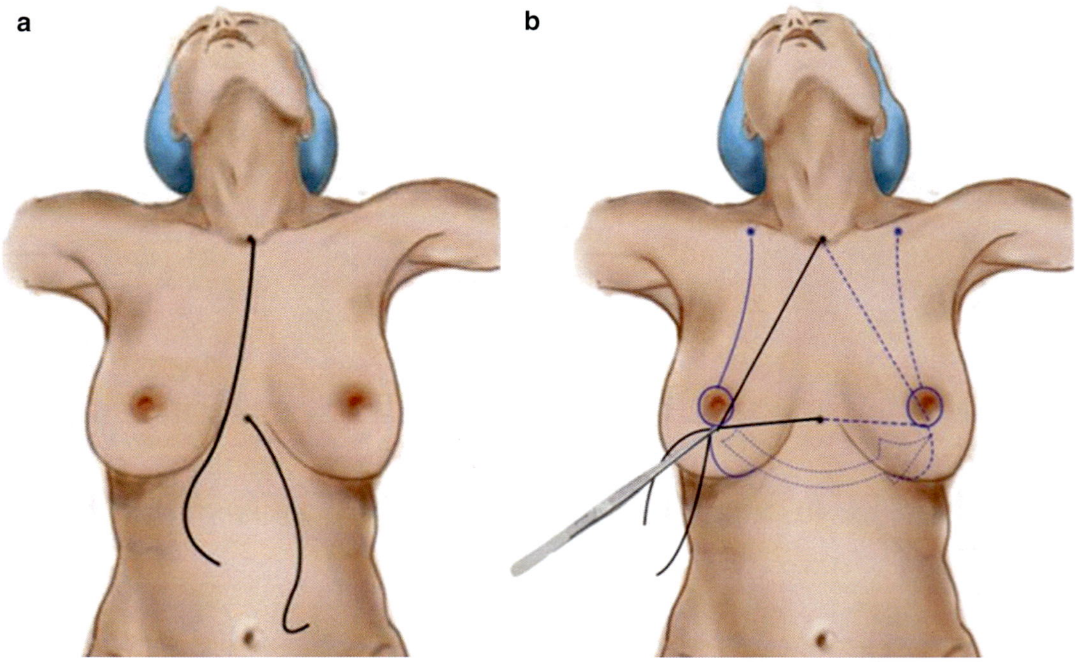

Fig. 7.2 Drawing to demonstrate surgical marking during surgery. (**a**) Two medial long stitches are made on the sternal notch and on the xyphoid process. (**b**) A vertical line is drawn from the midclavicular point, passing the nipple. The two long stitches showed in (**a**) are useful as a compass for a comparison of the two breasts before, during, and after the operation as well

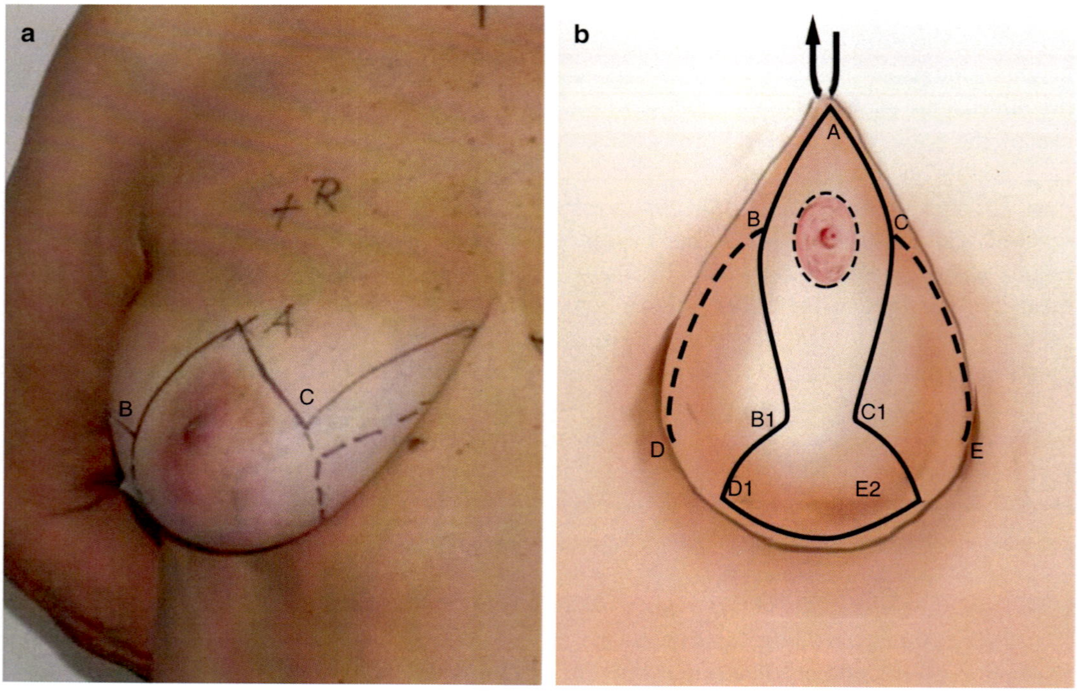

Fig. 7.3 Surgical marking in the operating room. (**a**) Photo of the patient with pre-marking to demonstrate my evolution: the points B and C are marked at the same level of the NAC according to Pitanguy's technique, but I make them much lower so that they cannot see them on the breast. (**b**) On the drawing, the points B1, C1, D1, and E1 can be seen marked according to my approach, in which the area for skin resection is similar to a rocket

these points are marked below, this resulted in a smaller area of skin resection. Consequently, the lower final scar is shorter and the area for skin resection is shaped like a rocket (Fig. 7.3b). This time, the horizontal segments on the medial and lateral breast are reduced, thereby leading to a decrease in the dimensions of the scars (Fig. 7.4). However, my goal has always been to achieve a good shape, with symmetrical volume and the nipple–areola complex (NAC) in harmony with the breast, but with short scars (Fig. 7.5).

Currently, the technical design of my surgery plays a part in the skin approaches and required glandular resection without much accuracy in the dimensions of the initial design. In fact, the demarcated area for skin resection is always smaller than I would like, as the excess skin is removed afterward.

Finally, it is worth saying that my method of marking allows me more freedom, with no fixed

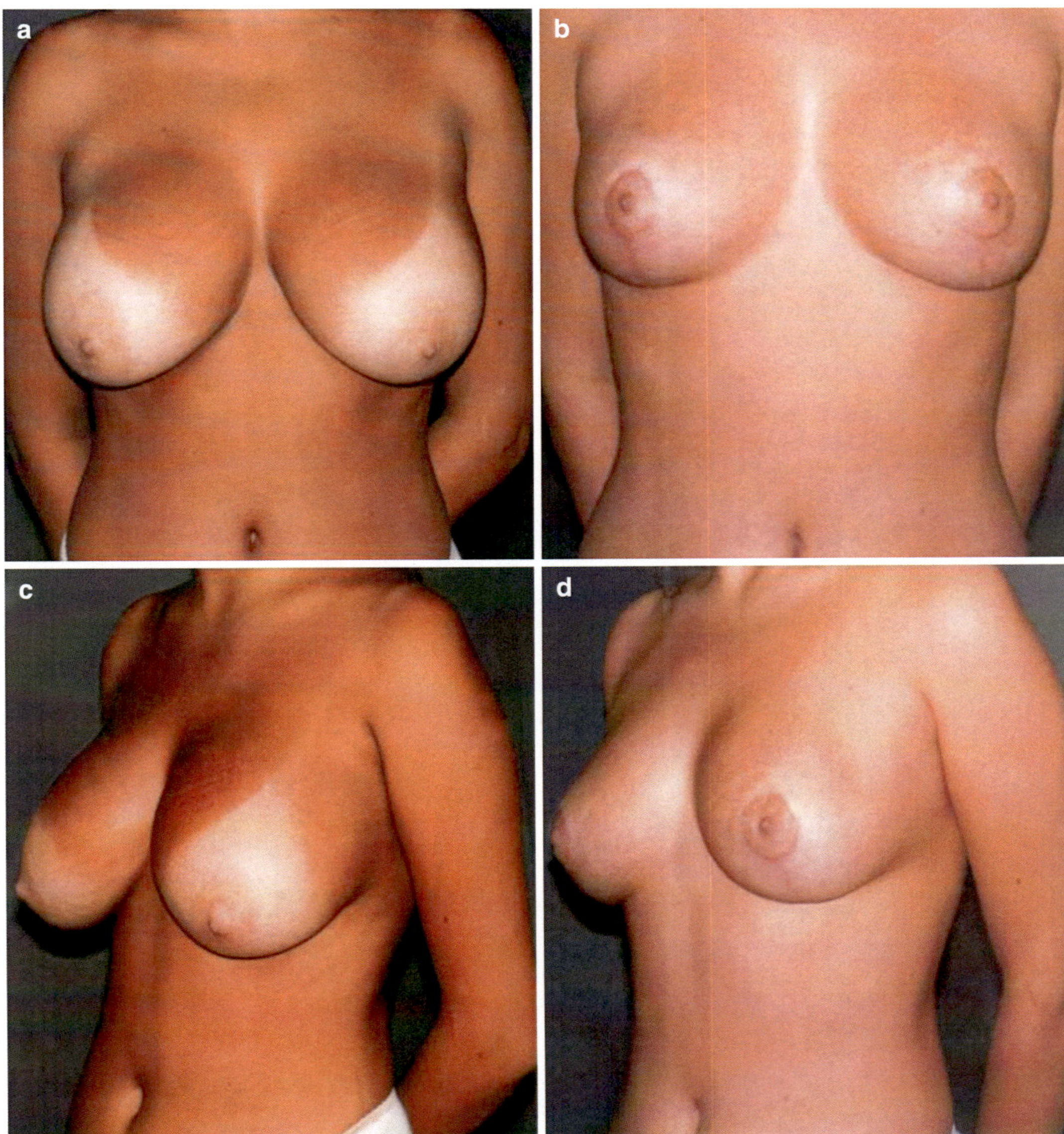

Fig. 7.4 A 20-year-old girl with hypertrophic breasts before and after reduction mastoplasty using my approach. (**a**), (**c**), and (**e**) Preoperative photos. (**b**), (**d**), and (**f**) Postoperative photos

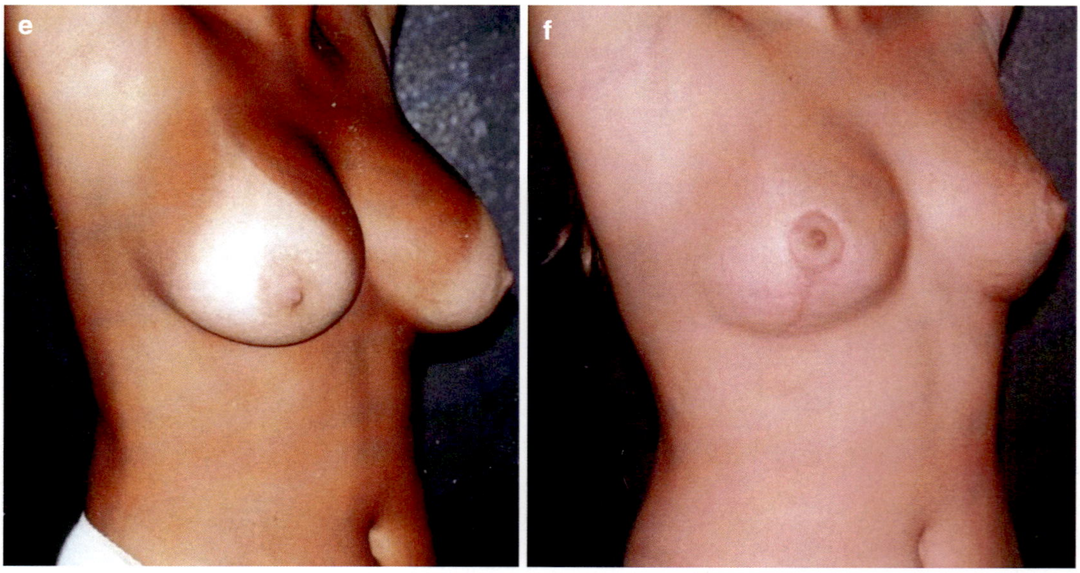

Fig. 7.4 (continued)

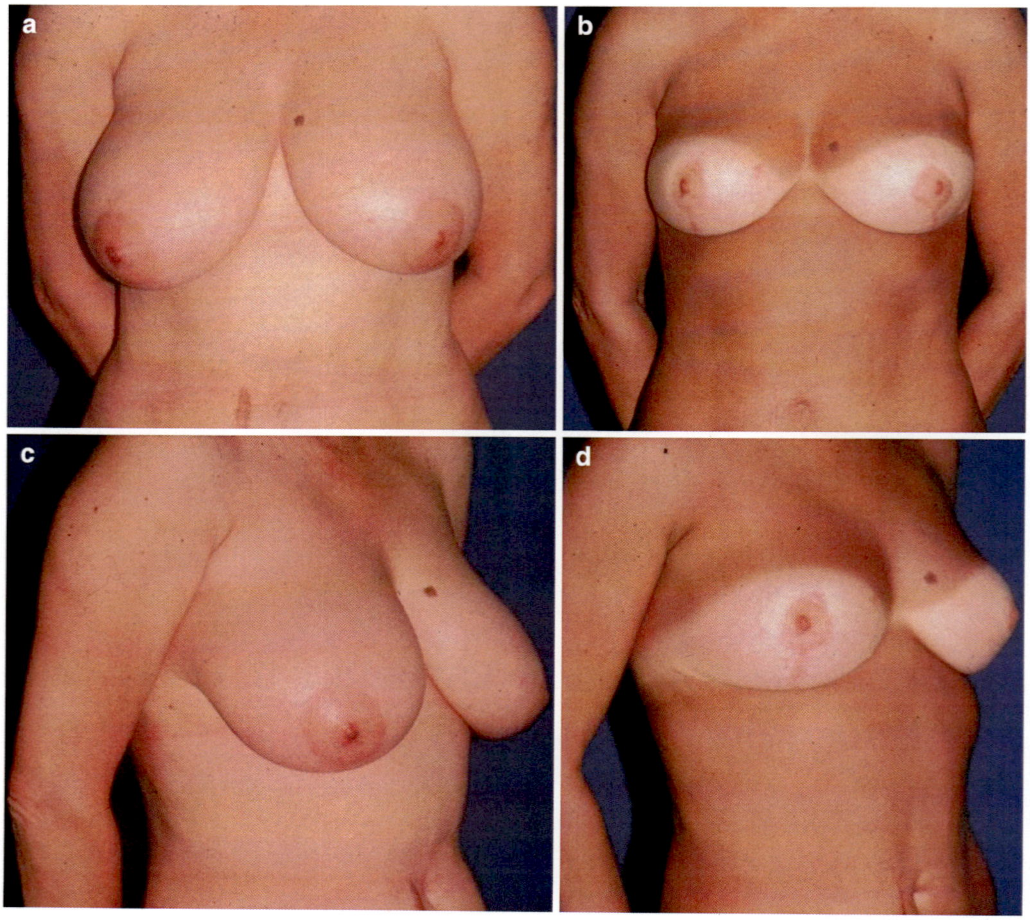

Fig. 7.5 A 34-year-old patient with large and ptotic hypertrophic breasts. (**a**) and (**c**) Preoperative photos. (**b**) and (**d**) Photos of the same patient after reduction mastoplasty

numbers and distances, but that all I have in mind is to create the volume and shape of the breast (Fig. 7.3).

Often, during mastoplasty, it is possible for me to perform extensive resections, leaving only a scar on the vertical line (Fig. 7.4). However, I have no desire to pursue such a result, or even promise to the patient that she will have only one scar. I am aware of the technical limitations and, above all, the huge variations in each case; thus I do not promise something that impossible to accomplish.

7.2.3.2 Anesthesia

Since the earliest years of my practice, I have performed mastoplasty employing local anesthesia combined with intravenous sedation under the care of an anesthesiologist. Even for large breasts, I have performed mammary gland resection of 1000 g on each side, following the same methodology. Currently, I do not face any difficulty in employing my methodology, as the patients themselves are informed by others before they come to the clinic for consultation.

7.2.4 Anesthetic Infiltration

The anesthetic infiltration is performed after the technical marking of the skin is done. My anesthetic solution is:

Lidocaine (2%) 40 mL
Distilled water 160 mL
Adrenaline (1/1000) 1 mL
Total solution 201 mL

This amount of anesthetic volume is enough to infiltrate both breasts, even in the case of large hypertrophy. It is worth emphasizing that the breast parenchyma should not be infiltrated, but only the base and at the subcutaneous level underneath the markings. For this reason, there is no relationship between breast volume and amount of anesthetic to be injected (Avelar 1993).

The first point to be infiltrated is the central segment of the inframammary crease followed by the subcutaneous layer of the external border of the breast. The lateral side of the chest and external border of the breasts are mainly innervated by the external branches of the intercostobrachial nerve.

Following the procedure, the base of the breast is then infiltrated, which means between the mammary tissue and the level of the pectoralis muscle. For good infiltration, I clamp the breast with one hand and at the same time a long needle is inserted using the other hand (Fig. 7.6a and b). This maneuver is very useful as the surgeon should feel the penetration of the needle at once. If there is any difficulty, insertion of the needle into the breast parenchyma should not continue, as it should be easily introduced into the connective tissue. Nevertheless, it is worth emphasizing that the parenchyma is heavily vascularized and any infiltration could reach a vessel and create an unpleasant situation.

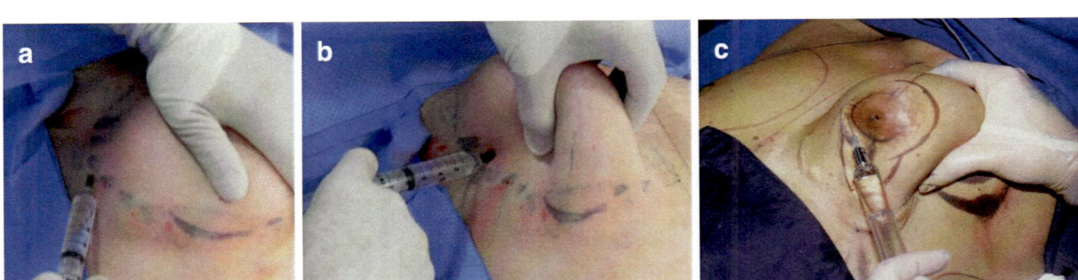

Fig. 7.6 Transoperative photos showing local infiltration on reduction mastoplasty. (**a**) Subcutaneous infiltration on external border of the breast to block endings of the intercostal branchial nerve as well as of the intercostal; (**b**) the breast is pulled foreword and using a long needle infiltration is done below the mammary gland and above the pectoralis muscle; (**c**) subdermal infiltration is done following surgical marking

As a final step, the subcutaneous plane corresponding to the technical markings below the areola are infiltrated, which is the most sensitive region (Fig. 7.6c). It is important to state that after infiltration, the period of analgesia lasts for a long time and the patient is not exposed to any suffering (Avelar 1993).

The other breast is infiltrated after the glandular resection has been performed on the first one. Following this systematization, infiltration is not overloaded, avoiding any risk of complications relevant to the methodology.

7.2.5 Glandular Resection

The base of the breast is grasped by the surgeon's assistant with two hands, but my preference is to employ an elastic rubber band all around to tie it up (Fig. 7.7).

I start the operation by making an incision circumscribing the areola followed by Schwartzman's (1930) procedure creating a massive and composite flap of the nipple–areola segment and mammary gland for maintenance of the blood supply to the nipple. Afterward, a 4-cm cutaneous incision is made with a knife into the submammary crease followed by dissection with scissors until the border of the glandular tissue is separated from the aponeurosis (Fig. 7.8). From this point, by gently digital undermining, the mammary gland is totally separated from the pectoralis muscle. This digital maneuver allows examination of breast tissue by direct palpation. Then, a wet compress is introduced through the opening to avoid bleeding during glandular resection. The breast is suspended by its top corner using a strong hulk, which is kept in the ideal position for glandular resection (Fig. 7.9). A curved incision is made below the nipple–areola region followed by two vertical incisions upward to separate the upper segment of the parenchyma, creating Pitanguy's "keel" with two wedges on each side (Fig. 7.9). Thus, consequently, two glandular columns are created, one medial and the other on the lateral side of the breast tissue (Fig. 7.10). The width of the "keel" and the thickness of the wedges at the base of the two columns show the degree of glandular resection provided (Fig. 7.11).

After glandular resection of one breast, anesthetic infiltration is performed on the opposite one according to the above description. Despite there being very little bleeding during such a pro-

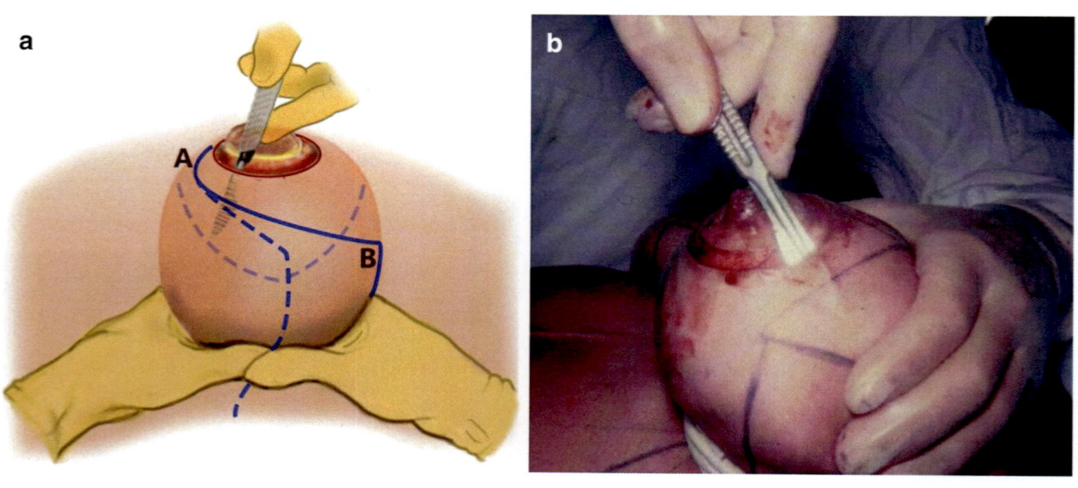

Fig. 7.7 Surgical marking is carried out and the base of the breast is held at its base to perform Schwartzmann's maneuver. (**a**) Drawing shows two hands holding the breast. (**b**) An elastic tape holding the breast while the maneuver is being performed with a knife

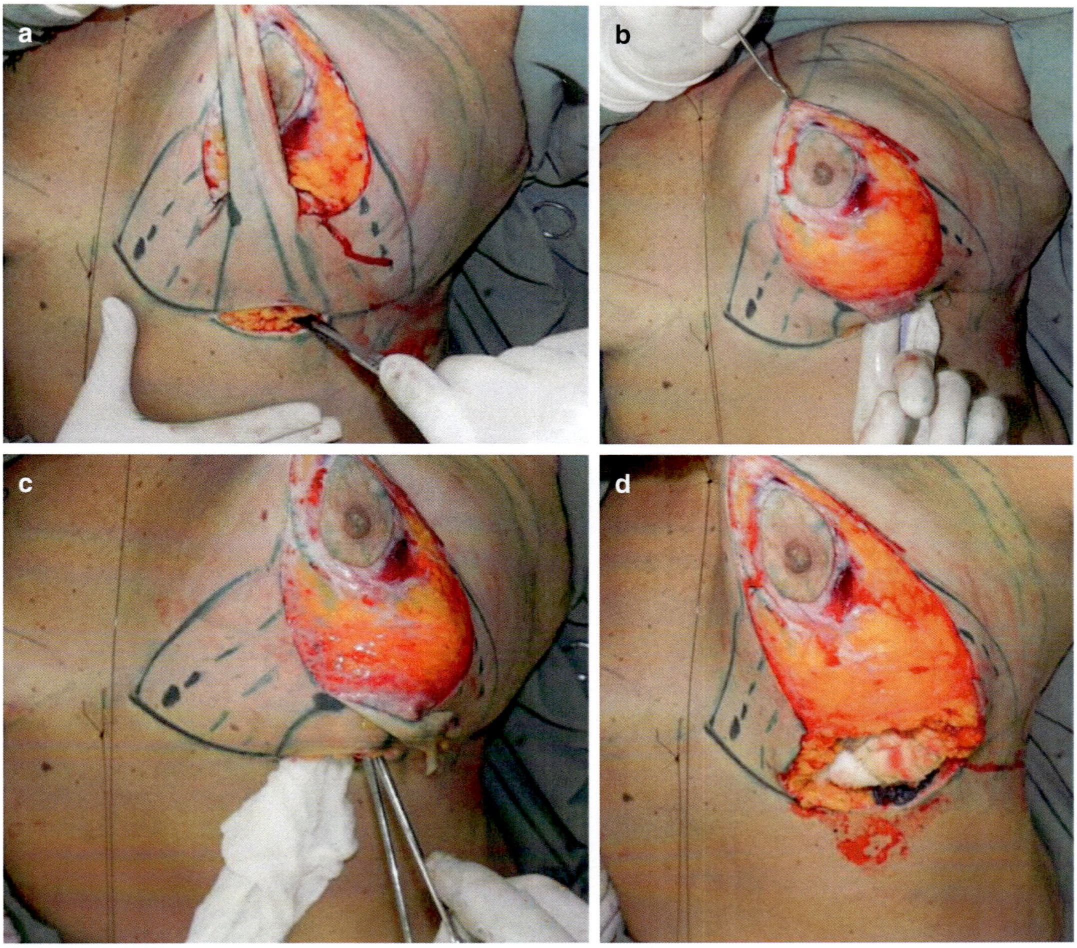

Fig. 7.8 Peroperative photos showing the area of skin, which is preserved according to my marking in comparison with Pitanguy's technique. The photos the undermining of the breast tissue from the pectoralis muscle. (**a**) A small incision is made in the submammary sulcus. (**b**) With a finger, undermining is carried out all over the submammary level. (**c**) Afterward, wet gauzes are introduced. (**d**) It can be seen that the skin is resected and the gauzes are placed below the mammary tissue and above the pectoralis muscle to avoid bleeding during surgery

cedure owing to anesthetic infiltration and to the digital dissection, hemostasis should be carefully performed. Following this systematization, no time is wasted and the volume of anesthetic infiltration is injected in two doses.

After careful hemostasis, the two columns are sutured. To facilitate closure my Z instrument is introduced under the remaining glandular tissue between the two columns (Fig. 7.12). The assistant pulls it up to suture the two columns to the aponeurosis of the pectoralis muscle. Afterward, a cutaneous temporary stitch is inserted to approximate points B and C on the midline of the submammary crease. Thus, it is possible to evaluate the size and shape of the future breast (Figs. 7.13 and 7.14). The excess skin is then pulled forward using special forceps to evaluate the amount to be removed (Fig. 7.13). I learned this maneuver from Pitanguy and Garcia (1972), as described by Noël (1928) and it is a very useful

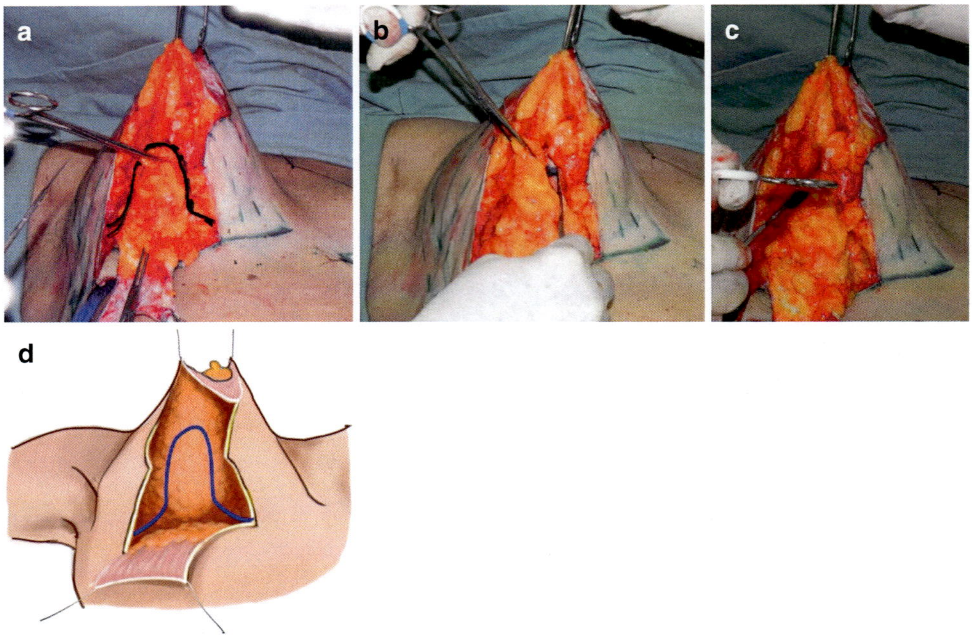

Fig. 7.9 Peroperative photos showing breast tissue resection as a "keel" following Pitanguy's technique. (**a**) Breast tissue to be resected is outlined. (**b**) The breast tissue is incised with a knife. (**c**) The "keel"-shaped resection. (**d**) Drawing shows the marking of breast tissue for a "keel" resection

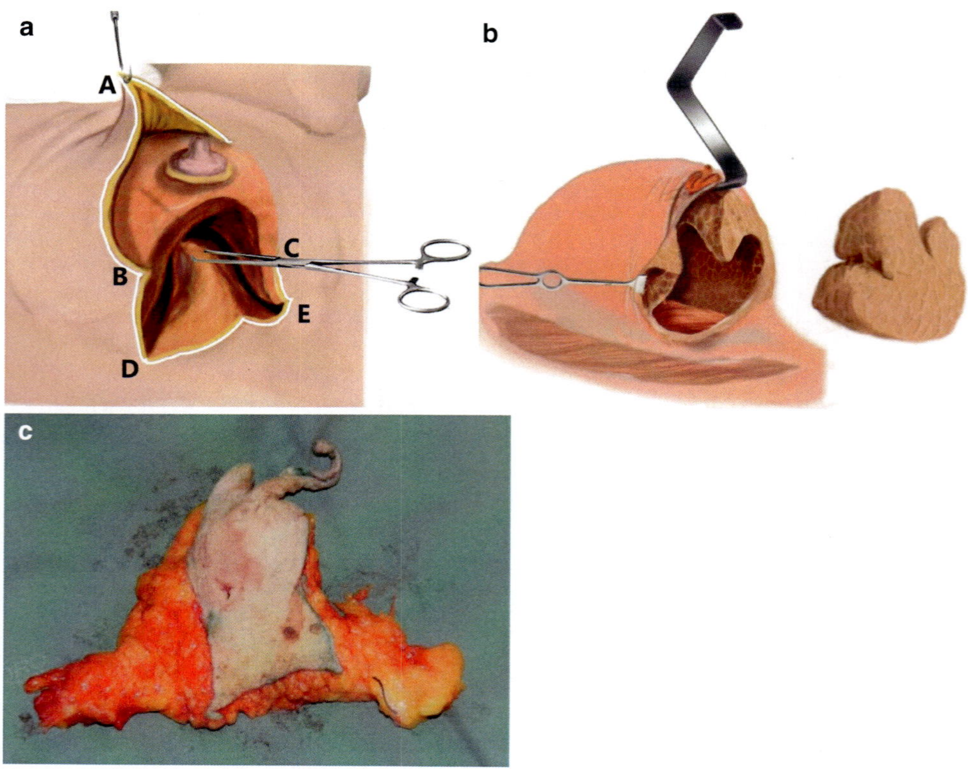

Fig. 7.10 Pitanguy's "keel" resection. (**a**) Drawing shows a "keel" resection held by forceps. (**b**) Drawing shows the breast after "keel" resection with my Z instrument introduced inside and pulling the breast upward. (**c**) Photo of the "keel" of mammary tissue and skin already removed

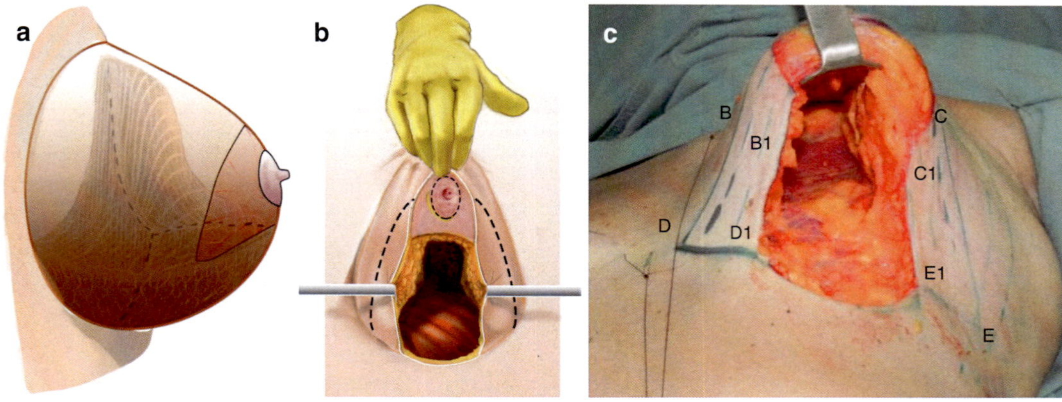

Fig. 7.11 Pitanguy's "keel" resection. (**a**) Drawing shows a perspective of the breast after "keel" resection in the center of the breast. (**b**) Drawing from the frontal view showing that through my marking, an extensive area of skin is not resected. (**c**) Per-operative photo from the frontal view where the inside of the breast can be seen after "keel" resection without any bleeding. The points B1, C1, D1, and E1 are marked according to my approach. The amount of skin that is not resected can be seen

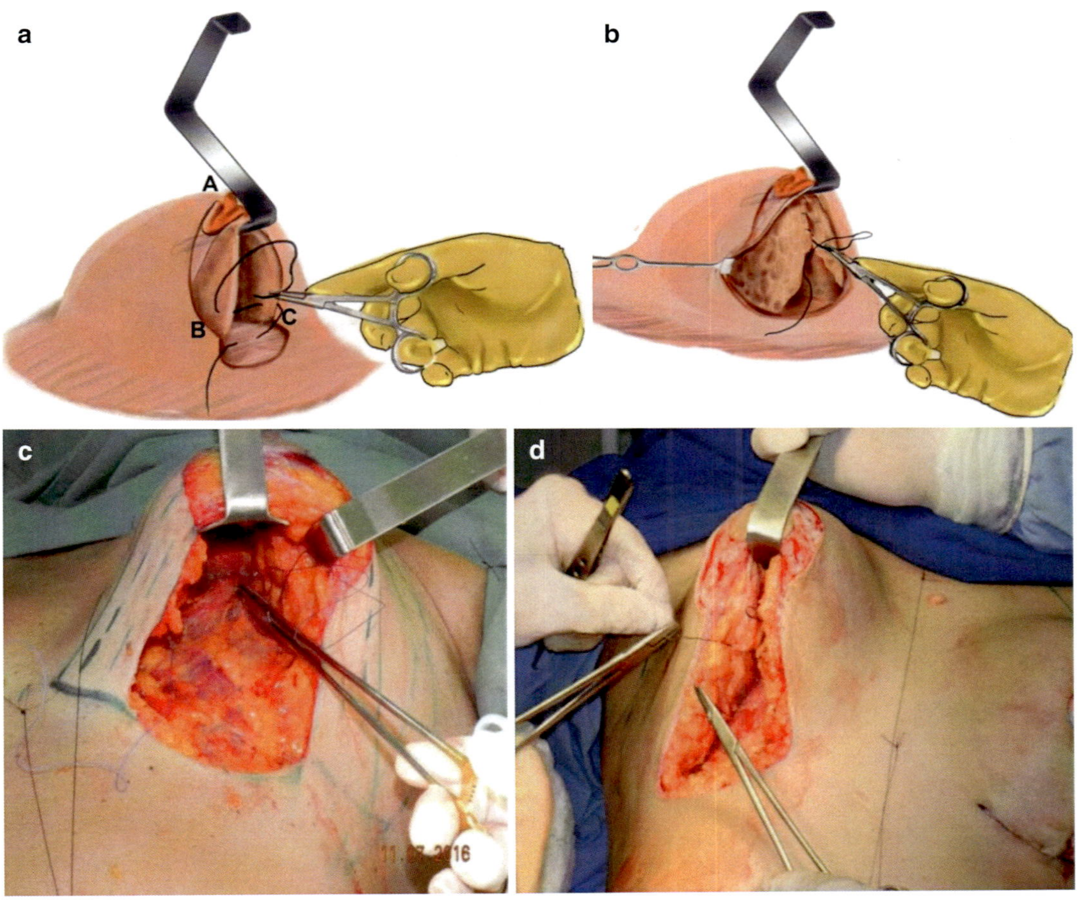

Fig. 7.12 Suturing of the two Pitanguy's columns created after resection of mammary tissue. (**a**) and (**b**) Drawings showing suture of the two columns. (**c**) and (**d**) Peroperative photos show the suturing of the two Pitanguy's columns created after breast tissue resection. (**e**) Scheme shows the suturing of the columns from the frontal view

e

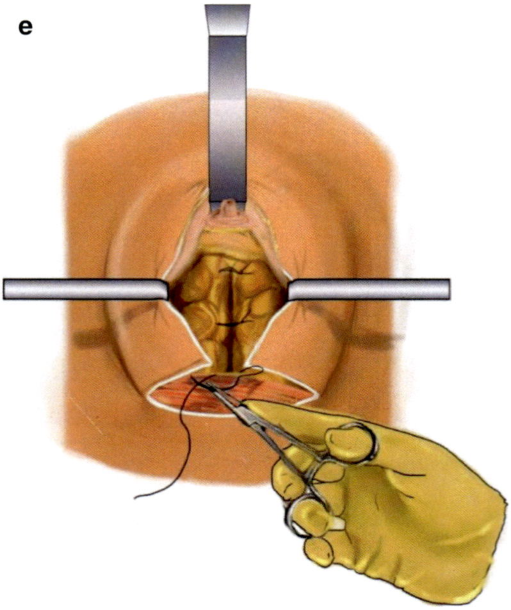

Fig. 7.12 (continued)

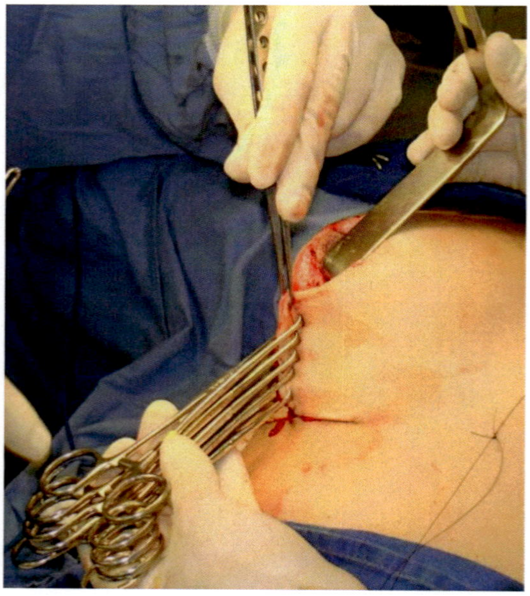

Fig. 7.13 Using my Z instrument introduced inside the breast, the NAC is pulled upward and the skin is de-epithelialized on both sides on vertical segment of the breast to create the dermal flap to be sutured. (**a**) Photo, oblique view of the right breast showing that the excess of skin was pulled forward and held by special forceps

procedure for adjusting content and container. I do not expect skin retraction, as described by Peixoto (1979).

Following the operation, I move to the other side of the operating table to perform the same procedure on the opposite breast. After inserting the temporary stitch on the opposite breast, it is mandatory to evaluate the two breasts concerning the size, shape, and position.

7.2.6 Repositioning the New Nipple–Areola Region

After temporary sutures are inserted, I perform dissection of the dermis to create two dermal flaps on each side of the vertical wound. The dermal flaps are sutured with isolated stitches, creating a dermal structure that works as a reinforcement of the vertical suture to adjust content and container (Avelar 1980, 1993). The dermal structure works as a plane to support the weight of the breast like a new skin brassiere. Afterward, using special forceps, the skin is pulled forward to evaluate the exact amount of excess to be resected according to Noël (1928) (Fig. 7.13). A running intra-dermal suture is inserted to close the wound. Afterward, the nipple–areola region is drawn on the vertices of the new breast using a special round marker. The new areolar area is de-epithelialized and the nipple–areola segment is then pulled from deep inside to the outside for suturing (Fig. 7.14).

7.2.6.1 Dressing After Surgery

Adhesive tapes are placed on the wound after internal suturing. Elastic tapes are applied covering both breasts similar to a brassiere and a garment is placed over it all. No drainage is used as there is no bleeding during surgery or “dead space”. Patients usually go home the next day with all postoperative instructions to avoid any strain on the upper limbs for at least 2 weeks. They return to my clinic 1 week after surgery when the first bandaging is removed and another one is placed and it is changed every 1 or 2 weeks

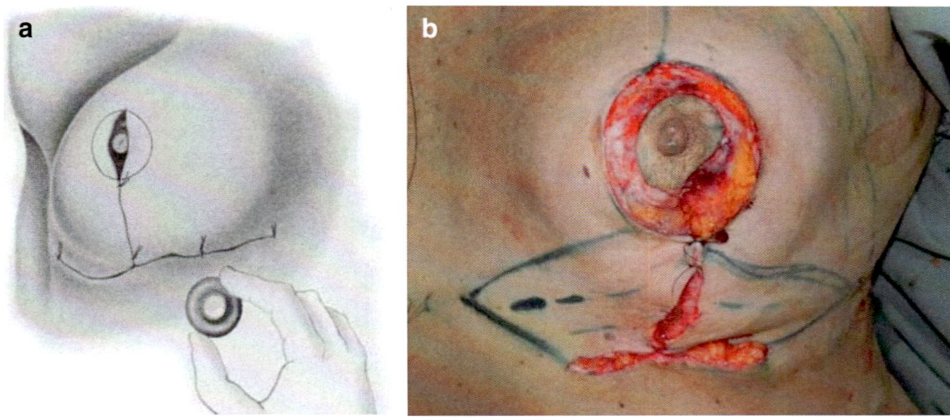

Fig. 7.14 Marking of the new NAC. (**a**) Drawing showing the technical marking. (**b**) On a peroperative photo the NAC can be seen already demarcated and a small scar on the submammary crease. Also, the extent of the skin that is preserved is demarcated

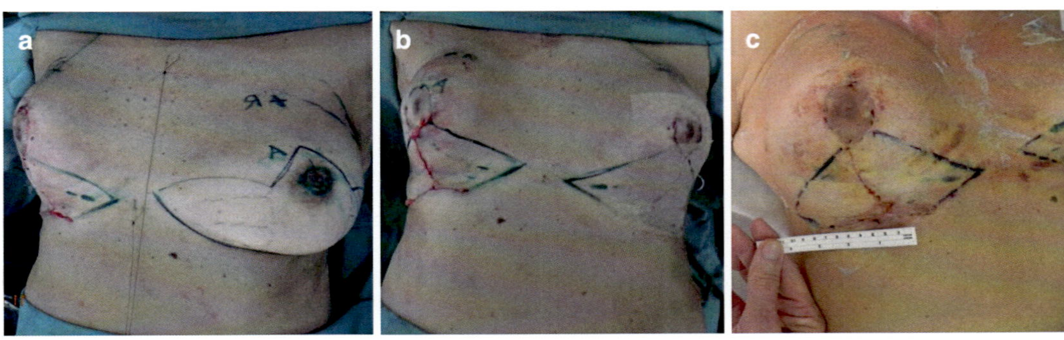

Fig. 7.15 Preservation of skin during reduction mastoplasty according to my approach in comparison with Pitanguy's technique. (**a**) Peroperative photo shows that reduction mastoplasty of the right breast has already been performed and on the left breast surgical marking can be seen. (**b**) Both breasts have been operated on, showing that an extensive area of skin has not been resected. (**c**) Same patient 1 week after the operation showing a very small scar on the submammary crease

for 2 months. No stitches are to be removed, as only internal suturing is performed.

7.3 Discussion

Every patient with breast abnormalities is looking for a better shape and size. On the other hand, it is a natural desire for a surgeon to expect to achieve those anatomical characteristics with reduced scars. It is important to emphasize that performing a mastoplasty with reduced scars should not jeopardize the size and shape of the breast after surgery. In fact, it is a balance between short scars and outstanding surgical results, as patients' are concerned about the shape of the breast and the surgeon is concerned with suitable final scars (Figs. 7.15 and 7.16).

Mastoplasty is an important field of plastic surgery that is constantly evolving, to fulfil not only the demands of the patients, but also the creativity of the plastic surgeons. Indeed, many past generations have left behind a fabulous arsenal of methods so that we can offer improved

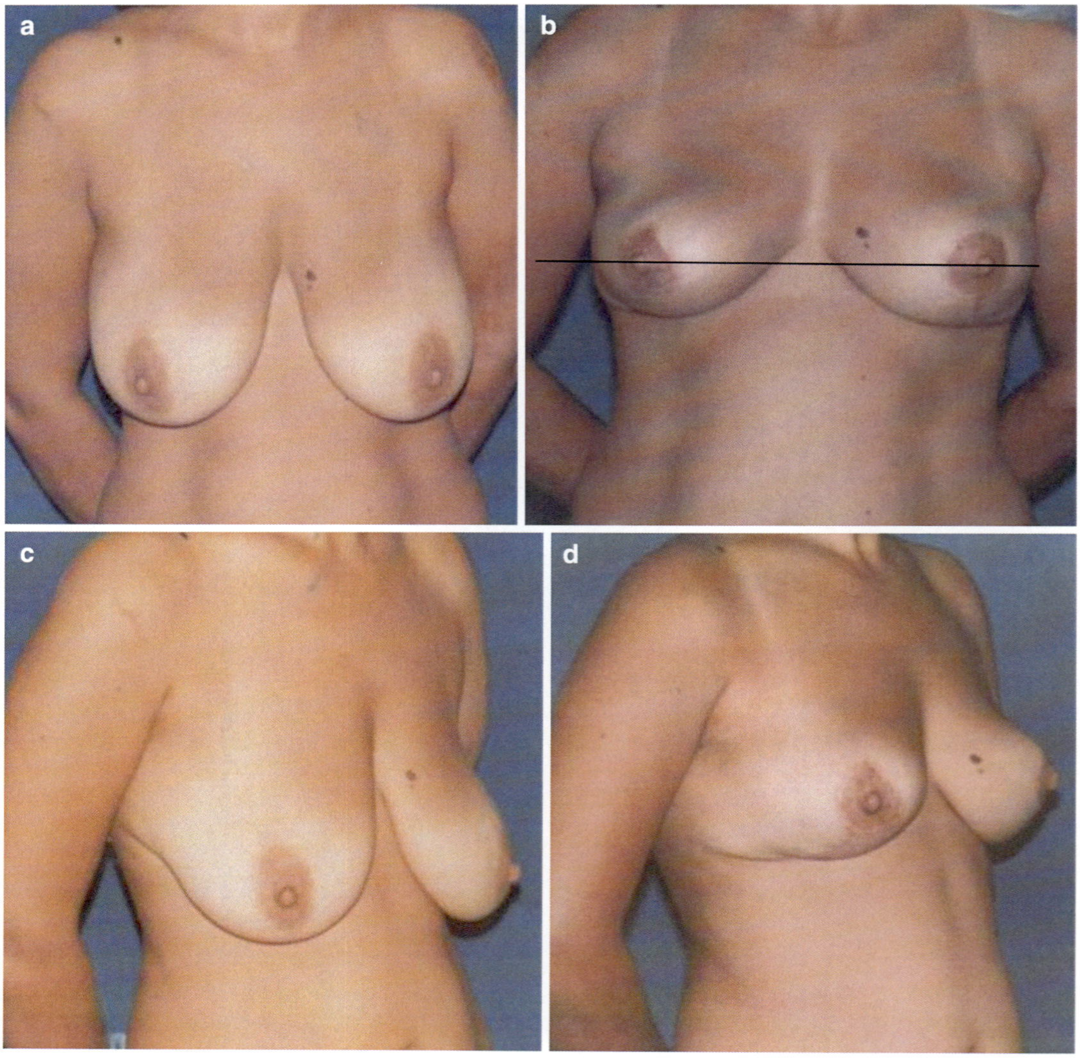

Fig. 7.16 A patient with very flabby, ptotic, and hypertrophic breasts before and after reduction mastoplasty. (**a**) and (**c**) Preoperative photos. (**b**) and (**d**) Photos of the same patient after the operation

results. Among the range of relevant factors, the struggle to reduce the scars resulting from mastoplasty can be highlighte. Nevertheless, despite the meritorious work and effort, a surgeon should not prioritize only one factor at the expense of achieving a good shape, external configuration, and especially preserving the functional aspects, where the sensitivity and lactation emerge with unusual meaning in the lives of patients (Figs. 7.17 and 7.18). Fortunately, this is bringing the universal notion of plastic surgeons who devote every effort to finding new operative solutions.

Blood transfusion used to be employed a long time ago, as heavy operative bleeding was reported by Maliniac (1945). However, since I started to employ local anesthesia combined with intravenous sedation under the care of an

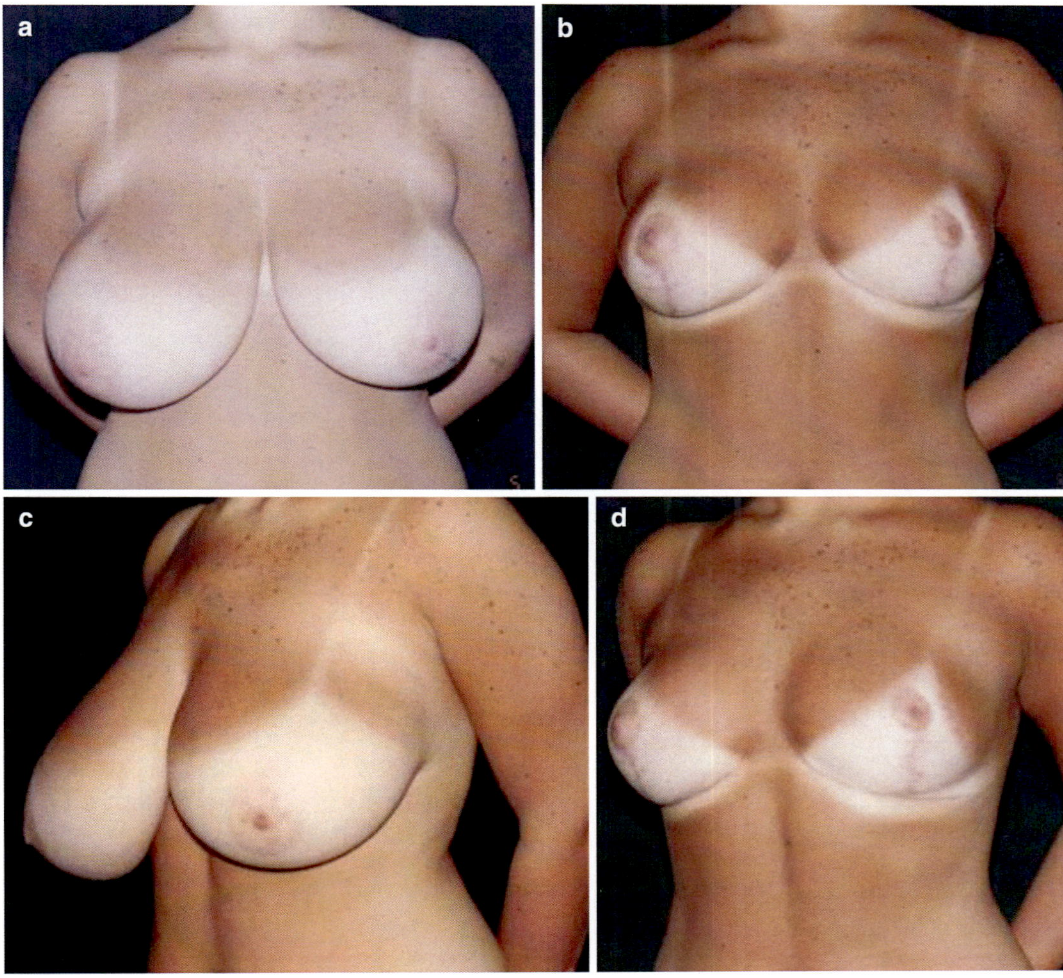

Fig. 7.17 A 21-year-old patient with very large hypertrophic breasts. (**a**) and (**c**) Preoperative photos. (**b**) and (**d**) Photos of the same patient after reduction mastoplasty showing a small scar on the submammary folds

anesthesiologist 35 years ago, I have not performed a blood transfusion. Another favorable situation is that I am not used to performing associated procedures through which patients may bleed too much during the operation.

No matter what the technique to be employed, the surgeon should aim to achieve harmony between the NAC and the breast, and this should be kept tightly balanced with the chest, and especially with the opposite breast. Here is a great challenge that is presented to us at each surgery and we need to achieve it every time. It is worth emphasizing that one failure in a single case may represent a small percentage in the wide sample of a surgeon, but for that patient it means 100%. Thus, we must work bearing in mind that it must always be achieved and that there are not many chances to repair any mistakes. Our great opportunity is the first time, and as such we incorporate all our knowledge, skill, attention, and care into all our surgical procedures.

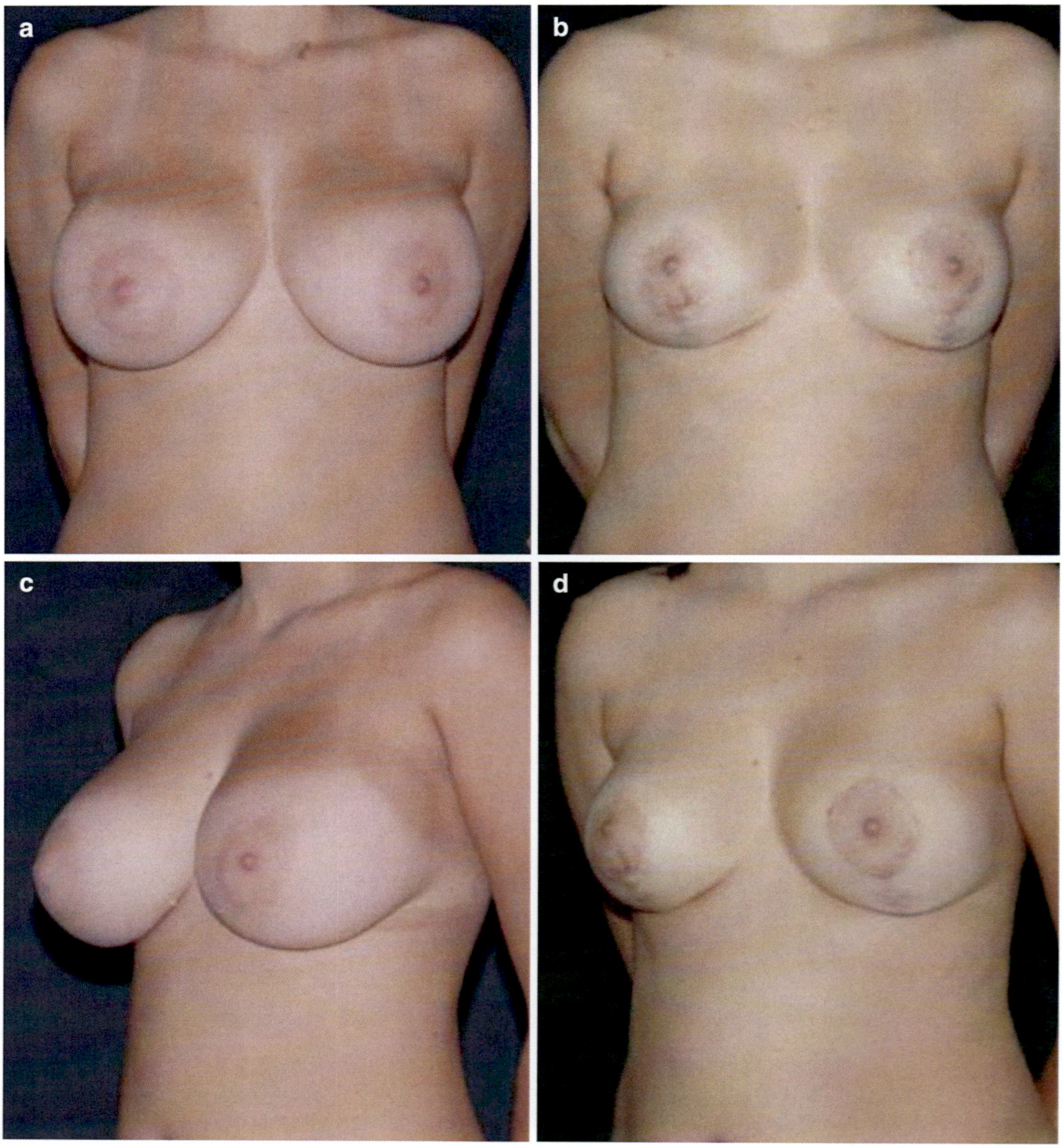

Fig. 7.18 A 24-year-old patient with hypertrophic breasts. (**a**) and (**c**) Preoperative photos. (**b**) and (**d**) Postoperative photos after reduction mastoplasty with small scars on the submammary folds

7.4 Complications

I described above that any surgeon may develop a new technique, but it is important to evaluate both the immediate postoperative complications and the long-term results. Fortunately, I had the privilege to be Prof. Pitanguy's resident during the period of my specialization when I had the opportunity to certify the efficiency of his technique. Thus, I bear testimony to the high level of his excellent results, which impressed me when I started my own practice. Therefore, some of the improvements in reduction mastoplasty I developed were based on his technique, which provided me with good surgical results. Probably for this reason, most of the major complications described in the medical literature did not occur in my patients. Among 1642 patients operated on during 43 years of my practice, some of the minor complications that occurred were: small hematoma formation (although careful hemostasis is achieved in all cases) and there is no "dead space," as there is never any undermining of skin flaps or other tissues; few patients presented sloughing of the areola (which healed secondarily, but in three patients, a skin graft from internal tissue as a donor area was performed); two patients with very fatty breasts presented nipple necrosis (which required reconstruction); some patients with very flabby breasts with excessive striae presented some degree of recurrent ptosis at later follow-up. Postoperative infection and dehiscence of the wound occurred in a few cases, although it has having take much care during surgery in addition to the routine use of prophylactic antibiotics.

Hypertrophic scars used to occur when I started my practice, but nowadays it is very rare because of the smooth suturing with no tension owing to internal stitches. Asymmetric breasts may occur after mastoplasty, but it is very rare among my patients, as surgical planning and marking are carefully carried out. A patient presented temporary alterations on the left arm due to too much stretching causing distention of the motor nerve, as the anesthesiologist exaggerated the position of the arms. The patient recovered all movement after a few days. It is advisable that the surgeon be attentive to the position of the arms during the operation.

As I have never utilized prefabricated patterns in my method, my final results achieve a good balance between the two breasts at the end of the operation, even in cases of severe asymmetry. I do not recommend employing prefabricated patterns as they do not take into consideration the individuality of the patients and the asymmetry of the skin, subcutaneous panniculus, and mammary gland.

Conclusions

The aesthetic appearance of the size and shape of the breasts in harmony with body contouring is the aim of mastoplasty procedures. These aspects of the breasts are related to historical and cultural factors of the time and to individual criteria. In this sense, when analyzing the aesthetic concept of the mastoplasty, which is performed to modify the shape of the breast, the focus should be on the subjective point of view of the patient and the surgeon's artistic creativity.

Reduction mastoplasty is performed under local anesthesia combined with intravenous sedation under the care of an anesthesiologist. The procedure is a variation of Pitanguy's technique leaving a short scar on the submammary crease, another vertical one with reinforcement of the dermis to provide adequate support of the weight of the breasts, and a periareolar scar. Resection of the mammary gland is performed as Pitanguy's "keel" in the central part of the breast and another segment on the base. There is no undermining of the panniculus and no "dead space". For this reason, there is no bleeding during or after the operation. No drainage is employed.

References

Avelar JM (1980) Creation of a dermoadiposeglandular flap with superior pedicle on mastopexy with or without silicone prosthesis inclusion. (Criação de retalho dermo-adiposo-glandular de pedículo superior nas mastopexia com ou sem inclusão de próteses de silicone). In: Brazilian symposium on breast surgery. sponsered by Brazilian society of plastic surgery—Region of São Paulo, August, São Paulo

Avelar JM (1993) Reduction mastoplasty under local anesthesia. (Mastoplastia redutora sob anestesia local) In: Avelar JM (ed) Loco-regional anesthesia on aesthetic surgery—(Anestesia Loco-regional em cirurgia estética)—Editora Hipócrates; São Paulo, pp 244–260

Avelar JM (2013) Surgical principles and planning for ear reconstruction. In: Avelar JM (ed) Ear reconstruction, vol 3. Springer, Heidelberg, pp 15–31

Avelar JM (2016) Surgical principles and classification of abdominolipoplasty or lipoabdominoplasty. In: Avelar JM (ed) New concepts on abdominoplasty and further applications, 3. Springer, Heidelberg, pp 31–43. doi:10.1007/978-3-319-27851-3_3

Maliniac JW (1945) Two-stage mammaplasty in relation to blood supply. Am J Surg 68:55

Noël A (1928) Aesthetische Chirurgie der Weiblichen Brust. Ein neues Verfahren zur Korrektur der Hängebrust. Med Welt 2:51

Peixoto GR (1979) Reduction mammaplasty: a personal method. In: Ely JF (ed) Transactions of the 7th international congress of plastic and reconstructive surgery, Cartgraf, São Paulo

Pitanguy I (1959) Breast hypertrophy. In: Wallace AB (ed) Transactions of the international society of plastic surgeons, 2nd congress, London and Edinburgh, E. & S. Livingstone

Pitanguy I (1960) Breast hypertrophy. In: Wallace AB (ed) Transactions of the international society of plastic surgeons, second congress. Edinburgh, E. & S. Livingstone, p 509

Pitanguy I, Garcia LC (1972) Important aspects of technical personnel in mammaplastia (Aspectos importantes de técnica pessoal em mammaplastia). Bol Soc Cir Plast Reconstr Cordoba 4:7

Schwarzmann E (1930) Technik der mammaplastik. Chirurg 2:932

Strömbeck JO (1960) Mammaplasty. Report of a new technique based on the two pedicle procedure. Br J Plast Surg 13(1):79

Wise RJ (1956) A preliminary report on a method of planning the mammaplasty. Plast Reconstr Surg 17:367

8 Reduction Mammaplasty in a Single Central Block

João Erfon, Claudio Mauricio M. Rodrigues, and Guilherme Teles

8.1 Introduction

In the 1980s, reduction mammoplasty procedures underwent a number of changes to reduce scarring, although these changes also resulted in a loss of form (Peixoto 1980, 1984). However, the concepts had a significant influence on the development of breast reduction surgery. New techniques have been investigated with the objective of achieving good breast shape with less scarring (Arié 1957; Bozola et al. 1987; Sepúlveda 1981). These techniques aim to reduce scarring and tension in the sutures by appropriately adjusting the new parenchyma with the skin that surrounds it (Erfon et al. 1989, 1992, 1996). However, the size of the scar is only reduced within the limits of possible skin contraction, which varies among patients.

Depending on the breast volume to be resected and the degree of ptosis of the breasts, incisions can be planned so that the scars end in an inverted T or vertical manner. The same principles of parenchyma resection use a single central block with the superior vascular pedicle and the nipple-areola complex (NAC) on the top. In this technique, the breasts are not modeled using tension on the skin but by proper fitting to the breast cone, which promotes more satisfactory results.

8.2 Method

We conducted a retrospective study of female patients who underwent breast reduction using the single central block technique from July 1985 to December 2015. Patients were classified into four groups according the size of the breast (Bozola et al. 1987; Franco and Rebello 1977), with the procedure adapted for each group. Three basic principles were followed: (1) modeling the breast parenchyma in a single central block, separated from the skin, without disconnecting the NAC; (2) creating a pedicle of the upper base, as described by Weiner et al. (1973) and modified by this author (Erfon et al. 1989, 1992); (3) reducing scarring using retraction of the skin and marking incisions that match the size and mounting of the parenchyma separated from the skin (Chiari 1992; Erfon et al. 1992, 1996).

Work performed at ArtClinic.

J. Erfon, M.D. (✉)
Department of Surgery, Walter Cantídio Hospital of the Federal University of Ceará, Rua Atilano de Moura, Fortaleza, CE 60810-180, Brazil
e-mail: erfon@artclinic.com.br

C.M.M. Rodrigues, M.D.
Unichristus University, Rua Atilano de Moura, Fortaleza, CE 60810-180, Brazil

G. Teles, M.D.
Defeitos da Face Hospital and Santa Cruz Hospital, Rua Atilano de Moura, Fortaleza, CE 60810-180, Brazil

J.M. Avelar (ed.), *Breast Surgery*, https://doi.org/10.1007/978-3-319-54115-0_8

8.3 Technique

The marking of the patient starts in an orthostatic position. A dotted line from the sternal notch to the xiphoid is marked and serves to verify the symmetry between the two breasts (Fig. 8.1a). The submammary sulcus is then defined. Point A, which is the uppermost point of the new NAC, is marked at 2 cm above the projection of the inframammary sulcus (Fig. 8.1a, b).

After the patient is anesthetized under sedation, in addition to local anesthesia or general anesthesia, her back is elevated to 45°. Starting at point A, two lines ranging from 5 to 9 cm in length are drawn toward each side of the NAC, thus defining the points B and C by forming a triangle (Fig. 8.1a, b). This marking defines the upper pedicle and vascular flap. The base of the pedicle can be expanded using a semi-circular line outside the "triangle," unifying points A, B,

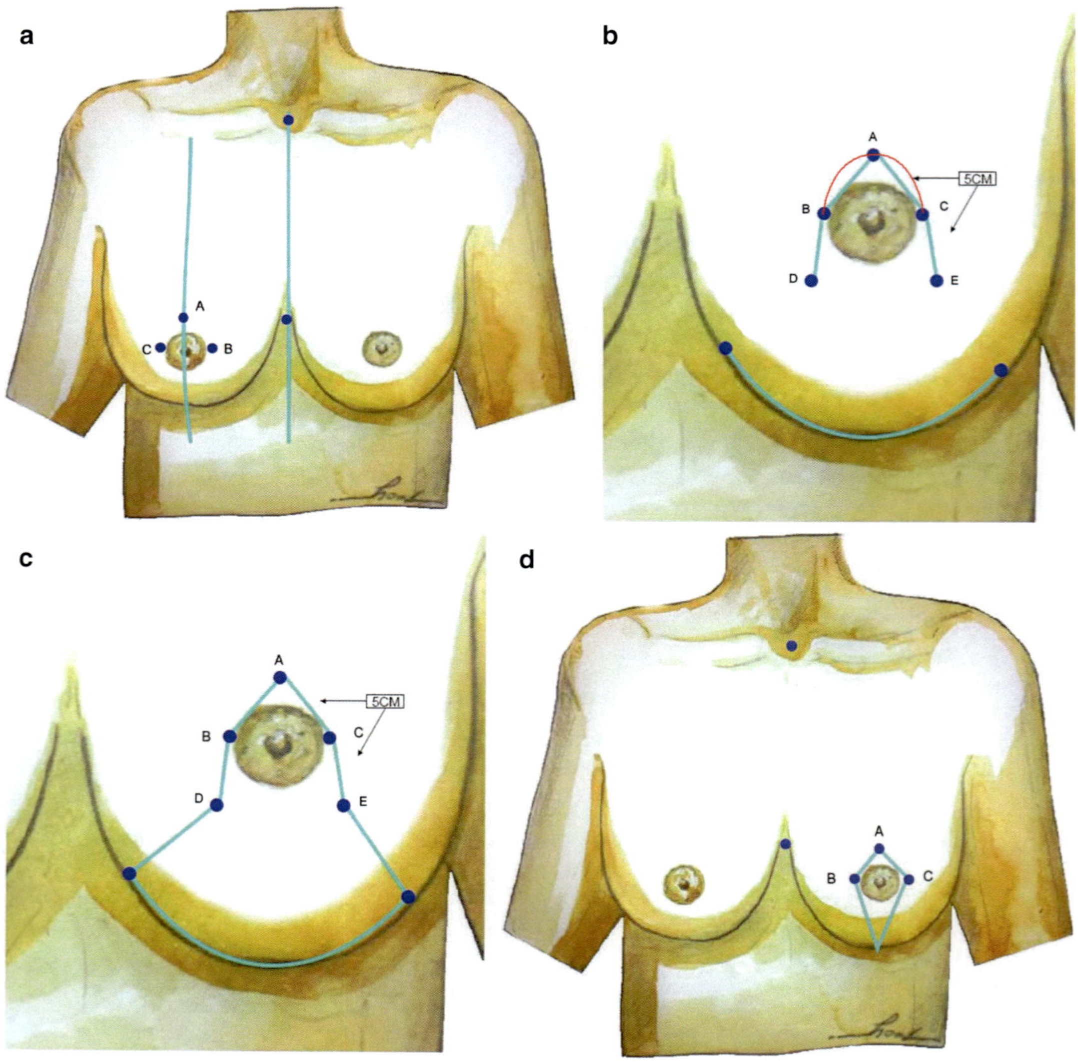

Fig. 8.1 Planning and marking the incisions. (**a**) Marking of the breasts while standing, starting with the previous midline of the body and points A, B, and C. (**b**) Marking the other incisions (see text). (**c**) Completed marking of the inverted T. (**d**) V marking for periareolar and vertical scars

and C (Fig. 8.1b). When the NAC is very lateralized the distance between A and C can be increased relative to the distance from A to B, allowing greater medial rotation of the same (Fig. 8.1c).

Two straight lines, each 5 cm in length, are marked starting from points B and C down, with a small inclination between them depending on the amount of skin to be resected (Fig. 8.1b). Two lines starting from the distal ends of these segments are joined to the submammary fold so that their dimensions, together, are approximately equal to the marking line in the same groove (Fig. 8.1b). The symmetry of the marking in the contralateral breast is created using the anterior midline of the body, keeping an equal distance between it and the medial incision of the drawing on each breast. This is the inverted T marking (Fig. 8.1c) .When the distal ends of the two straight 5-cm segments are very close to one another, the marking to the submammary sulcus can be concluded in a V (Fig. 8.1d).

In patients under general anesthesia, the retromammary space is infiltrated with a saline solution (adrenaline saline 1:500 mL). In patients who received a local anesthetic and sedation, the anesthesia solution used is one ampoule (1 mL) adrenaline (1:1000) in 160 mL saline in addition to 40 mL of 2% xylocaine.

The surgery begins with de-epithelialization of the area around the NAC, extending 2 cm below it. Then, a total skin excision is carried out in the previously marked area in the lower pole of the breast (Fig. 8.2c).The medial and lateral skin flaps (2 cm thick) are dissected. The dissection continues to 1 or 2 cm above points B and C, going to the muscle fascia (Fig. 8.2d). Dissection of the retromammary space is performed by completely freeing the breast from the thorax plate, resulting in a single central block that comprises the breast parenchyma and the NAC, maintained by the upper pedicle (Fig. 8.2c) (Davison et al. 2007).

The breast volume is reduced in the external and medial quadrants (in minor amounts) by keeping the entire distal and posterior extent of the single central block (Fig. 8.2c, d). This block needs sufficient tissue to create the new breast (Fig. 8.2a, b, e-h). Then, the single central block is attached to the thorax in the new planned position using two stitches with 3-0 colorless mononylon: one stitch at the distal end of the flap fixed to the center of the submammary fold and another on the back part of the block, securing it to the muscle fascia at the posterior projection of the NAC in the new position (Fig. 8.2c, d).The dermal suture is started with three stitches using 3-0 colorless mononylon, uniting the skin flaps using 5-cm straight lines, which form the vertical scar. The first stitch joins the distal ends of these two segments to the submammary sulcus, the second stitch joins points B and C, and the third stitch joins the middle part (Fig. 8.3g). The symmetry can be checked at this point of the surgical procedure because the NACs are fully positioned (Fig. 8.3g, h) (Lassus 1987).

The suture is concluded using subdermal stitches with 4-0 colorless mononylon in the skin flaps and 5-0 colorless nylon in the NAC. Monocryl can also be used. External sutures are rarely used. Bandaging is carried out with dry gauze and a special brassiere that is used for 2 months.

In cases of mastopexy, the same technique can be used to remove only the skin and retain all lipoglandular tissue for the formation of a new breast. In such cases, the tissue of the side quadrants is used and sutured to the central block of the breast to increase its volume (Fig. 8.3c-f).

8.4 Results

From July 1985 to December 2015, a total of 2005 mammoplasties were performed using this technique: 1531 reduction mammoplasties and 474 mastopexies. The average patient age was 46 years (range: 17–75 years). The average resected volume was 350 g per side, ranging from 0 g in mastopexies to 1550 g in breast reduction.

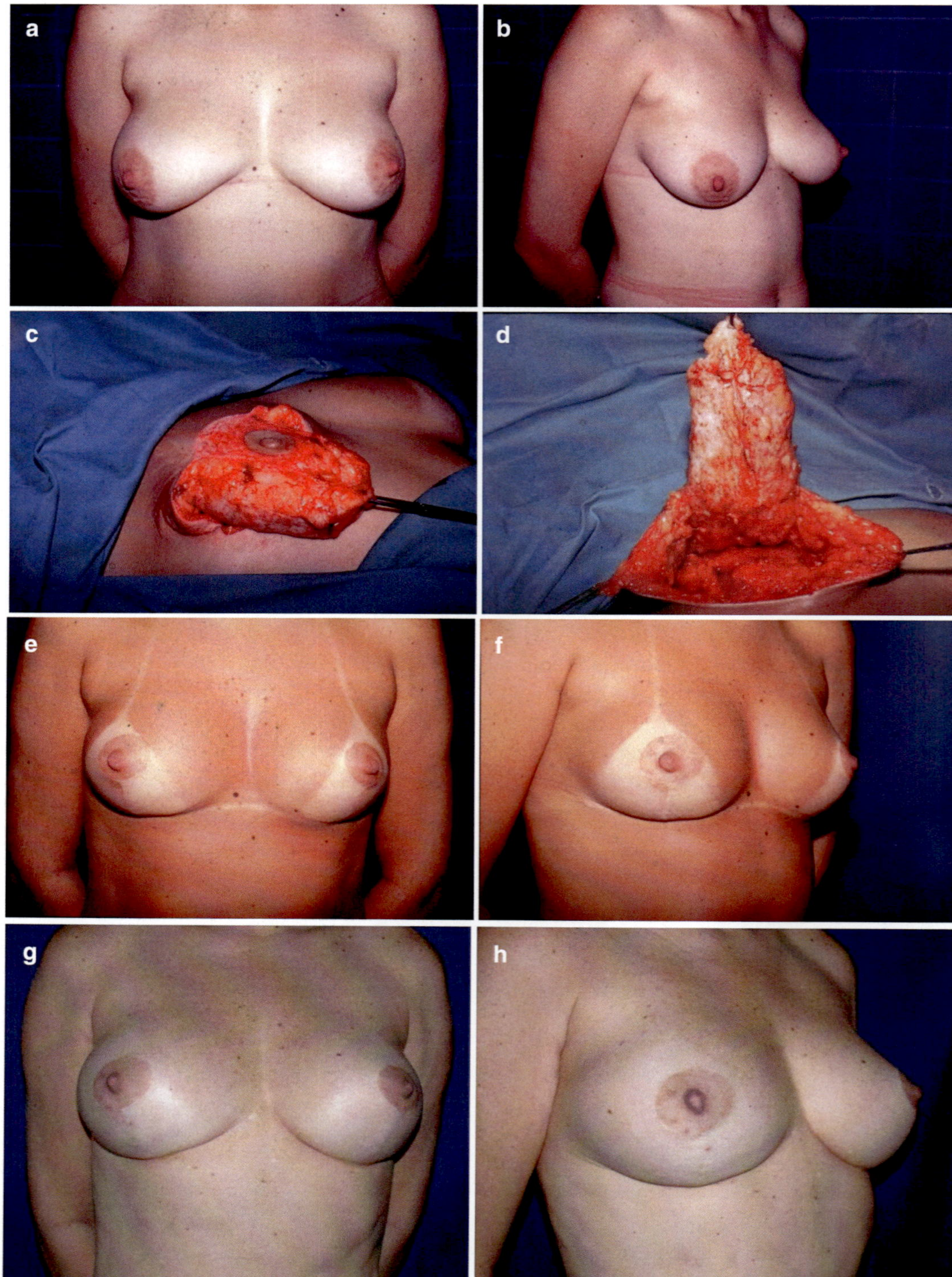

Fig. 8.2 Before, during, and after mammoplasty using a single block technique. (**a** and **b**) Preoperative breast hypertrophy. (**c** and **d**) Intraoperative showing a single central block of mammary parenchyma, with the NAC at the top. (**e** and **f**) Six months postoperative. (**g** and **h**) 19 years postoperative

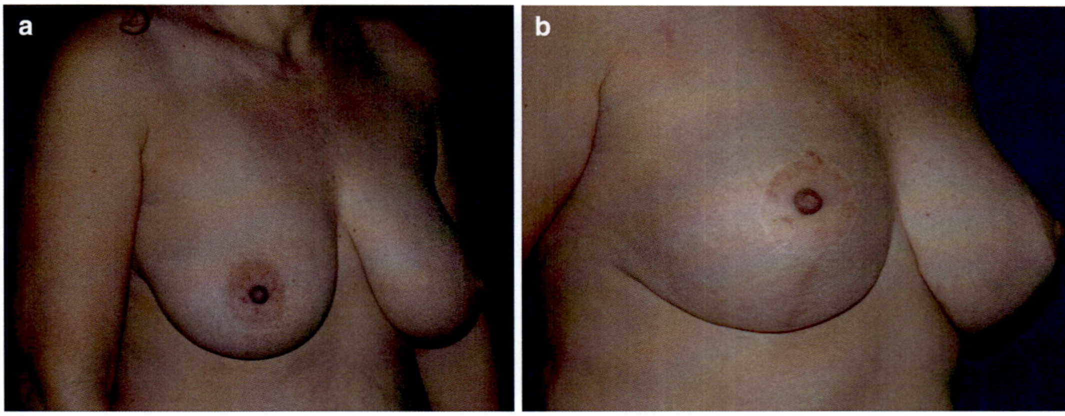

Fig. 8.3 Preoperative and late postoperative hypertrophy and ptosis mammary. (**a**) Preoperative hypertrophy and ptosis mammary. (**b**). Postoperative reduction mammoplasty, 6-month follow-up

The observed results are superior to those obtained previously using other techniques by the same author (McKissock 1972; Pitanguy 1967, 1976; Strombeck 1960). The benefits of this technique include the following: easy shaping of the breast into a conical form, good maintenance of the NAC and skin flap vascularization, preservation of breast sensitivity and the possibility of breastfeeding, good-quality scars, reduced stress on the skin flaps, and a natural and easy rise of the NAC, which is held in its new position by a breast tissue block posteriorly and inferiorly to it. An additional advantage is the possibility of greater resection of glandular tissue in the upper lateral quadrant, allowing for better shaping of the breast cone (Figs.8.2c, d).

8.5 Discussion

Providing patients with the desired physical and psychological change, with a seamless integration between body and mind, has been a constant concern of the senior author. Breast lift surgery is a body contouring technique that is able to provide aesthetic improvement, in addition to psychological and physical improvement related to ptosis and breast hypertrophy. Common complaints of back pain, bra indentations on the shoulders, and dermatitis in the submammary folds are resolved or mitigated after this procedure, thus improving the quality of life of these patients (Kececi et al. 2015; Spector and Karp 2007).

Mammoplasty techniques can be classified mainly by use of pedicle vascularization of the NAC and the final position of the scar. Ultimately, the choice of technique depends on the experience of the surgeon, the expectations of the patient, the positioning and extent of the scars, and the degree of hypertrophy and ptosis of the breasts.

Many techniques for breast reduction have been described, indicating the difficulty of this type of surgery (Erfon et al. 1992, 1996; Weiner et al. 1973). A group of authors emphasized the form and shape of the breast parenchyma (Lima 1979; McKissock 1972; Pitanguy 1967, 1976; Souza Pinto et al. 1983; Strombeck 1960), whereas others were concerned about the extent of the scars (Arié 1957; Peixoto 1980, 1984; Sepúlveda 1981). A third group most valued surgical planning and the marking of the skin (Benelli 1988, 1990; Bozola et al. 1987; Wise et al. 1963).

As a basis for techniques of modern mammoplasty, Lexer (1912) described partial resection of the inferior pole by implementing the NAC and final scar in an inverted T shape. In 1930, Schwarzman described periareolar de-epithelialization and the importance of preserving the dermis for vascularization of the NAC—concepts that are still used today. In 1942, Thorek carried out amputation of the lower pole of the breast and grafting of the NAC in large breasts, where the pedicle elevation of the NAC to its desired end position was considered unlikely. In 1957, Arié described the superior pedicle technique with periareolar de-epithelialization, NAC implementation, and closing in an inverted T shape. The latter has been modified and become better known through the publications of Pitanguy (1967, 1976), who described in detail the marking of the breast with predetermined lines, breast construction, and positioning of the NAC. In 1960, Strombeck introduced the concept of a bipediculated flap in a horizontal form—an idea that was later reinforced by McKissock (1972) who used a bipedicled flap in its vertical form. Skoog (1963) and Silveira-Neto (1976) described, respectively, the upper lateral and upper medial flaps. The inferior pedicle was first described in 1976 by Jurado (1979) and, soon after, by Robbins (1977); it then gained popularity because of its versatility and reliability. All of the above techniques underwent modifications from their original forms to become the currently most widely used techniques—each with its indications, advantages, and disadvantages. Weiner et al. (1973) described his technique with a higher single dermal pedicle to implement the NAC in cases of subcutaneous mastectomy, breast reduction, and breast lift (Weiner et al. 1973).

Breast reduction is one of the most difficult procedures in plastic surgery. It aims to obtain the result of a new breast with a beautiful shape, adequate volume, well-positioned NAC, and preserved vascularization and sensitivity (Orlando and Guthrie 1975). Many techniques have been described, but a movement in the direction of scar reduction began in the 1980s—sometimes at the expense of form and shape, which had always been prioritized by most authors, regardless of the extent of the scars (McKissock 1972; Pitanguy 1967, 1976). In 1985, the senior author of this chapter had a new idea, prioritizing not only the form and the scars, but also—and primarily—preservation of the functions of the breast (Erfon et al. 1989, 1992, 1996).

For Abramo (2012), maintaining the vascularization and the sensitivity of the NAC was primordial using the superior dermal pedicle (Abramo 2012). Agbenorku et al. (2012) concluded that breast reduction eased many of the physical and psychological symptoms in a group of patients with gigantomastia in Ghana (Agbenorku et al. 2012). Chiummariello et al. (2008) investigated the possibility of breastfeeding by comparing four different pedicles for breast reduction; the superior pedicle was more favored for postsurgical breastfeeding. His results showed that infants could be breastfed by 60.7% of patients whose technique used the superior pedicle, 55.1% of the lateral pedicle, 48% of the medial pedicle, and 43.5% of the inferior pedicle (Chiummariello et al. 2008).

Van Deventer et al. (2008) described necrosis of the NAC as a serious complication that can occur in the hands of experienced surgeons (Van Deventer et al. 2008). Other authors reported an incidence ranging from 0.8% to 2.1% for complete necrosis of the NAC and 7.3% for partial necrosis of the NAC (Van Deventer et al. (2008). Karsidag et al. (2011) suggested the use of a free graft of the NAC associated with a dermoglandular pedicle superior base to obtain better results in the shape of the breasts, as well as reduce necrosis of the NAC, in cases of gigantomastia and severe ptosis (Karsidag et al. 2011). Foustanos et al. (2011) advocated for a change in the upper pedicle of Pitanguy's technique to facilitate lifting of the NAC in cases of gigantomastia and dense breast parenchyma. This technique makes two flaps that overlap, a medial pedicle nourished by internal intercostal vessels on the other side and vascularized by the lateral thoracic vessels (Foustanos et al. 2011).

Mammoplasty using a central single block is easy to plan and perform, even for new surgeons. It allows for a final result that is within the preoperative expectations. The position of the NAC and other incisions may be easily changed during the procedure, if necessary, by the flexibility of the marking. Maintaining a single central block consisting of mammary parenchyma and NAC facilitates the modeling of a new breast and its rise (NAC), which occurs naturally in its new position without the need for traction as in other techniques. It is necessary, however, to leave enough tissue volume inferiorly and posteriorly to the NAC, because the skin flaps are very thin (about 2 cm in thickness) and do not add much to the new breast volume. The NAC is on top of the central single block, without tension, when the appropriate tissue volume is left (Fig. 8.3g, h).The single central block of tissue also helps obtain symmetry between the breasts because it is very easy to identify specific differences in these flaps. When a higher rise is necessary for the NAC, the single central flap should be longer, narrower, and thicker (Fig. 8.2c, d).

8.6 Complications

Mammoplasty has reported complication rates ranging from 5% to 30% (Fischer et al. 2014). Complications can be classified as early or late, as well as major or minor, depending on the need to revise surgical or invasive procedures. Typical early complications include bruising, partial necrosis of the skin or fat, slough of the NAC, wound dehiscence, and infection. The most common late complications are hypertrophic scarring, asymmetry, hypertrophy recurrence, abnormal sensitivity of the NAC, and breastfeeding failure. Clinical factors such as age, obesity, diabetes, hypertension, and smoking and surgical factors such as resected breast volume and duration of surgery are associated with higher rates of complications.

Using the technique described in this chapter, steatonecrosis was observed at the most distal end of the flap in 45 (2.24%) patients. There were no cases of NAC necrosis. Bruising occurred in 5 patients (0.24%) and seroma in 82 (4.08%) patients. Dehiscence in the inverted T was not very frequent because there is no tension over the skin flaps in this technique (compared with other techniques that shape the breasts with the skin flaps); it occurred in 65 (3.24%) patients. One case of infection led to a 2-cm necrosis of the skin on the edges of the vertical scar; it required reoperation for wound closure and adjustment according to the contralateral breast. The senior author of this paper experienced two cases (0.09%) of partial necrosis of the NAC to a minimum extent, which healed by secondary intention. Reoperations were performed in 95 (4.73%) patients for skin adjustments or further reductions in volume. In most cases, the review was prompted by the vertical incision scar.

Conclusion

Mammoplasty is one of the most difficult procedures in plastic surgery. The aim of this surgery is to achieve a new breast with a beautiful shape, adequate volume, a well-positioned NAC, and preserved vascularization and sensitivity. The technique described in this chapter uses a single central block with an upper vascular pedicle, incorporating the breast parenchyma with the NAC. The advantages of this procedure include ease of modeling the breast into a cone shape; ease of lifting the NAC; good preservation of vascularization in the NAC and skin flaps; preservation of breast sensitivity (which can be identified using simple tests of tactile sensitivity); preservation of breastfeeding function; good-quality scars; reduced stress on the skin flaps; and natural rise of NAC, which is kept in its new position by a breast tissue block that is left inferiorly and posteriorly to it. The surgery is easy to plan and perform, with very satisfactory aesthetic results. Thus, it can be an appealing surgical option for cases of breast reduction and/or mastopexy.

References

Abramo AC (2012) A superior vertical dermal pedicle for the nipple-areola: an alternative for severe breast hypertrophy and ptosis. Aesthetic Plast Surg 36:134–139

Agbenorku P, Agamah G, Agbenorku M, Obeng M (2012) Reduction mammaplasty in a developing country: a guideline for plastic surgeons for patient selection. Aesthetic Plast Surg 36:91–96

Arié G (1957) Una Nueva Técnica de Mastoplastica. Ver Lat Americana Cir Plástica 3:23–28

Benelli L (1988) Technique de plastie mamaire: le "round block". Rev Fr Chir Esthet 50:7

Benelli L (1990) A new periareolar mammaplasty: the "round block" technique. Aesthetic Plast Surg 14(2):93–100

Bozola AR et al (1987) Sistematização de Mamaplastia em "L". Revista Soc Bras Cir Plástica 2(1):13–33

Chiari A Jr (1992) The L short-scar mammaplasty: a new approach. Plast Reconstr Surg 90:233–246

Chiummariello S, Cigna E, Buccheri EM, Dessy LA, Alfano C, Scudery N (2008) Breastfeeding after reduction mammaplasty using different techniques. Aesthetic Plast Surg 32:294–297

Davison SP, Mesbahi AN, Ducic I, Sarcia M, Dayan J, Spear SL (2007) The versatility of the superomedial pedicle with various skin reduction patterns. Plast Reconstr Surg 120(6):1466–1476

van Deventer PV, Page BJ, Graewe FR (2008) The safety of pedicles in breast reduction and mastopexy procedures. Aesthetic Plast Surg 32:307–312

Erfon J, Barbosa V, Brasil AG Jr (1989) Reduction mammaplasty in central block. In: Annals of the international symposium recent advances in plastic surgery. São Paulo, pp 306–313

Erfon J, Barbosa V, Brasil A Jr (1992) Reduction mammaplasty in a single block. In: Hinderer UT (ed) Plastic surgery, vol 2. Elsevier, Madrid, pp 629–634

Erfon J, Hochberg J, Ardenghy M, Cols (1996) Central block reduction mammaplasty and mastopexy. In: Proceedings of the 65th annual scientific meeting of the American society of plastic and reconstructive surgeons, vol 19. Dallas, pp 176–178

Fischer JP, Cleveland EC, Shang EK, Nelson JA, Serletti JM (2014) Complications following reduction mammaplasty: a review of 3538 cases from the 2005-2010 NSQIP data sets. Aesthetic Surg J 34(1):66–73

Foustanos A, Panagiotopoulos K, Skouras G (2011) Intraoperative modification of Pitanguy technique of reduction mammaplasty for elevation of the nipple-areola complex in case of severe breast ptosis. Aesthetic Plast Surg 35:55–60

Franco T, Rebello C (1977) Cirurgia Estética, 1ª Edição. Atheneu, Rio de Janeiro, p 211

Jurado J (1979) The vertical dermal-glandular flap of inferior single pedicle in breast surgery. Presented at the 7th international congress of plastic and reconstructive surgery, Rio de Janiero

Karsidag S, Akcal A, Karsidag T, Yesiloglu N, Yesilada AK, Ugurlu K (2011) Reduction mammaplasty using the free-nipple-graft vertical technique for severe breast hypertrophy: improved outcomes with the superior dermaglandular flap. Aesthetic Plast Surg 35:254–261

Kececi Y, Sir E, Gungor M (2015) Patient-reported quality-of-life outcomes of breast reduction evaluated with generic questionnaires and the breast reduction assessed severity scale. Aesthetic Surg J 35(1):48–54

Lassus C (1987) Breast reduction: evolution of a technique. A single vertical scar. Aesthetic Plast Surg 11:107

Lexer E (1912) Hypertrophiebei der Mammae. Munch Med Wochen Chr 59:2702

Lima JC (1979) Breast reduction: new method and refinements. In: Ely JF (ed) Transaction of the seventh international congress of plastic reconstructive surgery. Cartigraf, Rio de Janeiro, p 508

McKissock PK (1972) Reduction mammaplasty with a vertical dermal flap. Plast Reconstr Surg 49(3):245–252

Orlando JC, Guthrie RH Jr (1975) The superomedial dermal pedicle for nipple transposition. Br J Plast Surg 28(1):42–45

Peixoto G (1980) Reduction mammaplasty: a personal technique. Plast Reconstr Surg 65(2):217–225

Peixoto G (1984) Reduction mammoplasty. Aesthetic Plast Surg 8:231–236

Pitanguy I (1967) Surgical treatment of breast hypertrophy. Br J Plast Surg 20(1):78–85

Pitanguy I (1976) Personal preferences for reduction mammaplasty. In: Goldwyn R (ed) Plastic and reconstructive surgery of the breast. Little Brown, Boston, p 167

Robbins TH (1977) A reduction mammaplasty with the areola-nipple based on an inferior dermal pedicle. Plast Reconstr Surg 59(1):64–67

Schwarzman E (1930) Die technik der Mammaplastik. Chirurg 2:932

Sepúlveda A (1981) Tratamento das Assimetrias Mamárias. Ver Bras Cirurgia 71:11–18

Silveira-Neto E (1976) Mastoplastia redutora setorial com pedículo areolar interno. In: XIII Congresso Brasileiro de Cirurgia Plástica, Porto Alegre, RS, Brazil
Skoog T (1963) A technique of breast reduction; transposition of the nipple on a cutaneous vascular pedicle. Acta Chir Scand 126:453–465
Souza Pinto EB et al (1983) Dermoadipose and adenoadipose flaps in mammaplasty. Aesthetic Plast Surg 7(7):101–108
Spector JA, Karp NS (2007) Reduction mammaplasty: a significant improvement at any size. Plast Reconstr Surg 120(4):845–850
Strombeck JO (1960) Mammaplasty: report of a new technique based on the two-pedicle procedure. Br J Plast Surg 13:79–90
Thorek M (1942) Plastic surgery of the breast and the abdominal wall. Charles C Thomas, Springfield
Weiner PL, Aiache AE, Silver L, Ttitanonda TA (1973) Single dermal pedicle for nipple transposition in subcutaneous mastectomy reduction mammaplasty or mastopexy. Plast Reconstr Surg 510(2):115–120
Wise RJ, Gannon JP, Hill JR (1963) Further experience with reduction mammaplasty. Plast Reconstr Surg 32(1):12

9 The Triple-Flap Interposition Mammaplasty: Personal Technique

Alberto M.L. Caldeira
and Yolotzin Mendez Aguilar

9.1 Introduction

The history of reduction mammaplasty from 1980 until the present day can be seen as a period of refinements of existing techniques that mostly focused on the reduction of the final scar. These existing techniques were established from the late 1950s to the late 1970s, a period defined as a "period of safety" (Psillakis and Cardoso de Oliveira 1990). Many of these techniques share the principle of Lexer and Kraske (Kraske 1923; Lexer 1925), that is, a central wedge dissection in the lower half and an approximation of the lateral poles to form the breast.

Almost all techniques reinforced an element that was felt to be neglected before and is nowadays associated with Schwarzmann (1930), that is, de-epithelialization of the skin around the areola and avoidance of skin separation from the gland to respect the cutaneous–glandular unity.

However, less consideration has been given to what we believe to be the fundamental principle in mammaplasty reduction. To produce a long-lasting aesthetically pleasing breast shape, the gland itself should be altered into the desired form. Some breasts need to be reduced at their base to control the height and form the conical projection. Thus, there may be a need for dissection of the gland from the pectoralis fascia.

Other breasts need a reduction in their axillary pole and should be put into a more medial position, with the areola on the apex of the newly created cone. To transform a pendulous breast into a cone-shaped one, there a method needs to be formulated that is versatile enough to allow this transformation.

The concept of glandular shaping goes back to Biesenberg (1928). However, in retrospect, the critical attention given to this approach focused on the complete dissection of the skin from the gland and the associated complications. Less attention was given to the merit of glandular shaping.

If the goal of the surgical procedure is to alter the form and volume of the breast, then the focus should be on the nature of the breast. This included analysis of skin quality, shape, and projection of the breasts, asymmetries, contouring of the surrounding areas (upper abdomen and lateral thorax), and content of the gland. Many of the existing techniques produce excellent results,

A.M.L. Caldeira, M.D., M.Sc., Ph.D., F.A.C.S. (✉)
Global Plastic Surgery Department—Casa de Saúde Portugal, Instituto de Pós-Graduação Médica Carlos Chagas, Universidade Santa Úrsula, Rio de Janeiro, RJ, Brazil

Plastic and Reconstructive Surgery Department, Caldeira-Roth Institute, Rua Visconde de Pirajá, 414—suite 1012, Ipanema, Rio de Janeiro, RJ CEP 22410-002, Brazil
e-mail: lottcaldeira@gmail.com

Y.M. Aguilar, M.D.
Global Plastic Surgery Department—Casa de Saúde Portugal, Universidade Santa Úrsula, Rio de Janeiro, RJ, Brazil

J.M. Avelar (ed.), *Breast Surgery*, https://doi.org/10.1007/978-3-319-54115-0_9

depending on the surgeon's ability to analyze the preoperative situation and to find a safe surgical solution for the required improvement in shape and thereby reduction in volume.

As many have pointed out, there is no one single technique for every patient. Consequently, the author suggests viewing the triple-flap interposition technique more as an approach, a base to start from, as the formation of three flaps offers variables that can change the breast shape.

9.2 History

The surgery of reduction mammaplasty was developed during this century, and is divided into five periods (Psillakis and Cardoso 1990):

1. Before (1900)
2. The pioneers (1901)
3. The trend period (1931–1960)
4. The period of safety (1961–1979)
5. The period of refinement (1980 until the present day)

9.2.1 The Pioneers (1901)

The most important contribution from this period was the improvement of different surgical methods.

Lexer (1925) described a technique with resection of the inferior pole, absence of the separation of the skin from the breast tissue, conification of the breast, and transposition of the nipple to a higher position (Kraske 1923; Lexer 1925).

Biesenberg (1928), after dissection of the skin, resected the other half of the breast parenchyma, using an S-shaped incision beginning in the axilla and extending to the lower pole under the areola. To rebuild the conical shape of the breast, the lower portion of the breast segment carrying the nipple was displaced upward and outward, the skin was replaced and the excess removed with a final inverted T-shaped scar (Biesenberg 1928).

9.2.2 The Period of Safety

Arié (1957) used a technique in cases of moderate ptosis and/or breast hypertrophy combined with skin excess, the lozenge or rhomboid technique, which yields good results and avoids a horizontal scar. It is indicated when the resection of only a quadrant of the mammary tissue is necessary to correct the breast. The incision along the inframammary fold would yield a more favorable scar. They believed that the technique predetermined the site of the nipple, and used resection of the upper pole, resulting in a flat breast with a quadrangular shape, and with diminished breast sensitivity (Pitanguy 1960, 1961; Pitanguy et al. 1984).

Liacir Ribeiro (1975) used several pedicles, and separated them into five groups; with the use of this new technique, vascularization would be from the lower breast pole, contrary to existing techniques at the time (Ribeiro 1975, 1989; Ribeiro et al. 1992).

9.2.3 The Period of Refinement

Peixoto's technique, published in 1980, was indicated in patients with simple and small breast ptosis and correction of moderate hypertrophy, with minimal skin resection and minimal breast tissue resection, resulting in smaller scars. It did not involve any changes of breast shape, it always maintaining the original form (Peixoto 1980).

The senior author returned to the concepts of Biesenberger, the opposite of Peixoto's technique. It was our belief that few techniques guarantee a conical breast base, and we developed a technique that guaranteed a conical-shaped breast and would facilitate placing the nipple–areola complex (NAC) at the apex of this cone. The first mammaplasties were performed in 1984 using the classical Pitanguy, Arié (1957), and Lozenge procedures (Pitanguy 1960, 1961; Pitanguy et al. 1984; Ribeiro 1975, 1989; Ribeiro et al. 1992).

A critical observation of the results, being in dialogue with other surgeons throughout the world, and reading critical publications, led to the conclusion that in many cases the results of these procedures did not meet the patient's and surgeon's expectations, especially in the long run, and sometimes also in the immediate postoperative state (Lassus 1986; Lima 1975; Maillard 1986; Marconi 1989; Marconi and Cavina 1993; Martins 1991; Mathes et al. 1980; McKissock 1972; Nicolle and Chir 1982).

The results were considered sometimes unfavorable because of the lack of conical shape of the breasts, pointing out that most procedures produce a round shape. Moreover, there was a consensus that many procedures do not provide adequate resection of the breast base and do not allow for medialization of the breast.

Most important was the observation that the operated breast tended to resume its previous shape in the late postoperative stage (Caldeira 1994a, b, c, 1995; Candiani et al. 1991; Peixoto 1980).

The triple-flap interposition technique was first presented in 1994 in the Annals of the 8th Congress on Senology (Breast Diseases), Rio de Janeiro. Follow-up was presented and published in the Transactions of the 11th Congress of the International Confederation for Plastic Reconstructive and Aesthetic Surgery in Yokohama, Japan, in April 1995. This approach was used by the senior author in his private practice with 1754 cases up to 1987 (Caldeira 1994a, b, c, 1995).

9.3 Triple-Flap Interposition Technique

The triple-flap interposition technique relies on an upper pedicle to the areola and is defined by the creation of three glandular flaps to shape a conical breast using skin resection that results in minimal scarring.

Glandular tissue is resected in a rhomboid or oblique manner, while creating a central, lateral, and medial glandular flap. The idea of the technique is to shape glandular tissue to create a conical breast, and to allow for, whenever necessary, the reduction of the mammary base and the axillary pole in addition to the medialization of the breast.

The areola is placed on the apex of the cone supplied by an upper pedicle. The interposition and suturing of the three glandular flaps promote the reformulation of the Cooper ligament system, thus resulting in a long-lasting conical breast configuration. Accordingly, the skin simply covers what has been shaped, free of traction or tension.

Skin glandular undermining takes place only in a limited area of the inferior hemisphere; the breast base is widely undermined from the pectoral fascia, although care should be taken not to injure the perforators of the internal and lateral thoracic arteries, which supply the glandular flaps. The triple-flap interposition is a mammaplasty technique that involves the following:

1. Shaping of glandular tissue to create a conical breast configuration.
2. Relocating the areola on a superior pedicle on the apex of the cone.
3. Skin undermining on the inferior hemisphere of the breast.
4. Undermining of the breast base from the pectoralis fascia.
5. Skin resection that results in minimal scarring.

The goals of the triple-flap interposition technique in mammaplasty can be outlined as the shaping of a conical, aesthetically pleasing breast, thereby reducing breast volume. The breast shape should be stable, the scars limited, and the procedure safe (Marconi and Cavina 1993; Nicolle and Chir 1982; Pitanguy 1960).

9.3.1 Markings and Skin Incision

The types of skin incision may vary depending on the skin condition and breast volume. Generally, apply the Lozenge (Fig. 9.1) (Ribeiro 1989), Peixoto's (1980), or circumferential techniques (Bustus and Loureiro 1985; Hinderer 1969). Alternatively, the marking of other short scarring techniques (Hollander 1924; Lalardrie and Mouly 1978), for example, the vertical mammaplasty of Lejour (1994), can be used (Fig. 9.2).

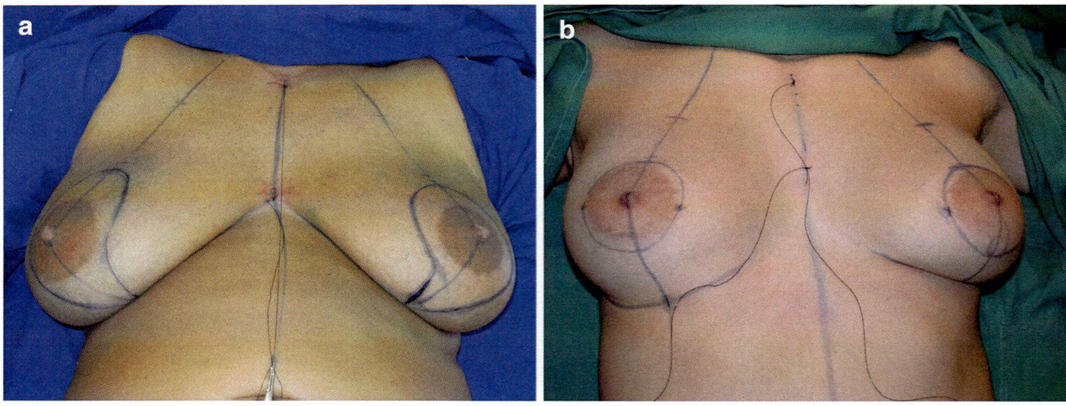

Fig. 9.1 Outline of incisions. (**a**) Lozenge and (**b**) circumferential marking

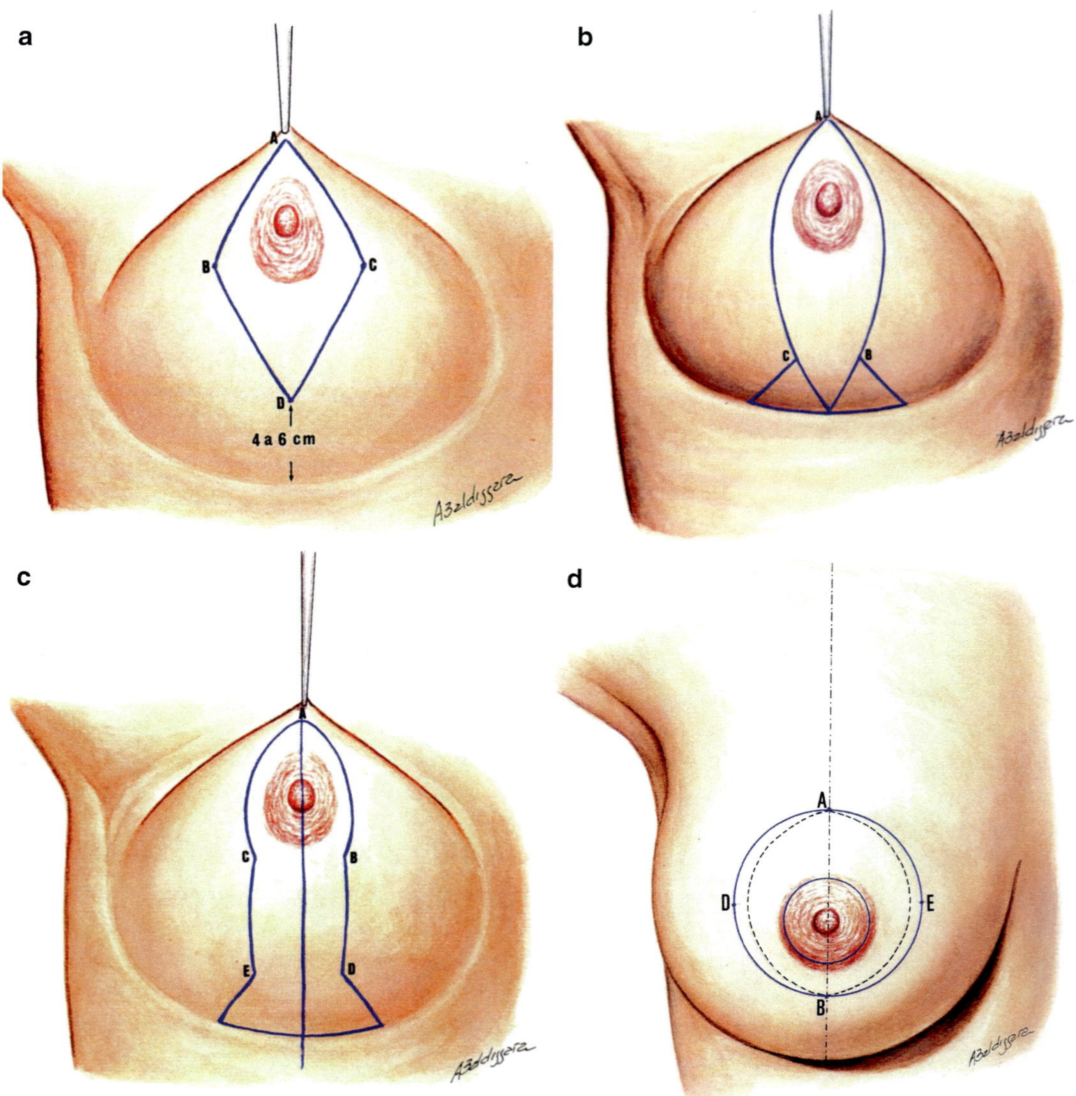

Fig. 9.2 (**a–d**) Diagram showing four marking examples used in this technique

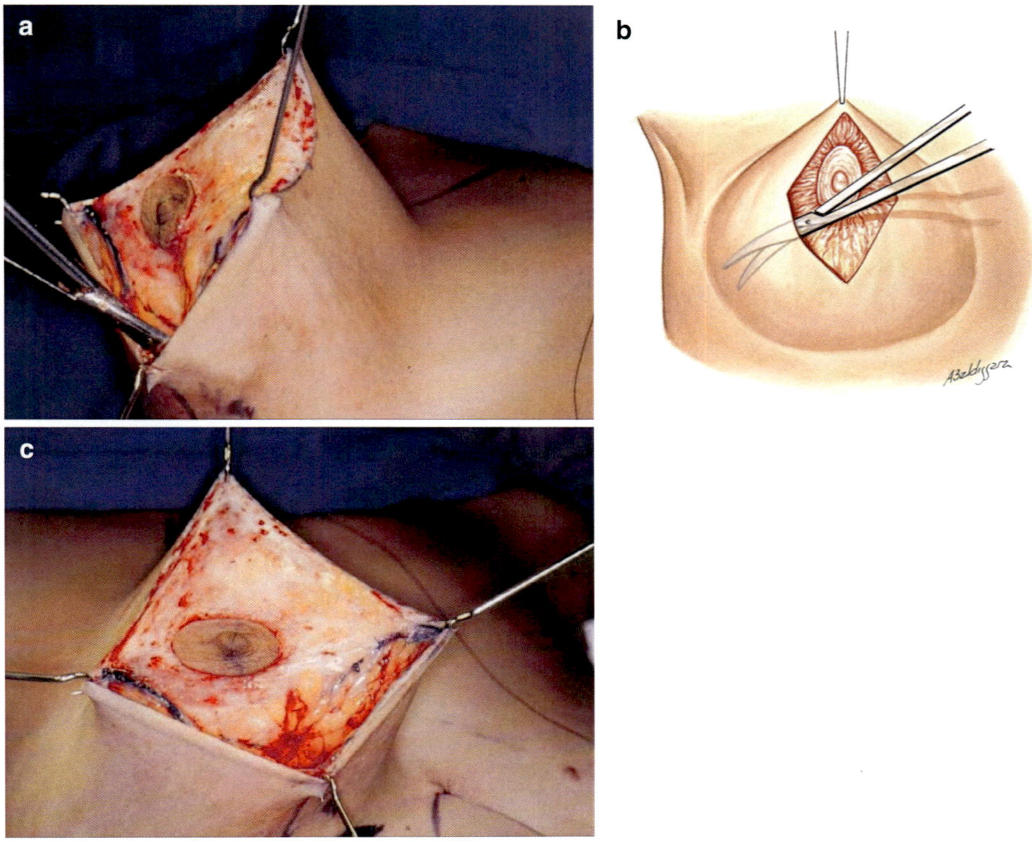

Fig. 9.3 (a–c) Skin–glandular undermining

After skin incision, de-epithelialization is carried out carefully to safeguard the NAC and the central flap, which will be formed later. Skin–glandular undermining of the interior hemisphere begins on the decorticated area and extends to the axillary region when necessary. This undermining should be carried out between the glandular and the areola tissue (Fig. 9.3).

The breast base is undermined from the pectoral fascia, and upon reaching the parasternal region, this should be done in a careful manner to preserve the perforators (second, third, and fourth rami) of the internal thoracic artery. The breast tissue is raised and two vertical incisions converging downward are made to create the central vertical flap with a base pedicle adequate for its extension. This flap is irrigated by the second perforator of the internal thoracic artery (Fig. 9.4) (Bertelli and Pereira 1994).

Two glandular tissue flaps corresponding to the medial and lateral pillars of the breast are created posteriorly. The medial horizontal flap is vascularized mostly by the third and fourth perforators of the internal thoracic artery and the lateral horizontal flap is vascularized by the ramification of the lateral thoracic artery and rami acromialis (Fig. 9.5) (Bertelli and Pereira 1994; Cardoso et al. 1984).

After comparing the total breast volume bilaterally, the glandular tissue is resected in a rhomboid, oblique manner (Pitanguy et al. 1984). Alternatively, the base of the gland can be removed in a disc-like fashion (Peixoto 1980). Thus, if the breast has a large base, it is easier to narrow and/or reduce the height of the projection of the new breast cone. In addition, the combination of both types of resection may be applied to achieve the desired shape (Caldeira et al. 1999).

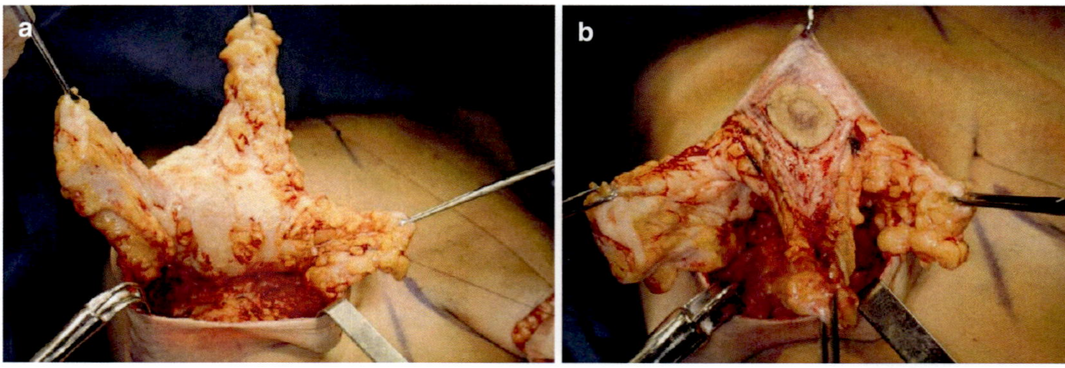

Fig. 9.4 (**a**, **b**) Central, medial, and lateral flaps

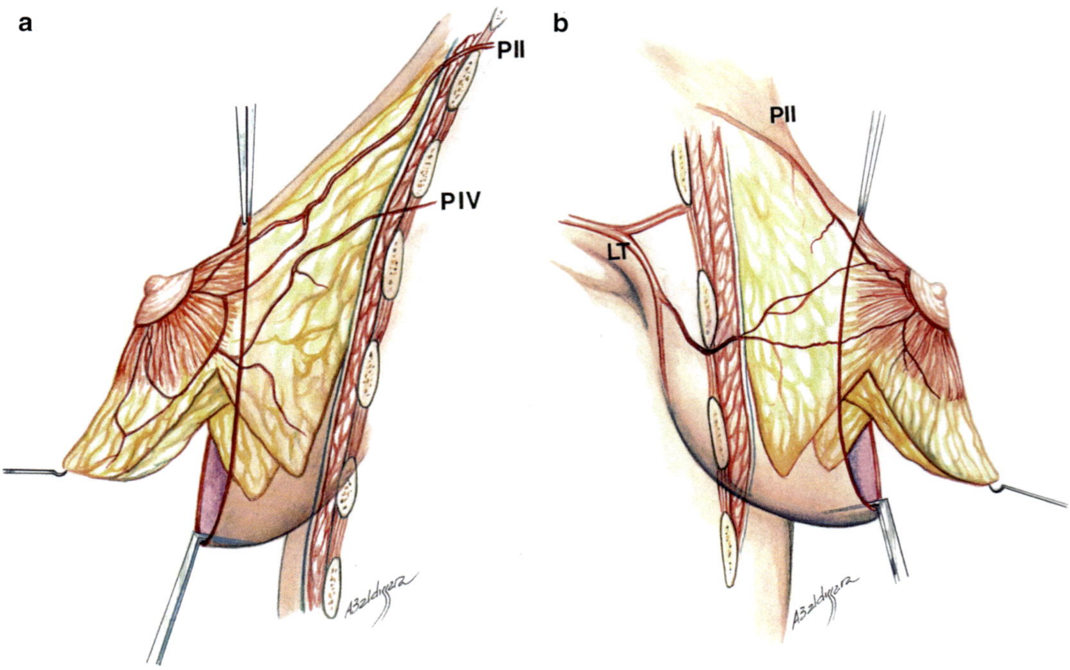

Fig. 9.5 (**a**) Medial view: the skin surface area and the glandular tissue are considerably vascularized by the second perforator. It includes the upper portion of the breast, the nipple–areolar complex (NAC), and the subjacent antero-medial region. (**b**) Lateral thoracic artery

Following careful hemostasis, the breast is raised by a hook placed at the apex that remains throughout the shaping of the breast. The distal end of the central flap is sutured to the fascia pectorals using three 2-0 Vicryl or Prolene sutures. The adequate length of the flap prevents the downward traction of the NAC (Fig. 9.6). The main purpose of this flap is to provide projection of the NAC and prevent a flattened aspect (Fig. 9.7). The two medial and

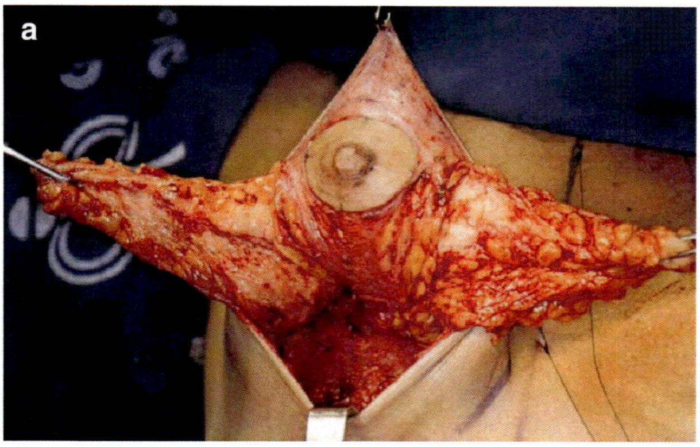

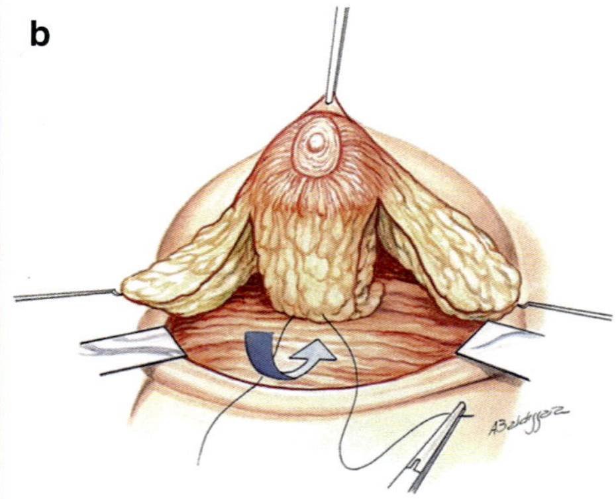

Fig. 9.6 (**a**, **b**) Fixation of the central flap

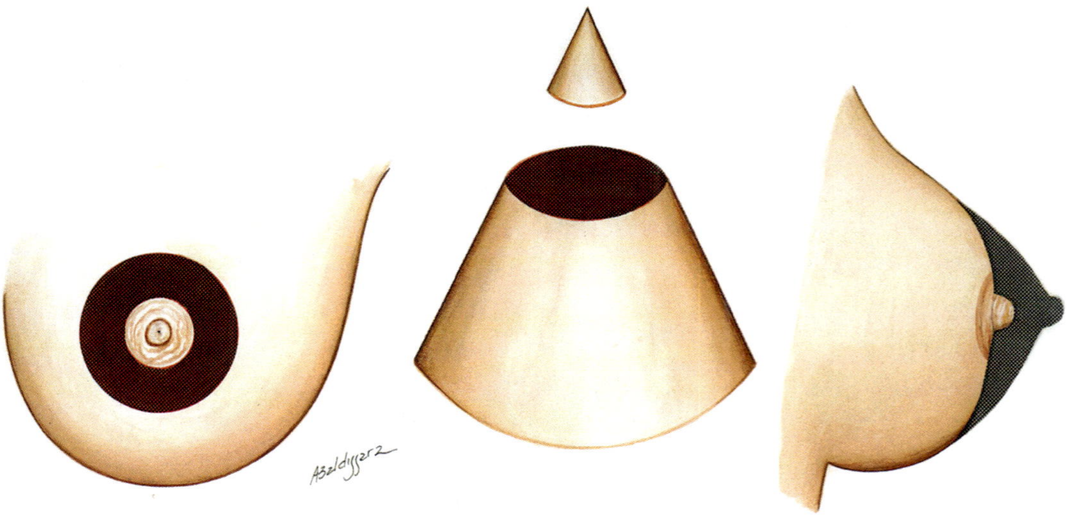

Fig. 9.7 The central flap has the function to improve the natural projection of the NAC

lateral horizontal flaps are rotated toward the midclavicular line and are transposed one over the over (Fig. 9.8).

The placement of these flaps determines the contour of the lower breast hemisphere, shapes the lateral and medial poles, and narrows the base. Moreover, this maneuver defines the new submammary fold, and helps to correct important breast asymmetries (Fig. 9.9). Positioning of the medial and lateral flaps depends on the need to provide more volume to either of these segments. Generally, the medial flap is deeply secured to the base of the lateral flap, which is rotated over the medial flap and sutured over its surface using 2-0 Vicryl or Prolene. Minor irregularities are corrected by trimming the fat tissue with scissors. Skin resection renders tension-free wound borders where the skin does not function as an outer brassiere. The areola is sutured using Gillies sutures with 6-0 Prolene (Fig. 9.10).

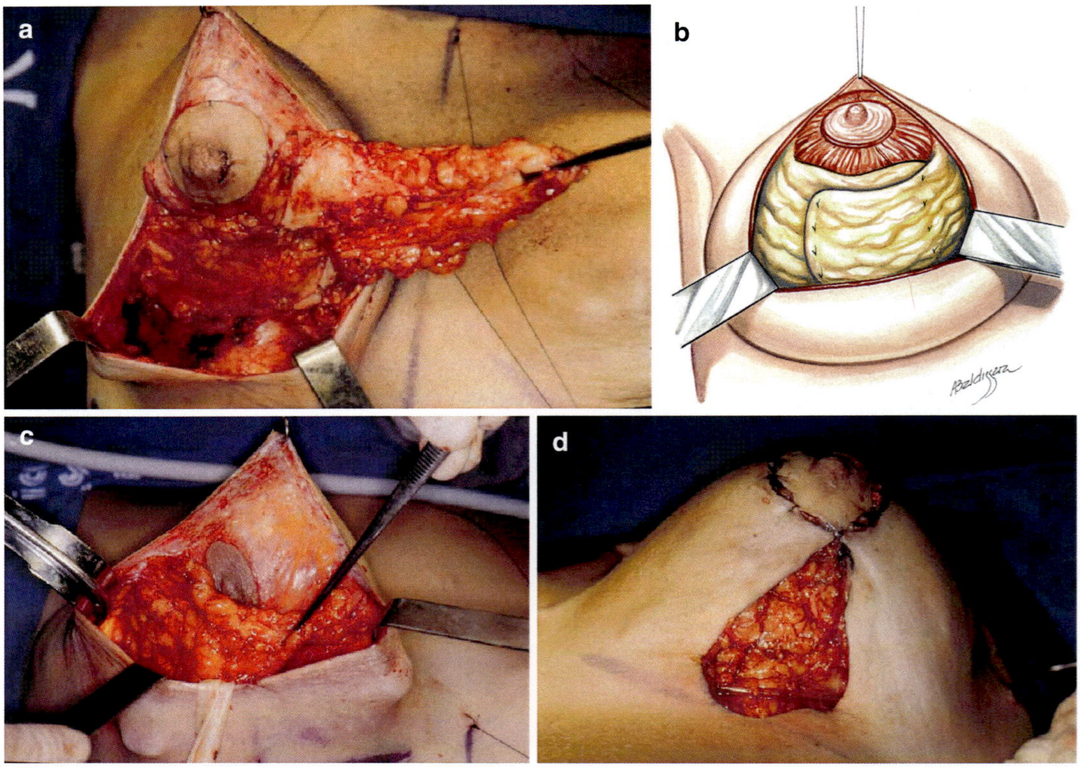

Fig. 9.8 Shaping the breast. (**a–c**) Interposition of the lateral and medial flaps. (**d**) The breast shape is sustained even before being sutured to the skin

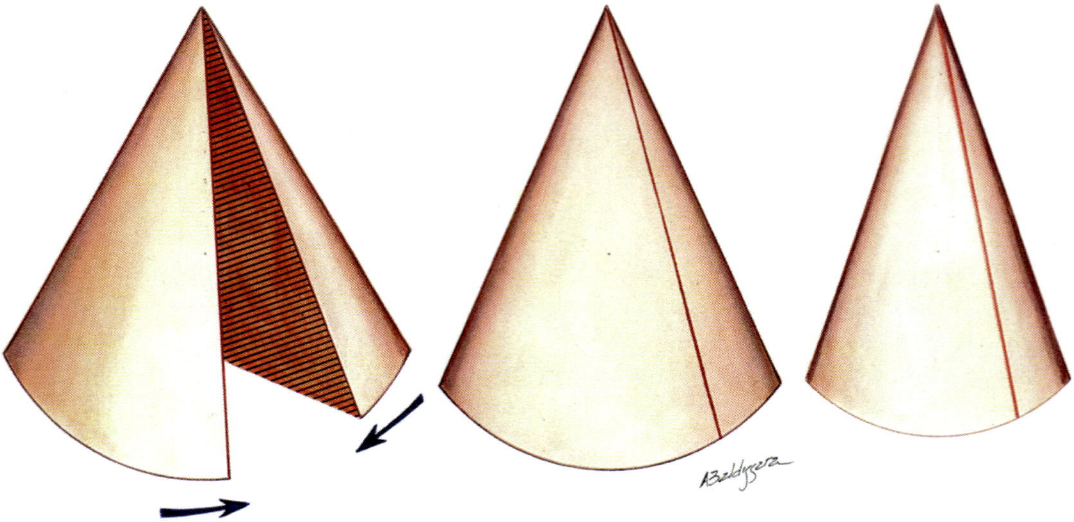

Fig. 9.9 Interposition of the lateral and medial flaps leads to a new breast shape through effective breast base reduction

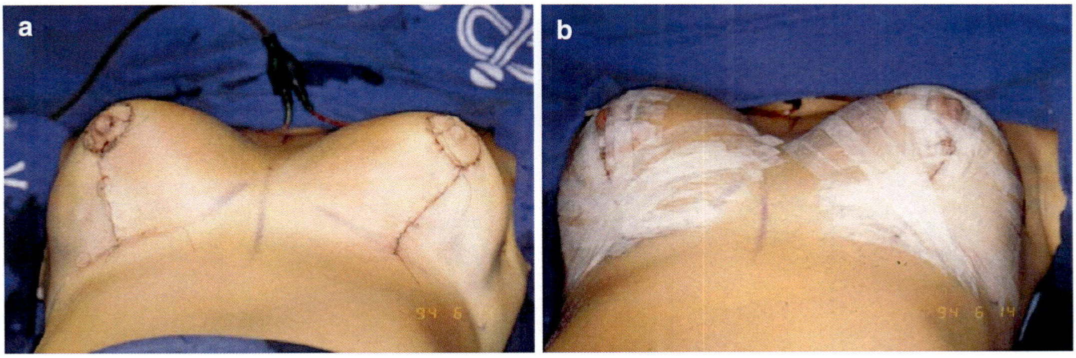

Fig. 9.10 (**a**, **b**) After the subcuticular and intradermal suturing, the new breast form is sustained by micropore tape remodeling and compressive dressing

9.4 Discussion

The goal of this technique is to provide breast stability by forming a glandular cone. Consequently, the skin covers what has been shaped, without tension, accommodating the ideal conditions for the scar to heal. Postoperatively, the reshaped breasts proved to be stable and maintained the desired conical shape in the long term (Figs. 9.11 and 9.12).

When used in a narrow-based or slightly wide breast, standard techniques generally produce good results. Many of these are Lexer–Kraske-type methods that approximate the lateral and medial pillars after wedge dissection (Cardoso et al. 1984; Lassus 1986; Lejour 1994; Lexer 1925; Strombeck 1961).

However, they often do not yield a satisfactory and stable result when applied to large-based, pendulous breasts with inelastic skin (Weiner et al. 1973; Williams and Hoffman 1981).

The reason why the breasts relapse to their former ptotic shape is because the nature of the shape has not been changed by these techniques. They have less volume, but the broad base and the glandular tissue have no "inner support" that prevents them from "falling down" (Hoffman 1986, 1987; Peixoto 1980; Pers et al. 1986).

The author believes that the forming of a narrow-based breast, together with interglandular suturing, provides a stable shape. One reason for this is that the Cooper ligaments are reorganized; thus, the gland is liberated from what could be called the "structural mammary memory." Another reason is that interglandular scarring leads to more fibrous content of the breast; the breast content will be firmer, especially in those cases where liposuction has been carried out to reduce the fat content of the gland.

Most importantly, the formation of the lateral and medial flaps, which are rotated toward the midclavicular line and are transposed over each other, creates an inner "brassiere," thereby giving the necessary inner support to prevent the breast from relapsing into their former shape. It may be argued that some of the heavy pendulous breasts have a substantial fat content and that the creation of a cone consisting of mostly fat tissue will not produce a long-lasting result. In these cases, we would extend the technique to a procedure that uses a strip of the pectoralis muscle to provide the "inner brassiere" (Fig. 9.13) (Caldeira et al. 1999).

The triple-flap interposition technique involves glandular undermining from the pectoralis fascia. The axial blood supply of the flaps should be respected; thus, the gland is not dissected completely and parts of the upper inner and outer quadrants remain untouched. There is a tendency for large adipose breast to atrophy in the postoperative period.

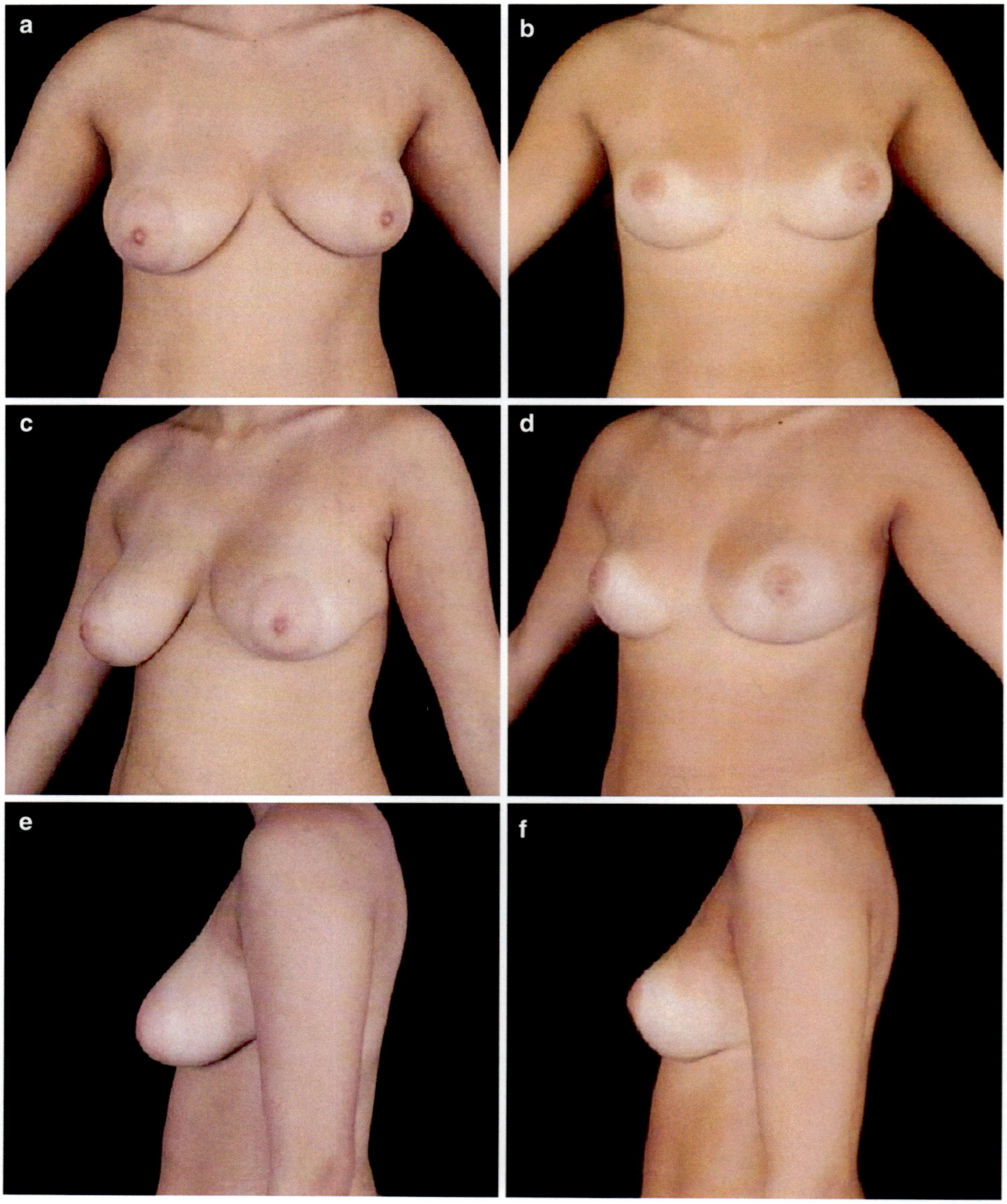

Fig. 9.11 A 20-year-old patient. Correction of moderate hypertrophy, ptosis, asymmetric breast volume and shaping. (**a**, **c**, **e**) Preoperative views. (**b**, **d**, **f**) Postoperative views. Evolution over 3 years

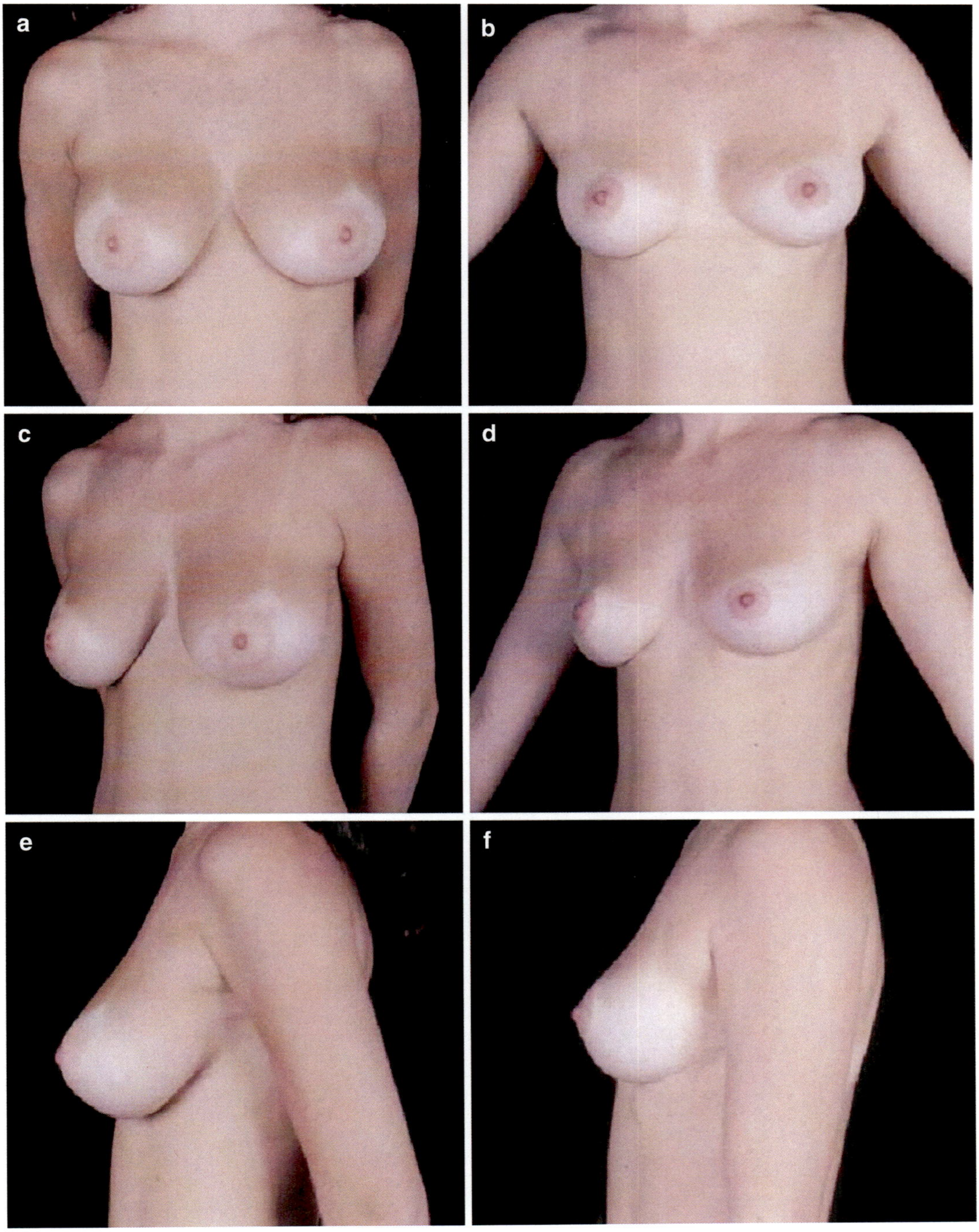

Fig. 9.12 A 23-year-old patient. Correction of moderate hypertrophy. (**a**, **c**, **e**) Preoperative views. (**b**, **d**, **f**) Postoperative views. Evolution over 4 years

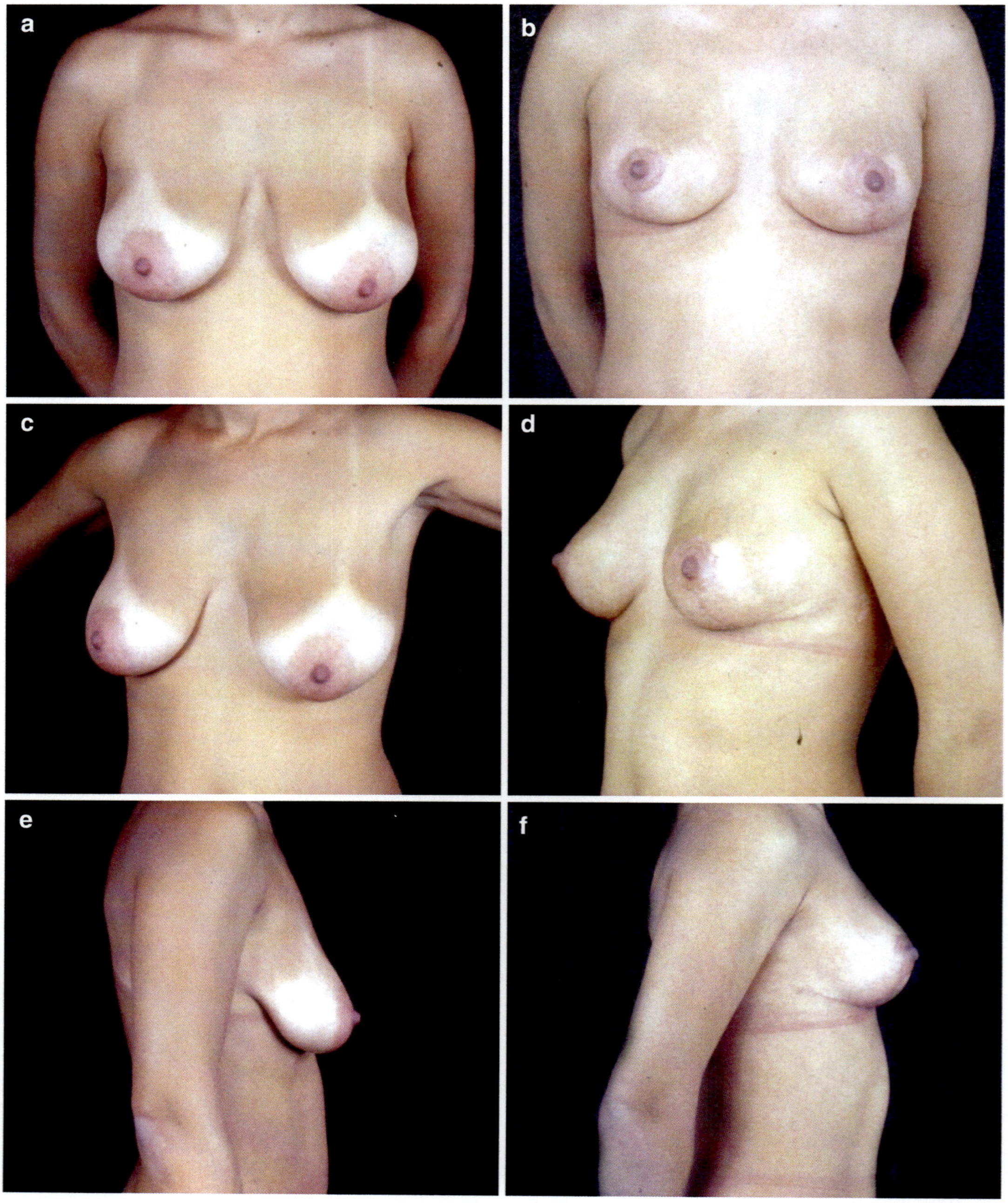

Fig. 9.13 A 31-year-old patient. Correction of moderate hypertrophy, ptosis, asymmetric breast volume, and shaping. (**a**, **c**, **e**) Preoperative views. (**b**, **d**, **f**) Postoperative views. Evolution over 5 years

This observation led the authors to reduce the breast and perform a second intervention when necessary after 6 months. This second procedure could be liposuction alone depending on whether the breast shape proved to be stable, or it could be a secondary reduction mammaplasty using the triple-flap interposition technique with or without the use of a pectoralis muscle flap (Caldeira and Lucas 2000).

The cutaneous–glandular undermining proposed by this technique allows complete visualization and manipulation of the various breast segments and consequently favors the treatment proposed.

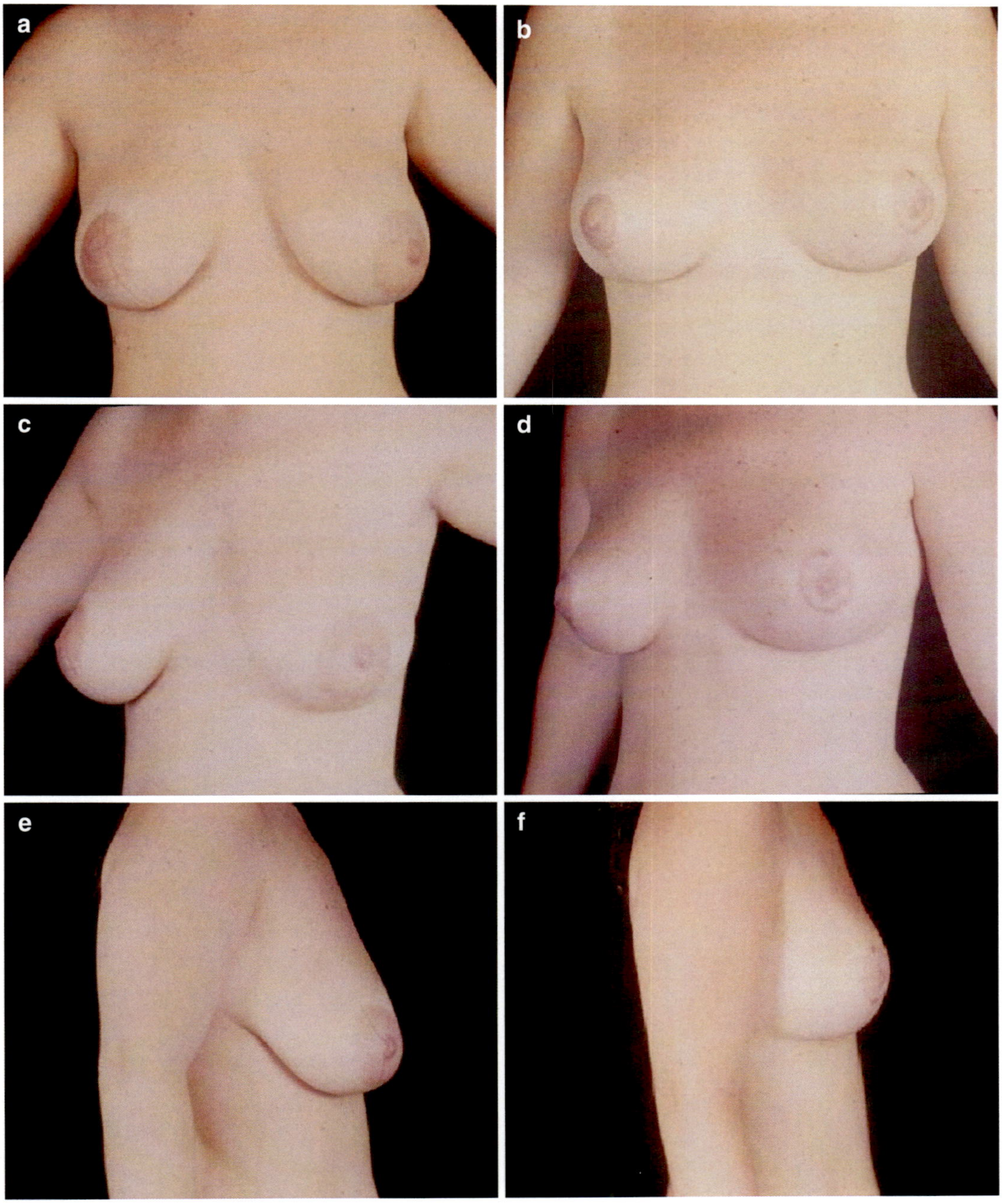

Fig. 9.14 A 19-year-old patient. Correction of mild hypertrophy and round breast shape. (**a**, **c**, **e**) Preoperative views. (**b**, **d**, **f**) Postoperative views. (**g**, **h**) Postoperative oblique and profile views. Evolution over 15 years maintaining the new conical shape

However, undermining the whole inferior hemisphere should be avoided per se. Specifically, when the skin resection yields and there is an inverted T scar, unnecessarily wide undermining causes skin necrosis in the conjunction area of the skin flaps (Fig. 9.14).

Consequently, the authors restrict the cutaneous–glandular undermining to an area that rarely exceeds the breast base. As a rule of thumb, undermining stops at approximately 1 cm away from the medial or lateral borders of the corresponding poles.

The use of a superior-based flap to the areola has proved to be safe in this specific technique and corresponds to the experience of other authors, who also rely on a superior-based flap.

The creation of the central flap that relies on the superior-based flap for blood supply provides the volume that is needed in the central and upper parts of the conical breast.

Thus, the fixation is not positioned superior to the future apex, but exactly under the future position of the areola. Plication of a central pedicle or flap to the pectoralis fascia alone does not provide sufficient long-lasting support for glandular tissue, that is, the breast will become ptotic again as the glandular tissue slides, along the pectoralis fascia, downward, as others authors have reported (De Souza Pinto et al. 1983; Hakme 1983; Nicolle and Chir 1984; Pers et al. 1986; Pitanguy et al. 1984; Ribeiro 1989; Rohrich et al. 2006). Stability of the breast shape is granted largely by interpositioning the three flaps with one another and not by plicating glandular tissue to the pectoralis fascia.

After the cutaneous–glandular undermining in the lower half, dissection of the gland from the pectoralis fascia, and creation of a conical gland, the new submammary fold ideally lies 2–3 cm above the old one. If not, there is a need for further reshaping and reduction.

The distance between the relocated areola and the new submammary fold should not exceed 6 cm. Underlying these statements is the observation that within the first 2 postoperative months, the breast descends by approximately 2–3 cm.

Consequently, the distance between the areola and the submammary fold enlarges as well. A distance of more than 8 cm is associated with a ptotic breast shape and thus the postoperative result would be less than ideal. The reason why the breast descends, that is, the submammary fold settles in a lower position, is subject to speculation.

The superficial fascial system needs 2–3 months to reorganize its collagen fibers, settling at a point where the gravitational pull is offset by the suspension given by the newly reorganized superficial fascial system; this "suspension" is also influenced, among other factors, by the shape of the breast, its content, and skin quality. In other words, a multitude of factors play a role in the descending of the submammary fold (Fig. 9.15). Therefore, the numbers described are the empirical answer to where the submammary fold settles and thus dictates the design of the breast intraoperatively.

Is the triple-flap interposition technique easy to learn? In the author's opinion, the technique is not more difficult to learn than other techniques.

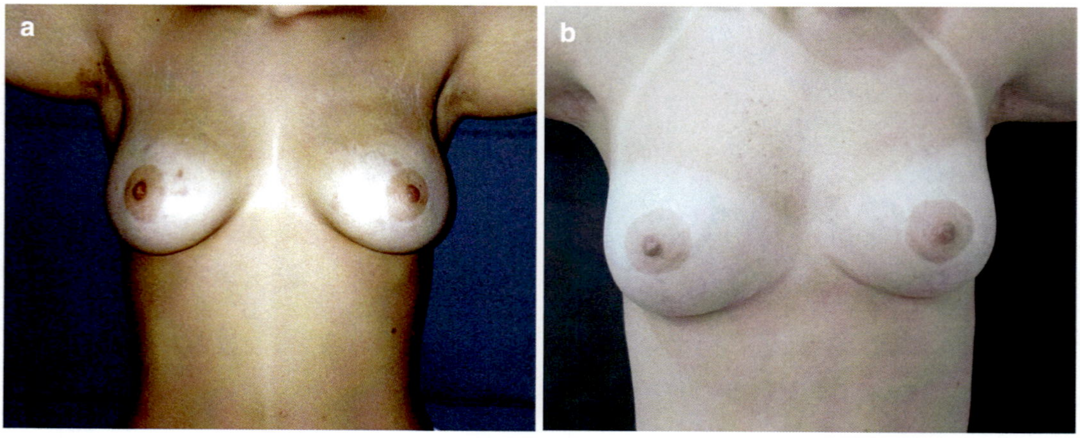

Fig. 9.15 A 34-year-old patient. Correction of moderate hypertrophy, ptosis, asymmetric breast volume, and shaping. (**a**, **c**, **e**) Preoperative views. (**b**, **d**, **f**) Postoperative views. Evolution over 8 years

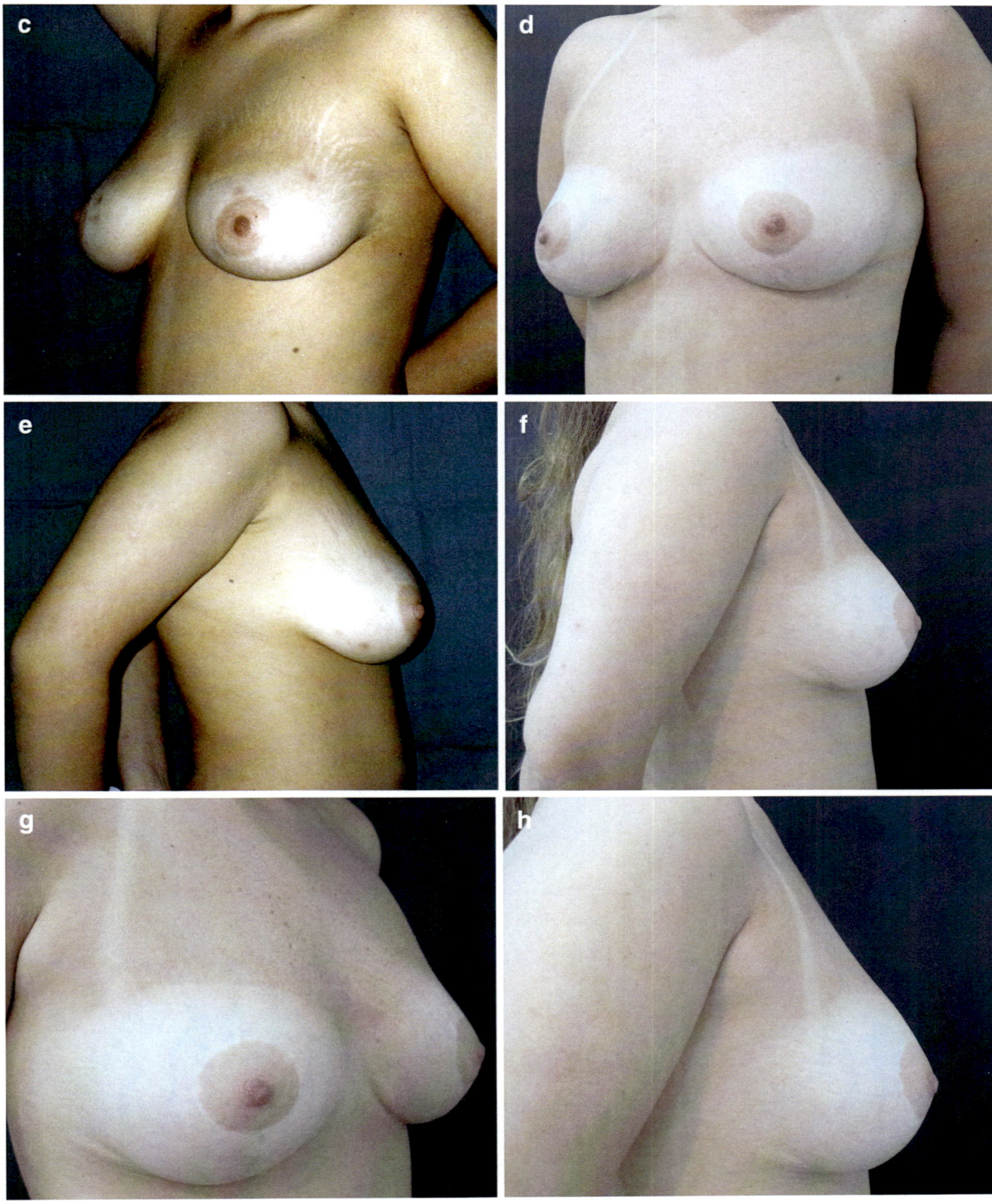

Fig. 9.15 (continued)

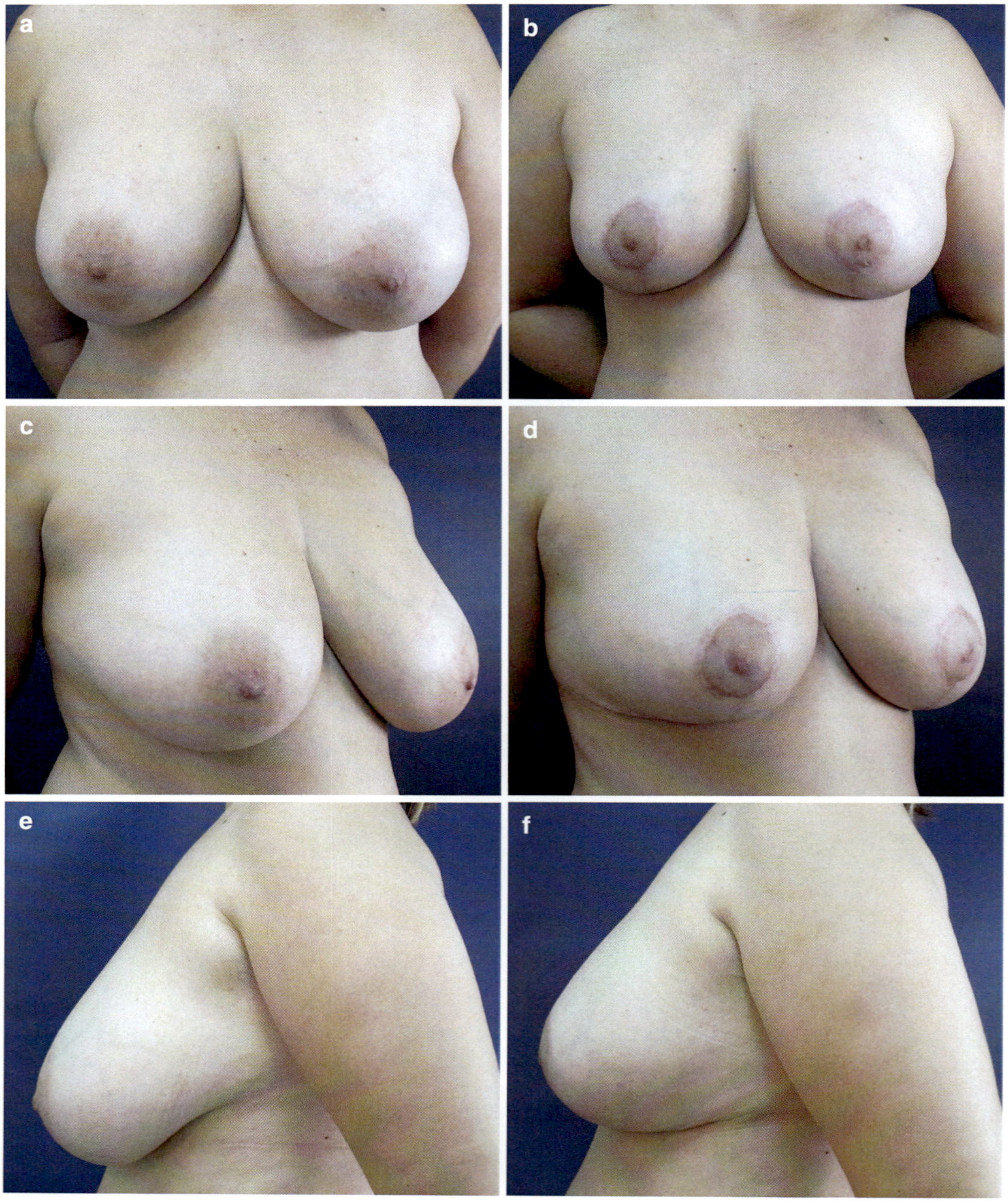

Fig. 9.16 A 43-year-old patient. Correction of severe hypertrophy, ptosis, asymmetric breast volume, and shaping, associated with body lipodystrophy. (**a**, **c**, **e**) Preoperative views. (**b**, **d**, **f**) Postoperative views. Evolution over 2 years

The creation of three flaps may sound complicated, but it only means that after dissection from the pectoralis fascia, the gland is divided into three parts. A fixed, predetermined tissue excision pattern is advocated by many authors, who often point out that the residents find it easier to adhere to fixed patterns during an operation (Caldeira et al. 1999; Lalardrie and Mouly 1978; Strombeck 1961) (Fig. 9.16).

However, it is exactly the "pattern" that often hinders the younger surgeon in grasping the operative technique, as she or he just needs to cut along the markings. With predetermined tissue excision patterns with no skin undermining, the skin tends to be excised during an early operation state, that is, before the gland has been reshaped. In the triple-flap interposition technique, skin excision takes place only after glandular shaping. In cases of asymmetric breasts, it is easier to obtain a symmetrical result with three flaps to shape the breast in comparison with techniques that use a wedge resection and approximation of two pillars (Caldeira and Roth 2008).

Conclusion

The triple-flap method has proved to be safe as long as the blood supply of the glandular flaps is respected. The results accomplished are long lasting and render the desired, aesthetically pleasing, conical breast. The Lexer–Kraske-type methods reduce the volume, but often fail to alter the nature of the breast form. Consequently, they tend to resume to their former shape in the long term; in other words, they are often subject to bottoming out. Reduction mammaplasty is about reshaping the gland into the desired form. Creating three glandular flaps to do this is suggested by the authors.

References

Arié G (1957) Una nueva tecnica de mastoplastia. Rev Lat Am Cir Plast 3:23

Bertelli JA, Pereira JFV (1994) The inframammary island flap: anatomical basis. Ann Plast Surg 32(3):315–320

Biesenberg H (1928) Eine neue Method der Mammaplastik. Zentralbl Chir 55:2382–2387

Bustus RA, Loureiro LEK (1985) Mamoplastia redutora de retalho glandular trilobulado de pedículo inferior por incisão periareolar. In: Transactions of the XXIV Congress of Plastic Surgery. Gramado, APLUB, p 484

Caldeira AML (1994a) New approach to breast surgery: a personal technique. In: Annals 8th International Congress on Senology, Rio De Janeiro, Brazil, p 1400

Caldeira AML (1994b) Nova abordagem de sustentação de mamoplastias. In: Comunication to the Jornada Paulista de Cirurgia Plástica. Brazilian Society Plastic Aesthetic and Reconstruction Surgery, São Paulo

Caldeira AML (1994c) Nova abordagem de sustentação de mamoplastias redutoras. In: Comunication to the X Congresso Iberolatinoamericano de Cirurgia Plástica, Vina Del Mar

Caldeira AML (1995) Triple-flap interposition technique. In: Communication to the 11th Congress of the International Confederation of Plastic, Reconstructive and Aesthetic Surgery, Yokohama

Caldeira AML, Lucas A (2000) Pectoralis major muscle flap: a new support approach to mammoplasty, personal technique. Aesthetic Plast Surg 24(1):58–70

Caldeira AML, Roth GB (2008) The triple-flap interposition mastoplasty. In: Shiffman MA (org.) Mastopexy and breast reduction: principles and practice, vol 1, 1st edn. Springer, Berlin, pp 103–113

Caldeira AML, Lucas A, Grigalek G (1999) Mastoplasty: the triple-flap interposition technique. Aesthetic Pas Surg 23(1):51–60

Candiani P, Campiglio GL, Signorini M (1991) Personal experience with the central pedicle reduction mammoplasty. Rev Soc Bras Cirplas:6–11

Cardoso AD, Pessanha MC, Peralta JM (1984) Three dermal pedicles for nipple-areola complex movement in reduction of gigantomastia. Ann Plast Surg 12(5):419–427

De Souza Pinto EB, Ferraz De Almeida AE, Reyes MF (1983) Dermoadipose and adenadipose flaps in mammoplasty. Aesthetic Plast Surg 7(2):101–108

Hakme F (1983) Técnica em “L” nas ptoses mamárias com confecção de retalhos cruzados. Rev Bras Cir 73:87

Hinderer UT (1969) Primera experiencia con una nueva tecnica de mastoplastia para ptosis ligeras. In: VI Reun Nac Soc Esp Cir Plasr Rep Madrid, vol 6, p 26

Hoffman S (1986) Recorrent deformities following reduction mammoplasty and correction of breast asymmetry. Plast Reconstr Surg 78(1):55–62

Hoffman S (1987) Reduction mammoplasty: a medicolegal hazard? Aesthetic Plast Surg 11(2):113–116

Hollander E (1924) Die Operation der Mammahyperthrophie und der Hängerbrust. Dtsche Med Wschr 50:1.400

Kraske H (1923) Die Operation der atrophischen und hypertrophischen Hängebrust. Munchen Med Wochenschr 70:672–673

Lalardrie JP, Mouly R (1978) History of mammoplasty. Aesthetic Plast Surg 2:167

Lassus C (1986) An “all-season” mammoplasty. Aesthetic Plast Surg 10(1):9–15

Lejour M (1994) Vertical mammoplasty and liposuction of the breast. Plast Reconstr Surg 94(1):100–114

Lexer E (1925) Zur Operation der Mammahypertrophie und der Hängebrust. Dtsch Med Wochenschr 51:26

Lima JC (1975) Our experience in breast reduction. In: VI Congress IPRS, Paris

Maillard GF (1986) A Z-mammaplasty with minimal scarring. Plast Reconstr Surg 77(1):66–76

Marconi F (1989) The dermal pursestring suture: new technique for a short inframammary scar in reduction mammoplasty and dermal mastopexy. Ann Plast Surg 22(6):484–493

Marconi F, Cavina C (1993) Reduction mammoplasty and correction of the ptosis. A personal technique. Plast Reconstr Surg 91(6):1046–1056

Martins PD (1991) Periareolar mammoplasty with a flap transportation. Rev Soc Bras Cir Plas 6:1

Mathes SJ, Nahai F, Hester TR (1980) Avoiding the flat breast in reduction mammoplasty. Plast Reconstr Surg 66(1):63–70

McKissock PK (1972) Reduction mammoplasty with a vertical dermal flap. Plast Reconstr Surg 49(3):245–252

Nicolle FV, Chir M (1982) Improved standards in reduction mammoplasty and mastopexy. Plast Reconstr Surg 69(3):453–459

Nicolle FV, Chir M (1984) Reduction mammoplasty and mastopexy: a personal technique. Aesthetic Plast Surg 8(1):43–50

Peixoto G (1980) Reduction mammoplasty: a personal technique. Plast Reconstr Surg 65(2):217–226

Pers M, Nielsen IM, Gerner N (1986) Results following reduction mammoplasty as evaluated by the patients. Ann Plast Surg 17(6):449–455

Pitanguy I (1960) Breast hypertrophy. In: Transactions of the international society of plastic surgeons, Second congress, London, Livingstone, p 502

Pitanguy I (1961) Mamaplastias. Estudo de 245 Casos Consecutivos E Apresentação de Técnica Pessoal. Ver Bras Cir 42:201

Pitanguy I, AML C, Alexandrino A, Martinez JG (1984) Mamoplastia redutora e mastopexia: técnica Pitanguy. Vinte e Cinco Anos de Experiência. Rev Bras Cir 74:265

Psillakis JM, Cardoso de Oliveira M (1990) History of reduction mammaplasty. In: Goldwyn RM (ed) Reduction mammaplasty, 1st edn. Little Brown, Boston. Chapter 1, pp 1–15

Psillakis JM, Cardoso de Oliveira M (1990) History of reduction mammaplasty. In: Goldwyn RM (ed) Reduction mammaplasty. Little, Brown and Company, Boston, pp 1–15

Ribeiro L (1975) A new technique for reduction mammoplasty. Plast Reconstr Surg 55(3):330–334

Ribeiro L (1989) Redução mamária. In: Cirurgia Plástica da Mama Medsi, Rio de Janeiro, pp 185–266

Ribeiro L, Mussy S, Accorsi JA (1992) Mamaplastía reductora: técnica circunferencial. Cir Plas Ibero Lat Am 18:249

Rohrich RJ, Gosmann AA, Brown SA, Reisch J (2006) Matopexy preferences: a survey of board-certified plastic surgeons. Plast Reconstr Surg 118(7):1631–1638

Schwarzmann E (1930) Die Technik der Mammaplastik. Chirurgie 2:932–943

Strombeck JO (1961) Mammaplasty: report of a new technique based on the two-pedicle procedure. Br J Plast Surg 13:79–90

Weiner DL, Aiache AE, Silver L, Tittiranonda T (1973) A single dermal pedicle for nipple transposition in subcutaneous mastectomy, reduction mammoplasty or mastopexy. Plast Reconstr Surg 51(2):115–120

Williams G, Hoffman S (1981) Mammoplasty for tubular breasts. Aesthetic Plast Surg 5(1):51–56

10 Reduction Mastoplasty: Personal Technique

Ramil Sinder

10.1 Introduction

The method we use is based on the Pitanguy's technique (Pitanguy 1961), which follows the principles of Lexer's technique (Lexer 1912): transposition of the nipple–areolar complex (NAC); resection of the excessive glandular tissue of the distal and infra-areolar segment of the breast, almost without any skin detachment and without using a prefabricated mold, resulting in peri-areolar and infra-areolar scars with an inverted T shape with the transversal branch at the level of the infra-mammary fold.

It is fundamental to mark the incisions, discount the distal displacement of the NAC and the infra-mammary fold owing to the weight of the severe hypertrophy of the breast.

10.2 Method

The technique described here has been already published, which has encouraged other surgeons to perform the operation (Sinder 1970, 1974, 1975).

R. Sinder, M.D.
Full Member of the Brazilian Society of Plastic Surgery, Av. Rui Barbosa, 532 Apto. 1501—Flamengo, Rio de Janeiro, RJ CEP 22250-020, Brazil
e-mail: ramilsinder@hotmail.com

Before the operation, it is mandatory to carry out surgical planning and the surgeon and patient should have a good understanding to achieve adequate results in a good balance between the breasts and with the body contour. First, the surgeon must discuss and listen to the patient's complaints concerning the size of the breast, with severe repercussions from a physical and psychological point of view. It is well known that several abnormalities of the chest and torso may occur, caused by deformities of the breasts.

10.2.1 Surgical Marking

To perform a breast reduction procedure, it is necessary to make surgical markings on the breasts for adequate orientation during the operation. For this reason, preoperative marking should be performed using methylene blue: the infra-mammary fold, the reference points of repair, and the skin incisions with the patient in the standing or sitting position. As recommended by Aufricht (1949), two stitches are done on the skin, one at the level of the sternal notch and the other at the base of the xyphoid process. Those reference points allow the transfer of symmetrical marks from the left breast to the right and vice versa. In the operating room, the patient is in a semi-sitting position.

First, the infra-mammary fold is demarcated. Afterward a trapezoid-shaped flap 4–5 cm in

J.M. Avelar (ed.), *Breast Surgery*, https://doi.org/10.1007/978-3-319-54115-0_10

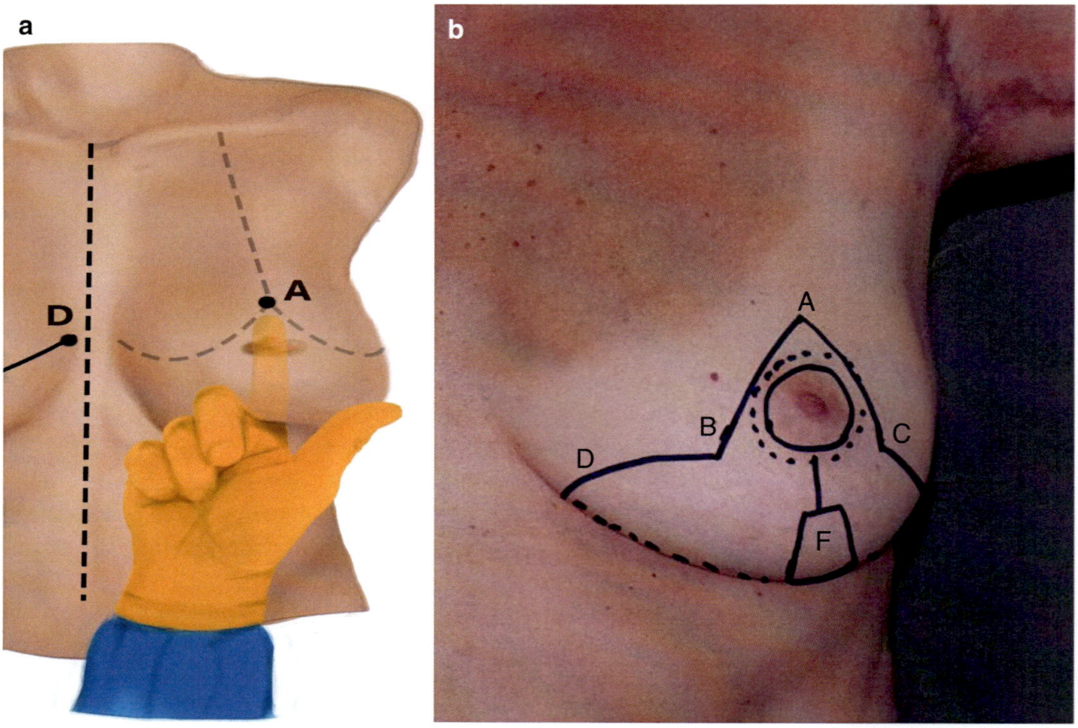

Fig. 10.1 Surgical marking. (**a**) Drawing shows Pitanguy's maneuver to determine point A. (**b**) After identification of point A, the other points B, C, D, and E are marked. The trapezoid flap (F) is drawn on the inframammary segment, with the base on the submammary fold

height based on the infra-mammary fold is drawn, equidistant from the nipple to the infra-mammary fold (Fig. 10.1).

Marking point A is the key to surgical marking before mastoplasty. From this reference point, all markings on the skin are made. There are various methods of marking point A during surgical marking, for example:

1. The geometrical or anatomical method: at the intersection of the hemi-clavicular or hemi-breast line with a transverse plane passing through the middle of the humerus (Penn 1955). The ideal position of the nipple is a little distal of this level.
2. A little higher than the crossing of the hemi-clavicular line, the proximal edge of a ruler is placed transversely behind the breast, close to the infra-mammary fold (Fernandes 1951)
3. With the surgeon's hand behind the breast, the tip of the index finger puts pressure on the middle of the infra-mammary fold (Fig. 10.1a) (Pitanguy 1961).
4. Using a plastic mold (Wise 1956; Strömbeck 1960)
5. When making the bi-digital pinch with traction toward the mid-mammary line, a supra-areolar bulge is formed with point A at the apex.

In the mid-clavicular line, just above the sub-mammary sulcus, we draw a circle of 4 cm in diameter (future position of the NAC). With manual and bi-digital maneuvers, we evaluate the excess tissue that must be resected and with the thumb and index fingers of both hands we "pinch" and we make a traction of the skin on each side of the circumference of the hemi-clavicular line until the areola is covered, which are the ends of the breast crease with points B and C respectively. We join points A to B, and A to C, and the ends of the infra-mammary fold with the D and E points respectively (Figs. 10.1b and 10.2).

When we mount the breast, this flap will be covered by the skin between the areola and the infra-mammary fold. Some stitches of the longitudinal infra-areolar and distal peri-areolar skin suture are made, transfixing the dermal face and the proximal end of the flap.

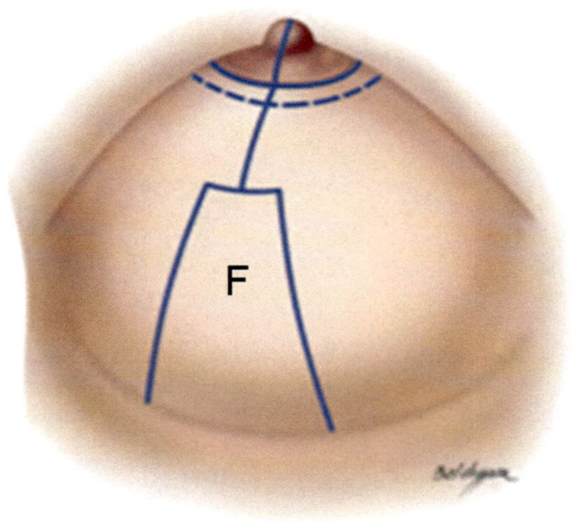

Fig. 10.2 Surgical marking before reduction mastoplasty. The drawing shows the trapezoid-shaped cutaneous flap (F) is demarcated, with its base on the submammary crease and the peri-areolar incision

10.2.1.1 The Operation

De-epithelialization of the skin around the areola by Schwarzmann's maneuver (Schwartzman 1930) is carried out and the trapezoid-shaped flap is made, following marking. The skin is incised all around the flap except on its base with its pedicle, which separated from the adipose–subcutaneous tissue.

10.2.1.2 Glandular Resection

Following previous evaluation and marking, the mammary tissue is resected according to the size of the breasts on both sides.

The resection of the infra-areolar tissue excess is performed via a flat incision in small and medium hypertrophy.

In larger breasts, the resection has a "keel" shape and forms two pillars that are sutured together to the aponeurosis of the pectoralis muscle; the mammary gland is largely detached from the pectoralis aponeurosis (Fig. 10.3).

Sometimes excision of the adipose–glandular tissue up to the base of the breast is carried out (Guinard 1903; Morestin 1907; Pontes 1973, 1981).

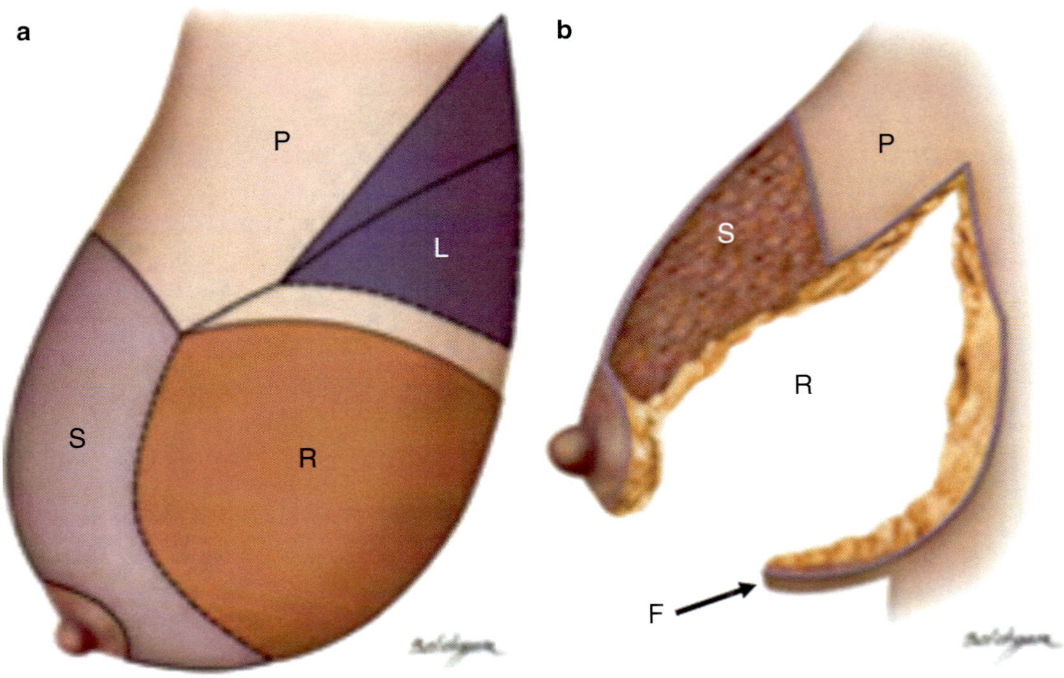

Fig. 10.3 Surgical markings. (**a**) Lateral view of the breast showing demarcated areas: *S* area for Schwarzmann's maneuver, *R* area for glandular resection, *P* remaining proximal segment of the breast with skin and mammary gland that will not be resected, *L* lateral prolongation of the mammary gland that may be resected in cases of large hypertrophic breasts. (**b**) Lateral view of the breast after glandular resection: the flap (F) indicated by the *arrow* is created before glandular resection

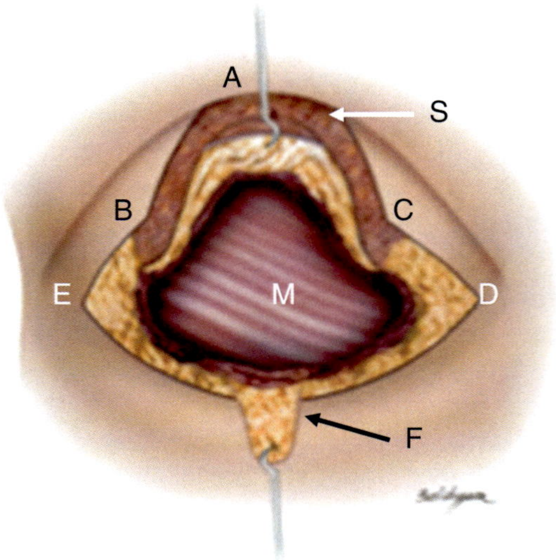

Fig. 10.4 Frontal view of the breast after glandular resection. The basic marking of points A, B, C, D, and E. The area S was de-epithelialized using Schwarzmann's maneuver with the nipple-areolar complex (NAC) being pulling upward by a strong hook. M pectoralis major muscle with its aponeurosis, F trapezoid-shaped flap is pulled downward by a small hook

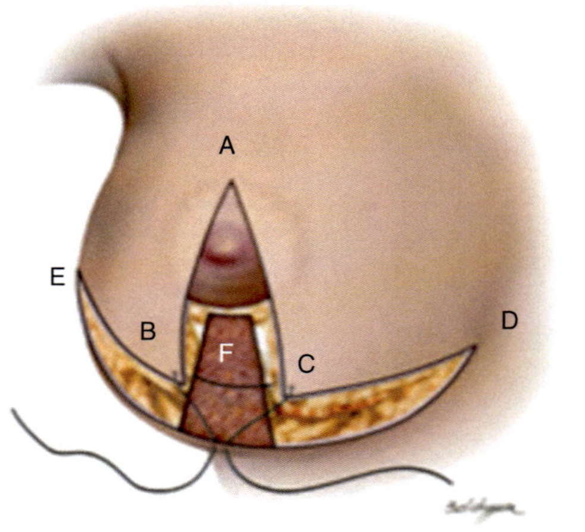

Fig. 10.5 Drawing shows the suture after glandular resection. A stitch is made to join point B to C on the midline of the breast covering the dermal–adipose flap F. Points D and E are placed at the submammary fold to indicate the ends of the areas of cutaneous and glandular resection

At this stage, we also perform excision of any excess fat and glandular tissue from the side of the breast on the axillary extension (Fig. 10.4). After rigorous hemostasis, we do the same on the other breast.

In gigantomasty we prefer the partial amputation of the breast, followed by modeling of the breast and NAC graft (Thorek 1942, 1946).

We check the shape and volume of the breast after glandular resection, supporting the breast with special forceps introduced under the NAC and two hooks, one at point B, the other at C that join at the inframammary fold, around the union of this medial third with the central third about 10 cm from the midline.

Breast suturing is carried out to fix the mammary gland to the aponeurosis of the pectoralis major (Malbec and Quaife 1957). The suturing is done in two planes between lines A–B and A–C (Fig. 10.5). Infra-areolar vertical or longitudinal suturing is done from the bottom up and with a hook, keeping the NAC close to point A to avoid invagination. The suturing of the inframammary fold should start by its ends and push the skin gently and progressively from the external ends toward the mid-clavicular line (Dowden et al. 1984) to prevent formation of "dog ears". The new NAC is drawn on top of the cone shape of the breast. The areola is sutured with U-shaped stitches (Gillies and Millard 1957; Lemos 1972).

A Penrose drain is used for 24 h. The wound is dressed using with microporous tape, long gauze, and a sterilized brassiere. The final surgical results may achieve natural aspects in good harmony with the body contour (Figs. 10.6 and 10.7).

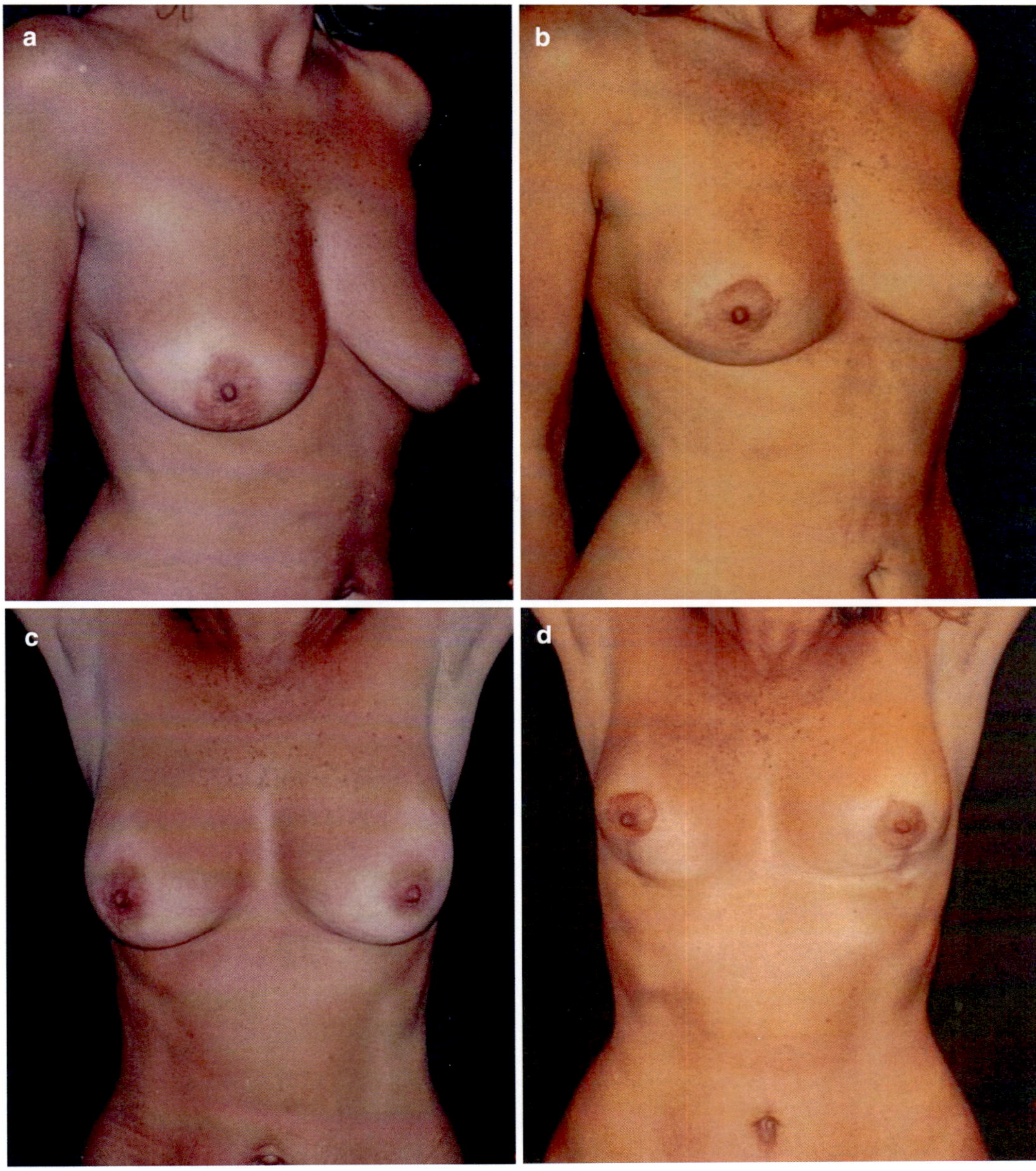

Fig. 10.6 A 48-year-old patient presented a ptotic breast. (**a**) and (**c**) Preoperative photos. (**b**) and (**d**) Post-operative photos 2 years after mammoplasty

10.3 Discussion

Nowadays, several techniques for reduction mastoplasty are described in the medical literature through which it is possible to achieve a very high rate of patient satisfaction with excellent aesthetic results. Since 1970, we have described a technique for creating a dermal–subcutaneous flap with its base on the submammary fold, which is a good support to the breast. The dermal–adipose flap is drawn during surgical marking and is introduced and sutured under the remaining mammary gland to avoid any sloughing of the junction of the inverted T scar (Figs. 10.4 and 10.5). The final scar is located peri-areolar and on the infra-mammary fold (Figs. 10.6 and 10.7). Surgical planning and markings are mandatory steps before operation (Fig. 10.1b). We prefer to

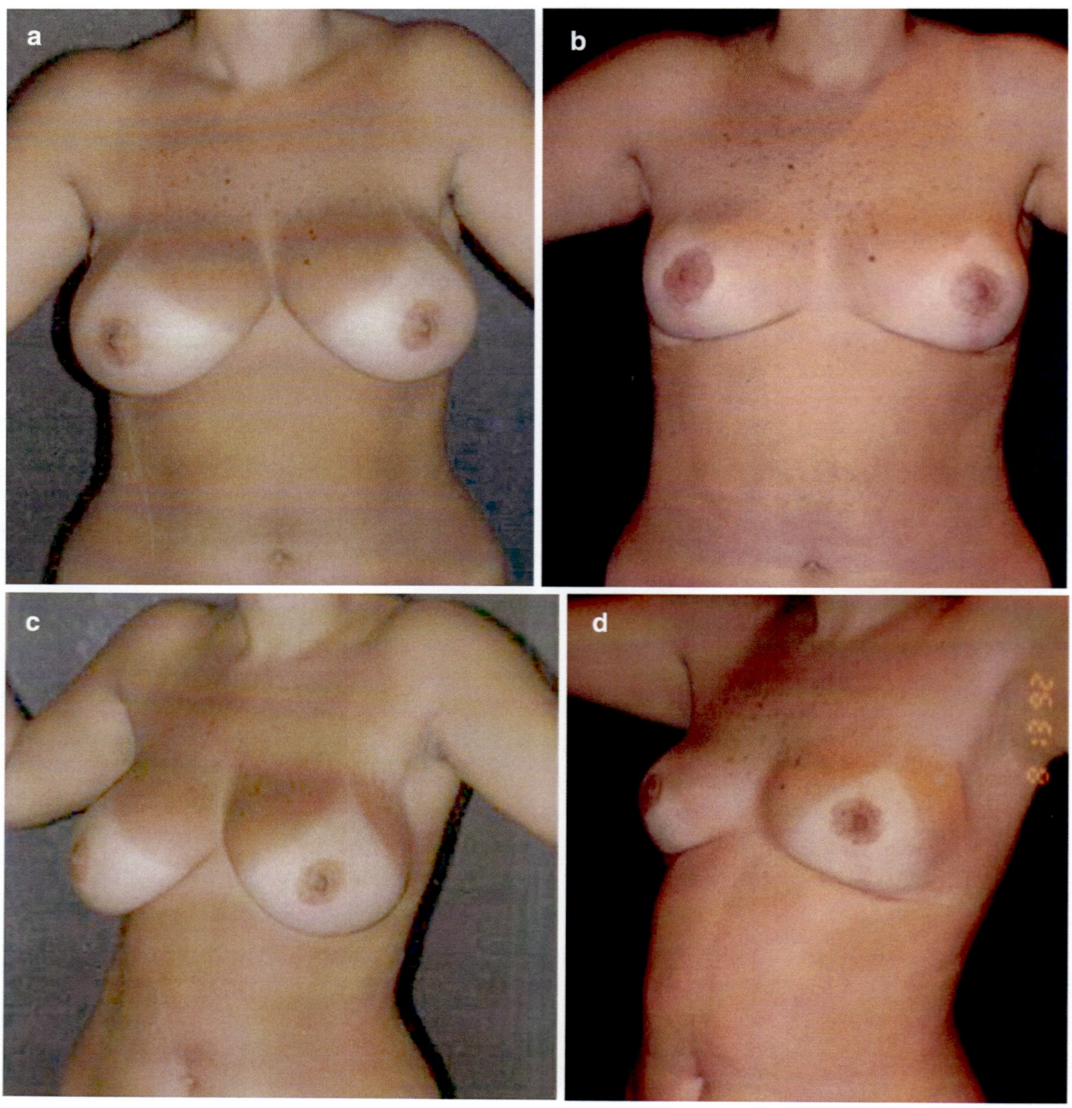

Fig. 10.7 A 43-year old patient presenting with hypertrophic and asymmetrical breasts. (**a**) and (**c**) Photos showing the preoperative aspect. (**b**) and (**d**) Photos 2 years after reduction mammoplasty

carry out marking of the patient in a standing or sitting position to mark the sub-mammary crease where the horizontal segment of the inverted T scar will be located.

Conclusions

To employ reduction mastoplasty through the technique described above may provide good aesthetic results with smooth scars located around the NAC and on the infra-mammary fold. The volume of the mammary glad to be resected is determined according to the surgical planning. The operation is performed with the patient in a semi-sitting position.

References

Aufricht G (1949) Mammaplasty for pendulous breast. Empiric and geometry planning. Plast Reconstr Surg 4:13

Dowden RV, Dinner M, Labandter HP (1984) Breast reduction for asymmetrical hypertrophy. Plast Reconstr Surg 73(6):928

Fernandes J (1951) Mastoplastias, nuestra experiência editorial universitária, Buenos Aires

Gillies HD, Millard DR (1957) Principles and art of plastic surgery, vol 2, 1st edn. Little, Brown & Company, Boston

Guinard A (1903) Semicirculares incisions par la resection discoide hypertrophie mammaire tratee. Bull Mem Soc Chir Paris 26:597

Lemos P (1972) Comunicação pessoal—first International Society of Aesthetic Plastic Surgery (ISAPS) Congress, January, Rio de Janeiro, Brazil

Lexer E (1912) Sitzungsbericht der Naturwissenschaftl–med Ges Jena München. Munch Med Wochenschr 59:2702

Malbec EF, Quaife JV (1957) Plastias mammarias. Nuestra experiências com inclusíones. Orientacián Médica 260:768

Morestin H (1907) Bilateral mammary hypertrophy corrected by discoid resection. Bull Mém Soc Chir Paris 33:201

Penn J (1955) Breast reduction. Br J Plast Surg 7:357

Pitanguy I (1961) Mammaplastias. Estudo de 245 casos consecutivos de mamaplastia e apresentação de técnica pessoal. Rev Bras Cir

Pontes R (1973) A technique of reduction mammaplasty. Br J Plast Surg 26:365–370

Pontes R (1981) Reduction mammaplasty—variations I and II. Ann Plast Surg 6(6):437

Schwartzmann E (1930) Die Technik der Mammaplastik. Chirurgie 2:932–943

Sinder R (1970) Tese apresentada à ex-Faculdade Nacional de Medicina, atual Universidade Federal Do Rio de Janeiro (UFRJ), Para concorrer à livre-Docência, Rio de Janeiro

Sinder R (1974) The use of dermo-adipose flap in abdominoplasty and mammoplasty—personal technique. (Uso de retalho dermo-adiposo em plásticas de mamas e de abdome—técnicas pessoais). XI Cong Bras Cirurgia Plástica. Belo Horizonte-MG

Sinder R (1975) Use of decorticated dermo-adipose flap in abdominoplasty and mammaplasty. VI International Cong Plastic Surgery. 24–29 August (page 58 of the abstract)

Strömbeck JO (1960) Mammaplasty: report of a new technique based on the two pedicle procedure. Br J Plast Surg 13:79

Thorek M (1942) Plastic surgery of the breast and abdominal wall. Charles Thomas, Springfield

Thorek M (1946) Plastic reconstruction of the breast and free transplantation of the nipple. J Int Coll Surg 9:194

Wise RJ (1956) A preliminary report on a method of planning the mammaplasty. Plast Reconstr Surg 17:367

11 Pectoralis Major Muscle Flap: A Support Approach to Mammaplasty, Personal Technique

Alberto M.L. Caldeira, Santos Espinal Gómez, Manuel Antonio Torreira Rios, and Walter Marrou Pautrat

11.1 Introduction

Breast ptosis is usually an acquired phenomenon resulting from an inadequate relationship between the breast container (skin) and its content (gland). Distention of the skin and/or glandular–adipose volume loss with posterior non-adaptation of the skin (elasticity and retraction capacity decrease) results in a container larger than its content.

There is a common and constant concern among many authors to avoid postoperative mammary ptosis. In 1882, Gaillard, Thomas et al. described an incision place at the level of the submammary fold to remove benign tumors, by which the breast was raised and attached to the second rib cartilage (Goulian 1976). There is significant concern among the various authors with regard to preventing breast ptosis.

In 1908, Dehner promoted an elliptical resection of the upper portion of the breast with posterior fixation to the rib periosteum (Dehner 1908).

Fixation of the gland to the thoracic wall by means of deep sutures, is used by many surgeons, having become widely known through works performed by Arié (1957) and Pitanguy (1962).

In 1987, the senior author began investigating the possibility of obtaining better aesthetic results through the modification of the breast architecture by means of three interposed breast tissue flaps (Caldeira 1994a, b; 1995a, b). The end in view was to provide reduction of the breast base and axillary pole and a more medial position of the lateral pole, which, besides conveying a substantial conification of the breast tissue, would also help project the areolo-mamillary complex to its apex. This technique favors a more effective and lasting breast shape besides maximal preservation of the skin covering and reduced postoperative ptosis.

Based on Milton Daniel's procedure, we began to associate the primary approach to breast tissue with a muscle approach for breast support and shape (Daniel 1993). This technique is based on the pars abdominalis of the major pectoralis muscle, which is positioned on the inferior breast pole Ribeiro (1975) and tractioned upward to restrain the action of gravity (Caldeira et al. 2008).

A.M.L. Caldeira, M.D., M.Sc., Ph.D., F.A.C.S., F.I.C.S. (✉)
Global Plastic Surgery Department, Casa de Saúde Portugal, Instituto de Pós-Graduação Médica Carlos Chagas/Universidade Santa Úrsula, Rio de Janeiro, RJ, Brazil

Plastic and Reconstructive Surgery Department, Caldeira-Roth Institute, Rua Visconde de Pirajá, 414 – suite 1012, Ipanema, Rio de Janeiro, RJ CEP 22410-002, Brazil
e-mail: lottcaldeira@gmail.com

S.E. Gómez, M.D. • M.A. Torreira Rios, M.D.
Global Plastic Surgery Department, Casa de Saúde Portugal, Instituto de Pós-Graduação Médica Carlos Chagas/Universidade Santa Úrsula, Rio de Janeiro, RJ, Brazil

W. Marrou Pautrat, M.D.
Instituto Ivo Pitanguy/Instituto de Pós-Graduação Médica Carlos Chagas, Rio de Janeiro, RJ, Brazil

J.M. Avelar (ed.), *Breast Surgery*, https://doi.org/10.1007/978-3-319-54115-0_11

11.2 Anatomical Considerations

Knowledge of certain anatomical details of the pectoralis major muscle leads to a better understanding of why this procedure does not substantially alter the anatomy and function of the referred muscle (Fig. 11.1).

The *pectoralis major* muscle has three main origins (clavicular, sternal, and abdominal) and fibers that emerge from the second to the sixth rib cartilages. The abdominal portion arises from the distal third of the stern, from the *rectoabdominal* muscle sheath and aponeurosis of the external oblique muscle (Gray 1935; Spalteholz 1923). In a lateral and cranial direction passing below the clavicular and sternal portions, the abdominal portion inserts on the intertubercular humeral groove at a deeper and more posterior position than the rest of the muscle fibers. The breast tissue in contact with the pectoral fascia presents a number of small prolongations that insert into the muscle (Fig. 11.2).

The blood supply in the pectoralis major muscle is type V, with one dominant vascular pedicle and a number of secondary segmental pedicles. The dominant pedicle is based on the thoraco-acromial artery and the secondary segmental pedicles are based on the internal thoracic artery. The fourth perforator of the internal thoracic artery and the terminal segment of the pectoral artery, a branch of the thoraco-acromial artery, supply the inferior third of the muscle. Besides this, other ramifications of the lateral thoracic artery and intercostal arteries contribute to the blood supply. The superior portion of the muscle is innervated

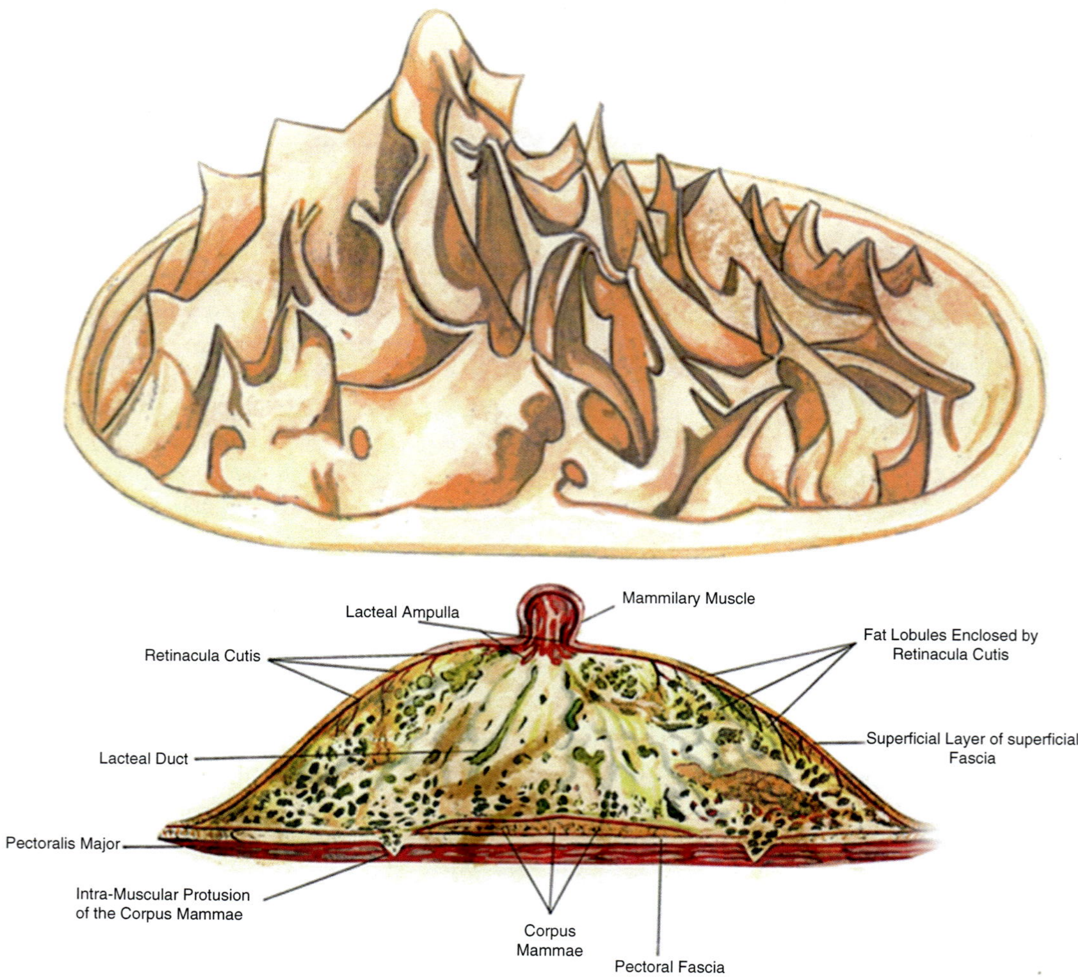

Fig. 11.1 *Top*: Cooper's ligaments of the breast. *Bottom*: Intramuscular protrusion of the corpus mammae

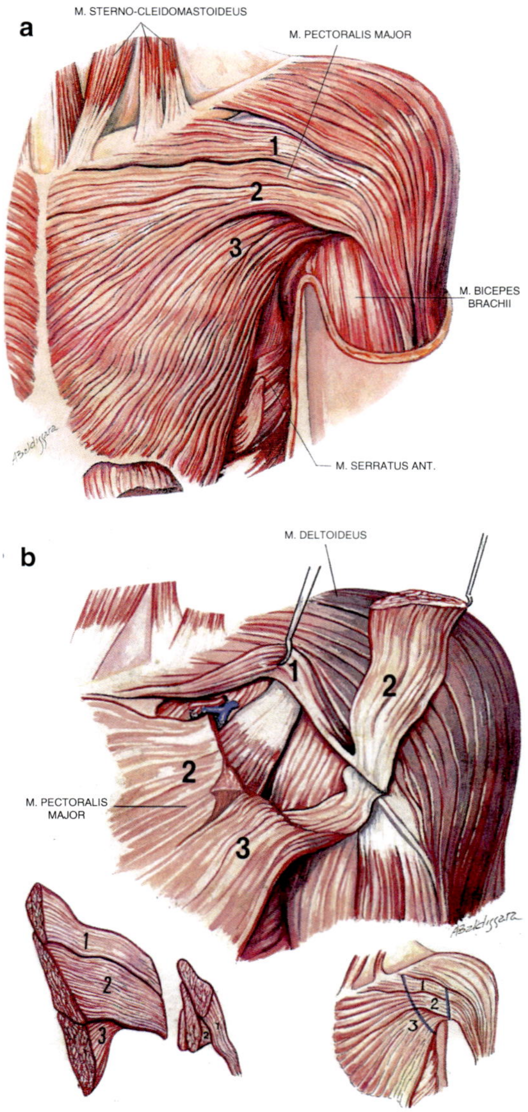

Fig. 11.2 (**a**) The three portions of the pectoralis major muscle converge like the leaves of a fan and present single insertions at the lateral border of the intertubercular sulcus of the humerus. (**b**) When the sternal portion (*2*) approaches the axillar, it progressively covers the abdominal portion (*3*). The two comprise a single body medially, but are individualized near the humerus

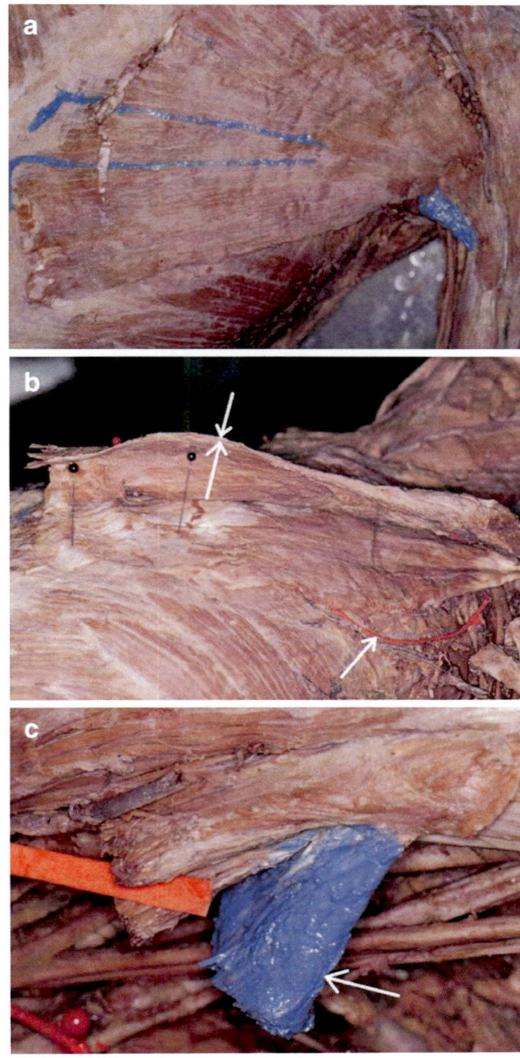

Fig. 11.3 Anatomical study showing (**a**) where the fourth perforator of the thoracic artery is based in relation to the parasternal border (*white dot*). The muscle incisions used to shape the flaps can be made at the superior or inferior limits related to the projection of this perforator. (**b**) The pectoral artery, a branch of the thoraco-acromial artery, slides over the deep surface of the pectoralis major muscle, penetrates the muscle, and is anastomosed with the perforating branches of the internal thoracic artery (*large arrow*). The lateral thoracic artery circles the lateral margin of the tendon of the pectoralis minor muscle and continues 4–5 cm along its lateral border before being buried in the pectoralis major muscle (*small arrow*). The thickness of the muscle defines the variant to be used. (**c**) Detail of the insertions of the pectoralis major muscle. The pars abdominalis penetrates the humeral intertubercular sulcus more posteriorly and deeply than the clavicular and sternal portions

by the medial pectoral nerve (C8 and T1), whereas the inferior third is innervated by the lateral pectoral nerve (C5, C6, and C7) (Ralph 1980).

The inferior third of the muscle promotes the final movement of adduction and internal rotation of the humerus, a function of little significance (Fig. 11.3).

11.3 Surgical Considerations

The senior author's surgical technique is based on the transformation of the lower segment of the pectoralis major muscle as a supportive element of the breast tissue. The lower third of the muscle (pars abdominalis) is used as a flap to various degrees. In this portion, the muscle thickness is relatively thin in women (0.5–0.8 cm), allowing mobilization and satisfactory handling (McCraw and Arnold 2007). The patient is placed in the supine position, with the dorsum at 45° and the arms abducted. This will allow visualization of the breast in a natural position. Skin marking will depend on the type of the breast, preference being given to skin resections that result in minimal scars and a tensionless wound closure.

With the breast firmly secured at its base, skin incision is carried out, followed by Schwarzmann's maneuver in a medial–dermal undermining, then cutaneous–glandular and muscle–glandular undermining of the inferior half of the breast.

Glandular resection will depend on the deformity to be corrected and on the resultant breast size desired. Reshaping the breast tissue begins by the preparation of three triangular flaps, medial, central, and lateral, posteriorly interposed, which produce a conical shape. Three types of pectoralis major muscle flaps can be prepared according to the anatomical type of the breast:

Type 1. The muscle is deeply incised in the same direction as its fibers. The incision is made in the inferior boundary of the fourth perforator of the internal thoracic artery. The muscle fibers are separated caudally with medial disinsertion of the muscles, thus forming the muscle pocket (Fig. 11.4). The inferior/lateral breast pole is inserted into this muscle pocket and secured with several sutures. This type is indicated for glandular breasts of moderate to large size with minor axillary projection (Fig. 11.5).

Type 2. Two parallel incisions are carried out on the pectoralis major muscle in the same direction of its fibers. The distance variation between these two parallels is 4–5 cm. The muscle flap is tractioned anteriorly and the borders of the pectoralis major are sutured with 3.0 mononylon (Fig. 11.6). The flap covers part of the inferior/lateral pole where it is secured. This type is indicated for breasts of glandular/adipose content with major axillary projection (Fig. 11.7).

Type 3. Similar to type 1, it consists of the preparation of a muscle pocket, although here the incision is performed in a cranial position to the projection of the fourth perforator of the internal thoracic artery (Fig. 11.8). Medial disinsertion of the muscle is carried out, in addition to ligature of the perforator. Type 3 is indicated for adipose breasts with discreet axillary projection (Fig. 11.9).

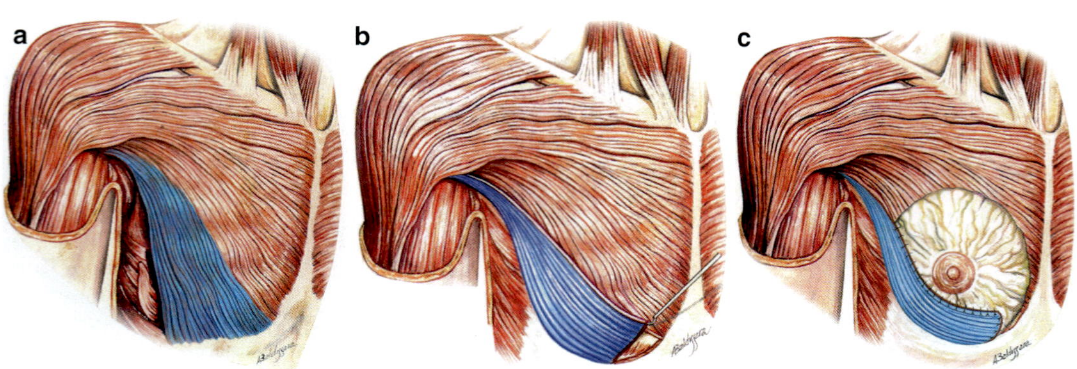

Fig. 11.4 (**a**) Procedure type 1 consists of using the muscle portion situated caudally to the fourth perforator of the internal thoracic artery. (**b**) By undermining and medial disinsertion of the muscle (**c**), the breast tissue pocket is shaped

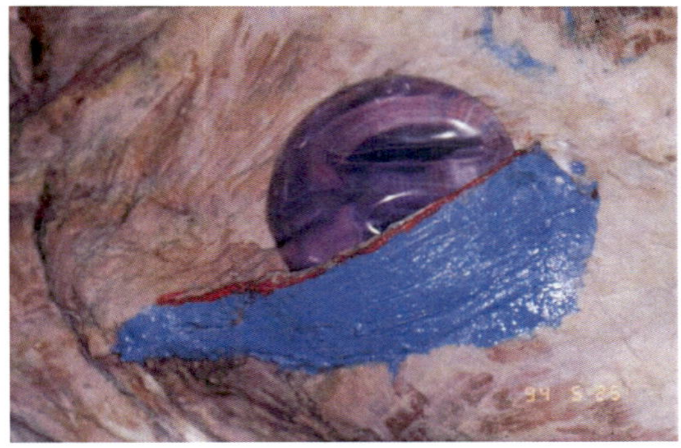

Fig. 11.5 Cadaver study of procedure type 1 simulating the resulting effect with a breast prosthesis

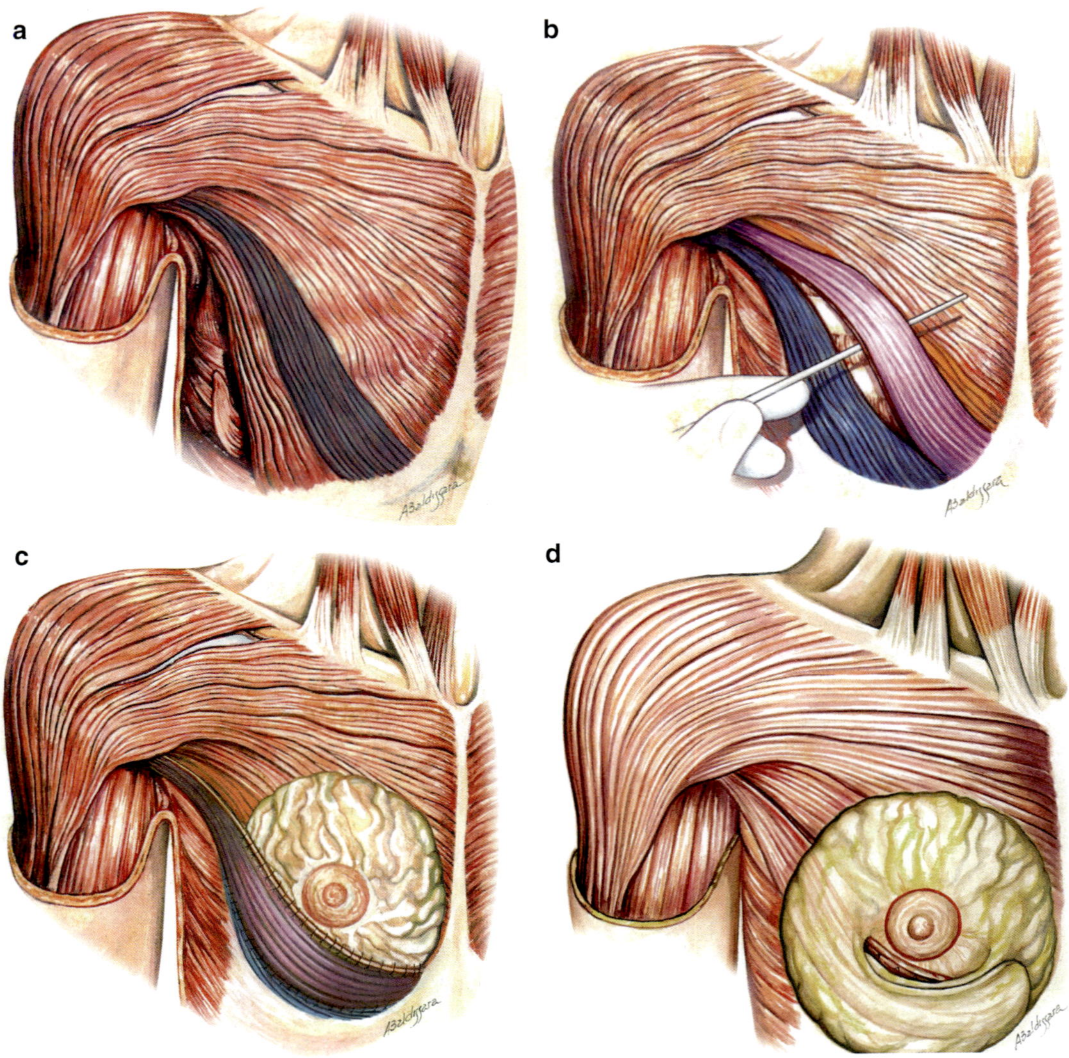

Fig. 11.6 (**a**) The muscle portion used in the type 2 procedure corresponds to a bipedicled flap (**b**), that, when ventrally tractioned (**c**), fully envelopes the breast assemblage (variant A) (**d**), or cover only the central glandulo-adipose flap (variant B)

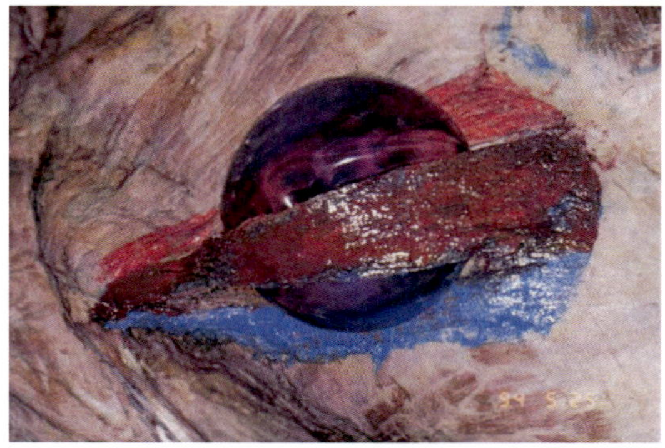

Fig. 11.7 The muscle segment in the type 2 procedure envelopes the breast gland, simulated in this example by a silicone gel breast implant

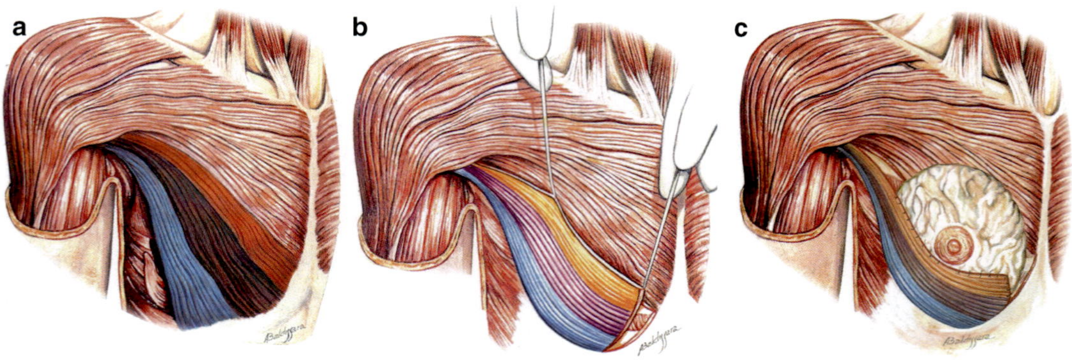

Fig. 11.8 (**a**) In the type 3 procedure the three portions of the pars abdominalis are used, (**b**) with its disinsertion compromising the fourth perforator of the internal thoracic artery. (**c**) A larger pocket that covers the inferior hemisphere and the breast tissue lateral pole is fashioned

The three types can be used in two ways.

Variant A: the muscle flap externally wraps the breast assemblage (lateral, central, and medial breast flaps) (Fig. 11.10). This variant is used when the muscle is underdeveloped (Fig. 11.11).

Variant B: The muscle flap is anchored directly onto the central flap of the breast tissue, which promotes internal support to the medial and lateral flaps. This variant is used when the muscle is thicker and larger (Fig. 11.12).

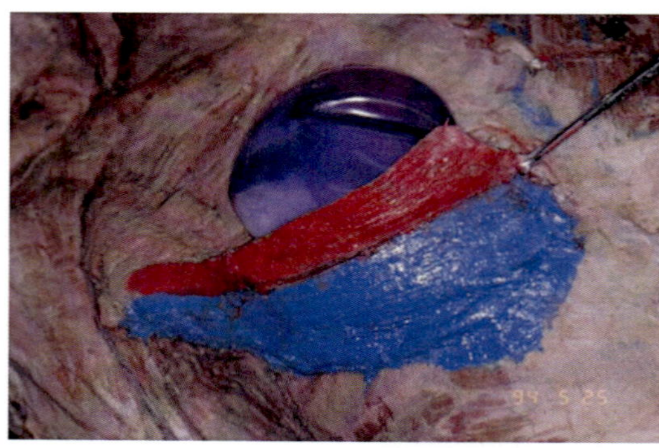

Fig. 11.9 Cadaver study of the type 3 procedure simulating the resulting effect with a breast implant

We use suction drains because of the wide glandular and muscle undermining. The subcutaneous tissue is sutured with separate 4.0 Vicryl stitches. Skin excess resection is carried out in such a way that closure of the wound borders is undertaken with no tension. The skin is distributed around the nipple with eight 4.0 Mononylon Gillies stitches followed by Monocryl intradermic continuous sutures. In the case of any vertical or horizontal incisions, closure is made with intradermic continuous sutures. We request patients to begin pectoral muscle contraction exercises after the 7th day, pulling the breast upward and thus eliminating any traction over the wounds.

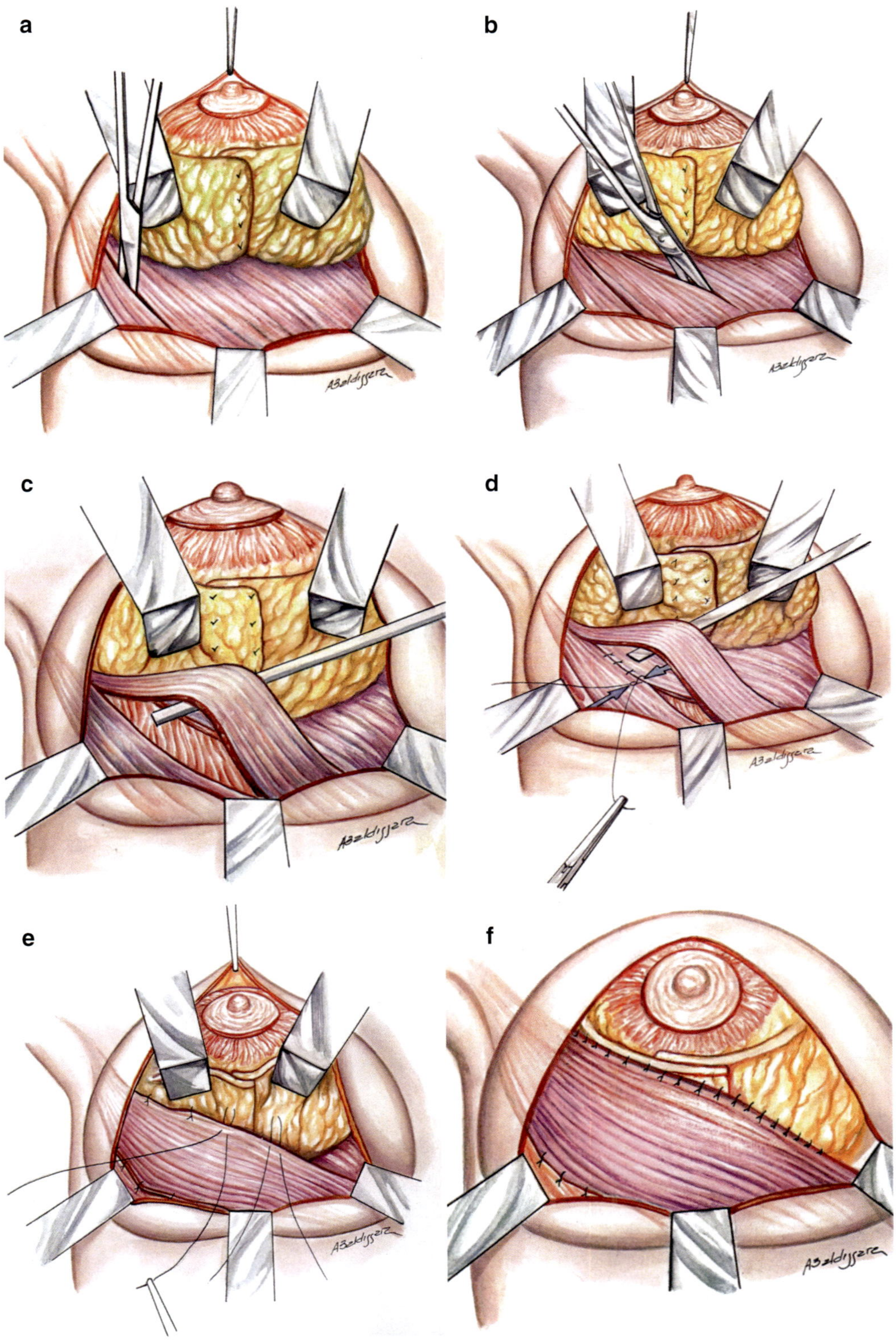

Fig. 11.10 (**a**, **b**) Drawings showing the variant A procedure and the type 2 procedure. Shaping of the bipedicled muscle flap. (**c**, **d**) The flap is raised and the borders of the pectoralis major muscle are sutured. (**e**, **f**) External fixation of the muscle flap to the glandulo-adipose tissue

Fig. 11.11 Transoperative views of how the muscle is approached in the type 2A procedure. The muscle is in place and covering the inferior breast pole

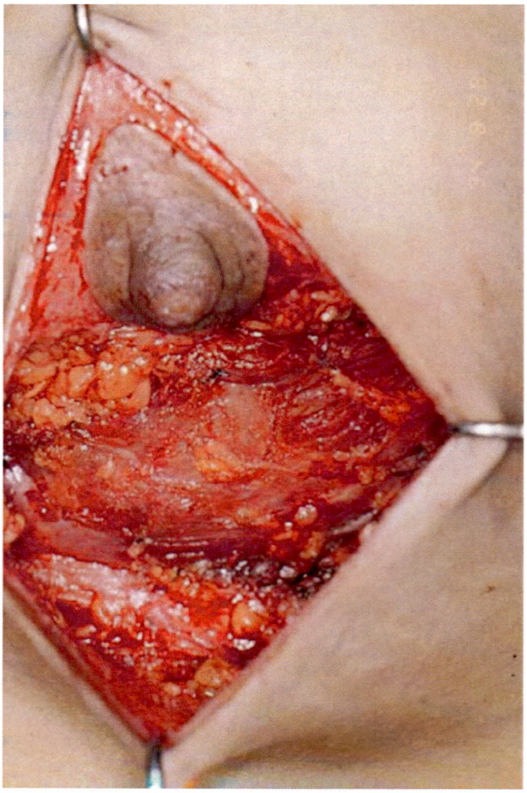

a

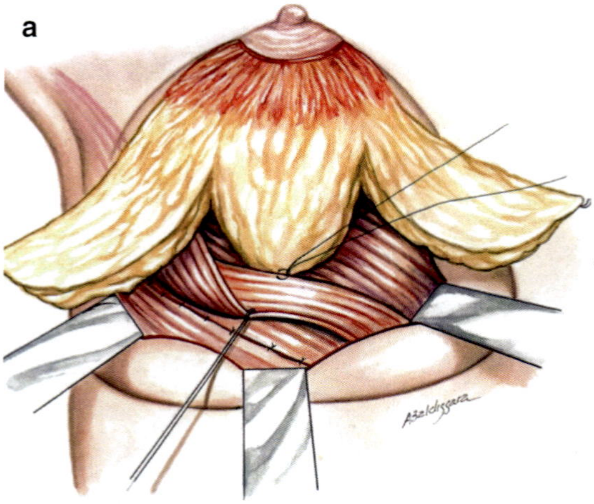

b

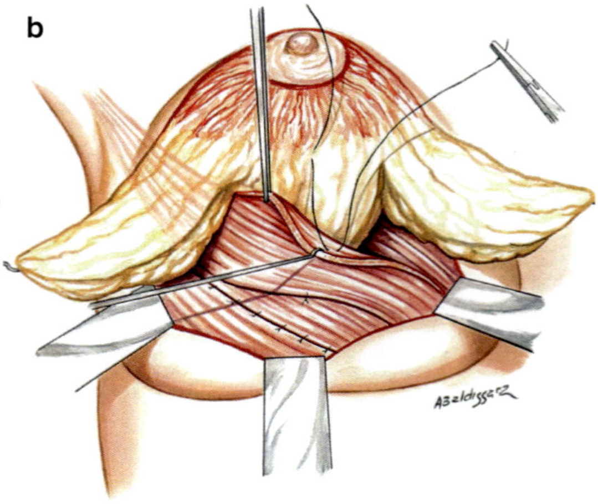

Fig. 11.12 (**a–c**) In the variant B procedure the muscle flap is sutured directly onto the central glandulo-adipose flap. (**d**, **e**) The medial flap is rotated and deeply secured to the muscle (**f**), and the lateral flap is transposed over the medial one

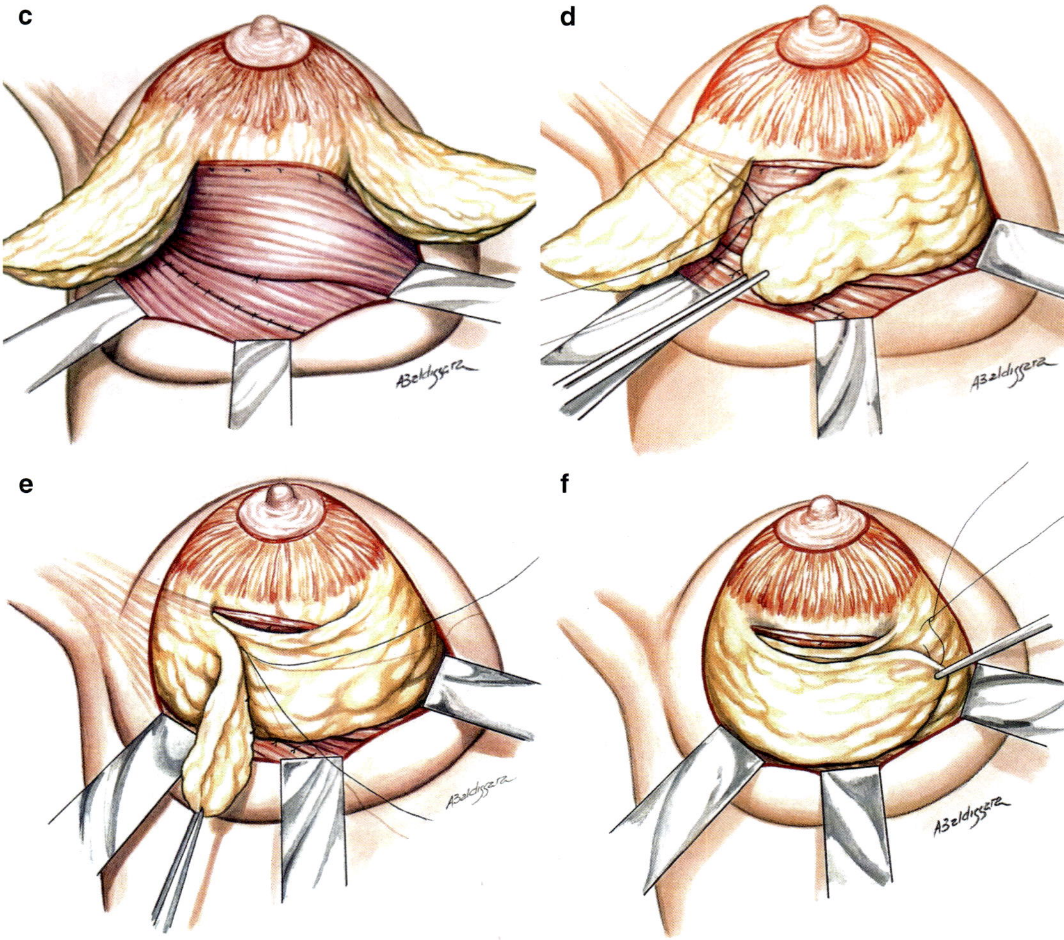

Fig. 11.12 (continued)

11.4 Discussion

The different techniques used in mastopexy and reductions have a temporary result in the medium and long term and sometimes also in the immediate postoperative period, as the breasts show a tendency to resume the anatomical configuration provided, even with traditional fastening methods of the gland over the pectoralis major muscle (Dehner 1908; Pitanguy 1962). The results were often considered unfavorable because of the lack of a conical shape of the breasts, pointing out that most procedures resulted in a rounded e breast (Candiani et al. 1991; Peixoto 1980).

Other authors employ dermal flaps of internal fixation needing enough dermis to allow anchoring of the flap in the pectoral muscle (Pitanguy 1962; Sampaio 1993). Furthermore, there is the disadvantage of limitations inherent to periareolar techniques.

The glandular nature of some breasts permits better maintenance of the superior breast pole shape and volume. Tissue redistribution and long-term support obtained with the technique we present here also achieve this objective in cases of breasts with a glandular–adipose content (Fig. 11.13).

The vertex of the breast is secured with the use of a pectoralis major flap, which avoids any

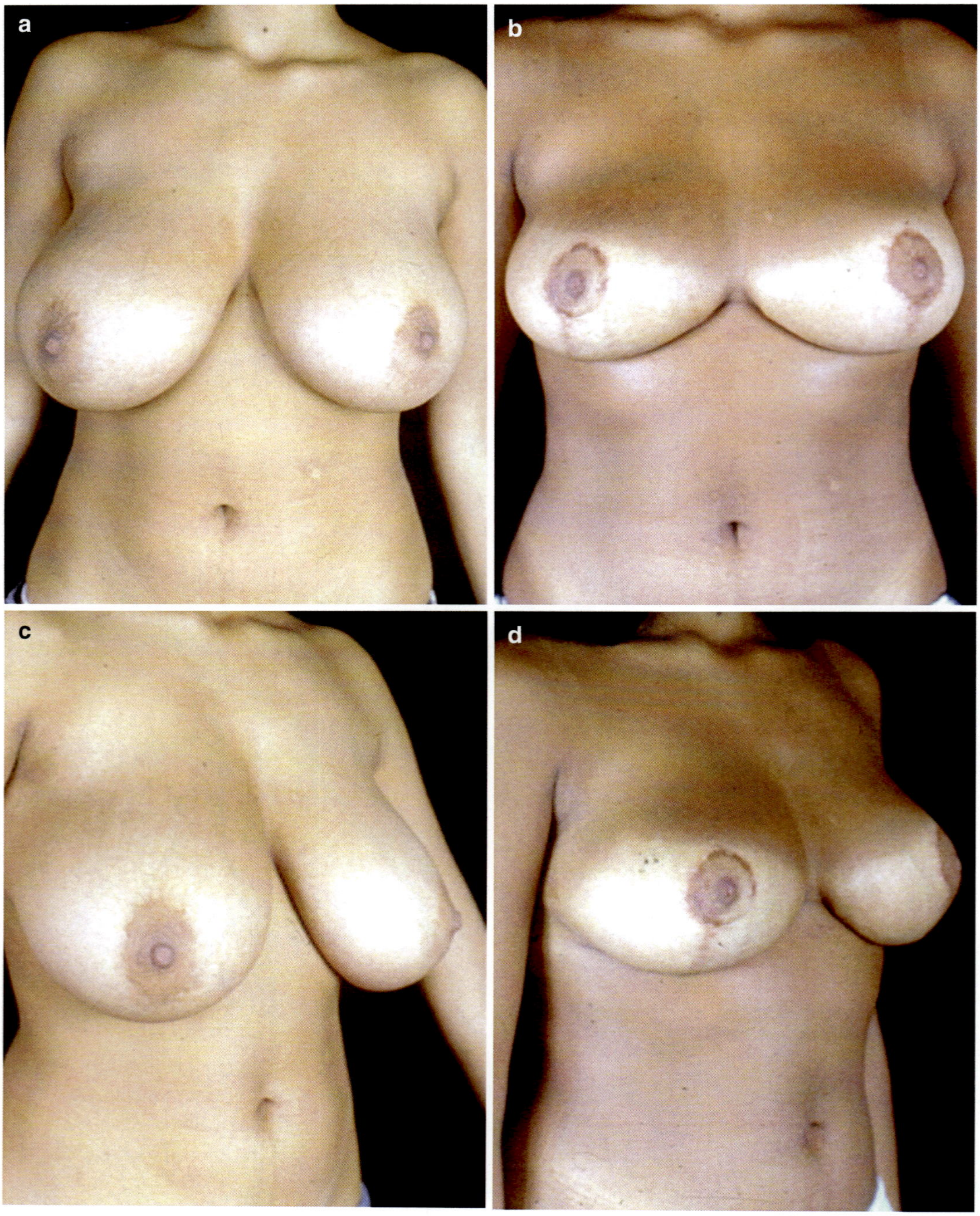

Fig. 11.13 (**a**, **c**, **e**) Preoperative views of an 18-year-old patient with bilateral large breast hypertrophy and ptosis. (**b**, **d**, **f**) Clinical checkup 8 months after surgery using the triple-flap interposition (TFI) technique and variant 3A (900 g was removed from the right breast and 850 g from the left one)

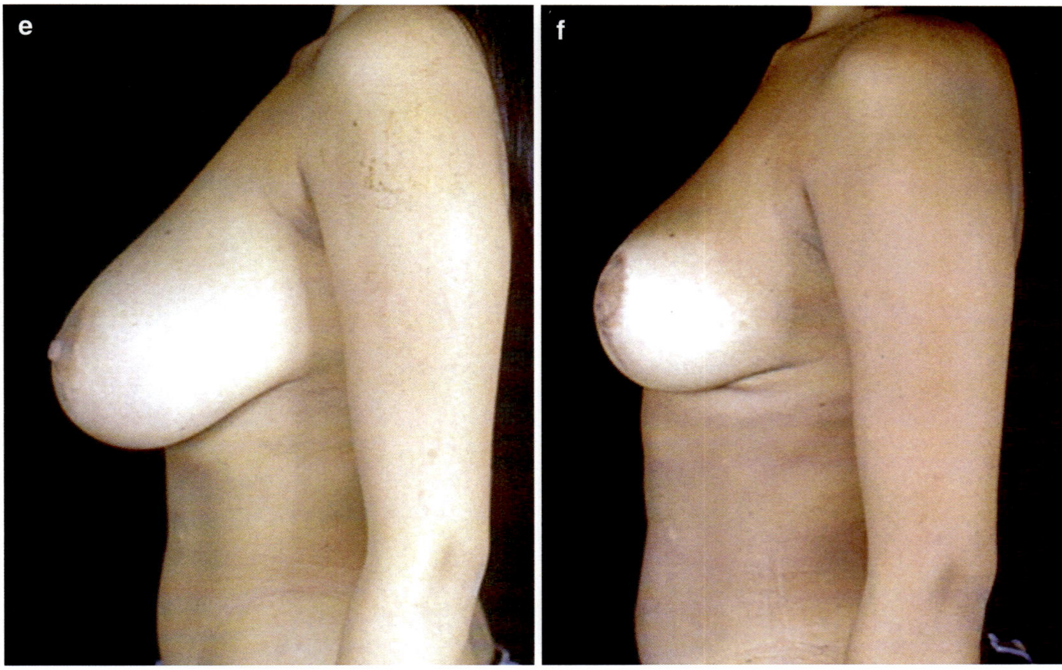

Fig. 11.13 (continued)

anterior–posterior flattening and prevents loss of the breast height; furthermore, when in the prone position, the breast does not slide laterally over the thorax and consequently eliminates breast and areolar deformity. In addition, the muscle avoids a definite sliding movement that usually occurs in the medium and long term with all the techniques presently in use (Fig. 11.14) (Dehner 1908; McKissock 1972; Skoog 1963).

Treatment of the axillary and lateral poles, which decreases and medializes the content, plus correction of breast asymmetries, present much more effective results. We believe that this technique also offers greater support and protection to breast implants.

One other advantage of the muscle flap is a decrease in postoperative complications. The muscle removes the weight of the breast over the scar and consequently prevents enlargement and formation of hypertrophic scars (Fig. 11.15).

Contraction of the muscle promotes an ascendant and harmonious movement of the mammary assemblage, which is more intense in women with marked muscular development.

We used type 2 and variant B more frequently, as most patients presented an important axillary component. Contrary to what was expected at the beginning of our study, although muscle medial disinsertion was carried out in types 2 and 3, muscular atrophy was unimportant in the postoperative period.

Contact of muscle and gland without fascia pectoralis mediation does not presuppose anatomical aggression, because under normal conditions the muscle is intimately related to the glandular parenchyma through glandular projections introduced into the muscular tissue (Daniel et al. 2015).

This technique proposes a muscular transposition for support of the mammary assemblage and

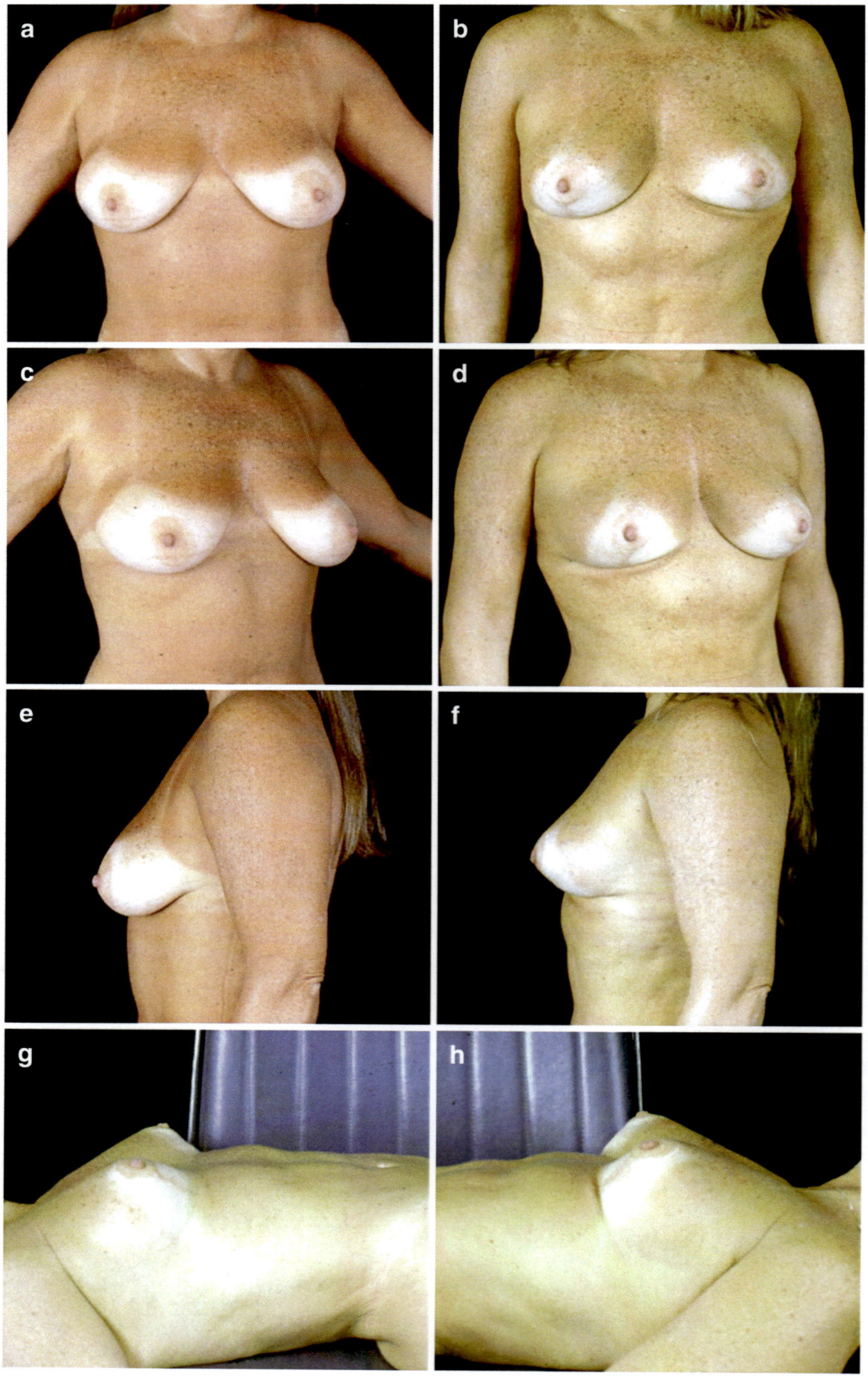

Fig. 11.14 (**a**, **c**, **e**) Preoperative views of a 42-year-old patient with moderate hypertrophy and a large base. (**b**, **d**, **f**) The 18-month result following the TFI technique and variant 1A. (**g**, **h**) In the prone position, note how the breast maintains its conical shape

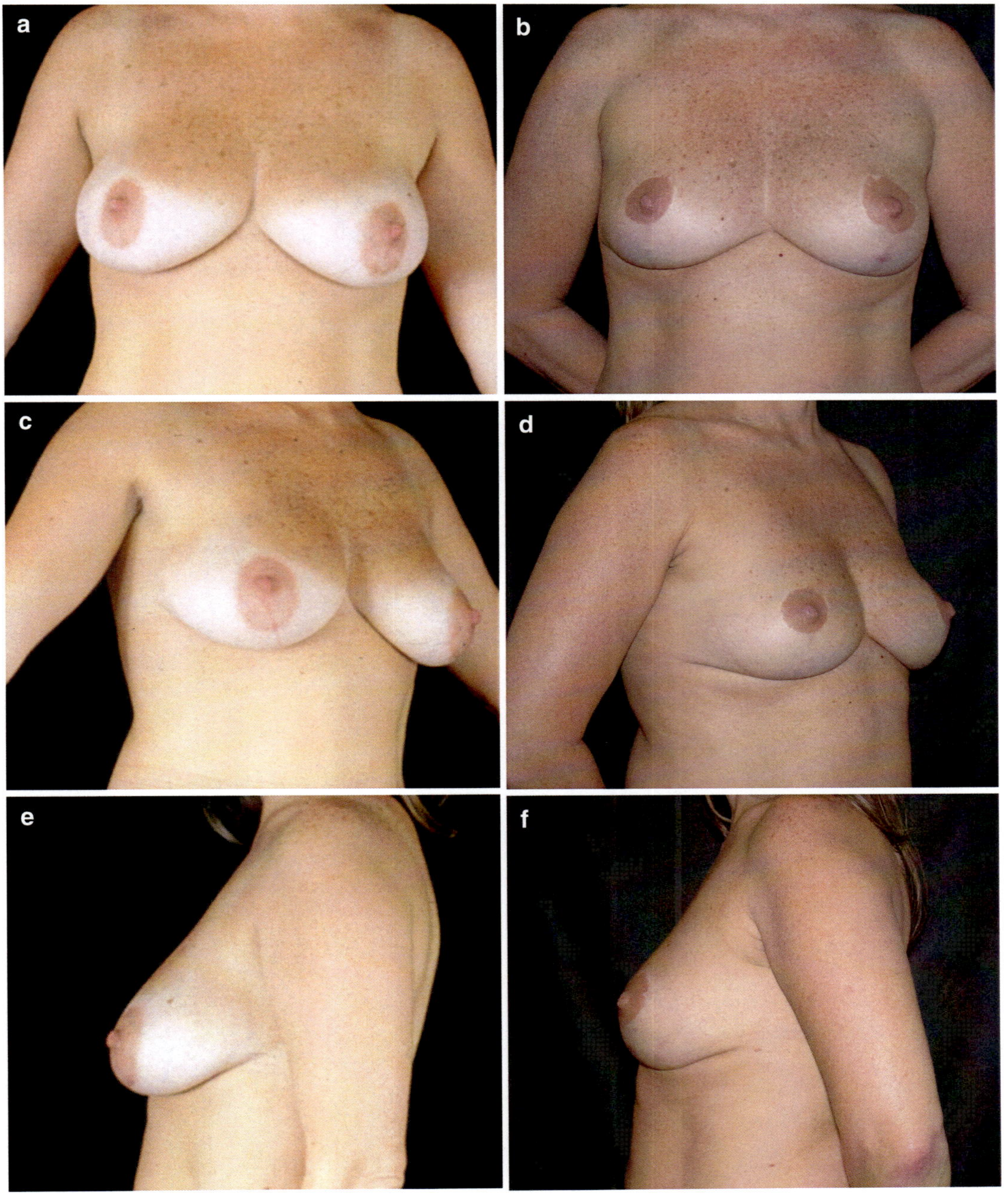

Fig. 11.15 (**a**, **c**, **e**) Preoperative views of a 38-year-old patient with mild breast hypertrophy and a considerable axillary and lateral pole. (**b**, **d**, **f**) Postoperative views 10 years after this approach, in which the surgical correction is maintained

consequent construction of an internal "brassiere," which avoids the complicating hazards that occur when alloplastic materials are used (Bustos 1992).

A dynamic breast deformity was the major complication observed with the use of the pectoralis major muscle. In patients operated on with the variants, the muscle excessively tractioned the lateral inferior portion of the breast. One of these patients underwent muscle resection under local anesthesia and in the other two the muscle was repositioned using variant B. We believe that this technique can even be used in athletes, in whom muscles are much more developed.

Variant B, in particular, promotes an overall upward traction of the breast assemblage that prevents breast ptosis. Figure 11.16 shows a female athlete with a predominantly adipose

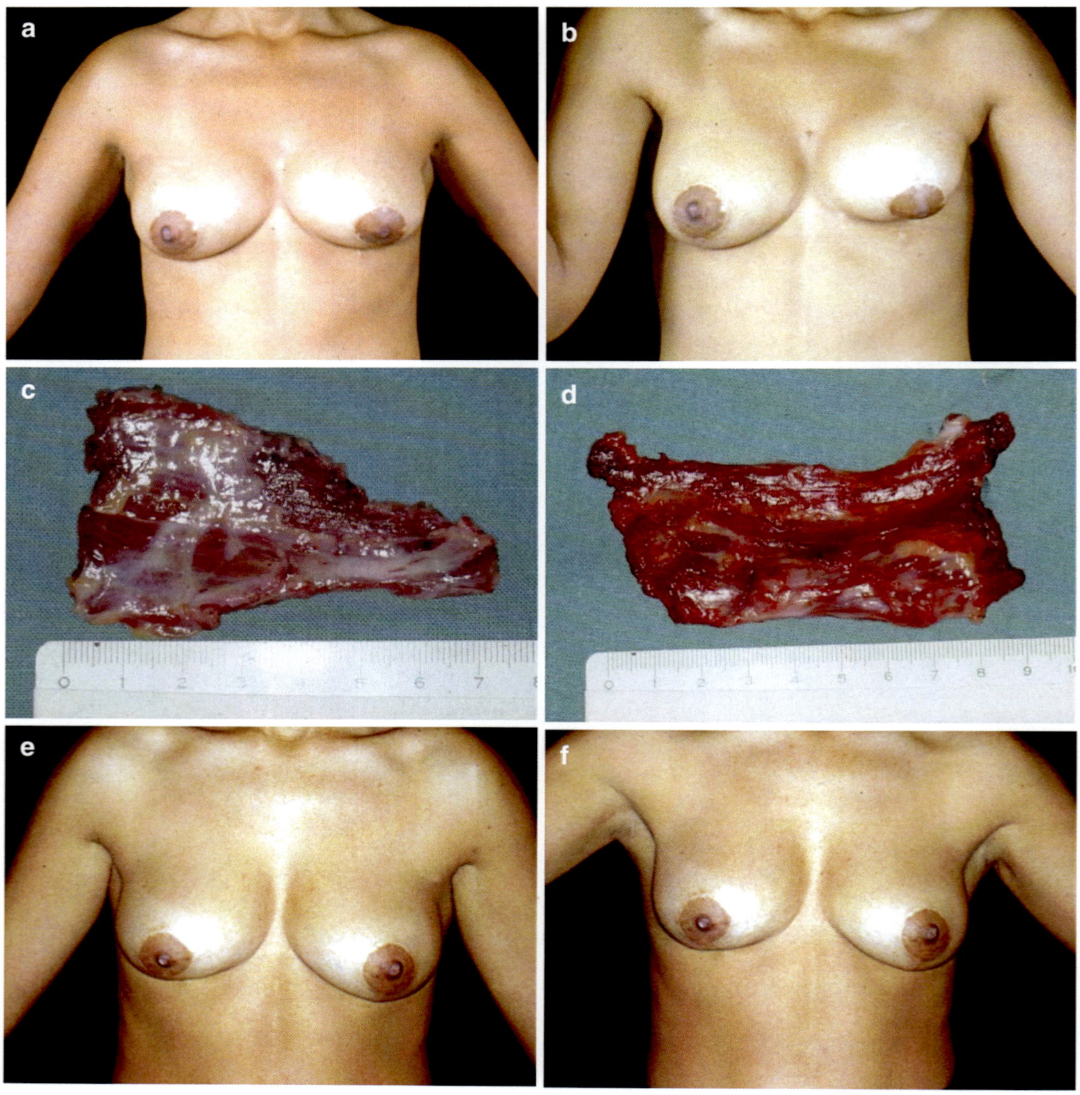

Fig. 11.16 (**a**) Athlete patient at rest and (**b**) contracting the pectoral muscles. A more conspicuous breast deformity can be observed on the left breast. (**c**) Muscle segment resected from the left breast. (**d**) Muscle segment resected from the right breast. (**e, f**) Postoperative views 3 years after the muscle flap resection with no compromising of the breast structure

breast and some preoperative asymmetry. The left breast was smaller than the right one, and as the patient did not wish to insert a breast prosthesis or decrease the size of the right and larger breast, we carried out the type 2A procedure on the right breast and the type 3A on the left one to increase its size. The excessive muscular mass on the left breast promoted excessive traction over the lateral inferior portion of the breast, appearing even more intense under voluntary contraction. The muscle segment was then resected on both breasts (Caldeira and Roth 2008).

We propose an integrated treatment of the mammary region with the interposition of three breast tissue flaps and a posterior approach to the pectoralis major muscle with any of the three types offered. The muscle flap provides a blood supply to the breast tissue flaps and, at the same time, preserves the new breast shape.

References

Arié G (1957) Una nueva tecnica de mastoplastia. Rev Lat Am Cir Plast 3:23

Bustos R (1992) Periareolar mammaplasty with silicone supporting lamina. Plast Reconstr Surg 89:646–657

Caldeira AML (1994a) New approach de Sustentação nas Mamoplastias. Personal technique. Annals 8th International Congress on Senology, Rio de Janeiro; p 1400

Caldeira AML (1994b) Nova Abordagem de Sustentação nas Mamoplastias Redutoras. Communication to the X Congreso Iberoamericano de Cir Plást Viña del Mar

Caldeira AML (1995a) A new support approach to mammaplasties; pectoralis major muscle flap. 11th Congress of the International Confederation of Plastic, Reconstructive and Aesthetic Surgery, Yokojama

Caldeira AML (1995b) Triple flap interposition technique. Communication to the 11th Congress of the International Confederation of Plastic, Reconstructive and Aesthetic Surgery, Yokohama; p 188

Caldeira AML, Roth GB (2008) The triple-flap interposition mastoplasty. In: Shiffman MA (ed) Mastopexy and breast reduction: principles and practice, vol 1, 1st edn. Springer, Berlin, pp 103–113

Caldeira AML, Barral SM, Araújo ID, Thomaz DR (2008) Aesthetic abdominal and breast reconstruction with reverse lateral thoracodorsal flap. Plast Reconstr Surg 121(5):346e–347e. doi:10.1097/PRS.0b013e31816b1188

Candiani P, Campiglio GL, Signorini M (1991) Personal experience with the central pedicle reduction mammaplasty. Rev Soc Bras Cir Plast 6:11

Daniel MJ (1993) Comunication to the 30th Brazilian Congress of Plastic Surgery, Curitiba

Daniel MJ, Ivan Maluf J, Alysson RM (2015) Mammoplasty with bipedicled flap from the pectoral muscle: 30 years of experience. Rev Soc Bras Cir Plast. doi:10.5935/2177-1235.2015RBCP0178

Dehner J (1908) Mastopexie zur Beseitigung der Hängebrust. Munch Med Wochenschr 55:1878–1886

Goullian D Jr (1976) Ptosis and its correction. In: Goldwyn RM (ed) Plastic and reconstructive surgery of the breast. Little Brown, Boston, pp 329–342

Gray H (1935) Anatomy: descriptive and applied. Longmans, London, p 456

McCraw JB, Arnold PG (2007) Atlas of muscle and musculocutaneous flaps. Interplast, Global-Help Publication; pp 97–689

McKissock PK (1972) Reduction mammoplasty with a vertical dermal flap. Plastic Reconstr Surg 49:245–252

Peixoto G (1980) Reduction mammaplasty: a personal technique. Plast Reconstr Surg 65(2):217–226

Pitanguy (1962) Une nouvelle technique de Plastie Mamaire. Ann Chir Plast 7:199–207

Ralph TM (1980) An anatomical study of the pectoralis major muscle as related to functioning free muscle tranplantation. Plast Reconstr Sur 65:610–615

Ribeiro L (1975) A new technique for reduction mammaplasty. Plast Reconstr Surg 55:330–334

Sampaio G (1993) Minimizing scars in the surgery. Perspect Plast Surg 7:59–85

Skoog T (1963) A technique for breast reduction. Transposition of the nipple on a cutaneous vascular pedicle. Acta Chir Scand 126:453–465

Spalteholz W (1923) Hand atlas of human anatomy, 7th English edn. Lippincott, Philadelphia

12 Reduction mammaplasty with Rotation of the Glandular Flap to the Superior Pole

Ewaldo Bolivar de Souza Pinto, Ana Paula Pimentel Spadari, Ilson Abrantes Rosique, Roosevelt Santos Oliveira Jr., and Priscilla Chiarello de Souza Pinto Abdalla

12.1 Introduction

The need to eliminate some of the extensive scars leads after surgery to the development of techniques with smaller incisions (de Souza Pinto et al. 1994). Reduction mammoplasty, with a vertical approach, is now more common, because it combines the improvement of the shape with a minor scar (Bozola 1982; Lejour 1994; de Souza Pinto et al. 1994).

Vertical mammoplasty allows minimal incision, good projection, and a better result throughout time, in comparison with an inverted T technique (Bozola 1982; Lejour 1994; de Souza Pinto et al. 1994).

The breast tissue can be excised without a large incision after careful liposuction improvement (Lejour 1994; de Souza Pinto et al. 1994), especially on the superficial layers, which is to be accomplished in any corporal region allowing skin retraction postoperatively (Avelar and Illouz 1986; Pitman 1993; de Souza Pinto et al. 1995). Liposuction has been acknowledged to be a good supporting technique for the removal of adipose tissue in both regions, which contributes to new remodeling (Avelar and Illouz 1986; de Souza Pinto et al. 1995). The purpose of this study is to show that the association of two modern techniques (vertical mammoplasty and superficial liposuction) allows for good aesthetic results in the patients (de Souza Pinto et al. 1994).

E.B. de Souza Pinto, M.D. (✉)
A.P.P. Spadari, M.D. • I.A. Rosique, M.D.
R.S. Oliveira Jr., M.D.
P.C. de Souza Pinto Abdalla, M.D.
Sociedade Brasileira de Cirurgia Plástica
(Brazilian Society of Plastic Surgery)—SBCP,
Santos, SP, Brazil

Dr. Ewaldo Bolivar de Souza Pinto Plastic Surgery
Service, São Paulo, SP, Brazil
e-mail: ewaldobolivar@uol.com.br

12.2 Method

12.2.1 Surgical Technique

We performed the marking of the inframammary fold, axillary, and thoracic regions in the orthostatic position, under light general endotracheal anesthesia, preceded by an adequate topical spray of lidocaine before intubation. The patient is kept in the semi-sitting position after completing the intubation procedures (Ribeiro 1989).

In a sequence, two notches are marked in the midclavicular line placed at 7 cm from the sternal furcula, depending on the thoracic width (Peixoto 1980; Pitanguy 1967; Ribeiro 1989). These notches give continuation to a perpendicular line that goes beyond the nipple as far as the inframammary fold (PDE 1994; de Souza Pinto et al. 1994).

J.M. Avelar (ed.), *Breast Surgery*, https://doi.org/10.1007/978-3-319-54115-0_12

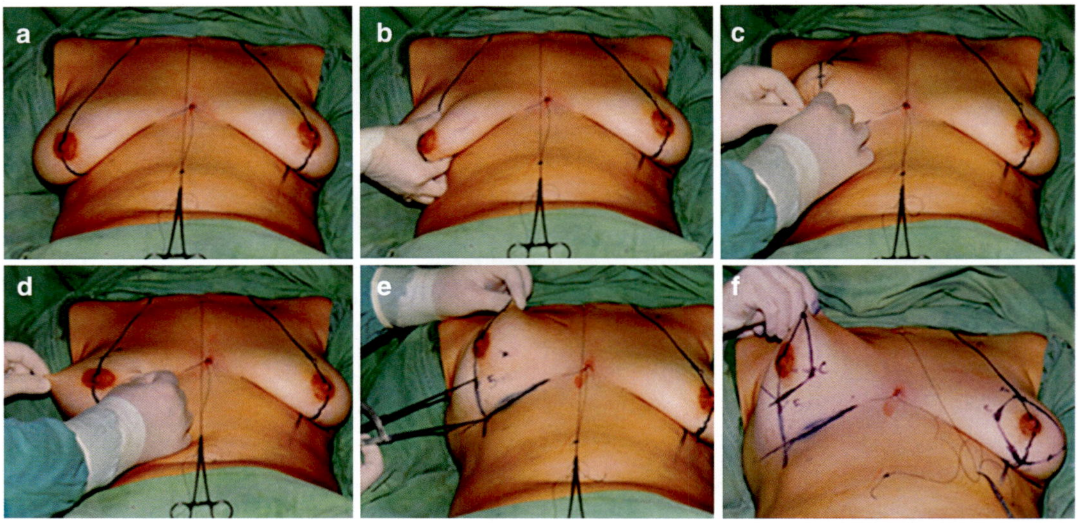

Fig. 12.1 (**a**) Markings. (**b**) Index finger maneuver. (**c**) Bidigital maneuver. (**d**) Points B and C. (**e**) Point D. (**f**) Marking inverted drop

After this, four extra notches are made.

- A: index finger maneuver corresponds to an inframammary fold projection, usually at distance ranging from 18 to 21 cm (Pitanguy 1967).
- B and C: medial and lateral of the nipple–areola complex, following an imaginary line approximately 1 cm below the nipple.

The distance between B and C is not supposed to go any further than 8 cm, especially if glandular hypertrophy exists. We always pursue confirmation of these two notches by measuring them using our hands, which should correspond in extent to the tissue to be removed.

- D: the lower marking, 5 cm above the inframammary fold at the projection of the midclavicular line.

To be more precise, we draw an ellipse by connecting A, B, C, and D, in an inverted drop (Fig. 12.1).

We initiate surgery by infiltrating axillary and thoracic regions in superficial and deep layers in a tumescent form with a standard solution along the afore-mentioned inverted drop, averaging 150 mL.

In sequence, we perform liposuction of the fat tissue with 4- or 5-mL perforated cannulas, from deep to superficial layers (Fig. 12.2).

Almost immediately, we notice the improvement of the mammary contour, with tissue retraction. We then mark a new areola and proceed with Schwarzmann's maneuver as far as approximately 1 cm below the line that connects B and C (Fig. 12.3).

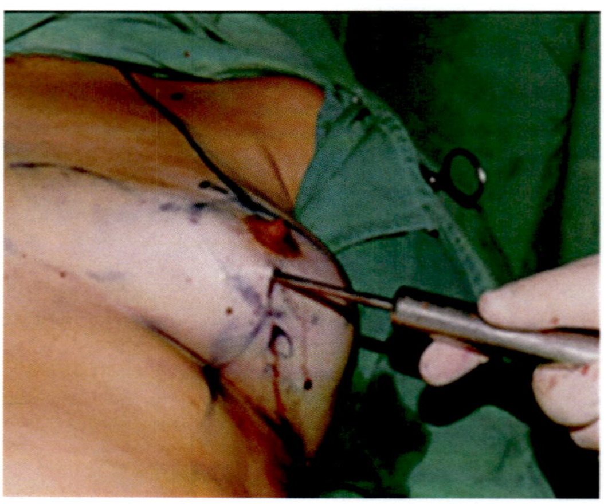

Fig. 12.2 Liposuction

Below this line, we perform a conical resection, perpendicular to the thorax (Fig. 12.4).

Next, the flap of the glandule is made by maintaining the superior pedicle (Fig. 12.4), aimed at increasing the upper mammary pole. This flap has the form of an inverted U, with the base near the thorax wall. When released, it revolves on its own axle, and then it is sutured onto the second or third costal arch, with to 2-0 mononylon (Figs. 12.4 and 12.5).

After hemostasis, the pillars are approached with three stitches using 2-0 mononylon. In the event of patients with a significantly laterally ptotic glandule, we mark the remaining skin with methylene blue, so that it can be resected, bearing in mind that the inferior extremity goes no further than 1 cm above the inframammary fold.

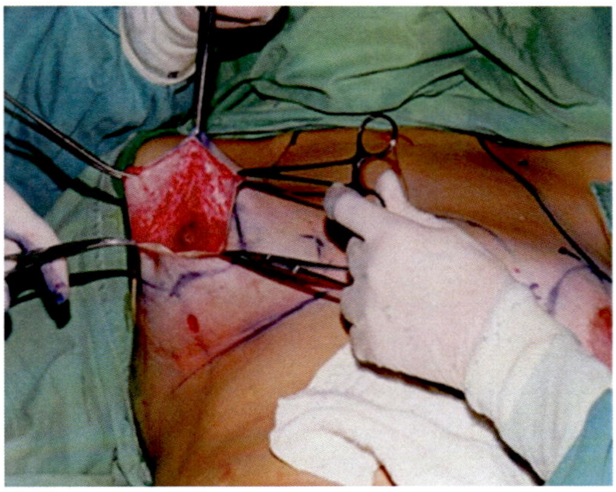

Fig. 12.3 Schwarzmann's maneuver

With upward breast traction, the closure begins with 4-0 non-absorbable sutures in the caudo-cranial direction and the final continuous intradermic sutures (de Souza Pinto et al. 1994).

A new areolar site is made with no tension, the suture is continuous with the 5-0 non-absorbable Gillies stitches. We often use a tubular drain for 24 h (Fig. 12.6).

12.3 Discussion

In cases treated with this technique, we observed a reduction of breast volume of 150 to 1000 g, maintaining the conical shape without changing the glandular function. The upper pole is maintained because we made a glandular flap (de Souza Pinto et al. 1994).

The superficial liposuction promotes a retraction of the skin generating a more harmonic contour in the inferior, medial and axillary pole.

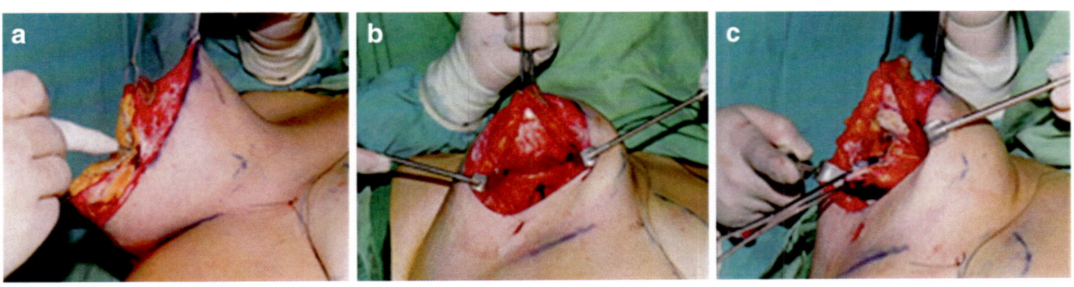

Fig. 12.4 (**a**) Conical resection. (**b**) Making a flap. (**c**) The flap

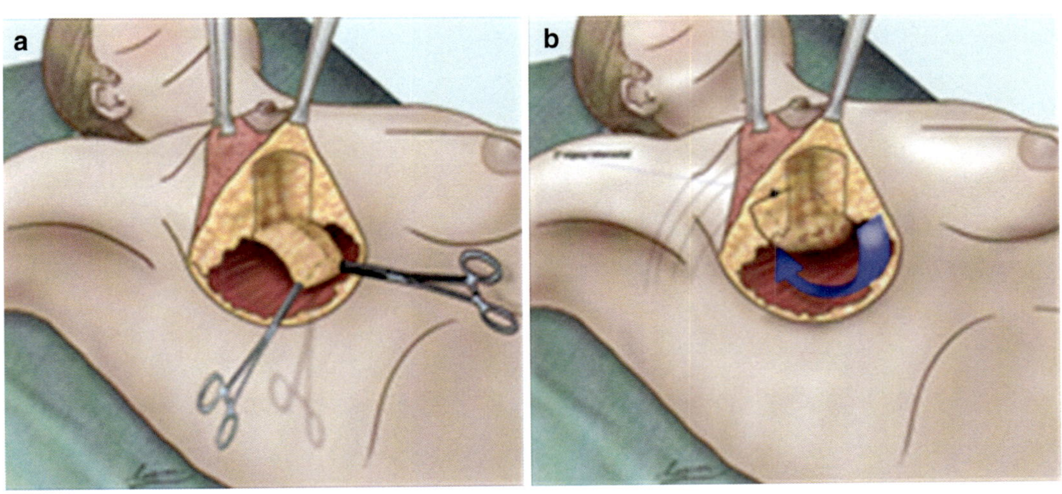

Fig. 12.5 (**a**, **b**) The inverted U form of the flap and rotation

This technique can be performed in cases of mild (grade I) to severe hypertrophy (grade IV), including cases of asymmetry and synmasty (Figs. 12.7, 12.8, and 12.9) (Avelar and Illouz 1986; Lejour 1994; de Souza Pinto et al. 1994, 1995).

12.4 Complications

Following the cases in this study, eight patients had scar tissue enlargement, one of which involved epitheliosis. We did not observe any cases of areolar necrosis or dehiscence of the surgery wound.

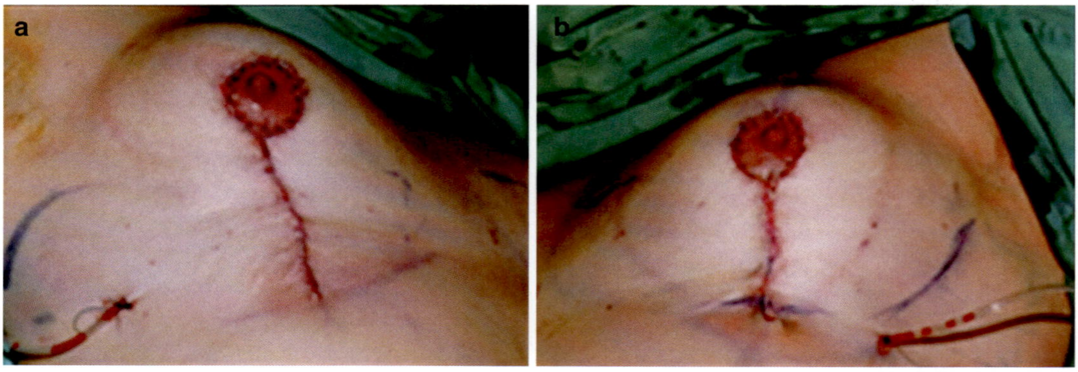

Fig. 12.6 (**a**, **b**) Tubular drain

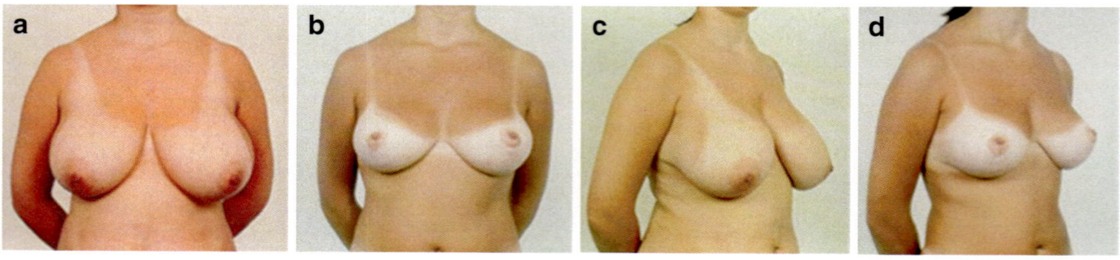

Fig. 12.7 (**a**, **c**) Preoperatively. (**b**, **d**) Five years postoperatively

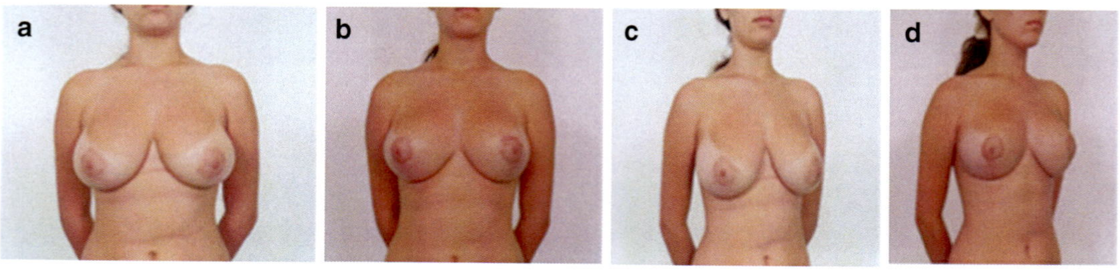

Fig. 12.8 (**a**, **c**) Preoperatively. (**b**, **d**) Nine months postoperatively

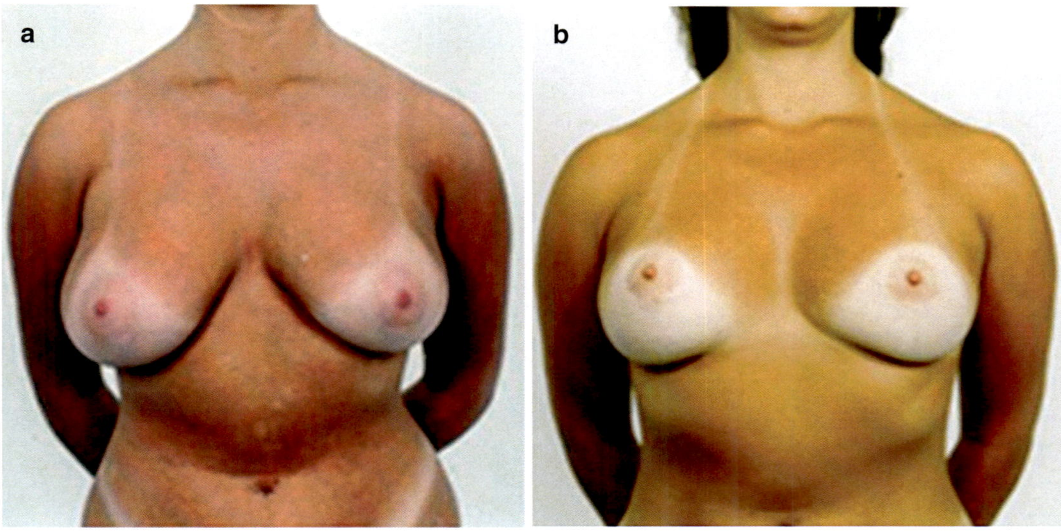

Fig. 12.9 (**a**, **c**, **e**) Preoperatively. (**b**, **d**, **f**) Five years postoperatively

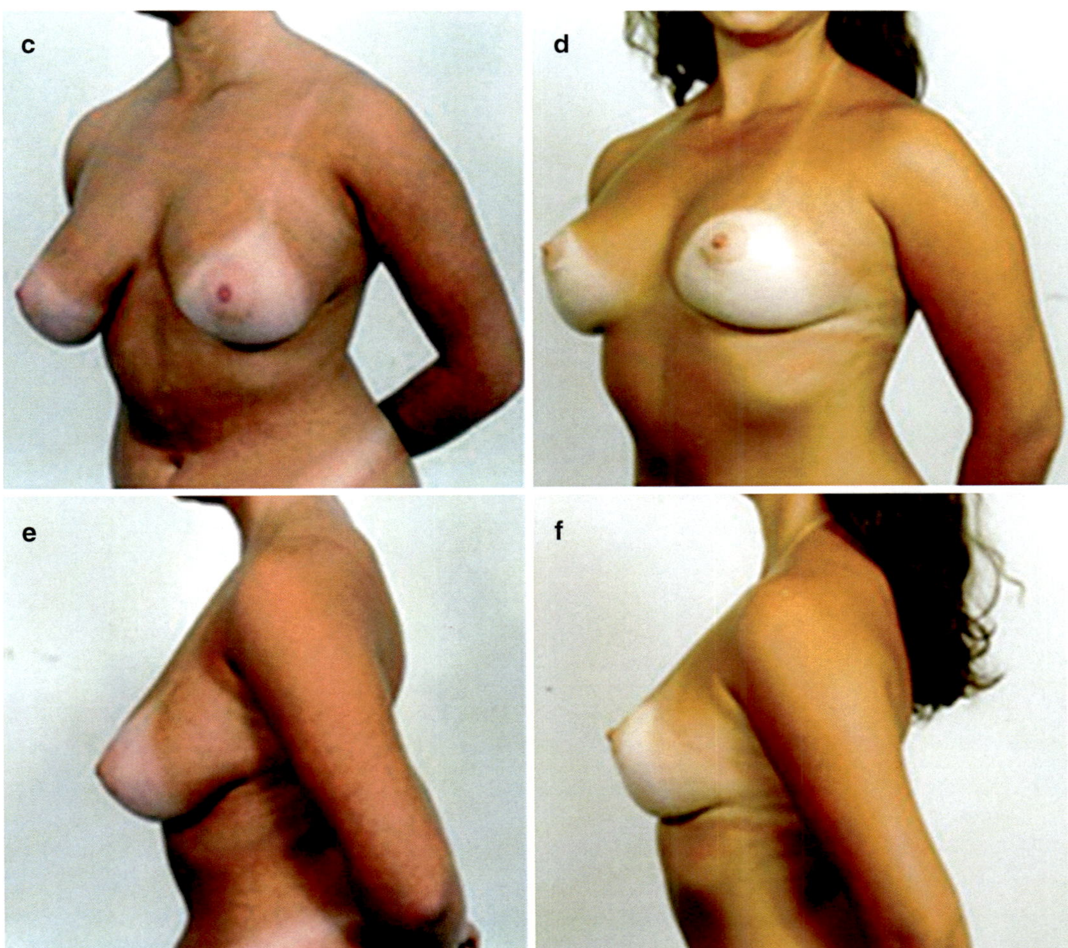

Fig. 12.9 (continued)

Conclusion

This technique comprises both breast reduction and harmonious mammary contours, in addition to maintaining the function and sensitivity. The form of the superior pole is also maintained owing to the flap. Superficial liposuction promotes skin retraction, both medially and laterally. It may be performed for different types of breasts, aiming for better results.

References

Avelar J, Illouz YG (1986) Lipoaspiração. Editora Hipócrates, São Paulo

Bozola AR (1982) Mamoplastia em L. Contribuição pessoal Ver AMRIGS 26:2007

de Souza Pinto EB, Queiroz FW, Erazo IPJ, et al (1994) Improving mammaplasty scars with lipoplasty. Scientific Display presented and published in ASPRS/PSEF/ASMS Annual Scientifc Meeting 1994; San Diego

de Souza Pinto EB, Erazo IPJ, Muniz AC, et al (1995) Superficial liposuction of the dorsal region. Transactions of the 11th Congress of the International Confederation; 1995 April 16–21; Yokohama, Japan. pp 134–137

Lejour M (1994) Vertical mammaplasty and liposuction. Quality Medical Publishing, St. Louis, MI

PDE M (1994) Mamoplastia por abordagem periareolar. Técnica Pessoal. In: AAB T (ed) Atualização em cirurgia plástica estética. SBCPER/Regional São Paulo. Editora Robe, São Paulo, pp 339–350

Peixoto G (1980) Reduction mammasplasty. A personal technique. Plast Rec Surg 65:217

Pitanguy I (1967) Surgical treatment of the breast hypertrophy. Br J Plast Surg 20:78

Pitman GH (1993) Liposuction and aesthetic surgery. Quality Medical Publishing, St. Louis, MI

Ribeiro L (1989) Cirurgia Plástica da mama. Medsi, Rio de Janeiro

Check for updates

13 Mammaplasty: Short Scar Breast Reduction

Roberto D. Basile

13.1 Introduction

In the 1980s, plastic surgeons already dominated with relative ease the techniques of reduction mammaplasty, some problems having been resolved, but others still awaiting a solution. At that time, I performed mammaplasty with good reductions, but with very long inframammary scars, especially in cases of large reductions in which the incisions ran from the axilla to the sternum. This occasionally caused problems for the nipple–areola complex (NAC) owing to excess traction (Pitanguy 1967; Skoog 1963; Strombeck 1960). Even when satisfied with their reductions, the patients inquired about the possibility of reducing the scars. It was on the basis of these requests that a group of surgeons who were not satisfied with the techniques that resulted in large scars started to look for a solution to this problem (Basile 1985; Marchac and DeOrlate 1982; Peixoto 1980). This trend motivated me to introduce technical modifications in my surgeries that resulted in a new procedure (Basile and Basile 2015).

R.D. Basile, M.D.
The American Society of Plastic Surgery, Arlington Heights, IL 60005, USA

The Brazilian Society of Plastic Surgery, São Paulo, SP, Brazil

Department of Plastic Surgery, Basile Day Hospital, Av. Prof Joao Fiusa, 2300, Ribeirao Preto, SP 14024-260, Brazil
e-mail: drbasile@gmail.com

Some problems had to be faced:

1. Reducing inframammary scars
2. Reducing NAC morbidity in cases of large reductions
3. Being able to remove large mammary volumes
4. Obtaining results with aesthetically pleasing shapes.

Experience and experimentation led to solutions that, after some refinement, resulted in a simple, efficient, and versatile technique (see Fig. 13.2).

The following solutions were developed:

1. Elevation of the mark of the new inframammary sulcus 3 cm above the original sulcus as the new breast is fully elevated and the sulcus needs to be higher (Fig. 13.1a).
2. Modification of skin removal by replacing horizontal resections with vertical compensations. Thus, all the excess skin is removed by pulling it upward in the cephalic direction. This procedure dramatically reduces the horizontal scar, leaving only a vertical scar in medium-sized and small breasts (Fig. 13.1d, e).
3. Total undermining of the breast based on the supramuscular areolar plane was routinely adopted. This procedure fully separates the breast from the thorax, facilitating glandular resection and elevation.
4. The concept was introduced that the most important feature in reduction mammaplasty

J.M. Avelar (ed.), *Breast Surgery*, https://doi.org/10.1007/978-3-319-54115-0_13

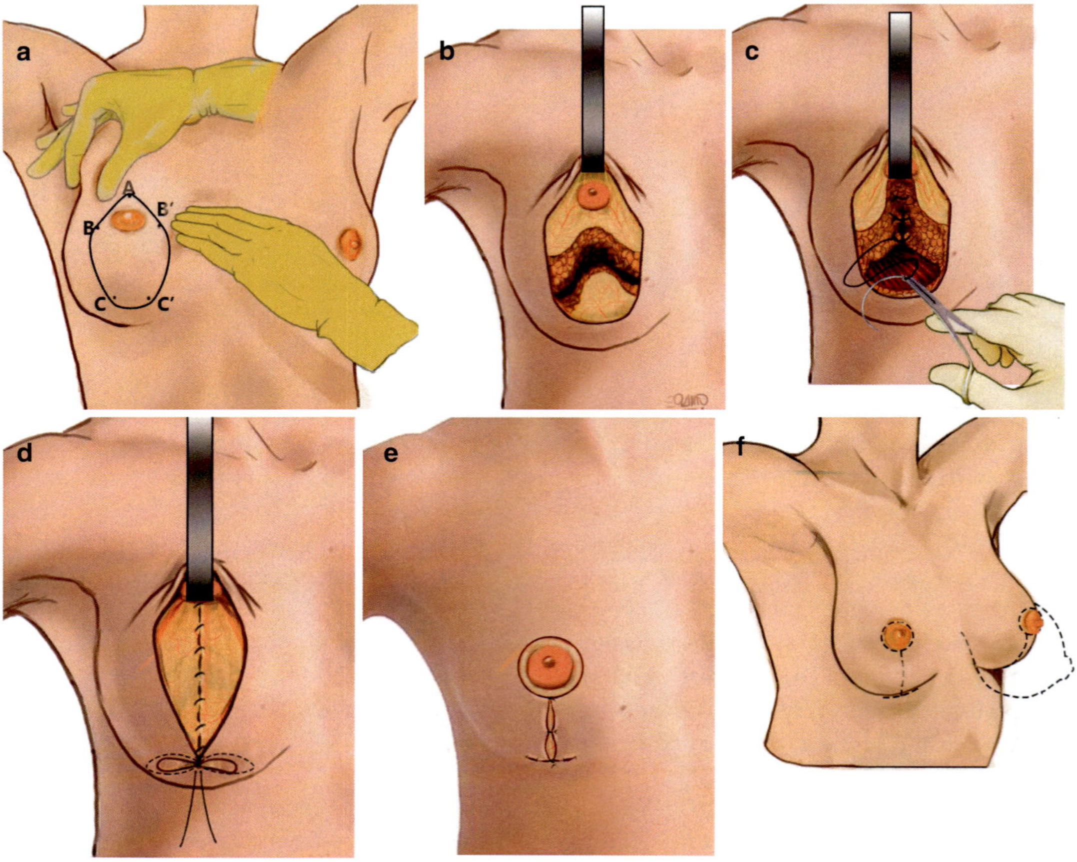

Fig. 13.1 (**a**) Dr. Basile's technique for reduction mammaplasty. Final drawing. (**b**) Beginning of the pyramidal bloc resection on the cubic base. (**c**) Final aspect of the resection and illustration of the pillars for construction of the breast. (**d**) Skin resection in the cephalic–vertical direction. (**e**) Position of the nipple–areola complex (NAC) on top of the breast. (**f**) Final suture, only vertical or minimally horizontal

is the remaining mammary shape and volume, as they form the new gland. Thus, my advice in large resections is to remove the gland by imagining a pyramid superimposed on a rectangular box as this shape permits the removal of volumes both in the height and in the base of the mammary cone without requiring skin resection (Fig. 13.1b).

5. The construction mode was modified using a simple concept that had never been used before. The new breast is constructed through its lateral pillars by pulling them separately to the center, without suturing them to each other. Three or four sutures are used to bring the glandular mass toward the middle and upward in a cephalic direction, and this traction is repeated on the sternal side, placing the pillars one in front of the other. This strategy molds the breast both along the axillary line and in the sternal region, resulting in a new mammary gland with a defined shape.
6. In other techniques, the NAC suffers due to the rotation of the pillars. Thus, in large reductions the pillars must be pulled for appropriate positioning. This construction permits the

NAC to be always on the top of the mammary cone and not buried. In other words, the gland is set up from the sides to the middle without rotation of the pillars (Fig. 13.1e).

7. Recently, I have been using this same technique to perform augmentation mastopexies. The implant is placed subpectorally and the gland is dissected from the pectoralis muscle and then elevated as described above. The glandular tissue is fixated to the pectoralis muscle in the same fashion as described above, with the implant protected by the muscle (Basile et al. 2012; Basile 2015).

13.2 Method

This technique is simple and does not require previous molds or marks. With the patient under general anesthesia and in a supine position on the surgical table, the clavicular midpoint is determined and extended to the inframammary sulcus. On this line point A is marked, the center of the future nipple, which is established by lifting the NAC upward and determining up to what point it may be lifted. In large breasts, this point is located on average 16 cm below the clavicle. Two points, B and B′, are then determined 1 cm below the line that cuts the nipples transversely. These points are determined by lifting the glands upward, invaginating the lower pole and evaluating the extent of the skin to be removed when an attempt is made to join them. Joining point A to points B and B′ form an isosceles triangle with a wider angle in large resections. Two centimeters above the inframammary sulcus, at the midpoint, I mark line CC′, parallel to the sulcus, which measures 2–4 cm depending on the gland volume. The tracing is completed by joining point B to point C and these lines are straight or curved according to the extent of resection. Lines BC and B′CI are external convex curves in large resections of skin and parenchyma, but always converge toward line CC′. Because of the short extent of the latter, small horizontal scars result.

In most of the cases operated upon, consisting of medium or small breasts, points C and C′ coincide.

This design provides a final result that eliminates the horizontal scar. A new areola is traced with molds and the periareolar incision is started, with de-epithelialization of the entire area of the triangle ABB′ using Schwarzmann's maneuver, continuing subcutaneously until reaching line CC′. The incision of the new inframammary sulcus, CC′ is made to a depth reaching the submammary areolar tissue, with undermining in the supra-aponeurotic region of the pectoralis major muscle. This extensive undermining is performed under virtually the entire gland, which is left practically isolated, although the irrigation and innervation emerging from the median intercostal spaces are fully preserved, with subcutaneous anastomosis with branches of the lateral thoracic artery. With the gland pulled upward, en bloc resection of the breast parenchyma is started with an incision 3 cm below the areola, which is the vertex of a pyramid that progressively widens downward until larger removal is performed horizontally in a rectangular block. This permits the extirpation of a large volume at the base of the mammary cone below the entire circumference, but preserves a cone that will be the new gland and that contains the NAC (Fig. 13.1b). The new breast is mounted with 2-0 nylon stitches that first attach it to the floor (the pectoral muscles). This suture positions the top of the gland approximately 15 or 16 cm from the line that joins the furcula to the clavicular midline (Fig. 13.1c). Three or four 2-0 nylon sutures are then used to take the axillary glandular mass to the middle and upward cephalically, a maneuver that projects the new breast and removes volume from the external axillary line, taking it to the upper medial pole. The same procedure is repeated in the external region so that the entire remaining part of the gland is directed medially and upward, placing the gland pillars one in front of the other. At this time, the gland is already formed, with the AMC on top. Any compensation is performed in an upward direction and only at this time are the pillars joined with sutures (Fig. 13.1c). After the mounting of the breast, subcutaneous suturing with colorless 4-0 nylon stitches is done in two layers, as I do not suture the skin. This stage of the mammaplasty is very important because the traction and direction of the sutures are from below to above, provoking skin compensation in the direction of the NAC. Thus, excess skin is removed in a vertical direction, a fact that greatly reduces or eliminates the horizontal incision (Fig. 13.1d–g). I started to use this technique in December 1979 and have been improving it gradually over the course of approximately 2000 cases, with minimal complications, which are listed below:

1. Scars with "dog ears" of excess skin, 10% of cases.
2. Recurrent breast ptosis, two cases of gigantomastia (0.22%).
3. Reoperation for further reduction, three cases (0.33%).
4. Breast asymmetries occurred in approximately 3% of cases, but were only noted by the surgeon, with no complaints on the part of the patients. Since using appropriate subcutaneous delipidation or liposuction in the region below the axilla, the "dog ears" phenomenon has no longer occurs.

13.3 Discussion

This method has left patients highly satisfied, as they value surgeries that leave minimal scars, which is demonstrated by an increased number of patients seeking mammaplasty and by the number of patients who express their desire to have

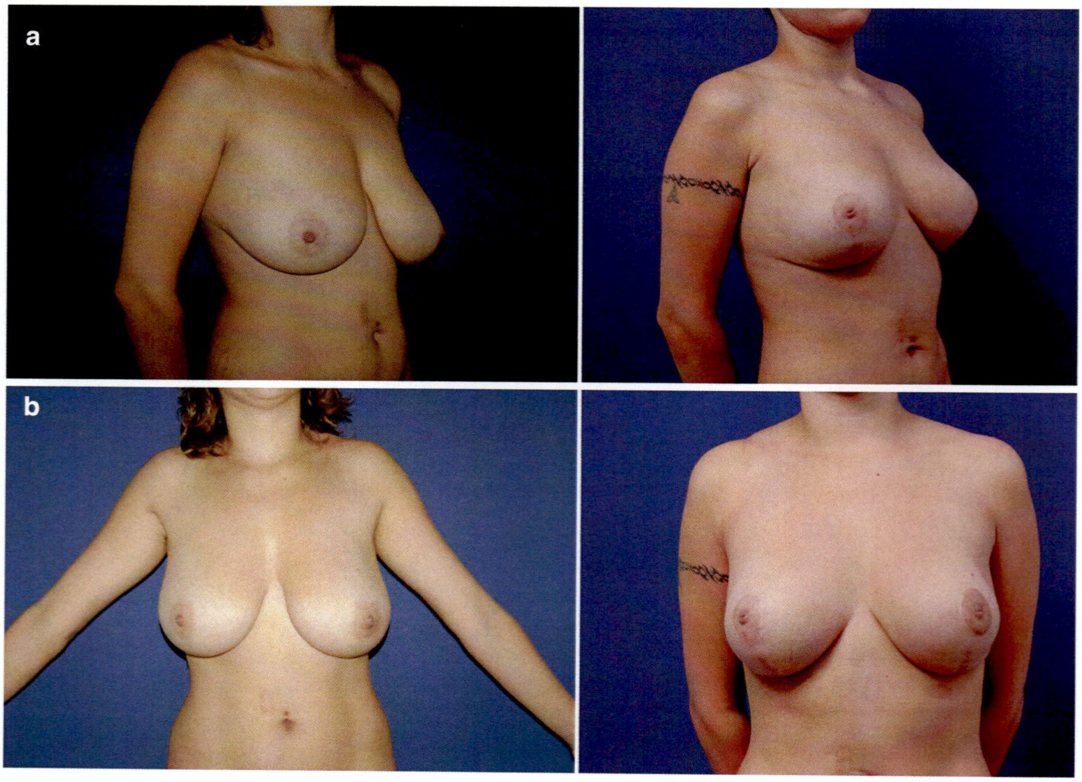

Fig. 13.2 (**a**, **b**) A 23-year-old patient with mammary hypertrophy and ptosis. Large reduction with a minimal horizontal scar

only vertical scars at their first visit (Figs. 13.2 and 13.3). In summary, I believe that the techniques directed at the elimination or the drastic shortening of horizontal scars satisfy both the surgeon and the patients and therefore should be continuously improved. Also, in view of the diversity and large number of mammoplasty techniques, those that are simpler incur fewer risks of surgical error and therefore provide greater patient satisfaction (Figs. 13.4 and 13.5). The technique permits breast reduction with pleasing shapes, minimal and only vertical scars or small horizontal scars in large breasts, with simple technical tracing.

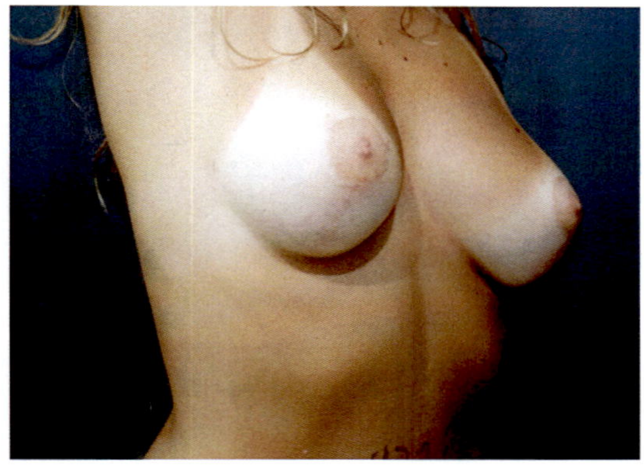

Fig. 13.3 A 20-year-old patient with mammary hypertrophy. Reduction mammaplasty without inframammary scars, with only a vertical suture. Close-up

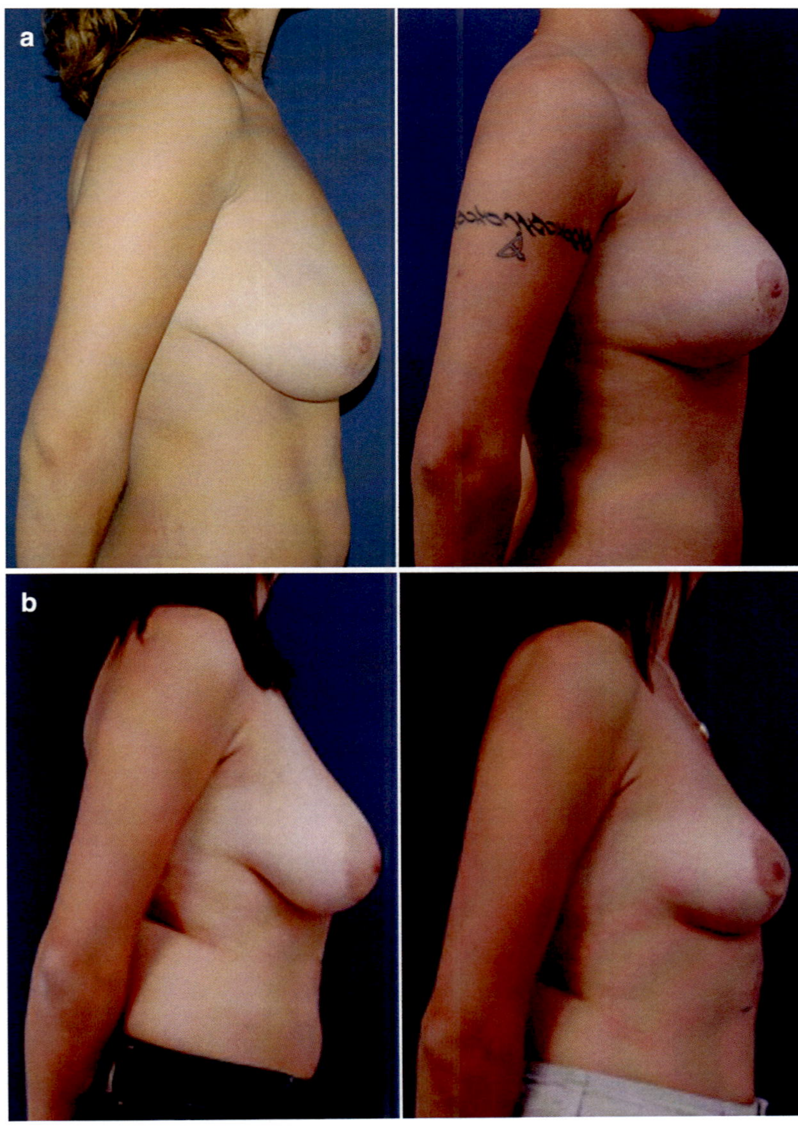

Fig. 13.4 (**a**, **b**) Two examples of severe mammary hypertrophy resulting in a minimal horizontal scar. Note in the profile view

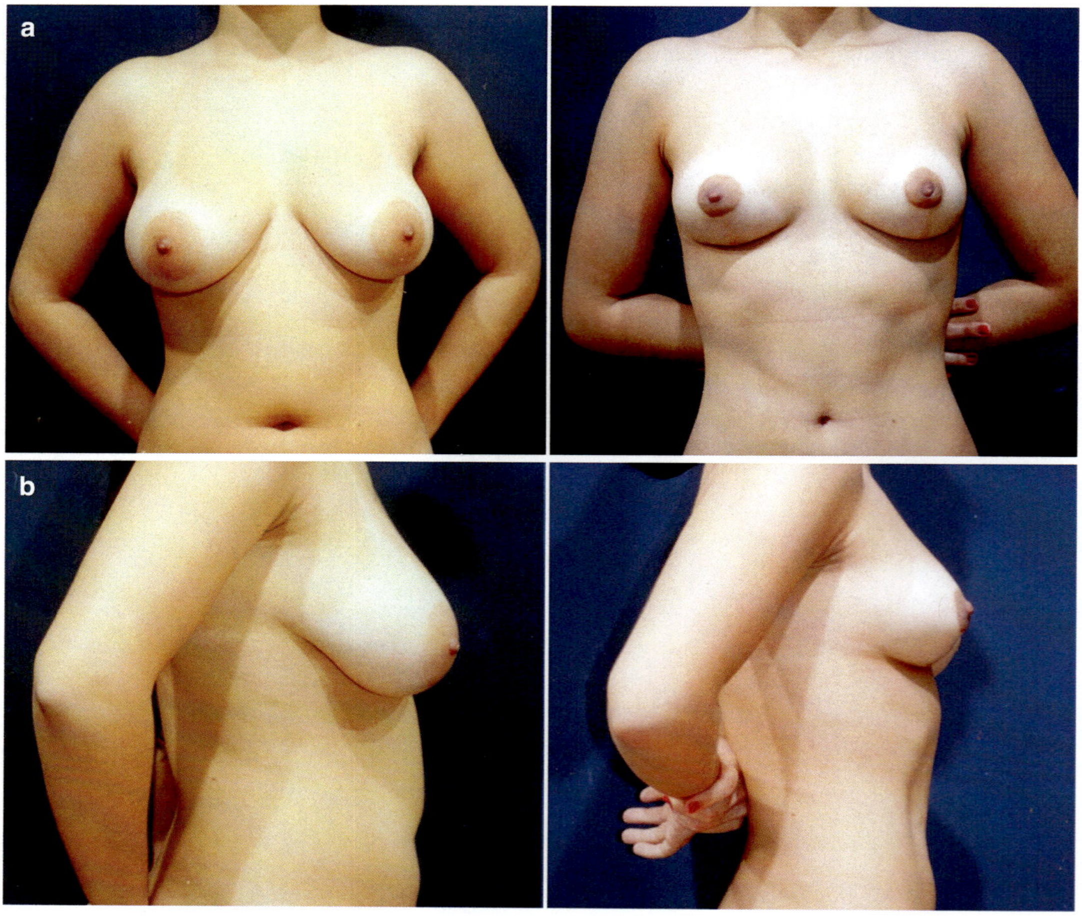

Fig. 13.5 (**a**, **b**) A 21-year-old patient with moderate hypertrophy. Front and profile views

Conclusion

Mammaplasty is quite a common procedure with very good aesthetic results. In fact, in the 1980s, plastic surgeons had already dominated with relative ease the techniques of reduction mammaplasty, some problems having been resolved, but others still awaiting a solution. Over the last few decades, I have developed a method through which it is possible to achieve good surgical results with short scars. A complete description of the technique is provided and details of the surgical methods are given. Our short scar breast reduction is effective at accomplishing good results with minimal scarring.

References

Basile AR (1985) Mammaplasty: large reduction with short inframanunary scars. Plast Reconstr Surg 76:130–135

Basile FV (2015) Evolutionary reasons for male preferences regarding the female breast shape. Plast Reconstr Surg Glob Open 3(10):e542

Basile FV, Basile AR (2015) Diagnosis and management of galactorrhea after breast augmentation. Plast Reconstr Surg 135(5):1349–1356

Basile FV, Basile AV, Basile AR (2012) Striae distensae after breast augmentation. Aesthet Plast Surg 36(4):894–900

Marchac D, DeOrlate G (1982) Reduction mammaplasty and correction of ptosis with a short inframammary scar. Plast Reconstr Surg 69:45–54

Peixoto G (1980) Reduction mammaplasty: a personal technique. Plast Reconstr Surg 65:217–226

Pitanguy I (1967) Surgical treatment of breast hypertrophy. Br J Mast Surg 20(1):78–85

Skoog T (1963) A technique of breast reduction. Transposition of the nipple on a cutaneous vascular pedicle. Acta Chir Scand 126:453–465

Strombeck JO (1960) Mammaplasty: report of a new technique based on the two-pedicle procedure. Br J Plast Surg 13:79–90

14 Reduction Mammaplasty with a Circular Folded Pedicle Technique

Waldir Teixeira Renó

14.1 Introduction

Every epoch and every culture has established a distinct concept of the ideal breast. As breast shape and size is unique to each individual and is largely determined by heredity, breast surgery is one of the most challenging and difficult procedures in plastic surgery. On the other hand, the patient's expectation is usually higher than what the surgeon can offer, only because breasts are the most prominent parts of the female silhouette. Even in a patient who is overweight, with large breasts and a projected abdomen, asking only for reduction with no interest in the cosmetic results, the surgeon must be prepared because the patient may demand sensual breasts.

The author presents a personal experience of over three decades based on a periareolar convergence of the breast tissues by a circumareolar dermo-glandular pedicle folded on itself to act as a central support and to promote the global mobilization of the breast and surrounding thoracic skin.

Only after completing the central support marking will the extension and direction of the scars be determined in the inferior pole. In this respect, the configuration of the scars can vary from periareolar, through vertical and oblique ones, up to an inverted T. In this respect, in young breasts with stretched skin, glandular content, and small to moderate hypertrophy, only one scar will extend from the areola to the submammary fold. However, in breasts with flaccid skin, lipomatous content, and moderate to severe hypertrophy, the resulting scar is an inverted T with a short medial branch that preserves the integrity of the skin for the medial-most part of the submammary fold.

The author observed an early ptosis of the inferior pole after reduction mammaplasty in patients with a thin and atrophic submammary fold. Therefore, over the last 15 years, the author has developed a *reverse flap* in the inferior pole to form a support pad in the submammary fold.

14.2 History

This technique was developed in the mid-1980s, as just a periareolar technique, and was named the "conical periareolar mammaplasty," characterized by a pocket suture in the de-epithelialized area of the periareolar pedicle (Renó 1985, 1986). It was later named the "round block" by Benelli (1988).

Already at that time, the author wanted a technique for various breast deformities. Therefore, an incision in the inferior pole was added and the pocket suture was replaced by U-shaped sutures to obtain better control over the distribution of

W.T. Renó, M.D.
Cirurgia Plástica D'America Clinica,
Plastic-Surgeon Santa Casa de Guaratinguetá,
Membro Titular da SBCP, Rua Paissandú, 368,
Guaratinguetá, São Paulo, SP, Brazil
e-mail: renosurg@uol.com.br

J.M. Avelar (ed.), *Breast Surgery*, https://doi.org/10.1007/978-3-319-54115-0_14

the breast tissue. The procedure was named the "circular folded pedicle technique" (Renó 1992a, b, 1996, 1999, 2009).

14.3 Technique

Preoperative markings are performed in the office and reinforced in the surgical room.

With the patient standing: the mid-sternum line, the anterior axillary line, vertical and transverse lines of the nipple, the submammary fold, and point A (a point between the sternal notch and the nipple at the level of the submammary fold), 17–23 cm from the sternal notch depending on the fat content and location, the muscular and skeletal chest wall contour, and the skin quality.

With the patient supine: the amount of skin to be de-epithelialized around the areola is estimated by the amount of skin that can be pinched between the thumb and middle finger while the index finger depresses the areola just below the nipple (Fig. 14.1a). The medial and lateral points pinched between the fingers are named points B and C respectively and will be connected to point A. This maneuver also puts back the glandular tissue in the superior pole, determining its shape.

Point B is medial and varies between 9 and 13 cm from the mid-sternum line. Point C is lateral and around 8–12 cm from the anterior axillary line. A circular line is drawn touching points A, B, and C. The final drawing varies from a circle to an ovoid design (such as the eye of a Cyclops).

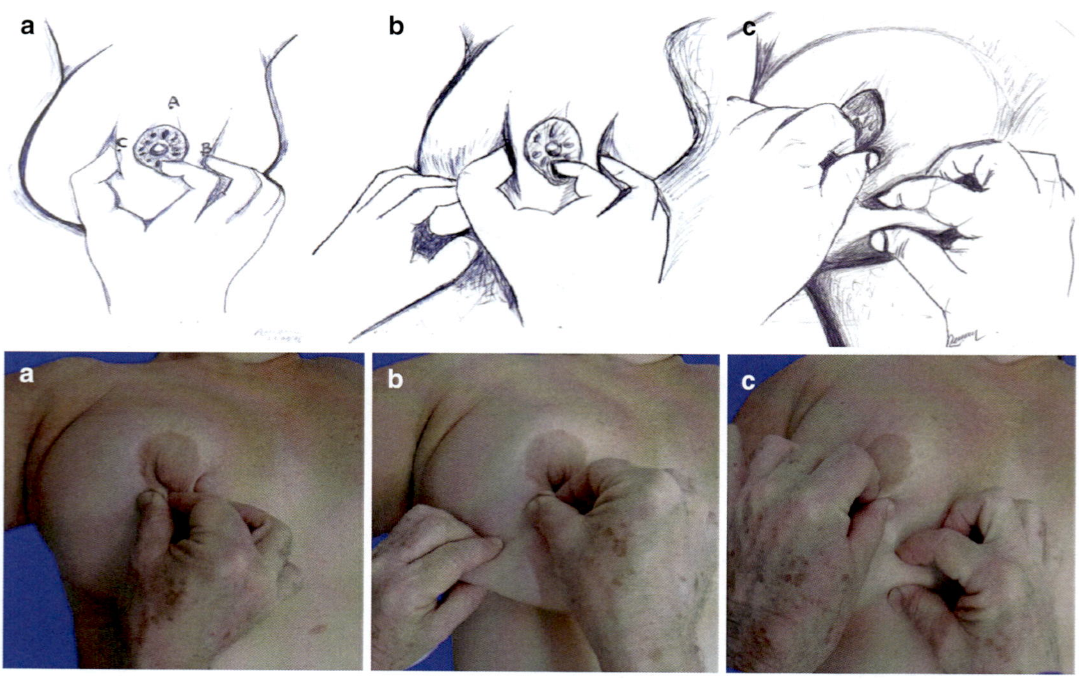

Fig. 14.1 (**a**) The periareolar marking. (**b**, **c**) The first pinching maneuver in the inferior pole is transverse, and determines longitudinal tissue excess in the lateral and medial inferior pole. A transverse fusiform marking is obtained. (**d**) The second pinching maneuver is longitudinal between the areola and the submammary fold, and determines the transverse tissue excess. A longitudinal fusiform marking is obtained. (**e**) Transverse tissue excess originates type 2 marking, a fusiform drawing varying between vertical and oblique, from the areola up to 1.0 cm above the submammary fold. (**f**) Longitudinal tissue excess originates type 3 marking, a drawing similar to a cyclops

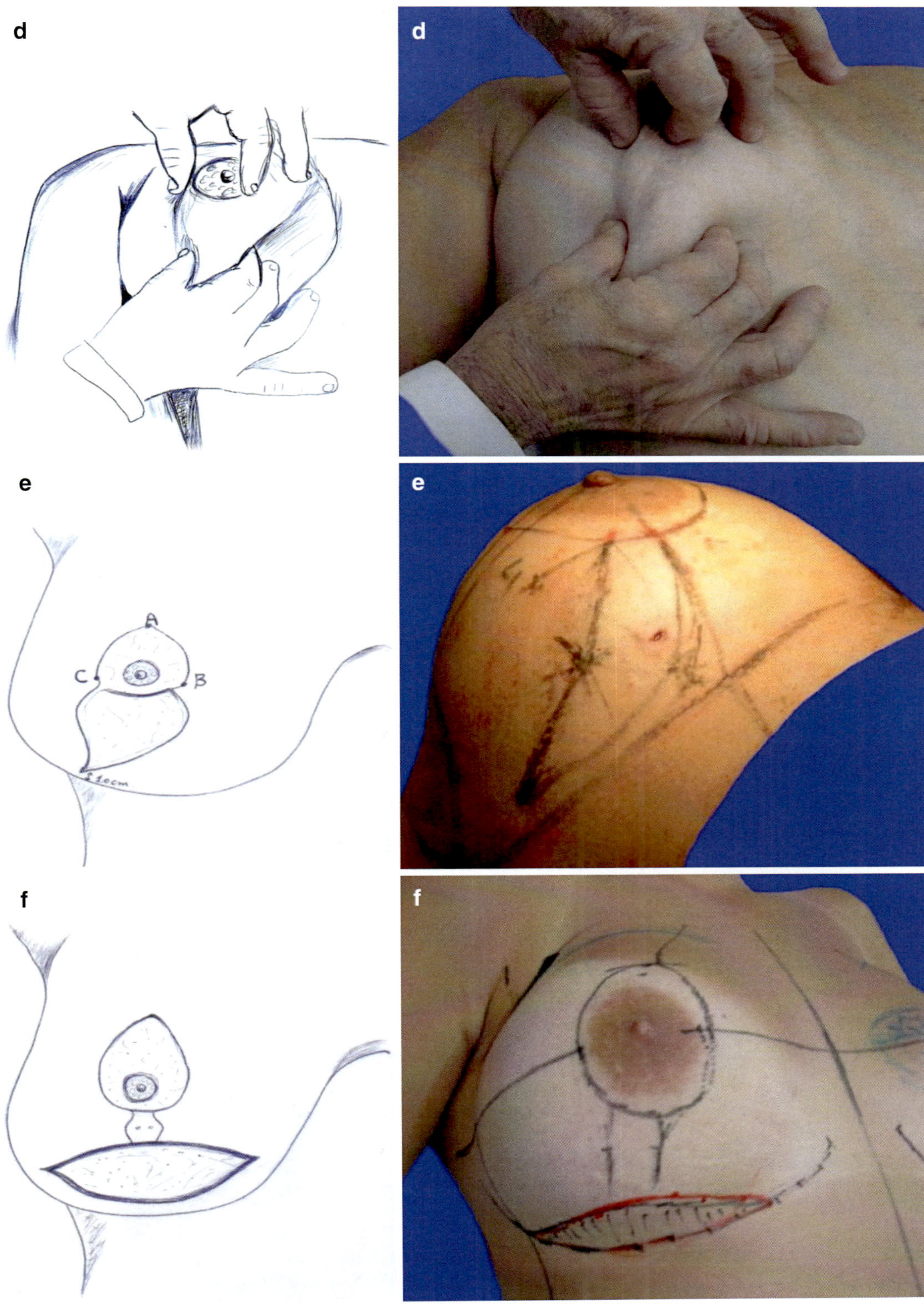

Fig. 14.1 (continued)

Maintaining the previous maneuver, the other hand pinches the inferior pole in two directions, longitudinal and transverse. The amount of skin to be marked is estimated by the amount of tissue that can be pinched between the thumb and the other fingers. The first pinching maneuver is transverse and above the submammary fold, and determines the longitudinal tissue excess (Fig. 14.1b, c). The superior and inferior points pinched between the fingers should be marked and a transverse fusiform marking is obtained. The second pinching maneuver is longitudinal between the areola and the submammary fold, and determines the transverse tissue excess (Fig. 14.1d). The medial and lateral points pinched between the fingers are marked and only a longitudinal fusiform marking is obtained, which may vary between the vertical and oblique ones according to the lateral and medial tissue excess. From these maneuvers three types of marking originate in the inferior pole:

Type 1: when these points form a coincident line, the scar will only be periareolar.

Type 2: when these points form a longitudinal fusiform marking (Fig. 14.1e), varying between vertical and oblique, only one scar will extend from the areola up to 1.0 cm above the submammary fold. The distance between the inferior edge of the areola and the submammary fold is around 5 cm.

Type 3: when these points form a transverse fusiform marking like the mouth of a Cyclops (Fig. 14.1f), the final scar will be an inverted T, with a short medial branch (Figs. 14.2 and 14.3). The distance between the inferior edge of the areola and the submammary fold will be around 5 cm.

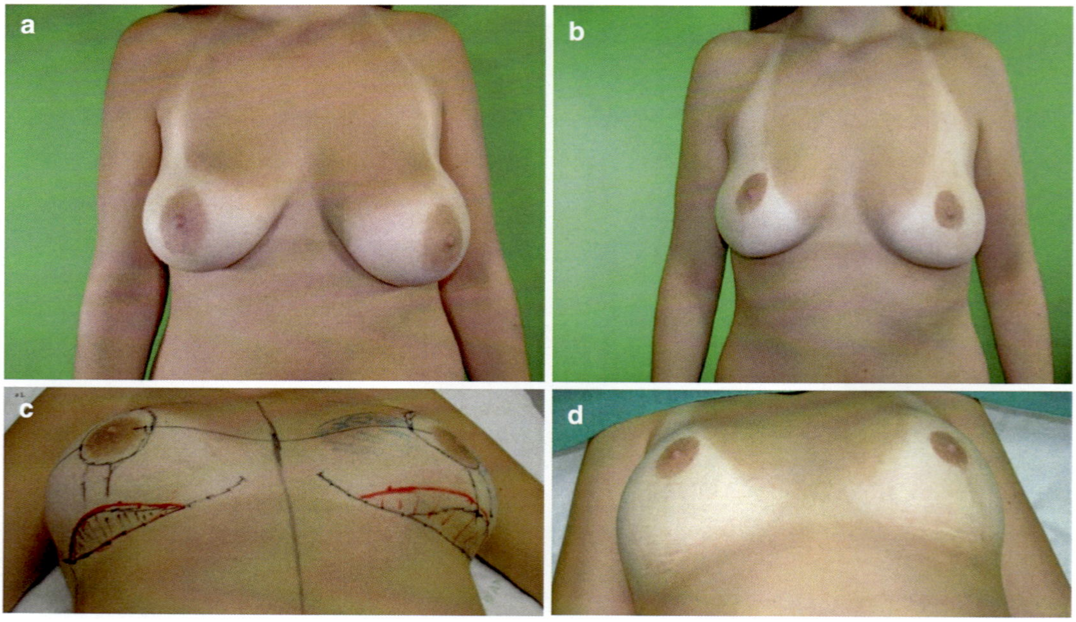

Fig. 14.2 (**a**) Preoperative 21-year-old patient with ptosis, hypertrophy, asymmetry, and a flattened superior pole. (**b**) Two years postoperatively following reduction mammaplasty with a circular folded pedicle type 3. (**c**) Preoperative marking is similar to a cyclops figure. In *green* (left breast) a medial glandular resection advances in the superior pole. (**d**) Two years postoperatively. The final scar is an inverted T with a short medial branch. (**e** and **g**) Preoperative 21-year-old patient with ptosis, hypertrophy, asymmetry, and a flattened superior pole. (**f** and **h**) Two years postoperatively following reduction mammaplasty with a circular folded pedicle type 3

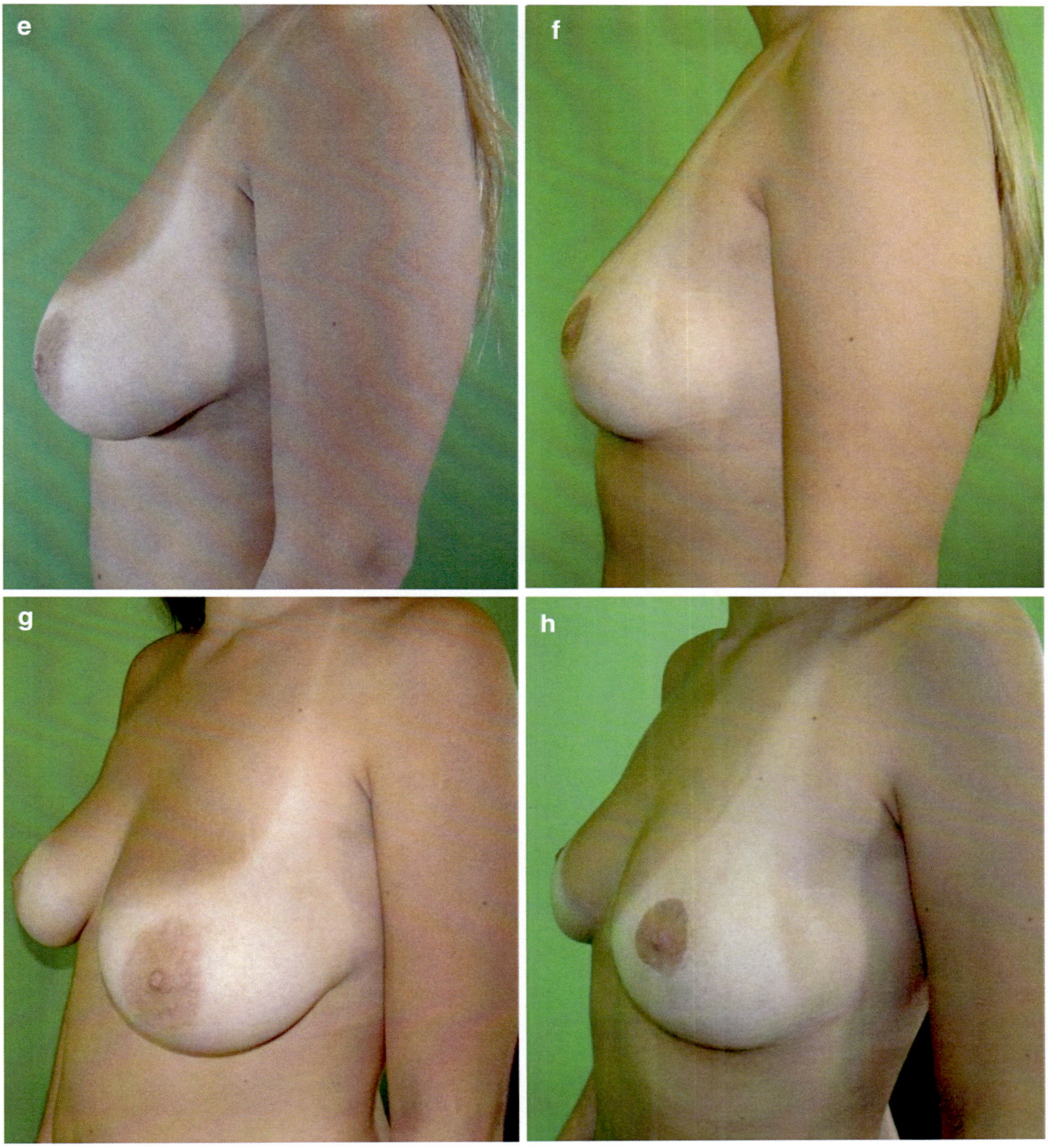

Fig. 14.2 (continued)

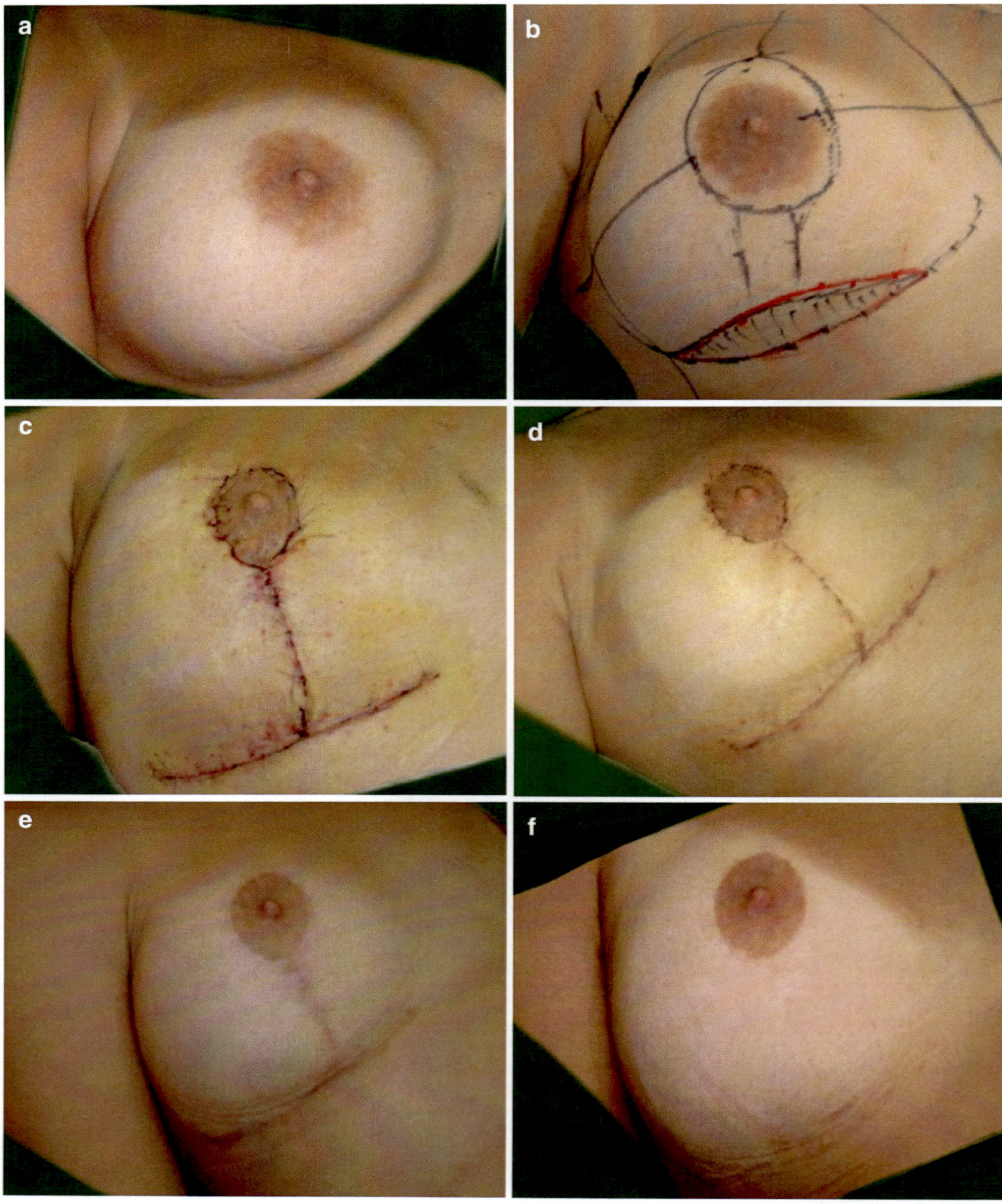

Fig. 14.3 Time evolution relative to the patient in Fig. 14.2. Preoperatively. (**b**) Preoperative marking. (**c**) Five days postoperatively. (**d**) Twelve days postoperatively. (**e**) Six months postoperatively. (**f**) One year postoperatively

If there is insufficient tissue to support the breast mound in the submammary fold owing to skin flaccidity and subcutaneous atrophy in this area, after the type 3 marking, a reverse flap is designed in the transverse fusiform marking to fill the submammary fold (Fig. 14.4). The final scar will be an inverted T as in type 3 (Figs. 14.5, 14.6, and 14.7).

The surgical maneuver step by step:

1. De-epithelialization around the areola (Fig. 14.8a).

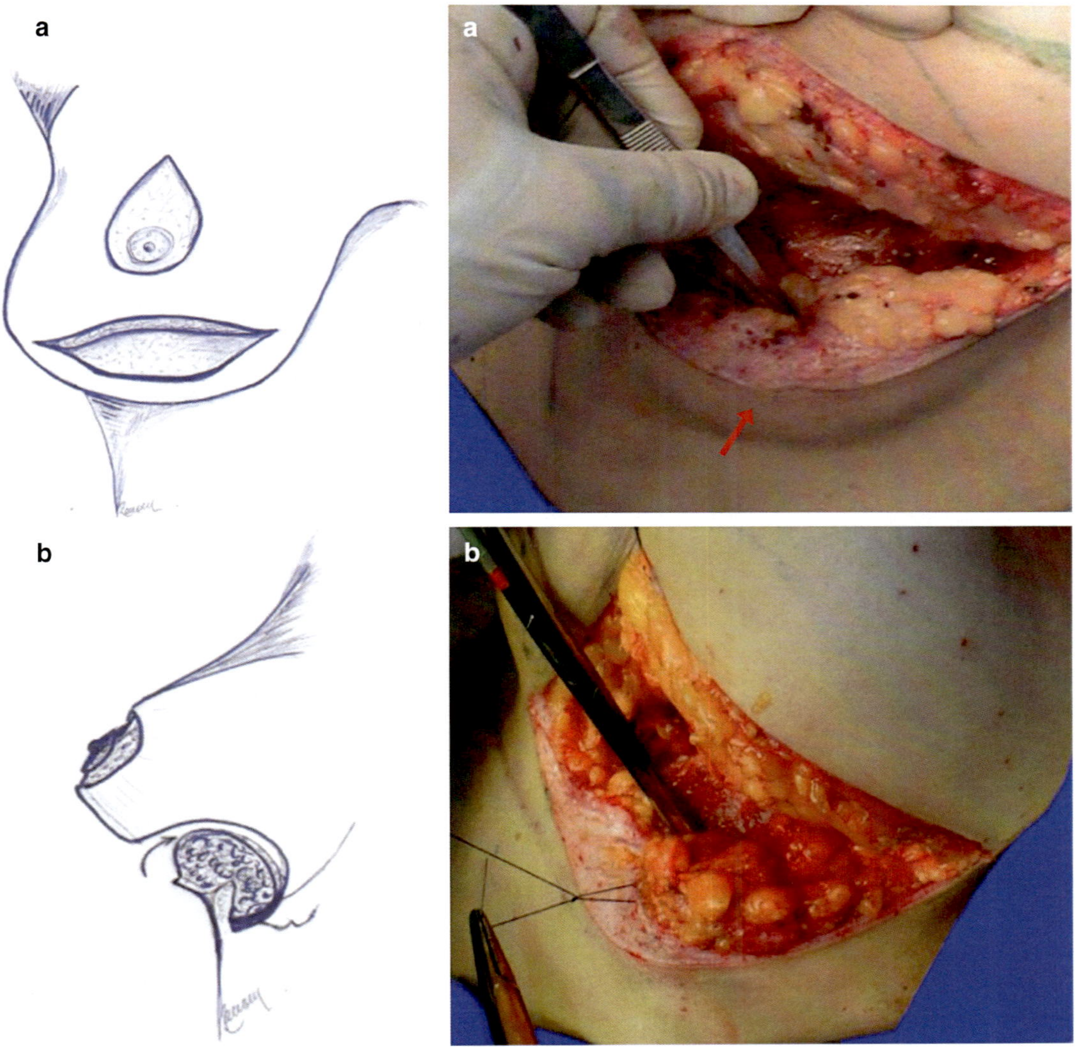

Fig. 14.4 (**a**, **b**) A reverse flap is designed to fill the submammary fold. (**a**) *Red arrow* indicates the bulking of the submammary fold

2. Semilunar incision of 2 cm thickness in the inferior edge of the periareolar de-epithelialization respecting the transverse nipple line (Fig. 14.9a).
3. From this incision, the de-epithelialized area around the areola is undermined using a special retractor to an extent that is variable between half and the apex of the periareolar flap, in accordance with the facility to raise the areola to the apex of this flap, and this is a priority maneuver (Fig. 14.8b).
4. Now, the de-epithelialized circle surrounding the areola is folded on itself and a stitch is made between the areola and the apex of the flap (point A) followed by some U-shaped sutures to stabilize the rise of the areola. Then, a simple skin suture is passed inferiorly to close the skin around the areola.
5. It is very important to observe that so far, only the periareolar flap procedure was performed. Therefore, the inferior pole approach is then defined: if the distance between the areola and the submammary fold is up to 6 cm, a longitudinal

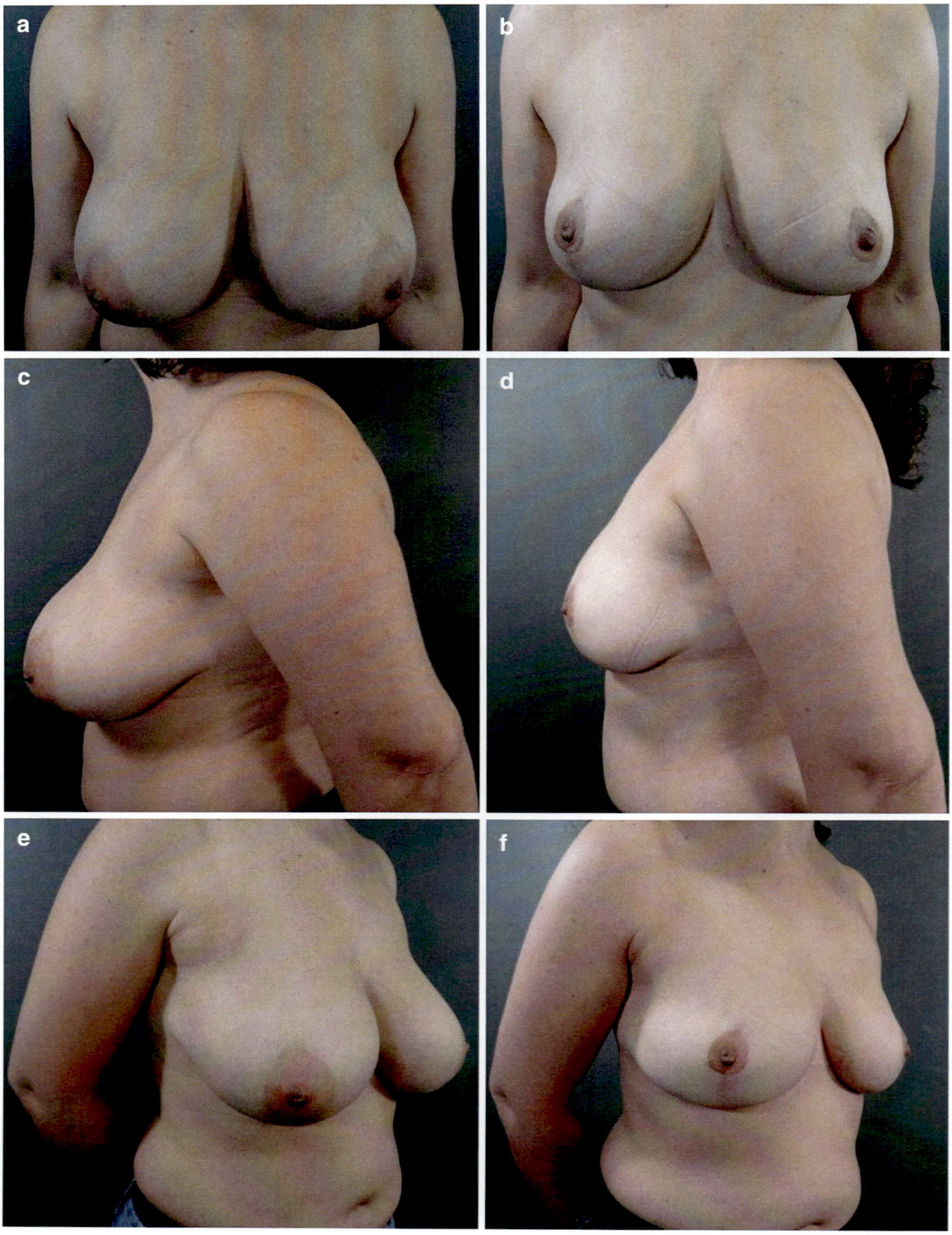

Fig. 14.5 (**a**, **c**, **e**) A preoperative 39-year-old patient with breast hypertrophy and ptosis (standing: nipple 27 cm from the sternal notch). (**b**, **d**, **f**) One year postoperatively after breast reduction of 330 g from the right and 360 g from the left breast following the circular folded pedicle technique with a reverse flap (standing: nipple 22 cm from the sternal notch)

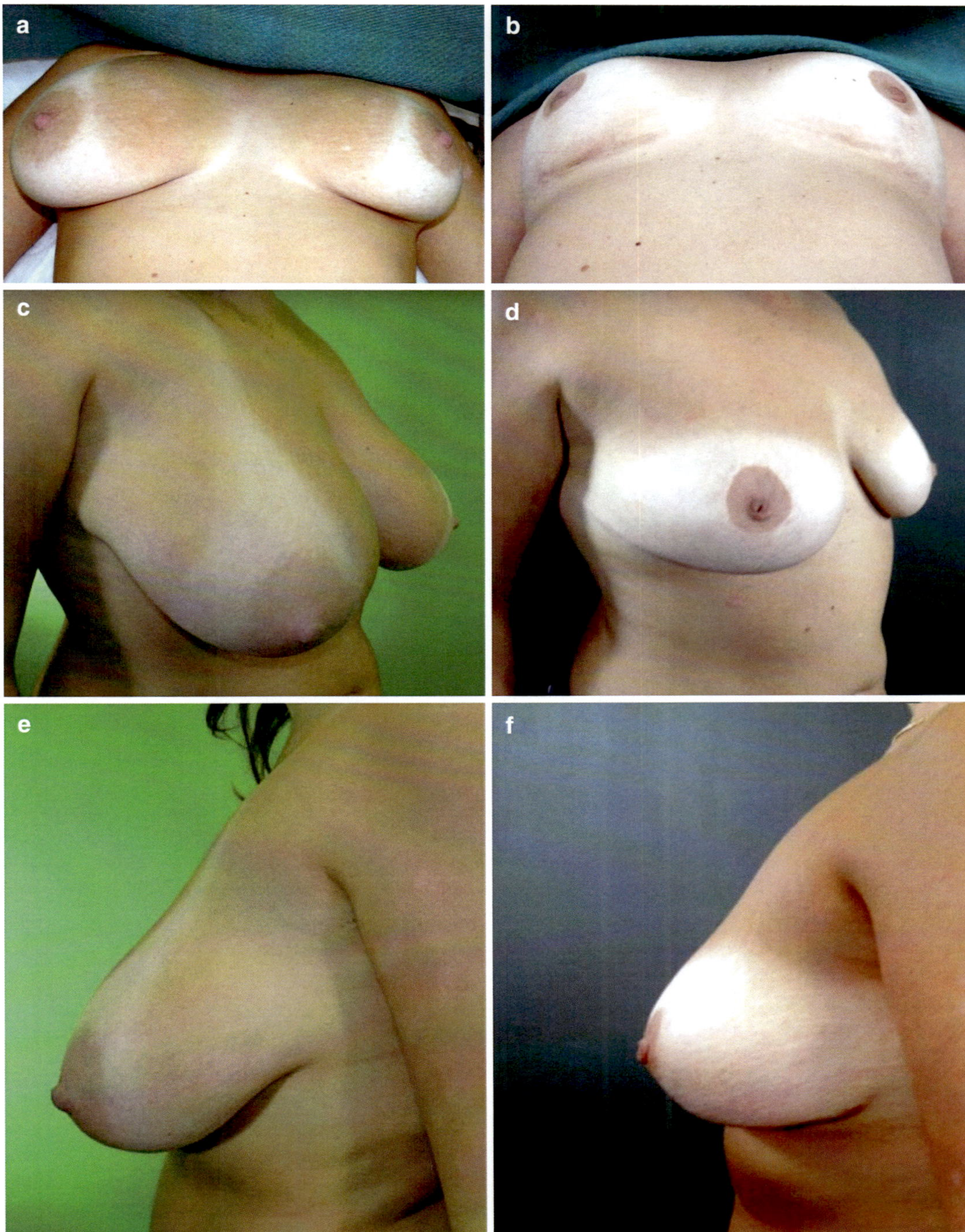

Fig. 14.6 (**a**, **c**) Preoperative view of a 22-year-old patient with hypertrophy, asymmetry, ptosis, lateralized nipple–areola complex (NAC), high and asymmetrical submammary fold, and skin flaccidity (standing: nipple 30.5 cm from the sternal notch). (**b**, **d**) Six years after reduction with circular folded pedicle and reverse flap (standing: nipple 22.5 cm from the sternal notch); breast reduction: right 780 g, left 650 g. (The same patient as in Fig. 14.13). (**e**) Preoperative view of a 22-year-old patient with hypertrophy, asymmetry, ptosis, lateralized NAC, high and asymmetrical submammary fold, and skin flaccidity (standing: nipple 30.5 cm from the sternal notch). (**f**) Six years after reduction with a circular folded pedicle and reverse flap (standing: nipple 22.5 cm from the sternal notch); breast reduction: right 780 g, left 650 g. (The same patient as in Fig. 14.13)

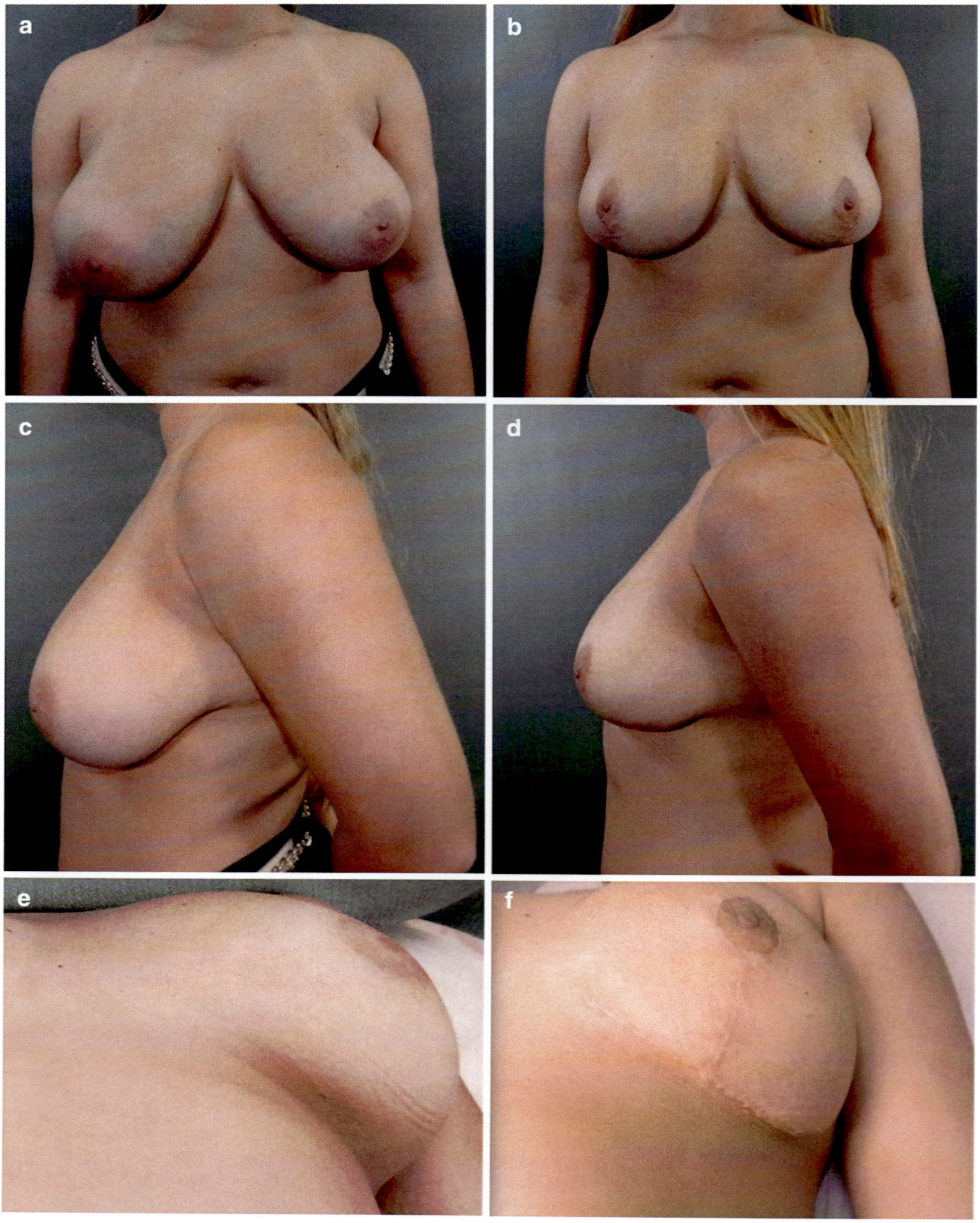

Fig. 14.7 (**a**, **c**) Preoperative view of a 26-year-old patient with hypertrophy, ptosis, asymmetry, lateralized NAC, and a high and asymmetrical submammary fold (standing: nipple 30 cm from the sternal notch). (**b**, **d**) One year and 2 months after reduction mammoplasty with a circular folded pedicle and reverse flap (standing: nipple 22.2 cm from the sternal notch)

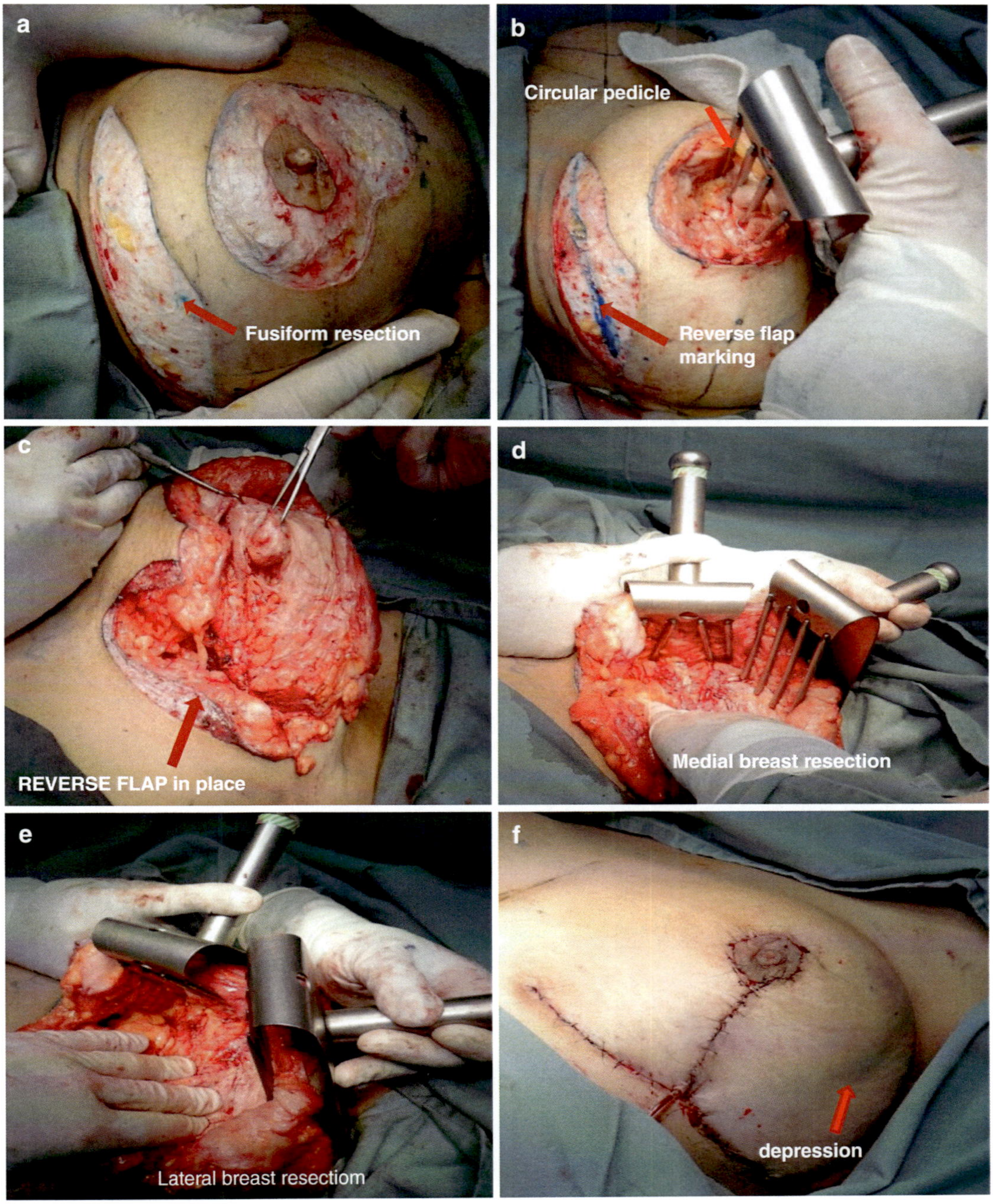

Fig. 14.8 Technical approach: (**a**) De-epithelialization. (**b**) Creation of the circular folded pedicle and demarcation of the reverse flap. Technical approach. (**c**) Reverse flap in place. (**d**, **e**) Breast resection. (**f**) Final aspect (*red arrow* indicates a temporary lateral depression caused by an internal anchorage suture fixed in the central axis)

(vertical or oblique) resection is feasible (Fig. 14.9c). However, if it is more than 6 cm, a transverse fusiform resection will be performed as explained in the type 3 marking (Fig. 14.9d).

6. If necessary, before the glandular resection, a reverse flap is developed (Fig. 14.8b, c). After the planned transverse fusiform marking is de-epithelialized, a curved transverse incision is made approximately 3 cm above its central inferior border. This incision goes down to the pectoralis fascia, and then the breast tissue is undermined caudally until the sixth intercostal space. Then, two or three sutures of 3-0 nonabsorbable suture are made between the de-epithelialized caudal border of the flap and the pectoralis fascia, pushing down the breast tissue to make the full submammary fold (Fig. 14.4a, b and see Fig. 14.11a).
7. Only then does the glandular resection start from caudal to cranial according to the previous marking. First, the glandular tissue is undermined in depth from the pectoralis fascia. Then, the glandular tissue is undermined 2 cm under the skin with a special retractor developed by the author (Fig. 14.9b). While the superior surface of the retractor slides over the skin, the inferior indented surface sticks to the breast tissue approximately 2 cm thick. Following the inferior surface of the indentation, the glandular tissue is incised and resected. This maneuver can be repeated as often as necessary, but care should be taken to avoid emptying the central area under the areola; on the contrary, the breast mound becomes flattened. The next step is the reinforcement of the suspensory ligaments of the mammary gland (Santos et al. 2016) and central pillar improvement using one main suture tied centrally and bringing together the remaining lateral and medial glandular wall (Fig. 14.8f). Other simple sutures are made between the gland and the fascia to close the dead spaces.

   In marking type 3, only after the glandular resection is the vertical skin excision performed in the inferior pole (Fig. 14.10a, b).
8. The closure is carried out from the deep to the superficial planes in the inferior pole. Fine U sutures between the skin and the areolar dermis involve gathering the skin around the areola and opening down to the approximately 3-cm diameter of the areola. After suturing, the nipple must be up to 6.5 cm above the submammary fold and the breast mound should look like a cone (Figs. 14.7f).
9. In summary, the technical sequence is as follows: the handling of the periareolar pedicle, the reverse flap procedure, and then the breast resection (Fig. 14.11a, b).

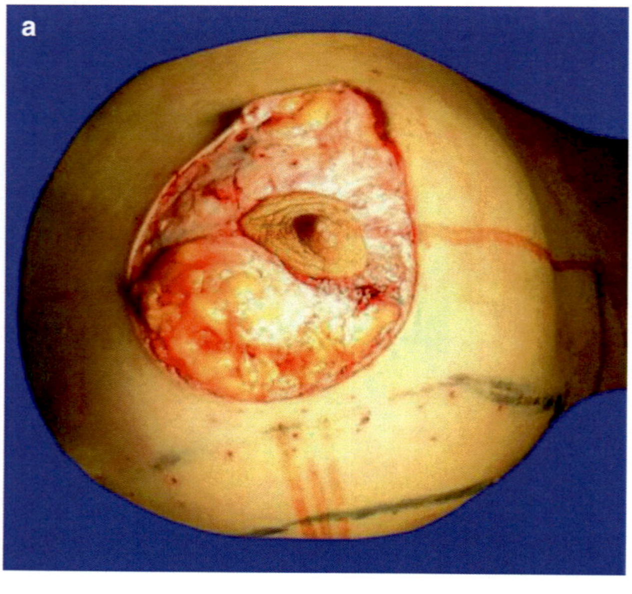

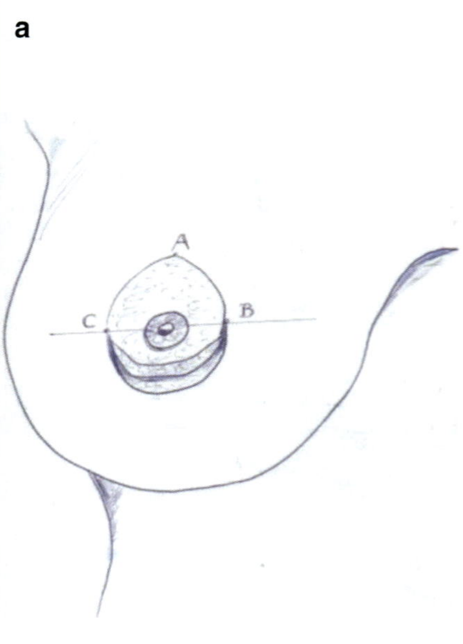

Fig. 14.9 Technical details. (**a**) Incision 2 cm thick. (**b**) A special retractor to undermine the periareolar pedicle, 2 cm thick. (**c**) Longitudinal (vertical to oblique) approach. (**d**) Transverse fusiform approach (Cyclops figure)

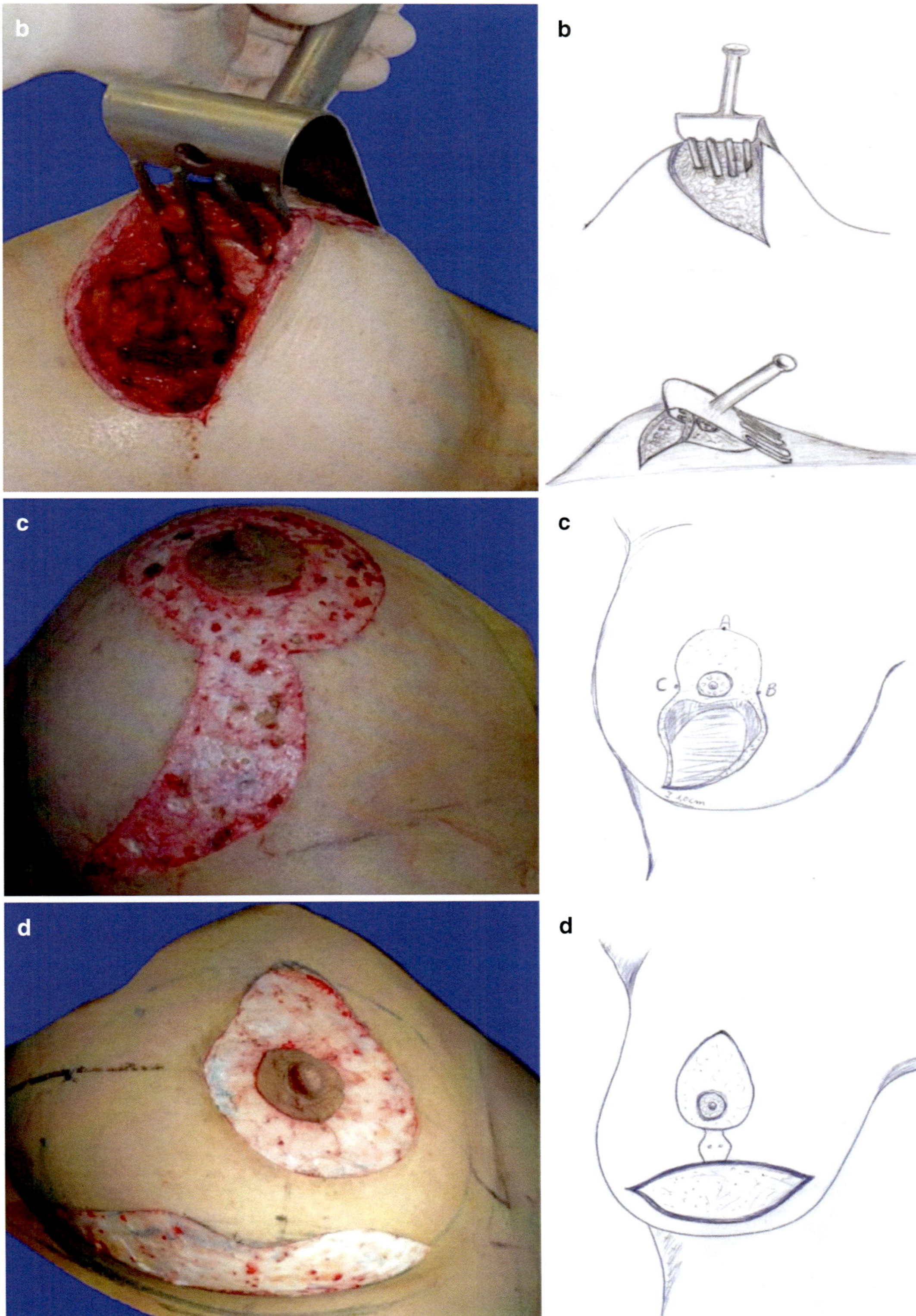

Fig. 14.9 (continued)

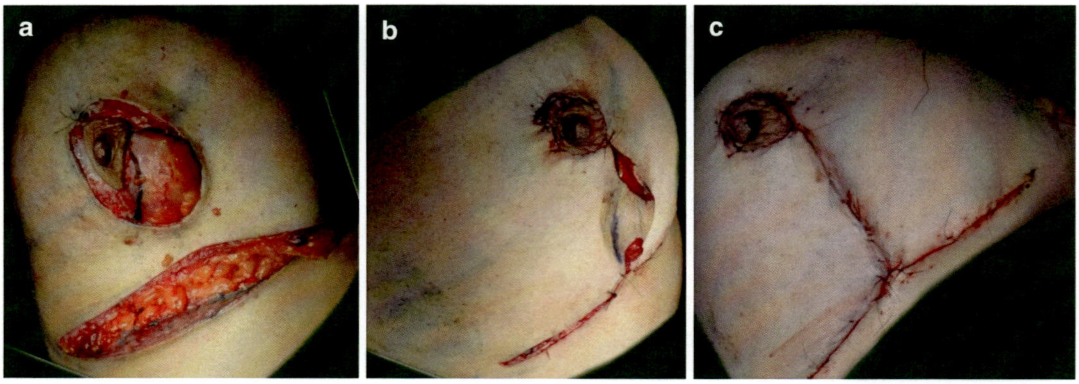

Fig. 14.10 Type 3 marking. (**a**) The glandular resection was carried out. (**b**) Only after the glandular resection was the vertical skin excision performed. (**c**) The skin is closed without tension. Same patient as in Fig. 14.5

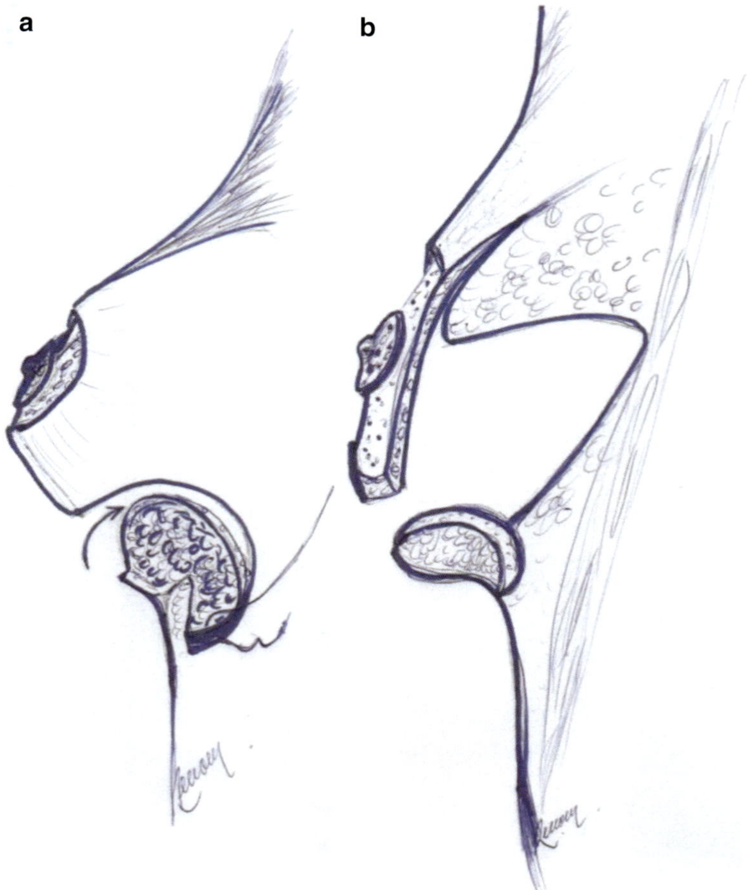

Fig. 14.11 The technical sequence is (**a**) the handling of the pedicle and the reverse flap procedure, (**b**) the breast resection

14.4 Complications

The rate of complications is low, because there is meticulous planning, and all dead space is sealed with sutures between the parenchyma and the pectoralis fascia.

Patient satisfaction with this technique has been good, but it is advisable to inform all of them about the postoperative time evolution (Figs. 14.3 and 14.12).

The most common complication was delayed healing due to minor wound separation less than

1.5 cm at the transition between the areola and the inferior scar and at the T junction. In severe hypertrophy and pendulous breasts, the nipples tend to depress (Fig. 14.12). The most severe complication that the author has experienced is one patient with total unilateral necrosis of the nipple–areola complex in a secondary mammaplasty. There were no cases of deep venous thrombosis in this series.

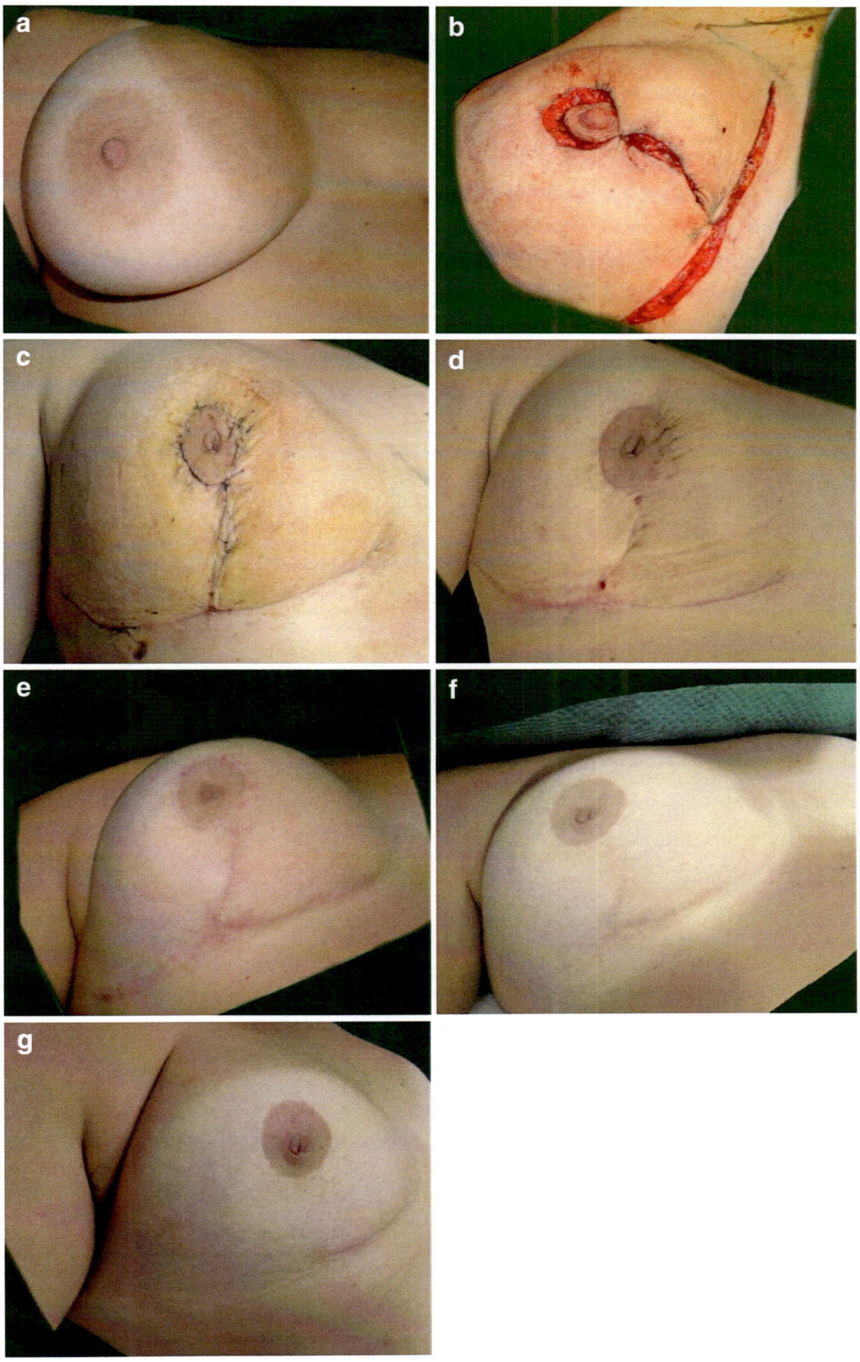

Fig. 14.12 Time evolution of the patient in Fig. 14.13. (**a**) Preoperatively. (**b**) Intraoperatively. (**c**) Five days postoperatively. (**d**) One month postoperatively. Time evolution of the patient in Fig. 14.13. (**e**) Four months postoperatively. (**f**) One year postoperatively. (**g**) Six years postoperatively

14.5 Discussion

This technique was developed with the aim of obtaining a good projection with better quality and a less extent of the scars. In tropical areas, dress code is very light and it is becoming difficult to hide long scars. Another problem is the mixing of races, which can generate severe scarring scars.

The trend over the last decades has been toward the transposition of dermal–glandular pedicles (Strombeck 1961; Skoog 1963; McKissock 1972; Ribeiro 1975). It is my opinion that in these Techniques the changes in the relationship of the breast mound to its overlying skin occur with time because of a lack of a central support, as the pedicle is stretched upward, whereas the remaining breast tissue is shaped downward. A distinct advantage of this technique is that the pedicle is folded on itself, carrying out a global movement of the breast directed around its central axis.

Up to now, mammaplasties have been classified according the configuration of the pedicle and a predetermined design of the scars. Thus, Dartigues (1925) was the first to describe the vertical technique, followed by Arié (1957), Lassus (1970), and Lejour et al. (1989). Dufourmentel and Mouly (1961) presented the oblique technique. Biesenberger (1928), Renó (2009) and Pitanguy (1959, 1961) popularized the inverted T technique. However, this classification is not applied to this technique. The reason is that the pedicle folded on itself generates several possible configurations of scars. This means that the accommodation and the shape planned for the new breast defines the necessary access and the resultant scar (Figs. 14.9c, d and 14.12). Thus, in the same patient, it is possible that the configuration of the scars will be different on each breast and we can say "a scar for each breast" (Figs. 14.14 and 14.15). The patient should be informed about this fact in advance.

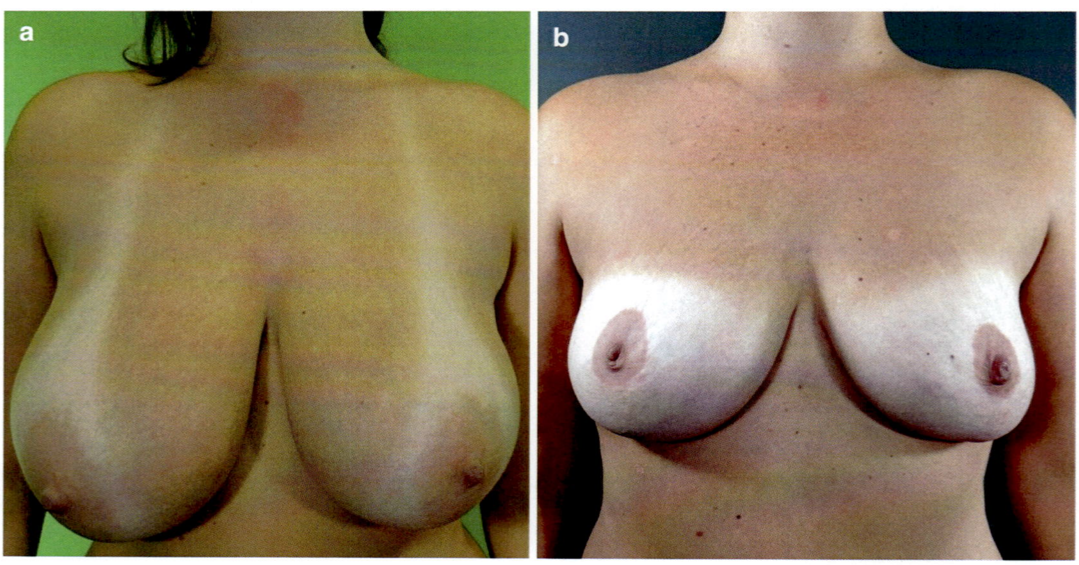

Fig. 14.13 (**a**) Preoperative view of a patient with severe hypertrophy and ptosis (standing: right nipple 30.5 cm and left 28.5 cm from the sternal notch). (**b**) Six years after a reduction of 1050 g with a circular folded pedicle technique and a reverse flap (standing: right and left nipples 22.5 cm from the sternal notch). The right nipple presents flattened with central inversion. (Same patient as in Figs. 14.6 and 14.12)

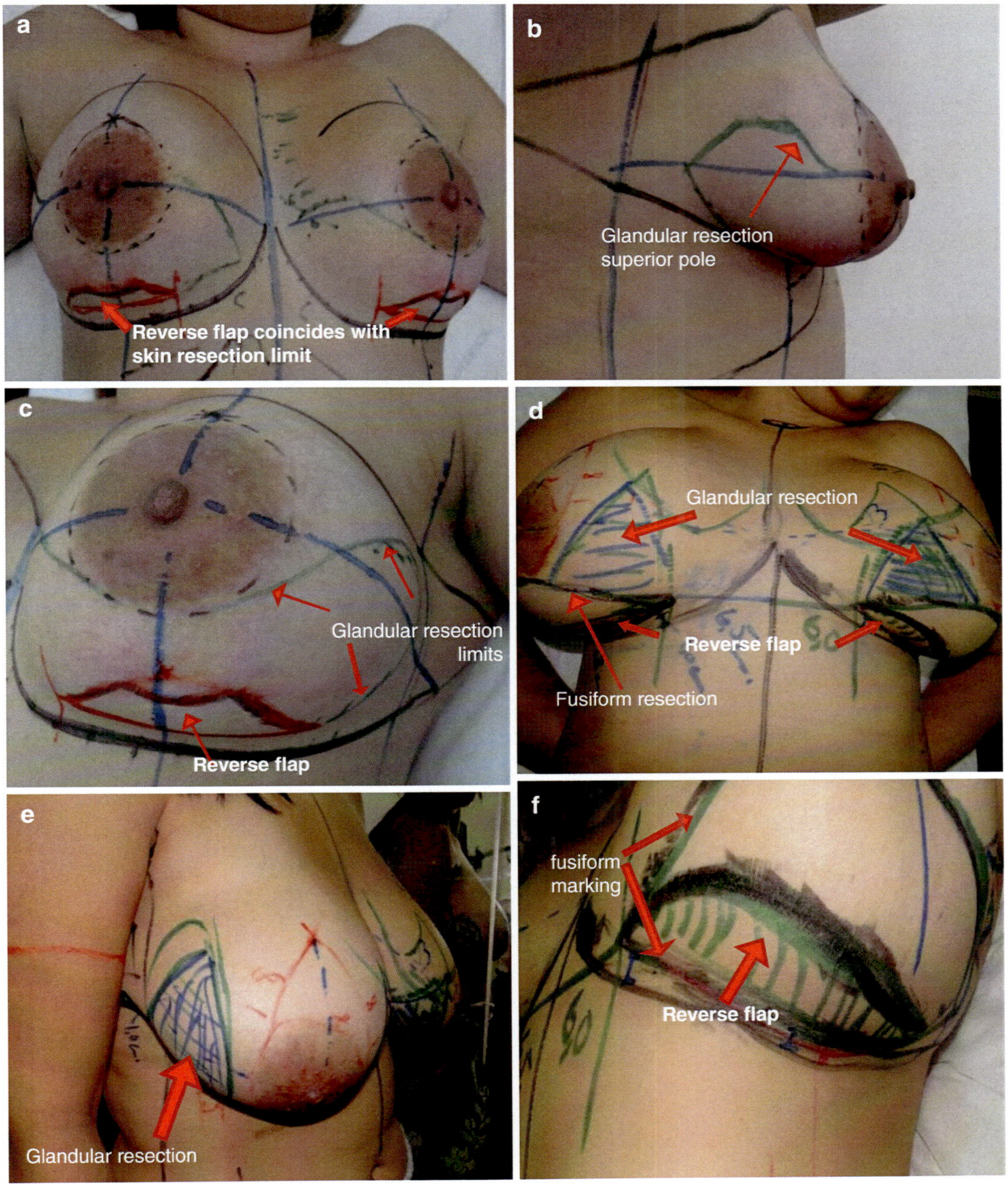

Fig. 14.14 Different designs for different breasts. (**a**–**c**) Small to moderate hypertrophy. The fusiform cutaneous resection is coincident with the reverse flap. *Green lines*, including the superior pole extension, represent the limits of glandular resection. Different designs for different breasts. (**d**–**f**) Severe hypertrophy. The fusiform resection is bigger than the reverse flap. *Green and blue lines* in the superior pole represent the glandular resection

Conclusion

The circular folded pedicle technique offers the versatility of dealing with various breast problems such as ptosis, hypertrophy, and asymmetry, while providing the possibility of minimal and excellent scarring, long-lasting results, and the option for surgical revision with the same approach, without lengthening the original scar (Figs. 14.15, 14.16 and 14.17).

The development of a reverse flap opens up the possibility of filling the submammary fold and acts as a pad that strengthens the central support (Fig. 14.18). The retractor developed for this technique makes the surgery easier, less traumatic, and is possibly the first step toward automation.

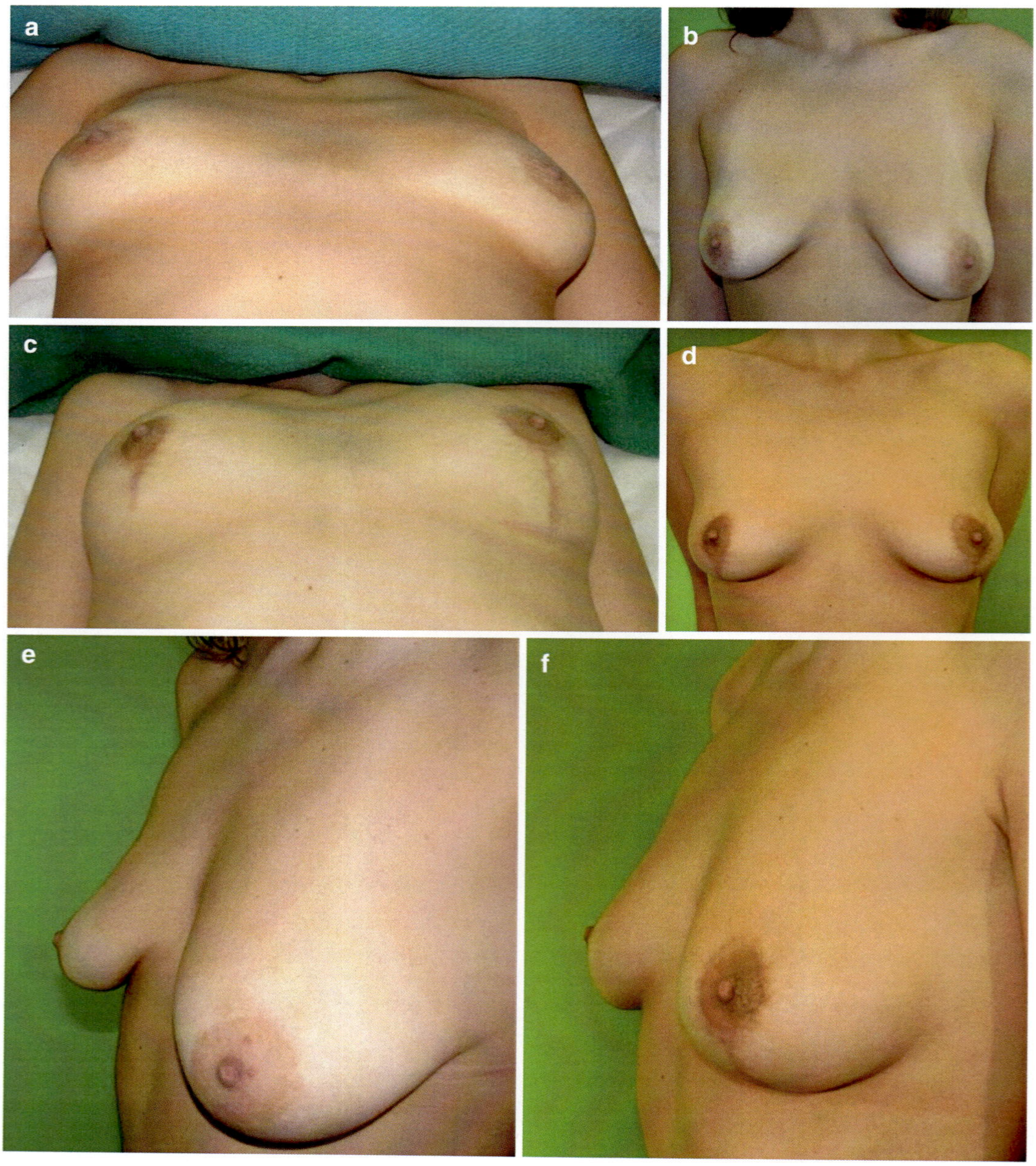

Fig. 14.15 A scar for each breast. (**a**, **b**, **e**) Preoperative view of a 30-year-old patient. (**c**, **d**, **f**) Four months postoperatively with a short vertical scar (type 2) on the right breast, and an inverted T (type 3) on the left breast. A scar for each breast

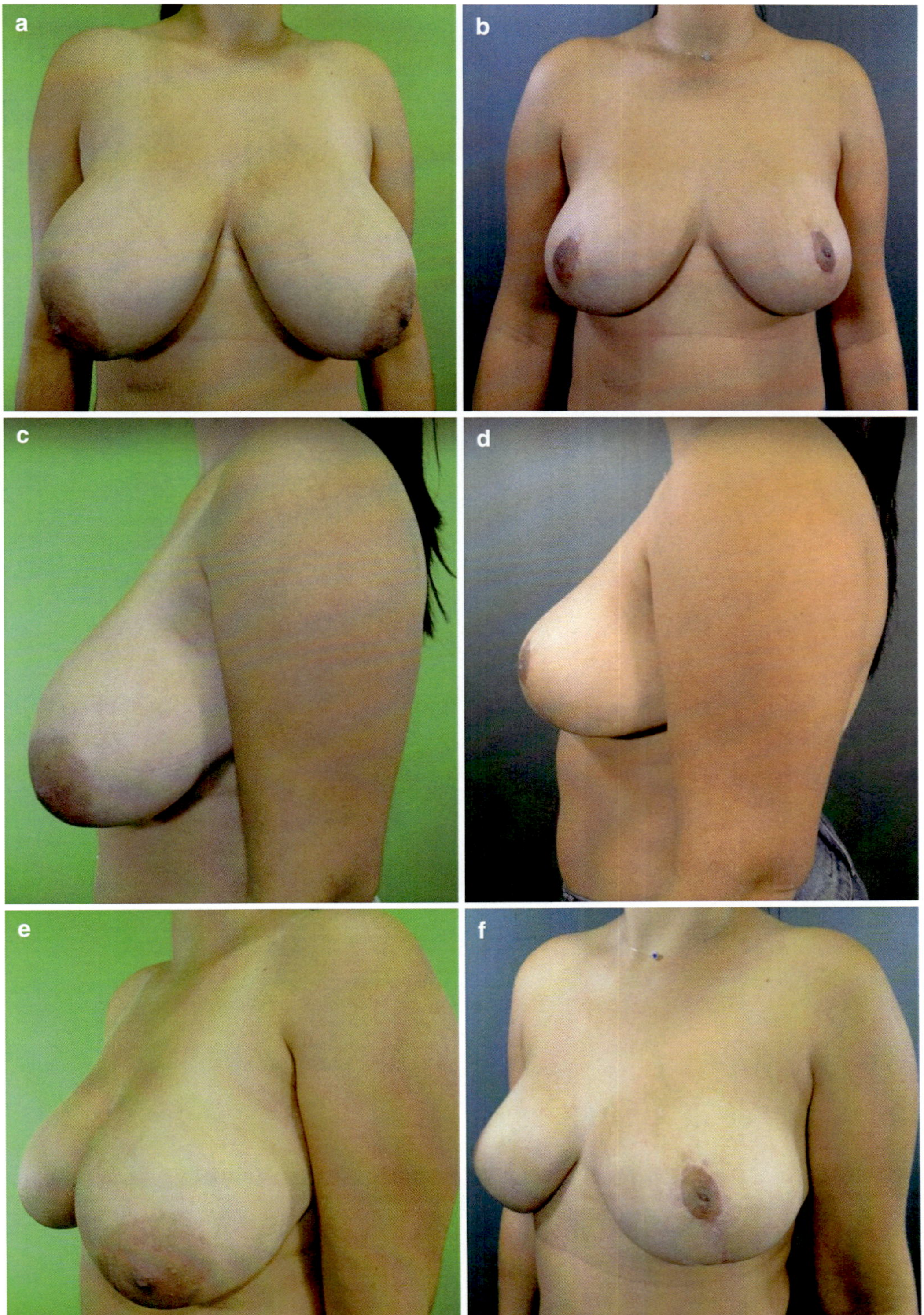

Fig. 14.16 (**a**, **c**, **e**) Preoperative view of a 26-year-old patient with hypertrophy, ptosis, and lateralized NAC (standing: nipple 30 cm from the sternal notch). (**b**, **d**, **f**) One year and 2 months after reduction mammaplasty with a circular folded pedicle and reverse flap (standing: nipple 22.2 cm from the sternal notch). Reduction of 500 g in the right and 560 g in the left breast

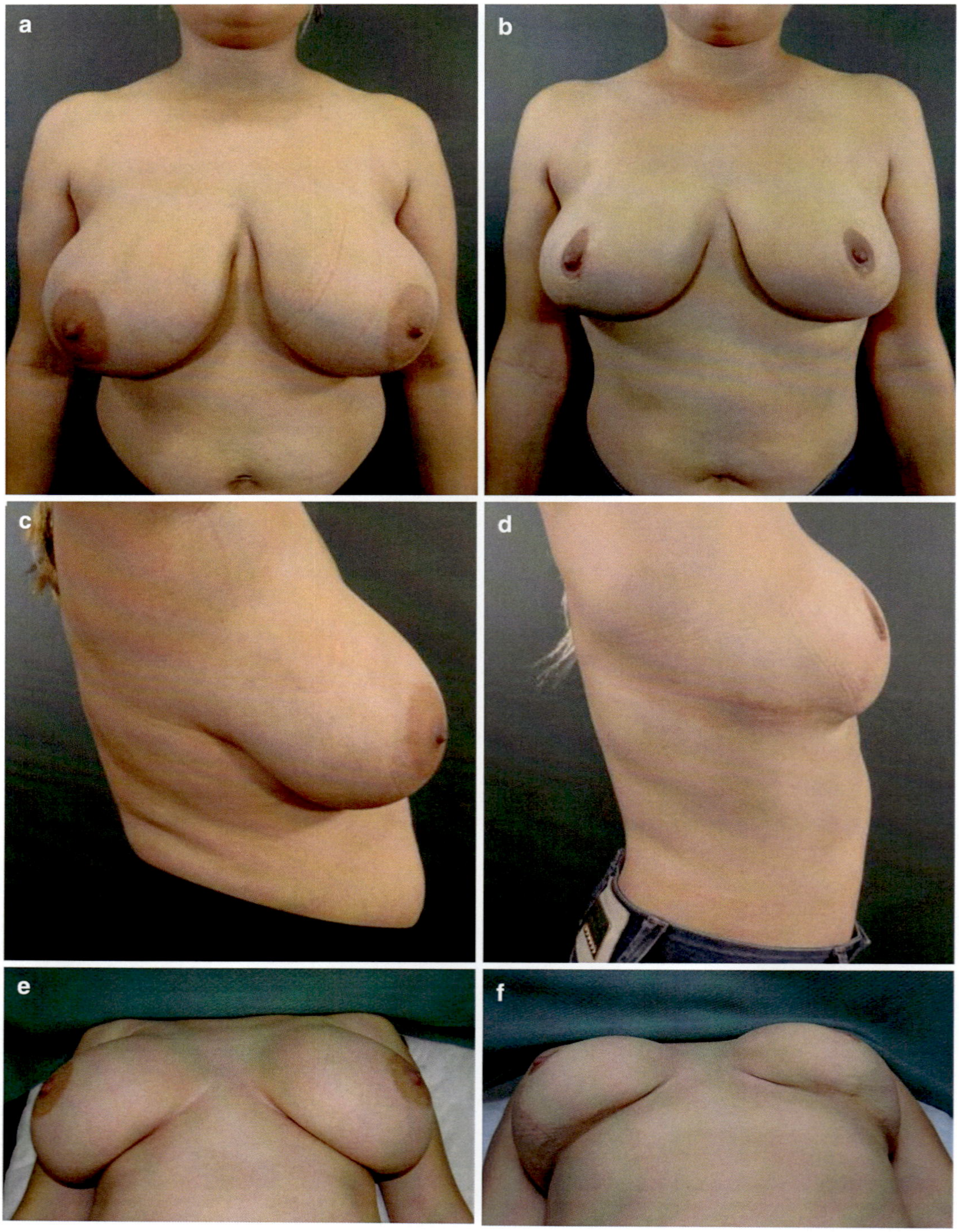

Fig. 14.17 (**a**, **c**, **e**) Preoperatively, a 24-year-old mother of three, with breast hypertrophy and ptosis (standing: nipple 27 cm from the sternal notch). (**b**, **d**, **f**) Four years postoperatively after breast reduction of 520 g in the right and 490 g in the left breast following the circular folded pedicle technique with a reverse flap (standing: nipple 21.5 cm from the sternal notch)

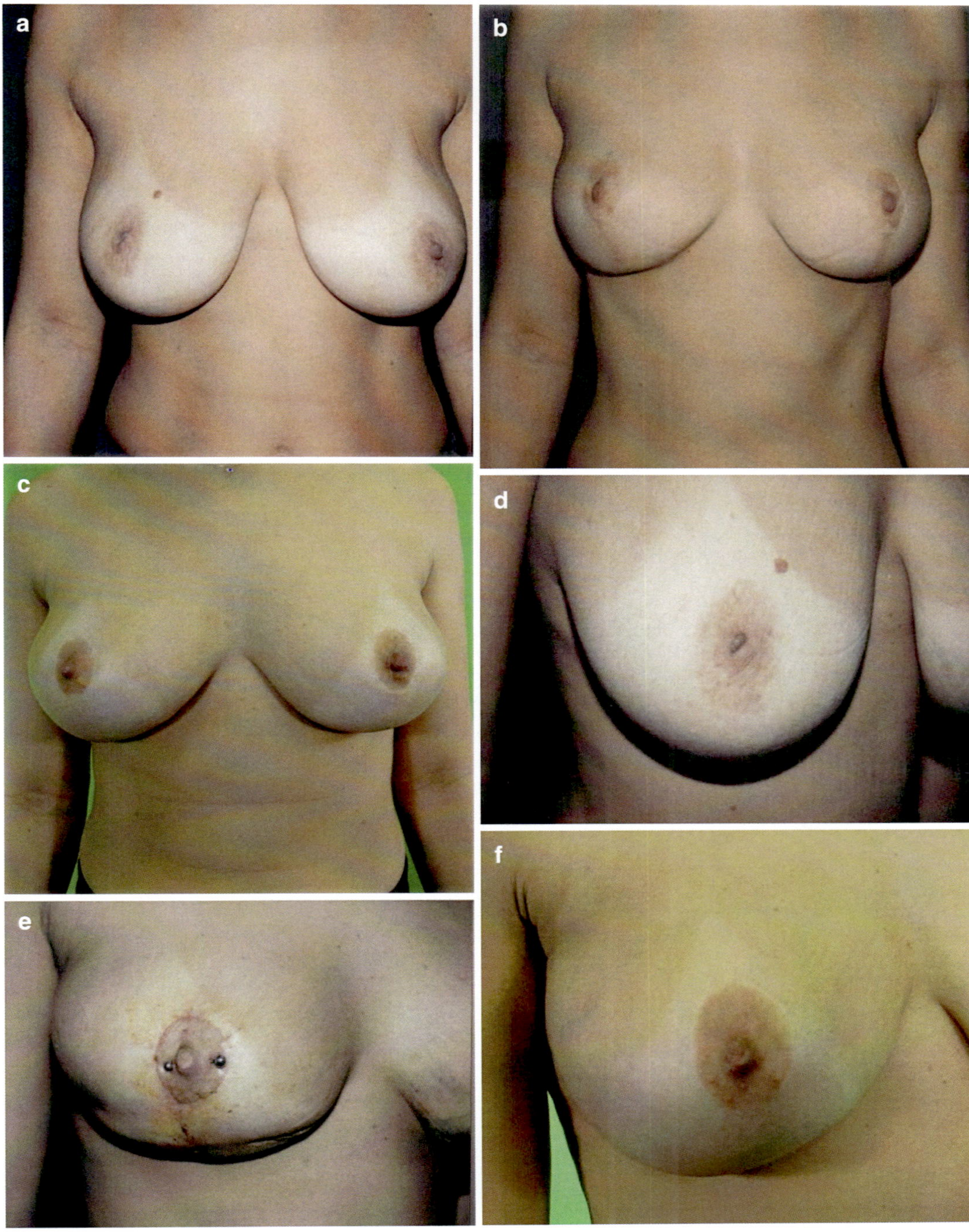

Fig. 14.18 (**a**, **d**) Preoperatively, a 25-year-old patient with ptosis, skin flaccidity, and right nipple inversion. (**b**) One year postoperatively. (**c**, **f**) Eight years postoperatively after a circular folded pedicle. (**e**) Nipple piercing for 3 months

References

Arié G (1957) Una nueva technica de mastoplastia. Rev Latinoam Cir Plast 3:23

Benelli L (1988) Technique de plastie mamaire: le "round Block". Rev Fr Chir Esthet 50:7

Biesenberger H (1928) Eine neue Methode der Mammaplastik. Zentralbl Chir 38:2382–2387

Dartigues L (1925) Traitement chirurgical du prolapse mammaire. Arch Franco-Belg Chir 28:313

Dufourmentel C, Mouly R (1961) Plastie mammaire par la method oblique. Ann Chir Plast 6:45–58

Lassus C (1970) A technique for breast reduction. Int J Surg 53(1):69–72

Lejour M, Abboud M, Declety A, Kertesz P (1989) Reduction des chicatrices de plastie mammaire de l'ancre courte a la vertical. Ann Chir Plast Esthet 35:369

McKissock PK (1972) Reduction mammaplasty with a vertical dermal flap. Plast Reconstr Surg 49(3):245–252

Pitanguy I (1959) Breast hypertrophy. Transactions of the Second International Congress of Plastic and Reconstructive Surgery, London

Pitanguy I (1961) Mammaplstias estudio de 245 casos consecutivos e apresentação de tecnica pessoal. Rev Bras Cir 42:201–220

Renó WT (1985) Mamaplastia periareolar em cone. Presented at 22nd Congresso Brasileiro de Cirurgia Plástica, Sessão Pinga-Fogo, Gramado, Brazil

Renó WT (1986) Mamaplastia Periareolar em Cone. III Jornada Sul Brasileira de Cirurgia Plástica, Porto Alegre, Brazil

Renó WT (1992a) Central support in mammaplasty. In: Hinderer UT (ed) Plastic Surgery, vol 2. Elsevier, New York

Renó WT (1992b) Reduction mammoplasty with a circular folded pedicle technique. Plast Reconstr Surg 90:65

Renó WT (1996) Reduction mammaplasty with a circular folded pedicle technique. In: Sperly A (ed) Mammaplasty brazilian procedures. Atlas CD-Rom, São Paulo

Renó WT (1999) Mammaplasty with a circular folded pedicle technique. Plast Reconstr Surg 104:1914

Renó WT (2009) Mammaplasty with a circular folded pedicle technique. In: Shiffman MA (ed) Mastopexy and breast reduction. Springer, Berlin, pp 471–481

Ribeiro L (1975) A new technique for reduction mammaplasty. Plast Reconstr Surg 55(3):330–334

Santos DC, Cardoso A, Barroso ML et al (2016) Suspensory ligament of the mammary gland: a case report. Aesth Plast Surg 40:98–101

Skoog T (1963) A technique of breast reduction: transposition of the nipple on a cutaneous vascular pedicle. Acta Chir Scand 126:453–465

Strombeck JO (1961) Mammaplasty: report of a new technique based on the two pedicle procedure. Br J Plast Surg 13:79–90

15 Arié's Technique: Surgical Principles and Its Historical Importance for Mastoplasty

Antonio Carlos Abramo

15.1 Introduction

Vertical scar mammaplasty for mastopexy was first described by Lötsch (Atiyeh et al. 2005) in 1923 followed by Dartigues (Dartigues 1925) in 1924. Arié (1957) popularized vertical reduction mammaplasty using a round de-epithelialized pedicle for the nipple–areola complex (NAC) with resection of the mammary tissue along the vertical axis of the breast, including the mammary tissue located underneath the areola. In 1959, the author added a stage to the previous technique resecting a small amount of glandular tissue underneath the NAC (Pitanguy 1960). Arié's concept regarding reduction mammaplasty for breast hypertrophy and ptosis differed radically from the classical concept from that time, which proposed extensive manipulation of the breast tissue (Penn 1955). As he had a background in breast cancer, Arié believed that it was possible to improve the size and shape of the breast, taking into account the biological type of the patient and the pathophysiological principles that have developed with regard to breast hypertrophy and ptosis. Bearing this in mind, and with the purpose of preventing complications, he developed a reduction mammaplasty with a vertical incision accompanied only by removal of the excess mammary tissue, restoring the original shape of the breast. No lateral or medial flap undermining was carried out. The main pedicle for the NAC was dermal and was located superiorly.

A simple modification of the vertical mammaplasty proposed by Arié was introduced by Pitanguy (1961), in 1960, to reduce the length of the incision below the inframammary fold, and was named the Arié–Pitanguy technique. According to Pitanguy, the simplicity of Arié's technique had the advantage of minimal tissue disturbance and avoided a scar in the inframammary fold where scar hypertrophy may occasionally occur (Rees 1967).

Since vertical mammaplasty was advocated by Arié, distinctive reduction mammaplasty using a vertical incision has been reported. More recently, several authors have published refinements of the vertical mammaplasty technique that have led to more predictable and reproducible results and, consequently, have increased the popularity of the procedure. Vertical mammaplasty excising tissue from both pillars, particularly laterally, provides tightness at the upper infra-areolar site, and has ensured the durability of the breast shape (Lassus 1987). In

A.C. Abramo, M.D., Ph.D. (✉)
Division of Plastic Surgery, General Hospital São Luiz Morumbi, Post Graduate Course of Plastic and Reconstructive Surgery, Institute of Assistance in Plastic Surgery of São Paulo, São Paulo, SP, Brazil
e-mail: acabramo@abramo.com.br

J.M. Avelar (ed.), *Breast Surgery*, https://doi.org/10.1007/978-3-319-54115-0_15

addition, reduction mammaplasty combining vertical and transverse approaches through a vertical incision have enhanced both upper and lower poles of the breast, with long-term recovery of the natural shape of the breast (Abramo et al. 2004).

Vertical mammaplasty has usually been indicated for young patients with mild or moderate degrees of both breast ptosis and hypertrophy. It has also been indicated for patients over 50 years of age with severe breast ptosis and large breast hypertrophy (Beer et al. 2002). To be effective, vertical mammaplasty must achieve results equal to or better than those achieved with conventional procedures, particularly the inverted T techniques (Nahai 1999).

Here we describe the relevance of the principles advocated by Arié for reduction mammaplasty through a vertical incision and its historical importance in the current aesthetic plastic surgery of the breast.

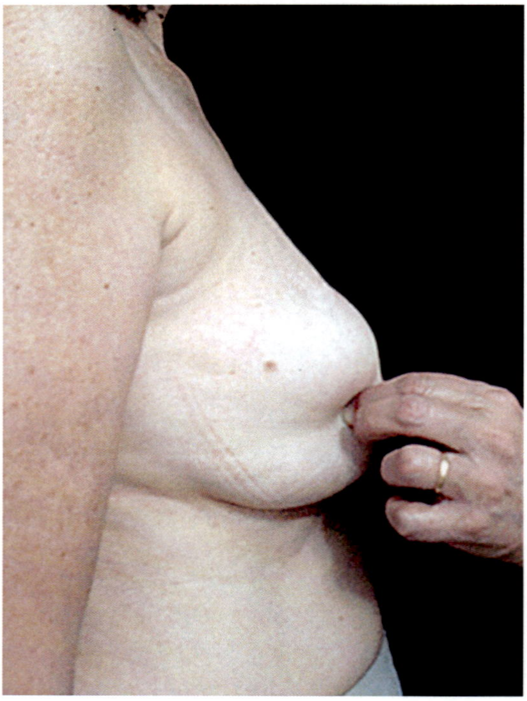

Fig. 15.1 Pinch test on the lower pole of the breast to achieve the distance between the major concavity of the vertical ellipse branches

15.2 Method: Operative Technique

With the patient in a half sitting position on the operating table, a vertical ellipse is outlined on the breast skin. Arié's original demarcation is made from the upper edge of the NAC to the inframammary fold by using a fixed suture in the mid-sternal line. According to Arié, this approach allows symmetry between the breasts and a symmetrical location for the NAC to be achieved. The opening between the branches of the vertical ellipse is performed regarding the degree of breast hypertrophy and ptosis. The distance between the branches of the vertical ellipse in the center of its concavity is achieved by a pinch test clamping the skin at the lower pole to establish nipple–areola displacement, breast elevation, and upper pole fullness (Fig. 15.1). A superficial periareolar skin incision is made, preserving the dermis. An intra-areolar incision is made only in cases of nipple–areola enlargement, to reduce the areolar diameter in accordance with the new shape of the breast. De-epithelialization of the periareolar region was 1–2 cm beyond the edge of the areolar incision accomplished according to Schwarzmann's maneuver, creating a round dermal

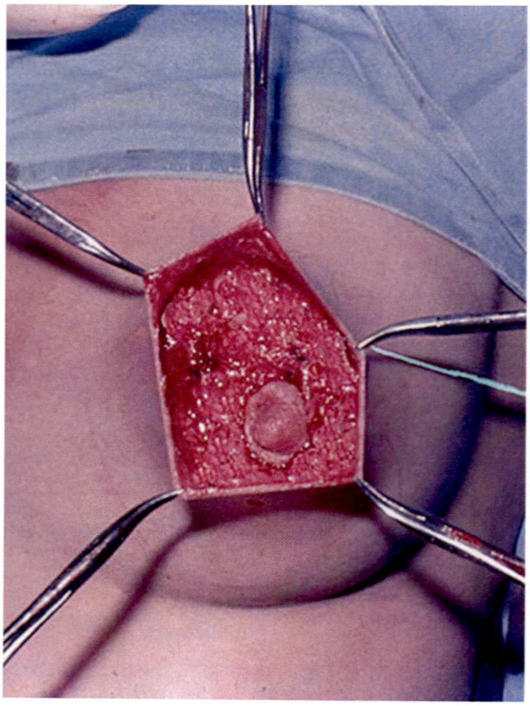

Fig. 15.2 De-epithelialization around the areola, creating a dermal flap for the nipple–areola complex (NAC)

bed to the NAC (Fig. 15.2). No further undermining is required. The extent of the periareolar detachment is just enough to carry the areola to its new position.

After that, the lateral and medial margins of the vertical ellipse are incised pulling the infra-areolar skin upward with the help of two hooks from the lower edge of the areola to the inframammary fold (Fig. 15.3). Next, an en bloc elliptical orange seed-shaped central wedge resection, as indicated by Arié in his original publication, involving skin and mammary parenchyma, is performed from below the areola to the inframammary fold (Fig. 15.4). Resection of the mammary parenchyma involves both adipose and glandular tissues. The en bloc orange seed-shaped resection also includes in its upper portion the glandular tissue located beneath the areola.

After resection of the mammary parenchyma, a superior pedicle for the NAC is established. The medial and lateral pillars of the remaining mammary tissue are approached together in the mid-line of the breast and anchored over the pectoralis aponeurosis with buried sutures from the second to the fifth intercostal space (Fig. 15.5). Anchorage in the pectoral aponeurosis raises the breast, filling its upper pole and providing a pleasant contour for the breast. The lateral and medial pillars of the breast are sutured together. Closure of the skin creates a vertical scar that crosses the inframammary fold, extending downward straight or laterally over the thoracic wall (Fig. 15.6).

To guarantee the surgical outcome, a brassiere-shaped dressing with plaster was applied over the entire chest wall beyond the anterior axillary line (Fig. 15.7). The brassiere-shaped bandage using plaster had the purpose of

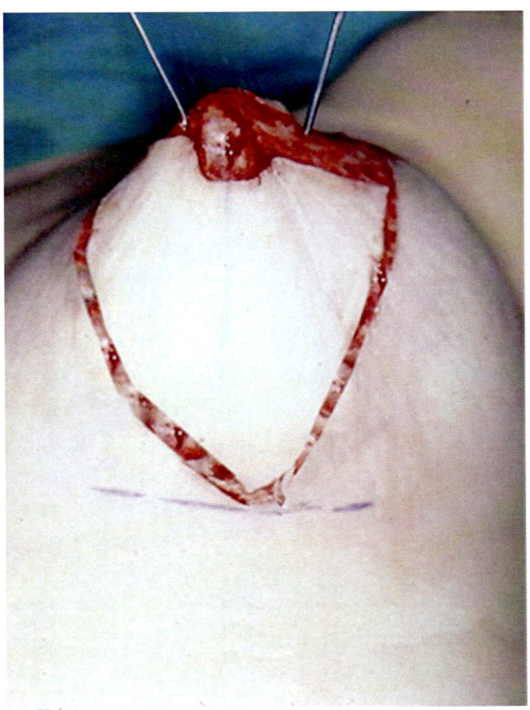

Fig. 15.3 The vertical ellipse is incised pulling the infra-areolar skin upward with the help of two hooks from the lower edge of the areola to the inframammary fold

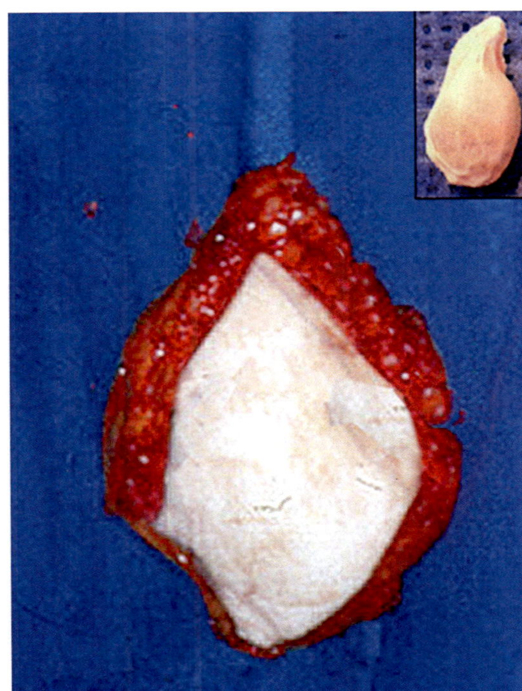

Fig. 15.4 Main image shows the en bloc orange seed-shaped resection, including the glandular tissue located beneath the areola on the upper tip. The smaller image shows an orange seed to compare with the shape of the en bloc resection

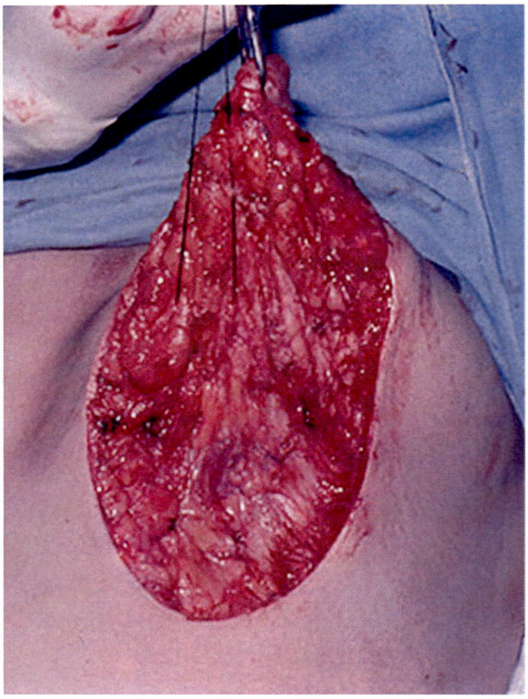

Fig. 15.5 The threat shows the medial pillar of the breast anchored over the pectoralis aponeurosis in the second intercostal space

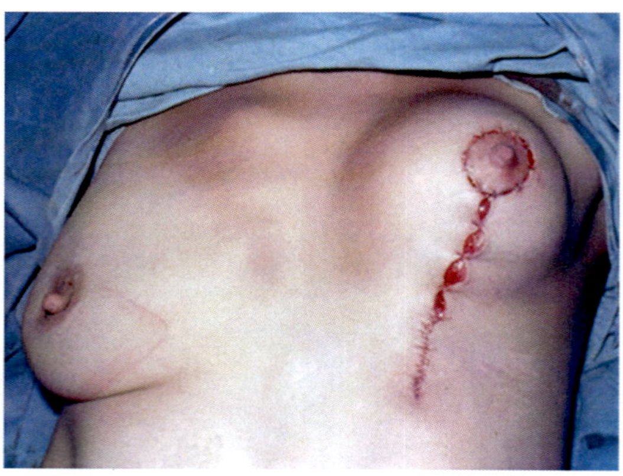

Fig. 15.6 After closure, the vertical scar is widely extended beneath the new inframammary fold. Reduction of the breast diameter with a well-located NAC and a balanced shape and projection of the breast were achieved on the left breast

modeling and ensuring the shape achieved for the breast after reduction mammaplasty through a vertical incision.

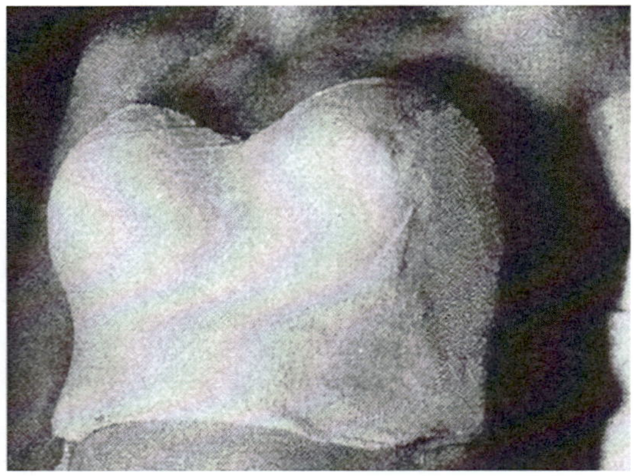

Fig. 15.7 A brassiere-shaped bandage with plaster was applied over the entire chest wall to model and ensure the shape of the breast after vertical reduction mammaplasty

15.3 Results

Reduction of the breast diameter with elevation of the breast and NAC was attained after reduction mammaplasty using the vertical approach proposed by Arié. A pleasant breast contour with an appropriate location for the NAC was achieved. In addition, a balanced shape, projection, and volume of the breast associated with the fullness of the upper pole was also achieved with the technique proposed by Arié (Fig. 15.8). Sensation of the NAC was not affected and dehiscence of the sutures was not usual with this technique.

Case Report: breast asymmetry characterized by moderate hypertrophy and ptosis on the right breast, and moderate hypertrophy with mild ptosis on the left (Fig. 15.9a, c). The opening between the branches of the vertical ellipse was performed regarding the degree of breast hypertrophy and ptosis. The distance between the branches of the vertical ellipse in the center of its concavity was 9 cm for the right breast and 7 cm for the left one. At 1 year postoperatively a balanced shape, projection, volume, and fullness of the upper pole are maintained (Fig. 15.9b, d).

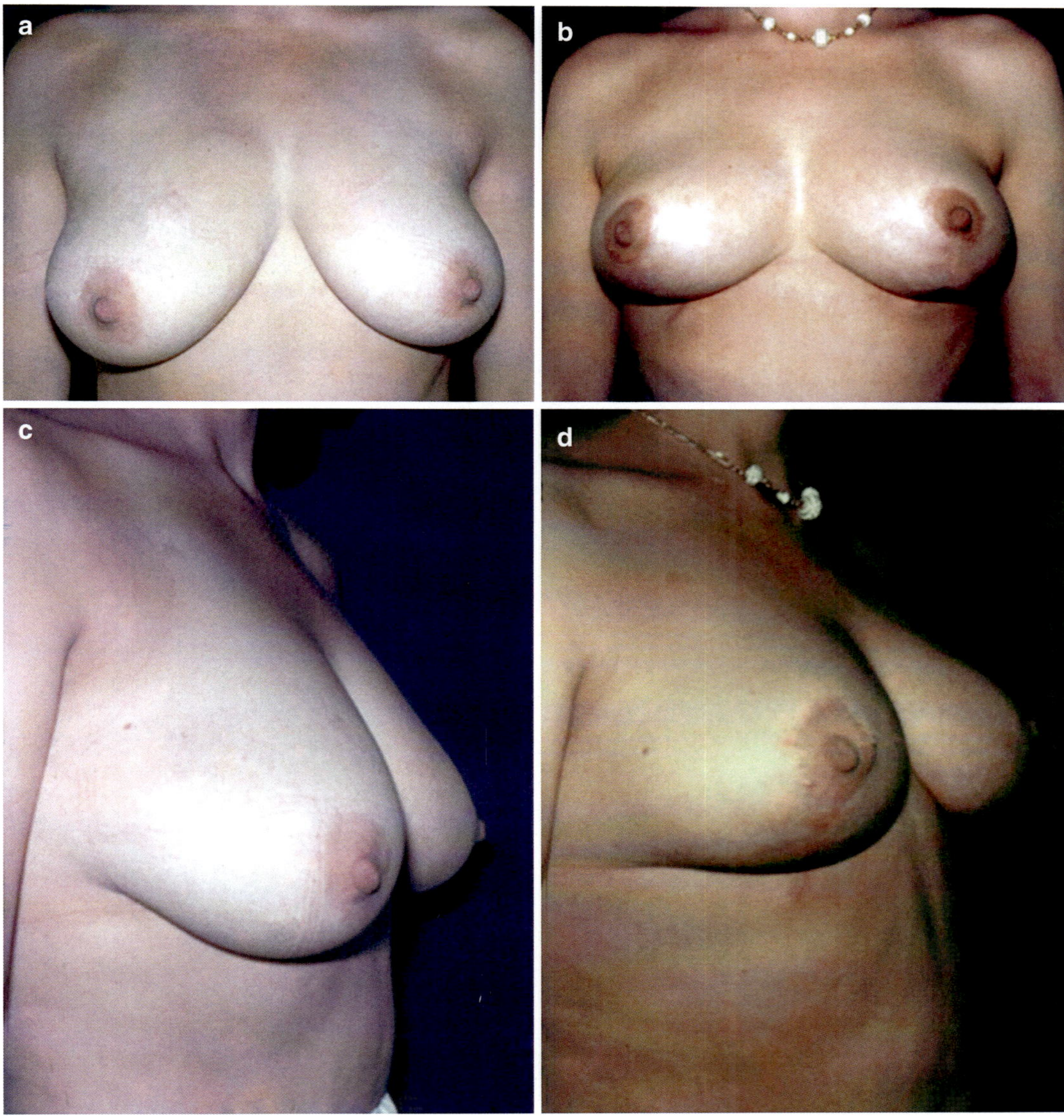

Fig. 15.8 (**a**, **c**) Severe breast ptosis and moderate hypertrophy on the right breast. Moderate breast ptosis and hypertrophy of the left breast. (**b**, **d**) At 1 year postoperatively. Vertical scar cannot be hidden by the overlap of the lower pole over the inframammary fold

15.4 Complication

Arié's technique, as it does not involve dissection of the lateral and medial pillars of the mammary parenchyma or of the skin flap, reduces the risk of breast tissue or skin necrosis. The vertical ellipse resection preserving the upper pole of the breast does not alter the sensitivity of the NAC. The brassiere-shaped bandage is more of a major discomfort than a complication, although it may become a complication when retained for over a week. The duration of its use increases the

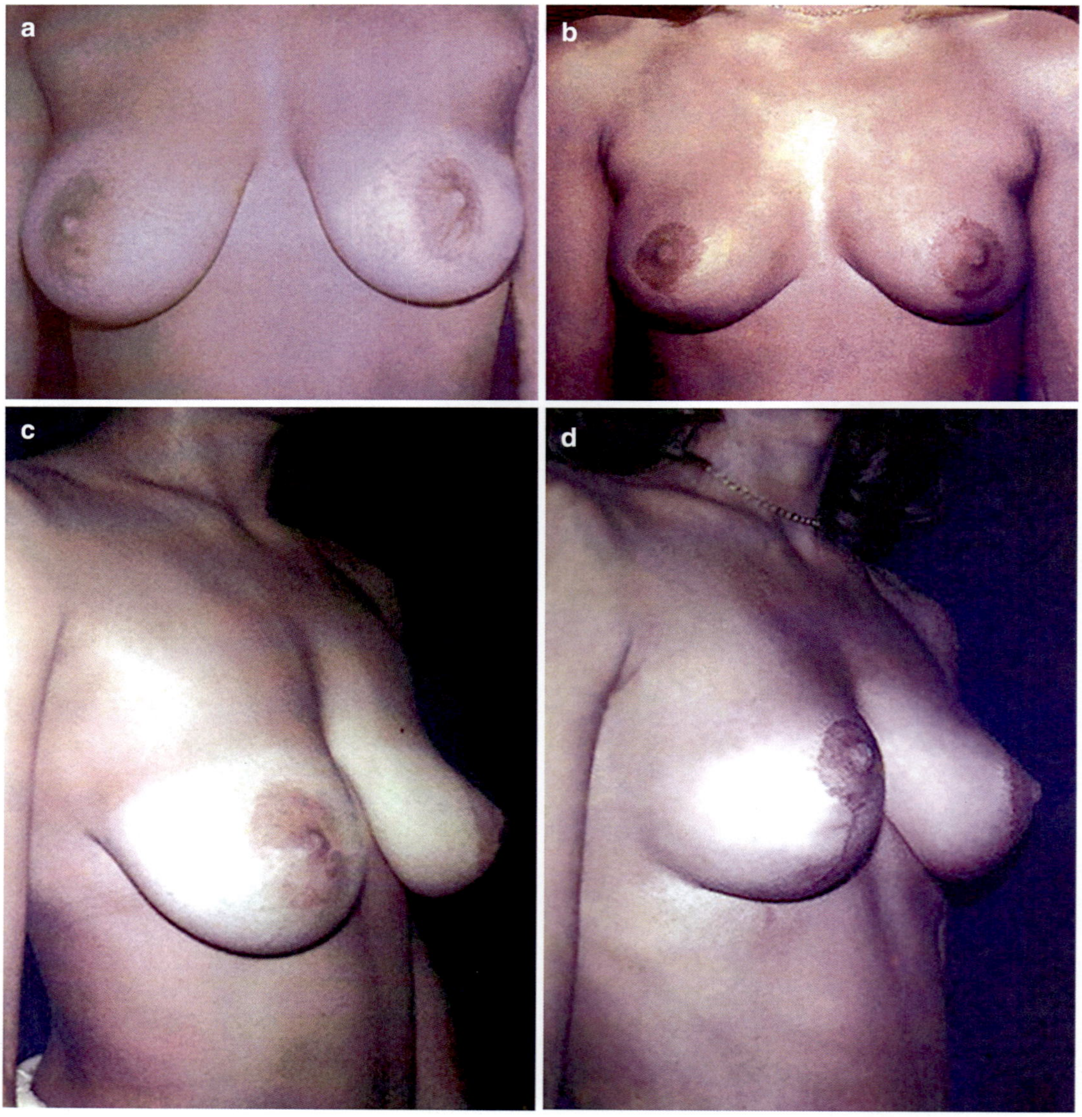

Fig. 15.9 (**a**, **c**) Preoperative view of asymmetrical breasts. (**b**, **d**) At 1 year postoperatively

risk of skin damage, particularly in patients with sensitive skin.

The main complication of the vertical mammaplasty proposed by Arié is the length of the vertical scar, which extends below the inframammary fold. Despite the vertical incision ending at the inframammary fold, the resulting scar always goes beyond the new inframammary fold created by the breast lift. The extent of the vertical scar below the inframammary fold can run linearly

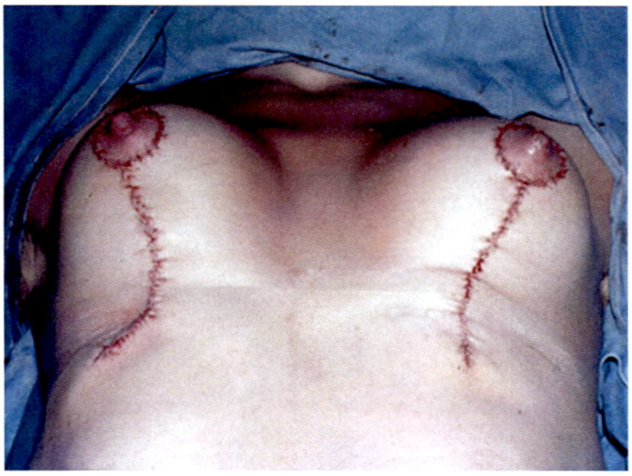

Fig. 15.10 The right vertical scar was extended laterally with a bulge at its distal end, whereas the left scar was extended in a straight line without distortion at its distal end

downward or be diverted laterally (Fig. 15.10). The length of the scar in the chest wall below the inframammary fold changes in accordance with the degree of breast deformity. The vertical scar may extend for a short distance below the inframammary fold in mild and moderate degrees of ptosis and may be hidden by the natural overlap of the lower pole of the breast over the inframammary fold (Fig. 15.11). However, in severe breast hypertrophy and ptosis and in some degrees of moderate breast hypertrophy and ptosis, the length of the vertical scar is more extensive, and is not hidden by the natural overlap of the lower pole over the inframammary fold (Fig. 15.12).

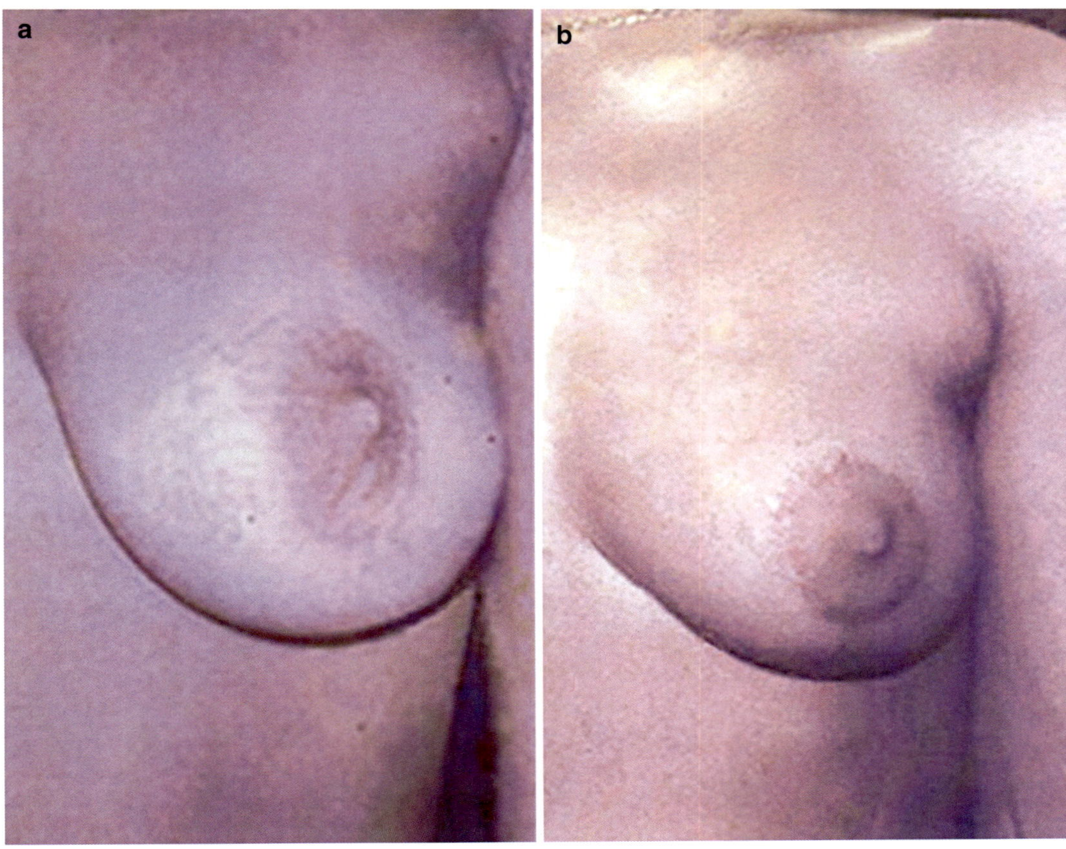

Fig. 15.11 (a) Preoperative view. (b) When the scar extends for a short distance below the inframammary fold, it may be hidden by the natural overlap of the lower pole over the inframammary fold

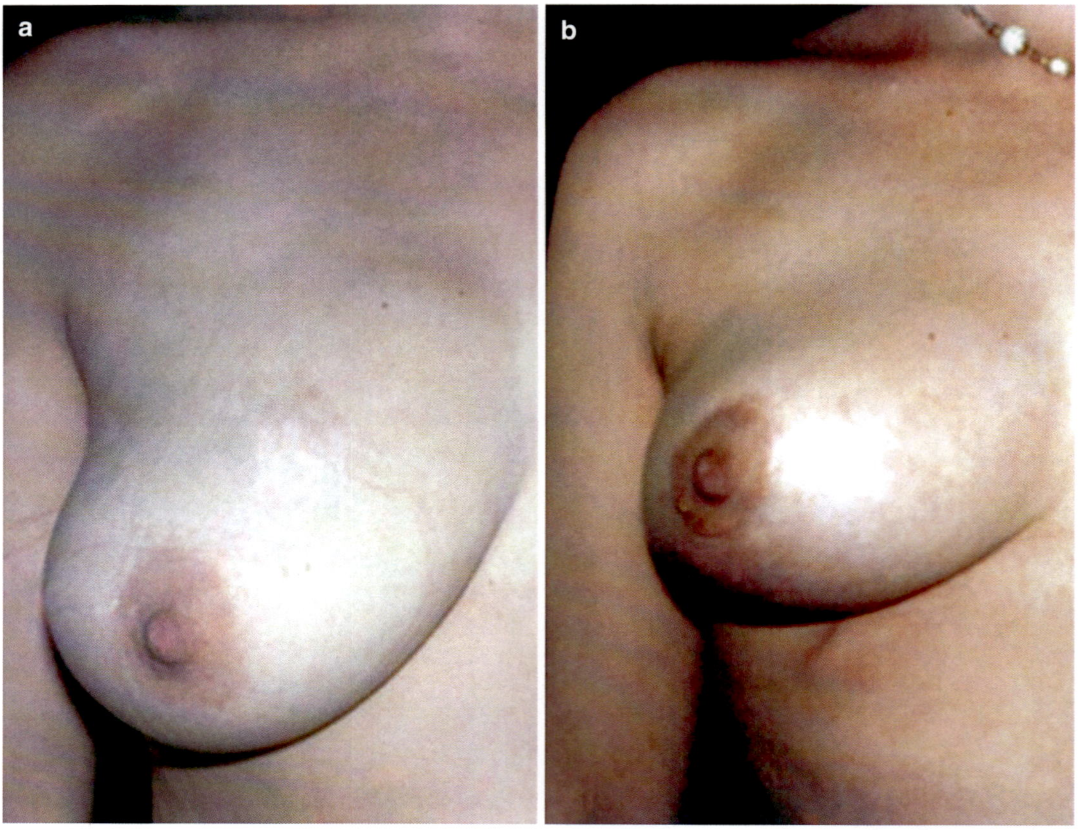

Fig. 15.12 (**a**) Preoperative view. (**b**) When the length of the vertical scar is widely extended below the inframammary fold, it cannot be hidden by the natural overlap of the lower pole over the inframammary fold

15.5 Discussion

A technique for breast reduction must be safe, reliable, reproducible, and easily performed. Arié was the first to report a simple aesthetic surgery for the breast in Latin America. Furthermore, he was also the first to develop a reduction mammaplasty through a vertical incision. His international contribution to plastic surgery of the breast was enormous, especially among Brazilian plastic surgeons. This is demonstrated by the number of aesthetic breast surgeries reported by Brazilian surgeons. His influence was also important in the development of aesthetic breast surgery in Latin America and Central America, also shown by several studies published from this continent. The simple principles of its technique in conjunction with the preservation of the nipple–areola sensation and the vascularization of the mammary parenchyma and skin were the starting points for new techniques.

These techniques were important not only for reduction mammaplasty through vertical incision, but also for reduction mammaplasty through techniques using distinctive incisions. The Pitanguy's attempt (Pitanguy 1961) to shorten the incision below the inframammary fold, known as the Arié–Pitanguy technique, gave rise to its inverted T reduction mammaplasty, which was disseminated and applied worldwide. His contribution also extended to Europe, being the starting point for the vertical reduction mammaplasty by Lassus (1987), in which a superior dermoglandular pedicle carries the NAC, whereas volume reduction is achieved through a central, en bloc segment resection without anchoring the gland to the pectoralis muscle. The simple principles of the vertical reduction mammaplasty of Arié's technique remained in

Europe until the arrival of Lejour (1994), who definitively popularized the technique.

Arié proposed a vertical mammaplasty to correct mild or moderate breast ptosis with distinctive degrees of breast hypertrophy. The technique provides a normal breast according to the patient biotype, not a virginal breast to a middle age or a fat woman (Arié 1957). The advantage of Arié's technique lies in the brevity of the surgical time and in its simplicity. No previous marking is necessary. The en bloc resection of skin, fat, and gland on the lower pole of the breast without lateral or medial dissection of the vertical pillars of the breast reduces the risk of suture dehiscence and necrosis at the vertical closure. Resection of the glandular tissue located beneath the areola, added in 1959 by the author, created a tissue gap at this level making easier the transposition of the NAC to its new location, avoiding distortions (Pitanguy 1960). The NAC is transposed on a superiorly based dermoglandular flap.

The dermal flap based superiorly for the NAC, as proposed by Arié, has been considered safe for nipple–areola transposition (Abramo 1991). The lateral and medial pillars of the breast are closed together centrally in a vertical scar on the breast meridian. Closure is done with separate and buried stitches at different levels to prevent suture dehiscence. No lateral or medial flap undermining is performed to avoid vascular compromise and consequently necrosis of the flaps. The brassiere-shaped bandage with plaster immobilizes the scar, preventing its dehiscence and therefore an infection at this level. Also, it maintains the shape of the breast obtained in surgery, modeling and ensuring its long-term maintenance.

Conclusion

Despite initial skepticism, vertical reduction mammaplasty has become increasingly popular in recent years because it best incorporates the two concepts of minimal scarring and a satisfactory breast shape. Currently, vertical scar techniques seem to be more popular in Latin America and Europe than in the USA. The technique, however, is not without major drawbacks, such as long vertical scars extending below the inframammary fold and a "dog-ear" at the lower end of the scar.

References

Abramo AC (1991) Pattern for reduction mammaplasty that uses a vertical dermal pedicle. Aesth Plast Surg 15:265

Abramo AC, Teixeira JC, Galindo A (2004) Mammaplasty combining vertical and transverse approaches through a vertical incision. Plast Reconstr Surg 113(2):508

Arié G (1957) Una nueva técnica de mastoplastia. Rev Iberolatinoam Cir Plast 3(1):23

Atiyeh BS, Rubeiz MT, Hayek SN (2005) Refinements of vertical scar mammaplasty: circumvertical skin excision design with limited inferior pole subdermal undermining and liposculpture of the inframammary crease. Aesthetic Plast Surg 29(6):519–531

Beer GM, Morgenthaler W, Spicher I, Meyer VE (2002) Modifications in vertical scar breast reduction. Br J Plast Surg 54:341

Dartigues L (1925) Traitement chirurgical du prolaspsus mammaire. Arch Franco Belg Chir 28:313

Lassus C (1987) Breast reduction: evolution of a technique. A single vertical scar. Aesth Plast Surg 11:107

Lejour M (1994) Vertical mammaplasty and liposuction of the breast. Plast Reconstr Surg 94:100

Nahai F (1999) Update on vertical mammaplasty (discussion). Plast Reconstr Surg 104:2299

Penn J (1955) Breast reduction. Br J Plast Surg 7:357

Pitanguy I (1960) Breast hypertrophy. In: Wallace AB (ed) Transactions of International Society of Plastic Surgeons, Second Congress, London, 1959. Livingstone, Edinburgh, p 509

Pitanguy I (1961) Aproximação ecletica do problema das mamoplastias. Rev Bras Cir 41:179

Rees TD (1967) Plastic surgery of the breast. In: Converse JM (ed) Reconstructive plastic surgery, The trunk, genitourinary system and experimental approaches, vol 5, p 1903

16 Sepúlveda's Technique for Reduction Mastoplasty

Mariangela Santiago

16.1 Introduction

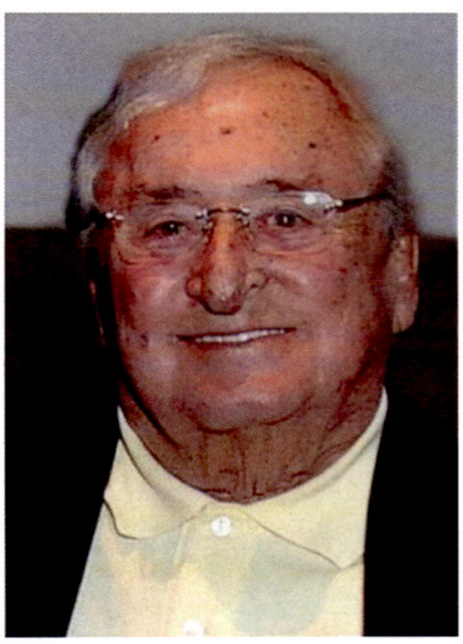

Dr. AntonioCarlos Aleixo Sepúlveda
1928–2015

Breast reduction is one of the most fascinating areas of plastic surgery. It involves several challenges, such as shape and volume, proportionality with the chest, preservation of erogenous sensitivity, which is very important in female sexual performance, symmetry, hidden/invisible scars, and lasting results.

Scars resulting from mammoplasties for the correction of hypertrophies and ptoses do not always satisfy the surgeon or the patients as they are extensive and sometimes approach the midsternal line and/or invade the anterior axillary line.

Analyzing the scars resulting from the techniques described, the ideal scar would be that in which the vertical segment would not surpass the submammarian sulcus and that would be short, with an average length of 4–5 cm, sufficient to provide a good shape to the breasts and good positioning of the areolas. The submammarian segment would truly need to be hidden in the sulcus, never surpassing the projection of the anterior axillary line.

The objective of the present project is to show a technique that could decrease scars, and that could be used in the various forms of breast hypertrophies and ptoses to obtain a good and aesthetically pleasing breast shape.

16.2 Method

Our technique evolved from the technique of Hollander (1924) and his followers, Dufourmentel and Mouly, Meyer and Kesselring, and Elbaz (Dufourmentel and Mouly 1961; Elbaz and Verheeck 1972), and others, and from the main surgical principles of Pitanguy's technique (Pitanguy 1967). We eliminate the medial segment of the submammarian scar of Pitanguy's technique.

16.2.1 Marking

The marking used for this method is shown in Fig. 16.1.

M. Santiago, M.D.
Brazilian Society of Plastic Surgery,
Rua Funchal 203, conj. 102, Vila Olimpia, São Paulo,
SP CEP 04551-060, Brazil

International Society of Aesthetic Plastic Surgery,
45 Lyme Road, Suite 304, Hanover, NH 03755, USA
e-mail: dramariangela@uol.com.br

J.M. Avelar (ed.), *Breast Surgery*, https://doi.org/10.1007/978-3-319-54115-0_16

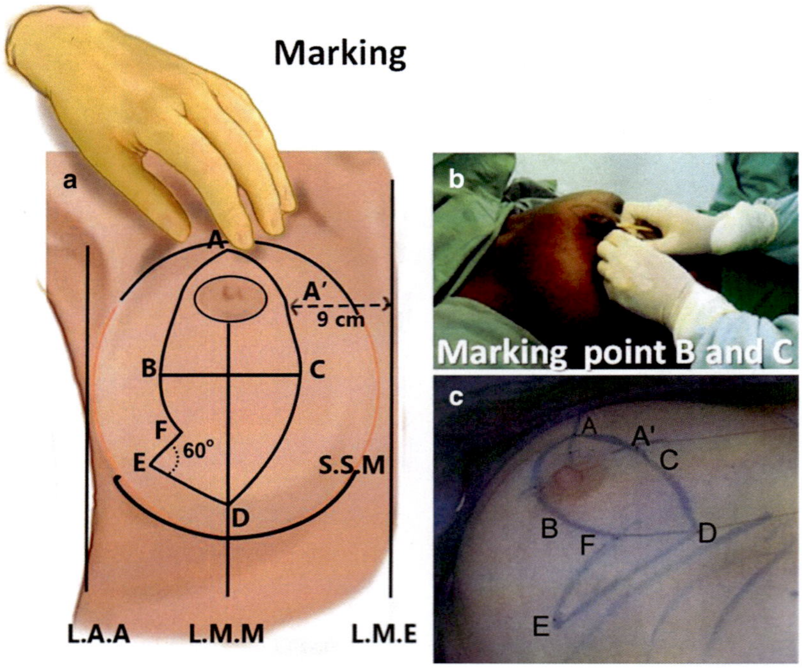

Fig. 16.1 Initial marking. Point A: placed along the midmammary line, slightly below the projection of the submammarian sulcus. Points B to C: marked according to each case, depending on the quantity of skin to be resected. They are situated slightly more than half the distance between the lower border of the areola and the submammarian sulcus. Point D: slightly above the submammarian sulcus, on the midmammary line, according to the degree of hypertrophy or ptosis. This marks the location of the new sulcus. Point E: 2–5 cm distant from point D in small and medium hypertrophies, but 1–2 cm higher. Greater distance in large hypertrophies. Point F: 2–5 cm distant from point E. Greater distance in large hypertrophies. Lines D–E and E–F form a 60°angle. The areolas are marked according to each case. In large hypertrophies and ptoses, the areolas should maintain a greater diameter

16.2.2 Resection

1. We conducted Schwarzmann's maneuver and decortication of the A-B-C triangle.
2. Glandular resection is carried out according to each case.

The type of resection chosen provides the height, volume, and contour of the breast.

We modify the resection of the glandular tissue obeying the criterion that the most important thing is "not what comes out, but rather, what stays," which is what will provide the new breast shape. Removal of breast tissue is ample (Fig. 16.2).

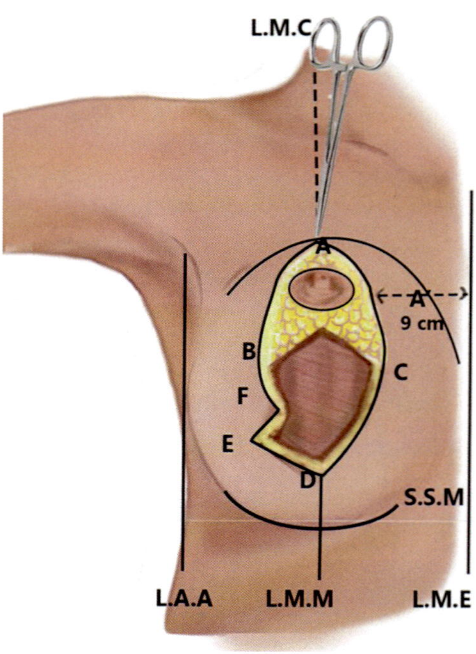

Fig. 16.2 Schwarzmann's maneuver and decortication of the A–B–C triangle. Glandular resection according to each case

16.2.3 Dynamics

The F point is approximated and sutured to the D point, which elevates. The distance A–F becomes even smaller than the distance A–D (Fig. 16.3).

The A point is deviated inwardly to obtain equality between the two margins of the wound. The A–A′ distance is variable. The new A point cannot be less than 9 cm from the midstream line to avoid convergence of the areolas (Fig. 16.4).

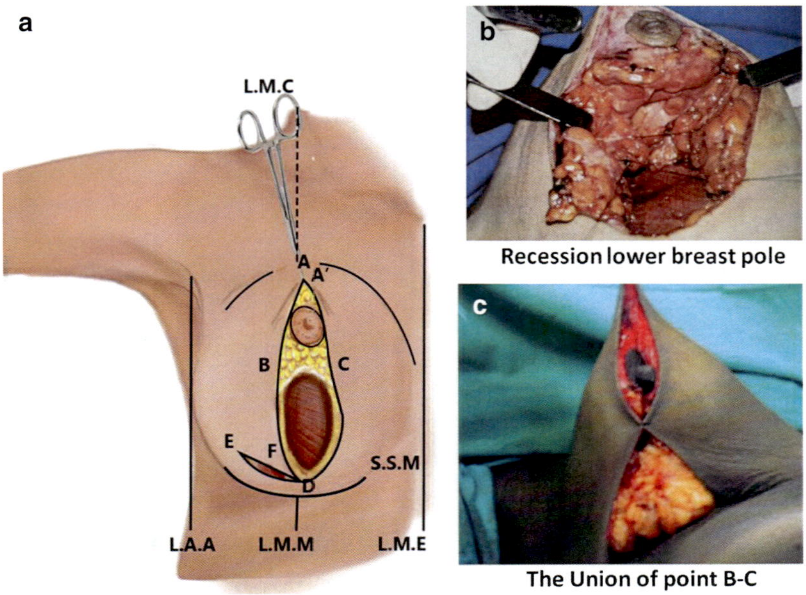

Fig. 16.3 (a) Point F is approximated and sutured to point D, which elevates. The distance A–F becomes even smaller than the distance A–D. (b) Resection of the lower mammary pole. (c) Union of points B and C

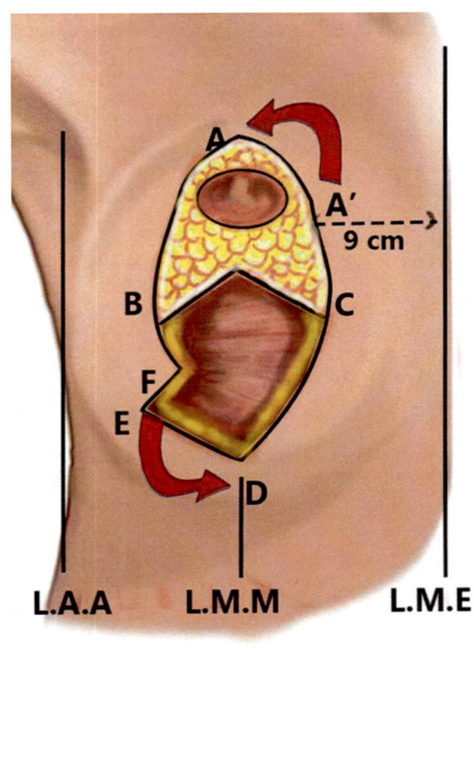

Fig. 16.4 Point A is deviated inward to obtain equality between the two margins of the wound. The distance A–A′ is variable

16.2.4 Content–Container Adjustment

Marking is not definitive. After the breast resection, a new mark is made to remove the excess skin from the external margin. The skin is strongly tractioned toward the midstream line and provides a good content–container ratio and the attainment of a new breast shape (Fig. 16.5).

The skin is gently tractioned laterally to avoid dislocation of the midstream line and carefully resected so as not to approximate the mammary eminences and the areolas too much (Fig. 16.5).

We always decorticate the margins of the wound at the level of the vertical suture, thus constructing a dermal pseudoligament that reinforces the suture, acting in the future as an obstacle to ptosis.

16.2.5 Suturing and Marking of the Areolas

Initially, suturing of the submammarian segment is carried out. On the vertical segment, suturing is carried out from the bottom upward, 4–5 cm from the margins. Above this point, a purse-string suture is performed.

16.2.6 Marking of the Areolas

1. The areola is marked with its inferior border 4.5–5 cm from the new submammarian sulcus, and its medial border at least 9 cm from the sternal line.
2. Decortications of the areas traced and implantation of the areolas (Fig. 16.6).

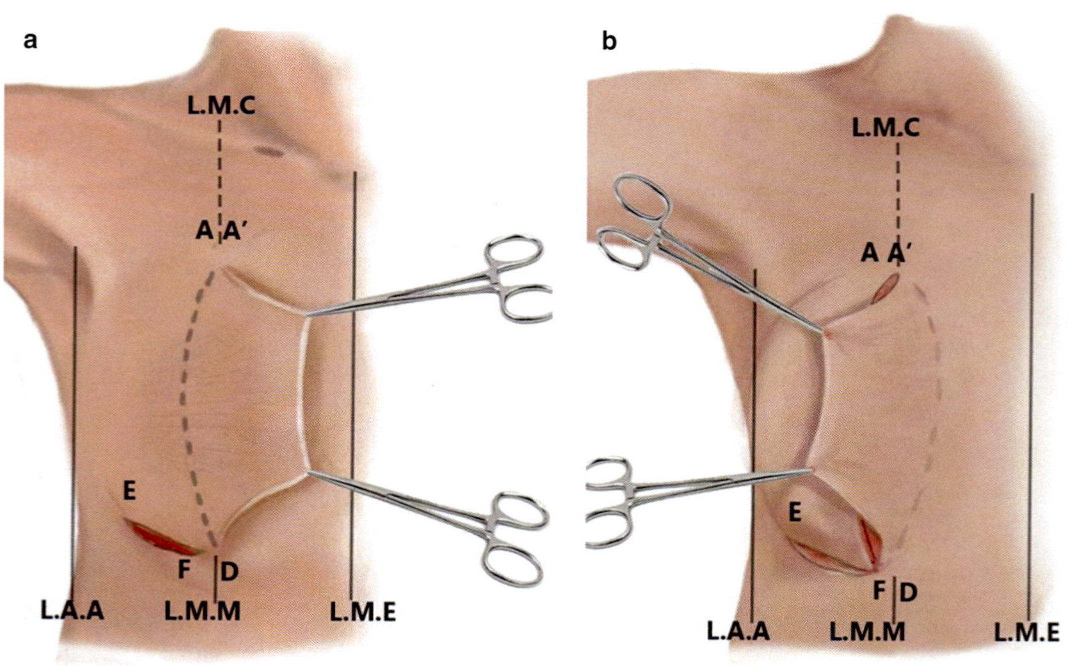

Fig. 16.5 (**a**) Resection of the excess skin from the external margin. (**b**) Resection of the excess skin from the internal margin

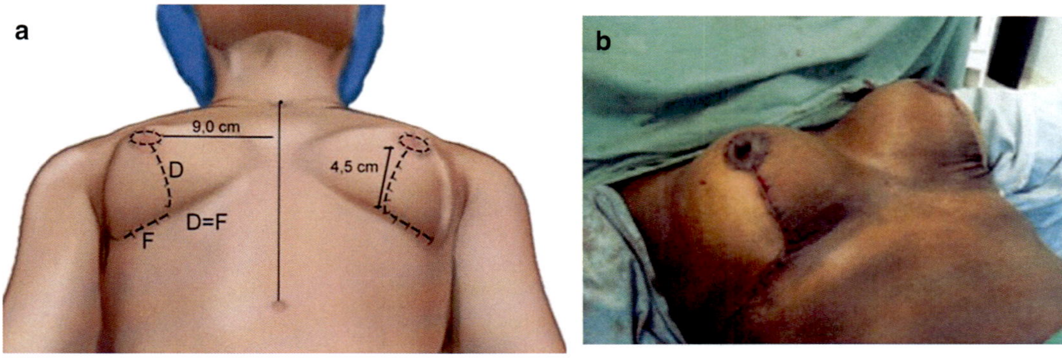

Fig. 16.6 (**a**) The areola is marked with its inferior border 4.5–5 cm, and its medial border at least 9 cm from the sternal line. (**b**) Finished look of the surgery

16.3 Discussion

The mastoplasty with an L-shaped scar, has the benefit of eliminating the medial segment of the horizontal scar. It has excellent indications in young patients with breasts with more glandular components and skin quality.

The techniques described by Bozola (1982), Chiari (1992) and Chaves et al. (1988), have similarities with regard to markings, and also in glandular resection and assembly of the breast.

A breast with a natural aspect is obtained, with the areola at the vertex of the cone, which elevates very little during the postoperative phase. Resection is done from underneath, according to each case, allowing the removal of more than 1 kg from each side. Adjustments are easily made. The approximated columns fill in the dead space. Resection of the second breast is carried out before shaping the first, to allow removal of breast tissue, identical in quantity and symmetrical in placement. The new breast will be maintained and supported by the skin "brassiere."

It is necessary for a correct relationship to exist between the content formed by the glandular adipose tissue and the container represented by the skin. Insufficient removal of the content leads to breakage of the resistance of the container and the formation of exaggerated bulging of the inferior pole, elevation of the areola above the normal position, and widening of the scar. The skin resection must be exact, with no exaggerated tension or flaccidity at the level of the vertical suture.

In general, patients are satisfied with the results when the technique is executed perfectly.

16.4 Result

We obtain a small scar in the shape of a comma, J, or inverted L. The vertical segment is 4–5 cm long in all cases. The horizontal segment never surpasses the anterior axillary line and is of variable length, depending on the case. In small and medium hypertrophies or ptoses, its average length is 2–5 cm. In large hypertrophies, it is longer, though without extending beyond the anterior axillary line.

During the immediate postoperative period, the breasts present with an elevated upper pole and flattening at the level of the vertical suture.

Next, they undergo accommodation and modification determined by scarring, by adjustment of the container to the content, and by the action of gravity. There will be lowering of the upper pole with inferior bulging and formation of the submammarian sulcus. The breasts then acquire a natural aspect with the areolas elevating slightly and occupying the vertex of the cone, and the submammarian scar is totally hidden in the sulcus (Figs. 16.7, 16.8, 16.9, and 16.10).

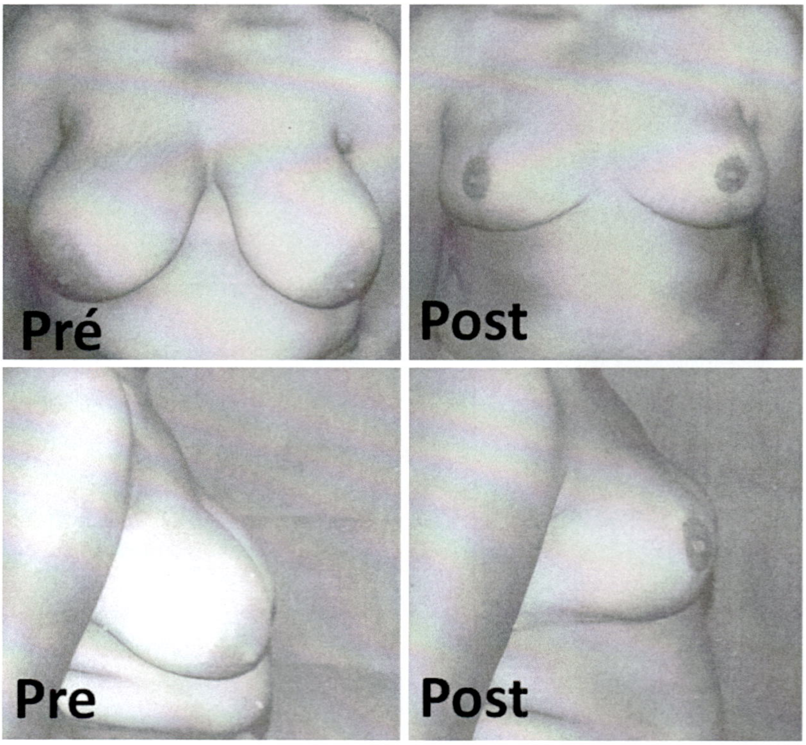

Fig. 16.7 Results of the patient operated on by Prof. Aleixo in 1980. Our tributes to the teacher

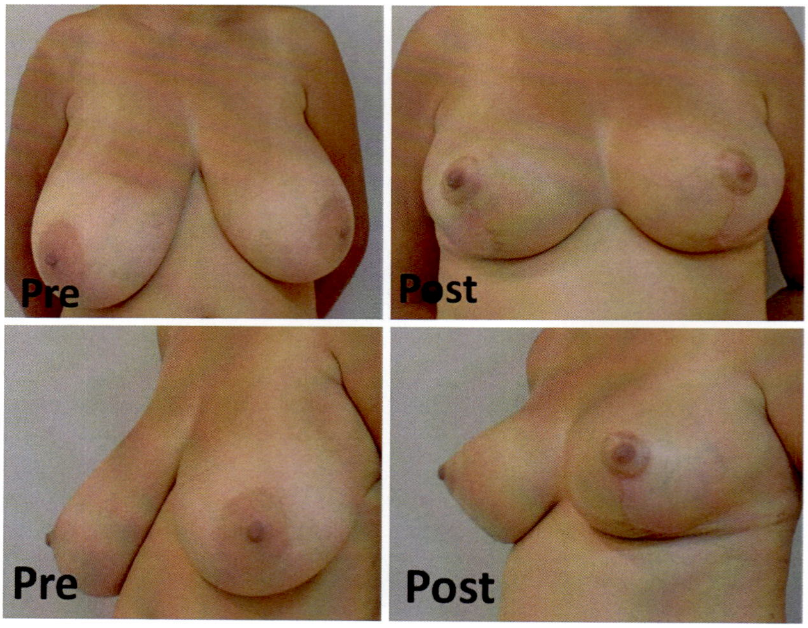

Fig. 16.8 Patient with grade III hypertropy by Berrocal Revueltas classifications. Breast reduction, by the described technique. Pre- and postoperative results of Dr. João Portocarrero, who kindly provided illustrations for this chapter. Our acknowledgments

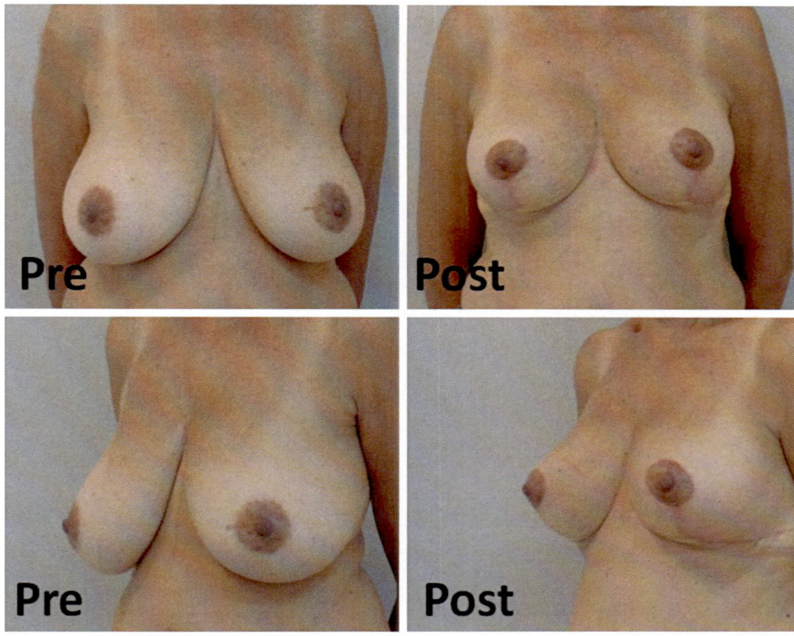

Fig. 16.9 Patient with grade III breast ptosis. Result after being submitted to the described technique. Our acknowledgments to Dr. João Portocarrero

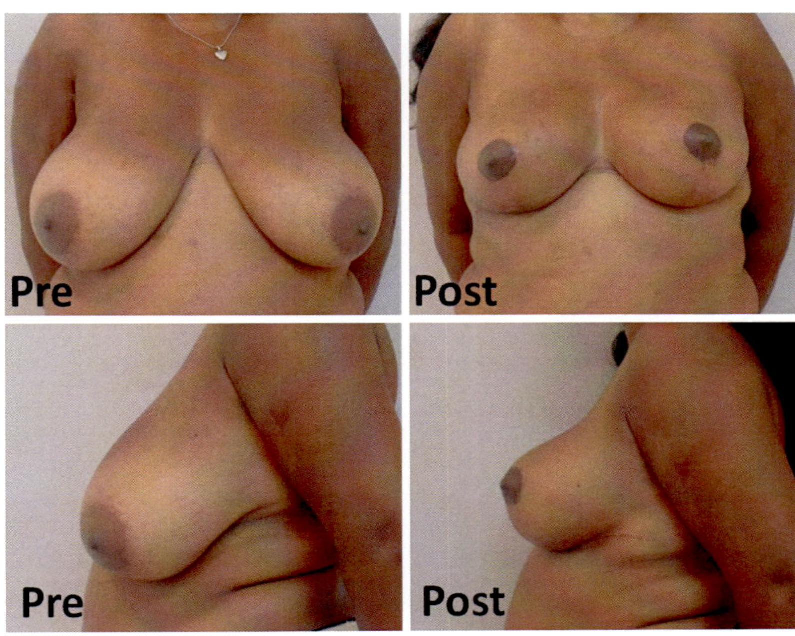

Fig. 16.10 Pre and postoperative of a patient with grade II hypertrophy and grade III Ptosis. Our acknowledgments to Dr. João Portocarrero

16.5 Complications

Complications are the same as those described for mammoplasty using other techniques, such as hematoma, dehiscence, seroma, areolar necrosis, and keloids.

Conclusion

The author carried out a critical study of the scars resulting from the most commonly used mammoplasties in the correction of breast hypertrophy and ptosis. He analyzed their location and shape, together with the advantages and disadvantages. He proposes a technique, which besides achieving a good breast shape, reduces the length of the scars. As small scar is left, in the shape of a comma, a J, or an inverted L.

Acknowledgements "The path of the righteous is like the light of dawn, which shines brighter and brighter until full day." ("Proverbs", 4:18).

Thus was Aleixo Sepúlveda, plastic surgeon, scientist and teacher, whose work expanded the horizons of Brazilian Plastic Surgery.

Those who, like me, have had the privilege of working alongside him, witnessing his knowledge and talent, received the special exemplary behavior of geniality, wisdom, humility, and generosity.

Dear Prof. Aleixo: wherever you are, receive our love, admiration, and our eternal gratitude.

Special thanks to his family, on behalf of his daughter, Candida Duarte Sepúlveda, who offered us unlimited access to the essential material for creation of this chapter.

Thanks to Dr. João Portocarrero Costa Sobrinho, who kindly provided the pre- and postoperative illustrative pictures.

References

Bozola AR (1982) Mamoplastia em L: contribuição pessoal. Rev AMRIGS 26(3):207–214

Chaves L, Ceceau MA, Magalhães HGA (1988) Mastoplastia em "L": um novo desenho. Rev Soc Bras Cir Plást 3(1):40–48

Chiari A Jr (1992) The L short-scar mammaplasty: a new approach. Plast Reconstr Surg 90(2):233–246

Dufourmentel CL, Mouly R (1961) Plastic mammaire par la méthode oblique. Ann Chir Plast 6:45–58

Elbaz JS, Verheeck G (1972) La cicatrice em L dans les plastie mammaires. Ann Chir Plast 17:283

Hollander E (1924) Die Operation der Mamma hypertrophie und der Hängebrust. Deutsch Med Wochenschr 50:1400

Pitanguy I (1967) Surgical treatment of breast hypertrophy. Br J Plast Surg 20(1):78–85

Sobrinho JBPC, Portocarrero ML, Portocarrero ML, Campos JHO (2012) Avaliação de técnica de mastoplastia redutora com cicatriz em "L" nas hipertrofias mamarias. Rev Bras Cir Plást 27(4):51–60

17 Costa Lima's Technique in Breast Hypertrophy

Humberto Campos and Ana Carolina Guimarães Rocha

17.1 Introduction

Gigantomastia, whether or not associated with ptosis and aesthetic discomfort, shows clinical symptoms directly related to the size and weight of the breasts. Pain in the neck and shoulders that often present as creases due to the straps of bras, premenstrual pain, trapezius muscle hypertrophy, dorsal kyphosis with compensatory lumbar lordosis, and trophic skin changes of the inframammary fold by maceration and venolinfáticas circulatory changes of the skin of the lower pole of the breast caused by ptosis.

Because of the difficulty in raising the nipple–areola complex (NAC) in major hypertrophy and gigantomastia, especially cases associated with severe ptosis, the wide base of the breasts, and the fibroglandular content, Costa Lima (1980, 1996) (Fig. 17.1) developed a technique applied in almost 4,000 cases of breast hypertrophy with retrotriangular resection in a solid triangular pyramid or tetrahedron, defining a flap of soft dermoglandular thinness containing the NAC (Cunha et al. 1996; Franco 2002). The technique further facilitates elevation of the NAC when used in cases of ptosis.

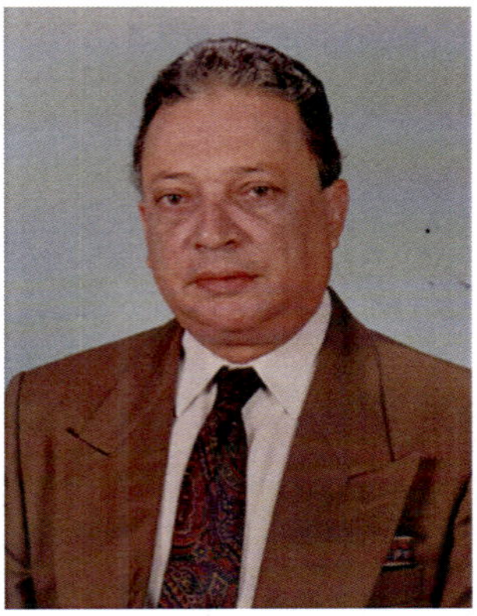

Fig. 17.1 Author photograph of the technical teacher Costa Lima

H. Campos, M.D. (✉)
Bahia School of Medicine and Public Health, Salvador, BA, Brazil

Brazilian Society of Plastic Surgery, São Paulo, SP, Brazil
e-mail: hc@humbertocampos.med.br

A.C.G. Rocha, M.D.
Brazilian Society of Plastic Surgery, São Paulo, SP, Brazil

17.2 Method

The marking of the skin used follows the standardization of Pitanguy (1963, 1981, 1994) (Fig. 17.2). The procedure with incisions begins with the markings and periareolar scarification (Ferreira et al. 1995; Gilles and McIndoe 1939; Hinderer 1994; Maliniac 1943; Schwarzmann 1930). First, resection of the median glandular portion is carried out using a transverse incision 1 cm below the lower edge of the NAC in a flat

J.M. Avelar (ed.), *Breast Surgery*, https://doi.org/10.1007/978-3-319-54115-0_17

section dividing the breast into two parts followed by an upward dissection of the breast up to the pectoral fascia, at the level of the second intercostal space, extending the dissection to the medial and lateral portions (Fig. 17.3).

Resection of the base of the breast leaves the glandular tissue in a shape of an equilateral triangle from a horizontal line parallel to the lower edge of the NAC with a dermal thickness of 0.5–1 cm and a variable length around 8 cm, depending on the width of the breast and the desire to narrow it (the higher the base of the triangle, the greater the narrowing of the base of the breast) Mark the figure of an equilateral triangle with the vertex at point A. Draw the figure of an equilateral triangle with the apex facing down (Fig. 17.4). From this triangle, the incisions are made using the scalpel to create a solid tetrahedron or triangular pyramid with its upper base (Fig. 17.5). Overcoming the lactiferous ducts, dissection is continued in a blunt manner, with a digital maneuver to Pitanguy's point A, with care so as to preserve a glandular bridge of 0.5–1 cm thick between the medial and lateral columns they formed. By removing this fragment, a space in the shape of a triangular pyramid or tetrahedron and two columns, medial and lateral, and symmetrical, are achieved (Fig. 17.6).

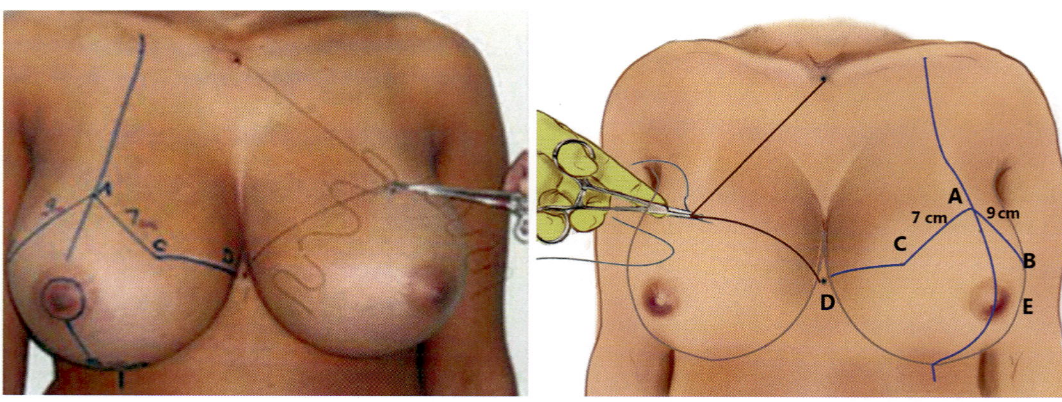

Fig. 17.2 Marking the points A, B, C, D, and E according to Prof. Pitanguy's technique

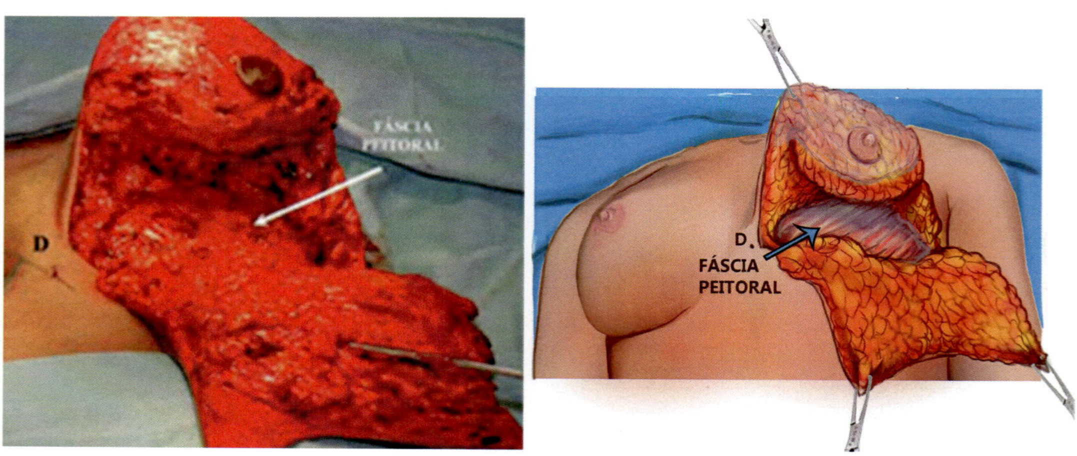

Fig. 17.3 Cross incision 1 cm below the lower edge of the nipple–areola complex (NAC) in the flat section and obliquely upward bipartindo the breast to the pectoral fascia, at the level of the second intercostal space

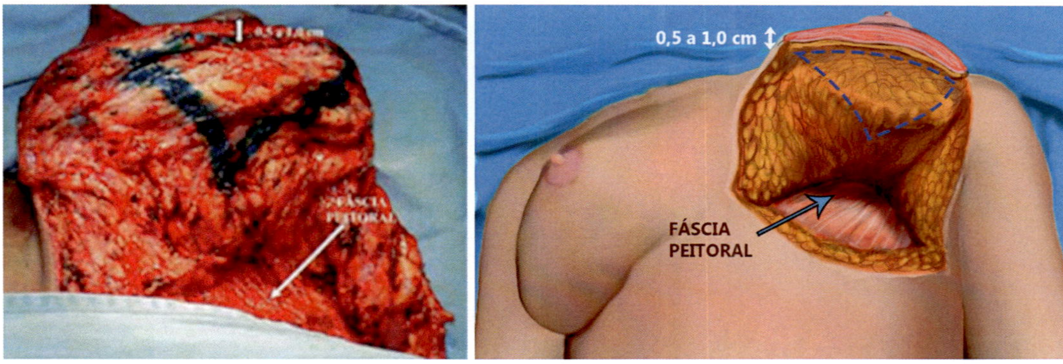

Fig. 17.4 Marking an equilateral triangle from a horizontal line parallel to the lower edge of the NAC with a dermal thickness of 0.5–1 cm and a variable size of about 8 cm, depending on the width of the breast and the desire for narrowing

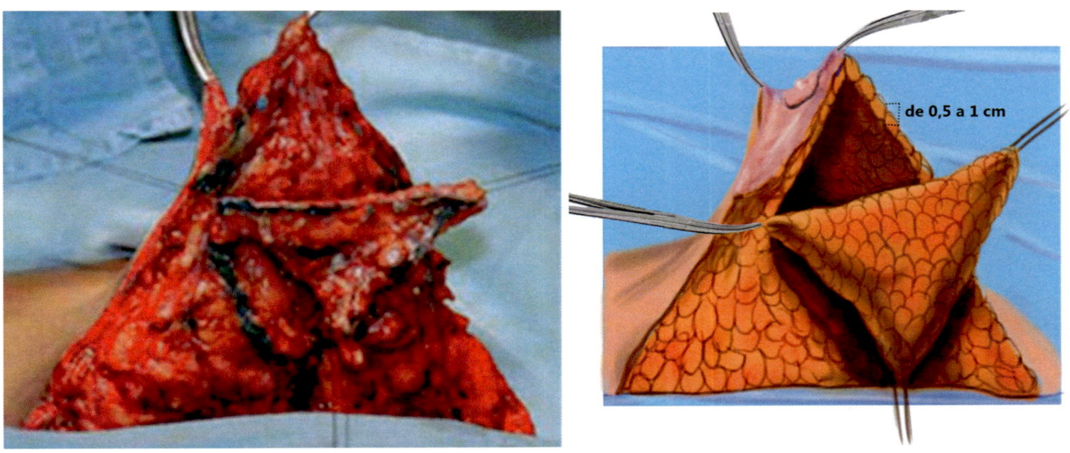

Fig. 17.5 Incision and resection of a solid tetrahedron or triangular pyramid with its upper base

The approach of these columns with simple points allows filling of the retro-areolar space and the rise of the NAC without tension or deformities (Fig. 17.7). Thus, the narrowing cone of the breast is achieved, modeling the breast in a natural way, which ensures a satisfactory NAC projection. Thus, the height of the breast was reduced by removing the base and its width was reduced by approximation of the medial and lateral columns. The NAC remains in the dermoglandular flap and can be migrated to the most convenient position without tension (Fig. 17.8) (Lima 1980, 1996).

In Fig. 17.9, we can see a sequence of technical execution of the movements performed by Prof. Costa Lima in the first presentation at scientific events.

The results of the correction of large mammary hypertrophy with severe ptosis, if using the technique of Prof. Costa Lima, are well observed on photographs of the preoperative and postoperative evolution after 6 months in Figs. 17.10, 17.11, 17.12, 17.13, 17.14, and 17.15.

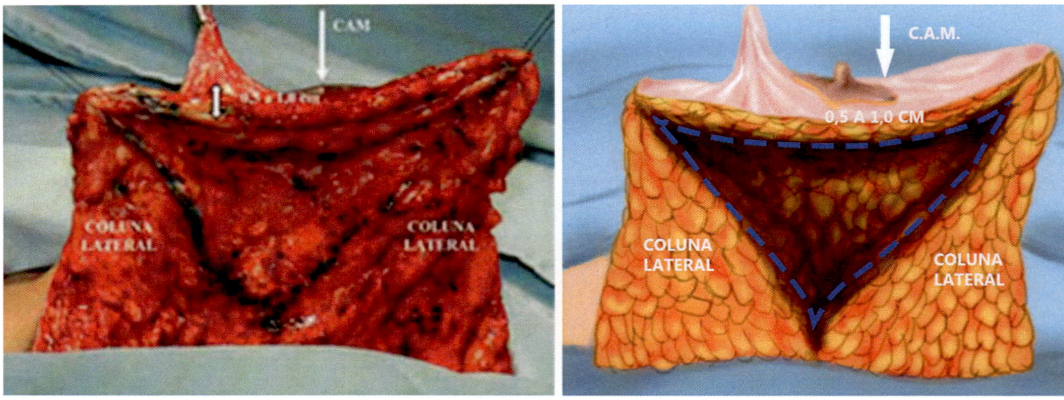

Fig. 17.6 Space in the form of a triangular pyramid or tetrahedron and two columns, medial and lateral, and symmetrical, resulting after removal of the fragment

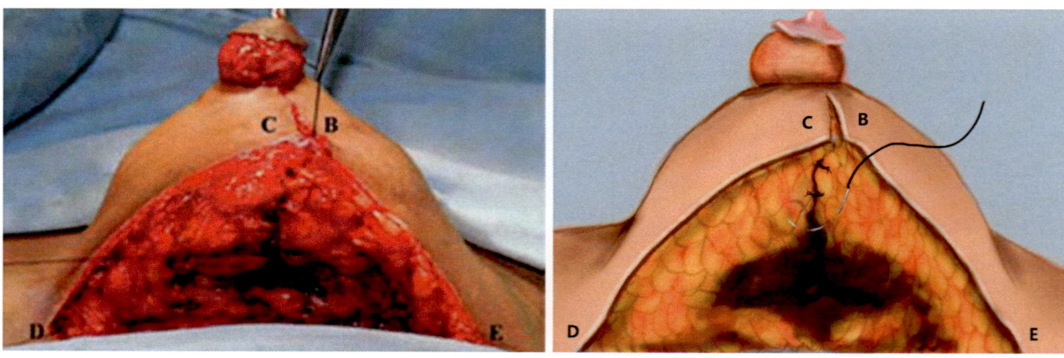

Fig. 17.7 Approximation of columns with simple points allows filling of the retro-areolar space and the rise of the NAC without tension or deformities

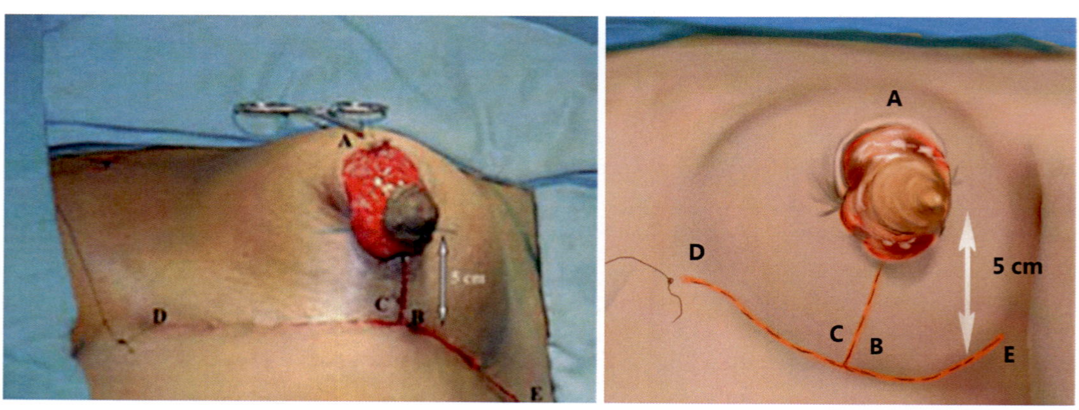

Fig. 17.8 The NAC remains in the dermoglandular flap and can be migrated to a more convenient position without any tension

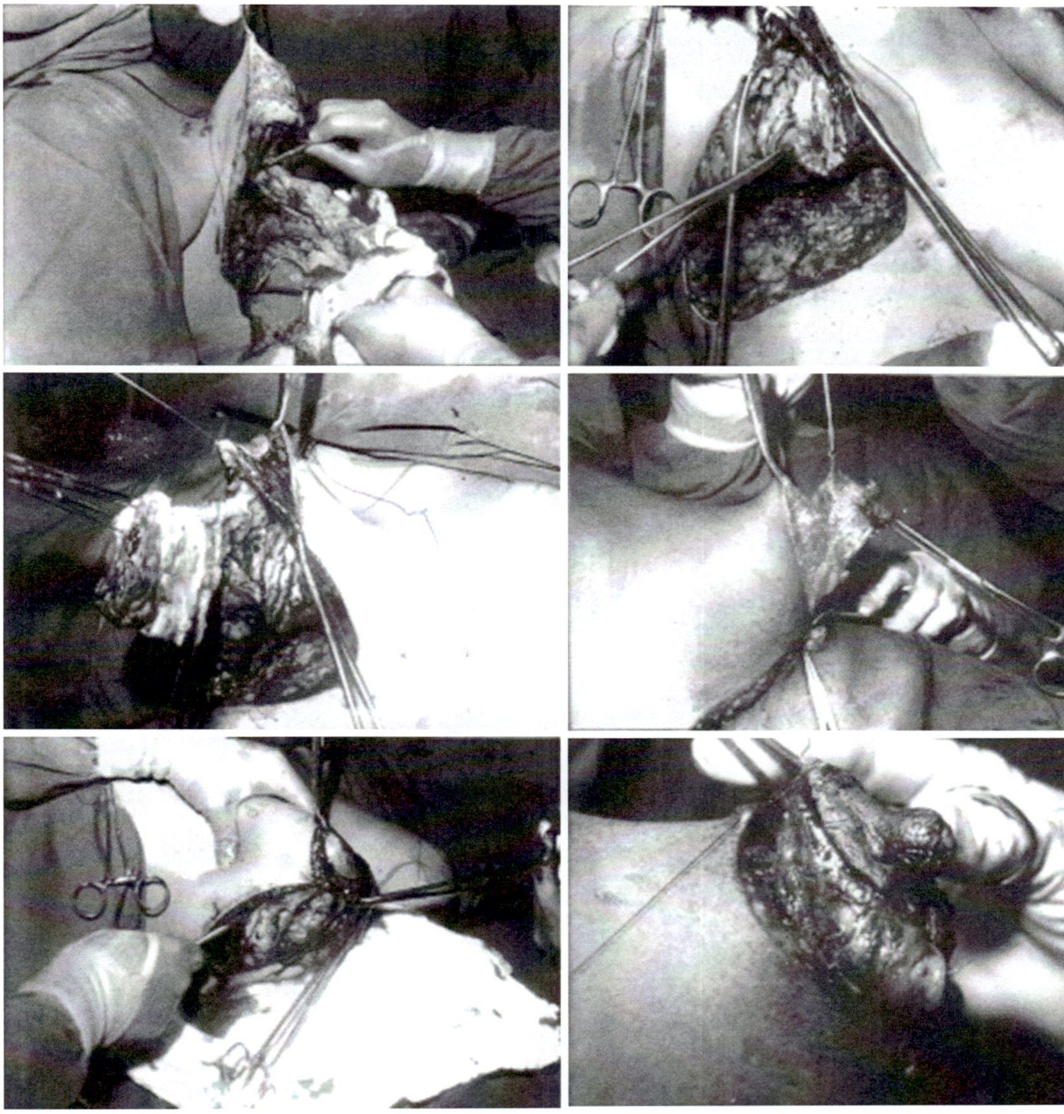

Fig. 17.9 Sequence surgery performed by the author of the technical teacher Costa Lima

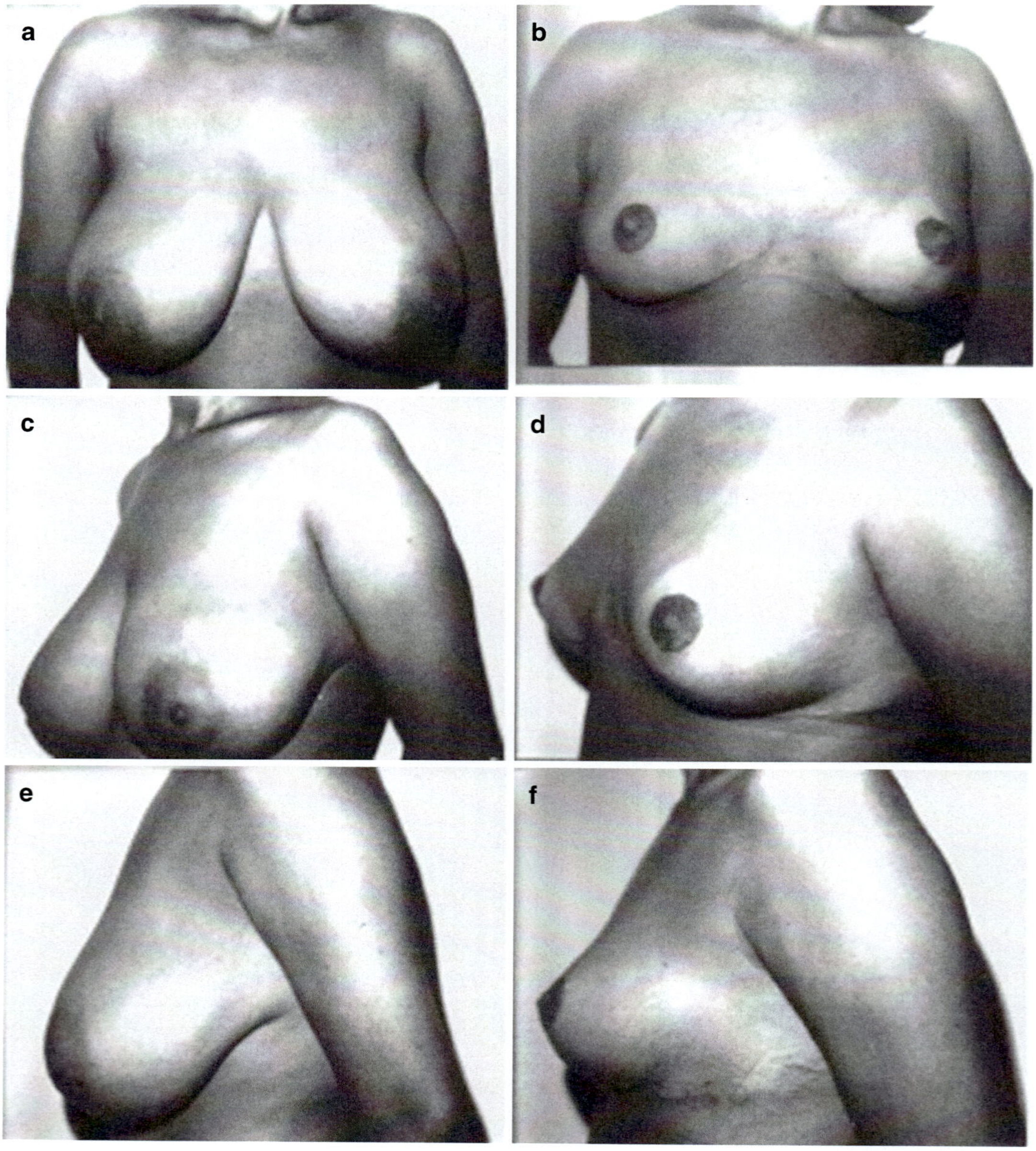

Fig. 17.10 Pre- and postoperative photos of the procedure performed by Prof. Costa Lima

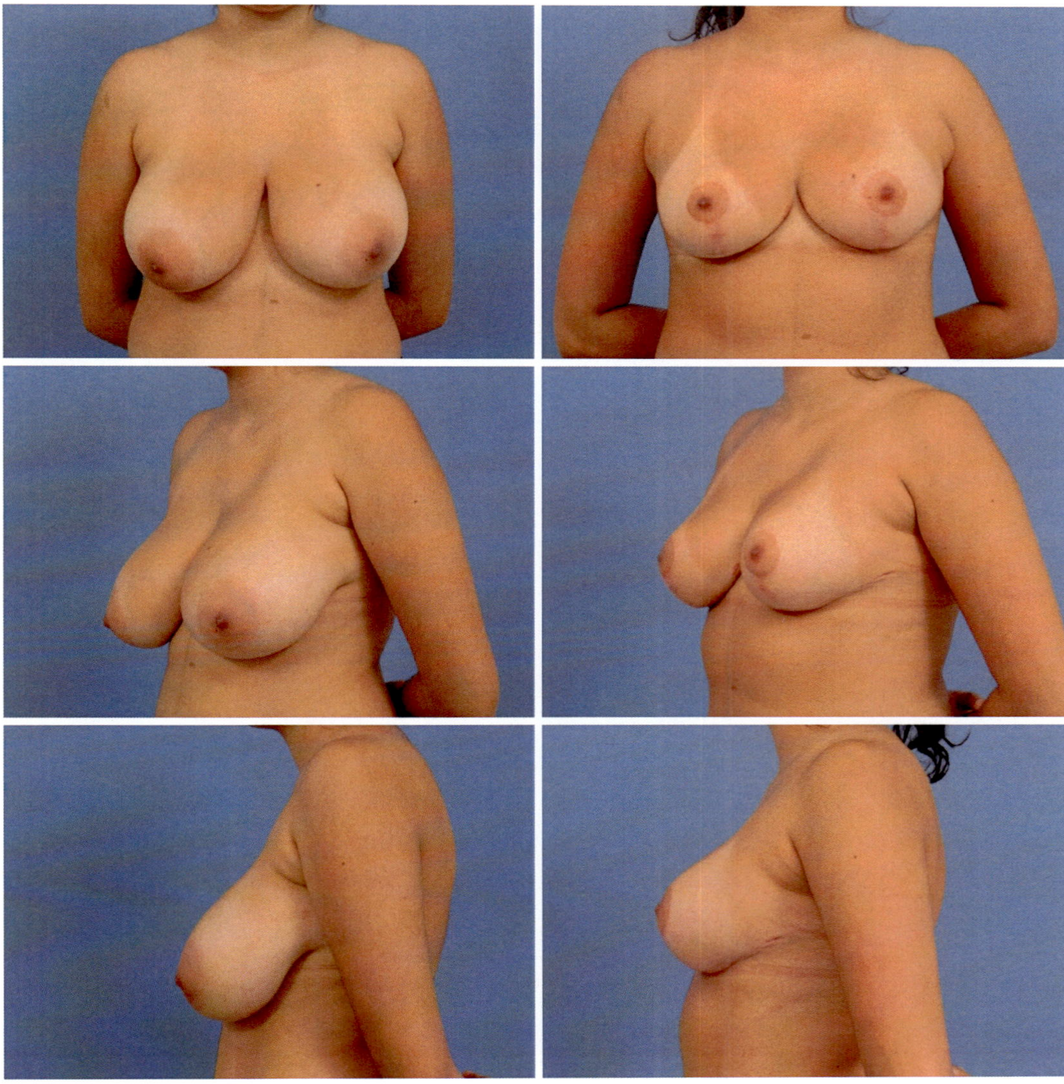

Fig. 17.11 Patient A. Pre and postoperative photos after 6 months

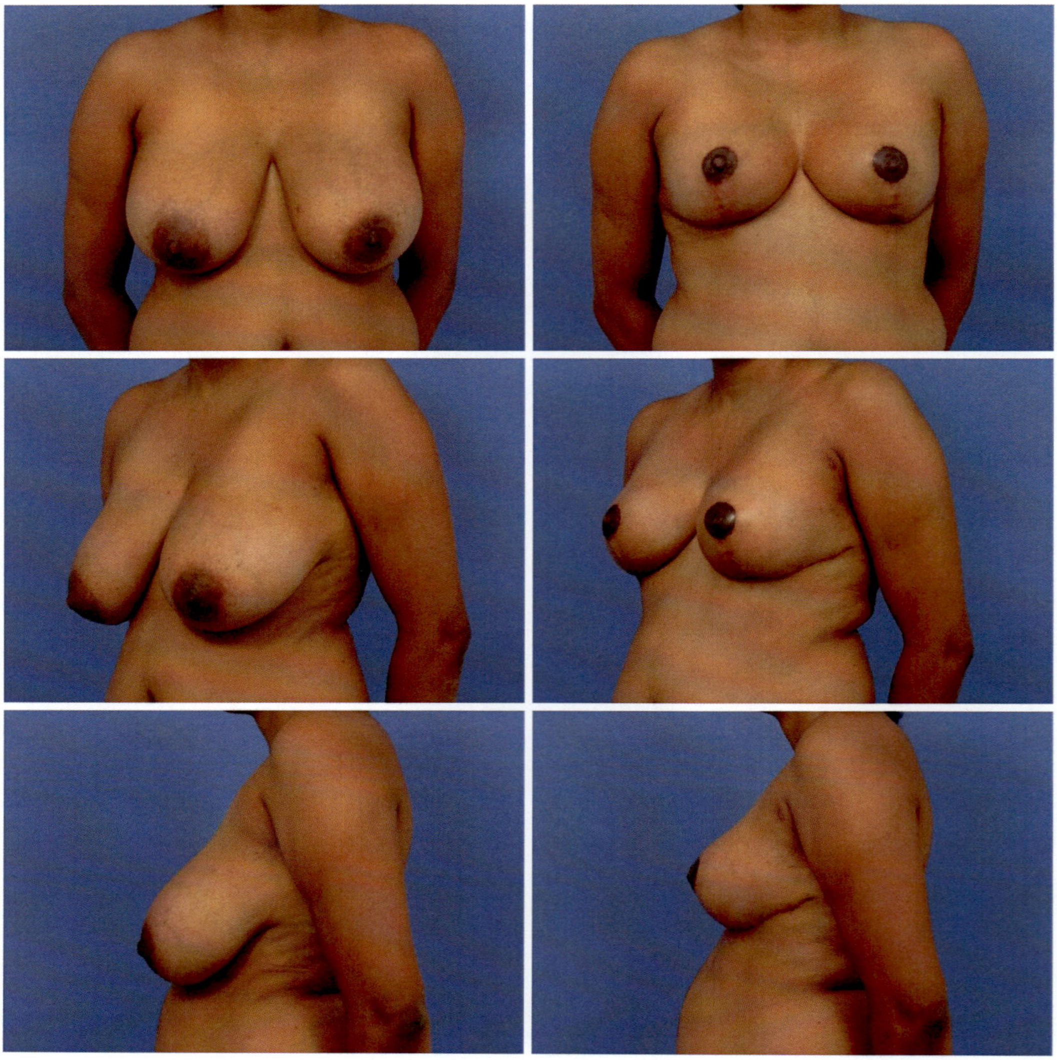

Fig. 17.12 Patient B. Pre and postoperative photos after 6 months

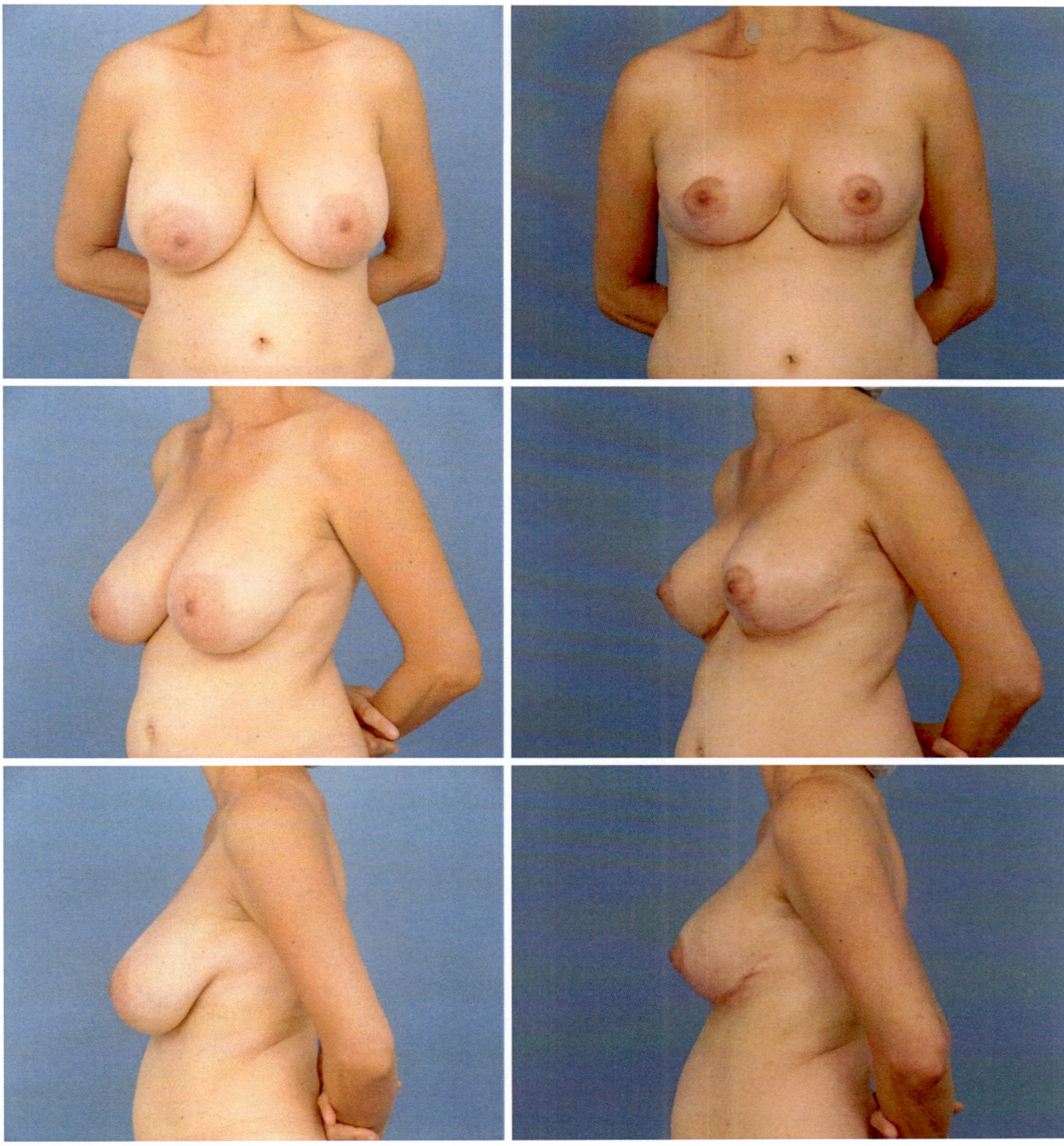

Fig. 17.13 Patient C. Pre and postoperative photos after 6 months

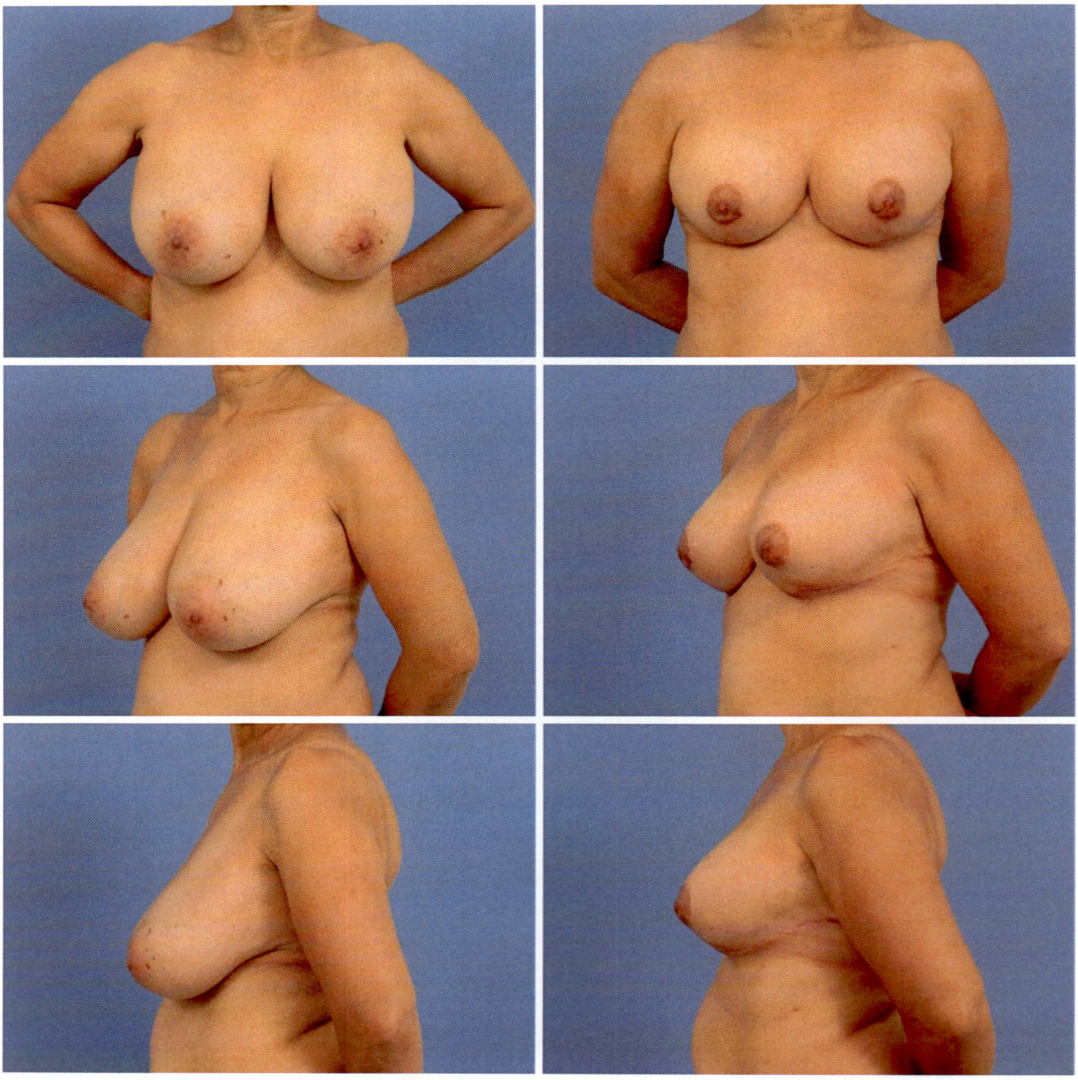

Fig. 17.14 Patient D. Pre and postoperative photos after 6 months

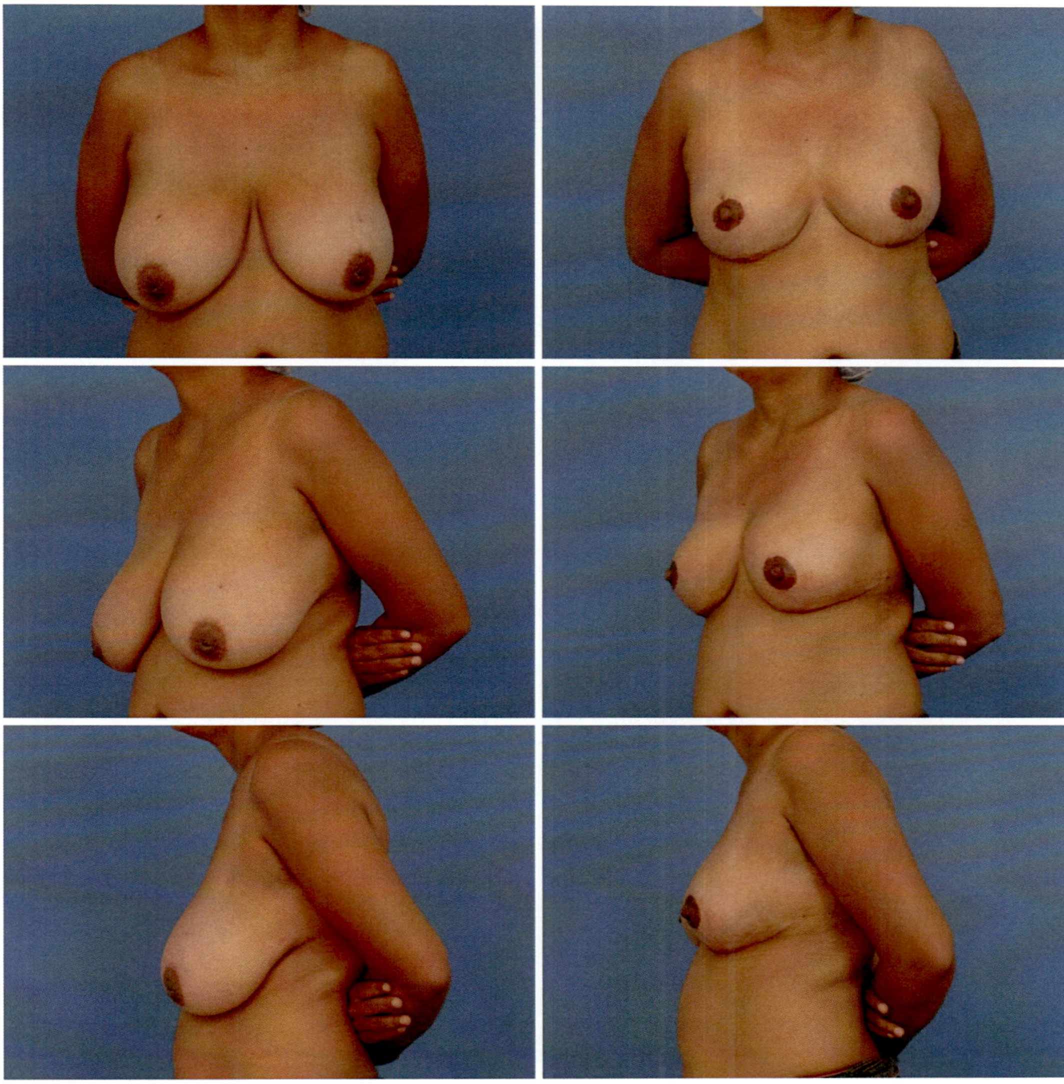

Fig. 17.15 Patient E. Pre and postoperative photos after 6 months

17.3 Discussion

Based on the studies of Salmon (1936), from 1973 Costa Lima (1980, 1996) devised this technique to perform large breast reductions while raising the NAC without difficulty: resection of the breast base, thus reducing its height, associated with decreased width by the withdrawal of medial and lateral breast prolongations and a tetrahedron- or triangular pyramid-shaped retroareola that is inversely proportional to the final width of the breast, resulting a thin and malleable vascular pedunculated flap.

The pedicle raises the NAC with vascularization guaranteed by a circular plexus width of 2–5 cm formed by branches of the internal mammary artery, from the inner upper lateral thoracic artery quadrant in the upper outer quadrant and intercostal branches (70–74%), or its variations: a plexus loop (20%) formed predominantly of the lateral thoracic artery or the radiated plexus (6%); i.e., when there are no anastomoses between the internal mammary arteries and lateral chest (Almeida 1991; Ferreira et al. 1995; Hinderer 1994; Pitanguy 1963; Schwarzmann 1930). In the latter case in particular, the risk of suffering of the NAC is increase (Rock et al. 2010). The creation of this flap requires a relatively short learning curve to make it as thin as possible, reducing vascular compression problems and allowing less risks of necrosis due to venous stasis.

The main suturing of the medial and lateral pillars forms an upper pole topping, occupies the space emptied by the outgoing segment of the tetrahedron or triangular pyramid and designs the NAC, which prevents retraction to deeper levels seen in 30% of cases by Strombeck (1960), a technique criticized by Ramirez (1994) as a point to be revised.

The Costa Lima technique does not require resection of the cylinder formed by upper areolar gland neither partial section of the pedicle, as it makes it safer from a vascular point of view, and does not provide any type of retraction to the NAC. However, with regard to scars, there are no differences between the two.

The Skoog (1963) technique is essentially the Strombeck procedure with a transected medial pedicle, forming a laterally based single pedicle carrying the NAC in an exclusively dermal flap to its ideal location by rotation. A delayed breast bascule movement is frequently reported in this surgery. Silveira Neto also describes a similar flap, but with a medial base carrying the NAC. However, in both techniques, the more twists determine the difficulty of the venous return also observed in Costa Lima's flap, where it is left thicker.

Several authors performed studies about NAC implementation by a dermoglandular flap inferior pedicle technique that is gaining more supporters owing to secure vascularization and retention of NAC sensitivity provided to maintain a thick flap and a broad base (Cunha et al. 1996). Sometimes this results in a larger breast, different from what is obtained with Costa Lima's flap.

This technique, despite the need for a slightly steeper learning curve, gives the surgeon a safe option for NAC implementation in a large ptosis, thereby facilitating their work and achieving placement of the NAC in an ideal position without major complications, leading to a good-quality final scar.

17.4 Complications

According to the technical author's experience of nearly 4,000 surgical cases, it is recommended to pay special attention to the fat hypermastia and the associated large ptosis, due to both the thickness of the dermoglandular flap for variations in the distribution of the vascular plexus that can lead to impaired vascularization of the NAC. Costa Lima also signaled that as thinner is the flap maintaining the NAC, it will occur less vascular complications due to an equilibrium between adequate venous return and also less vascular compression, recalling the importance of maintaining the integrity of pedicle flap vascularization (Lima 1980, 1996).

When this technique was first performed, there were some cases of partial and total necrosis of the NAC, always venous stasis, but with care taken with regard to decreased compression, only a few cases of epitheliosis were observed. Complications related to the general procedure were coincident with each other vigentes (Rock et al. 2010) techniques.

Rocha et al. (2010) used this technique in 118 patients, and showed four cases of necrosis of the inferior pole of the NAC (3.39%), not coincident with smoking, but the reports were related to obesity, which hindered the making of a pedicle thin enough. These complications arose during the first procedures performed, starting with congestion and cyanosis that gradually improved to result in a loss of 25–30% of the semicircular lower areolar border in a month, and after the second intention healing, the final deformity was not as serious as it initially appeared, and was treated by a wedge resection and suturing.

Rocha et al. (2010) also referred to three cases (2.61%) of hematoma in this work, one spontaneous and the other two occurred in the group of patients with medications for prevention of deep vein thrombosis/thromboembolic prophylaxis (Marchi et al. 2005) from the first day after surgery. They were resolved by draining after opening one or two stitches.

There were two (1.69%) cases of dehiscence of partial suture epitheliosis and skin necrosis owing to sharp tension in the suture line, excessive skin removal, one of which was related to the prophylactic use of radiation therapy for keloids. There were also two cases of lipolysis (1.69%), which, although unilateral, did not lead to asymmetry that was evident in the late postoperative period. The volume of operated breasts did not allow small scars to be achieved, the goal of many authors and, in some cases, even with the help of liposuction, they went beyond the anterior axillary line (Rock et al. 2010).

Conclusions

This technique is effective in the migration of the NAC, especially in breast hypertrophy with severe ptosis (Lima 1980, 1996).

References

Almeida RA (1991) Short scars reduction mammaplasty. Plast Reconst Surg 88(6):1112

Cunha FI, Carpaneda CA, Pepper C, Massid R, Matos W, Gama LHP (1996) Mastoplasties: use of later breast flap. In: Tournieux AAB, Curi M (eds) Update on plastic-surgery SBCP. Rone Editorial, Sao Paulo, pp 325–330

Ferreira LM, Castilho HT, Duarte IS, Andrees JM (1995) Aesthetic surgery. In: Ferreira LM (ed) Plastic surgery guide. Atheneu, Sao Paulo, pp 287–291

Franco T (2002) Aesthetic surgery of the breast. In: Franco T, Franco D, Gonçalves LFF (eds) Principles of plastic surgery. Atheneu, Sao Paulo, pp 671–697

Gilles H, McIndoe A (1939) The technique of mammaplasty in conditions of hypertrophy of the breast. Surg Gynec Obst 68:658–665

Hinderer UT (1994) Reducción of mammary plasty. Basic principles. Tecnicas personales. In: Coiffmann F (ed) Cirurgia Plastica, Estetica y Reconstrructiva, 2nd edn. Massom-Salvat, Barcelona, pp 3350–3385

Lima JC (1980) Breast reduction: new method and refinements. In: Ely JF (ed) Transactions of the VII Cong IPRS-1979. Cartgraf, Rio de Janeiro, pp 518–521

Lima JC (1996) Large breast reductions: personal technique. In: Tournieux AAB, Curi M. editores Atualização in plastic surgery-SBCP. Sao Paulo: Robe Editorial;.p. 301–309.

Maliniac J (1943) Arterial blood suply of the breast. Arch Surg 7:329

Marchi C, Schlup IB, Lima CA, Schlup HA (2005) Prophylaxis assessment of deep vein thrombosis in a General Hospital. J Vasc Bras:171–175

Pitanguy I (1963) Breast hypertrophy: contribution to its treatment. Rev Lat Am Cir Plast 7(3):142–164

Pitanguy I (1981) Breast reduction mammoplasty: surgical technique. In: Pitanguy I (ed) Aesthetic plastic surgery of head and body. Springer, Berlin, pp 9–11

Pitanguy I (1994) Tratamiento de las anomalies her mammary gland: technical personales. In: Coiffmann F (ed) Plastic surgery Reconstructiva y Estetica, 2nd edn. Masson-Salvat, Barcelona, pp 3327–3343

Ramirez MA (1994) Mammoplasty reductora by bipedicled vertical colgajo. In: Coiffmann F (ed) Surgery plastic, reconstructive aesthetic y, 2nd edn. Masson-Salvat, Barcelona, pp 3396–3399

Rock ACG, Costa CS, Campos H (2010) Costa Lima technique in breast hypertrophy associated with lower retail vascular pedicle. Rev Bras Cir Plast 25(1)

Salmon M (1936) Les artères de la peau, vol 29. Masson, Paris, p 137

Schwarzmann E (1930) Die Technik der Mammaplastik. Chirurg 2:932–943

Skoog RT (1963) Tecnhique for breast reduction: transposition of the nipple on the cutaneous vascular pedicle. Acta Chir Scand 26:453–465

Strombeck OJ (1960) Mammoplasty: report of a new technique based on two pedicles procedure. Br J Plast Surg 13:79–90

18 Peixoto's Technique for Reduction Mastoplasty

Marcus Vinicius Alfano Moscozo
and Rafael Andrade Alves

18.1 Introduction

Dr. Gerardo do Rego Peixoto (Fig. 18.1) was born in Carape-Redenção, in the state of Ceará, but it was in Salvador/Bahia that he obtained his medical degree from the prestigious Faculdade de Medicina da Bahia in 1956. For a few years, he practiced medicine as an acknowledged general surgeon, but was soon seduced by the new and puissant medical specialty that was flourishing, mainly because of Prof. Ivo Pitanguy in Rio de Janeiro. Therefore, he went to Rio to become specialized under Prof. Pitanguy in the mid-1960s and returned to Salvador in 1968, when his winning trajectory as a plastic surgeon began.

His concerns about the results and complications of reduction mastoplasty techniques existing at the time, especially regarding the extent of the final scars and the vascular compromise of the skin and nipple–areolar complex, in addition to the difficulty of applying one technique out of the variety that were available for all types and mammary volumes (Peixoto 1979) induced him to propose a new procedure for the treatment of mammary hypertrophies and ptosis. He presented his ideas for the first time at the Sixth International Congress of Plastic and Reconstructive Surgery in 1975 (Paris) and published them in the main international scientific journals in the specialty (Peixoto 1980, 1984).

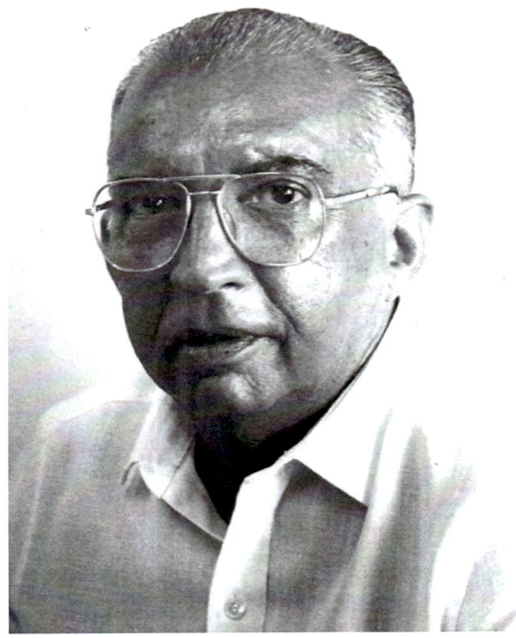

Fig. 18.1 Dr. Gerardo Peixoto. (Copyright - Collection of the Peixoto's family)

I worked with Dr. Peixoto for more than 11 years until his death, and was able to

M.V.A. Moscozo, M.D. (✉)
Brazilian Society of Plastic Surgery, Hospital São Rafael, Salvador, BA, Brazil

Ibero-Latin American Society of Plastic Surgery, Punta del Este, Uruguay
e-mail: moscozo@uol.com.br

R.A. Alves, M.D.
Brazilian Society of Plastic Surgery, Hospital São Rafael, Salvador, BA, Brazil

J.M. Avelar (ed.), *Breast Surgery*, https://doi.org/10.1007/978-3-319-54115-0_18

experience the evolution of his concept and ascertain the great versatility and applicability of his technique for reduction mastoplasty. I now present his procedure, being faithful to his own description, but also adding my interpretation.

18.2 Principles and Substantiation of the Technique

The main propositions of the new procedure were:

1. Reduction of the extent of the final scar, if possible eliminating the horizontal segment. For that reason, he proposed four designs that were applied to each breast specifically depending on the volume, skin quality, and content that were previously evaluated as the following (Fig. 18.2):

(a) Vertical incision without skin removal for cases in which the skin has good elasticity and only requires reduction of the breast content (predominantly glandular tissue, without ptosis) (Fig. 18.3a);

(b) Vertical incision with skin removal, indicated for breasts with grade I ptosis, but still with good skin elasticity, few or no stretch marks (striae distensae) and small resection of glandular tissue (Fig. 18.3b);

(c) Vertical and periareolar incisions—in 90% of indications (Peixoto and Goldwyn 1990), it is advised for patients with ptosis of grade II

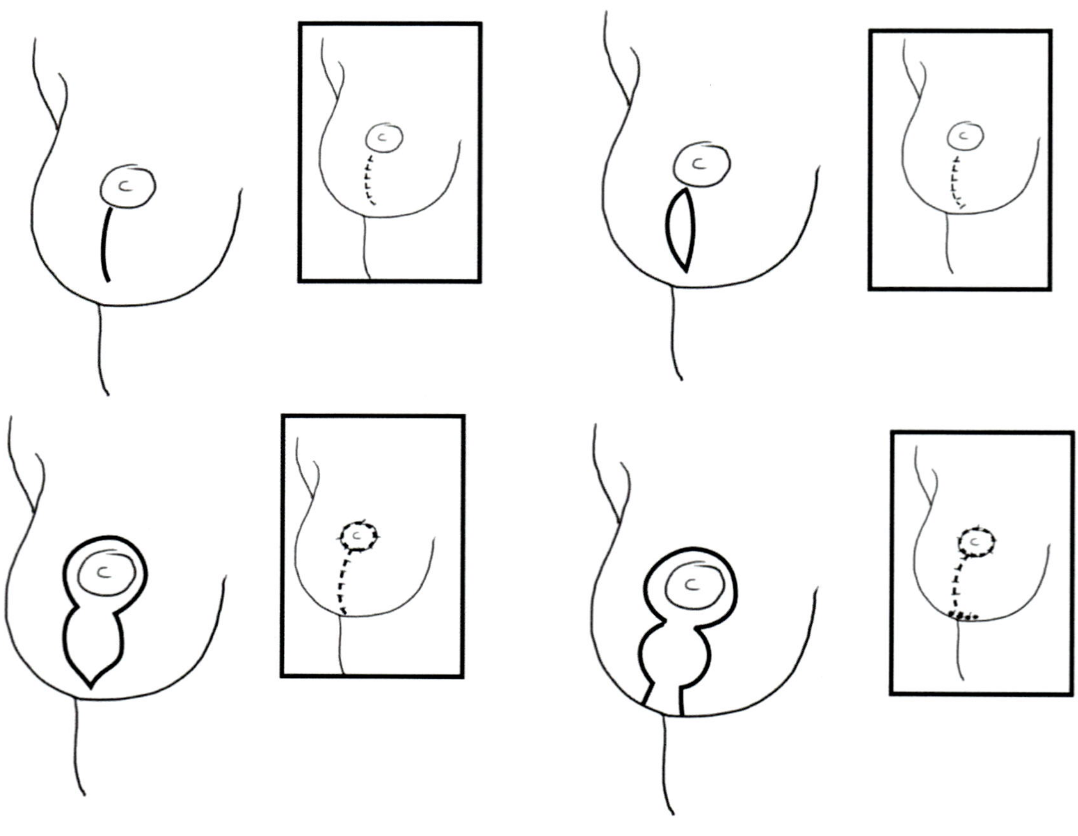

Fig. 18.2 Four designs and corresponding scars

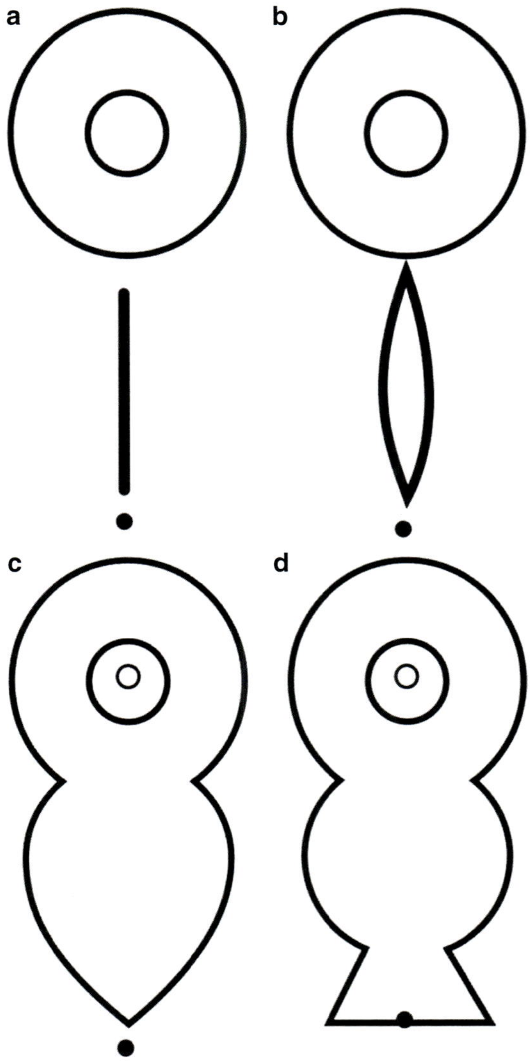

Fig. 18.3 Incisions. (**a**) Only a vertical incision in a breast without ptosis. (**b**) Vertical incision with skin removal. (**c**) Vertical and periareolar incisions used in small to large hypertrophy. 90% of indications. (**d**) Vertical, periareolar, and small horizontal incisions, indicated for giant hypertrophy

or higher to increase the volume from small to large when the distance from the lower edge of the areola to the inframammary fold is between 7 and 10 cm (Fig. 18.3c);

(d) Vertical, periareolar, and small horizontal incisions, indicated for giant hypertrophy (Fig. 18.3d).

2. The breast is completely freed from the muscular aponeurosis system underneath and the preservation of vascular pedicles from internal mammary, subclavian, and lateral thoracic arteries.
3. Excision of excess mammary tissue, which varies depending on previous evaluation of skin quality and breast content (mainly glandular tissue) aiming for container/content balance (Fig. 18.4).
4. Resection of the base and lower pole of the mammary cone, with the intention of reconstructing or building a smaller cone, leaving 5–7 cm from its original height (Fig. 18.5).
5. To trust the skin's ability to retract.

These prepositions were substantiated by anatomical and physiological knowledge, especially in studies by Salmon and Maliniac (Maliniac 1943; Salmon 1939) on mammary vascular anatomy and physiological skin qualities: elasticity and contractility.

As the mammary gland is derived from the differentiation and specialization of sweat glands and its blood supply is distributed by a subcutaneous net coming from the above-mentioned vascular pedicles, it is possible to dissociate it from the deep layer over the aponeurosis of the pectoralis major without compromising its nutrition and preserving its function.

Nowadays, the skin's ability to retract is considered a fact and we count on it for liposuction, rhinoplasties, and other procedures, but when it comes to this technique it is not considered to be an easily manageable variable, as it directly depends on the skin's elasticity, the presence of stretch marks or fibrotic scars, and also on the balance of the resection and glandular/fatty tissue proportions, which are influenced by the surgeon's experience.

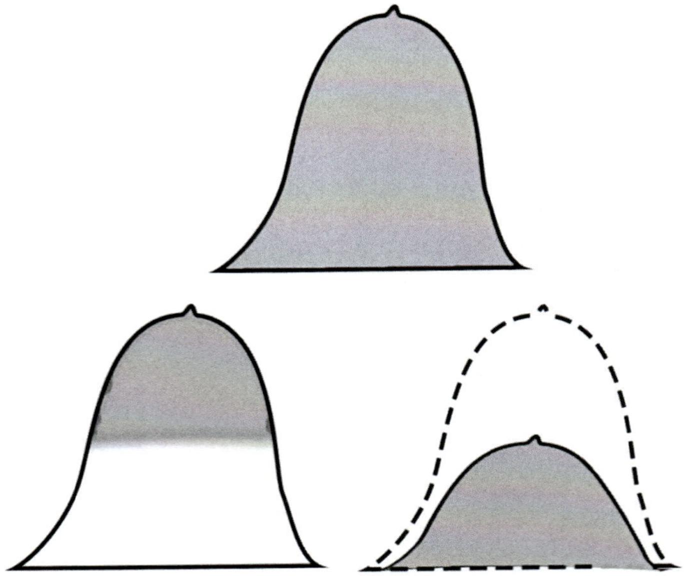

Fig. 18.4 Excision of excess tissue. It shows the breast after skin retraction and adjustment on the thorax

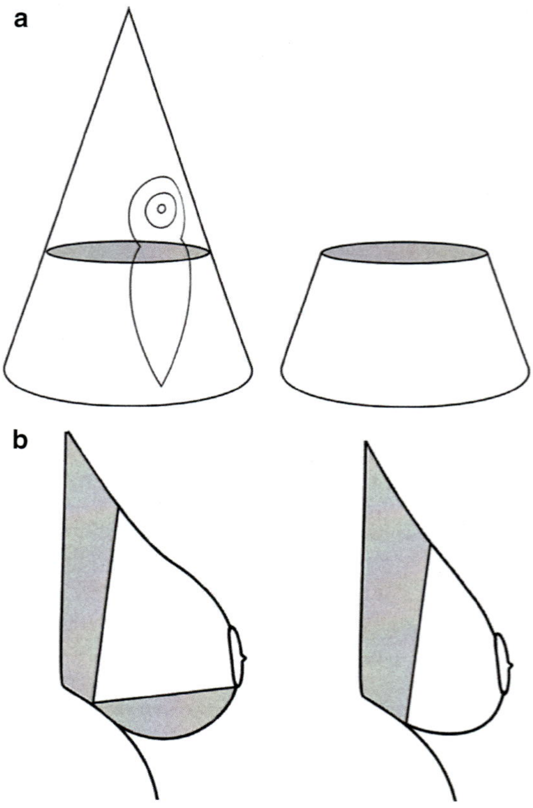

Fig. 18.5 (**a**) Resection of the base of the mammary cone, retaining its original form. (**b**) Resection of the cone's base and lower pole in the turgid and glandular breast or only the base, used in all cases

18.3 Description of the Technique

1. Anesthesia and body positioning: the technique should be the one best known by the team with the patient in the supine position with a 30° inclination of the thorax and abducted arms.
2. Marking: after skin quality and glandular content evaluation, the design can be chosen, among the four proposed, according to the criteria detailed on item 18.2.1. We describe design (Fig. 18.3c) because it is the most commonly used.

It begins with the marking of point A via a bidigital maneuver, clamping the excess skin at the upper pole toward the mid-clavicular line and point E (marking 1 cm distance from inframammary fold B to avoid the scarring extending beyond that), subtracting 1–2 cm depending on the skin's flaccidity; the more flaccid the skin, the smaller the amount subtracted to determine point "b" (this subtraction represents the amount of skin between the fingers during the bidigital maneuver). The distance between the base of the nipple (point C) and point B determines a radius that is transferred with a compass circularly around the nipple–areola complex (NAC), up to half of it (Fig. 18.6).

Then, the bidigital maneuver is performed again immediately below the NAC in the lower pole and

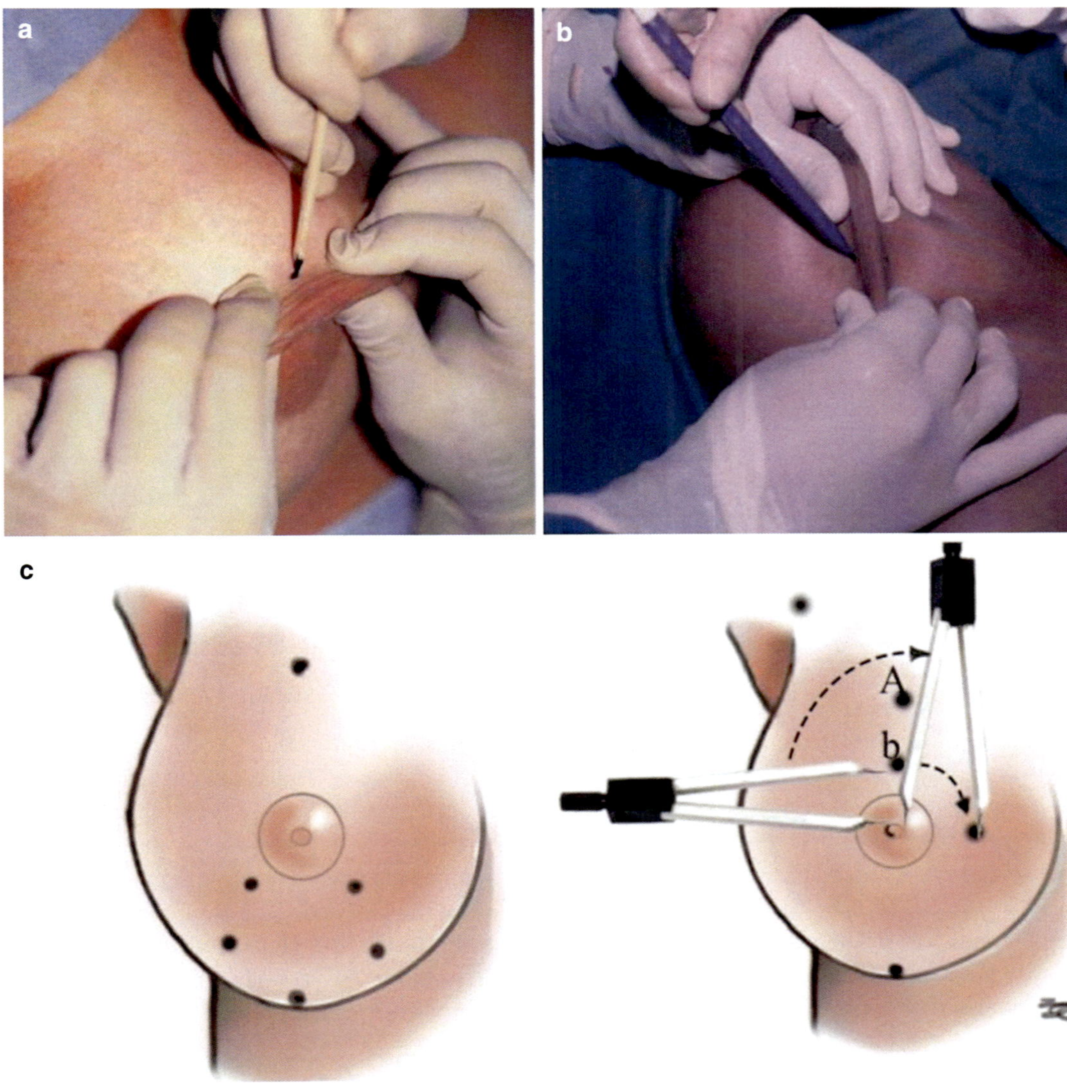

Fig. 18.6 Marking. Bi-digital maneuvers clamping the skin excess in superior (**a**) and inferior (**b**) pole. (**c**) Distance between the nipple's base and point "b" is transferred with a compass circularly around the nipple–areola complex

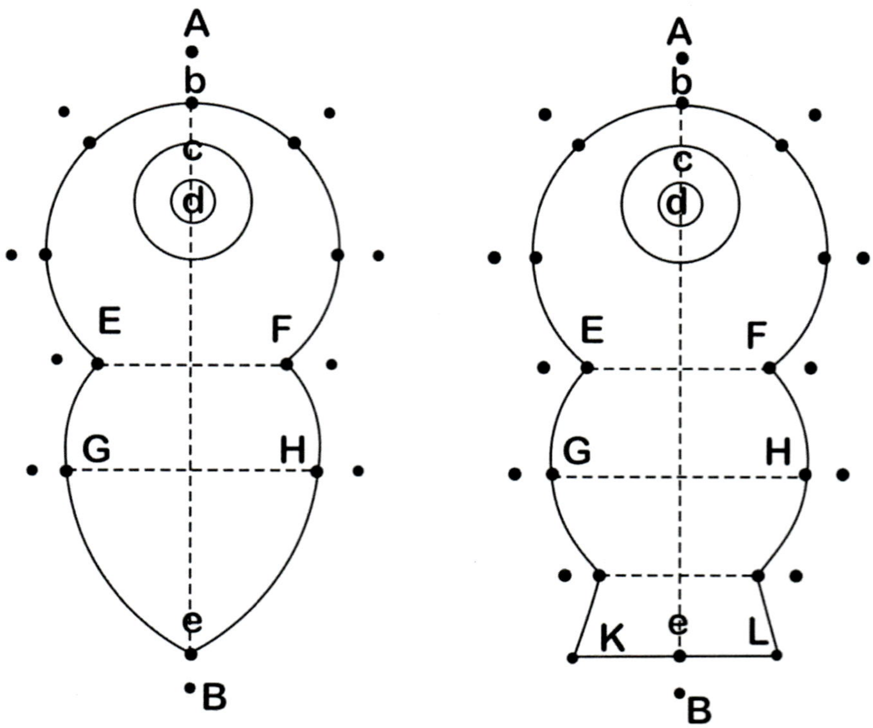

Fig. 18.7 Final markings

with the same subtraction (1–2 cm) the following points are marked: E, F, G, and H. The periareolar circle is completed by connecting the previously determined points to E and F and then to H and G. Lastly, all marked lines meet at point E (Fig. 18.7).

1. Initial maneuvers: Schwarzmann's maneuver is applied to a delimited periareolar area, except for designs (Figs. 18.3a, b and 18.8). The lower pole is incised within the outline until the deep layer is reached (the fascia between the dermoglandular tissue and the aponeurosis of the pectoralis major and serratus anterior muscles), and the whole breast is dissected over this layer to free the base of the mammary cone.
2. Resections are carried out according to specific requirements in each case, varying from no resection to a large resection. Most commonly, we start with a lower pole resection, then a mammary cone base on a linear ascending oblique line and approximately 30° inclination to force a bascule to the chest (Fig. 18.9) and a lateral descending oblique line corresponding to the chest curvature. The amount of tissue removed from the base depends on the initial volume and is determined by the mammary cone height that will remain, approximately 5–7 cm (Fig. 18.10).
3. Assembly is carried out by approximating the pillars with the help of a hemostat, using absorbable or non-absorbable sutures, as many stitches as necessary (Fig. 18.11).

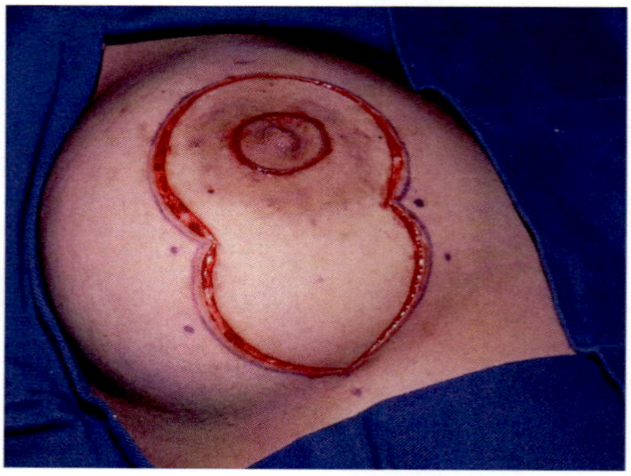

Fig. 18.8 Incision and Schwarzmann's maneuver

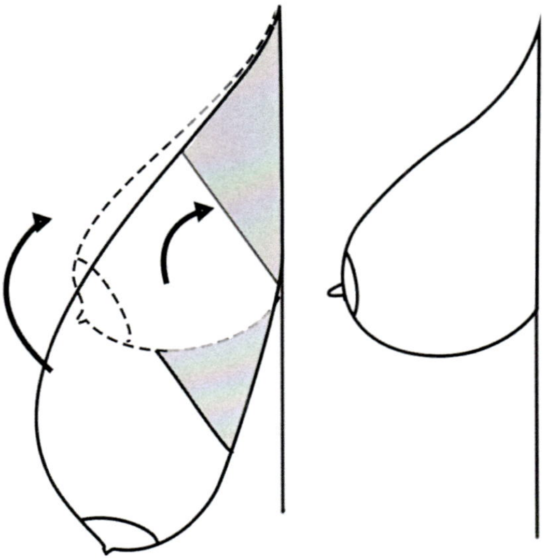

Fig. 18.9 Repositioning and bascule of the breast on the thorax after cone base resection

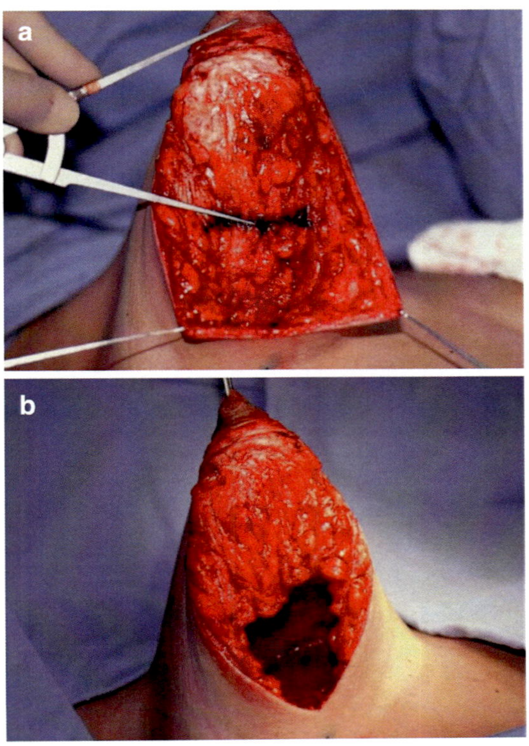

Fig. 18.10 (**a**) Marking and (**b**) resection of the base of the cone, leaving 5–7 cm of the height

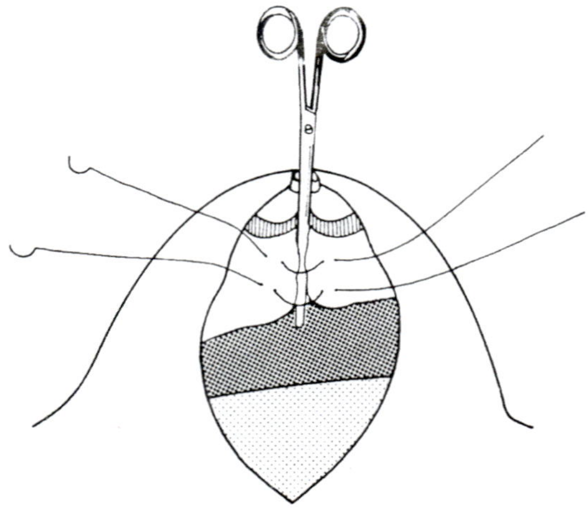

Fig. 18.11 Approximation of the pillars with the help of a hemostat

4. Closure: after rigorous homeostasis review, a two- or three-layered closure is initiated, approximating the lower layer with a non-absorbable suture. Usually, there is no tension over the suture line.
5. Drainage and bandaging: aspiration drainage by counter-opening is routinely performed. A simple bandage with gauze is then placed over the wound and a triangular-shaped external mounting is applied using adhesive tape that can be changed whenever necessary and retained for 30 days or more, as it is auxiliary to the skin's retraction process.

18.4 Complications and Unsatisfactory Results

Vascular complications such as areolar or flap necrosis are almost non-existent owing to careful observation of the vascular anatomy in this technique. In giant breasts, because of chronic vascular stretching, epidermolysis is more common, but still rare. Also, in those cases, the need for surgical reviews is more common owing to insufficient skin removal or retraction. In cases of large hypertrophy, there is also a higher incidence of NAC enlargement.

18.5 Final Considerations

Peixoto's technique for breast reduction is without any doubt a good option for those who value smaller scars. Also, the technique's safety is an important factor in its application. Unfavorable aspects include a long learning curve contrasting with the current immediacy, as this technique requires patience from doctor and patient in cases of large hypertrophy cases, in which skin retraction and accommodation takes months, causing mutual insecurities.

Dr. Peixoto advised his technique for all breast volumes, as long as one of the four designs is chosen, but he admitted that it is best indicated for breasts with mild to moderate hypertrophy, with predominantly glandular content and skin with preserved elasticity, without stretch marks, as in those cases, the skin retraction is more predictable.

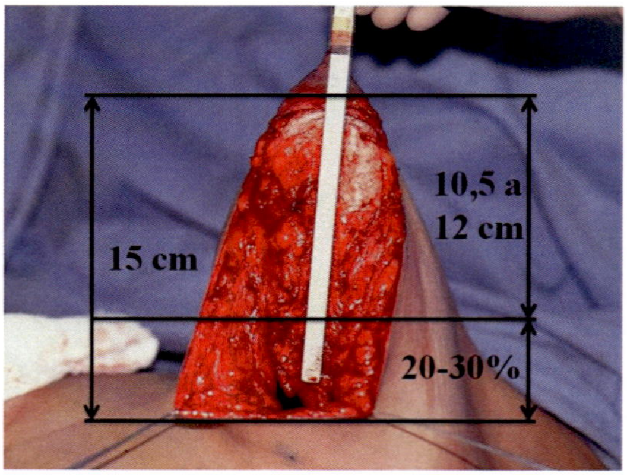

Fig. 18.12 Proportional resection of the base of the mammary cone, removing up to 20% of the height of the mammary cone

18.6 Personal Contribution

As a contribution to the technique, we propose that the resection of the base of the mammary cone is carried out proportionally, removing up to 20% of the height of the mammary cone. The substantiation is that when 20% of the base of a cone is removed, 50% of its volume ends up being removed (Fig. 18.12), which results in a more central projection. In Peixoto's procedure, the removal is performed by leaving 5–7 cm from the original height of the mammary cone.

During assembly, a Brito–Moscozo curved needle can be used (Fig. 18.13) (Brito and Moscozo 2016), an adaptation of the Stocchero needle (Stocchero 2001, 2007), making the process easier. See some results of patients operated trough this technique by the author (Figs. 18.14, 18.15 and 18.16) and by Dr. Peixoto (Figs. 18.17 and 18.18).

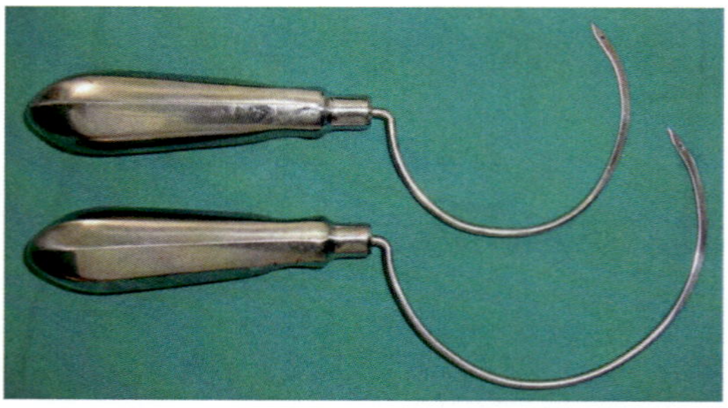

Fig. 18.13 Brito–Moscozo curved needle

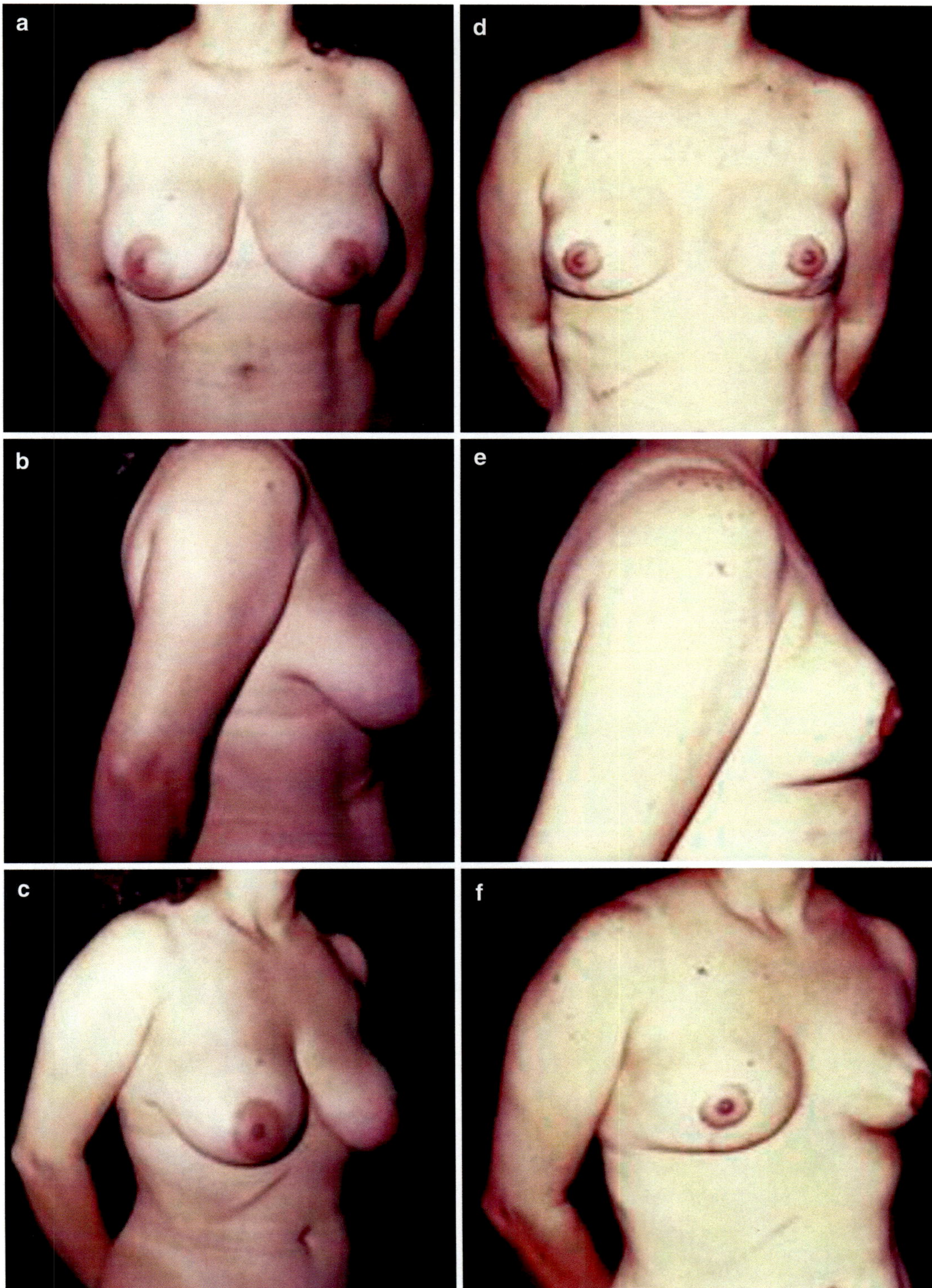

Fig. 18.14 Author's archive. (**a–c**) Preoperatively. (**d–f**) One month postoperatively. For the marking used, see Fig. 18.3c

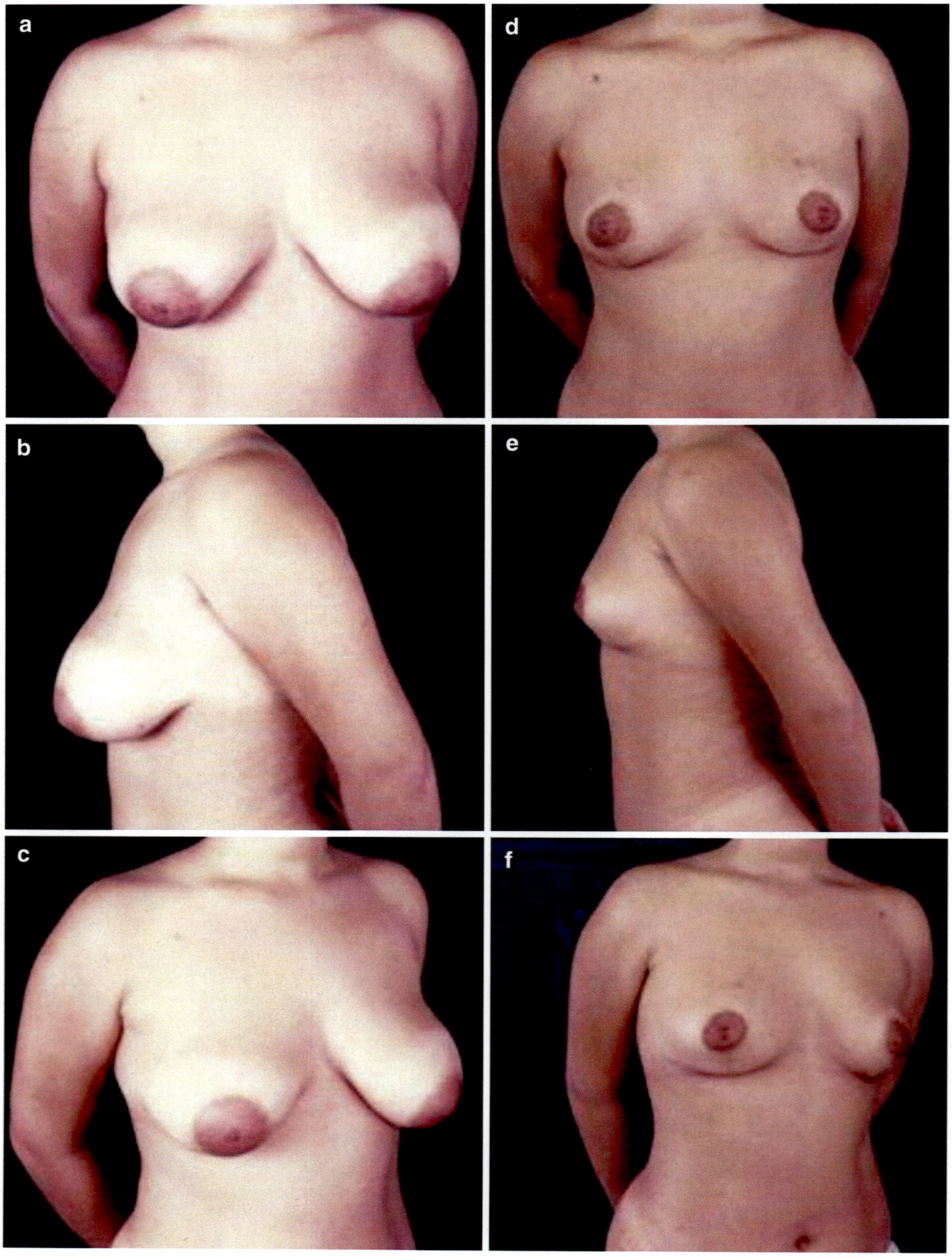

Fig. 18.15 Author's archive. (**a–c**) Preoperatively. (**d–f**) One year postoperatively. For the marking used, see Fig. 18.3c

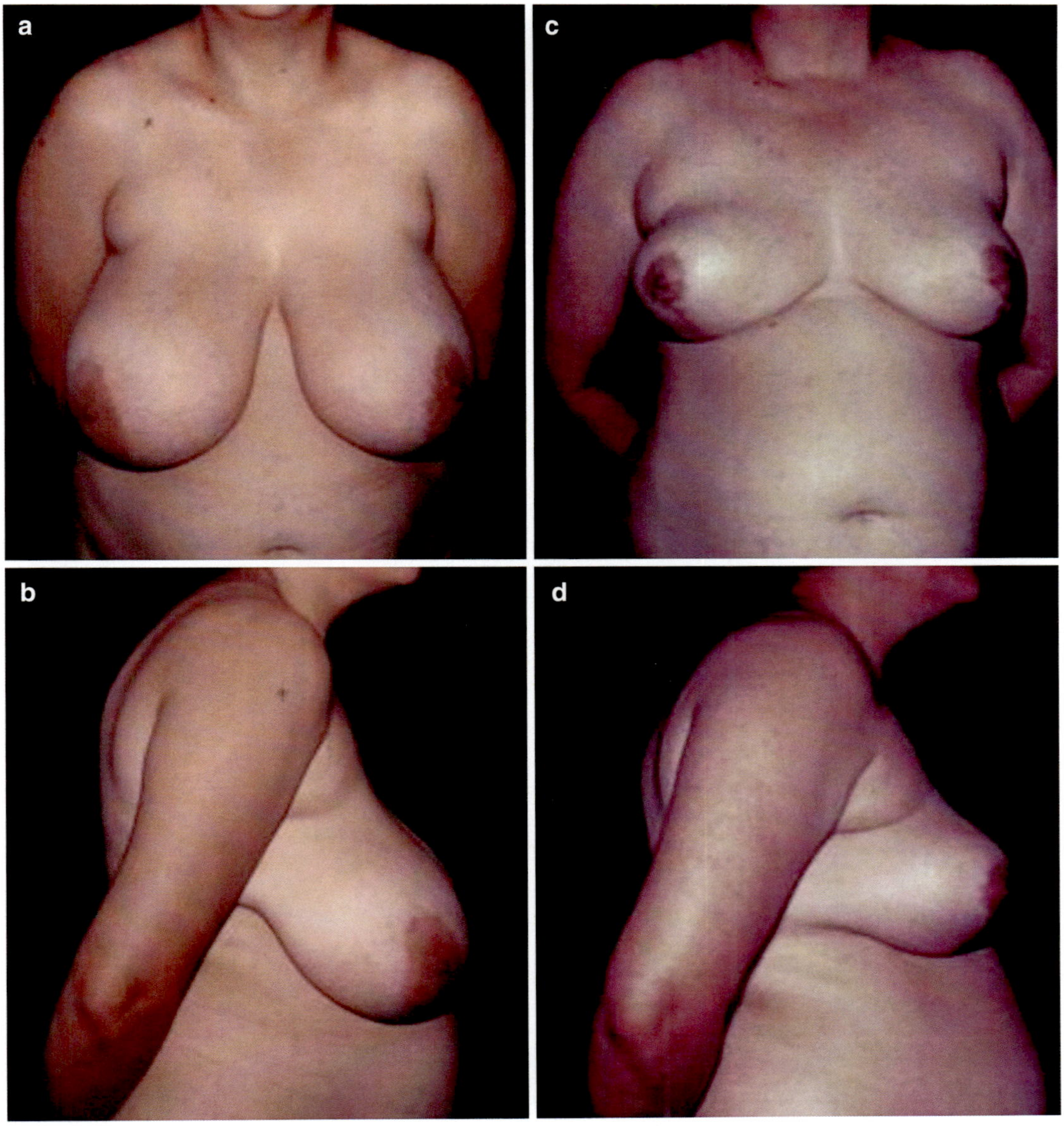

Fig. 18.16 Author's archive. (**a**, **b**) Preoperatively. (**c**, **d**) Six months postoperatively. For the marking used, see Fig. 18.3c

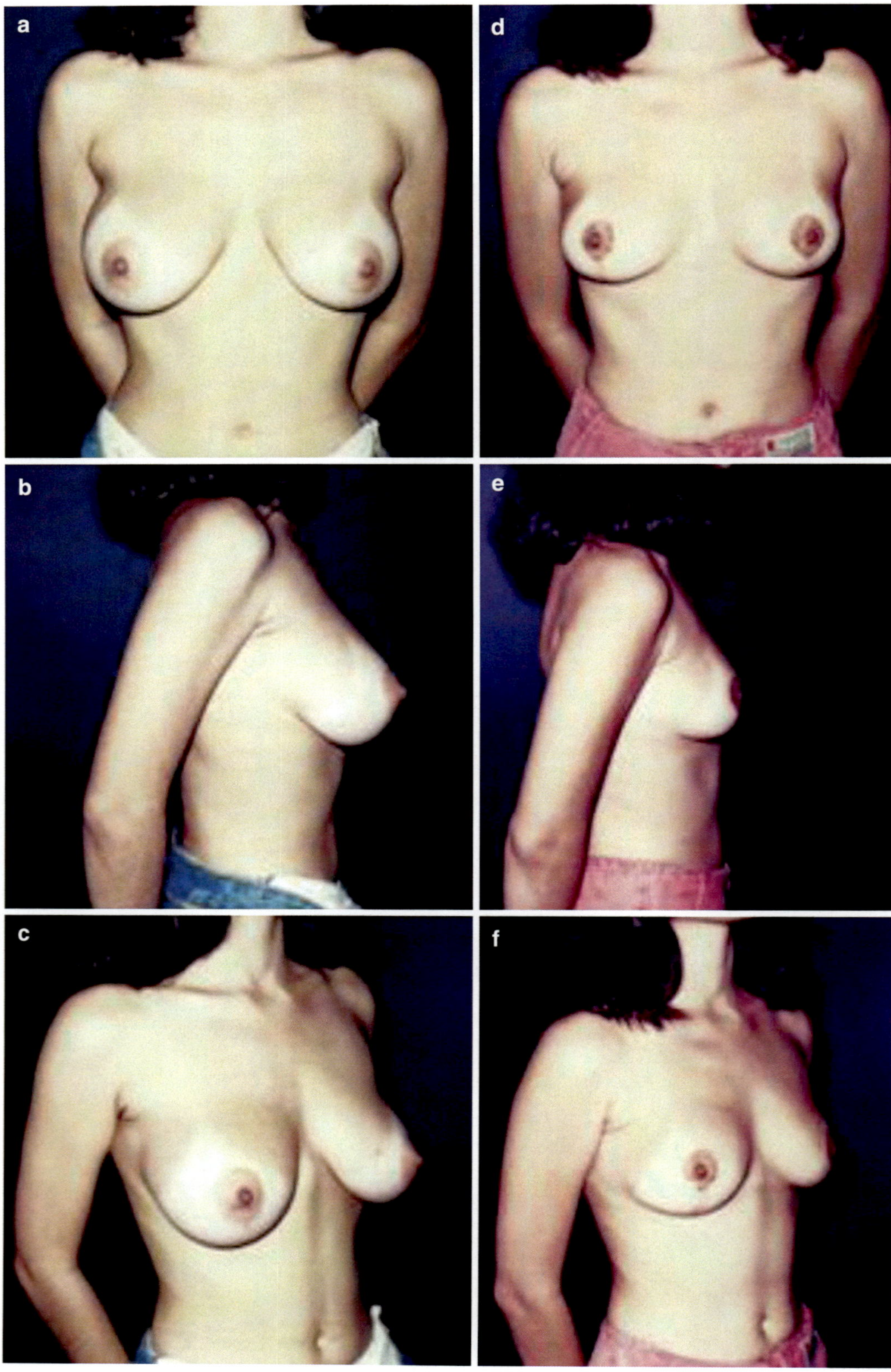

Fig. 18.17 Peixoto's archive. (**a–c**) Preoperatively. (**d–f**) Three months postoperatively. For the marking used, see Fig. 18.3c

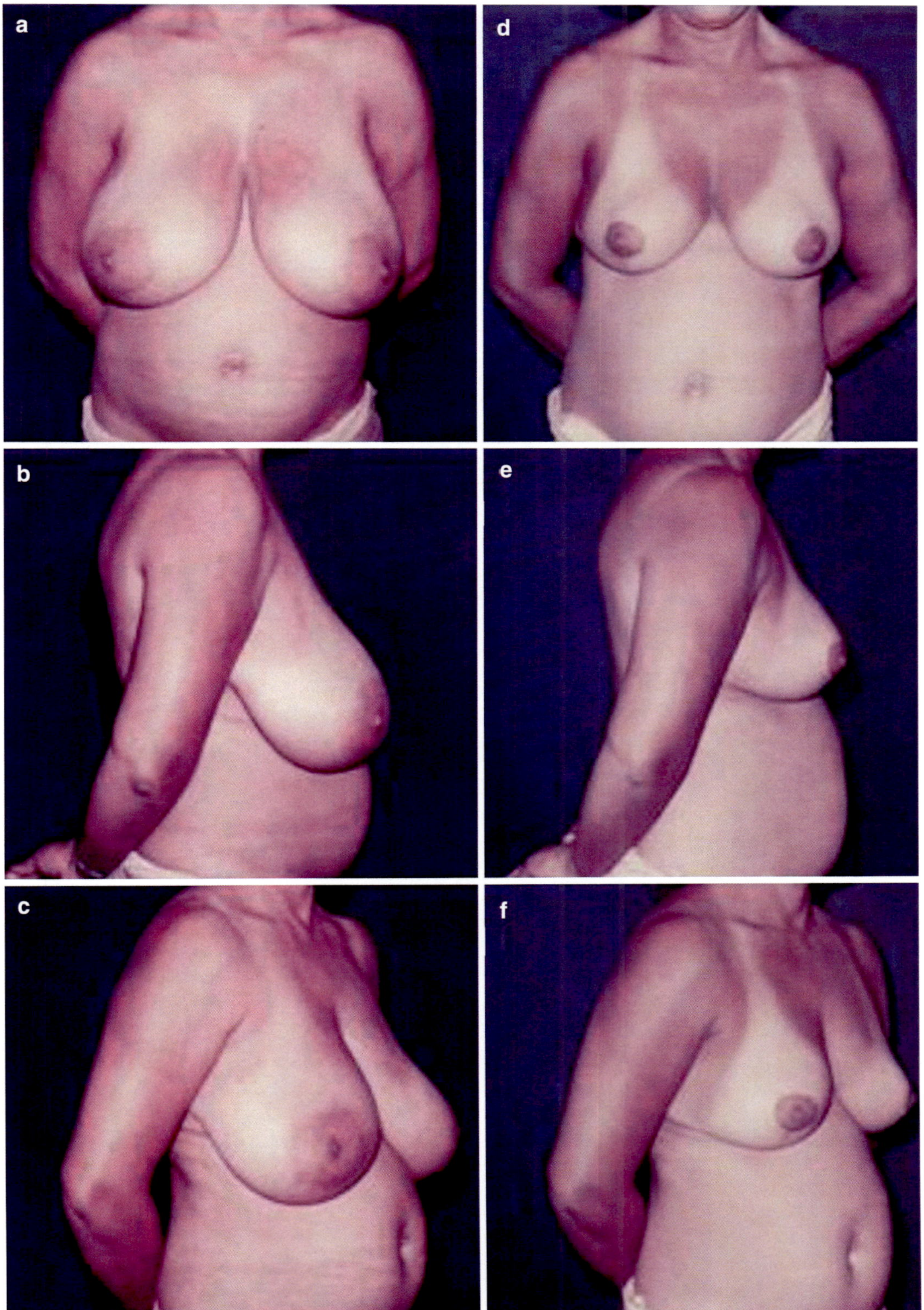

Fig. 18.18 Peixoto's archive. (**a–c**) Preoperatively. (**d–f**) One year postoperatively. For the marking used, see Fig. 18.3c

References

Brito FAP, Moscozo MVA (2016) Sutura circumferential da mama com agulha de Brito-Moscozo: técnica alternativa para sutura dos pilares nas mamoplastias. Rev Bras Cir Plást 31(1):19–24

Maliniac JW (1943) Arterial blood supply of the breast. Arch Surg 47:329

Peixoto G (1979) Reduction mammaplasty. A personal method. Translation of Seventh International Congress of Plastic and Reconstructive Surgery. Rio de Janeiro

Peixoto G (1980) Reduction mammaplasty: a personal technique. Plast Reconstr Surg 65(2):217–226

Peixoto G (1984) The infra-areolar longitudinal incision in reduction mammaplasty. Aesth Plast Surg 9:1

Peixoto G (1990) Reduction mammaplasty: a personal view. In: Goldwyn RM (ed) Reduction mammaplasty. Little Brown, Boston, p 337

Salmon M (1939) Les artères de la glande mammaire. Ann Anat Pathol 16:477

Stocchero IN (2001) The roundblock SMAS treatment. Plast Reconstr Surg 107(7):1921–1923

Stocchero I (2007) Shortscar face-lift with the round block SMAS treatment: a younger face for all. Aesth Plast Surg 31(3):275–278

Pigossi's Technique for Reduction Mastoplasty

19

Moacyr Pires de Mello Filho,
Antonio Carlos Herrmann de Andrade,
and Alessandra Grassi Salles

19.1 Introduction

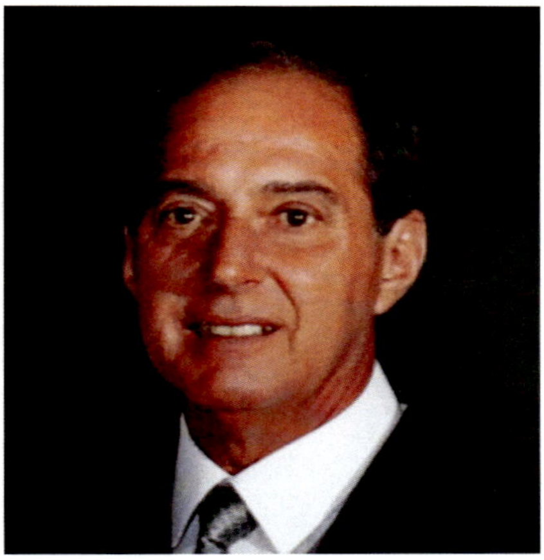

Prof. Dr. Nelson Pigossi
03/03/1932–18/01/1998

M.P. de Mello Filho, M.D. (✉)
Cirurgica, De Mello Cirurgia Plástica,
Av. Pedroso de Morais, 1619 Sala 805 Alto de Pinheiros, São Paulo, SP CEP 05419-001, Brazil
e-mail: piresmello@terra.com.br

A.C.H. de Andrade, M.D.
Rua Joaquim Floriano, 466, cj.1616, São Paulo, SP 04534-002, Brazil

A.G. Salles, M.D., Ph.D.
Plastic Surgery, Hospital das Clínicas da Faculdade de Medicina da Universidade de São Paulo,
Rua Joaquim Floriano, 466, cj.2102, São Paulo, SP 04534-002, Brazil

The period from the 1960s to the 1980s was characterized by the significant development of new tactics for surgical approaches to the breasts (Arie 1957; Bartels et al. 1976; Dufourmentel and Mouly 1968; Erol and Spira 1976; Figallo 1977; Goulian 1971; Hrivnakova 1980; Johnson 1981; Kahn et al. 1968; McKissock 1972; North 1975; Strombeck 1960). Various authors focused their efforts on improving the safety (Peixoto 1967; Pitanguy 1967; Ribeiro 1975; Skoog 1983; Strombeck 1960) and the results of breast surgery, which until that time had been very precarious (Andrews 1984; Bozola et al. 1982; Gruber and Jones 1976; Hinderer 1976; Ship et al. 1989).

One of these surgeons was Dr. Nelson Pigossi (Pigossi 1980), who since the 1970s had progressively developed principles and tactics for approaching breast surgery, as he treated a large number of patients at the Universidade de São Paulo's Hospital das Clínicas; his work drew attention from the medical community and from patients because of the quality and durability of his results, with scars that were always discreet.

This technique is characterized by resection of the volume from the base of the breast, bipartition of the mammary tissue and the remaining dermis below the areola, and the interconnection of the dermoglandular flaps; the medial is used for the middle of the mammary cone and next the lateral is mobilized medially and attached to the tendon tissue near the sternal insertion of the lower ribs to give stability to the shape of the breast.

J.M. Avelar (ed.), *Breast Surgery*, https://doi.org/10.1007/978-3-319-54115-0_19

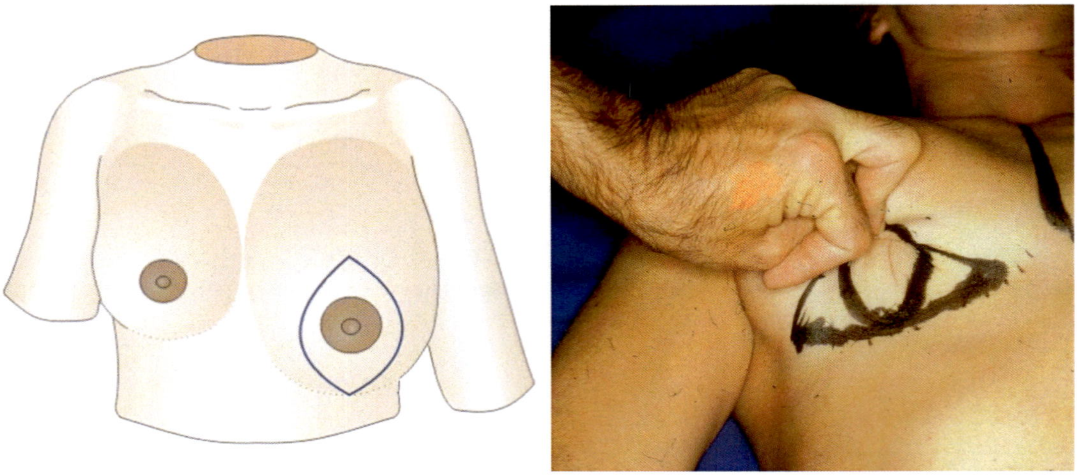

Fig. 19.1 Demarcation of the vertical spindle and pinch test

19.2 Description of the Technique

Marking is based on two spindles of skin, one vertical and the other horizontal.

The highest point of the vertical spindle is at the midpoint of the patient's humerus or above, which is where the upper part of the new areola will be located, and the lowest point corresponds to the future mammary crease. The amount of skin to be mobilized medially determines the width of this oval, considering the breast tissue to be resected (using the "pinch test"), skin flaccidity and resistance, in addition to the possibility of including the associated volume if the procedure is an augmentation mammaplasty. The surgeon cannot try to "economize" with the width of the skin resection, which should be tight or else the firmness of the future breast will be compromised (Figs. 19.1 and 19.2).

The horizontal spindle is determined in its lower arch by the position of the future mammary crease and the upper arch by the height of the mammary pyramid to be resected. The extremities are marked as a function of the remainder of the lateral and medial skin to avoid residual ear-like flaps of skin. The greater the need for rotation and resection of breast tissue in this area, the higher the lateral triangle will be (Figs. 19.3 and 19.4).

The surgery begins with the circumcision of the areola and the de-epithelialization of the area marked by the vertical spindle, which will be used as a dermoglandular flap in the future.

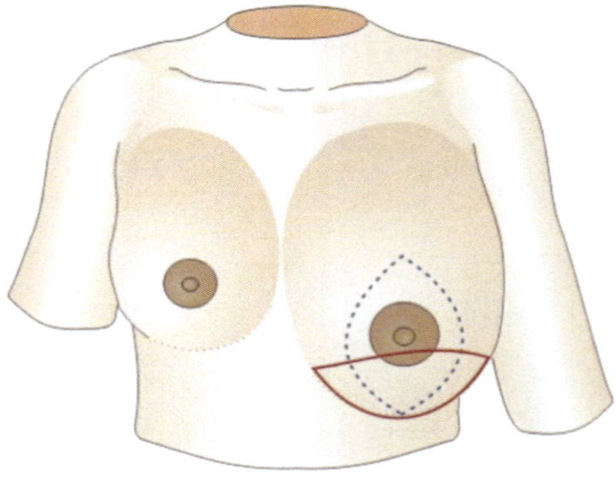

Fig. 19.2 Appearance of the demarcation in a patient with a large reduction of volume

The line of the future mammary crease is incised up to the muscle plane, completely separating the base of the breast from the muscular fascia. The muscular fascia must remain intact so that we can later establish suture points. The separation should extend to the height of the first intercostal space, particularly on severely ptotic breasts (Figs. 19.5 and 19.6).

When it is necessary to resect the breast tissue, preference is initially given to denser or more cystic areas to improve the pathophysiology of the remaining breast tissue.

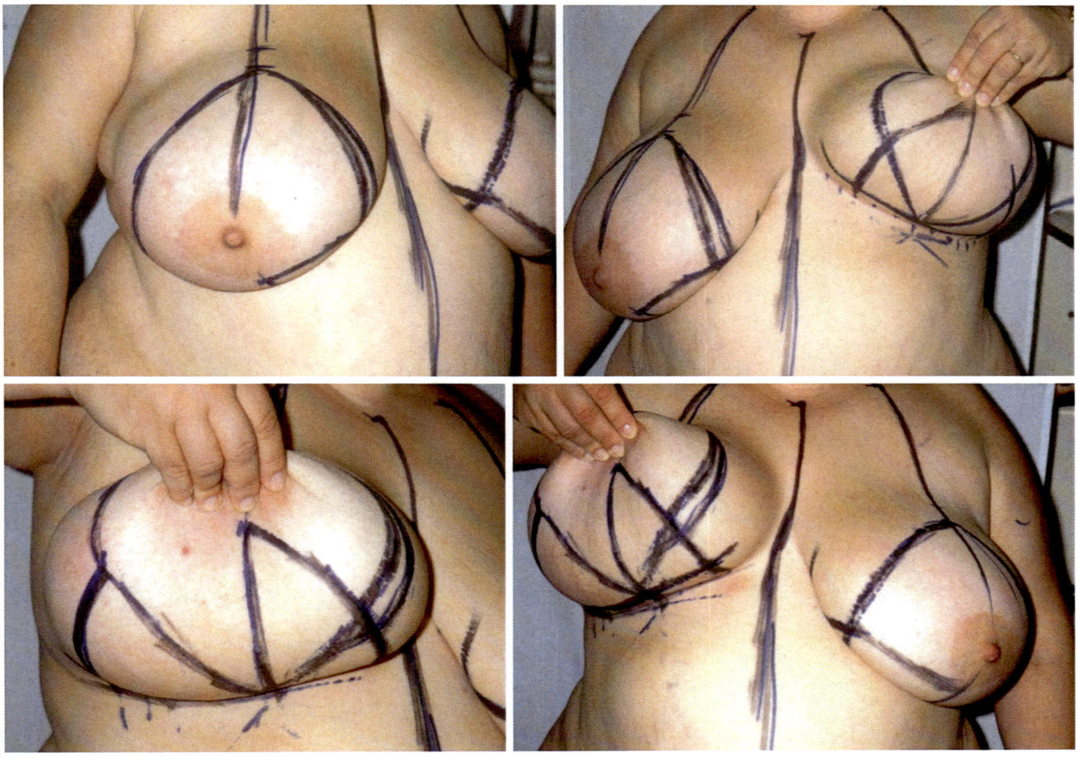

Fig. 19.3 Demarcation of the horizontal spindle and possible variations in demarcation according to the variation in volume and ptosis of the breast

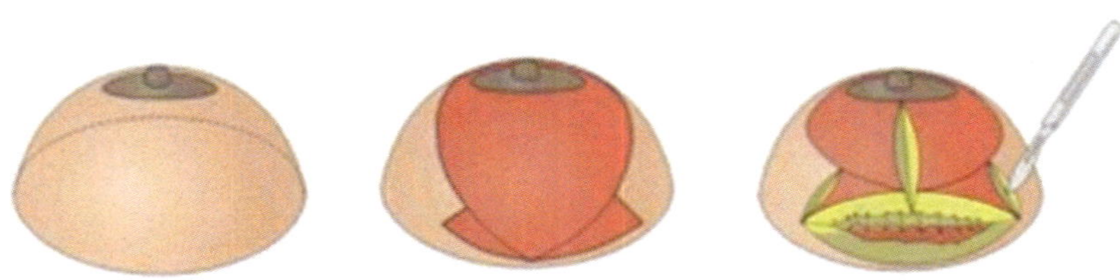

Fig. 19.4 Deepidermization and bipartition of the flaps after separation of the parenchyma

For vertically long breasts with a normal diameter (normal or narrow base), the base of the breast is resected; for breasts with a wide base, the lateral and medial tissue is resected and narrowed, and for gigantomastia the resection is combined.

Technically, we begin the resection by emptying the medial flap, followed by the lateral flap and finally the base of the breast. Complementary resections for further narrowing of the base are made after most of the tissue mass has been removed.

After resection is complete, the abundant perfusion of the flaps and the residual mammary tissue is visible, because the lateral and medial vascular chains of the breast are preserved.

If it is necessary to resect more breast tissue, the extent of the lateral and medial flaps that will touch is reduced, always preserving part of the lateral flap for the medial rotation at the base of the breast.

At times, the medial flap is completely removed in very large resections, or even extends to the resection above the level of the areola.

Assembly begins with two or three sutures between the breast tissue in the upper quadrants and the uppermost exposed portion of the muscular fascia of the pectoralis major, raising the

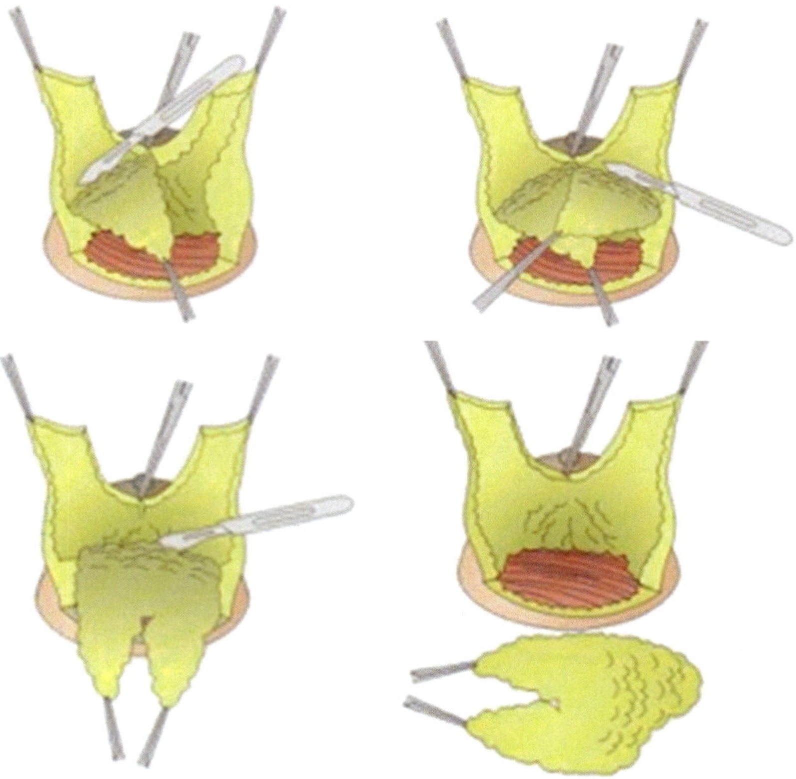

Fig. 19.5 Resection of the volume of the lateral and medial flaps and the base of a left breast

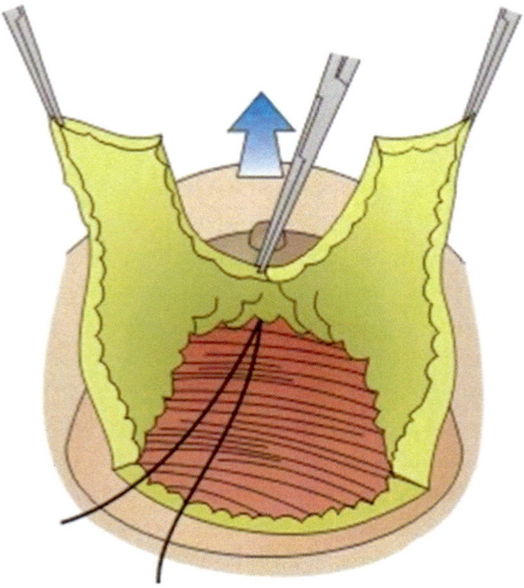

Fig. 19.6 Sutures in the upper pole

tissue in the neck of the breast upward (hypercorrection) so that after a few months the volume will remain in this region (Figs. 19.7 and 19.8).

The medial flap is mobilized toward the center of the breast, or more laterally when necessary, with a stitch in the muscular fascia of the pectoralis major to fill this area and to project the areola.

Next, the lateral flap is mobilized medially, fixing it with a stitch in the insertion of the pectoral muscle in the ribs, reducing the diameter of the base of the mammary cone and reducing the tension and the weight of the breast on the skin.

The skin is then sutured around the exterior of the areola without necessarily following the previous markings to perceive the balance of the tensive forces between the skin and the nipple–areola complex and consequently achieve a rounded and regular areola.

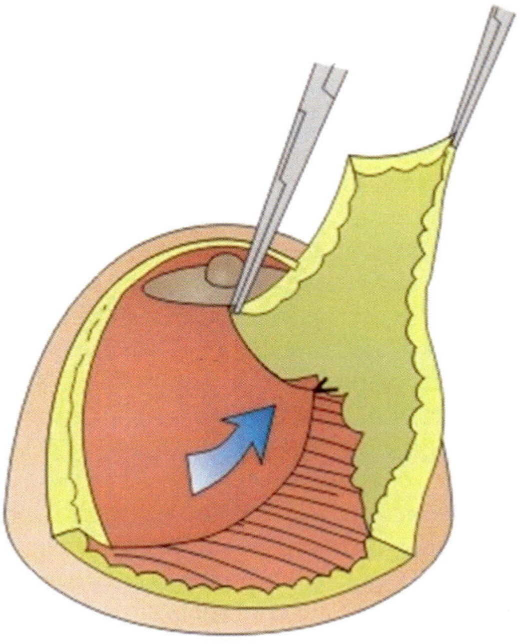

Fig. 19.7 Fixation of the medial flap of a left breast

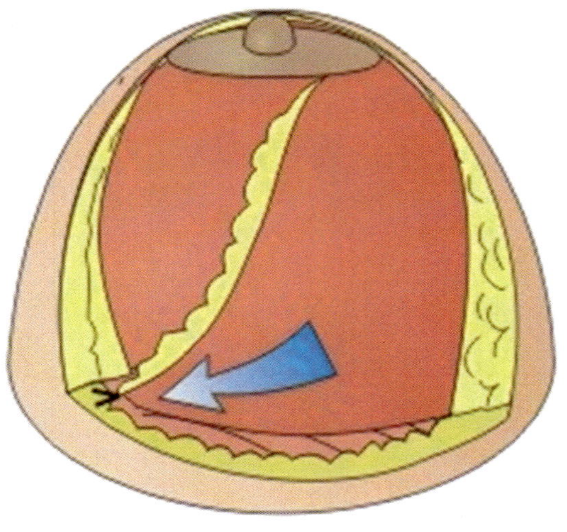

Fig. 19.8 Fixation of the lateral flap of a left breast

The final appearance of the breast displays a peculiar format: the lower pole appears flattened, the upper pole appears hyper-corrected, inserted into the upper portion of the neck of the breast, with the flattened areola turned downward.

The results of this technique rely heavily on the balance between the forces that act during the healing process, obtaining the counterweighting of the breast by 6 months after the procedure. The force of gravity and the tension of the resected skin act on the breast cone in equilibrium with the way the flaps are fitted together, reducing tension and preserving the shape of the breast pyramid. The reduced tension on the skin sutures permits good scarring. These dermoglandular flaps are the base of the breast support rather than the skin, which is the case in some techniques in which a significant descent of the breast and a loss of shape can be observed.

The medial flap fills the resected areas, and can be positioned more medially or laterally depending on the resected area, and can even be sacrificed in cases of excess volume without damage to the areolar circulation.

The lateral flap is the support flap, and its preservation is essential; it may vary in thickness or length according to each case.

Perfusion of the residual breast tissue arrives through the lateral and medial chain of the breast, which provides a very high degree of security for the areas used in the assembly process.

19.3 Discussion

Plastic surgeons have increasingly emphasized the pathophysiological treatment of the breasts, and this technique meets all the basic requirements. It is often indicated only for resection of fibro-cystic changes in the breast when patients seek surgical relief for premenstrual pain that does not respond to treatment and when they are not concerned about the outcome of the surgery.

A characteristic of this technique is the fact that the surgeon is not limited to a single resection pattern, allowing tissue to be removed from all quadrants of the breast where necessary, with good ease of assembly and final shape.

Even in patients with large losses of mass, in most cases this technique avoids the need for mammary prostheses by projecting the breast cone. We oppose the current widely-held opinion that advises resection of healthy breast tissue and replacement with mammary implants to confer rigidity to the breast. In our opinion, behind this concept lie ignorance and the inability to use techniques that assemble the mammary cone so well.

In this technique, we noticed a very small prevalence of necrosis of the T (the junction of the two lower breast scars, the vertical and horizontal). We believe that this results from the elliptical shape of the skin resection, the absence of skin detachment, and structuring with the medialization of the lateral flap, leading to a decrease in the tension of the sutures at this point and consequently less postoperative ischemia.

In the last two decades, there has been an overemphasis among many surgeons on making an exaggerated effort to reduce the size of the scars (Arufe et al. 1977; Aryan 1980; Bustos 1987; Marchac and Olarte 1982; Tamerin 1963; Wray et al. 1975). As a result, the skin was excessively separated from the subcutaneous tissue, liposuction was used excessively as a complement to breast reconstruction techniques, and the use of all types of meshes and fabrics was introduced into the assembly process, leading to major catastrophes in the outcomes of some patients and insufficient results in others. With this in mind, the ascent of the areola was spared, along with the ideal resection of the volume, greatly limiting patient satisfaction. Scars were seen as the enemy of the plastic surgeon. We see scars in a variety of ways; good scarring, which is inevitably present in cases of severe ptosis and volumes, do not greatly hamper the life of a patient who has received good guidance and a good procedure. This technique allows a minimal incidence of hypertrophic scarring, even in high-risk groups, making the surgery very safe in terms of the predictability of scar quality (Figs. 19.9, 19.10 and 19.11).

We are also very concerned about the late appearance of skin separation in the techniques that separate the skin from the mammary parenchyma. We have perceived a great loss in elasticity and potential atrophy of the dermal layer, which is seen to be flaccid and to contain telangectasias because of dilation of the dermal vessels.

This technique is quite flexible; thus, we can change the shape of the hypertrophic breast, creating a better height and width ratio. In cases where the breasts have large bases the surgeon

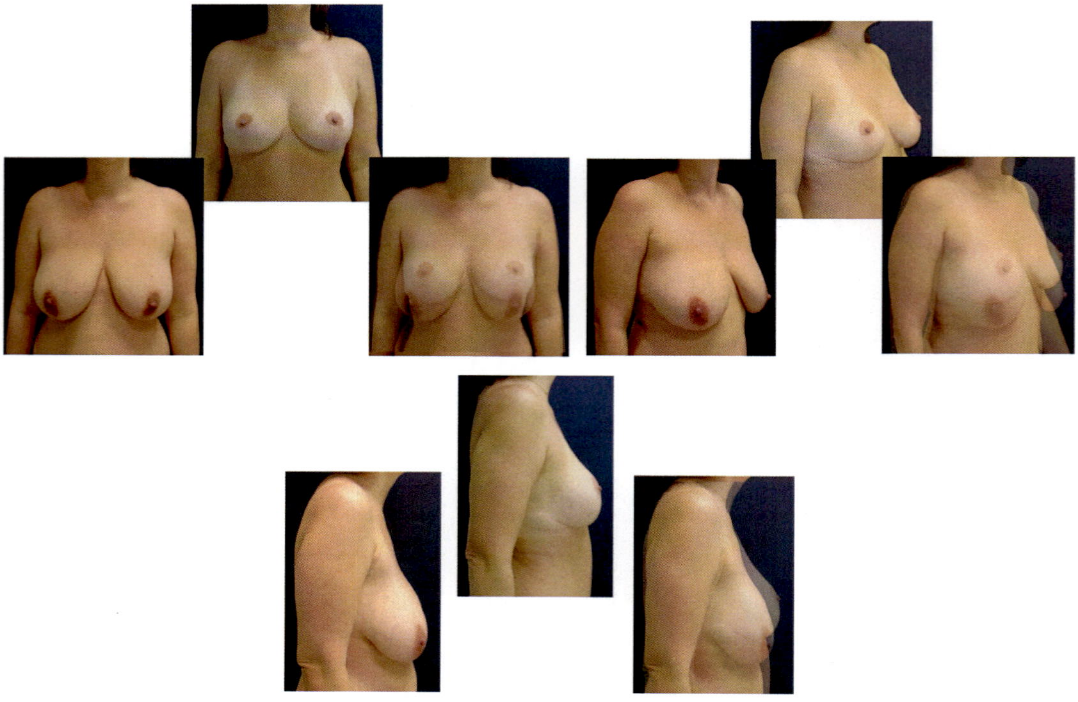

Fig. 19.9 Patients pre- and post-procedure

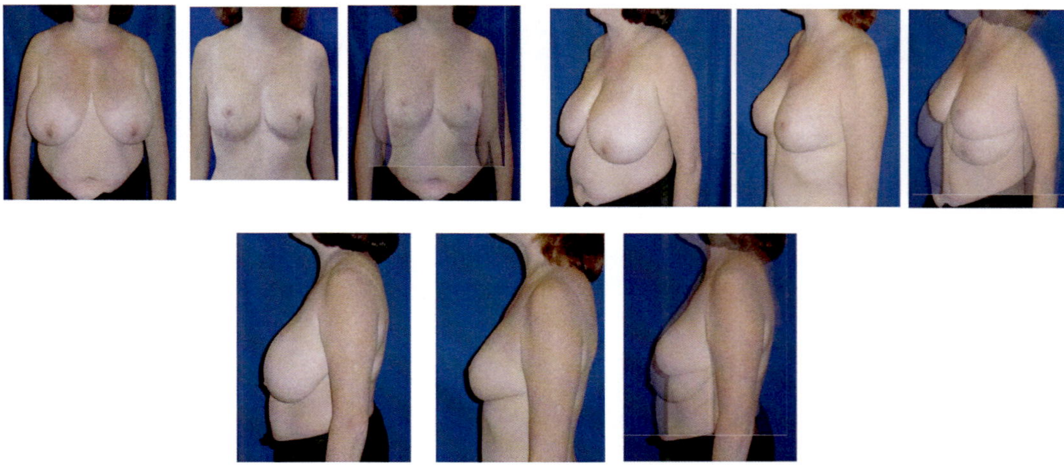

Fig. 19.10 Patients pre- and post-procedure

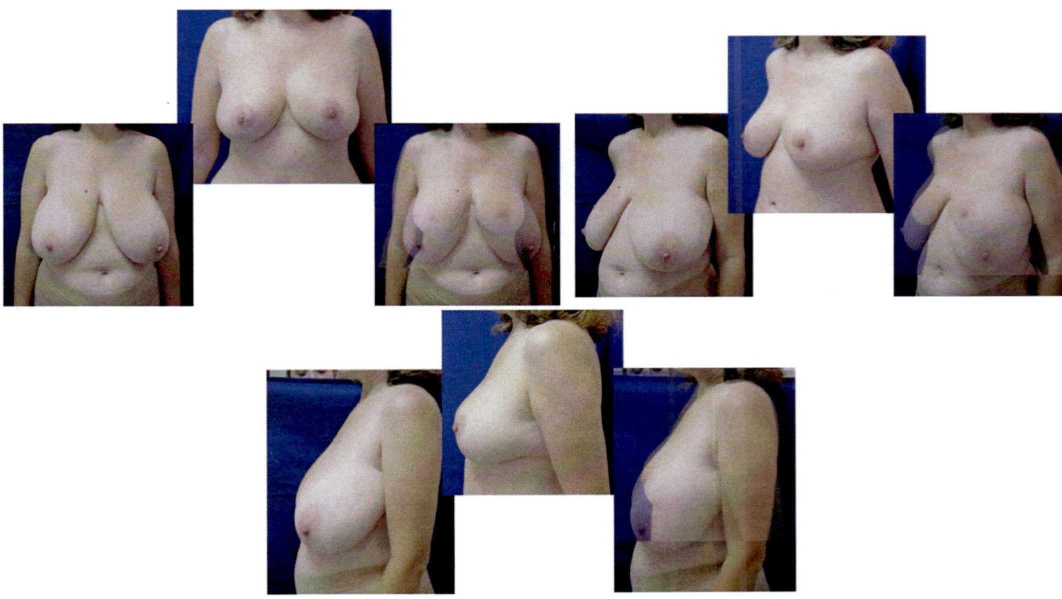

Fig. 19.11 Patients pre- and post-procedure

can resect the medial and lateral portions of the breast in a curved shape, greatly decreasing the diameter of the base of the breast (Silva 1964).

After 2–3 months the breast begins to move in a counterweighted manner. The neck of the breast partially yields by 4–6 months, and then remains for several years. These changes are the result of a balance in the acting forces and the rigidity of the breast scarring in this phase.

Breastfeeding is preserved even after large resections, because the way in which the parenchyma is removed does not destroy the continuity of the remaining glands to the breast duct. Mastitis and mammary abscesses are not seen during lactation. The authors have been using this technique since 1967.

A constant in this technique is the lack of damage to the areola; the dermis is always released along what remains of the de-epithelialized edge of the vertical oval, even in very ptotic breasts, which demonstrates the effective circulation of the remaining tissue in extreme situations. In this way, we avoid the use of radical techniques such as free grafting of the nipple–areola complex.

This technique requires some years of apprenticeship alongside a more experienced surgeon, as some small variations are used for various types of breasts.

These results with minimal complications position this technique as one of the safest for obtaining good breast cone shapes and securing perfusion of the mammary tissue and the nipple–areola complex, excellent quality in scar progress, and durable results.

Note that this technique has been used for more than 50 years by various surgeons, and is still current and safe with very predictable results; essentially, it has undergone very few modifications over the years.

References

Andrews JM (1984) A technique for reduction mammoplasty. Aesth Plast Surg 8:55–58

Arie G (1957) Uma nueva técnica de Mamoplastia. Rev Latinoam Cir Plast 3:23

Arufe HN, Erenfryd A, Saubidet M (1977) Mammaplasty with a single vertical, superiorly based pedicle to support the nipple-areola. Plast Reconstr Surg 60:221–226

Aryan S (1980) Reduction mammaplasty with the nipple-areola carried on a single inferior pedicle. Ann Plast Surg 5:169–177

Bartels RJ, Strickland DM, Douglas WM (1976) A new mastopexy operation for mild and moderate breast ptosis. Plast Reconstr Surg 57:687–691

Bozola AR, Oliveira MC, Sanches WM, Kurimori NS, Chaen LHT (1982) Mamaplastia em "L", contribuição pessoal. Rev Amrios 26:207–217

Bustos R (1987) Mamaplastia periareolar. Tema livre apresentado no XXIV Congresso Brasileiro de Cirurgia Plástica, São Paulo

Dufourmentel C, Mouly R (1968) Modification of "periwinkleshell operation" for small ptotic breasts. Plast Reconstr Surg 41:523

Erol OO, Spira M (1976) A mastopexy techique for mild to moderate ptosis. Plast Reconstr Surg 65:603–609

Figallo E (1977) Surgical treatment of mammary ptosis without hypertrophy. Plast Reconstr Surg 60:189

Goulian D (1971) Dermal mastopexy. Plast Reconstr Surg 47:105

Gruber RP, Jones HW (1976) The "donut" mastopexy: indications and complications. Plast Reconstr Surg 65:34–38

Hinderer UT (1976) The dermal brasserie mammaplasty. Plast Reconstr Surg 3:349

Hrivnakova J (1980) A new modification of Bigg's operation for the correction of ptotic brasts. Acta Chir Plast 22:93

Johnson GW (1981) Central core reduction mammaplasties and Marlex suspension of breast tissue. Aesthetic Plast Surg 5:77

Kahn S, Hoffman S, Simon BE (1968) Correction of non-hypertrophic ptosis of breasts. Plast Reconstr Surg 41:244

Marchac D, Olarte G (1982) Reduction mammaplasty and correction of ptosis with a short inframammary scar. Plast Reconstr Surg 469:45

McKissock PK (1972) Reduction mammaplasty with a vertical dermal flap. Plast Reconstr Surg 49:245–252

North JF (1975) Mammaplasty hyperinvolution and ptosis. Br J Plast Surg 28:310

Peixoto G (1967) Reduction mammaplasty: a personal technique. Plast Reconstr Surg 20:78–85

Pigossi N (1980) New technique for reduction mammoplasty. Presented at the Brazilian Symposium on Breast Surgery. Sponsered by Brazilian Society of Plastic Surgery—Region of São Paulo, August, São Paulo

Pitanguy I (1967) Surgical treatment of breast hypertrophy. Br J Plast Surg 20:78–85

Ribeiro L (1975) A new technique for reduction mammaplasty. Plast Reconstr Surg 55:330–334

Ship AG, Weiss PR, Engler AM (1989) Dual-pedicle dermoparenchymal mastopexy. Plast Reconstr Surg 83:281

Silva G (1964) Mastopexy with dermal ribbon for supporting the breast and keeping it in shape. Plast Reconstr Surg 34:4

Skoog T (1983) A technique of breast reduction mammaplasty. Acta Chir Scand 126:453–457

Strombeck JO (1960) Mammaplasty: report of a new technique based on the two-pedicle procedure. Br J Plast Surg 13:79–90

Tamerin JA (1963) The Lexer-Kraske mammaplasty: a reaffirmation. Plast Reconstr Surg 31:442

Wray RC Jr, Holtman B, Weeks PM (1975) Factors in the production of inconspicuous scars. Plast Reconstr Surg 56:266

20 Reduction Mastoplasty for Mammary Hypertrophy Using a Thin Superior Lateral Pedicle

Márcio Paulino Costa,
Guilherme Cardinal Barreiro,
and Nuberto H. Teixeira

20.1 Introduction

When the plastic surgeon prepares for a breast reduction, he or she has to evaluate certain characteristics, including breast size, breast shape, and the degree of ptosis. Heavier breasts with excessive ptosis can be a surgical challenge. For example, the surgeon may have difficulty transposing the nipple-areola complex (NAC). In these cases, we find that a reduction mammoplasty using a superior medial thin pedicle technique (Costa et al. 2008) is one of the best options. This technique can safely reduce large breasts with good aesthetic results (Costa et al. 2008).

In this chapter, we present a new technique that uses a thin superior lateral pedicle, which may be of particular interest for patients with breast cancer. Over the years, we have been faced with tumors in the superior medial quadrant in patients with large breasts. In these cases, the breast must be reduced using an aesthetic reduction mammoplasty to reconstruct the breast but without the superior medial pedicle. Therefore, the options are to use the inferior pedicle or the superior lateral pedicle. We prefer to use the superior lateral pedicle, because we find it difficult to shape the breast with the inferior pedicle. However, when using the superior lateral pedicle as described by Skoog (1963), we had another problem: the pedicle was too thick and the transposition of the NAC to its new position was difficult.

Armed with the knowledge of reduction mammoplasty based on a superior medial thin pedicle technique described by Costa et al. (2008), we used the same principles but changed the source of the pedicle to the lateral area. Utilizing a thin superior lateral pedicle (1.5–2.0 cm gross), the resection was performed in two steps: (1) resecting the base excess at a plane perpendicular to the breast (which determines the cone's height) and (2) removing the central half keel (which determines the breast's diameter).

20.2 Methods

Eighty patients with mammary hypertrophy underwent surgery in our clinic in the last 10 years. Severe mammary hypertrophy was defined by cup size, the weight of resected breast tissue, and the height of nipple elevation

M.P. Costa, M.D., Ph.D. (✉)
Brazilian Society of Plastic Surgery, ISAPS, FILACAP, ASPS, Hospital das Clínicas, University of São Paulo Medical School, Rua Gabriel dos Santos, 759 12° andar, Santa Cecília, 01231-011 São Paulo, SP, Brazil
e-mail: marciopaulino@bol.com.br

G.C. Barreiro, M.D., Ph.D.
Brazilian Society of Plastic Surgery, University of Campinas (UNICAMP), São Paulo, SP, Brazil

N.H. Teixeira, M.D.
Brazilian Society of Plastic Surgery, University of São Paulo Medical School, São Paulo, SP, Brazil

J.M. Avelar (ed.), *Breast Surgery*, https://doi.org/10.1007/978-3-319-54115-0_20

(Melega et al. 1992; Rees 1971; Rees and LaTrenta 1994). The breast shape of all patients was type 2 according to Rees' classification (Melega et al. 1992; Rees 1971; Rees and LaTrenta 1994). According to Regnault, all patients had third-degree ptosis (Regnault 1974).

Forty patients had breast tumors; of these, 50% were malignant tumors, for which the patients underwent quadrantectomy. In 20 patients, the medial portion of the breast was larger than the lateral. In 20 patients, the option to use the superior lateral pedicle was the surgeon's choice.

20.2.1 Preoperative Markings

In this procedure, demarcation of the breast is done with the patient erect. The new desired position of the areola is estimated by projecting the inframammary crease to a line that crosses the clavicular midpoint, while the future location of the nipple is determined by the index finger (point A; Fig. 20.1). Points B and C are determined using the pinch test: With the thumbs and index fingers, the skin of the breast is pinched together approximately at the inferior border of the areola (Fig. 20.1).

According to the degree of hypertrophy and the amount of tissue resection, the length of the arm and the angle of the wedge resection vary. The length of the medial arm (AB) is between 8 and 9 cm, whereas the lateral arm (AC) is between 10 and 12 cm (Fig. 20.1) in most patients. The breast is then elevated and inframammary crease marked.

With the thumb and index finger of one hand pinching the breast skin at the level of points B and C, the base limit of resection is determined. The medial and lateral lines are marked, connecting point B to the medial and point C to the lateral junctures of the inframammary crease (points D and E; Fig. 20.1). Point F depends on the base width, ranging from 10 to 12.5 cm (approximately the midpoint of the distance between points D and E; Fig. 20.1).

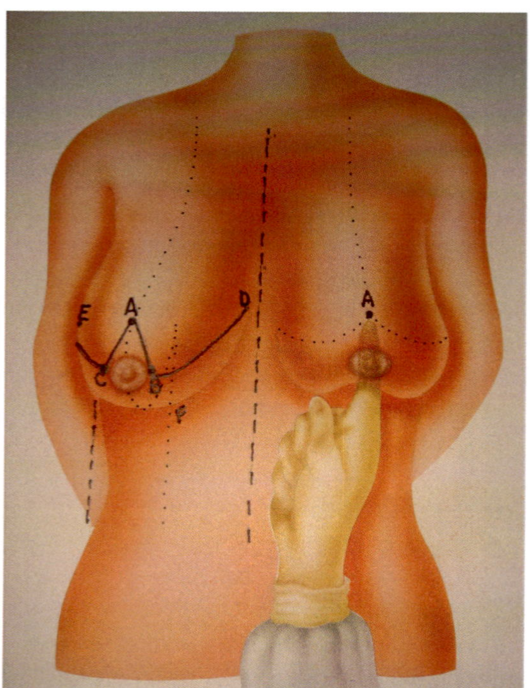

Fig. 20.1 Procedure for preoperative markings

20.2.2 Surgery

The patient is evaluated and the markings are done in the preoperative period (Fig. 20.2). Incisions are made in the upper V and around the areola markings. The upper V and the subdermal plexus surrounding the nipple are de-epithelialized.

The operation begins with the patient in the supine position and arms adducted. The inframammary

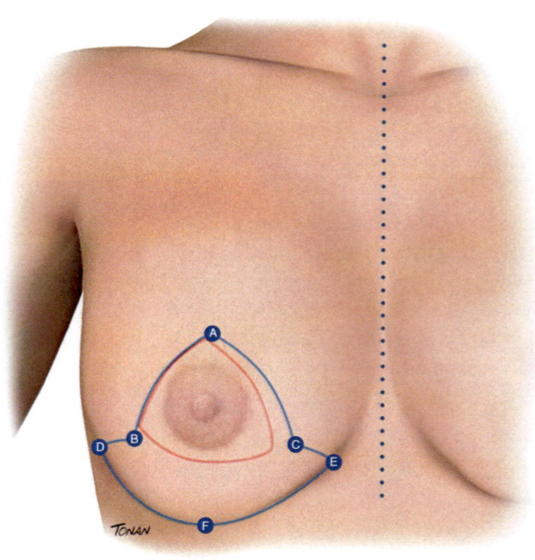

Fig. 20.2 Procedure for preoperative markings

crease incision is made. The breast is lifted off the deep surface of the superficial fascia over the pectoralis major (medially until the projection of point B over the pectoralis and laterally far from the projection of point C over the pectoralis major).

The superior lateral pedicle is marked. The width of the flap base is between 6 and 7 cm, leaving 1 cm in the upper part and the lower part of the V. A line is drawn passing near the areola. Therefore, the flap is undermined with 1.5 cm of thickness and is made progressively thicker at the base. While undermining the flap in the subcutaneous layer, it is important to include some glandular tissue beneath the areola (Fig. 20.3).

Next, resection of the excessive mammary tissue is accomplished with the patient in an elevated position of 80°, in two steps. First, the base excess is resected at a plane perpendicular to the breast, which determines the cone's height (Fig. 20.4). Second, the central half keel

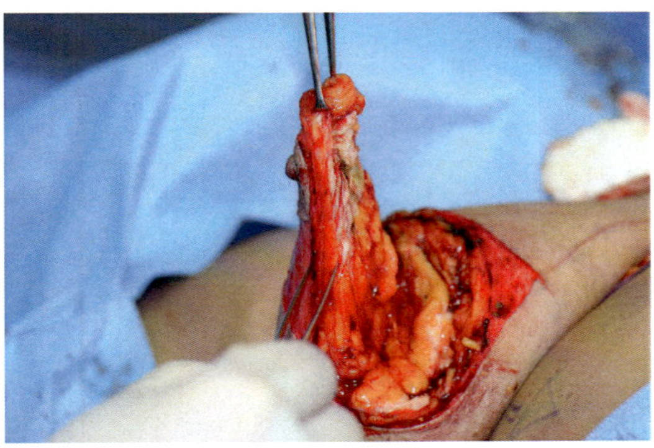

Fig. 20.3 Thin lateral superior pedicle

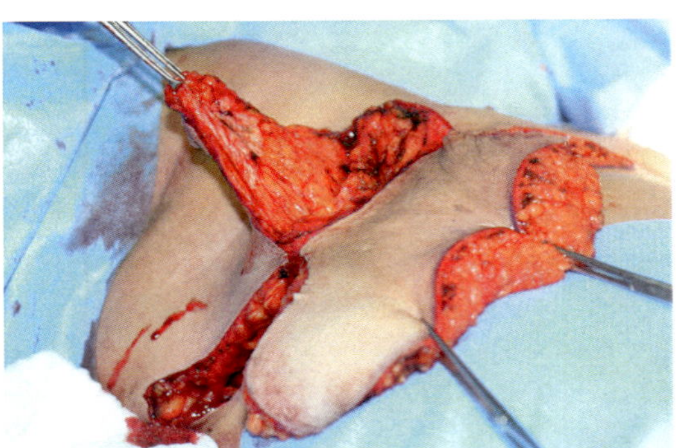

Fig. 20.4 Cone height

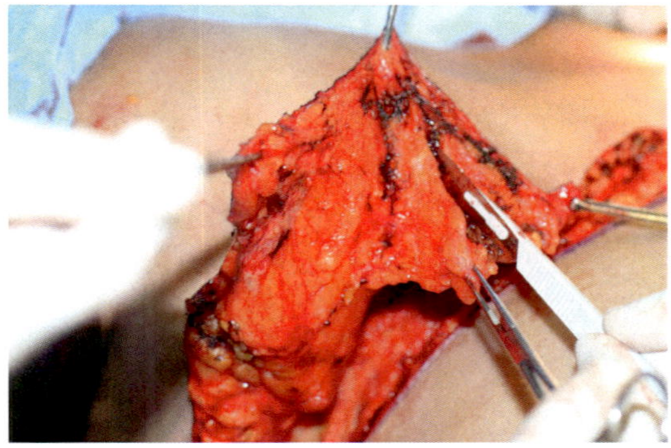

Fig. 20.5 The central half keel, which determines the breast diameter

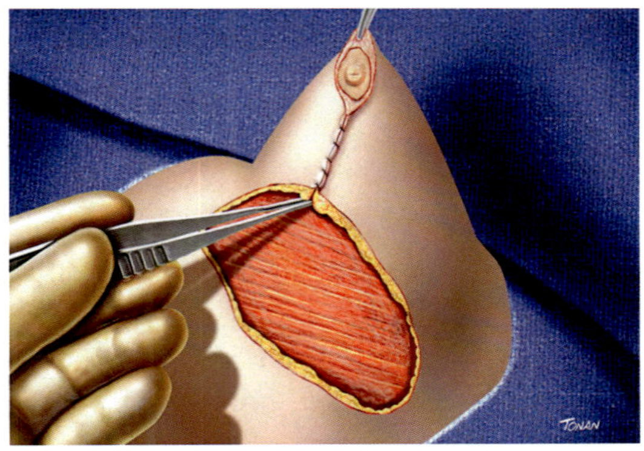

Fig. 20.6 The sutures approximate the medial and lateral pillars for a greater projection of the areola

is removed, which determines the breast's diameter (Fig. 20.5).

The NAC is moved upward to its new position. An incision of approximately 1 cm can be made on the lateral portion of the V at point B if it is necessary to enhance the areola's transposition distance.

The breast segments are approximated at the midline using 3-0 monocryl sutures. Sutures of 2-0 mononylon are used to approximate the medial and lateral pillars and for a greater projection of the areola and nipple (Fig. 20.6).

A trifurcation suture of 3-0 monocryl is used between points B, C, and F. If more skin needs to be removed, it can be taken along AB and BC. Then, the skin is closed. The patient is drained (Fig. 20.7).

Surgical results are demonstrated in Figs. 20.8, 20.9, 20.10, 20.11, 20.12, 20.13, 20.14, 20.15, 20.16, and 20.17.

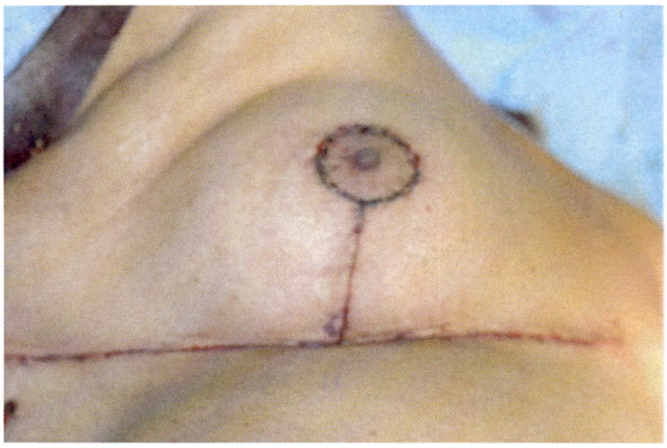

Fig. 20.7 The final aspect of the breast

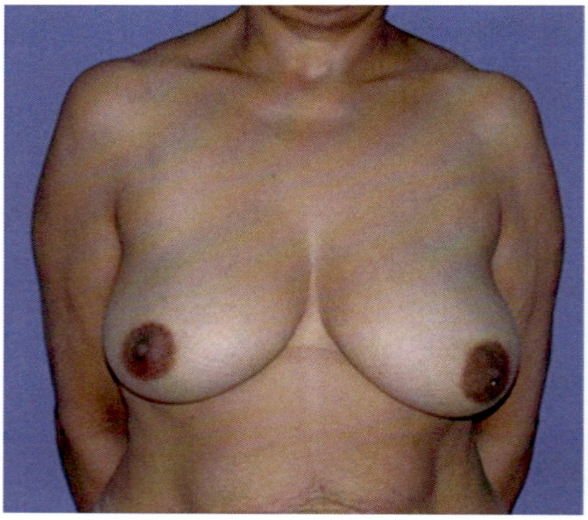

Fig. 20.8 Patient A: preoperative

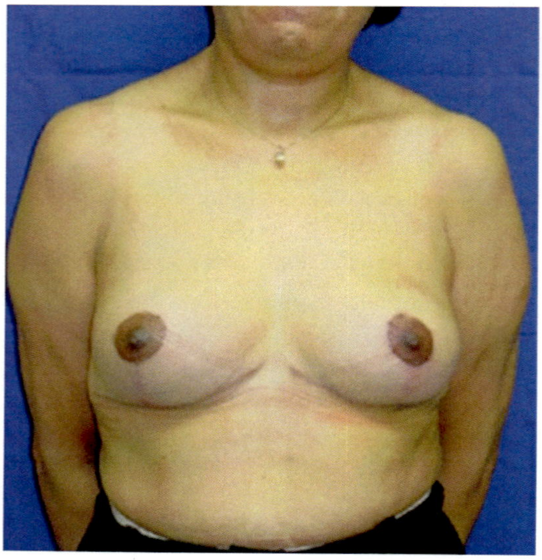

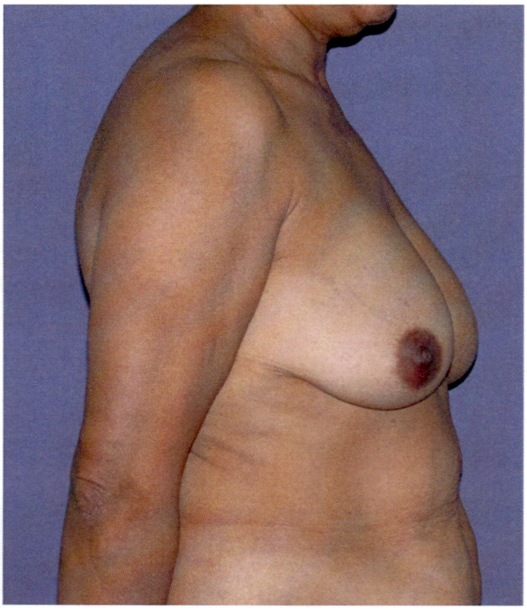

Fig. 20.10 Patient A: preoperative

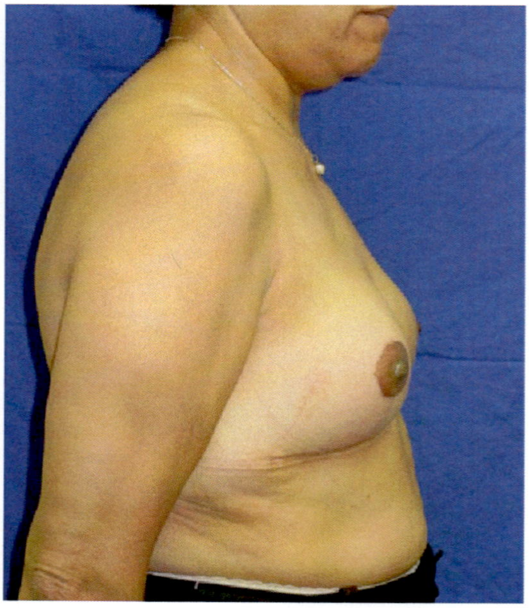

Fig. 20.11 Patient A: postoperative lateral view

Fig. 20.9 Patient A: 9 months postoperative, with 950 g removed from the left breast and 800 g from the right breast

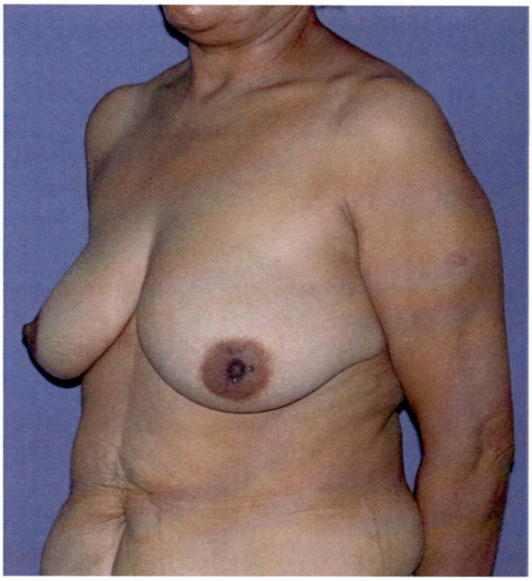

Fig. 20.12 Patient A: preoperative

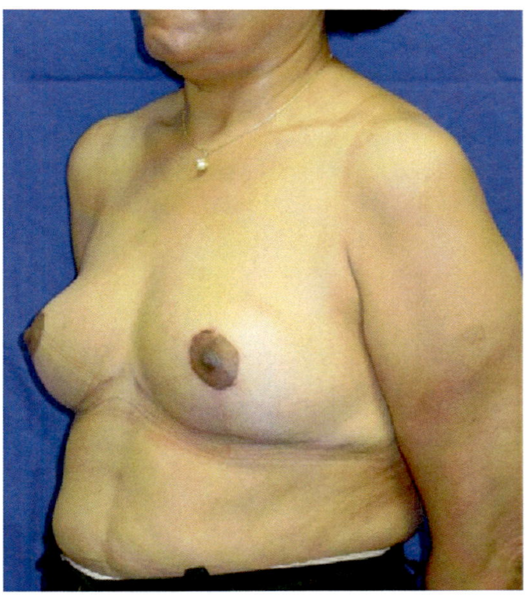

Fig. 20.13 Patient A: postoperative 3/4 view

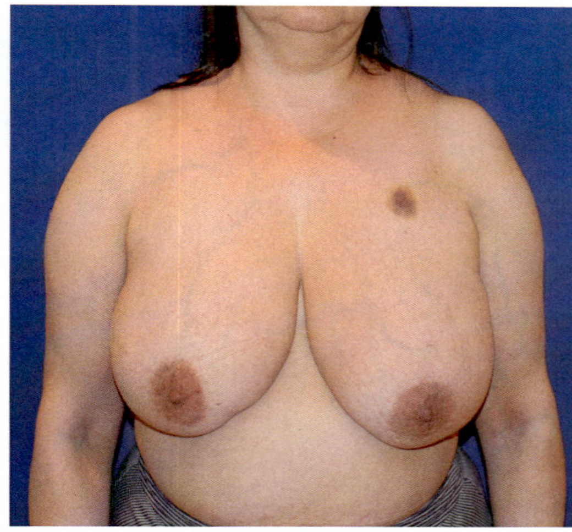

Fig. 20.14 Patient B: preoperative

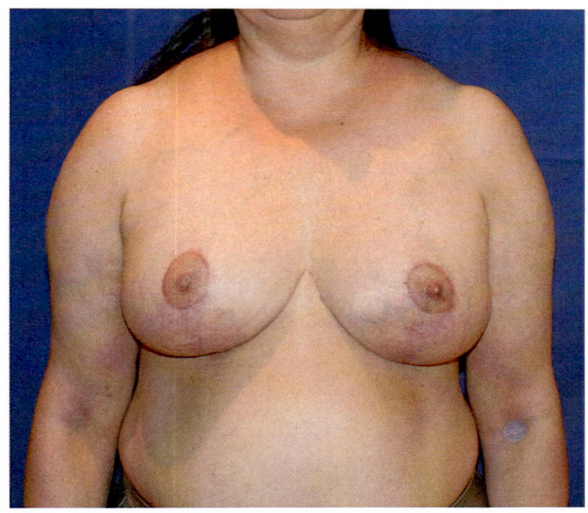

Fig. 20.15 Patient B: 18 months postoperative, with 1350 g removed from the right breast and 1500 g from the left breast and the nevus

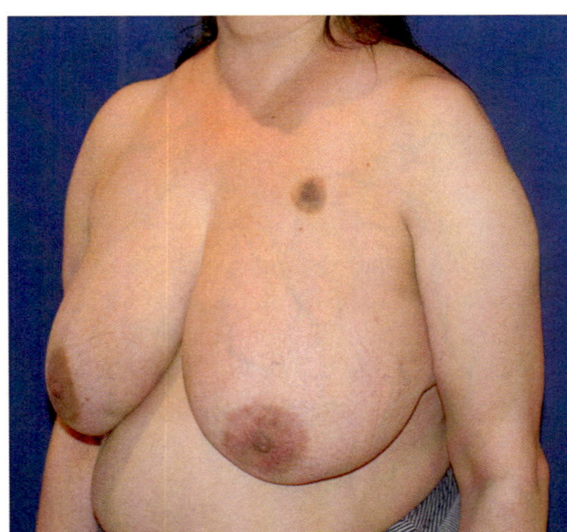

Fig. 20.16 Patient B: preoperative

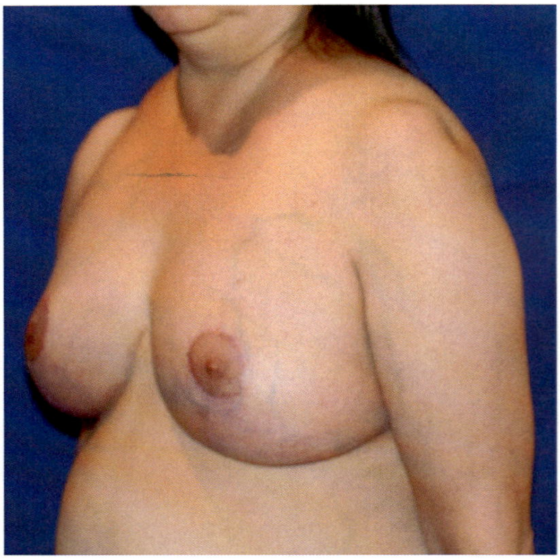

Fig. 20.17 Patient B: postoperative 3/4 view

20.3 Discussion

Multitudes of plastic surgery procedures are used to correct hypertrophic breasts (Bames 1948; Baroudi and Lewis 1976; Biesenberger 1931; Born 1994; Bustos 1988; Brauman 1994; Conway 1952; Courtiss 1993; Courtiss and Goldwym 1977; Costa et al. 2005, 2008; de Benito and Sanza 1993; de Castro 1976; Dufourmentel 1939; Farina 1972; Ferreira et al. 1995; Gillies and McIndoe 1939; Hawtof et al. 1989; Johnson 1976; Shin et al. 1996; Koger et al. 1994; Lassus 1996; Lejour 1994; May 1956; McKissock 1972; Meijer 1974); Pitanguy 1960. The idea to use a superior lateral pedicle for reduction mammoplasty started with the thin superior medial pedicle (Costa et al. 2008). As described in the literature (Skoog 1963), the thicker superior medial pedicle and lateral pedicle have a problem: it is difficult to transpose the NAC. Furthermore, there are issues with blood flow, which can compromise the viability of the NAC.

These problems have been solved by thinning the pedicle. With a thin pedicle, transposition is easier. Furthermore, the problem with blood circulation in the NAC (an excess of arterial flow and poor venous drainage) are eliminated. Decreasing the width of the pedicle reduces the arterial flow comparing with the venous drainage, thus preventing thrombosis and necrosis of the areola.

When the thin superior medial pedicle is used, the nutrition comes from the internal mammary arteries and their branches. When the thin superior lateral pedicle is used, the nutrition comes from the lateral thoracic and thoracodorsal arteries and their branches. Which is the best pedicle? Theoretically, the internal mammary arteries provide better nutrition. However, we performed breast reconstructions for oncoplastic surgery using the thin superior medial pedicle on one side and the thin superior lateral pedicle on the other side with no differences in results between the two sides.

Although our technique uses a thin pedicle, similar outcomes can be achieved in different hands (Figs. 20.8, 20.9, 20.10, 20.11, 20.12, 20.13, 20.14, 20.15, 20.16 and 20.17). Patient satisfaction following this procedure was high.

20.4 Complications

Considering the large volume of tissue removed and the size of the operated breasts, few complications were observed. The complications were similar to those reported for other techniques described in literature (Costa et al. 2005; de Benito and Sanza 1993; Lassus 1996; McKissock 1972; Pandeya 1995; Sampaio Goes 1996).

Complications for the 80 patients who underwent this procedure between 2006 and 2016 are listed in Table 20.1. One patient developed seroma (1.1%) without further problems. There was one case (1.1%) of small volume hematoma, which was evacuated by punctures with no need for reoperation. In

Table 20.1 Complications

Complications	Number of cases	%
Seroma	1	1.2
Hematoma	1	1.2
Infection	0	0
Areola necrosis	0	0
Skin ischemia	2	2.4
Radiodermitis	40	50
Fat necrosis	45	56.2

three patients (3.3%) with inverted T scars, superficial skin ischemia occurred and healed by secondary intention. There were no cases of areola infection or necrosis. The cases with radionecrosis and fat necrosis were patients with breast cancer treated by radiotherapy.

Conclusion

The results of this study clearly demonstrate that thin superior lateral pedicle reduction mammoplasty is a viable option for patients with severe mammary hypertrophy.

References

Bames HO (1948) Reduction of massive breast hypertrophy. Plast Reconstr Surg 3:560

Baroudi R, Lewis JR (1976) The augmentation-reduction mammaplasty. Clin Plast Surg 3:301

Biesenberger H (1931) Deformitaten und Hosmetishe Operationen der weiblichen Brust. Maudrich, Vienna

Born G (1994) The "L" reduction mammaplasty. Ann Plast Surg 32:383

Brauman D (1994) Reduction mammaplasty by suction alone. Plast Reconstr Surg 94:1095

Bustos R (1988) Mamaplastia periareolar. Communication to the XXVth Brazilian Congress of Plastic Surgery. Salvador

Conway H (1952) Mammaplasty: analysis of 110 consecutive cases with end-results. Plast Reconstr Surg 10:303

Costa MP, Tuma P Jr, Ferreira MC (2005) Reduction mammaplasty with resection of a trapezoid base prism and adduction of the arms. Plast Reconstr Surg 116(1):242–250

Costa MP, Ching AW, Ferreira MC (2008) Thin superior medial pedicle reduction mammaplasty for severe mammary hypertrophy. Aesthet Plast Surg 32(4):645–652

Courtiss EH (1993) Reduction mammaplasty by suction alone. Plast Reconstr Surg 92:1276

Courtiss EH, Goldwym RM (1977) Reduction mammaplasty by the inferior pedicle technique. An alternative to free nipple and areola grafting for sever macromastia or extreme ptosis. Plast Reconstr Surg 59:500

de Benito J, Sanza IF (1993) Periareolar techniques for mammary reduction and elevation. Aesthet Plast Surg 17:311

de Castro CC (1976) Mammaplasty with curved incisions. Plast Reconstr Surg 57:596

Dufourmentel L (1939) Chirurgie reparatrice et correctrice des téguments et des formes. Masson, Paris

Farina R (1972) Reduction mammaplasty with free grafting of the nipple and areola. Br J Plast Surg 25:393

Ferreira MC, Ishida J, Gemperli R, Monteiro AA Jr, Tuma PT Jr (1995) Reduction mammoplasty with shortened scars: surgical technique. Rev Hosp Fac Med São Paulo 50:22

Gillies H, McIndoe AH (1939) The technique of mammaplasty in conditions of hypertrophy of the breast. Surg Gynecol Obstet 68:658

Hawtof DB, Levine M, Kapetanski DI, Pieper D (1989) Complications of reduction mammaplasty: comparison of nipple-areolar graft and pedicle. Ann Plast Surg 23:3

Johnson CF (1976) New technique for reduction mammaplasty. Plast Reconstr Surg 57:372

Koger KE, Sundle D, Press BH, Hovey LM (1994) Reduction mammaplasty for gigantomastia using inferiorly based pedicle and free nipple transplantation. Plast Reconstr Surg 33:561

Lassus C (1996) A 30-tear experience with vertical mammaplasty. Plast Reconstr Surg 97:373

Lejour M (1994) Vertical mammaplasty and liposuction of the breast. Plast Reconstr Surg 94:100

May H (1956) Breast plasty in the female. Plast Reconstr Surg 17:351

McKissock PK (1972) Reduction mammaplasty with a vertical dermal flap. Plast Reconstr Surg 49:245

Meijer R (1974) A modified Aufricht reduction mammaplasty. Plast Reconstr Surg 53:129

Melega JM, Zanini SA, Psillakis JM (1992) Cirurgia Plástica Reparadora e Estética, 2nd edn. Medsi, Rio de Janeiro, pp 707–724

Pandeya NK (1995) Another technique for reduction mammaplasty. Plast Reconstr Surg 95:774

Pitanguy I (1960) Breast hypertrophy. In: Transactions of the International Society of Plastic Surgeons, Second Congress, London 1969. Edinburgh, Livingstone, p 509

Rees TD (1971) An historical review of mammaplasty. In: Transactions of the Fifth International Congress of Plastic and Reconstructive Surgery. Butterworths, Glen Waverley, Australia pp 1167–1173

Rees TD, LaTrenta GS (1994) Aesthetic plastic surgery, vol 2, 2nd edn, pp 925–1002

Regnault P (1974) Reduction mammaplasty by the "B" technique. Plast Reconstr Surg 53:19

Sampaio Goes JC (1996) Periareolar mammaplasty: double skin technique with application of polyglactine or mixed mesh. Plast Reconstr Surg 97:959

Shin KS, Chung S, Lee HK, Lew JD (1996) Reduction mammaplasty by central pedicle with short submammary scar. Aesthet Plast Surg 20:69

Skoog T (1963) A technique of breast reduction: transposition of the nipple on a cutaneous vascular prdicle. Acta Chir Scand 126:453

Strombeck JO (1971) Reduction mammaplasty. Surg Clin North Am 51:453

21 Reduction Mastoplasty and Mastopexy: Personal Approach Based on Other Techniques

José Carlos de Miranda and Miriam Fialka

21.1 Introduction

Surgeries for mammary reduction and mastopexy have evolved greatly over the decades.

In the literature, there is an enormous number of publications and scientific works, with a great diversity of behaviors, but there are some determined maneuvers that are basic in their execution. However, it is difficult to clarify the initial authorship of these techniques, tactics or approaches (Ribeiro 1975).

Reviewing the techniques on which the personal approach we use is based, we see that some techniques are very old. The better knowledge of the anatomy of the breasts that ensures safer in surgical behaviors requires more recent techniques that brought the author to his current personal surgical approach.

Thus, in this retrospective study, we see the importance of Villandre—1911, with the transposition of the nipple–areola complex (NAC) (Schwarzmann 1930); Lexer—1912, who left periareolar and subareolar scars in the shape of an inverted T, but without Schwarzmann's maneuver (Fernandez 1951).

Also worthy of citation is the technique of Lotsch—1923, with final scars to the periareolar and infra-areolar vertical line (Lexer 1912); Schwarzmann—1930, with the maneuver of the transposition of the NAC, through a dermal–adipose–glandular pedicle, (Sinder et al. 2012).

One of the techniques that influenced our current marking was established by Arié, who demonstrated his technique using Schwarzmann's maneuver an infra-areolar resection in a wedge shape and transposition of the NAC (Arié 1957).

Our current approach was influenced by the technique with which we initiated our mammaplasty surgeries, idealized by Pitanguy—1961, with individualized dermal–adipose–glandular resection in each case that, after Schwarzmann's maneuver, was dependent on factors such as volume, elasticity of the skin, and consistency of the breast (Lotsch 1925; Pitanguy 1977, 1978).

The technique of Pontes, with the section of the breast at a right angle with the thoracic wall, 2 cm below the NAC complex, allowed the breast to have better fullness with regard to the skin–fat relationship and of the mammary gland, with a firmer consistency after surgery, bringing support to our personal approach (Toledo 1989).

Ribeiro and Backer, who had conceived a decorticated flap based on an inferior pedicle, to the level of the submammary fold, that is, fixed in the fascia of the pectoralis major muscle, with the objective of providing a more voluminous and persistent superior mammary pole, brought the possibility of, when necessary, adjusting this remnant in our personal approach (Pontes 1981).

J.C. de Miranda, M.D. (✉) • M. Fialka, M.D.
Plastic Surgery, Clinica Miranda,
Curitiba, PR, Brazil
e-mail: j.miranda@uol.com.br

J.M. Avelar (ed.), *Breast Surgery*, https://doi.org/10.1007/978-3-319-54115-0_21

Bozola, with his technique, allowed a simplified vision of the mammary excess to be resected (Bozola et al. 1982).

Chidid, with the use of denuded triangular flaps in the distal portion of the flaps sutured below the areola, provided us, in our approach, with reinforcement in the union of the vertical scar (Chidid 1984).

Benelli, with a periareolar suture in the "tobacco pouch" of the cutaneous incision, allowed better periareolar cutaneous distribution, in addition to the reduction of the tension on the scar to this level, bringing to our personal approach a touch of the "foreign author," which results in a final scar of better quality (Benelli 1990).

Toledo, using liposuction in reducing periareolar mammaplasty, brought a contribution to our personal approach, in the case of small asymmetries, after surgery (Peixoto 1985).

Avelar, in 1993, with the publication of his book showed the advantages of a smaller scar and the possibilities of carrying out the surgery under local anesthesia (Avelar 1993).

Peixoto, who made a small cutaneous incision, even in large glandular resections, based on the concept of the contractility of the skin. The cutaneous envelope is readjusted to the content that was reduced (Peixoto 1979, 1980, 1984).

21.2 Objective

The objective of the present chapter is to present the author's personal approach to breast reduction surgery and mastopexy, based on the techniques that the author has observed over four decades of comment and experience in his professional life.

21.3 Technique

The approach used by the author is based primarily on the techniques attributed to Schwarzmann, Arié, Pitanguy, Peixoto, Pontes, Ribeiro, Chidid, and Benelli, with additional influence from the experience of other professional specialists from Brazil, and the acquired personal experience throughout the years of professional life.

Peixoto's technique, on which we rely too much in our personal approach, is based on the concept of contractility of the skin, Thus, in hypertrophy, amputation of the base of the breast is carried out, by a volume that seems appropriate (Fig. 21.1a), with the security of knowing that the irrigation and innervation will be supplied within the thickness proposed for the cutaneous–adipose remnants (Fig. 21.1b). For the mastopexy cases, the mammary parenchyma is retained as considered necessary.

In the assembly of the breast, with or without glandular resection, the portion of previous mammary cone that was retained is adapted to the thoracic wall, and the excess cutaneous–adipose remnant suffers from a process of retraction and readjustment to the new content (Fig. 21.1c, d).

The marking of the skin resection of the breast obeys the rules divulged by Peixoto's technique, where point A is marked using a simple bidigital maneuver, usually corresponding to the projection of the submammary fold, in the midline of the mammary cone. The confluence of points BC is also marked by a bidigital maneuver. Point D can be marked 1–3 cm from the submammary fold, according the excess tissue (Fig. 21.2a, b).

The marking of segment BCD is also made using a bidigital maneuver (Fig. 21.2c).

The diameter of the ABC marking, the distance between B and C, and the longitude of the segments BD and CD are changeable, in agreement with the volume and consistency of the breast, and the elasticity of the mammary skin. In breasts with pronounced flaccidity, the marking is directly effected using bidigital maneuvers; in more compact and more glandular breasts, the final marking will be about 1 cm inside the area previously marked (Fig. 21.2d).

Initiating the surgery, we proceed to Schwarzmann's maneuver in the periareolar region, with decortication of the marked region. In cases in which a more voluminous superior pole is necessary, we can use the remnant of Ribeiro's inferior pedicle, and proceed to decorticate the skin from the whole area demarcated in the mammary skin. The resultant remnant is sutured

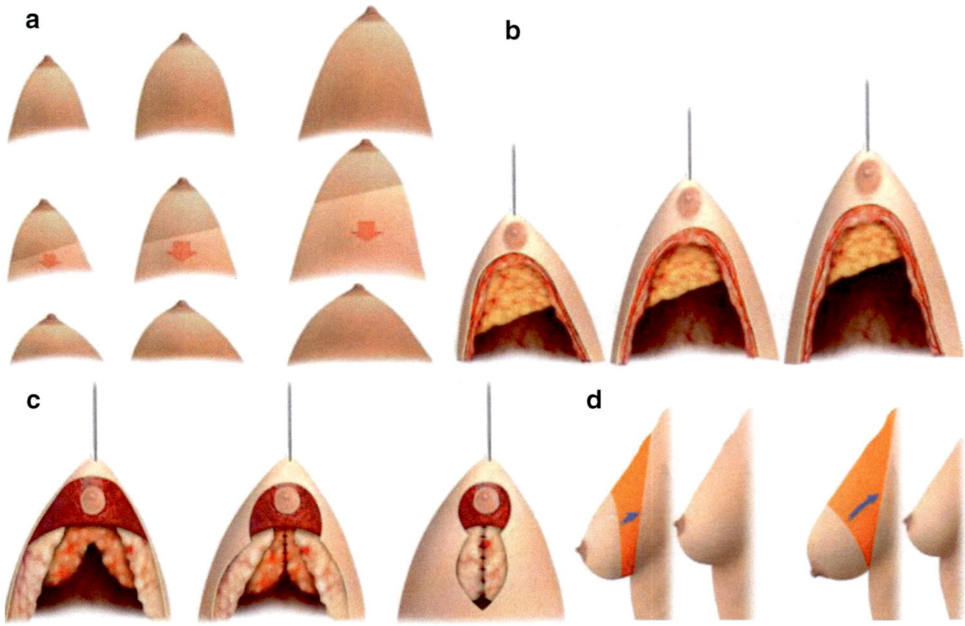

Fig. 21.1 Concepts of Peixoto's technique. (**a**) Amputation of the base of the breast, by appropriate volume. (**b**) Nerves, artery and vein are in the thickness of flaps (**c**), (**d**) In the reconstruction of the breast, the portion of the remaining mammary cone fits at the thoracic wall, with retraction of skin and better adaptation of the remaining dermal–adipose tissue

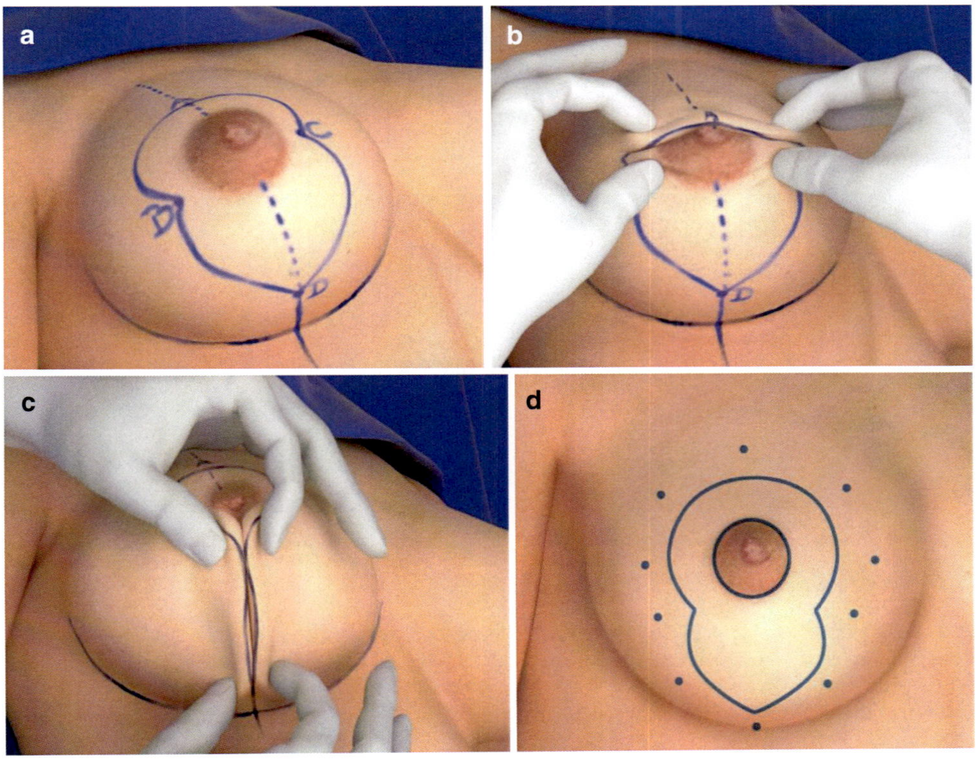

Fig. 21.2 Marking of the breast for the personal approach. (**a**) Breast already marked with its points ABCD. (**b**) Bidigital maneuvers in the marking of the breast. (**c**) Marking of the cutaneous excess in the inferior polar region of the breast. (**d**) Final configuration of the marking, according to the cutaneous flaccidity and consistency of the breast

to the aponeurosis of the pectoralis major muscle (Fig. 21.3a).

The dermal incision that we make in the segments that will result in the vertical scar is made about 1 cm inside the incision effected in the superficial portion of the skin (Fig. 21.3b).

In cases in which Ribeiro's pedicle is not used, we proceed to the detachment of the mammary tissue content, including the remaining lateral and medial flaps, up to the corresponding level of what would be the area of incision of the remaining medial and lateral flaps of Pitanguy's technique (Fig. 21.3c, d).

The lateral and medial skin and fat flaps that are detached in the transition between the fat tissue and glandular tissue must have a thickness of about 1.5 to 2.5 cm, depending on the thickness of the existing skin flap, which it will make with the vascular track that will provide a blood supply to the remaining flap of tissue (Fig. 21.4a).

The amputation of the base of the breast and its lateral and medial flaps, in addition to the excision of excess conforms to the corporeal proportionality, but respecting the criteria for personal and patient proportionality. Another possibility is to retain all the content, to comprise what after the surgery will be the final mammary volume (Fig. 21.4b).

The excision of the excess could be carried out selectively from its remaining lateral, medial, and inferior pole region, in addition to the base of the breast, respecting the Pitanguy's excision tech-

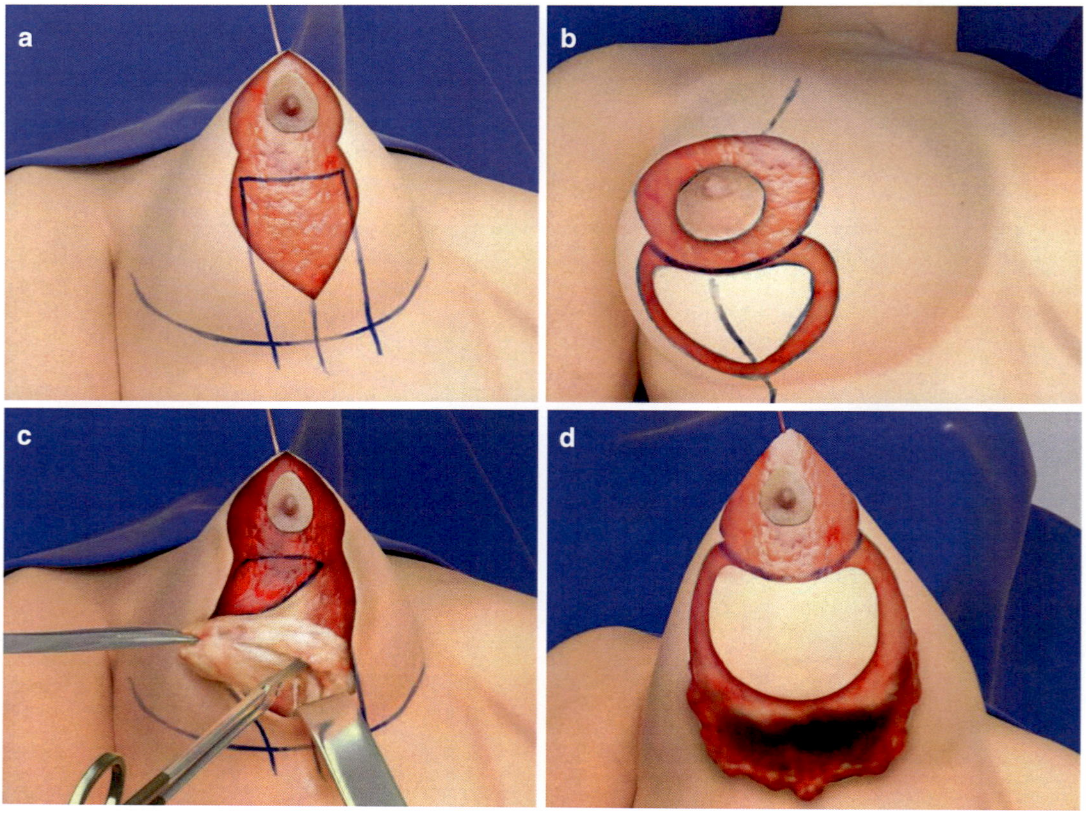

Fig. 21.3 Beginning of the surgery. (**a**) Periareolar or total decortication of the demarcated area, configuration of Ribeiro's pedicle when necessary. (**b**) In cases in which we do not use a pedicle, we make an incision in the inferior segment 1 cm inside the cutaneous incision, preserving a little of the dermis. (**c**), (**d**) Detachment of the breast at its base

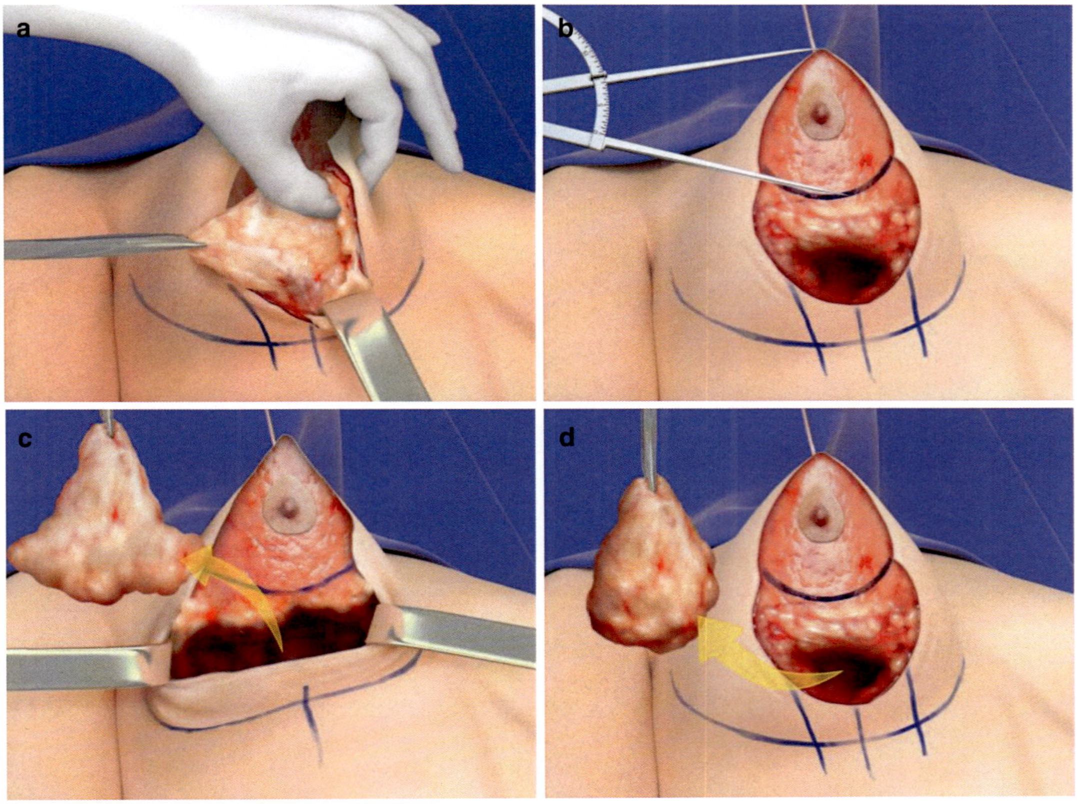

Fig. 21.4 Detachment and choice of tissue to be preserved. (**a**) Lateral and medial flaps with a thickness of 1.5–2 cm. (**b**) Measurement of tissue to be preserved. (**c**) Selective excision of excess tissue attributed to Pitanguy. (**d**) Resection attributed to Pontes

nique in its central portion, when we want to reduce the width of the mammary base (Fig. 21.4c), or the excision attributed to Pontes, when we want a more compact breast (Fig. 21.4d).

The volume of the mammary tissue remaining after the resection of the affected tissue varies in accordance with the above-mentioned proportionality criteria (Fig. 21.5a). The dermal periareolar flap will have an infra-areolar prolongation, which, when pulled and sutured, will serve as reinforcement, as a brace, to the mammary cone to be restored in agreement with the technique attributed to Chidid (Fig. 21.5b).

In the assembly of the breast, we proceed with the approach from the medial and lateral flaps for the medial line, through the points of nylon suture 2–0 or 3–0, in addition to the personal criterion of whether or not to carry out the suturing of the flap to the aponeurosis of the pectoralis major muscle at the level of the second costal arc, also with two the three wire points of nylon 3-0 (see Fig. 21.9). These steps will cause the breast to rise, determining a new position next to the chest wall (Fig. 21.1d).

After reconstitution of the breast cone, in its glandular and fat tissue, we proceed to make a dermal tape in accordance with Chidid's technique, as the figure has already demonstrated, using an inverted suture with nylon 3-0 (Fig. 21.5c–d).

Suture of periareolar area, in a "tobacco pouch" shape with nylon 3–0, using Benelli's technique, causing a reduction of the diameter of the NAC to be sutured, with consequent traction and better accommodation of the dermal–adipose

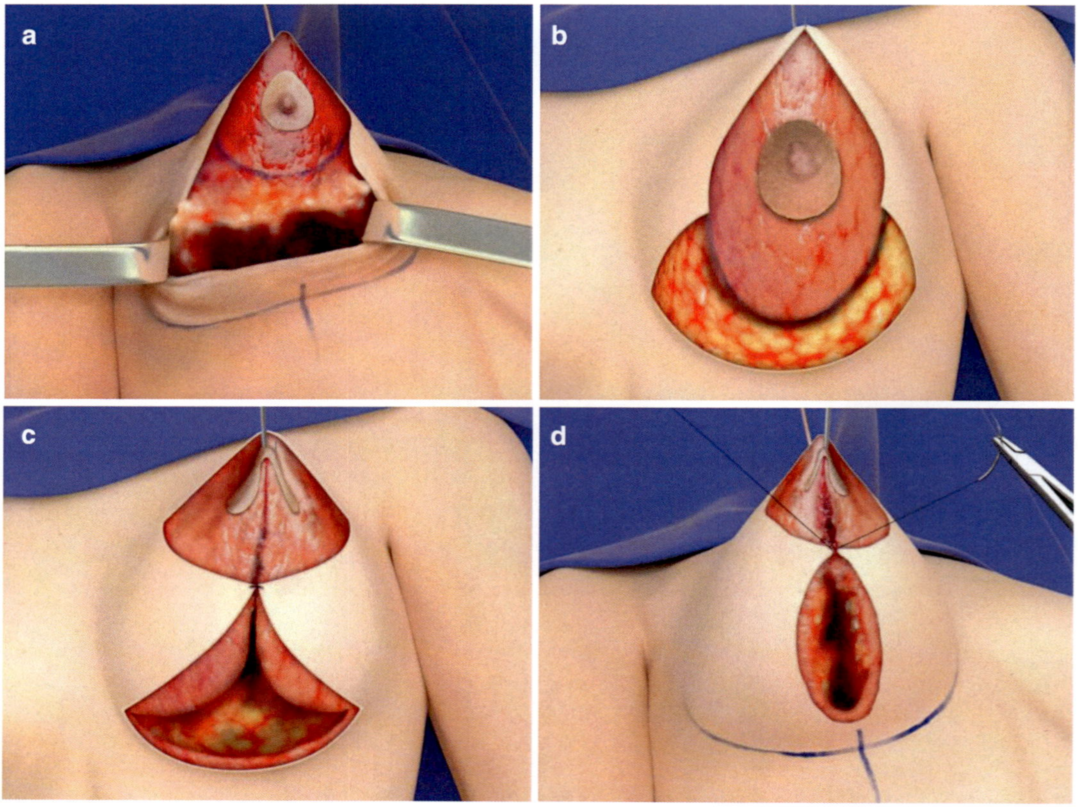

Fig. 21.5 (**a**) The remaining cutaneous tissue obeys the proportionality criteria and (**b**) the dermal periareolar flap has a sub-areolar prolongation. (**c**, **d**) Reconstruction of the breasts using the dermal fat flap to effect a dermal brace to reinforce the inferior polar region, according to Chedid

flap around the mammary cone, in addition to less tension in the scar, preventing a posterior widening of the scar to the periareolar area (Fig. 21.6a). The suturing of the cutaneous tissue is complemented by an intra-dermal suture with polyvicryl no. 3 (Fig. 21.6b).

In cases of intense cutaneous flaccidity, where we observe the presence of redundant skin in the inferior portion of the vertical scar ("dog ear"), we can make an immediate correction by carrying out a small longitudinal cutaneous resection (Fig. 21.6c). If there is only a small amount of redundant skin, correction is not effected immediately; therefore, the excess that is initially present may spontaneously resolve in the subsequent weeks or months (up to 4 months). After this period, if necessary, we carry out the correction of a smaller area of tissue excess, resulting in a minor longitudinal scar (Fig. 21.6d).

As final procedure, we carry out superior traction of the breast with a strengthened hook, Micropore tape is then placed on the breast where it is retained for 7–10 days, contributing to the adequacy of the remaining dermal–adipose tissue around the mammary cone (Fig. 21.7).

The operative sequence is demonstrated in (Figs. 21.8, 21.9, 21.10, 21.11).

21.4 Results

In the surgeries we have carried out since concluding our post-graduate studies, that is, 40 years, we observed that in the first 7 years we used solely

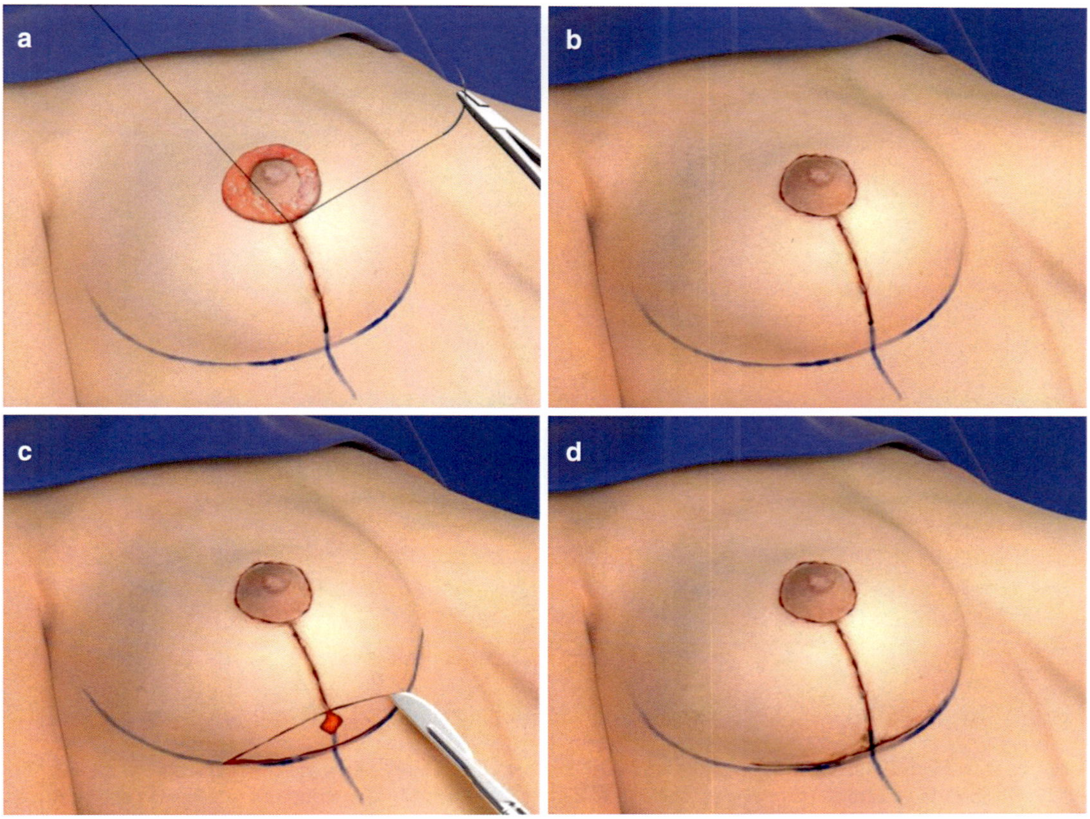

Fig. 21.6 (**a**) Benelli's maneuver for periareolar suture. (**b**) Intra-dermal cutaneous suture. (**c**), (**d**) In cases of tissue excess to the level of the mammary sulcus, the correction can be effected immediately or the patient can wait for 4–6 months for spontaneous resolution or minor correction retrospectively

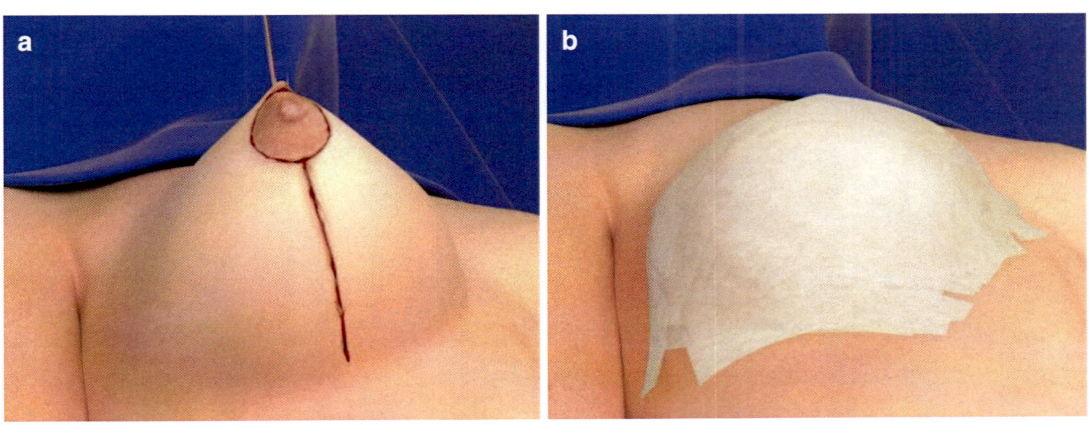

Fig. 21.7 (**a**, **b**) Elevation with a reinforced hook and held in place by Micropore tape for 7–10 days

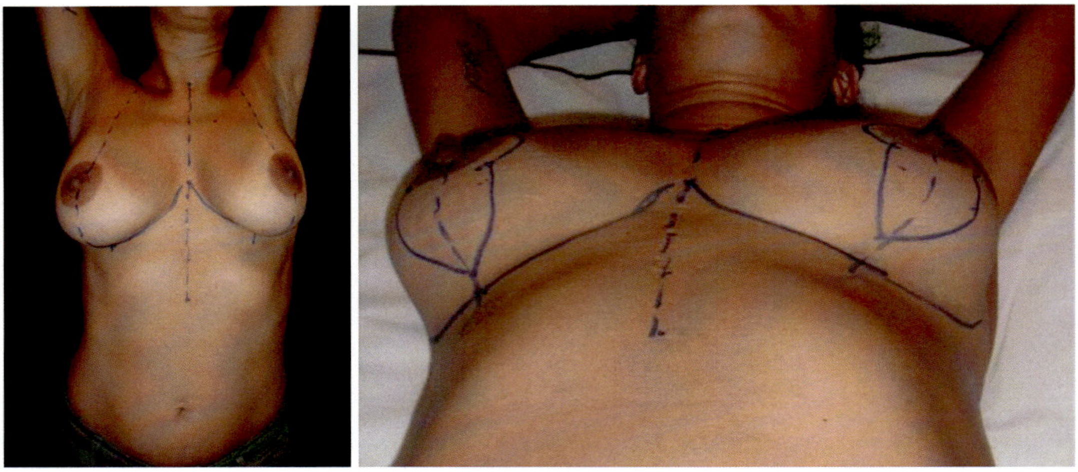

Fig. 21.8 (a) Breast hypertrophy with ptosis and asymmetry. (b) Breast marked as previously explained

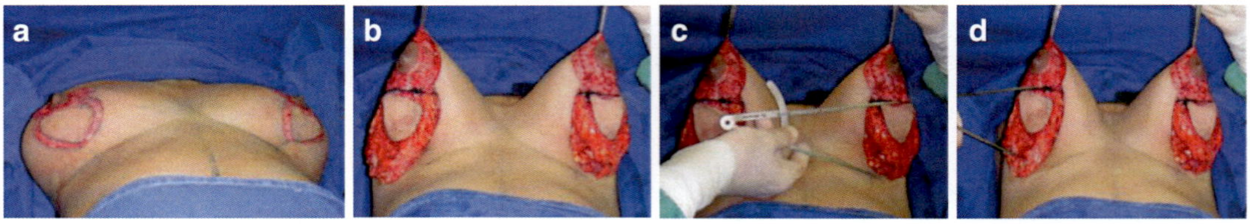

Fig. 21.9 Decortication and detachment of the breast. (a) Decortication with narrow maintenance of dermal remnant 0.5–1.5 cm in width. (b) Detachment of the breast with the existing asymmetry and marking of the area to be dried. (c), (d) Measuring the resection to perform in the breasts.

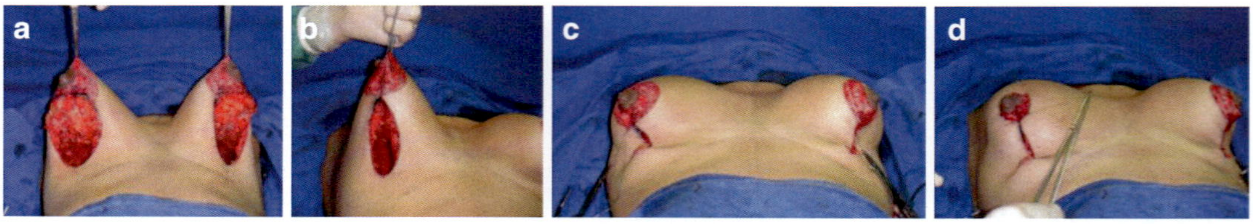

Fig. 21.10 (a) Glandular and fat tissue already dried up. (b), (c) Assembly of the breast using the approach already described in the text and the images. (d) Periareolar suture using Benelli's technique

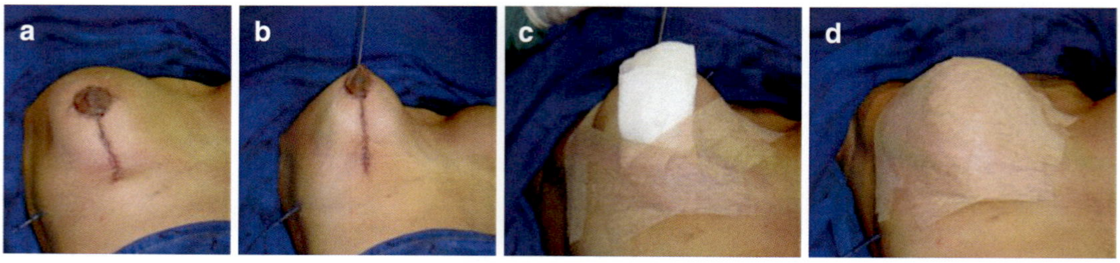

Fig. 21.11 (a) Assembly of the finished breast. (b) Elevation of the breast with use of a strong hook. (c), (d) End of the bandage with Micropore tape on the breast

the marking technique attributed to Pitanguy. Since then, with the greater spread of new approaches and techniques, we have added and incorporated new tactics that have resulted in the way in which we currently approach cases of breast hypertrophy and mastopexy.

In case 1, we have a patient with breast hypertrophy degree 2 pre- (Fig. 21.12a–c) and 6 months postoperatively (Fig. 21.12d–f).

In case 2, we have a patient with mammary ptosis with intense flaccidity and large weight loss of the patient preoperatively (Fig. 21.13a–c) and 6 months postoperatively, with conservation of all the mammary tissue in the plastic repair (Fig. 21.13d–f).

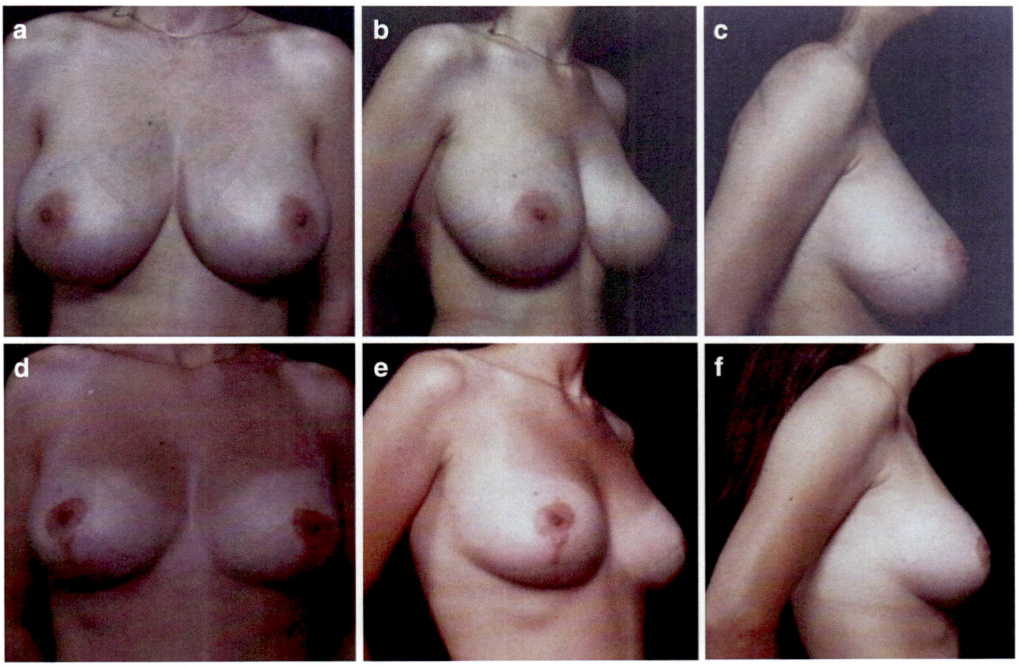

Fig. 21.12 (**a–c**) Preoperative photos of medium hypertrophy. (**d–f**) Results 6 months postoperatively using our personal approach

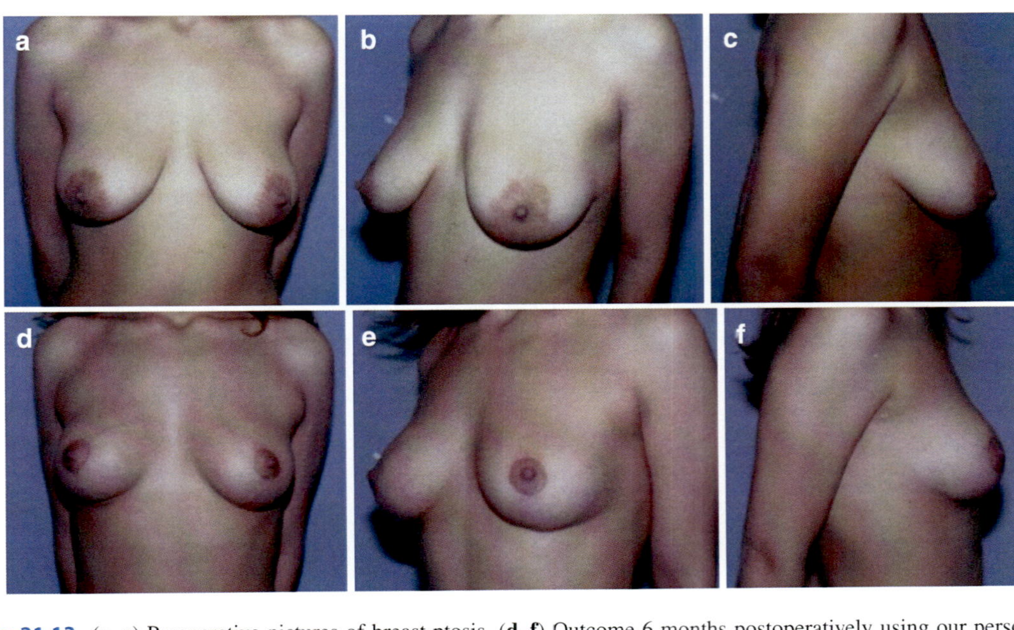

Fig. 21.13 (**a–c**) Preoperative pictures of breast ptosis. (**d–f**) Outcome 6 months postoperatively using our personal approach

In case 3, we present a patient with breast hypertrophy degree 1 (Fig. 21.14b, c), 6 months postoperatively (Fig. 21.14d–f), 1 year, 9 months postoperatively (Fig. 21.14g–i), and 6 years, 9 months postoperatively when the patient had regained weight (Fig. 21.14j–l).

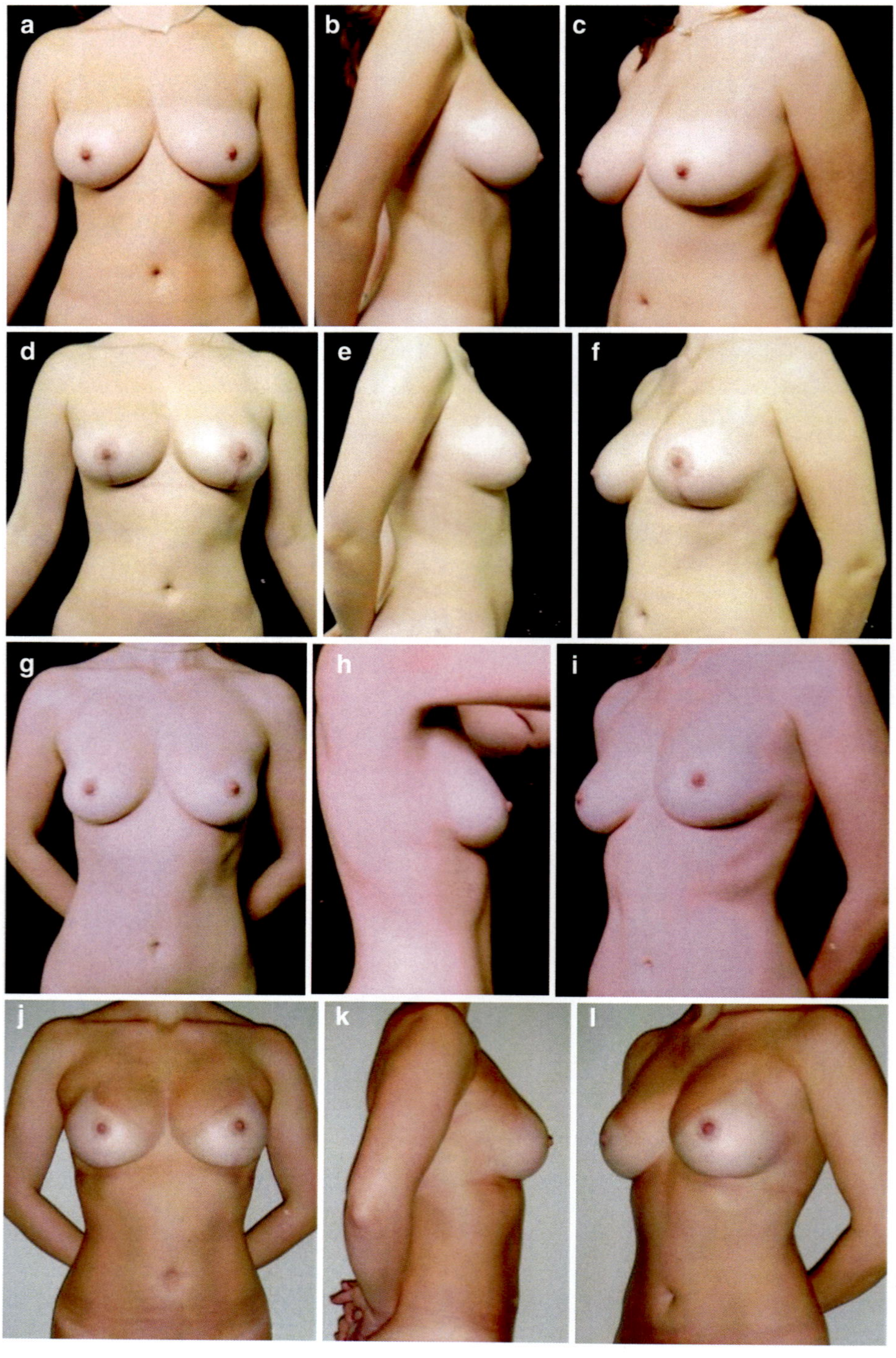

Fig. 21.14 (**a–c**) Preoperative pictures. (**d–f**) Photos after 6 months postoperatively using our personal approach. (**g–i**) Photos of the same patient 1 year and 9 months postoperatively, after thinning and reduction of breast volume. (**j–l**) Photos of the same patient 6 years and 9 months postoperatively, after regaining her usual weight

21.5 Complications

The complications were in accordance with those observed by other authors, corresponding to the possible occurrence of hematomas, seromas, and cutaneous infectious processes in small areas.

As unfavorable results, we had in some cases the presence of redundant cutaneous tissue in the region of the submammary fold, which needed to be corrected in agreement with the demonstrated procedure already shown, resulting a small longitudinal scar (Fig. 21.11a, b).

21.6 Discussion

Breast reduction surgery and/or mastopexy have been described since the end of the nineteenth century (Ribeiro 1975; Sinder 1970) and in agreement with the authors there was a scientific spread of the various techniques that have been carried out by innumerable colleagues with the opening the clinics and hospitals to other colleagues for demonstration of all techniques.

Still, according to Ramil, "the true authorship of numerous surgical maneuvers is often difficult to clarify, some being attributed to a number of surgeons. In some cases there may be a genuine coincidence, but in others, it has accidental or intentional distortions, overshadowing or erasing completely the names of modest surgeons of creative spirit. Also, the trend to forget or to ignore the past ends up creating controversies or a trend of showing as something new surgical maneuvers that have been carried out already." (Sinder 1970).

The techniques currently used for breast reduction have been in existence for more than 50 years, and continue to be executed. From the greatest knowledge of the mammary anatomy, new alternatives appeared, with the use of various techniques, to of improve the shape and consistency of the breasts, or to facilitate the migration of the NAC complex in cases of severe hypertrophy.

At the present time, greater evolution is difficult.

We have to evaluate this, because of the great variability of breast shapes, volumes, localizations, mammary gland tissue consistency, and elasticity of the skin, in addition to the fact that women have varying conditions of weight, lean or fat, or have undergone bariatric surgery or pregnancy, and others in whom the surgical procedures executed for mastopexy or reduction will vary. One single procedure does not exist that is ideal for all situations, and at the same time, it is impracticable to use a different technique for each patient.

We need to think about the balance of the volumes of the upper pole of the breast, about the position of the NAC complex, about the position of the breast itself, and about the implantation and consistency of the breast. However, what can be deduced, it is that an ideal breast is not possible.

Some considerations of the technique attributed to Peixoto who in our opinion did not have in his professional career did not receive the recognition he deserved, lad us to think about the key factors for optimal surgery:

(a) Systematic detachment of the base of the breast, leaving behind the deep planes; no damage of the vascular circulation; allows good visualization for the resection of the excess tissue; facilitates hemostasis, and makes possible the location of the new base in its normal plane.
(b) The procedure of amputation of the base of the mammary cone in various amounts, depending on how much to leave for the final volume; if the approach used is to give the breast a cone shape, after amputation, a smaller cone remains.
(c) Taking into account the elasticity of the skin, which allows its retraction on the remaining content, with consequent readjustment of the shape if intended; it must be observed that the skin suffers from the phenomenon of retraction, because of its diverse variability (age, presence of stretch marks, weight loss, etc.).
(d) Attempting to retain the integral function of the organ, preventing anatomical injuries to the breast; the presence of multiple flaps, crossed or under other anatomical structures, certainly will cause damage in future interventions, or the analysis of complementary examinations of the breast.
(e) The extent of the scar is very important, how much smaller and better; when the scar remains inside the mammary area proper,

the quality is better; it has the aesthetic advantage of the longitudinal scar being on the horizontal line.

One of the basic principles of surgical tactics in the personal approach presented here is the reduction in the number of incisions, with the consequent lesser perception of the resultant scars, in addition to a shape that will be compromised little over the years.

Conclusion

The proposed personal approach allows the less correction of large breast hypertrophy, and mastopexy, where the resultant cutaneous scar is as small as possible, with no effect on the shape, an issue that has already been discussed for several decades, that is, scars versus shape of the breasts.

Each time it is performed, our personal approach becomes more applicable to the requirements of a modern world, which places people in a more competitive circle, where the time for the recovery from surgical procedures requires less and less time. When inappropriate scars and the currently artificial aspects of excellent surgery are questioned each time, we have to take care of a sector of the population that requires surgeries with less scarring without having an inappropriate effect on the shape, and fewer sequelae.

References

Arié G (1957) Nova técnica em mamaplastia. Rev Lat Amer Cir Plast 3:28

Avelar JM (1993) Mastoplastia redutora sob anestesia local: Anestesia Loco Regional em Cirurgia Estética. Editora Hipócrates, p 244–260

Benelli L (1990) A new periareolar mammaplasty: the "round block" technique. Aesth Plast Surg 14: 93–100

Bozola AR, Oliveira HC et al (1982) Mamoplastia em L: contribuição pessoal: R. AMRIGGS, Porto Alegre 26(3):207

Chidid N et al (1984) Cinta Dérmica em mamaplastia: Anais de Temas Livres—XXI Cong, Bras De Cir Plast, p 42

Fernandez O (1951) Mamaplastia redutora: Cirurgia Plástica da mama. MEDSI, Editora Medica Científica LTDA: Histórico, p 12

Lexer (1912), E Muenchen Med. Wchnscher. Nr p 49 Cited in Mamaplastia redutora: Cirurgia Plástica da Mama, 2ª Edição, Ribeiro L; Medbook – Editora Científica; Chapter 1- Mamaplastia redutora: Histórico, p 3

Lotsch G M (1925) Operationen und der Weiblichen Brust, In: Bier A, Braun H and Kummel (Eds), cited in Mamaplastia redutora: Cirurgia Plástica da Mama 1989. MEDSI – Editora Medica Científica LTDA: Histórico, p 5

Peixoto G (May 1979) Reduction mammaplasty: a personal method. In: Transactions of the 7th International Congress of Plastic and Reconstructive Surgery, Rio de Janeiro, Brazil, p 551–553

Peixoto G (1980) Reduction mammaplasty: a personal technique. Plast Reconst Surg 65:217

Peixoto G (1984) Reduction mammaplasty. Aesth Plast Surg 8:231–236

Peixoto G (1985) The infra-areolar longitudinal incision in reduction mamaplasty. Aesth Plast Surg 9:1–5

Pitanguy I (1967) Surgical treatment of breast hypertrophy. Br J Plast Surg 20:78

Pitanguy I (1977) The Pitanguy Procedure, Cited in: Reconstructive Plastic Surgery, Converse, Vol. 7 Second Edition; W. B. Saunders Company: p 3677–3680

Pitanguy I (1978) Mamaplastia. Editora Guanabara Koogan S. A., Rio de Janeiro, Capítulo 4, Técnicas Operatórias, p 50–52

Pontes R (1981) Reduction mammaplasty – variations I & II. Ann Plast Surg 6(6):437

Ribeiro L (1975) A new technique for reduction mammaplasty. Plast Reconstr Surg 55(3):330

Schwarzmann (1930), E. Die Technik der Mammaplastik. Der Chir. 2(932)

Sinder R (1970) Mamaplastia, Tese apresentada à Faculdade de Medicina para concorrer à Livre Docência, Rio de Janeiro, Brasil

Sinder R et al cited in Mamaplastia redutora: Cirurgia Plástica da Mama, Liacyr Ribeiro (2ª Edição), MEDSI – Editora Medica Científica LTDA, Histórico; p 1

Toledo L et al (1989) cited in Mamaplastia redutora: Cirurgia Plástica da Mama, Liacyr Ribeiro. MEDSI – Editora Medica Científica LTDA: Histórico, p 32

Villandre C (1925) Cited by Dartigues, L.: Arch Franco-Belges Chir, 28: 325

Personal Technique: Reduction Mastoplasty in Gigantomastia with Thin Superior Medial Pedicle

22

Márcio Paulino Costa, Guilherme Cardinal Barreiro, and Nuberto H. Teixeira

22.1 Introduction

There are many techniques used to correct hypertrophic and pendulous breasts using plastic surgery (Bames 1948; Baroudi and Lewis 1976; Biesenberger 1931; Born 1994; Bustos 1988; Brauman 1994; Conway 1952; Courtiss 1993; Courtiss and Goldwyn 1977; Costa et al. 2005, 2008; Dartigues 1935; de Benito and Sanza 1993; de Castro 1976; Dufourmentel 1939; Farina 1972; Ferreira et al. 1995; Gillies and McIndoe 1939; Hawtof et al. 1989; Johnson 1976; Shin et al. 1996; Koger et al. 1994; Lassus 1996; Lejour 1994; May 1956; McKissock 1972; Melega et al. 1992; Pontes 1973; Rees 1971; Rees and LaTrenta 1994; Regnault 1974; Ribeiro 1975; Robbins 1977; Sampaio Goes 1996; Schatten et al. 1971; Varotto 1996; Skoog 1963; Strombeck 1971, 1960). In cases of gigantomastia, amputation with a free nipple graft is most frequently used. In such cases, its aesthetic limitations of loss of nipple projection, partial or total nipple necrosis, hypopigmentation of the nipple–areola complex (NAC) and loss of sensitivity are frequently present (Gillies and McIndoe 1939).

In patients with heavier and ptotic breasts, who need large resections of breast tissue, where the suprasternal notch-to-nipple distance is long, the use of nipple–areola transposition techniques is a challenge for the surgeon.

With the aim of solving these problems, the superior medial technique with a thin pedicle has been used by me and the gigantomastia group at the Hospital das Clinicas, USP School of Medicine, with excellent results (Costa et al. 2008).

This technique of reduction mammoplasty is based on the following principles: mammary reduction utilizing a thin superior medial pedicle (1.5–2.0 cm thick) and resection performed in two steps: (1) the base excess at a plane perpendicular to the breast (this determines the cone's height) and (2) a central half keel (this determines the reduction in the breast diameter).

22.2 Methods

More than 800 patients with breast hypertrophy have been operated on at Hospital das Clínicas, São Paulo University Medical School over the last 17 years. Definitions of severe breast hypertrophy are varied and include cup size, weight

M.P. Costa, M.D., Ph.D. (✉)
Hospital das Clínicas, University of São Paulo Medical School, Brazilian Society of Plastic Surgery, ISAPS, FILACAP, ASPS, Rua Gabriel dos Santos, 759 12 andar, Santa Cecília, 01231-011 São Paulo, SP, Brazil
e-mail: marciopaulino@bol.com.br

G.C. Barreiro, M.D., Ph.D.
University of Campinas (UNICAMP), Brazilian Society of Plastic Surgery, São Paulo, SP, Brazil
e-mail: guilhermecardinali@hotmail.com

N.H. Teixeira, M.D.
University of São Paulo Medical School, Brazilian Society of Plastic Surgery, São Paulo, SP, Brazil
e-mail: nubertoneto@uol.com.br

J.M. Avelar (ed.), *Breast Surgery*, https://doi.org/10.1007/978-3-319-54115-0_22

of the resected breast tissue, and the height of nipple elevation (Meijer 1974; Pitanguy 1965; Rees 1971).

Regarding breast shape, 100% of the patients belonged to type 2 according to Rees' classification (Meijer 1974; Pitanguy 1965; Rees 1971). According to Regnault, 100% had third-degree ptosis. (Rees and LaTrenta 1994). Neck pain, back pain, and bra strap indentations were reported by all patients. Breast measurements were obtained with the patient standing.

22.2.1 Preoperative Markings

Marking of the breast is done with the patient erect. The new, desired position of the areola is estimated by projecting the inframammary crease to a line that crosses the clavicular mid-point, whereas the future nipple is determined by the index finger (point A) (Fig. 22.1).

Points B and C are determined by the pinch test (using the thumbs and index fingers the skin of the breast is pinched together near the inferior border of the areola. The postoperative breast result could be visualized using this preoperative pinching maneuver (Fig. 22.1).

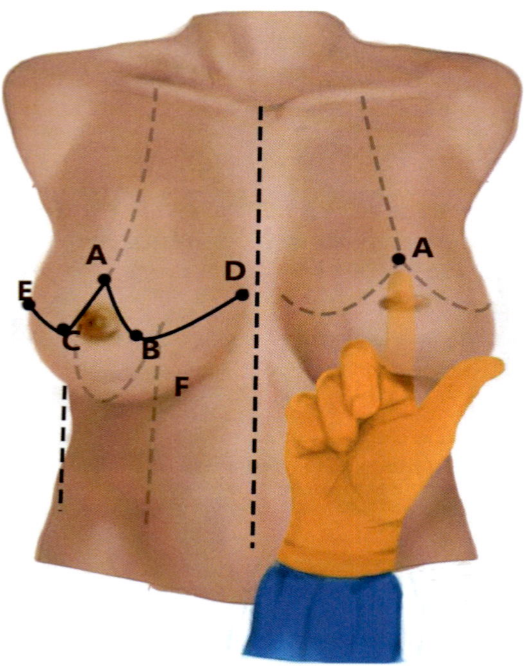

Fig. 22.1 Preoperative markings

According to the degree of hypertrophy and the amount of tissue resection, the length of the arm and the angle of the wedge resection are varied. The length of the medial arm (AB) is between 8 and 9 cm and the lateral arm (AC) is between 10 and 12 cm (Fig. 22.1) in most patients.

The breast is elevated and the inframammary crease marked.

With the thumb and index finger of one hand pinching the breast skin at the level of points B and C, the base limit of the resection is determined. The medial and lateral lines are marked connecting the points B to the medial and C to the lateral junctures of the inframammary crease (points D and E) (Fig. 22.1). Point F depends on the base width and may range between 10 and 12.5 cm (approximately half way between D and E) (Fig. 22.1).

22.2.2 Surgery

The patient is evaluated preoperatively (Figs. 22.2 and 22.3) and the marks are made (Fig. 22.4).

Incisions are made in the upper V and around the areola markings. The upper V and the subdermal plexus surrounding the nipple are de-epithelialized (Fig. 22.5).

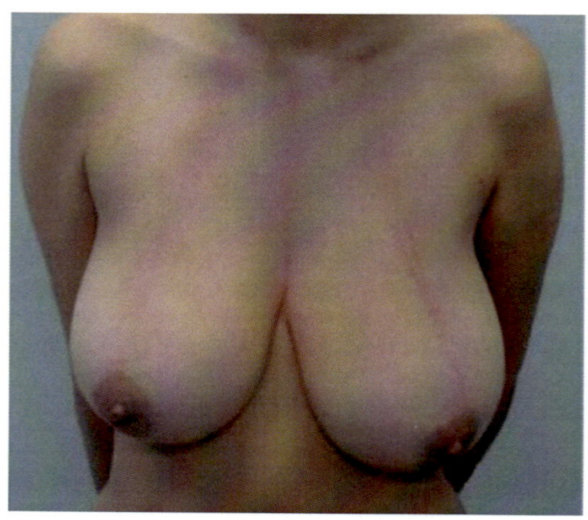

Fig. 22.2 Photo of the preoperative breast

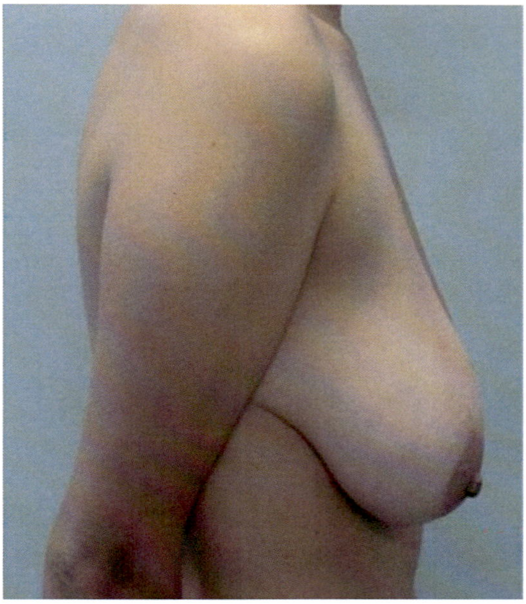

Fig. 22.3 Photo of the preoperative breast

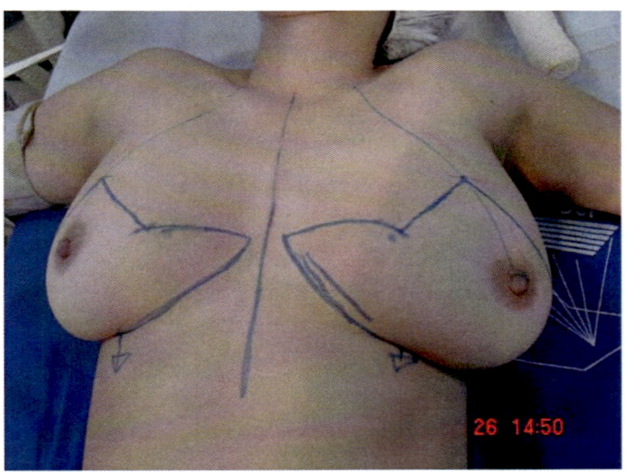

Fig. 22.4 Photo showing the preoperative markings

The operation begins with the patient in the supine position and arms adducted. The inframammary crease incision is made, and the breast is lifted off the deep surface of the superficial fascia over the pectoralis major (medially until the projection of point B over the pectoralis and laterally, far from the projection of point C over the pectoralis major).

The superior medial pedicle is marked. The width of the flap base is between 6 and 7 cm, leaving 1 cm in the upper part of the V and in the lower part of it. A line is drawn passing near the

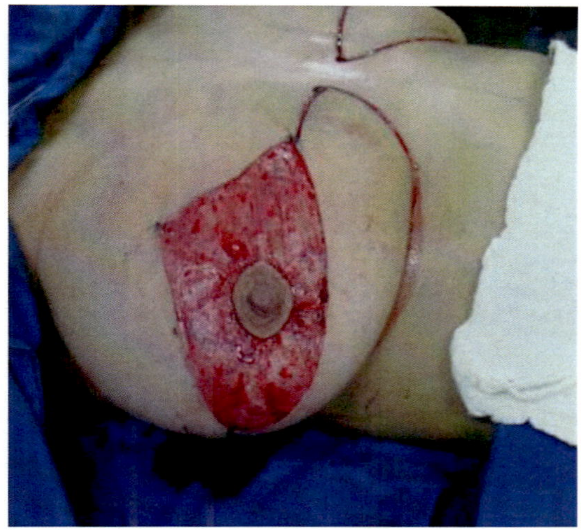

Fig. 22.5 Photo showing the upper V and the subdermal plexus surrounding the de-epithelialized nipple

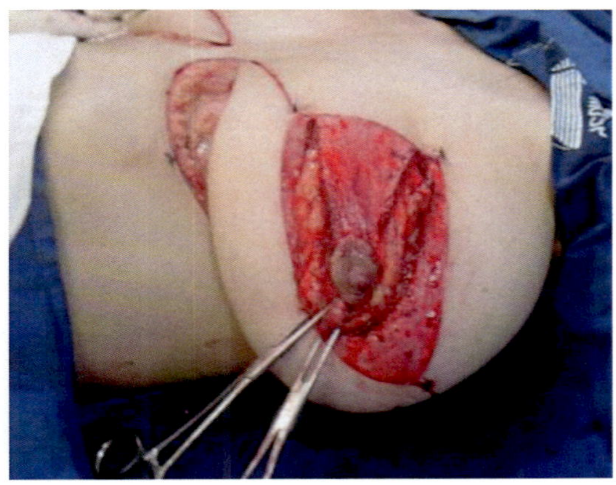

Fig. 22.6 Photo showing the undermined superomedial pedicle

areola. Therefore, the flap is undermined with 1.5 cm of thickness and is made progressively thicker at the base. While undermining the flap in the subcutaneous layer, it is important to include some glandular tissue beneath the areola (Fig. 22.6).

Next, resection of the excess mammary tissue is accomplished with the patient in an elevated position of 80 ° (nearly sitting up), in two steps: (1) the base excess at a plane perpendicular to the breast (this determines the height of the cone) (Fig. 22.7) and (2) a central half keel (this determines the reduction of the breast diameter) (Fig. 22.8).

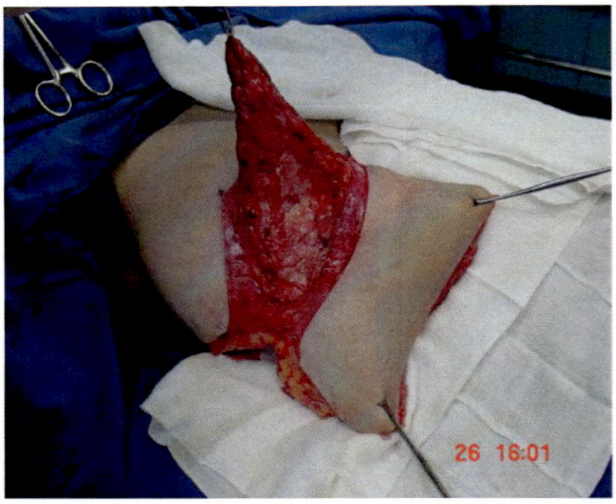

Fig. 22.7 Photo showing the base excess resection at a plane perpendicular to the breast (this determines the height of the cone) and the thickness of the pedicle

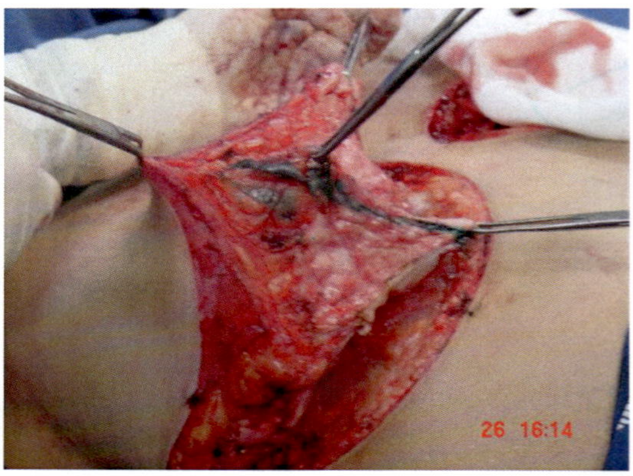

Fig. 22.8 Photo showing the central half keel resection

The NAC is moved upward to its new position. A cut of about 1 cm can be made on the medial portion of the V at point B if it is necessary to enhance the transposition distance of the areola.

The breast segments are approximated at the midline using sutures of 3-0 monocryl. Sutures of 2-0 mononylon are applied to approximate the medial and lateral pillars and a greater projection of the areola and nipple occurs (Figs. 22.9 and 22.10). A trifurcation suture of 3-0 monocryl is inserted among points B, C, and F. If more skin is needed to be removed, it can be taken along AB and BC. Skin closure is carried out (Fig. 22.11) and drainage performed. The results of the thin superior medial technique are demonstrated in (Figs. 22.12–22.29).

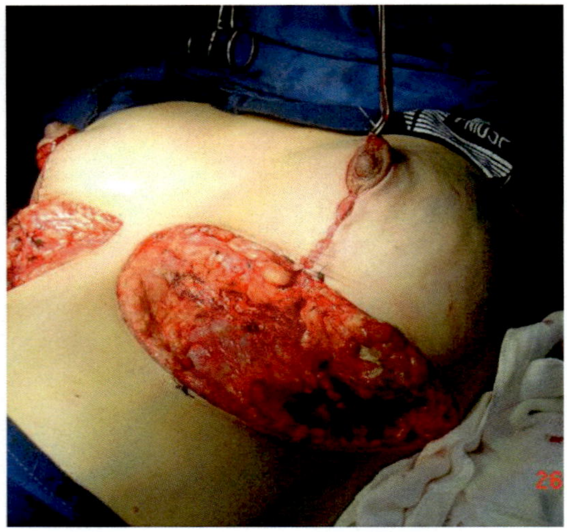

Fig. 22.9 Photo showing the lateral and medial segments of the horizontal scar sutured after the transposition of the nipple–areola complex

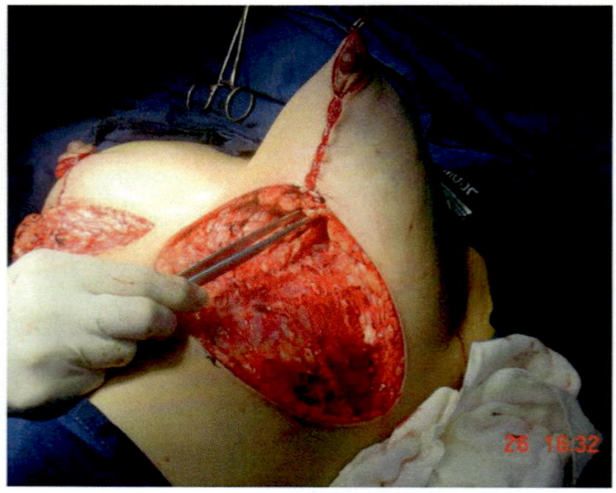

Fig. 22.10 Photo showing the sutures of lateral and medial pillars

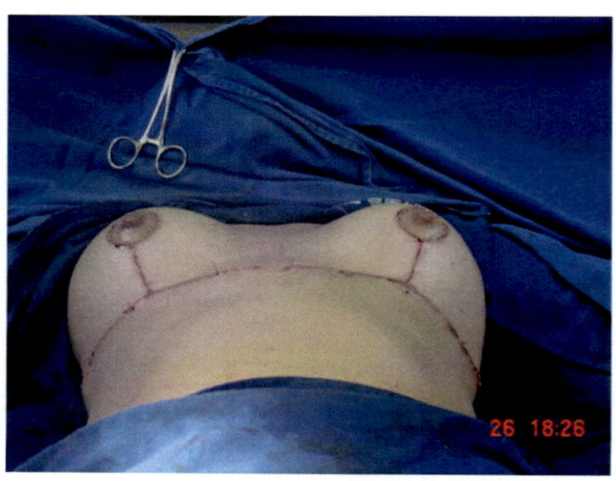

Fig. 22.11 Photo showing the final aspect of the surgery

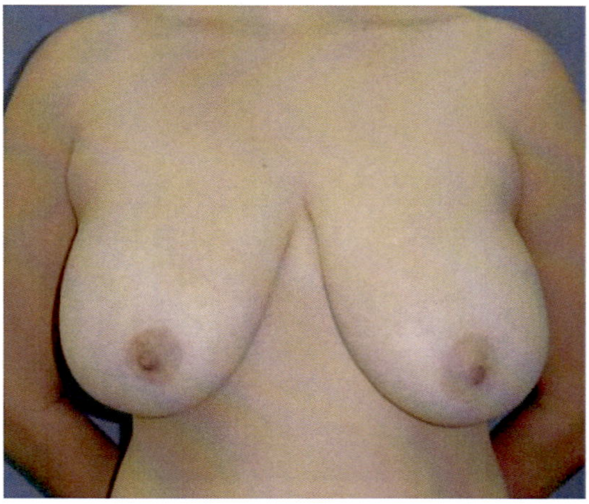

Fig. 22.12 Patient A preoperatively

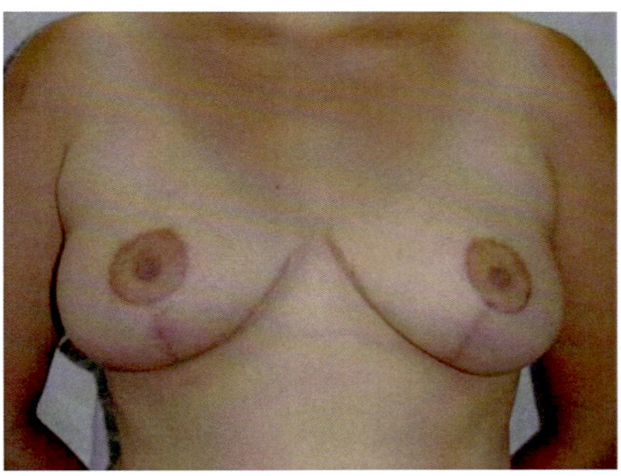

Fig. 22.13 Nine months postoperatively, 1050 g removed from the left breast and 1000 g from the right breast

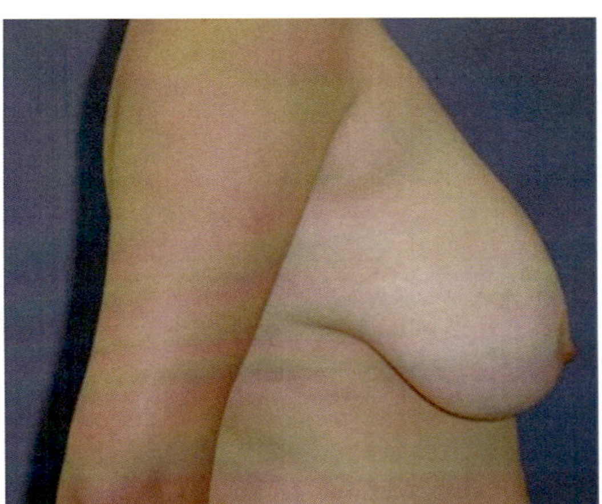

Fig. 22.14 Patient A preoperatively

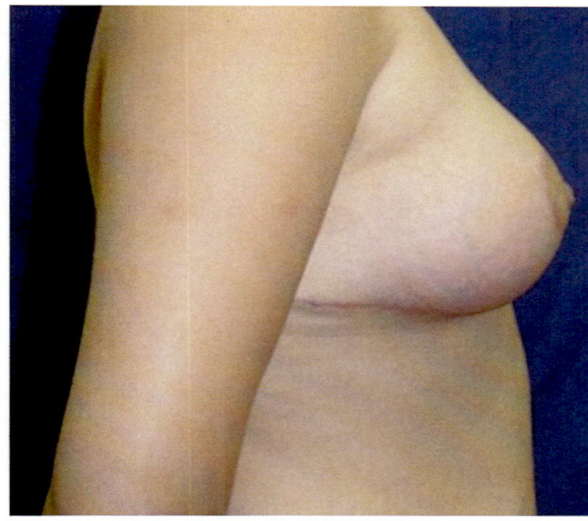

Fig. 22.15 Postoperative lateral view

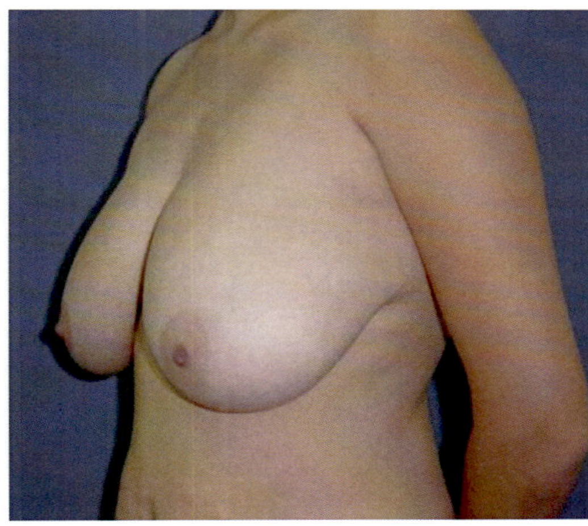

Fig. 22.16 Patient A preoperatively

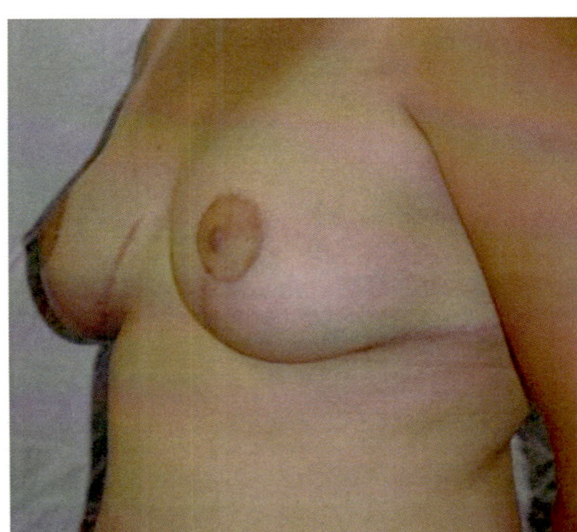

Fig. 22.17 Postoperative 3/4 view

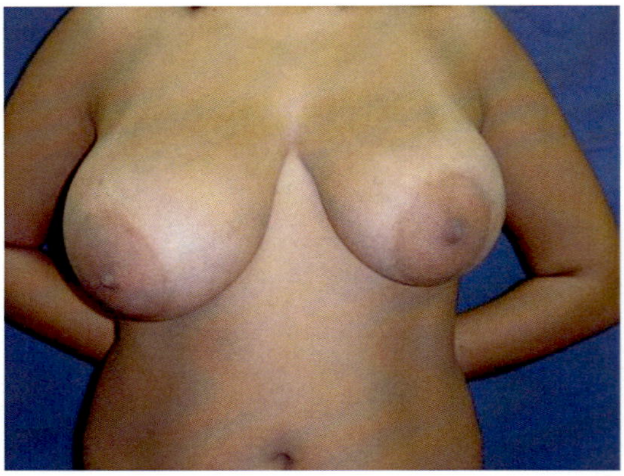

Fig. 22.18 Patient B preoperatively

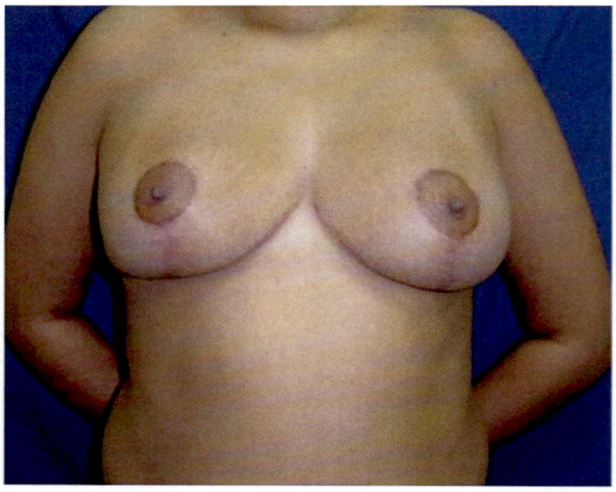

Fig. 22.19 One year and 6 months postoperatively, 1250 g removed from the right breast and 800 g from the right breast

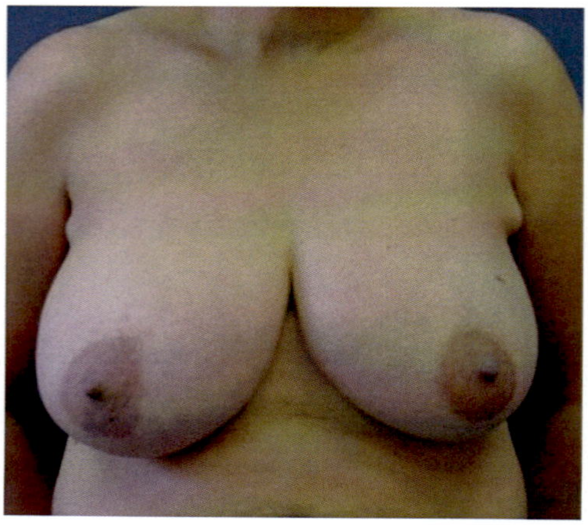

Fig. 22.20 Patient C preoperatively

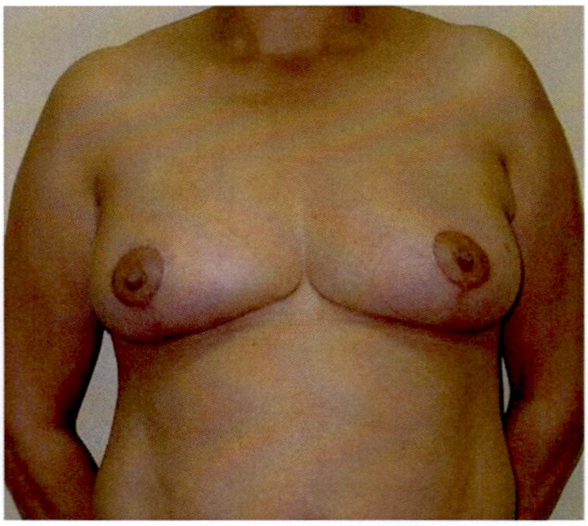

Fig. 22.21 One year and 6 months postoperatively, 1900 g removed from the right breast and 1700 g from the right breast

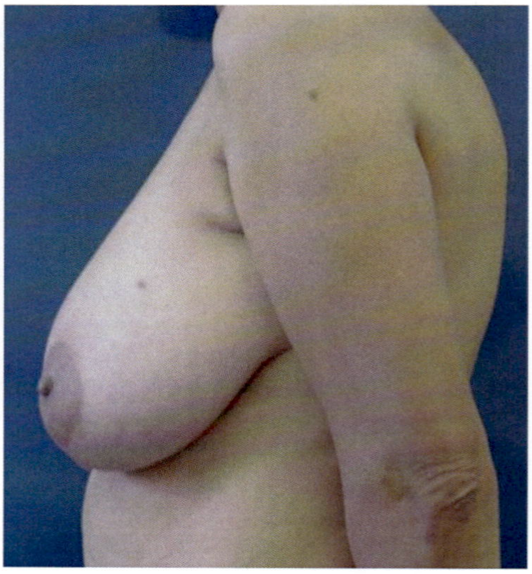

Fig. 22.22 Patient C preoperatively

22.3 Discussion

There are a multitude of procedures used to correct hypertrophic breasts with plastic surgery (Bames 1948; Baroudi and Lewis 1976; Biesenberger 1931; Born 1994; Bustos 1988; Brauman 1994; Conway 1952; Courtiss 1993; Courtiss and Goldwyn 1977; Costa et al. 2005, 2008; Dartigues 1935; de Benito and Sanza 1993; de Castro 1976; Dufourmentel 1939; Farina 1972; Ferreira et al. 1995; Gillies and McIndoe 1939; Hawtof et al. 1989; Johnson 1976; Shin et al. 1996; Koger et al. 1994; Lassus 1996; Lejour 1994; May 1956; McKissock 1972); Pitanguy 1960.

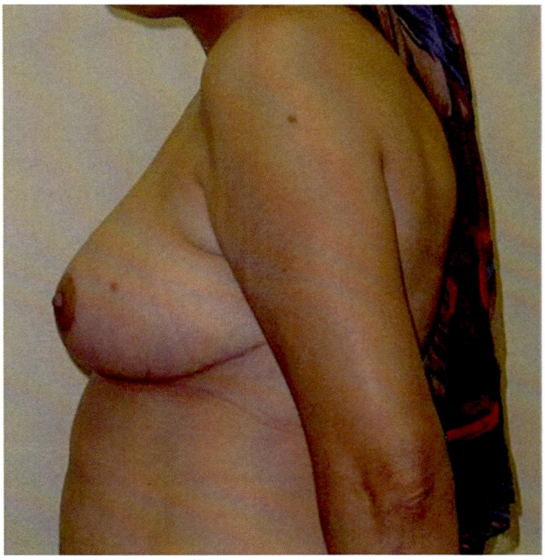

Fig. 22.23 Postoperative lateral view

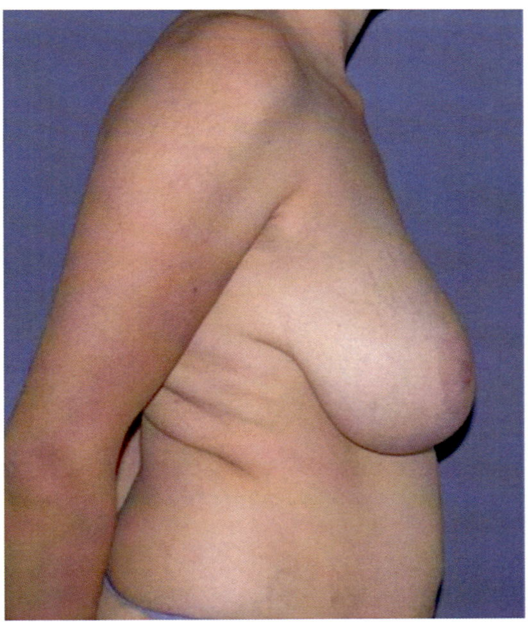

Fig. 22.24 Patient D preoperatively

The superior medial pedicle reduction mammoplasty with a thin pedicle is a safe surgical option for severe mammary hypertrophy, which could solve problems such as when the distance between the new, desired position of the NAC is too long.

The advantages of a superior medial pedicle include reliable circulation with the capacity of a long transposition distance of the NAC. Results such as a mean change in nipple position of

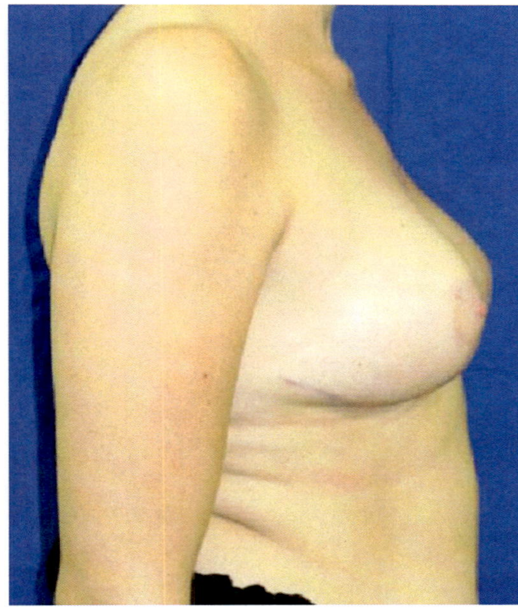

Fig. 22.25 Two years postoperatively, lateral view, 1000 g removed

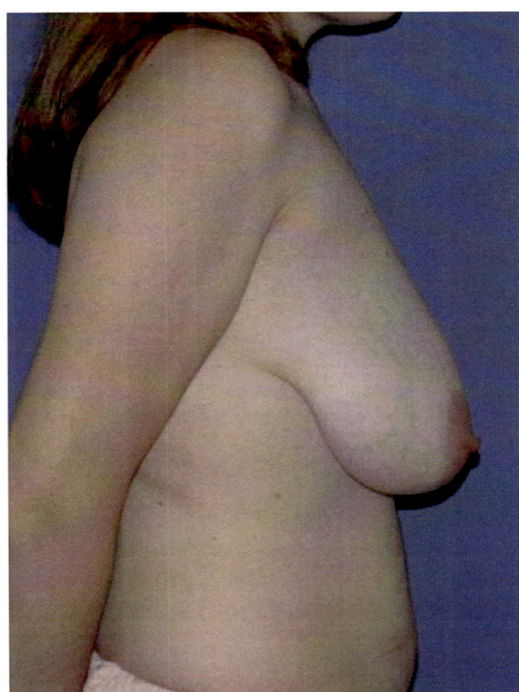

Fig. 22.26 Patient E preoperatively

16 cm (range 12–21 cm) and a mean weight of each breast of 1400 g (range 750–3000 g) have been shown in a study with 90 patients carried

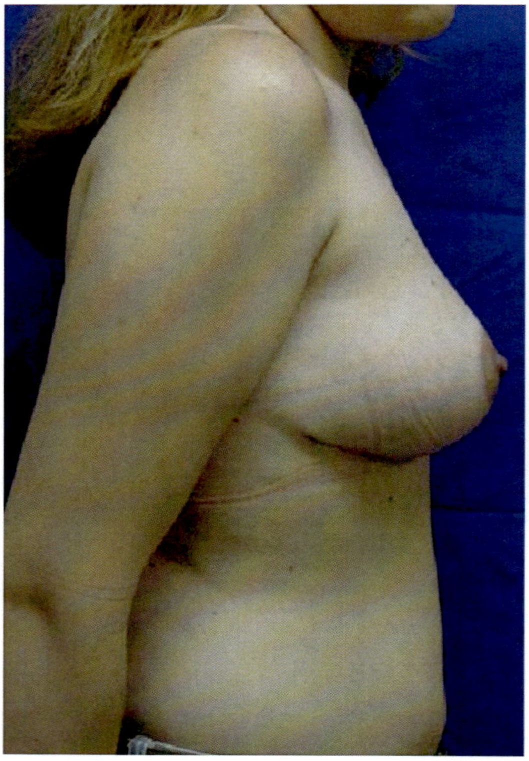

Fig. 22.27 Two years postoperatively, lateral view, 1050 g removed

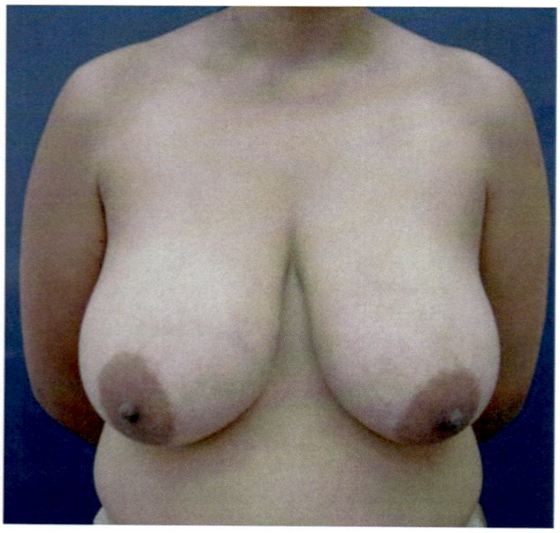

Fig. 22.28 Patient F preoperatively

out between 2000 and 2005 at Hospital das Clinicas, University of São Paulo.

From an anatomical standpoint, a thin pedicle with adequate blood supply avoids problems with

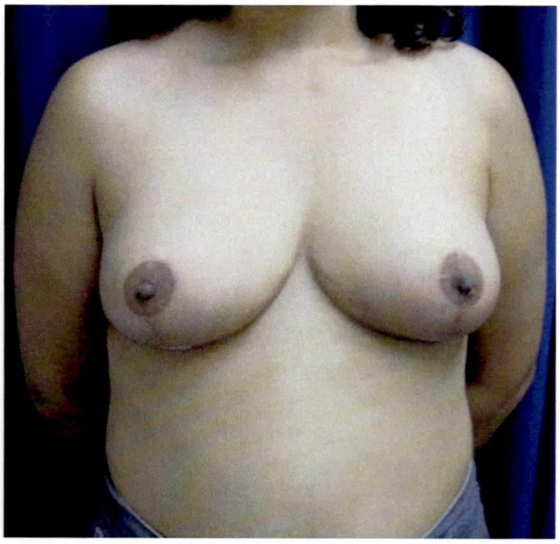

Fig. 22.29 Two years, 1250 g removed

venous drainage. A thicker pedicle would bring an excess of arterial flow without competent venous drainage, causing areolar necrosis.

Although the technique uses a thin pedicle, in different hands, similar outcomes can be achieved. Residents of São Paulo's University Medical School are performing this surgery well.

Considering the large volumes removed and the size of the operated breasts, only a few complications were observed, and were similar to those reported following other techniques described in the literature (Costa et al. 2005; Dartigues 1935; Koger et al. 1994; May 1956; Orlando 1975; Robbins 1977). Patient satisfaction following this procedure was high.

Another important detail is that the same principle of the thin superior medial pedicle can be used for a superior lateral one. The markings are the same, but instead of using the medial area, the lateral area would be used. The importance of this assertion is that in an oncological breast with a tumor in a superior medial position, a superior lateral pedicle can be used.

22.3.1 Complications

The complications arising in a series of 90 patients treated between 2000 and 2005 are shown in Table 22.1.

Table 22.1 Complications

Complications	Number of cases	%
Seroma	1	1.1
Hematoma	1	1.1
Infection	0	0
Areolar necrosis	0	0
Skin ischemia	3	3.3

There were only a few complications. One patient developed seroma (1.1%) but had no further problems. There was one case (1.1%) of a small volume hematoma, which was evacuated by punctures with no need for re-operation. In three patients (3.3%) with inverted T scars superficial skin ischemia occurred and healed with secondary intention. There were no cases of areolar infection or necrosis.

Conclusion

The results of this study clearly demonstrate that thin superior medial pedicle reduction mammaplasty is a safe and reliable technique in cases of severe breast hypertrophy.

References

Bames HO (1948) Reduction of massive breast hypertrophy. Plast Reconstr Surg 3:560

Baroudi R, Lewis JR (1976) The augmentation-reduction mammaplasty. Clin Plast Surg 3:301–308

de Benito J, Sanza IF (1993) Periareolar techniques for mammary reduction and elevation. Aesthet Plast Surg 17:311

Biesenberger H (1931) Deformitaten und kosmetische Operationen der weiblichen Brust. Maudrich, Vienna

Born G (1994) The "L" reduction mammaplasty. Ann Plast Surg 32:383–387

Brauman D (1994) Reduction mammaplasty by suction alone. Plast Reconstr Surg 94:1095–1096

Bustos R (1988) Mamaplastia periareolar. In: Communication to the XXVth Brazilian congress of plastic surgery, Salvador

de Castro CC (1976) Mammaplasty with curved incisions. Plast Reconstr Surg 57:596

Conway H (1952) Mammaplasty: analysis of 110 consecutive cases with end-results. Plast Reconstr Surg 10:303

Costa MP Tuma P Jr, Ferreira MC. (2005) Reduction mammaplasty with resection of a trapezoid base prism and adduction of the arms. Plast Reconstr Surg;116(1):242–250

Costa MP, Ching AW, Ferreira MC (2008) Thin superior medial pedicle reduction mammaplasty for severe mammary hypertrophy. Aesthetic Plast Surg 32(4):645–652

Courtiss EH (1993) Reduction mammaplasty by suction alone. Plast Reconstr Surg 92:1276

Courtiss EH, Goldwyn RM (1977) Reduction mammaplasty by the inferior pedicle technique. An alternative to free nipple and areola grafting for severe macromastia or extreme ptosis. Plast Reconstr Surg 59:500

Dartigues L (1935) Les anomalies du sein en dehors des hypertrophies et des prolapsus. Bull Mem Soc Méd Paris 139:575

Dufourmentel L (1939) Chirurgie reparatrice et correctrice des téguments et des formes. Masson, Paris

Farina R (1972) Reduction mammaplasty with free grafting of the nipple and areola. Br J Plast Surg 25:393

Ferreira MC, Ishida J, Gemperli R, Monteiro AA Jr, Tuma PT Jr (1995) Reduction mammoplasty with shortened scars: surgical technique. Rev Hosp Fac Med São Paulo 50:22

Gillies H, McIndoe AH (1939) The technique of mammaplasty in conditions of hypertrophy of the breast. Surg Gynecol Obstet 68:658

Hawtof DB, Levine M, Kapetanski DI, Pieper D (1989) Complications of reduction mammaplasty: comparison of nipple-areolar graft and pedicle. Ann Plast Surg 23:3

Johnson CF (1976) New technique for reduction mammaplasty. Plast Reconstr Surg 57:372

Koger KE, Sundle D, Press BH, Hovey LM (1994) Reduction mammaplasty for gigantomastia using inferiorly based pedicle and free nipple transplantation. Plast Reconstr Surg 33:561

Lassus C (1996) A 30-tear experience with vertical mammaplasty. Plast Reconstr Surg 97:373

Lejour M (1994) Vertical mammaplasty and liposuction of the breast. Plast Reconstr Surg 94:100

May H (1956) Breast plasty in the female. Plast Reconstr Surg 17:351

McKissock PK (1972) Reduction mammaplasty with a vertical dermal flap. Plast Reconstr Surg 49:245

Meijer R (1974) A modified Aufrich reduction mammaplasty. Plast Reconstr Surg 53:129

Melega JM, Zanini SA, Psillakis JM (1992) Cirurgia Plástica Reparadora e Estética, 2ª Edição Edit. Rio de Janeiro, Medsi, pp 707–724

Orlando JC (1975) The superomedial pedicle for nipple transposition. Br J Plast Surg 28:42

Pitanguy I (1960) Breast hypertrophy. In: Transactions of the International Society of Plastic Surgeons, Second Congress, London, Livingstone, p 509

Pitanguy I (1965) Reduction mammaplasty with preservation of nipple glandular continuity. J Am Med Womens Assoc 20:942–945

Pontes R (1973) A technique of reduction mammaplasty. Br J Plast Surg 26:365

Rees TD (1971) An historical review of mamaplasty. In: Transactions of the fifth international congress of plastic reconstructive surgery, Butterworths, Melbourne, p 1167–1173

Rees TD, LaTrenta GS (1994) Aesthetic plastic surgery, vol II, 2nd edn. Piccin, Padova, pp 925–1002

Regnault P (1974) Reduction mammaplasty by the "B" technique. Plast Reconstr Surg 53:19

Ribeiro L (1975) A new technique for reduction mammaplasty. Plast Reconstr Surg 55:330

Robbins TH (1977) A reduction mammaplasty with the areola-nipple based on a inferior dermal pedicle. Plast Reconstr Surg 59:64

Sampaio Goes JC (1996) Periareolar mammaplasty: double skin technique with application of poliglactine or mixed mesh. Plast Reconstr Surg 97:959

Schatten WE, Hartley JH Jr, Hamm WG (1971) Reduction mammaplasty dy the Dufourmentel-Mouly method. Plast Reconstr Surg 48:306–310

Scutari M, Varotto S (1996) A nest swallow's technique in reduction mastoplasty and mastopexy. Acta Chir Ital 52:169

Shin KS, Chung S, Lee HK, Lew JD (1996) Reduction mammaplasty by central pedicle flap with short submammary scar. Aesthet Plast Surg 20:69–76

Skoog T (1963) A technique of breast reduction: transposition of the nipple on a cutaneous vascular pedicle. Acta Chir Scand 126:453–465

Strombeck JO (1971) Reduction mammaplasty. Surg Clin North Am 51:453

Strombeck JO (1960) Mammaplasty: report of a new technique based on two-pedicle procedure. Br J Plast Surg 13:79–90

23 Reduction Mastoplasty: Personal Technique

Angela Maria Fausto Souza, Paulo Roberto Botica do Rêgo Santos, Marcio Milman

23.1 Introduction

The breasts are organs of great relevance to a woman's female identity. The concepts related to their ideal shape and volume are full of variation, according to time and culture. An example of this is the huge amount of production on the theme in the different areas of knowledge, such as fine and literary arts and science. In the latter are included psychoanalytical issues and those related to medical therapy, where pathology of the breast and plastic surgery are included. Both types of surgical treatment are so intricately related that one cannot separate them. The breast also has a reproductive function, such as breast feeding. This aspect increases the complexity and value of its treatment.

Therefore, breast reduction (BR) involves an individualized aesthetic perception related to shape, volume, and symmetry, other than the relationship between the breast and body. The choice of surgical tactics that will best lead to the desired result has as its goal the challenge of attending not only the patient's, but also the surgeon's expectation, who with his technical knowledge and creativity indicate the most appropriate surgery (Fig. 23.1a, b; case 1).

The techniques used in BR are based on different concepts and approaches that reside in the planning of the skin excision, in the different methods of volumetric reduction, and in the maneuvers for nipple–areolar (NAC) repositioning (Pitanguy 1967).

There are many classifications of the size of breast hypertrophy (BH) in the literature, based on the volume or weight of the breast to be reduced. The one that seems to us to be the most logical is that which classifies them as follows: small, i.e., removal up to 200 g; moderate, i.e., from 200 to 500 g; large, i.e., from 500 to 1500 g; and gigantomastia, i.e., more than 1500 g. Physical and psychological distress caused by excessive volume may be aggravated when associated with other deformities such as asymmetries, distant or unaesthetic positioning of the NAC, and poor skin quality.

A.M. Fausto Souza, Ph.D. (✉) • P.R.B. Rêgo Santos, M.D.
M. Milman, M.D.
Gynecology Department, Oswaldo Cruz Foundation, Rio de Janeiro, RJ 22461-220, Brazil
e-mail: angelafausto@cirurgiaplast.com.br

J.M. Avelar (ed.), *Breast Surgery*, https://doi.org/10.1007/978-3-319-54115-0_23

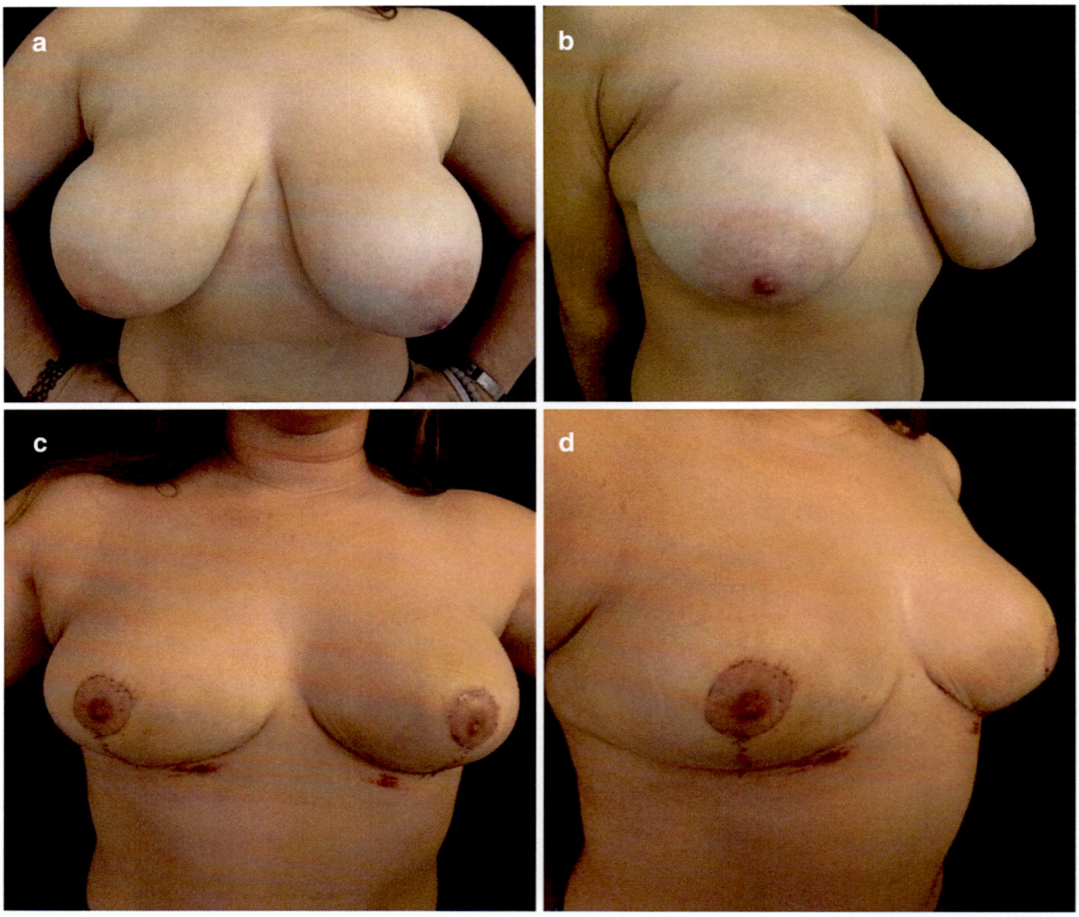

Fig. 23.1 Case 1. (**a**) Preoperative, frontal view. Breast hypertrophy with Vertical dimension predominance. (**b**) Preoperative. Oblique view. Submammary fold with very high implantation. (**c**) Postoperative. Frontal view Image. (**d**) Postoperative. Oblique view showing new submammary fold implantation, lower than preoperative. (**e**) Intraoperative marking of points A, B, C, D and E, highlighting the differences in the height of the implantation of the submammary fold. (**f**) Intraoperative bidigital maneuver to estimate the amount of skin and parenchymal removal. (**g**) Intraoperative markings of the surgical plane incisions in the approach of the breast with vertical dimension predominance. Points A, B, C, D and E. Delimitation of the area to be de-epithelized in the inferior projection of points B and C until the submammary fold. Here we show the temporary stitch of the areola at point A. (**h**) Intraoperative. Inferior pedicle individualization showing the marking of the estimated parenchymal resection

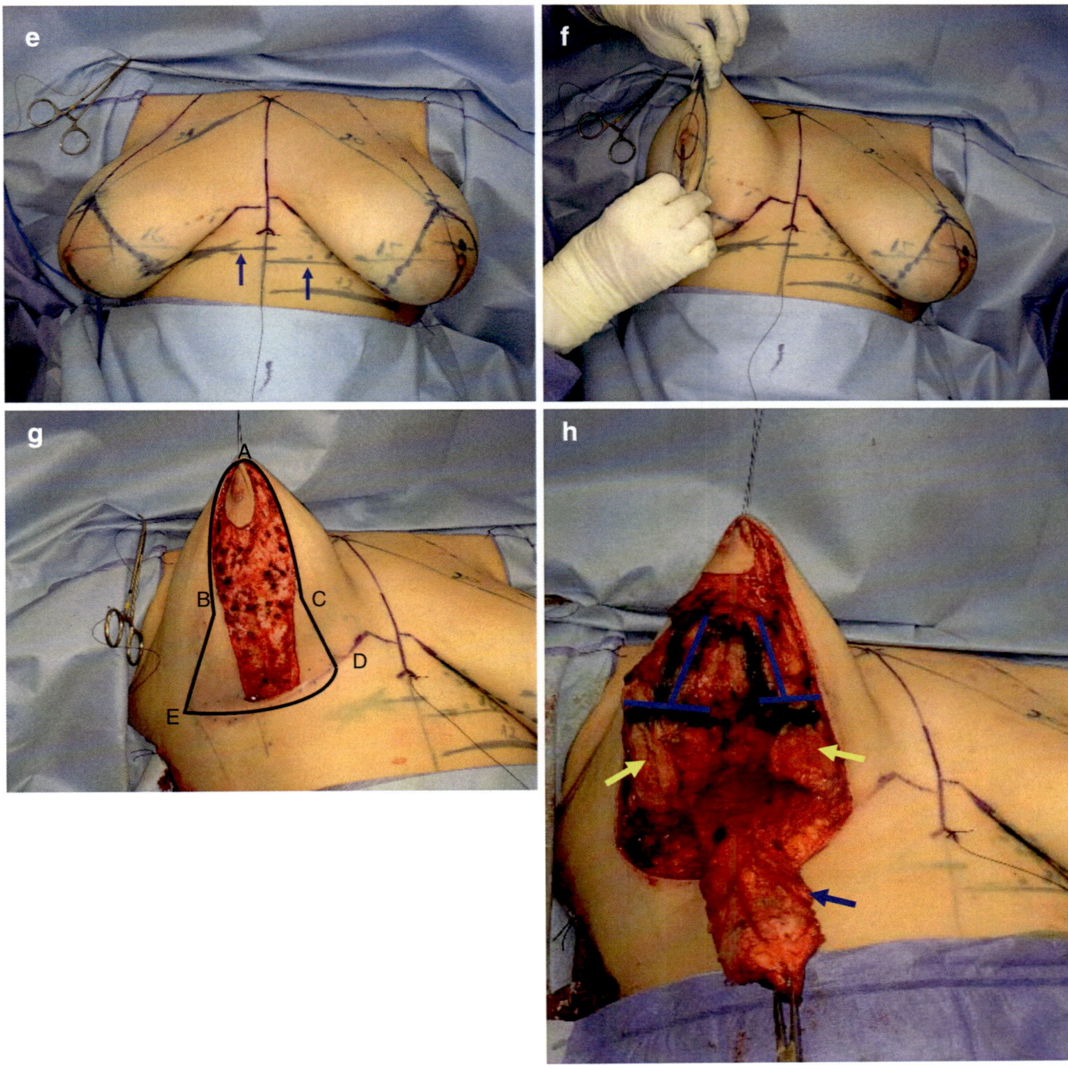

Fig. 23.1 (continued)

23.2 Method

We perform laboratory tests, imaging evaluation of the breasts, and detailed photographic pre-operative registering. The photographs are important in the analysis of data and surgical planning. Our systematization in the approach of candidates for BR is divided into three groups: teenagers and young nulliparous, post-pregnancy, and at climacterium (Skoog 1963).

In the first group, we perform BR surgeries from adolescence, at 14 years of age, with no associated obesity. The surgical indications occur when BH is present with great body disproportion or is psychologically affecting the patient in her development. We must alert the parents to the possibility of a second procedure, in case the breast grows again after surgery. In young women, we should preserve lactation, when possible.

Post-gestational women comprise the second segment, in which BR sought with greater frequency. Some of these patients previously had BH or became hypertrophic after breast-feeding. They request restructuring of breast shape and projection, and are greatly concerned about the scar size.

Patients of the third group are at climacterium. They may present with severe BH and, usually, have orthopedic postural complaints and great discomfort. Chronic skin disorders are frequent, owing to contiguous contact of the breasts over the superior abdomen or on the intermammary space. In this group, the greatest demand is for a significant reduction in breast volume.

23.3 Evaluation Parameters

The patient's breasts should be inspected in the supine position, according to the following aspects: breast shape and size; texture of the skin and the tissues that comprise the breast; position and mobility of the NAC; and submammary sulcus implantation.

23.3.1 Shape and Size of the Breast

(A) Horizontal dimension predominance: In these situations, we may find synmastia and/or the external quadrants of the breast may project beyond the lateral thoracic limit, when in the patient is in the orthostatic position. The NAC may be located away from the breast's middle axis, in a divergent or convergent position. The possibility of scar union in the midline must be informed to the patient (Fig. 23.1e; case 1).

(B) *Vertical dimension predominance*: they are usually larger breasts with greater NAC dystopia, which creates a huge degree of difficulty for its elevation. The skin suffers greater and continuous stretching with a consequent increase in cutaneous laxity. The scars tend to be of a larger size and breast feeding may be compromised (Figs. 23.1a and 23.2; cases 1 and 2).

23.3.2 Skin Texture and the Tissues That Comprise the Breast

In BH, the skin rarely has good elasticity. Frequently, the breast shows laxity and stretch marks, which cause an unequivocal loss in its elasticity, reducing breast support. This fact must be considered in surgical planning.

The quality of the tissues that comprise the breast parenchyma varies according to age and body development throughout life. In a young patient, a glandular component is frequent, conferring a denser texture to the gland. On the other hand, when the gland completes its development, during pregnancy and at advanced ages, the glandular tissue goes through a process called liposubstitution, on average from 35 years of age. Regarding surgery, those breasts with dense glandular tissues have reduced flap mobilization compared with liposubstituted breasts. However, in those with higher densities, the mammary cone projection tends to maintain a long-lasting result.

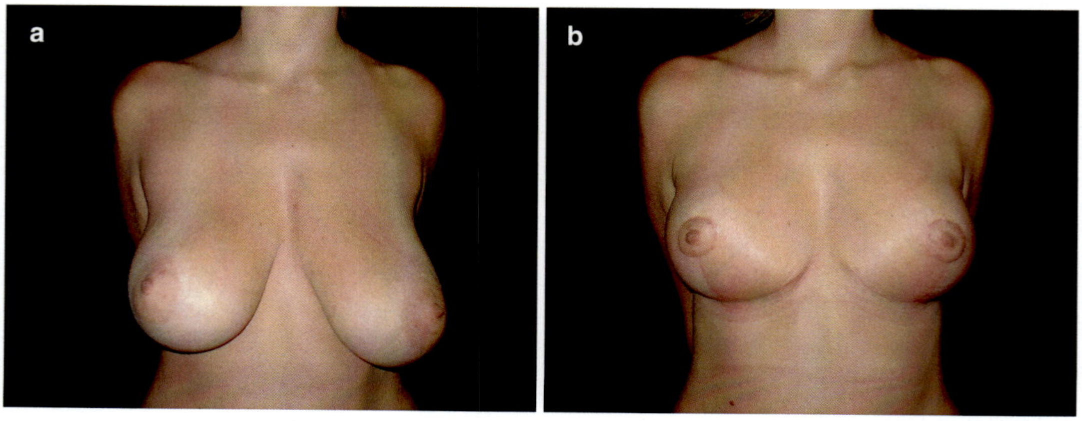

Fig. 23.2 Case 2. (**a**) Preoperative images. Pre-op. Frontal. Vertical hypertrophy and asymmetry of the breasts. (**b**) Two years Postoperative. Result after using inferior pedicle for superior pole projection

23.3.3 NAC Position and Mobility

The NAC distance in the mid-line, in relation to the sternal furcula, is of great relevance as a pre-surgical parameter. The NAC may be well placed, without the need for long transposition. In other situations, it may be completely dystopic, independently of the degree of BH, being so distant that the creation of areolar flaps is necessary, based on different vascular sectors of the breast. In our practice, we prefer the superior or medial pedicles for they possess a greater blood supply, although other alternatives may be indicated (Figs. 23.3d and 23.3; cases 3). Free grafting is rarely indicated.

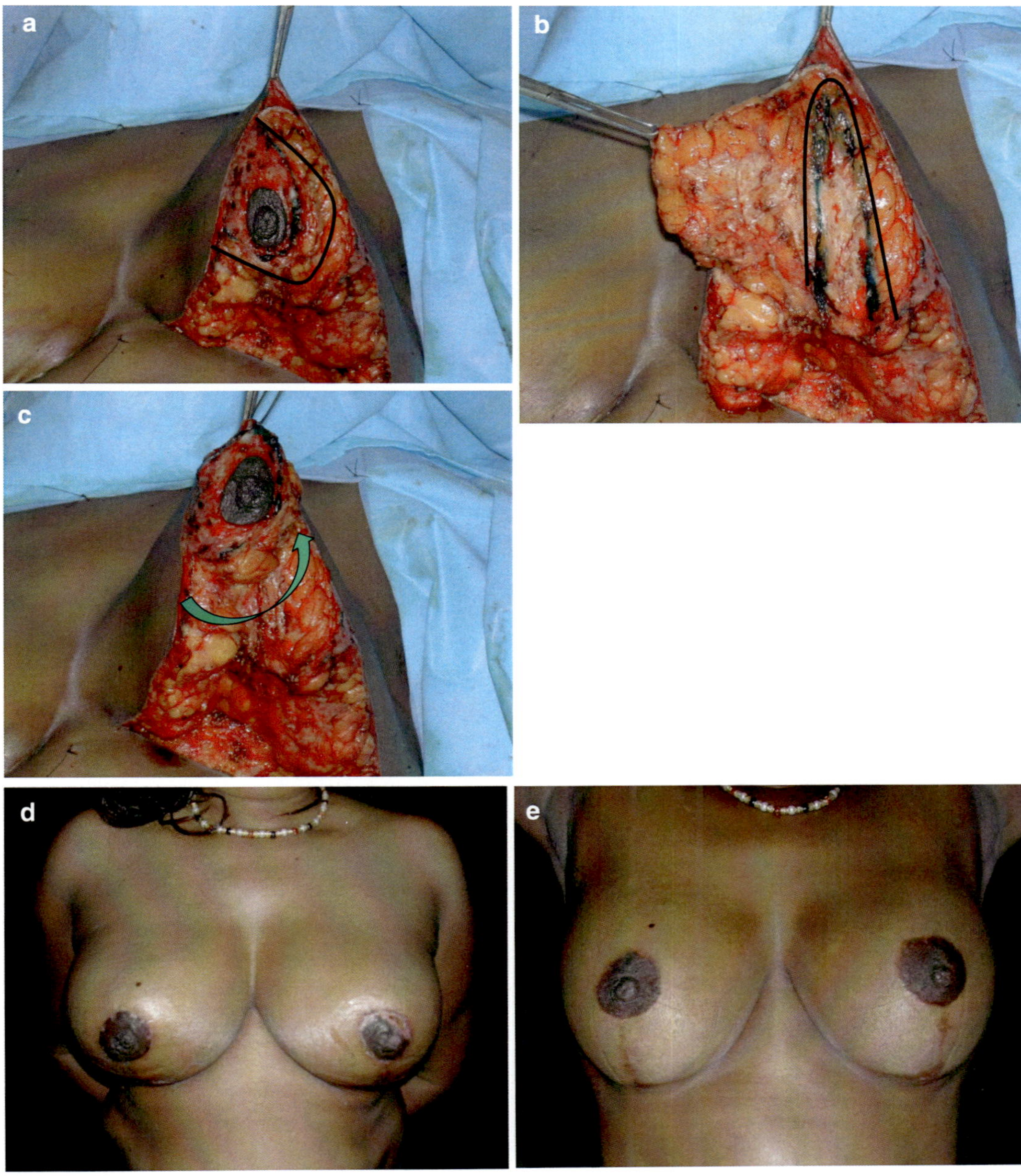

Fig. 23.3 Case 3. (**a**) Marking of the supero-medial areolar flap. (**b**) Keel- type resection of the breast's center showing the areolar flap being pulled laterally. (**c**) New areolar position at point A through flap rotation. (**d**) Postoperatively. Epidermolysis of left areolar tissue. (**e**) Two years postoperatively. Complete healing and good pigmentation of epidermolysis

23.3.4 Submammary Fold

The submammary folds are structures of great relevance as a parameter for the evaluation of symmetry. They may present with various alterations, among them the asymmetrical submammary fold and those with very high implantation are highlighted. In the former, the breast is presented with significant ptosis (Fig. 23.1b; case 1). In this case, the sulcus should be repositioned to a lower location, longitudinally widening the breast base. With this approach, we can achieve a more balanced cone in the two dimensions and harmonize the proportions between the quadrants.

23.4 Surgical Planning

Preoperatively, with the patient in the orthostatic position, we perform the marking of point A in the right and left mammary midline, as described in the evaluation parameters, based on Pitanguy's technique. Point A is estimated through digital projection of the finger placed in the mammary fold, on the superior pole. Immediately, we compare this point A evaluation, observing it in relation to another parameter of positioning, which is the medial line of humeral bone reference. The latter is valued by us mainly in cases of submammary fold dystopia. The distance from point A to the sternal furcula is programmed at an average distance of 18–19 cm. Next, we mark points B and C. Their position is determined by pulling point A superiorly and by using a bidigital maneuver, we estimate the volume reduction and excess skin in the vertical dimension (Fig. 23.3; case 3) (Pitanguy 1967).

Two lines are drawn following the inferior projections of points B and C up to the submammary fold. Next, we mark points D and E, extremely medial and lateral respectively, on the submammary fold line. After the marking, we proceed to the maneuver of de-epithelializing around the areola among points A, B, and C, and, in the contiguous inferior area inside the inferior vertical projection of points B and C up to the submammary fold marking (Fig. 23.1; case 1). We liberate the NAC through a transverse incision between points B and C. Then, we immediately individualize the area of the inferior flap with two vertical incisions at the projections of points B and C up to the submammary fold and preserve this inferior flap. We fix the NAC at its superior limit, using a traction stitch, at point A. This maneuver informs us, in a practical way, about the degree of difficulty for NAC ascension, which directs us to the need for the creation of an areolar pedicle. Afterward, we proceed with the resection of the excess glandular tissue, in the vertical and horizontal dimensions of the breast, delimiting the lateral and medial pillars, which form the new breast cone. On average, we leave 8–10 cm in the T vertical dimension between the base and point A. This dimension is related to the final size of the breast (Fig. 23.3d; case 3).

In a sequence, we fix with a temporary stitch the lateral and medial pillars to the submammary fold, in its new position, in the breast midline. At this moment, the final horizontal scar extension is re-evaluated with the removal of the excess skin medial and lateral flaps contained between segments C–D and B–E. We then complement the volumetric reduction in the vertical dimension of the breast (Peixoto 1980).

We strongly try to ensure that the medial extent of the scar does not reach the sternal region and, in the lateral region that it does not surpass the new breast cone limit or that it is not prolonged in the axillary direction. The remaining inferior pedicle flap, if indicated to help in the structural composition of the breast cone, should be made with an average base of 4 cm in width and approximately 2 cm thick, in its superior portion, and with a greater thickness at the base, so that it includes a larger number of perforator vessels. Its fixation is done in the pre-pectoral fascia, at the superior breast limit, when we wish to regain volume, to increase superior pole projection (Dufourmentel and Mouly 1961).

In younger patients with BH with a horizontal dimension predominance, elastic skin, and well-positioned NAC, we use another surgical approach. The marking of point A is similar. We proceed to the planning of skin removal in the vertical dimension superiorly with an arched circled line external to the

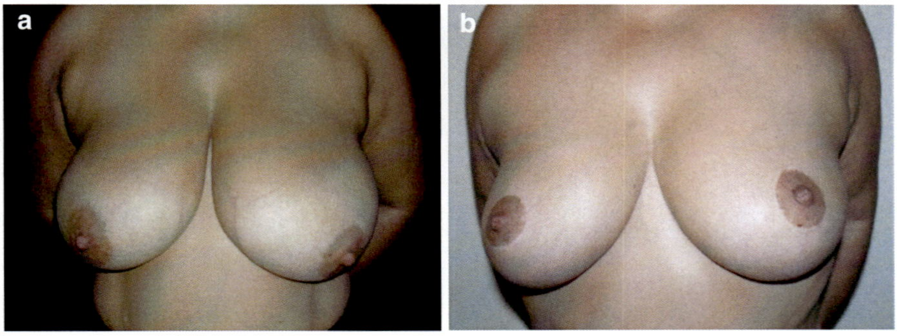

Fig. 23.4 Case 4. (**a**) Preoperatively. Frontal view. Severe ptosis, hypertrophy, asymmetry and diverging NAC. (**b**) Five years postoperatively. Frontal view. Performed with supero-medial areolar flap

NAC (Fig. 23.4) The marking of points B and C and their inferior projection in the direction of the submammary fold are performed in the same manner as described above. The difference resides in the marking of a higher new position of the mammary fold. We elevate it, on average 2 cm, as a plan to reduce the extent of the medial (C–D) and lateral (B–E) components of the horizontal scar. In these cases, we use the principles of Peixoto's and Marchac's techniques (Figs. 23.1 and 23.5a–e; case 5).

We position NAC during the final mounting of the breast, in both approaches, leaving a vertical measurement between the inferior limit of the NAC to the submammary fold of 5–7 cm. This variation is related to the size of the new breast.

23.5 Discussion

Although we always attempt to aim for a significant reduction of volume with good symmetry and shape, the result depends on the quality of the tissues and the degree of deformity to be treated.

The final size of the scars is a factor directly connected to the breast volume reduction and to skin laxity. It does not seem to us to be good conduct to lose breast shape to get a reduced scar. Rarely, the elimination or excessive reduction in the horizontal component of the T will produce a favorable aesthetic result. In our opinion, a harmonious shape of the breast cone is paramount in relation to the extreme concepts of scar elimination or reduction. However, there are parameters that should be avoided, when possible, such as invasion of the scar into the pre-sternal region with union of the horizontal scars. When exceeding the lateral breast limit, the scar should be oriented in the direction of the horizontal sulcus, avoiding directing it toward the axilla (Regnault 1974).

The previous location of the NAC determines the technique to be used. The surgeon's experience and analysis of the surgical plan directs the best choice. The breast flaps are extremely well vascularized, according to the method. Although we should have in mind that anatomical variations exist, which could lead to a partial or total loss of flaps. These situations may occur in long flaps, at NAC transposition. In young women, we must pay attention to the preservation of the ductal network. One important parameter is the repositioning of the NAC in the breast cone. The presence of stretch marks, excessive laxity, and greater fatty content in the breast parenchyma have a negative impact on the result (Ribeiro et al. 2002).

23.6 Complications

Although breast reduction is considered to be a major surgery, the number of complications is relatively low. According to Strombeck, the larger the resected volume, the higher the complications rate. Such complications are intimately related to the size of the breast, the relationship between the glandular and adipose tissue, the position of the NAC, in addition to the quality of the skin.

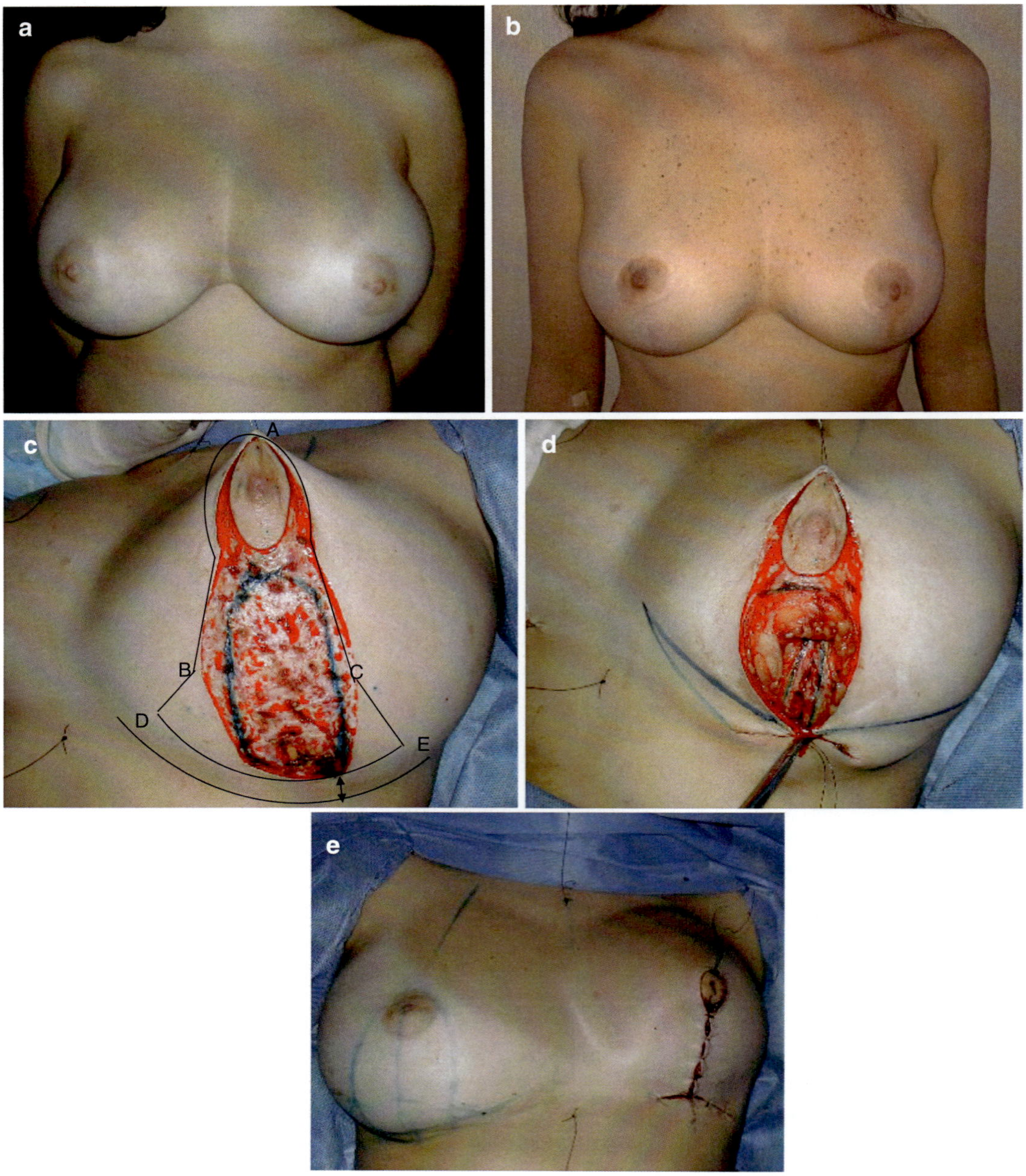

Fig. 23.5 Case 5. (**a**) Preoperatively. Frontal view Breast hypertrophy showing horizontal dimension predominance. (**b**) Five years postoperatively, frontal view. (**c**) Intraoperatively. Detail of the marking with raising of the submammary fold, reduced horizontal scar (I did not understand) and marking of the inferior pedicle flap. (**d**) Intraoperatively. Temporary stitch between points B and C to the submammary fold midline showing the amount of avoided skin resection in the horizontal scar (*blue markings*). (**e**) Intraoperatively. Significant breast reduction with a reduced horizontal scar, preserving a good breast cone shape

The intercurrences may be divided basically into two groups. One is related to the aesthetic result of the breast and the other is related to the complications inherent to the surgical act, which makes us wonder if we could have avoided them. Thus, detailed surgical planning is of utmost importance.

In the case of cosmetic complications, the most frequent is related to the insufficient reduction of breast volume. The frustration in not reaching the expectation of a volumetric reduction of the breast is the main complaint and some of the patients request reoperation. This may be related to the non-comprehension, by the surgeon, of the patient's demands. Another relevant cosmetic complication is the presence of breast asymmetry. It is known that, frequently, the breasts are asymmetrical, which obliges the doctor to inform the patient about it. This difference may be in the mammary structure, with different volumes and shapes, or in body structure asymmetries, which will not be solved by BR. In volumetric asymmetries, evaluation becomes entirely the surgeon's responsibility during the operation (Lejour 1994).

Other cosmetic problems are related to position, form, sensitivity, and color alterations of the NAC. They are complications inherent to the surgical procedures and we cannot guarantee that they will not happen. We should consider the superior rotation of the breast goes through in late postoperative period. Implantation in an abnormally high or low position causes significant dissatisfaction for the patient and is frequently difficult to resolve (Finger et al. 1989).

Skin problems are very rare in our experience and are mostly related to NAC epidermolysis, when maneuvers for NAC transposition with areolar flaps or grafts are performed (Fig. 23.5; case 5). Liponecrosis of the flap extremities is uncommon and may evolve into calcifications, seen posteriorly on breast imaging (Le Roux 2011).

Scars, when malpositioned, may interfere with the perception of symmetry between the breast cones. The type of scarring of the patient and, secondarily, the tension exerted on it within the content of the breast cone, may lead to dehiscence and hypertrophic or widened scars, which, in general, are treated in a conservative manner.

Conclusions

A detailed evaluation of the patient candidate for BR surgery is fundamental. The psychological, postural comfort, and better body relation benefits are evident and dramatic. Obtaining a good result in the breast cone is more important than the scars. The need for areolar flaps for the comfort and safety of NAC transposition in BH should always be considered. It is very important to inform the woman about the durability and limitations of her surgical result, in addition to any possible alterations in sensitivity, which may be definitive or temporary. We use approaches that retain a larger amount of glandular tissue contiguous to the NAC, prioritizing breast-feeding.

The new breast shape is like a photograph of time, as it will continue to develop and modify throughout the patient's life. Body changes such as weight variation, pregnancy, and aging all alter the result obtained.

References

Chiari A Jr (2002) The L short-scar mammaplasty. Clin Plast Surg 29:401–409

Dufourmentel C, Mouly R (1961) Plastie mammaire par la méthode oblique. Ann Chir Plast 6:45–58

Finger RE, Vasquez B, Drew GS et al (1989) Superomedial pedicle technique of reduction mammaplasty. Plast Reconstr Surg 83:471–480

Lejour M (1994) Vertical mammaplasty and liposuction of the breast. Plast Reconstr Surg 94:100

Le Roux CM et al (2011) Preventing venous congestion of the nipple-areola complex: an anatomical guide to preserving essential venous drainage networks. Plast Reconstr Surg 127:1073–1079

Peixoto G (1980) Reduction mammaplasty: a personal technique. Plast Reconstr Surg 65:217–226

Pitanguy I (1967) Surgical treatment of breast hypertrophy. Br J Plast Surg 10:78

Regnault P (1974) Reduction mammaplasty by the "B" technique. Plast Reconstr Surg 53:19–24

Ribeiro L, Accorsi A Jr, Buss A et al (2002) Creation and evolution of 30 years of the inferior pedicle in reduction mammaplasties. Plast Reconstr Surg 110:960–970

Skoog T (1963) A technique of breast reduction: transposition of the nipple on a cutaneous vascular pedicle. Acta Chir Scand 126:453–465

24 Technique and Approaches for Different Breasts

Claudio Cardoso de Castro
and Sheyla Maria Carvalho Rodrigues

24.1 Introduction

Various philosophical concepts have been involved in breast reduction and mastopexy and were also thought to be an important determinant of the procedure's success. First, the volume, the skin, the tissue quality, and the blood supply to the breast. Second, the patient's age and expectations. And, third, but not least, the surgeon's experience and his capacity for a sound operative strategy with regard to sculpting of an artistic breast with minimal scarring.

24.2 Operative Strategy

When you are planning to operate on breasts, it is necessary to analyze the similarities between the breasts, not forgetting, however, that they are not identical. Requirements of an ideal breast reduction must take into consideration: (a) breast size and consistency, (b) grade of ptosis, (c) distance between the suprasternal notch and the nipples, (d) location of the nipple on the breast, (e) the blood supply and the nerve supply, (f) skin quality, and, most importantly, (g) the relationship between the breast tissue and skin.

C.C. de Castro, M.D. (✉) • S.M.C. Rodrigues, M.D.
Department of Plastic Surgery, University of the State of Rio de Janeiro, Rua São Francisco Xavier, Rio de Janeiro, RJ, Brazil
e-mail: ccardosodecastro@gmail.com

Based on these factors, it is our opinion that each breast deserves individualized skin markings (Cardoso de Castro 1984) (not patterns) and individualized tissue resection. Overall, the greater the skin excess in relation to the breast tissue, the more skin is removed. The amount of skin resected determines the length of the scar. When a surgeon tries to reduce the length of the scar by limiting skin removal, the shape and appearance of the breasts are usually compromised.

Step-by-step, the ideal surgery needs to be planned so the breasts attain a natural form in proportion to other parts of the body. Symmetry between the breasts, preservation of sexual function and breastfeeding, and scars that are not visible through normal clothing are desired.

In this chapter, skin markings and the different methods of tissue removal are described.

24.3 Positioning and Anesthesia

The patient is operated on in a sitting position with the arms extended at 70–90° on an arm board. The preferred anesthesia for breast reductions is general anesthesia supplemented with local anesthetic infiltration, although small mastopexies and reductions are possible under local anesthesia and sedation. The infiltration is performed with a solution of 0.9% saline, lidocaine, ropivacaine, and epinephrine 1:200,000, the latter used for local vasoconstriction.

J.M. Avelar (ed.), *Breast Surgery*, https://doi.org/10.1007/978-3-319-54115-0_24

24.4 Skin Resection

With the patient in a sitting position, a line is drawn from the midclavicle to the submammary sulcus passing through the nipple. At the projection of this line, a point is marked on the submammary fold. This point, A, corresponds to the new position of the nipple–areola complex (NAC). It can be placed lower in some cases when the breast tissue is firm and the surgeon notices that lifting the nipples will be difficult. Sometimes it is easier to elevate the nipple and areola several centimeters and other times even 2 cm is very difficult (Fig. 24.1) After determining the position of point A, the angle of the vertical limbs is marked by placing the thumb and index finger of one hand and pinching the breast (Fig. 24.2). The positioning of the points B and C should not be much greater than 7 cm from point A. The definition of these points depends on the relationship between skin and breast tissue, and on the surgeon's skill, experience, and common

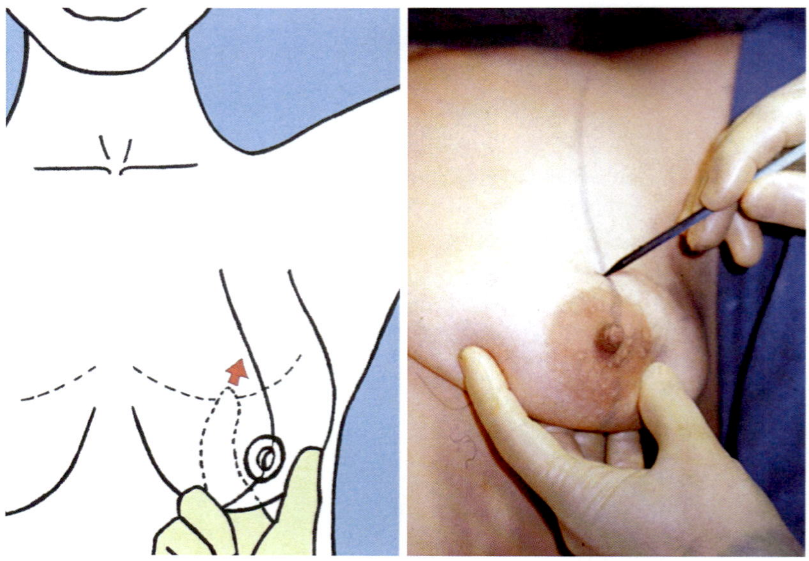

Fig. 24.1 Schematic representation and preoperative view of the marking of point A

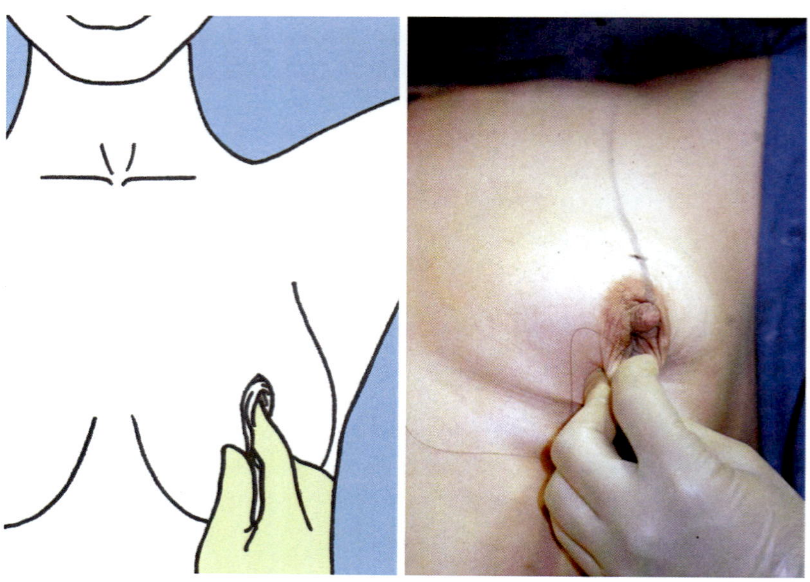

Fig. 24.2 Schematic representation and preoperative view of evaluating the location of points B and C

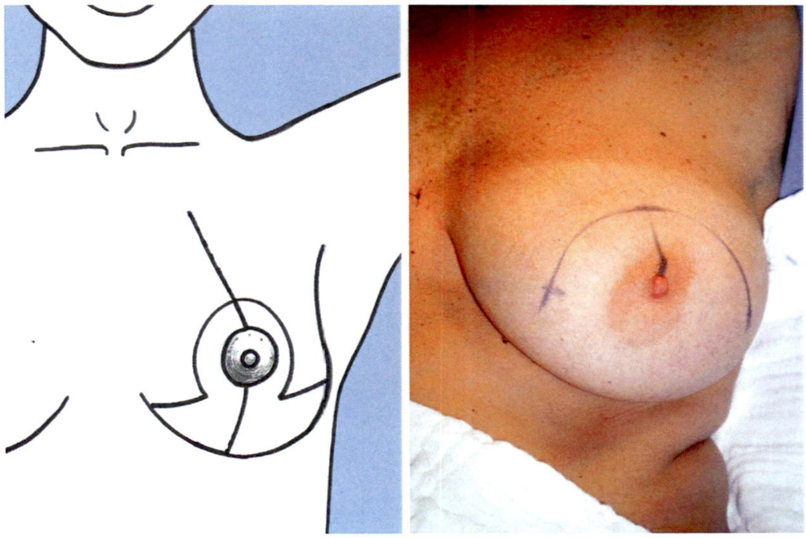

Fig. 24.3 Schematic representation and preoperative view of the marking of curved lines AB and AC

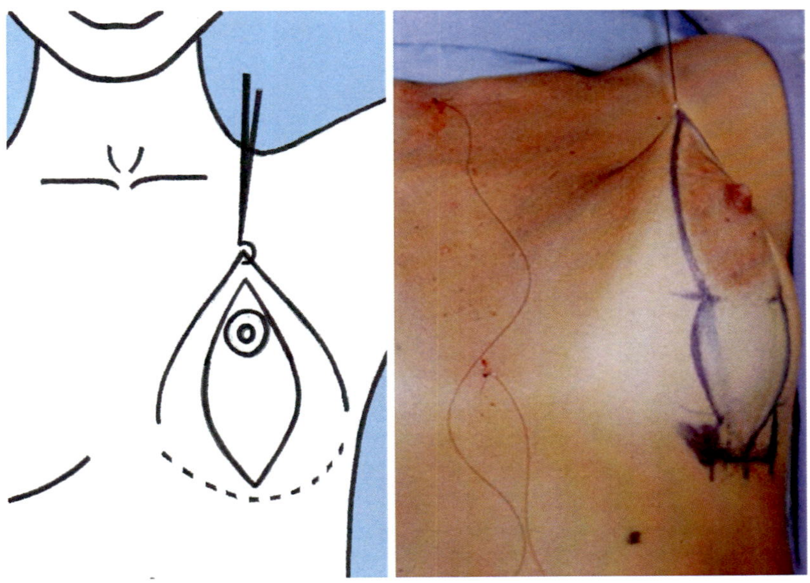

Fig. 24.4 Schematic representation and preoperative view of point D

sense. The angle decides the amount of resection, the new form and consistency of the "new breast." The lines AB and AC can be more or less curved depending on the skin excess (Fig. 24.3) (Cardoso de Castro 1976). The greater the skin excess, the more curved the lines AB–AC should be. Points B and C are then linked to the lateral and medial extremities of the inframammary fold.

When the skin resection area is marked in the form of an ellipse this should not extend beyond the inframammary sulcus. The congruence of these lines is marked 2.5–3 cm above the inframammary sulcus on the meridian line of the breast (Fig. 24.4). This is point D. The excess is marked, and care should be taken not to extend the line of resection beyond the inframammary sulcus.

The vertical scar does not extend beyond the submammary fold, but if too much skin is taken, not enough remains to accommodate, and an inverted-T-shaped marking is designed. The extent of the inframammary incision depends on the size of the breast and chiefly on the relationship between the skin and breast tissue. If there is an excess of skin, this excess must be eliminated. The final scar may be long, but if the skin excess is not treated with the purpose of minimizing the scar, the end result will certainly not be good. The surgeon must avoid joining the incision in the median line.

If the patient presents mild hypertrophy and a good skin quality, a vertical scar with or without a small compensation in the inframammary fold is recommended. An important precaution is to not take too much skin. The role of the final sutures is closed without tension of any kind. The sutures without tension yield imperceptible scars regardless of length.

With these principles in mind (Pitanguy 1967, 2000), we have three different types of skin markings and three different types of final scars: (a) a vertical scar, (b) an inverted T with a small horizontal scar at the inframammary fold, and (c) a classic inverted scar (Figs. 24.5, 24.6, and 24.7). All these techniques leave a periareolar and a vertical scar. The appearance of these scars varies according to each individual patient.

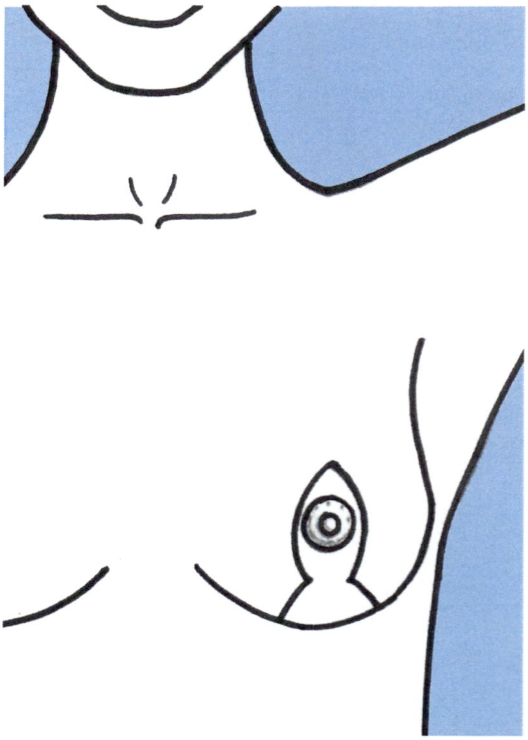

Fig. 24.6 Schematic representation of the inverted T with a small horizontal scar at the inframammary fold

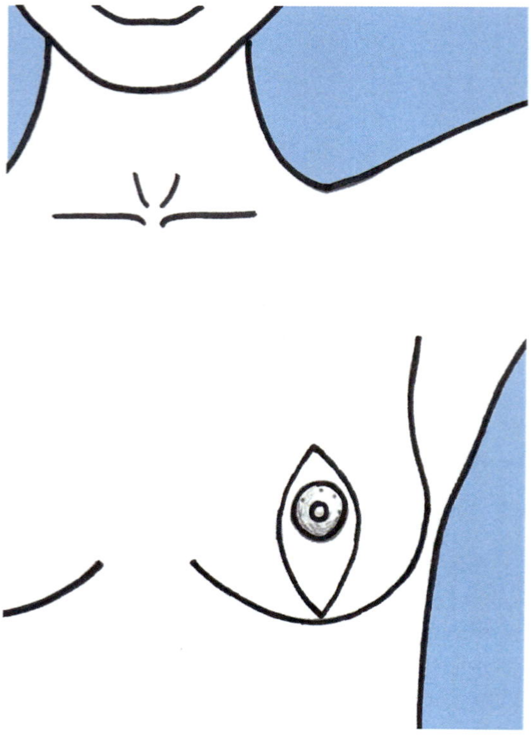

Fig. 24.5 Schematic representation of the vertical scar

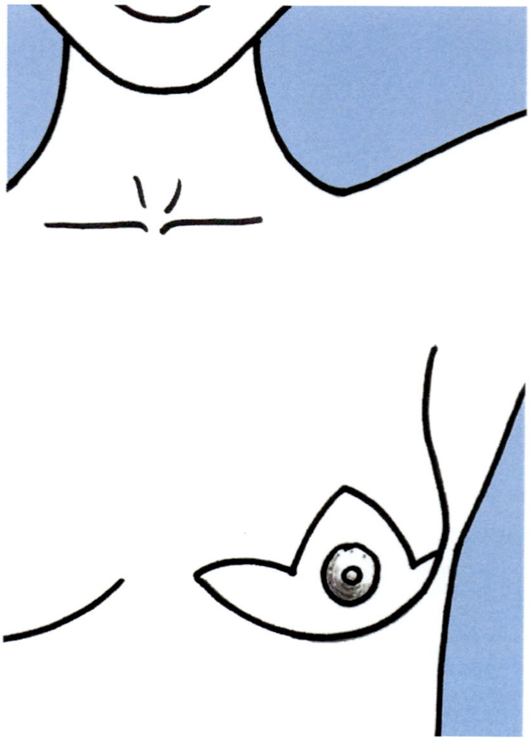

Fig. 24.7 Schematic representation of the classic inverted scar

24.5 Tissue Resection

The key is to realize that the type of tissue resection depends on the size, consistency, and shape of the breast and mainly on the relationship between the breast tissue and skin. It is important to remember that resection of the mammary parenchyma determines its shape. The extent of the breast tissue resection is planned using three different types of resection: (a) a plane resection (Pontes 1981), (b) a posterior resection (Pontes 1981), and (c) a keel resection (Figs. 24.8, 24.9 and 24.10) (Pitanguy 1967).

The author recommends plane resection for cases of hypertrophy where the superior pole is flat and the patient needs her breasts reduced, but requires tissue in the upper pole (Fig. 24.8). The posterior resection is ideal for breasts with hypertrophy with excess tissue in the superior pole and in addition allows removal of a large amount of tissue in the posterior resection (Fig. 24.9), and the keel resection is the best option for an overall breast reduction (Fig. 24.10).

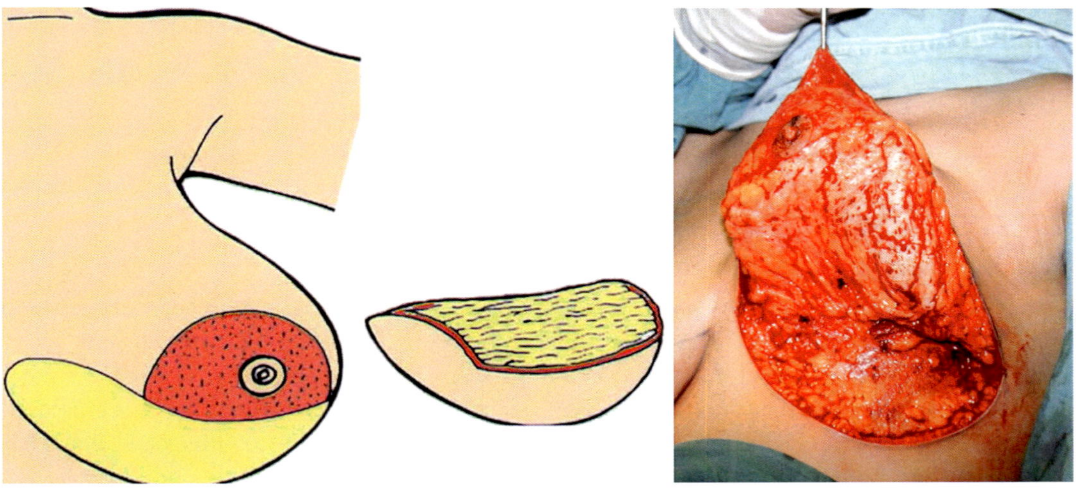

Fig. 24.8 Schematic representation and preoperative view of plane resection

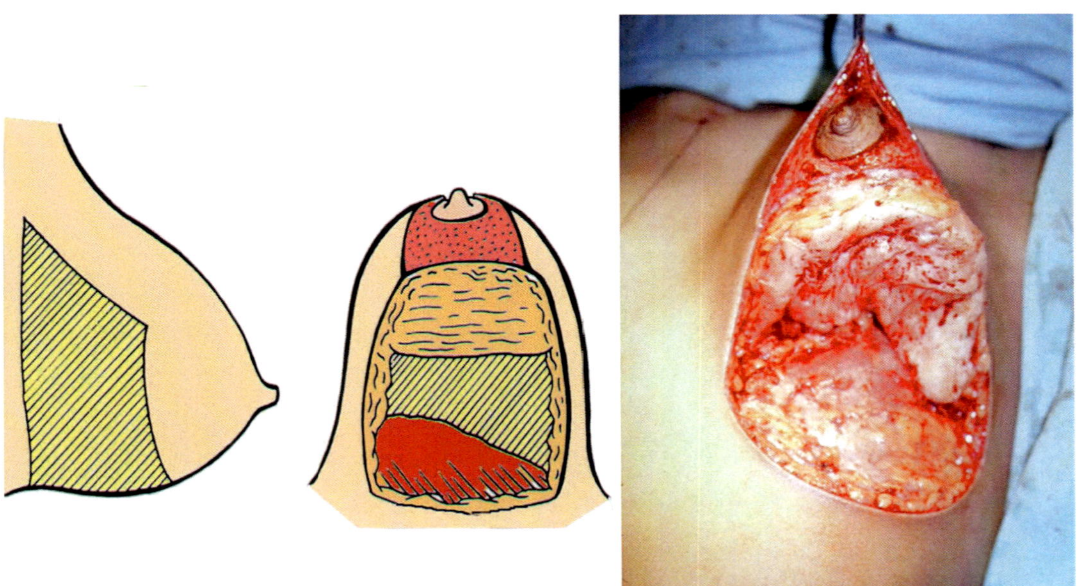

Fig. 24.9 Schematic representation and preoperative view of posterior resection

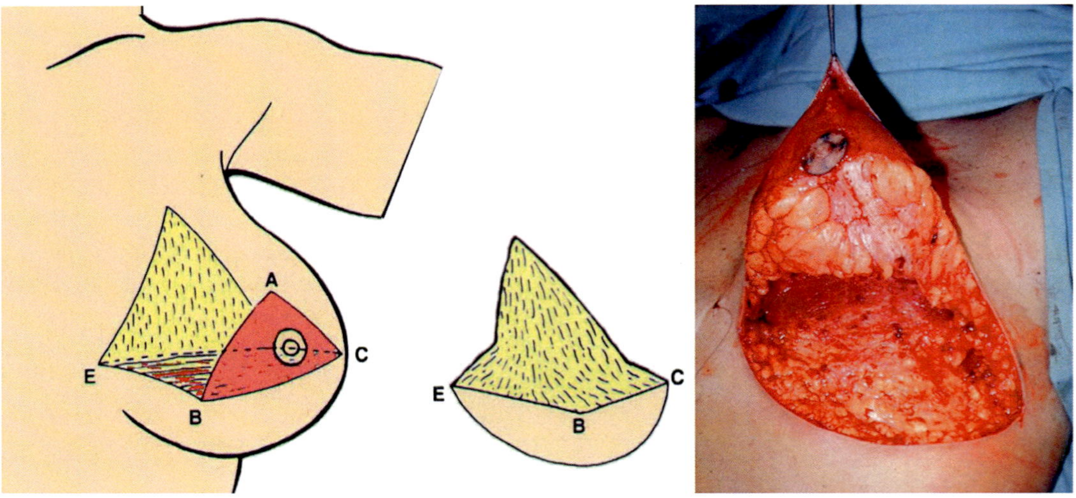

Fig. 24.10 Schematic representation and preoperative view of keel resection

24.6 Complications

Reductive mammoplasty, like any surgical intervention, is not exempt from the possibility of complications. Although the risk is considerably reduced, early or late complications may occur, such as nipple necrosis, infection, fat necrosis, wound dehiscence, hematoma, asymmetries, and unsightly scars (Lejour 1999).

24.7 Discussion

Surgeons have had a tendency to reduce the final scar of a mammaplasty (Lassus 1996; Lejour 1994; Marchac and Olarte 1982; Peixoto 1980); however, the relationship between breast tissue and skin should be a great guide. When a woman demands breast surgery, she desires to improve her appearance regardless of scars. We have had no complaints concerning the extent of the scars, but many concerning their quality and appearance. Sometimes patients complain about the size or form of their breasts. If it is necessary to increase the extent of the scar to improve the appearance of the breast, all patients agree with this course of action. Every breast has the scar it deserves (Figs. 24.11, 24.12, 24.13, and 24.14).

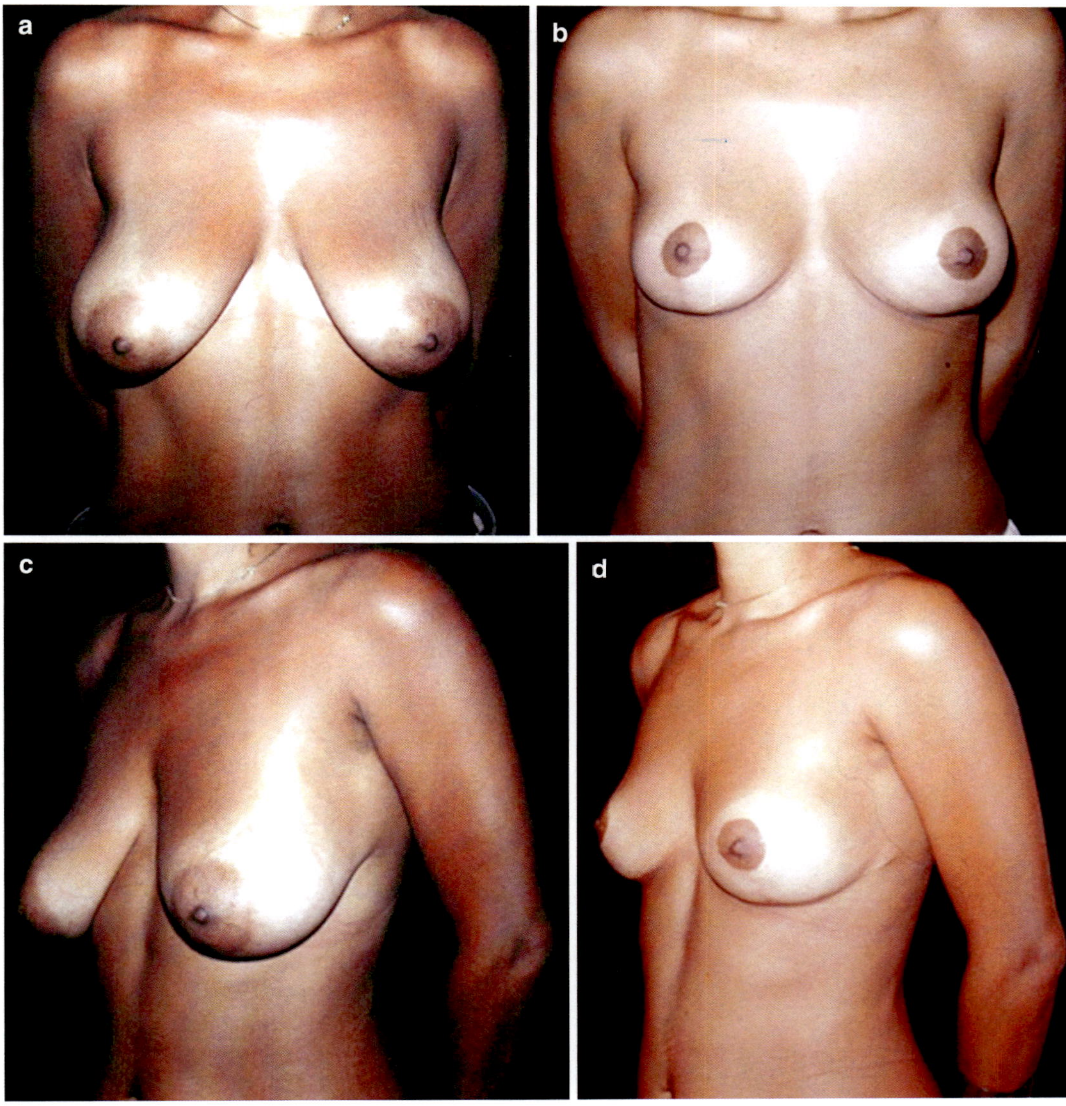

Fig. 24.11 (**a–c**) Middle-aged patient with ptosis and no tissue on the upper mammary pole before and (**b–d**) 1 year after only skin excess was removed. No scars are visible

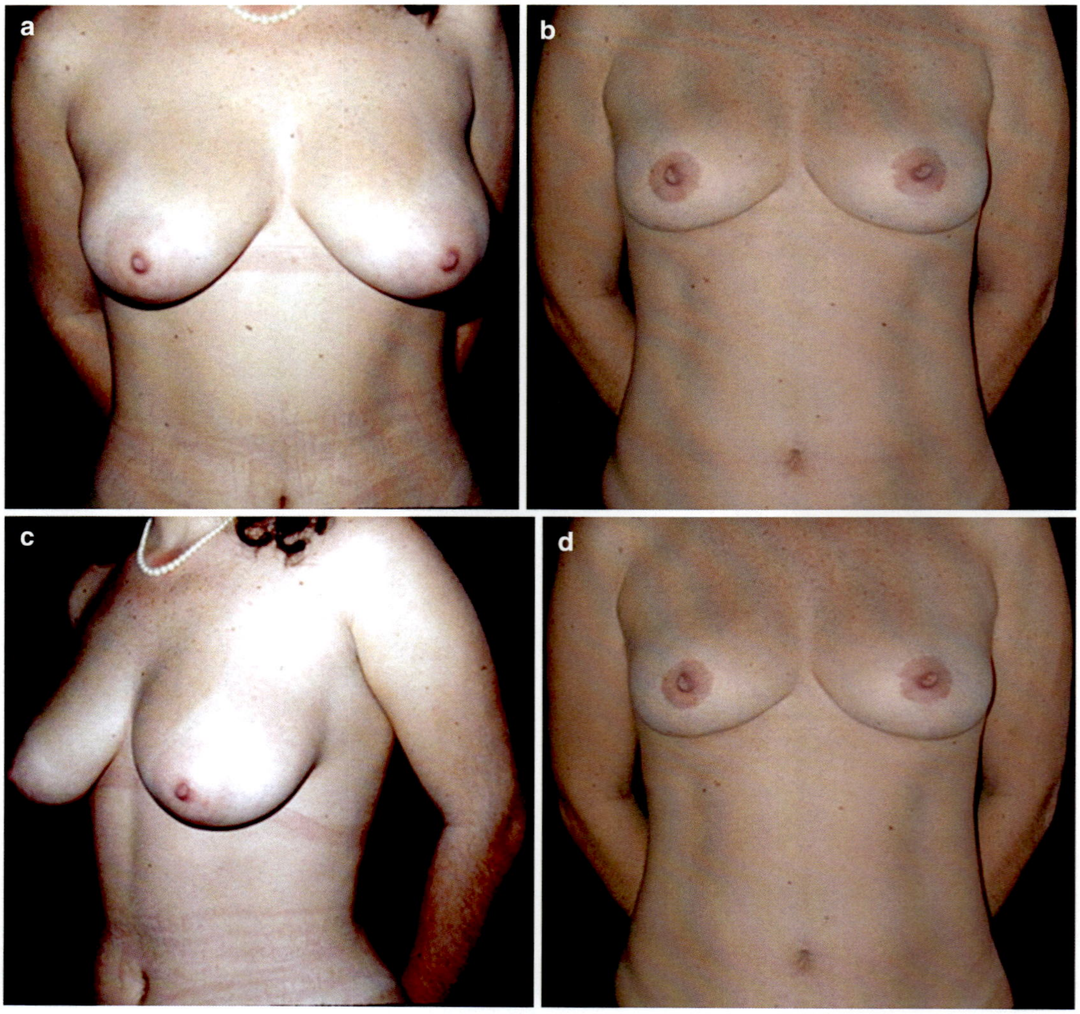

Fig. 24.12 (**a–c**) Young patient with ptosis and hypertrophy before and (**b–d**) 10 years after plane resection of 120 g on the right breast and 170 g on the left breast

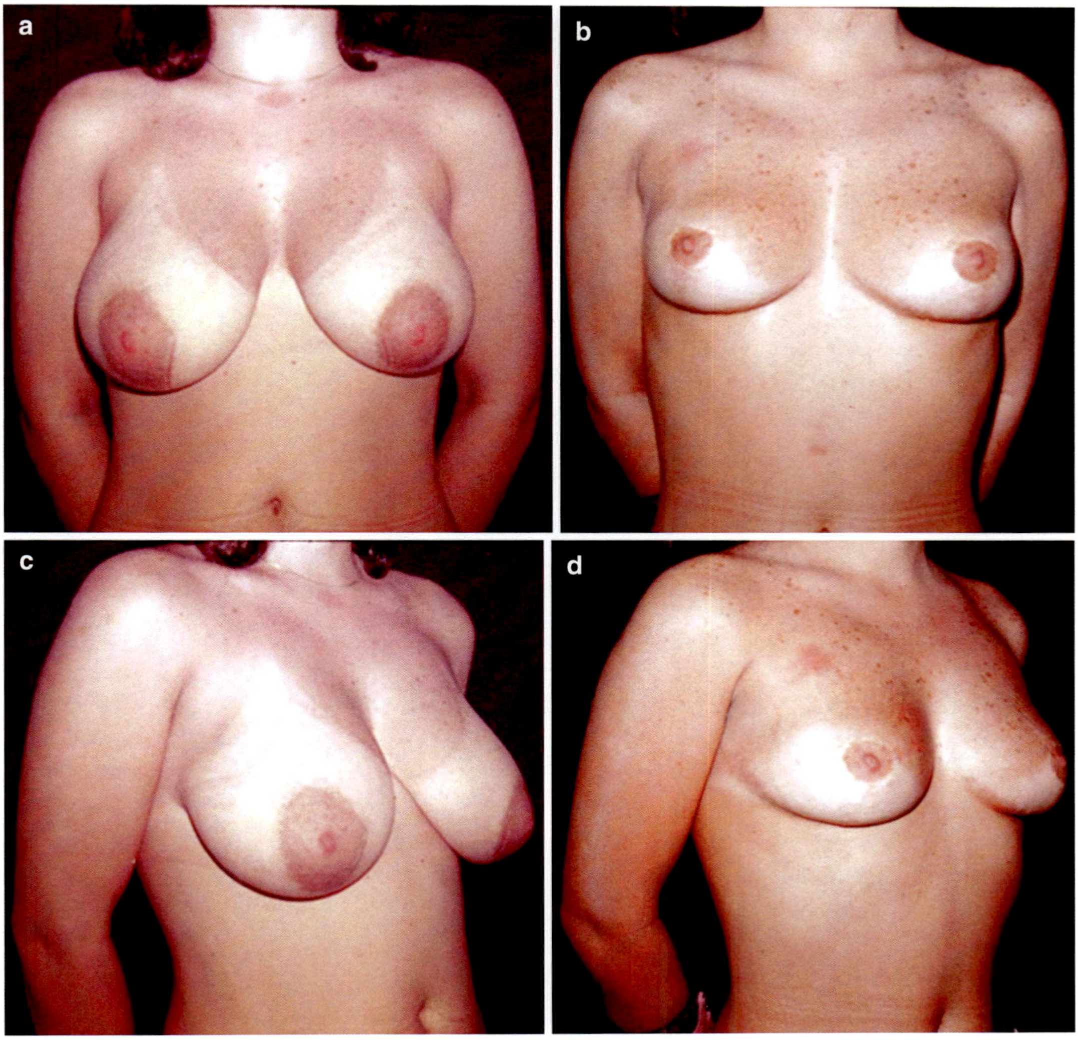

Fig. 24.13 (**a–c**) Young patient with hypertrophy and asymmetry before and (**b–d**) 5 years after breast reduction with posterior resection

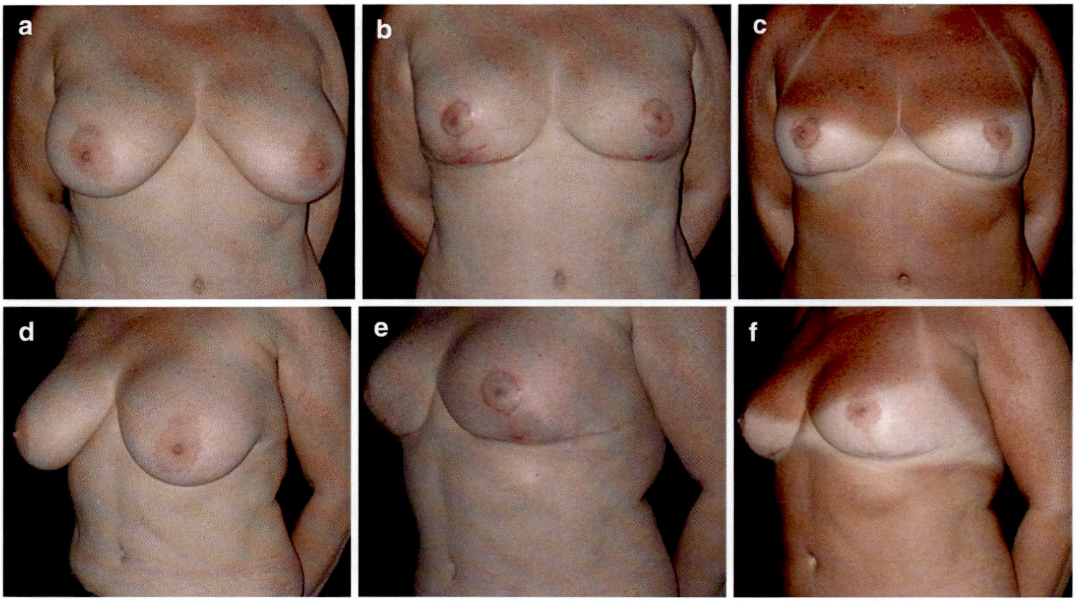

Fig. 24.14 (**a–d**) Middle-aged patient with moderate hypertrophy before and (**b–e**) 44 days and (**c–f**) 14 months after keel resection of 370 g on the right breast and 490 g on the left breast

Conclusion

The authors believe that the surgical principles and the philosophical concepts have been the state of the art in reduction mammaplasty so far. Several approaches to breast reduction have been attempted to combine the "natural form and appearance" with the appeal of short-scars, with a high level of satisfaction and a small number of complications. Patients are concerned with scar quality, not the extent of the scar. If the quality is good, success is guaranteed.

References

Cardoso de Castro C (1976) Mammaplasty with curved incisions. Plastic Reconstr Surg 57:596–600

Cardoso de Castro C (1984) The value of non-prefixed marking in reduction mammoplasty. Aesthet Plast Surg 8:237–241

Lassus C (1996) A 30 year experience with vertical mammaplasty. Plast Reconstr Surg 97:373–380

Lejour M (1994) Vertical mammaplasty and liposuction of the breast. Plastic Reconstr Surg 94:100–114

Lejour M (1999) Vertical mammaplasty: early complications after 250 personal consecutive cases. Plast Reconstr Surg 104:764–770

Marchac D, Olarte G (1982) Reduction mammaplasty and correction of ptosis with a short inframammary scar. Plastic Reconst Surg 69:45–55

Peixoto G (1980) Reduction mammaplasty: a personal technique. Plastic Reconstr Surg 65:217–226

Pitanguy I (1967) Surgical treatment of breast hypertrophy. Br J Plast Surg 20:78–85

Pitanguy I (2000) Evaluation of body contouring surgery today: a 30-year experience. Plastic Reconstr Surg 105:1499–1516

Pontes R (1981) Reduction mammaplasty—variations I and II. Ann Plast Surg 6:437

Reduction Mastoplasty with Prismatic Resection on a Trapezoid Base for Median Hypertrophic Breasts and Breasts with a Large Base

25

Márcio Paulino Costa,
Guilherme Cardinal Barreiro,
and Nuberto H. Teixeira

25.1 Introduction

Many techniques are currently employed to promote breast reduction, but all have in common the fact that the operation is performed with the patient's superior limbs abducted (Bames 1948; Baroudi and Lewis 1976; Biesenberger 1931; Born 1994; Bustos 1988; Brauman 1994; Conway 1952; Courtiss 1993; Courtiss and Goldwyn 1977; Dartigues 1935; De Benito and Sanza 1993; Costa et al. 2005, 2008; Dufourmentel 1939; Farina 1972; Ferreira et al. 1995; Gillies and McIndoe 1939; Hinderer 1979; Johnson 1976; Shin et al. 1996; Koger et al. 1994; Lassus 1996; Lejour 1994; May 1956; McKissock 1972; Melega et al. 1992; Rees and LaTrenta 1980; Regnault 1974; Ribeiro 1975; Robbins 1977; Sampaio Goes 1996; Schatten et al. 1971; Scutari and Varotto 1996; Skoog 1963; Strömbeck 1971, 1960; Thorek 1942).

The breast is a dynamic structure, as its shape and position vary according to the different movements and postures of the human body (Meijer 1974; Letterman and Schurter 1965; Rees 1971).

When comparing the position of the breast with the arms abducted and the arms at the side of the body, it can be observed that in the former situation the breasts are less ptotic, more projected, and the nipples are also laterally deviated. Similarly, the breast's shape is altered when the woman is standing versus a supine position. The action of gravity in the latter situation results in less ptosis and more widely spread breasts. The breast is a three-dimensional structure; thus, the way in which the excess tissue is removed determines the final shape.

The reduction mastoplasty technique with prismatic resection on a trapezoid base is based on the following principles: mammary reduction using adducted arms associated with a resection performed in two steps: (1) a central trapezoid prism (similar to a gold bar); (2) the base excess at a plane perpendicular to the breast (this determines the cone's height).

M.P. Costa, M.D., Ph.D. (✉)
Hospital das Clínicas, University of São Paulo Medical School, Brazilian Society of Plastic Surgery, ISAPS, FILACAP, ASPS,
Rua Gabriel dos Santos, 759 12o andar, Santa Cecília, 01231-011 São Paulo, SP, Brazil
e-mail: marciopaulino@bol.com.br

G.C. Barreiro, M.D., Ph.D.
University of Campinas (UNICAMP), Brazilian Society of Plastic Surgery, São Paulo, SP, Brazil

N.H. Teixeira, M.D.
University of São Paulo Medical School, Brazilian Society of Plastic Surgery, São Paulo, SP, Brazil

J.M. Avelar (ed.), *Breast Surgery*, https://doi.org/10.1007/978-3-319-54115-0_25

25.2 Methods

25.2.1 Surgical Technique

25.2.1.1 Markings

The breast is marked with the patient standing. The new desired position of the areola is determined by projecting the inframammary crease to a line that crosses the clavicular mid-point, whereas the future nipple is determined by the index finger (point A; Fig. 25.1).

An ellipse is drawn starting from point A and following the areolar border up to a point located 2 cm above the mammary inframammary crease (previously demarcated with the patient supine), and at a distance of 10 (±2) cm of the line that crosses the thoracic center (from the sternal notch to the umbilicus; Fig. 25.2). Measurements may vary depending on breast positioning (if more or less lateralized), and mammary volume.

The patient is positioned on the table in a supine position and with the arms adducted. Infiltration with vasoconstrictors was performed in patients to reduce bleeding.

De-epithelialization is carried out in the area previously marked by the ellipse. The skin of the mammary parenchyma is detached laterally and medially, and is also separated from the pectoralis major muscle enough to excise the excess mammary tissue. This technique approaches the skin and glandular tissue separately (Fig. 25.3).

Resection of the exceeding mammary tissue is accomplished with the patient in an elevated position, nearly sitting up, in two steps: (1) prism with a central trapezoid base (similar to a gold bar) (Figs. 25.4, 25.5, and 25.6), followed by suturing of the lateral and medial pillars (Fig. 25.7); (2) the base excess located on a plane perpendicular to the breast (height of the cone; Figs. 25.8 and 25.9).

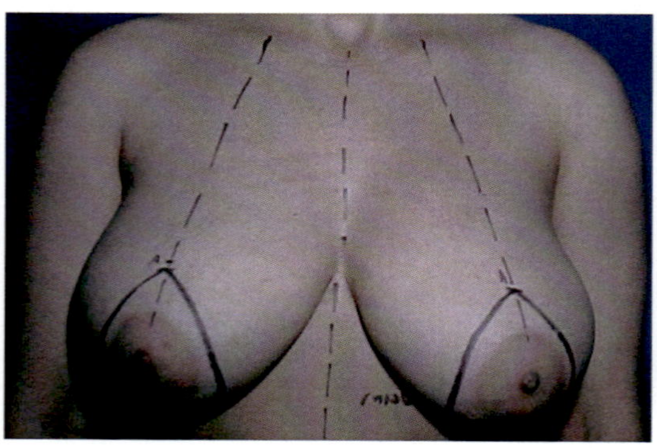

Fig. 25.1 Photo demonstrating the marking of the future position of the areola

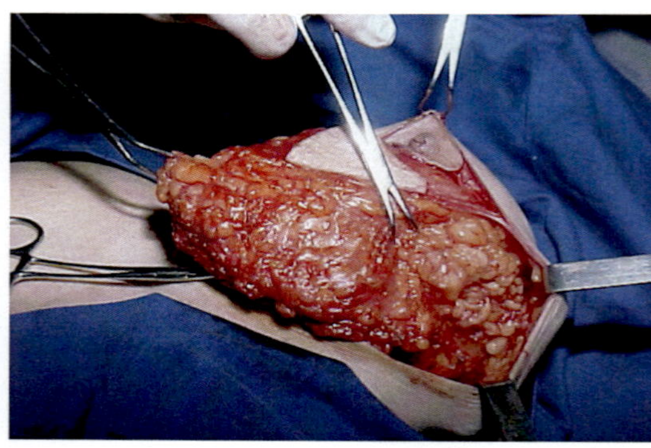

Fig. 25.3 Photo demonstrating extensive detachment of the skin of the mammary parenchyma. The pincers exert traction upon the lateral prolongation of the mammary tissue to obtain extensive mobility

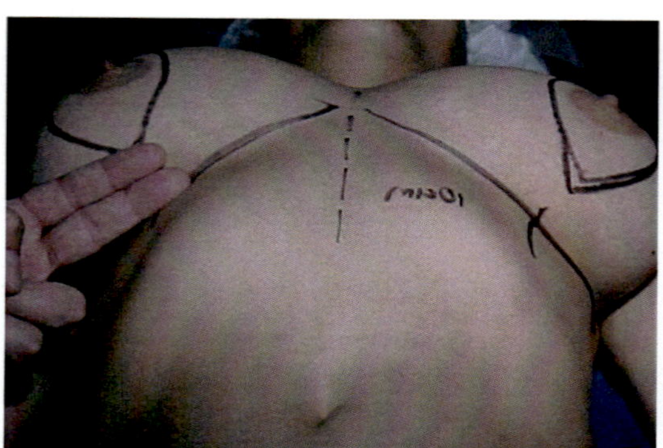

Fig. 25.2 The ellipse following the areolar border and attaining a ± 2 cm distance from the inframammary crease

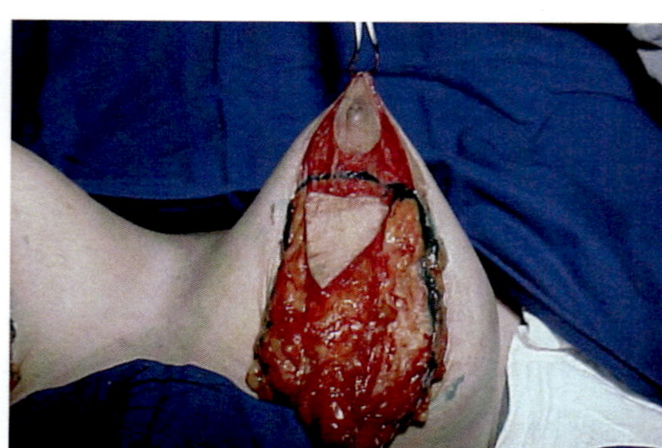

Fig. 25.4 Photo and drawing demonstrating marking of the trapezoid base prism to be removed

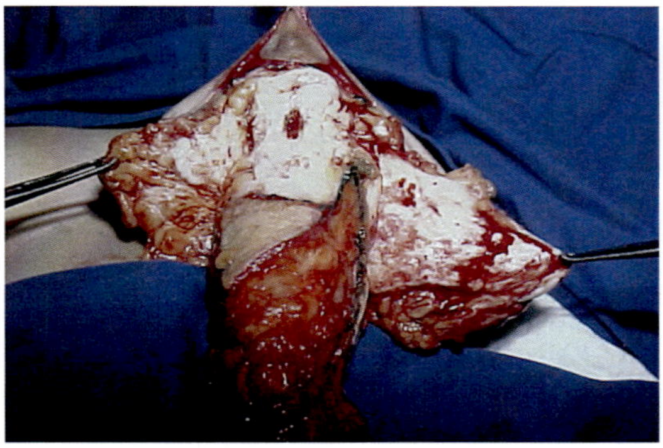

Fig. 25.5 Photo demonstrating resection of the excess mammary parenchyma with the form of a trapezoid base prism

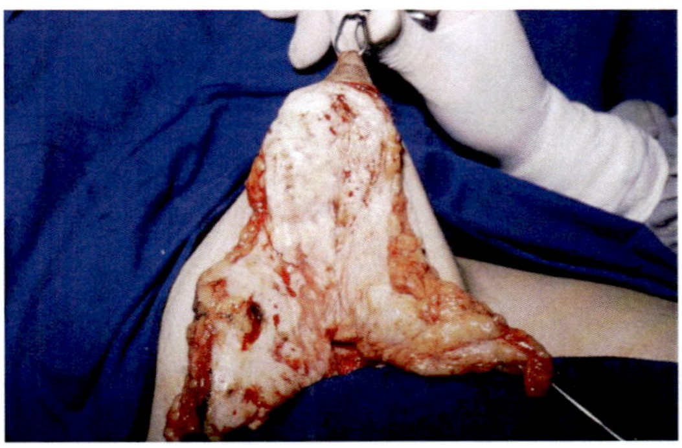

Fig. 25.6 Photo and drawing demonstrating the final aspect after removing the prism

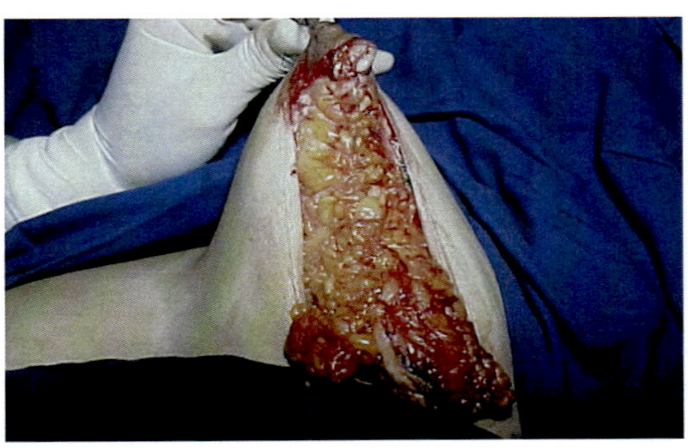

Fig. 25.7 Photo taken after suturing of the two pillars and marking of the resection of the mammary parenchyma base

After resection of the base, a stitch is made to fixate the breast at its new position. When the medial and lateral pillars are sutured, a greater projection of the areola and nipple occurs. The next step includes the fixation of the entire mammary base to the pectoralis major muscle.

The volume of fat that remains between the novel mammary position and the inframammary crease previously marked is removed.

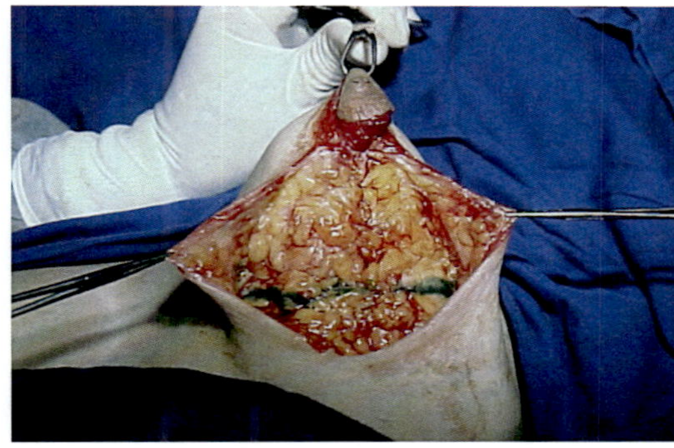

Fig. 25.8 Photo demonstrating base resection in a plane perpendicular to the breast

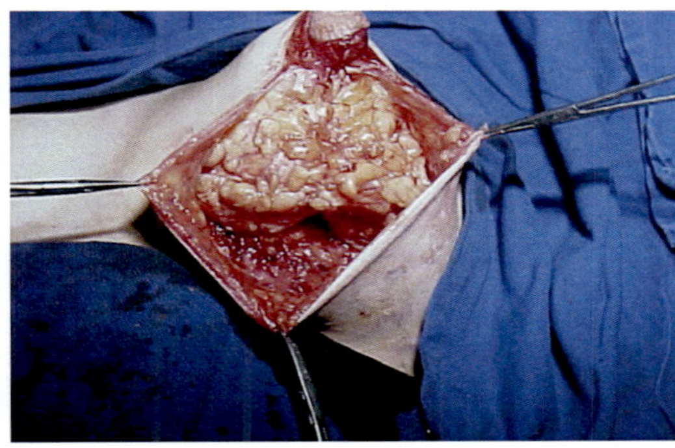

Fig. 25.9 Photo demonstrating the aspect after the base resection

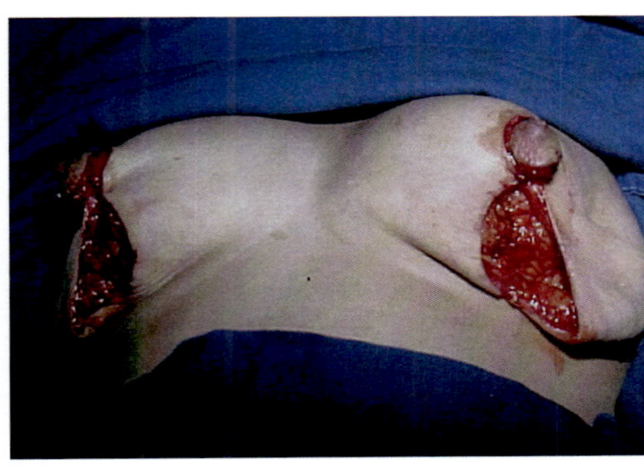

Fig. 25.10 Photo demonstrating skin excess after resection of the mammary tissue

The new position of the areola, which will be irrigated by the superior pedicle, is determined. This position may vary in relation to point A (medial, lateral, or superior) according to the need.

The excess skin to be removed is marked in a downward to upward direction to obtain a vertical scar (Figs. 25.10, 25.11, and 25.12).

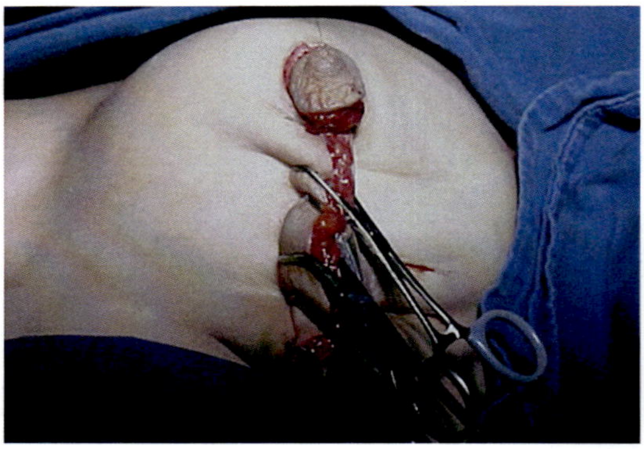

Fig. 25.11 Photo demonstrating marking for the posterior resection of the excess skin, which follows an upward direction

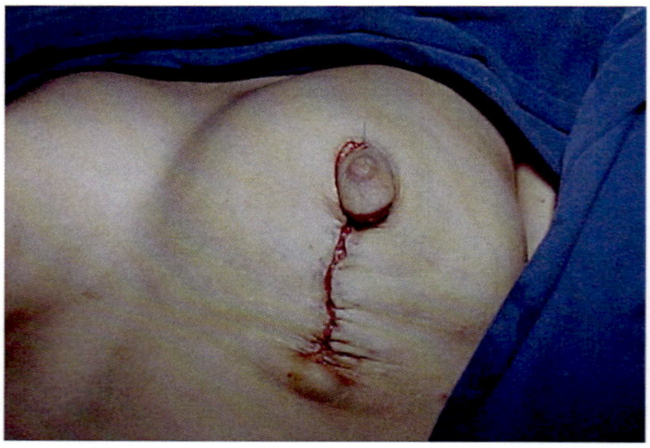

Fig. 25.12 Compensation for the excess skin to obtain a vertical scar

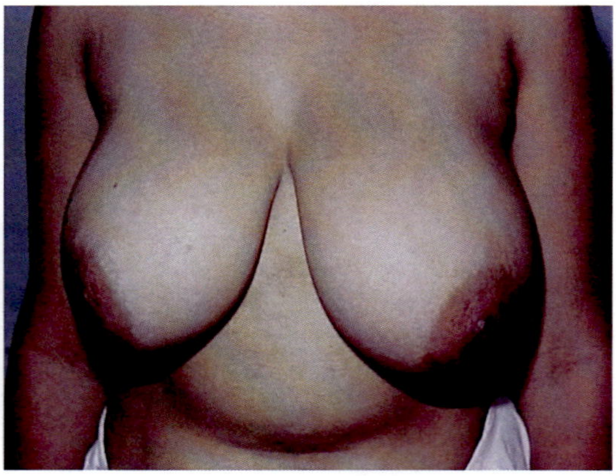

Fig. 25.13 Patient A, preoperatively

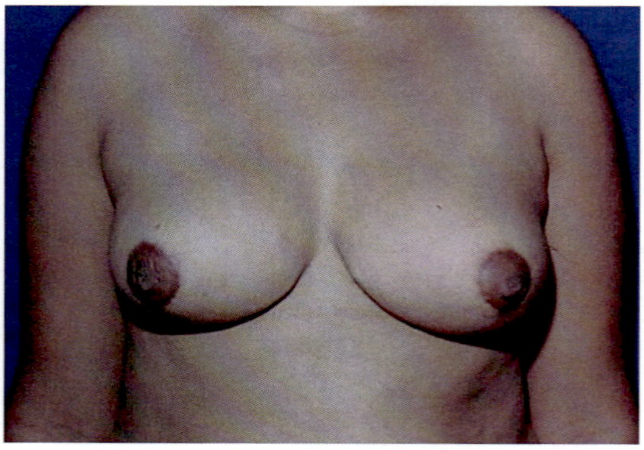

Fig. 25.14 Four years postoperatively, 900 g removed from the left breast and 780 g from the right breast

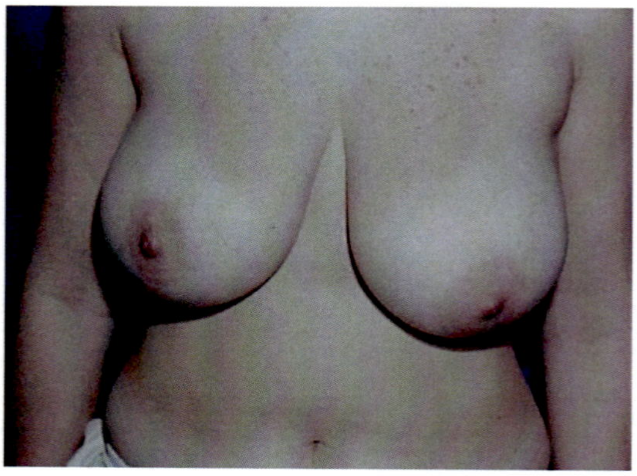

Fig. 25.15 Patient B, preoperatively

25.3 Discussion

In a series of 310 mammary reductions performed at Hospital das Clínicas University of São Paulo, mammary tissue resection ranged from 500 to 1300 g, with a mean value of 650 ± 20 g on each side. The highest distance determined by areolar transposition in the operated patients was of 13.5 cm, with a mean of 6.5 cm. The resulting scar ranged from a vertical one (90.0%) to a small inverted T (10%), never exceeding the mid-sternal or anterior axillary line (Figs. 25.13, 25.14, 25.15, 25.16, 25.17, and 25.18).

The way in which the resection is done leads to a comparatively larger reduction of the superior mammary diameter in relation to the base, thus allowing better support, which is offered by a base with a proportionately larger diameter (Fig. 25.19). This tends to diminish mammary

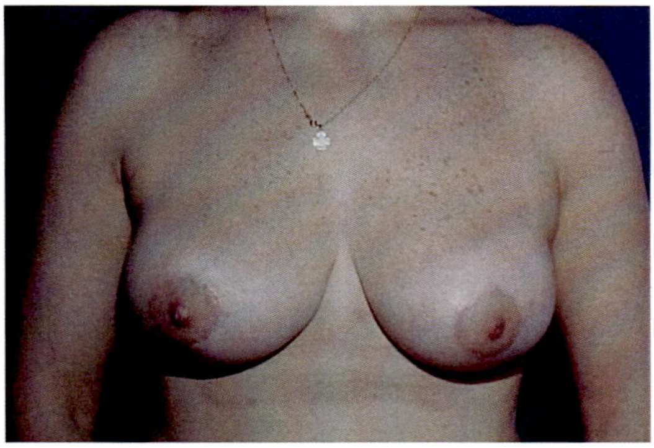

Fig. 25.16 One and a half years postoperatively, 820 g removed bilaterally

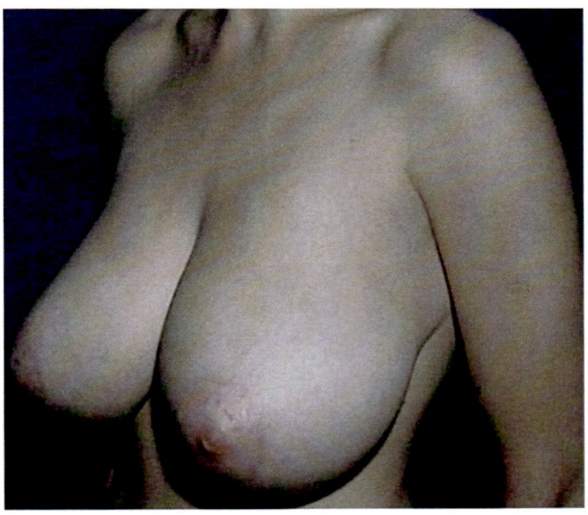

Fig. 25.17 Patient C, preoperatively

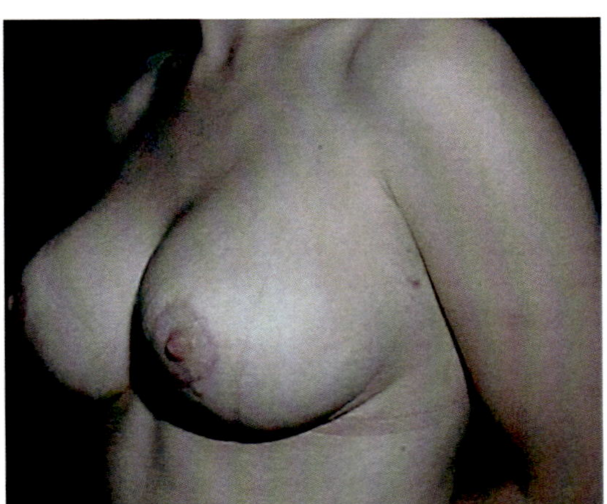

Fig. 25.18 Two years postoperatively, 1180 g removed bilaterally

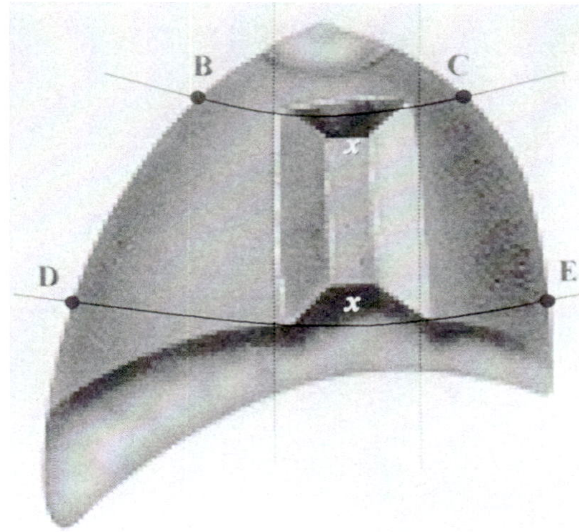

Fig. 25.19 Comparing weather the diameter measurents: BC/DE=K , BC-X/DE-X <K

falling during the postoperative period, and also prolongs the result.

In addition, the technique favors areolar projection as the pillars are approximated.

The areolar projection is very important to obtain good aesthetic results (Sampaio Goes 1996). In techniques in which a keel-shaped resection is carried out (Farina 1972; Pontes 1973), or in which the trapezoid base prism is made, the pillars are approximated. However, in the latter, better areolar projection is obtained because the space to be filled in by the mammary tissue below the areola is larger and so is the resulting vector (Fig. 25.20).

Reduction mastoplasty with prismatic resection on a trapezoid base approaches the skin and mammary tissue separately. The resulting shape at the end of the surgery depends on the mode of excess tissue resection, but does not depend on the tension applied to the skin. In fact, the skin is used only for covering and not for shaping the breast. This procedure contributes to increments in the longevity of breast reduction surgeries.

Considering the preoperative breast size and the volume removed, results concerning the final shape can be seen after 3 or 4 months. The small folds observed in most cases during the immediate post-surgical period (Fig. 25.12) accommodate until the fourth week. In a small number of

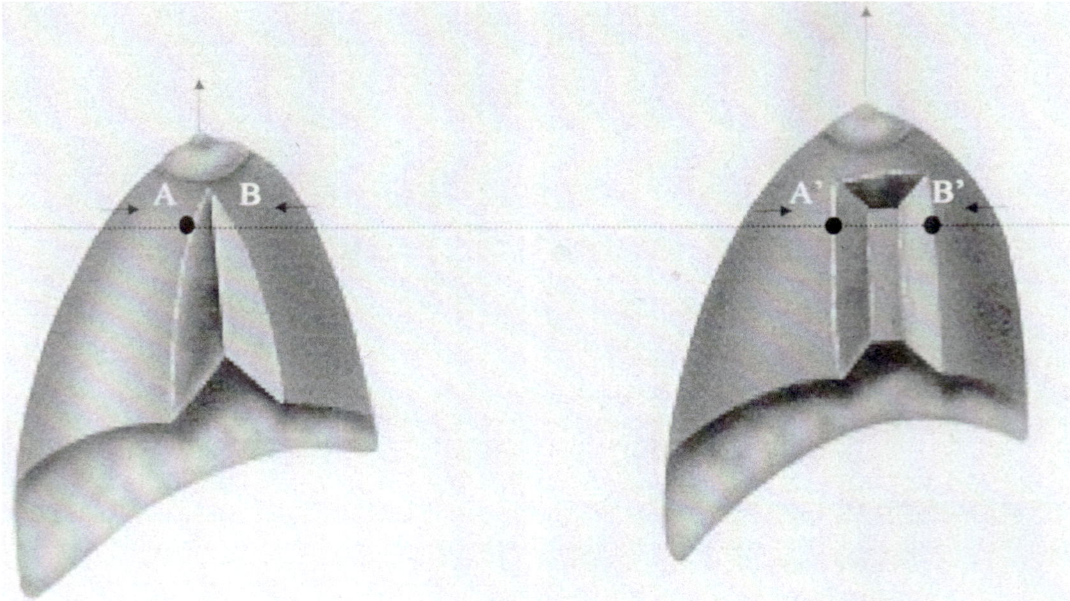

Fig. 25.20 Comparison of techniques: keel-shaped, with the trapezoid base prism. Distance A′B′ > AB

cases, redundant skin persists at the level of the infra-mammary crease for more than 4 months, and can be corrected by a small T-shaped incision. It is important to emphasize that the above-mentioned complication occurred in resections of more than 800 g. However, we prefer a small late correction to obtain a shorter scar with no impairment of the final aesthetic result.

Although the technique is new, in different hands similar outcomes can be achieved. Residents of São Paulo's University Medical School are performing this surgery well.

Considering the large volume removed and the size of the operated breasts, few complications were observed, and were similar to those for other techniques described in the literature (Costa et al. 2005; Lassus 1996; McKissock 1972; Orlando 1975; Pitanguy 1960; Robbins 1977).

The technique has some emblematic characteristics: (a) It is a versatile technique as it may be applied to small, medium, or large breasts; (b) final results may be predicted with good levels of accuracy, as the patient is operated in an anatomical position; (c) short scars are obtained; (d) good projection of the areola is achieved; (e) large breast reductions are permitted; (f) the manner in which the excess tissue is removed results in less falling during the postoperative period; (g) stretching of the brachial plexus nerves is minimized, as the patient's arms are adducted; (h) a large decrease in the breast's diameter is permitted.

When the plastic surgeon plans breast surgery, he must know the main problems to be solved. In the case of heavy, ptotic, and asymmetric breasts, there is a large height or a large diameter. This technique allows large decreases in breasts with wide diameters. It is one of the most important characteristics that can solve one of the challenges that we have in breast surgery: changing the shape of breasts with wide diameters. With the decrease in the breast's diameter, its appearance seems to be younger and more beautiful.

Often, the reduction mastoplasty with prismatic resection on a trapezoid base is used to reduce the contralateral breast of patients reconstructed using a transverse rectus abdominis myocutaneous (TRAM) flap.

25.3.1 Complications

There were few complications observed in the series of 310 patients operated on at Hospital das Clinicas. Five patients developed seroma (1.61%)

without further problems. There were five cases (1.61%) of small volume hematoma, which were evacuated by punctures, with no need for re-operation. In ten patients (3.22%) with inverted T scars, superficial skin ischemia occurred and healed by secondary intention. There were no cases of areolar infection or necrosis.

Concerning areola sensitivity, 15 patients complained of diminished sensitivity for a period longer than 6 months, but all improved after 1 year. These patients underwent mammary tissue resections of more than 900 g and had shown severe ptosis preoperatively.

Conclusions

Reduction mastoplasty with prismatic resection on a trapezoid base is an adequate therapeutic option for mammary hypertrophy. It is an excellent choice for breasts with large diameters.

References

Bames HO (1948) Reduction of massive breast hypertrophy. Plast Reconstr Surg 3:560

Baroudi R, Lewis JR (1976) The augmentation-reduction mammaplasty. Clin Plast Surg 3:301

Biesenberger H (1931) Deformitäten und kosmetische Operationen der weiblichen Brust. Maudrich, Vienna

Born G (1994) The "L" reduction mammaplasty. Ann Plast Surg 32:383

Brauman D (1994) Reduction mammaplasty by suction alone. Plast Reconstr Surg 94:1095

Bustos R (1988) Mamaplastia periareolar. In: Communication to the XXVth Brazilian congress of plastic surgery, Salvador

Conway H (1952) Mammaplasty: analysis of 110 consecutive cases with end-results. Plast Reconstr Surg 10:303

Costa MP, Tuma P Jr, Ferreira MC (2005) Reduction mammaplasty with resection of a trapezoid base prism and adduction of the arms. Plast Reconstr Surg 116(1):242–250

Costa MP, Ching AW, Ferreira MC (2008) Thin superior medial pedicle reduction mammaplasty for severe mammary hypertrophy. Aesthetic Plast Surg 32(4):645–652

Courtiss EH (1993) Reduction mammaplasty by suction alone. Plast Reconstr Surg 92:1276

Courtiss EH, Goldwyn RM (1977) Reduction mammaplasty by the inferior pedicle technique. An alternative to free nipple and areola grafting for severe macromastia or extreme ptosis. Plast Reconstr Surg 59:500

Dartigues L (1935) Les anomalies du sein en dehors des hypertrophies et des prolapsus. Bull Mem Soc Méd Paris 139:575

De Benito J, Sanza IF (1993) Periareolar techniques for mammary reduction and elevation. Aesthetic Plast Surg 17:311

Dufourmentel L (1939) Chirurgie reparatrice et correctrice des téguments et des formes. Masson, Paris

Farina R (1972) Reduction mammaplasty with free grafting of the nipple and areola. Br J Plast Surg 25:393

Ferreira MC, Ishida J, Gemperli R, Monteiro AA Jr, Tuma PT Jr (1995) Reduction mammoplasty with shortened scars: surgical technique. Rev Hosp Fac Med São Paulo. 50:22

Gillies H, McIndoe AH (1939) The technique of mammaplasty in conditions of hypertrophy of the breast. Surg Gynecol Obstet 68:658

Hinderer UT (1979) The dermal brasserrie mammaplasty. Clin Plast Surg 3:349

Johnson CF (1976) New technique for reduction mammaplasty. Plast Reconstr Surg 57:372

Koger KE, Sundle D, Press BH, Hovey LM (1994) Reduction mammaplasty for gigantomastia using inferiorly based pedicle and free nipple transplantation. Plast Reconstr Surg 33:561

Lassus C (1996) A 30-year experience with vertical mammaplasty. Plast Reconstr Surg 97:373

Lejour M (1994) Vertical mammaplasty and liposuction of the breast. Plast Reconstr Surg 94:100

Letterman G, Schurter M (1965) Reduction mammaplasty with preservation of nipple glandular continuity. J Am Med Womans Assoc 20:942

May H (1956) Breast plasty in the female. Plast Reconstr Surg 17:351

McKissock PK (1972) Reduction mammaplasty with a vertical dermal flap. Plast Reconstr Surg 49:245

Meijer R (1974) A modified Aufricht reduction mammaplasty. Plast Reconstr Surg 53:129

Melega JM, Zanini SA, Psillakis JM (1992) Cirurgia Plástica Reparadora e Estética, 2ª Edição. Edit Medsi, Rio de Janeiro, p 707–724

Orlando JC (1975) The superomedial pedicle for nipple transposition. Br J Plast Surg 28:42

Pitanguy I (1960) Breast hypertrophy. In: Transactions of the international society of plastic surgeons, second congress, London 1969. Livingstone, Edinburgh, p 509

Pontes R (1973) A technique of reduction mammaplasty. Br J Plast Surg 26:365

Rees TD (1971) An historical review of mammaplasty. In: Transactions of fifth international congress of plastic and reconstructive surgery. Butterworths, Melbourne, pp 1167–1173

Rees TD, LaTrenta GS (1980) Aesthetic plastic surgery, vol II, 2nd edn, pp 925–1002

Regnault P (1974) Reduction mammaplasty by the "B" technique. Plast Reconstr Surg 53:19

Ribeiro L (1975) A new technique for reduction mammaplasty. Plast Reconstr Surg 55:330

Robbins TH (1977) A reduction mammaplasty with the areola-nipple based on an inferior dermal pedicle. Plast Reconstr Surg 59:64

Sampaio Goes JC (1996) Periareolar mammaplasty: double skin technique with application of polyglactine or mixed mesh. Plast Reconstr Surg 97:959

Schatten WE, Hartley JH Jr, Hamm WG (1971) Reduction mammaplasty by the Dufourmentel-Mouly method. Plast Reconstr Surg 48:306

Scutari M, Varotto S (1996) A nest swallow's technique in reduction mastoplasty and mastopexy. Acta Chir Ital 52:169

Shin KS, Chung S, Lee HK, Lew JD (1996) Reduction mammaplasty by central pedicle with short submammary scar. Aesthetic Plast Surg. 20:69

Skoog T (1963) A technique of breast reduction: transposition of the nipple on a cutaneous vascular pedicle. Acta Chir Scand 126:453

Strömbeck JO (1971) Reduction mammaplasty. Surg Clin North Am 51:453

Strömbeck JO (1960) Mammaplasty: report of a new technique based on two-pedicle procedure. Br J Plast Surg 13:79

Thorek M (1942) Plastic surgery of the breast and the abdominal wall. Thomas, Springfield

26 Reduction Mammaplasty: McKissock's Technique, a Personal Approach

Emília Silva Klein and Joel Araújo Silva

26.1 Introduction

In the twentieth century, many surgeons initiate different approaches to the existing surgery techniques. These approaches would now prioritize physiology, shape, aesthetics, and lasting results. Among the many possible types of mammaplasty, the reduction of hypertrophy and gigantomastia is the most complex. The previously available techniques were difficult to execute and led to some unsatisfactory results. Among the unpleasant characteristics related to those techniques are the difficult positioning of the nipple–areola complex (NAC), the resulting breast shape, and postoperative complications. When employing Strömbeck's, Pitanguy's, Skoog's and Weiner's techniques. I was introduced to McKissock's technique (1972) in 1978. This technique introduced the bipedicle bridge flap and it proved to be safer for cases of mild and moderate mammary hypertrophy and for those of ptosis, providing similar results to the previously adopted techniques. Nevertheless, for the patients with severe hypertrophy whose first option would be to employ Thorek's technique (1942), the results achieved were unsatisfactory. Thorek's technique, once used in young patients, led to some unfavorable aspects such as loss of nipple–areolar sensitivity and sectioning of galactophore ducts, and these complications undermined its use. The experience acquired by employing McKissock's technique encouraged us to propose adaptations to it and to use it for cases of major hypertrophy. Dr. Liacyr Ribeiro's (1969–1971) description and classification of the mammary pedicles with regard to vascularization, structure, and usage constituted major facilitators to the comprehension in addition to a stimulus to the introduced tactic. This tactic may be manipulated on a case by case basis.

Breasts not only play an important role in women's femininity, but also in women's psychological and physical wellbeing. Shape, size, and body harmony constitute a great challenge for the surgeon. Treating severe mammary hypertrophy, where large skin, fat, and glandular resection is needed, nipple–areola repositioning at a more elevated spot, and smaller and more aesthetic scars are still reasons for study and there is still a lot to find out.

The surgical tactic addressed here employed in larger resections preserves the T-shape scar,

E.S. Klein, M.D. (✉) • J. Araújo Silva, M.D.
Hospital Belo Horizonte, Av. Pres. Antônio Carlos, 1694, Belo Horizonte, MG, Brazil
e-mail: emilia.klein@gmail.com

J.M. Avelar (ed.), *Breast Surgery*, https://doi.org/10.1007/978-3-319-54115-0_26

as this one offers greater reliability in the postoperative period. This chapter discusses aspects regarding the modification of McKissock's flat vertical bipedicle as an option in the surgical treatment of cases of large and severe mammary hypertrophy.

26.2 Method

Various modifications to the original McKissock's technique have been introduced. In our hands, the bipedicle vertical flap described by McKissock is modified. The original 3.0-cm thickness (Fig. 26.1) bridge flap is transformed in a continuous or partially continuous massive block. If it is completely fixed to the pectoralis major muscle the result is a continuous block. It may also be fixed at three-quarters distally, resulting in a partially continuous massive block. In cases in which a partially continuous block is used, parenchyma is removed to form a keel shape, similar to Pitanguy's technique, to better accommodate the flap, thus avoiding the folding effect observed in the original technique, which could lead to postoperative complications. The upper portion of the flap receives blood supply from the dermal plexus. The distal portion receives blood supply from the subdermal plexus, from the fourth and fifth intercostal arteries, and the intercostal veins. Along all its extension, the flap is supplied by intercostal trunks, thus its great reliability. We have been using this modified dermal flap not only for treating patients with severe mammary hypertrophy, but also at all degrees of hypertrophy and flaccid and/or ptotic breasts when the patient refuses mammary implants.

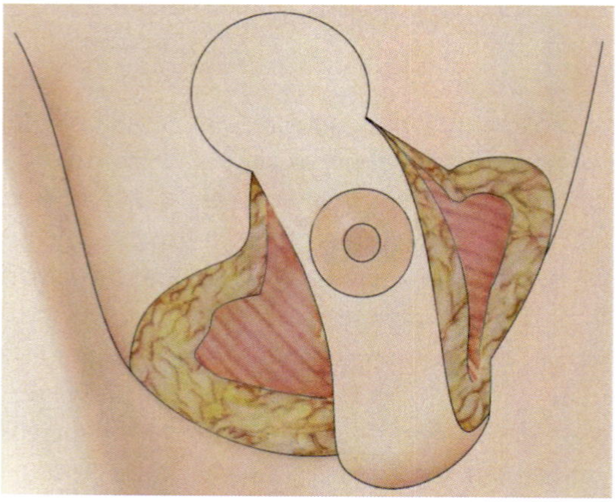

Fig. 26.1 McKissock's original bridge flap

Inverted T-shaped scars are our most frequent result, but we do not exclude the possibility of inverted L-shaped, J-shaped or comma-shaped scars in smaller breasts with no skin excess.

Preoperative marking is key for a good execution. The parameters used for preoperative marking are the usual ones. Wise's pattern may be used or we may draw it hands-free. Marking begins with the patient in a full upright position. A midsternal line is drawn and the inframammary fold is marked. From the furculum's midpoint a 5.0–7.0 cm distant point is marked at the clavicle. The next point is marked by drawing an imaginary horizontal line passing through the midsternal line toward the nipple. The point is marked 9.0–10 cm from the midsternal line. Then, a line is drawn uniting the last two points described and down to the inframammary fold. This line does not necessarily cross the nipple. Point A is found using a middle finger's projection at the inframammary fold (Fig. 26.2a). Points B and C are marked by using a bidigital pinch maneuver measuring 5.0–5.5 cm downward from the base of the new NAC location. Points B and C are then united to the new inframammary fold, which is drawn 0.5–1.0 cm upward from the original one (Fig. 26.2c). The bipedicle vertical flap is then drawn beginning at the point where the line descending from the clavicle crosses the new inframammary fold. From this

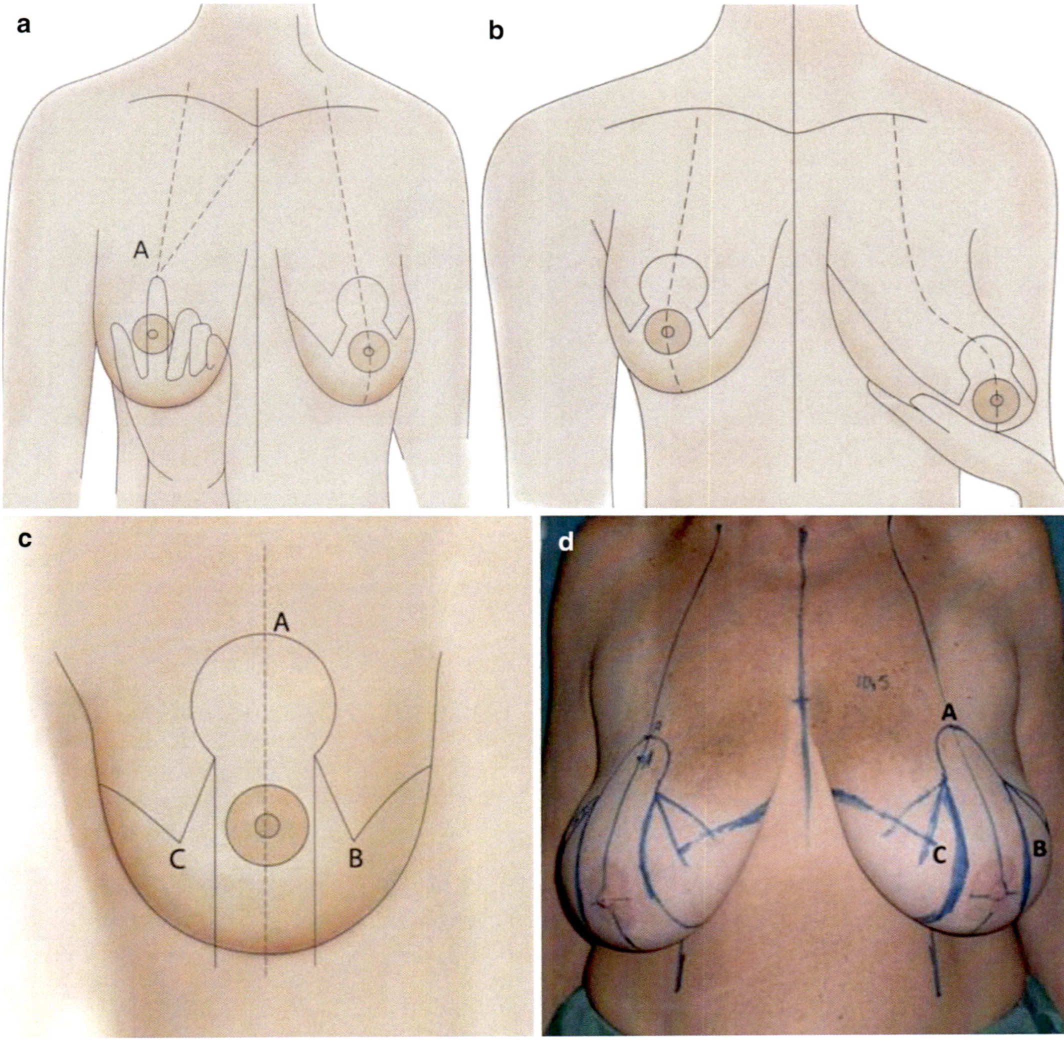

Fig. 26.2 Planning. (**a**) Point A marking. (**b**, **c**) Points B and C and vertical bipedicle flap marking. (**d**) Standard preoperative markings

point, two points are marked laterally and medially 4.0–5.0 cm in each direction. From the base of the nipple two other points are marked laterally and medially 1.5 cm in each direction. The end points are found at the lateral and medial base of the new NAC site. Last, the three points laterally and medially should be united (Fig. 26.2b, d).

26.2.1 Operative Technique

Surgery follows the previous markings. The areola is determined by using areola markers with a diameter of 3.5–4.0 cm. Flap decortication is carried out according to the previously made markings. Incisions should be carefully made through its medial and lateral margins.

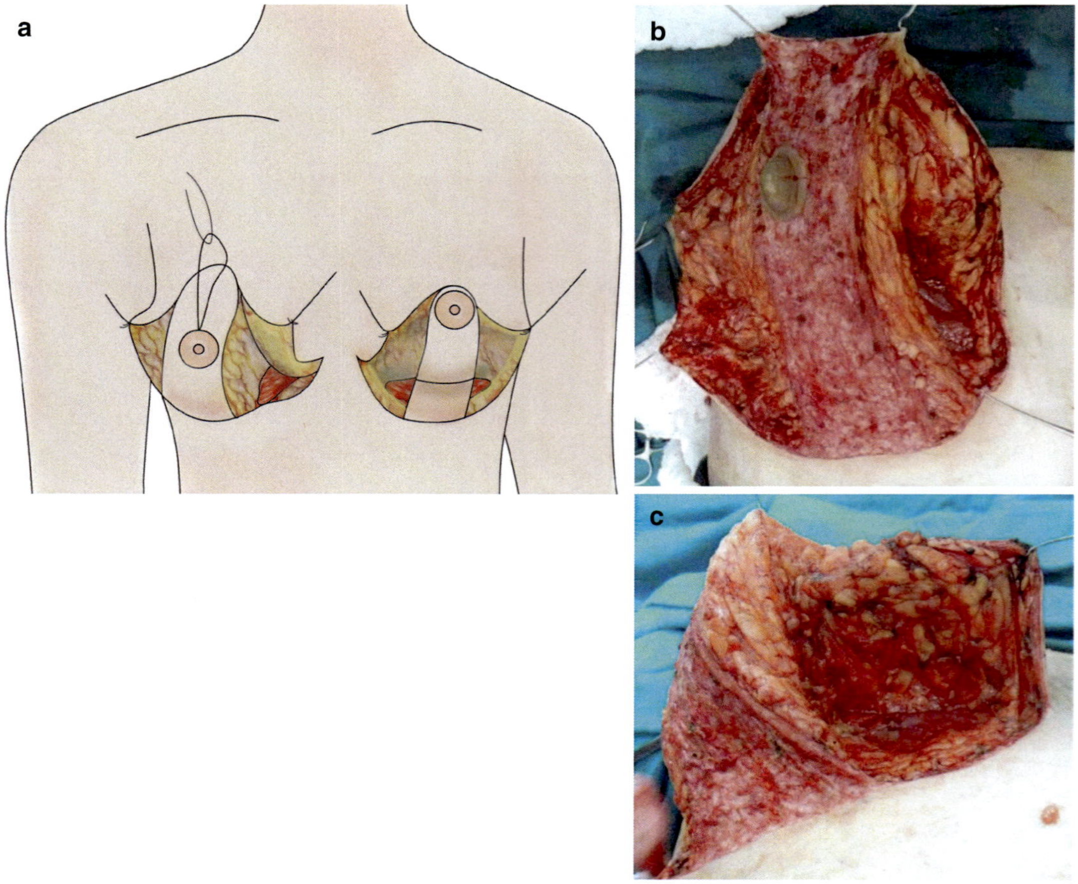

Fig. 26.3 Modified bipedicular vertical flap—the block is fully attached to the pectoralis major muscle

The dermal flap is tailored and kept completely or partially fixed to the pectoralis major muscle (Fig. 26.3). Excess parenchyma is resected laterally and medially. For better accommodation of the flap or when the flap length exceeds 50 cm, additional resection should extend to the lateral and medial quadrants. Occasionally, keel-shaped resection, as proposed by Pitanguy may be employed. Following hemostasis, closure begins by fixing the areola to point A using a slow absorbable suture. Then, the breast should be elevated to allow the identification of the breast conus. Once identified, non-absorbable 2-0 sutures should be employed to join the lateral and medial pillars to the base of the bipedicle flap, forming the breast conus (Fig. 26.4). Points B and C are then approximated and sutured with slow absorbing 3-0 suture. For greater breast projection, a second stitch with either absorbable or non-absorbable 3-0 suture is inserted approximately 1.0 cm away from the B and C union points. The flap may be kept in its position or it may be shifted and medially fixed for around 3.0 cm of its lower implantation for better definition of the breast's medial contour. Closure of the

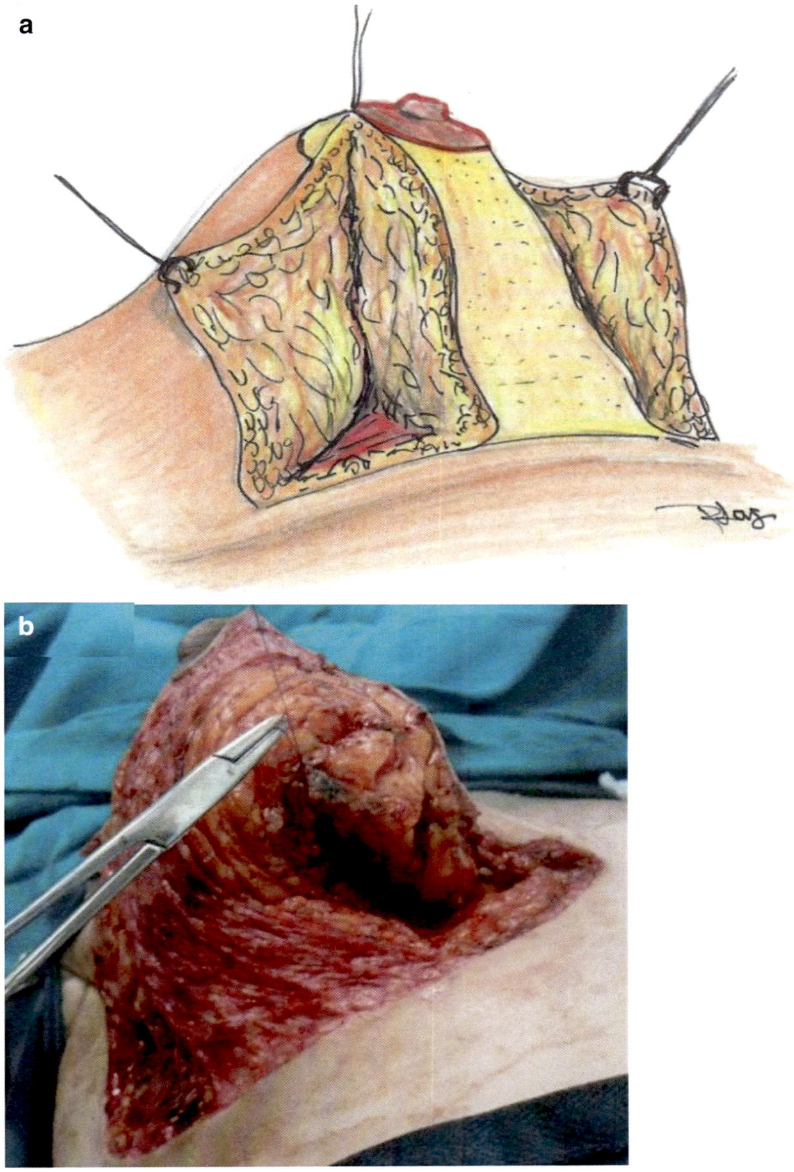

Fig. 26.4 Breast closure. Fixing the lateral and medial pillars to the base of the bipedicle flap forming the breast conus

bleeding areas including the areolar area is carried out in layers with slow absorbing 3-0 sutures. At the lower bleeding area, closure is performed from its lateral and medial extremity toward the vertical line of the inverted T-shaped scar (Fig. 26.5). The skin is closed with intradermal slow absorbing 4-0 sutures. Dry gauze and Micropore tape are applied as dressing, and a bra is immediately put on (Figs. 26.6 and 26.7).

Fig. 26.5 Final aspect of the sutured breasts. Immediately postoperatively

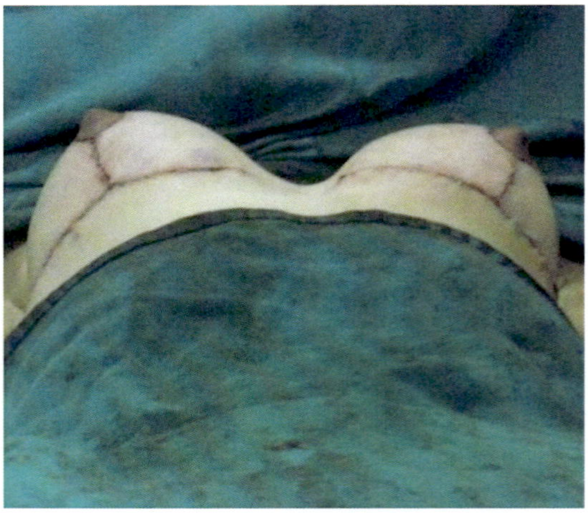

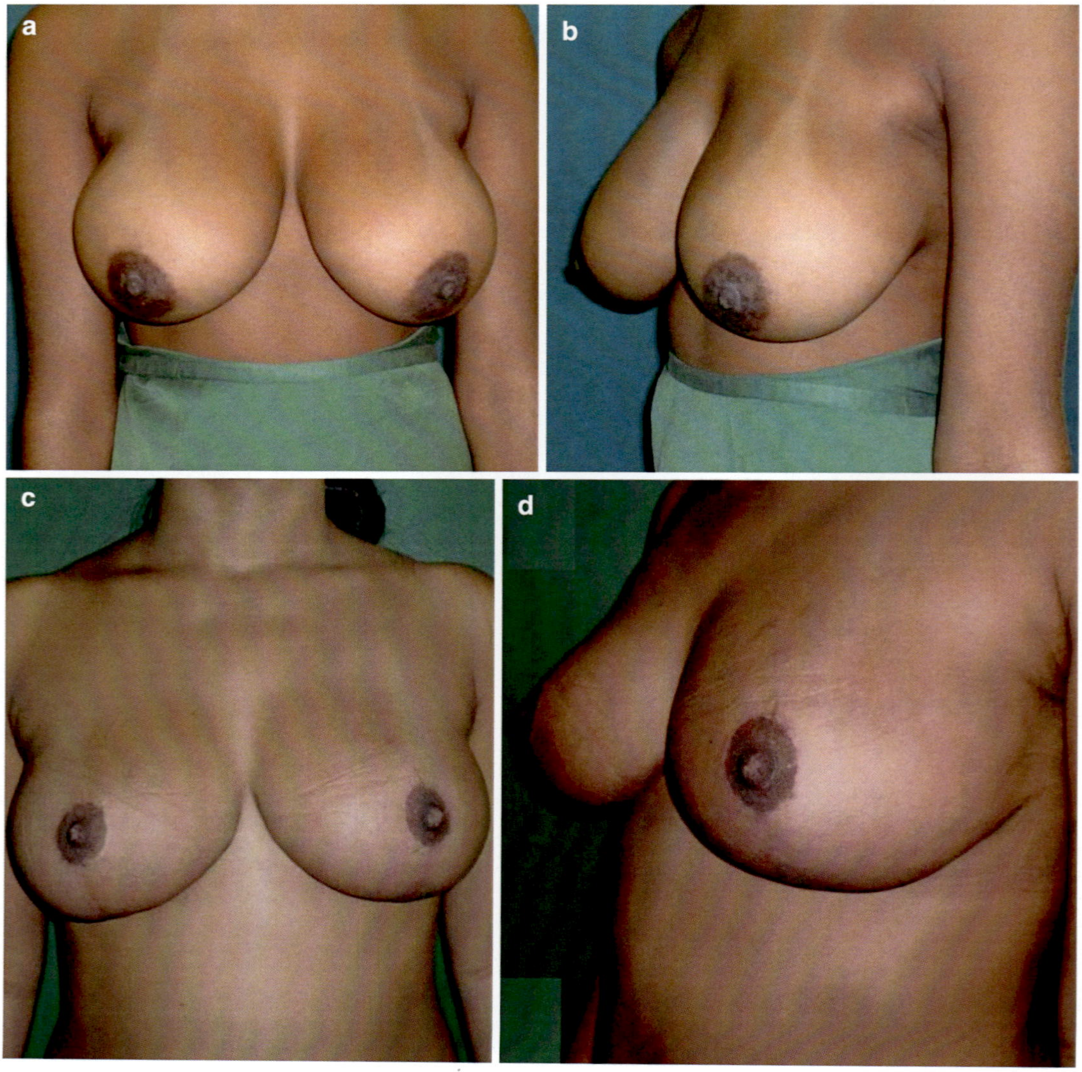

Fig. 26.6 A 34-year-old patient. (**a**, **b**) Preoperative views. (**c**, **d**) Six months postoperatively

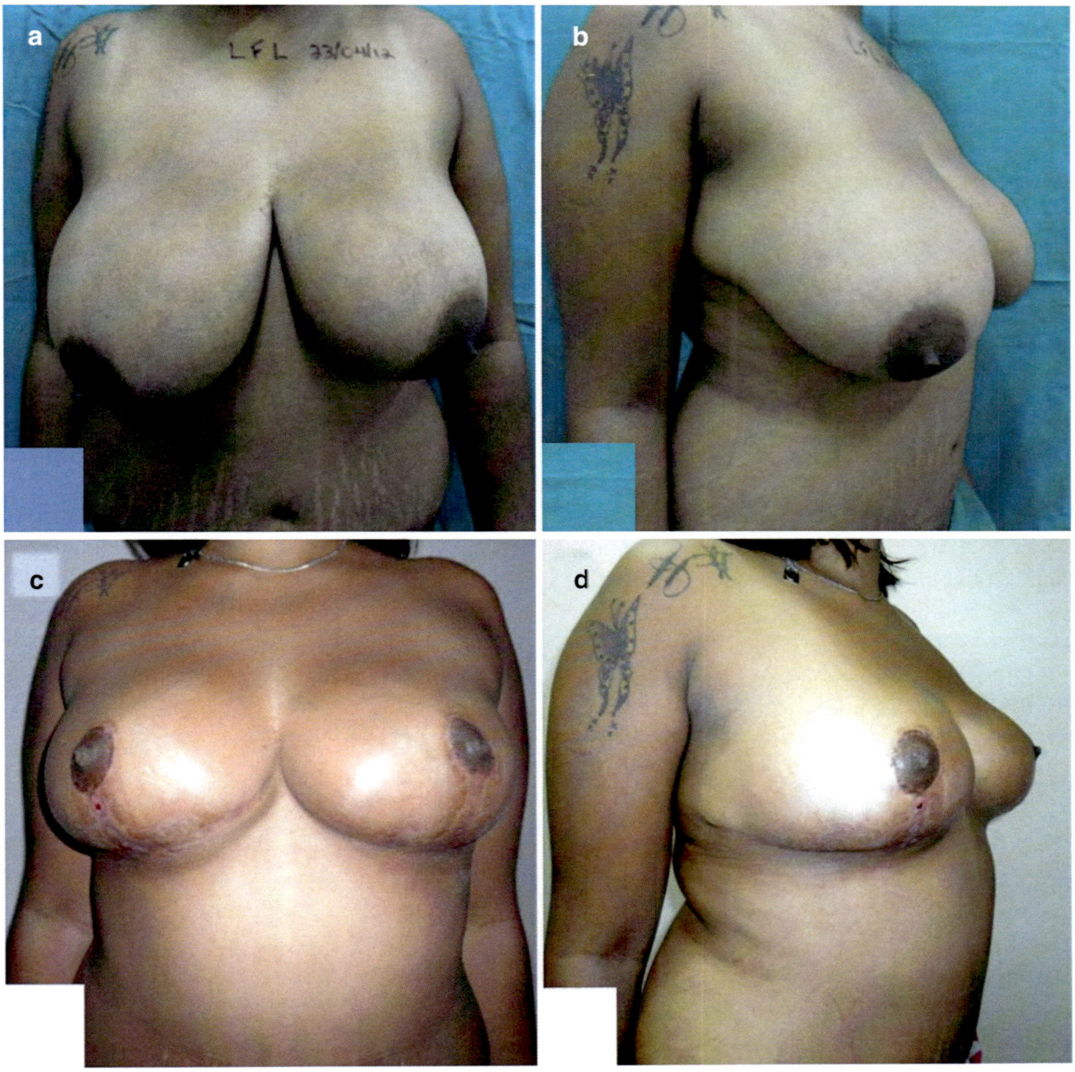

Fig. 26.7 A 27-year-old patient. (**a**, **b**) Preoperative views. (**c**, **d**) Three months postoperative views. Wound dehiscence may be observed in an inverted T-shaped scar close to the areola

26.3 Discussion

Seeking harmonious and long lasting results, many techniques have been approached by authors. McKissock's original technique applied to small and moderate hypertrophy yields similar results once compared with other techniques. Unfavorable factors regarding McKissock's technique are usually noted to be flap elbowing, epidermolysis, areolar depigmentation, and partial or total necrosis of the NAC. Long-term inadequate breast projection is also noted.

For severe hypertrophy, Thorek's technique presents well-accepted results. It allows greater parenchymal resection and reduced surgery duration. Remarkable unfavorable factors regarding Thorek's technique are the loss of nipple sensation once the NAC has been grafted and the sectioning of the galactophore ducts, especially in young patients. Preservation of NAC sensation is also important as an erogenous stimulus. Therefore, employing a bipedicular dermal flap attached to the pectoralis major muscle as a massive block allows a greater blood supply, reduced flap elbowing, reliable and immediate results, satisfactory breast projection, a sensitive NAC, preserved galactophore ducts, and finally a lower complication rate compared with the original technique. The unfavorable factors of this approach remain related to the amount of surgeon's experience and the patients' demand for sensitivity, steeper learning curve and the need for the surgeon to have experience in other techniques so as to better adapt the shape of the flap according the patient's biotype. Size and shape asymmetries need to be corrected in a new surgery (usually 4 months' postoperatively). Gigantomasty, in some cases needed to be treated in a two-step surgery with 6- to 12-month intervals.

Patients who have undergone reduction mammaplasty employing block or partial block flaps reported a sensitive NAC and satisfactory mammary consistency compared with breast implants. Long-lasting results with good breast projection have also been noted. This modification to McKissock's technique has been proved feasible and its results were satisfactory.

26.4 Complications

I have been using this approach for 25 years. I have treated around 500 cases of severe mammary hypertrophy and the most frequent complications arose from the junction of the vertical portion of the inverted T-shaped scar and the inframammary fold scar and from the junction of the vertical portion of the T-shaped scar and the areola. These complications were more frequent in smokers and were usually characterized by small areas of dehiscence (Fig. 26.7) or necrosis. Dehiscence healed by secondary intention. Discrete epidermolysis at the areolar border was infrequent and upon healing could lead to depigmentation. In such cases, we indicated micropigmentation at the sites. A rare complication was breast asymmetry, which was corrected thereafter. Owing to the racial mixing observed in Brazilian women, keloids were frequent, but healed with the use of triamcinolone (20 mg). For the most severe keloids, resection and radiotherapy were required.

Conclusion

The reduction mammaplasty demands imaginative thinking to adapt the technique to each specific breast size and shape, and to the patient's expectations. There is no one ideal technique. Plastic surgeons are constantly seeking constantly harmonious and long-lasting results, smaller scars and fewer complications. The vertical bipedicle flap, totally or partially fixed to the pectoralis major muscle, affords a desirable vascular supply, which aids in preventing avascular complications and better breast shaping. This technique resulted in a better and safer postoperative period, firm and well-projected breasts, and patients reported a high level of satisfaction.

References

McKissock PK (1972) Reduction mammaplasty with a vertical dermal flap. Plast Reconstr Surg 3(49):245

27 Adaptations of Techniques and Tactics in Mammaplasty

Irene Coelho de Souza
and Vera Tatiana Coelho de Souza

27.1 Introduction

As the breasts are the most outstanding sexual attributes of the female silhouette, it is natural that the plastic surgeons have created innumerable techniques for their remodeling in an attempt to recreate attractive shapes, or in many cases, to make them acceptable within what society considers to be beauty. Unfortunately, there is no standard technique to resolve all cases. Because of the various types of breasts, it depends on the surgeon's vast experience in this area as to whether the technique is applied adequately.

In the course of our experience, we have been able to create tactics and adapt them to ideal techniques for each type of mammaplasty, to offer shape and size in accordance with the biotype of the patient, a firm consistency, the conservation of glandular and erotic functions, imperceptible scars, and patient satisfaction.

I.C. de Souza, M.D. (✉) • V.T.C. de Souza, M.D.
Cirurgia Plastica, Clinica Cirurgica Drs. Irene e Carlos Souza, Belém, PA, Brazil
e-mail: clinicasouza@ig.com.br

27.2 Method

27.2.1 Preoperative Care

Routine laboratory examinations, X-ray of the thorax, cardiology check-up, and mammography after the age of 35 should all be carried out preoperatively.

27.2.2 Local Examination

We verified the shape, size, asymmetry, spots, skin type, container-container relationship and the presence of tumors.

With our experience, at this time, we make the appropriate statement with a prediction of postoperative results.

Technique and have a prevision of the postoperative results.

27.2.3 Technical Indication

Because of our training, when we began to operate, we only used Pitanguy's techniques for large and medium hypertrophy, and the Arié–Pitanguy techniques on small hypertrophy and ptosis. Thirty years ago, we began to make a few modifications to these techniques, perfecting them each day (Fig. 27.1).

On large hypertrophic breasts in older patients, and in moderate hypertrophy with accentuated flaccidity, where the container is larger than the

J.M. Avelar (ed.), *Breast Surgery*, https://doi.org/10.1007/978-3-319-54115-0_27

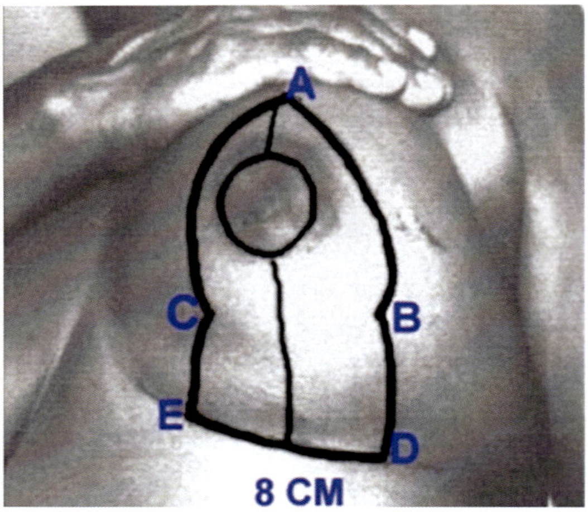

Fig. 27.1 Photo shows marking in the modified Pitanguy technique, with the horizontal incision reduced

content, we advocate Pitanguy's technique with the following modifications: marking is independent of this; we always place the patient in an orthostatic position, which in our opinion gives greater precision. We mark the points of reference that are common in all techniques: manubrium of the sternum, the xiphoid cartilage, and the midclavicular line.

27.3 Modified Pitanguy's Technique

Point **A** is marked on the midclavicular line on the projection of the mammary sulcus. The distances **AB** and **AC** are extended not less than **9 cm**, as we find that the larger these distances, the smaller the horizontal incision **DE**. The distance **BC** is determined by digital pinching.

We use the ancillary lipoaspiration procedure, in the axillary and median portions to diminish the horizontal marking we made at about **8 cm**. Pitanguy I (1971), (1984), (1996).

After Schwarzmann's classic maneuver, glandular resection is carried out, always weighed, which could be in a shape of a keel, rhomboid, or flat depending on the case. We do not empty the upper pole, always leaving it full to prevent its flattening later.

We fix the mammary tissue to the muscle wall. Suturing is begun in the vertical incision, after decortication of the borders, where we create a dermal support to prevent the widening of the scar and ptosis. The horizontal suture is pulled away in the direction from out to in to prevent flaps, with prolongation of the inferior demarcation. We use intradermic Mononylon 4-0, and separate sutures with Mononylon 6-0.

The position of the nipple–areola complex (**NAC**) should be in accordance with the newly formed breast, always in the vertex of the cone, suturing with Mononylon 5-0 in **U**-shaped stitches. Its distance from the mammary sulcus should never be less than **5 cm**, as in the bascule movement observed postoperatively, only the submammary sulcus of the inferior portion of the **NAC** is increased. While the distance of the manubrium of the sternum would not be modified. We use plaster of Paris dressings and drains for 24 h.

We have not observed any major complications; only cutaneous wounds on suture lines in **3**% of cases, and hypertrophic scars in **4**% of cases (Figs. 27.2 and 27.3).

30 years—old patient presenting hypertrophie mammary 5 years liter

In cases of large juvenile hypertrophy, moderate hypertrophy, and ptosis, we use the L technique, based on the technique of Aleixo Sepúlveda (1981), with some modifications.

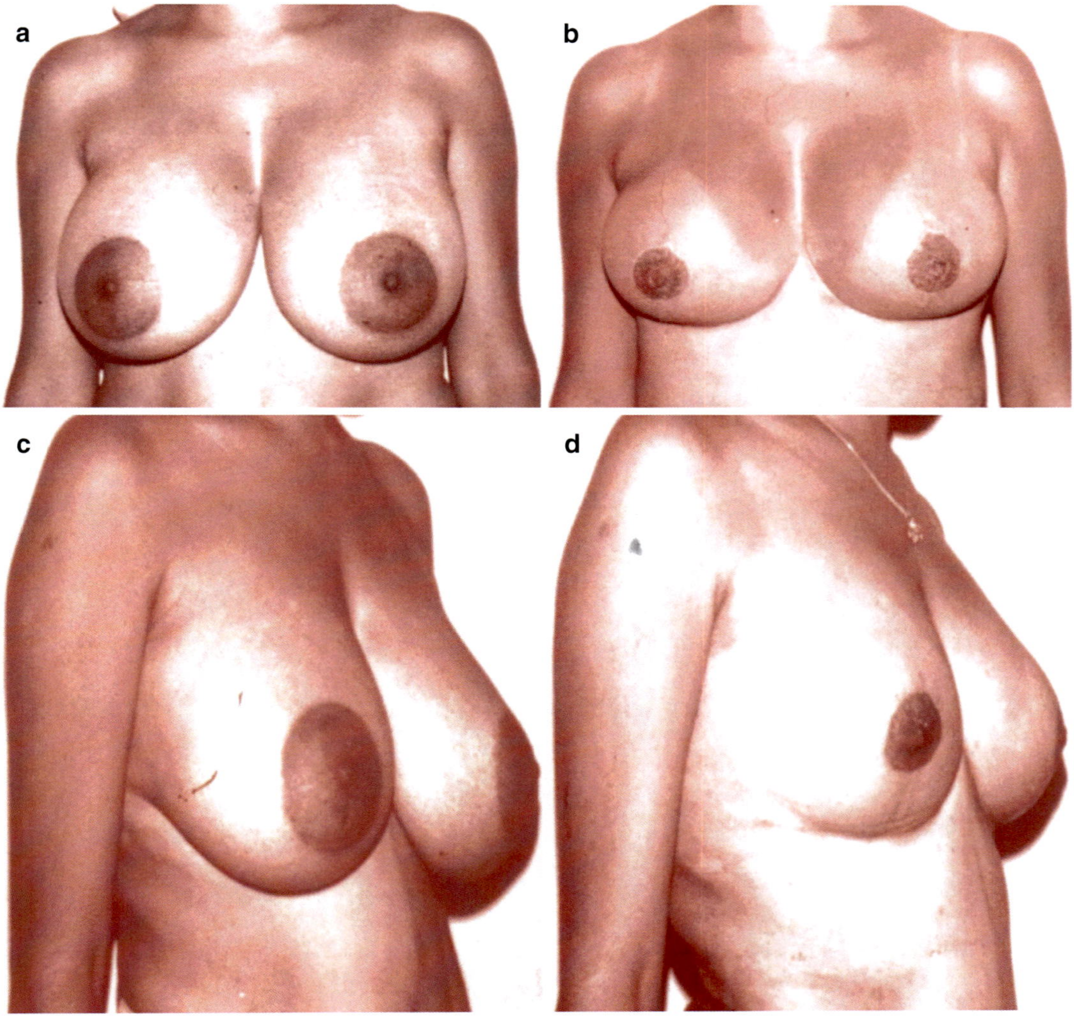

Fig. 27.2 (**a**, **c**) Preoperative image of a 40-year-old patient showing breast hypertrophy and ptosis with posture alterations. (**b**, **d**) Postoperative reductive mammaplasty using the modified Pitanguy technique and ancillary lipoaspiration in the axillary and medial region

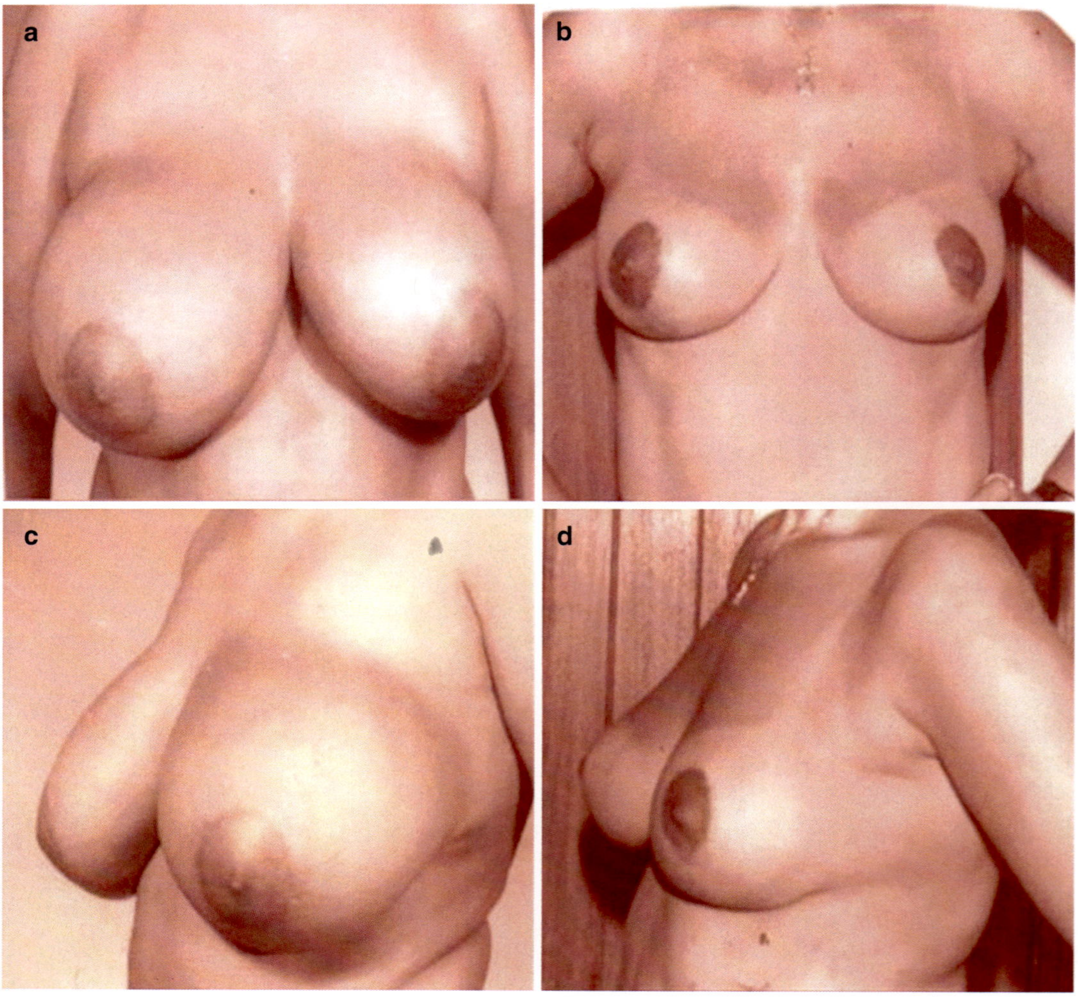

Fig. 27.3 (**a**, **c**) Pre-operative view of 30 years old patient showing large breast hypertrophy with asymmetry and, (**b**, **d**) pós operative with modified Pitanguy technique and procedure of ancillary lipoaspiration in the axilary and medial region

Technique of Aleixo Sepúlveda

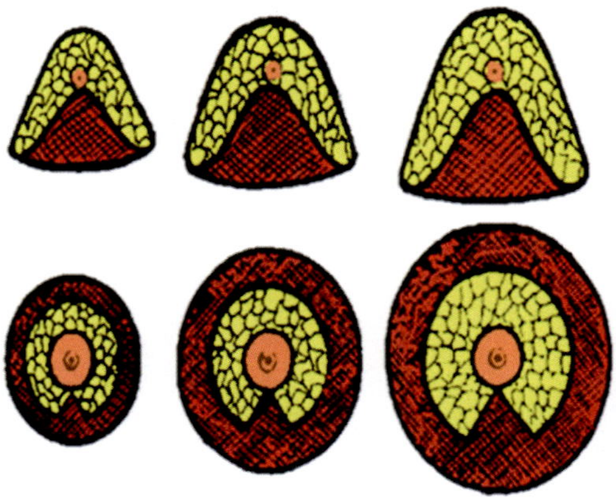

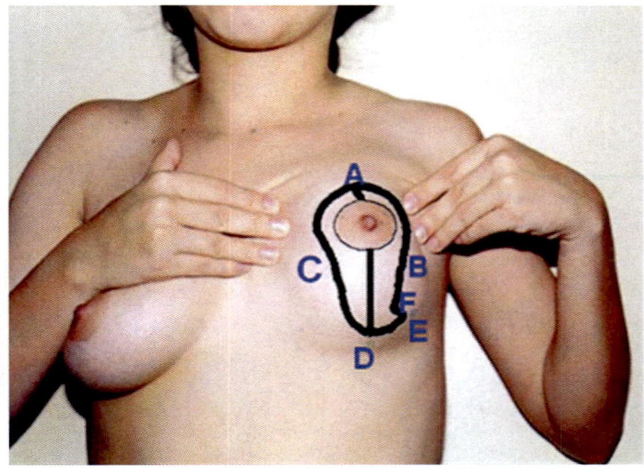

Point **A** is placed on the midclavicular line on the projection of the submammary sulcus.

Points **B–C** vary in each case. It is determined by digital pinching between the submammary sulcus and the lower borders of the **NAC**.

Point **D** is placed 1.5 cm from the submammary sulcus on the mid-mammary line.

Point **E** in accordance with the size of the breast, could be **2–5** cm from point **D**, and **1** cm higher than this.

Point **F**: the distance from point **E**, would depend on the size of the breast.

The Schwarzmann maneuver is made in the **ABC** area, the glandular resection would vary in each case and up to **1.2 kg** could be removed from each side. The skin is remarked after the glandular removal to remove the excess.

The **NAC** will be marked in accordance with the case, as it is larger in severe hypertrophy, a minimum of **5 cm** from the new submammary sulcus. The suturing and dressing techniques are carried out, as previously described.

The index of patient satisfaction shows that **80**% consider the results excellent, **15**% good, and **5**% satisfactory (Figs. 27.4, 27.5 and 27.6).

We find that the final shape fulfils and at times exceeds the expectations of the patients, and the resultant scar never reaches the anterior auxiliary line.

Because there is no horizontal incision toward the xiphoid cartilage, but a demarcation of the breast toward the middle mammary line, the results are more lasting. The index of asymmetry is observed in the same cases that were described in the Schwarzmann maneuver.

For the past 30 years, we have used Peixoto's demarcation technique on the skin in cases of mammary ptosis with a flattened superior pole internally. We perform a fatty skin resection of the superior pedicle that encloses the lower pole of the breast positioning it laterally within it, based on the technique of Longrace (1959). The resected part is rotated and fixed to the muscle wall with Mononylon 2-0 sutures (Fig. 27.7).

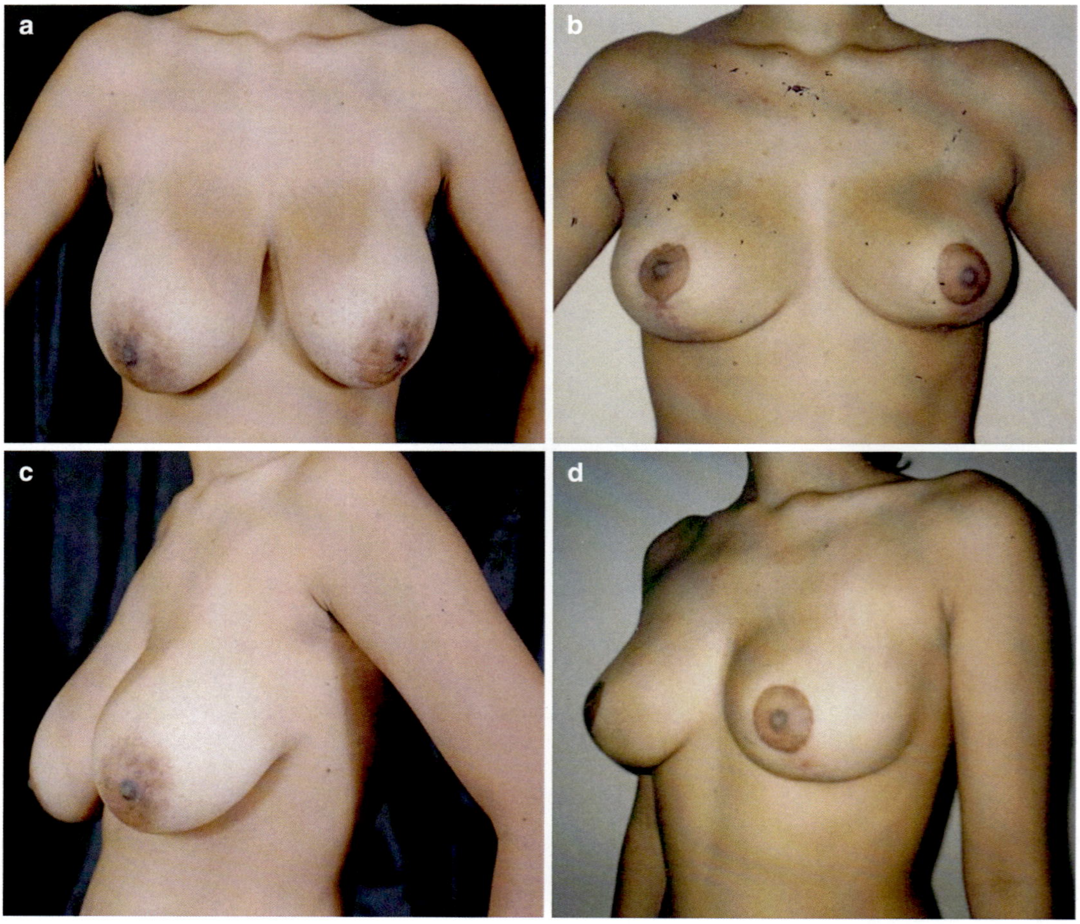

Fig. 27.4 (**b**, **d**) Post operative view of the same patient 2 years later after surgery with modified Pitanguy technique and procedure of ancillary lipoaspiration in the axillary and median region

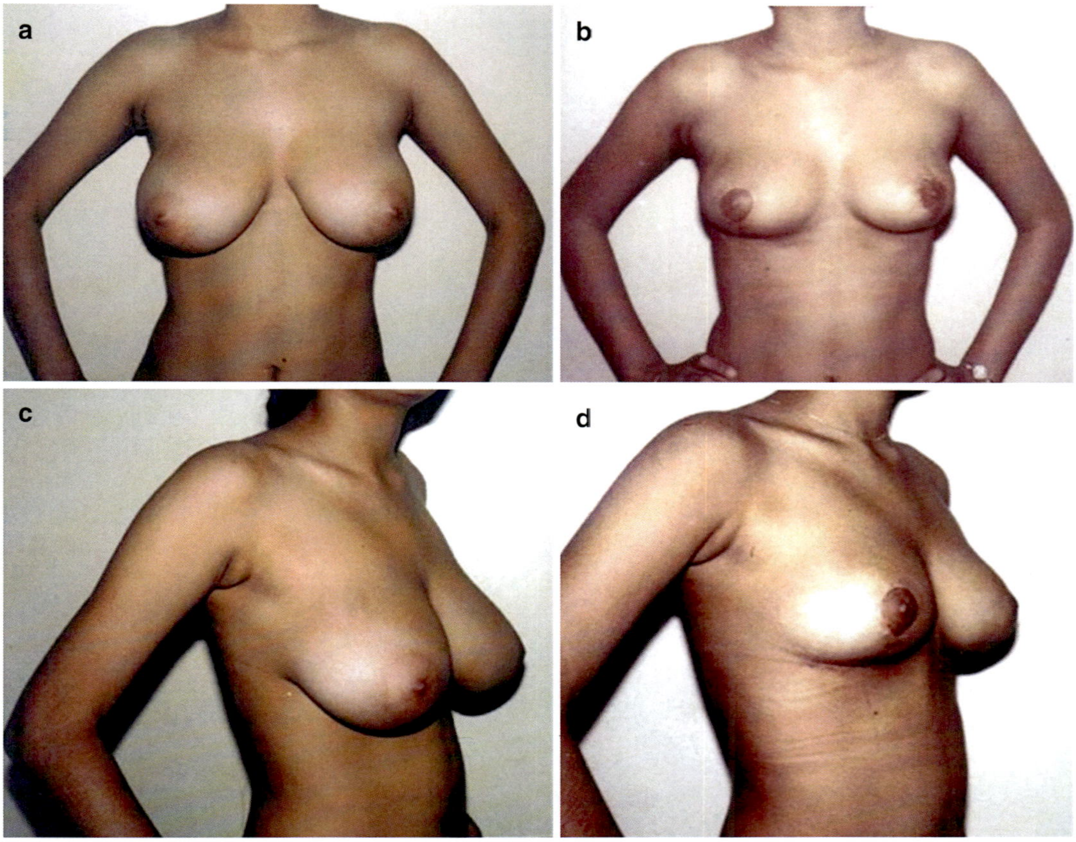

Fig. 27.5 (**a**, **c**) A 19 year-old patient preoperatively, presenting hypertrophy with asymmetry. (**b**) The same patient postoperatively 19 years after surgery using the **L** technique

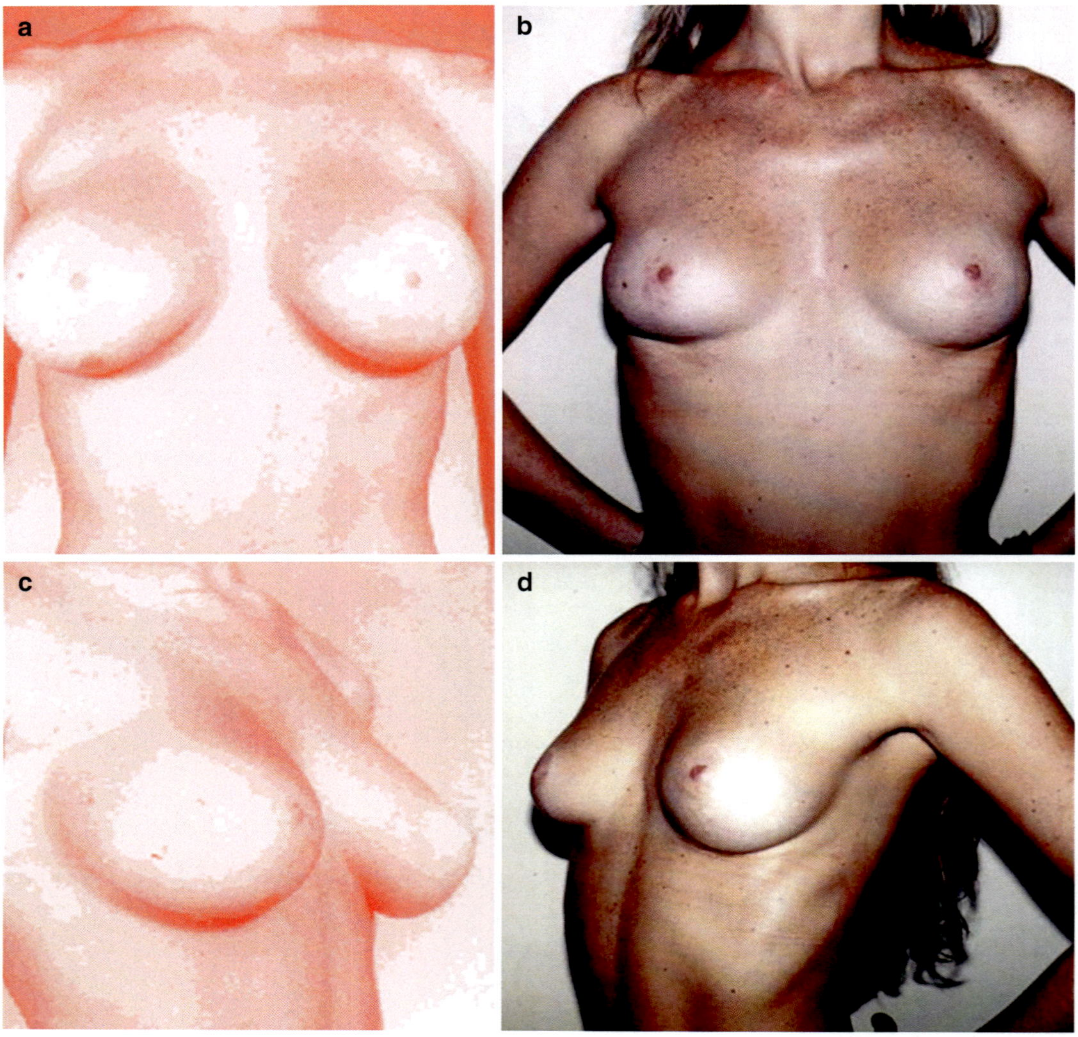

Fig. 27.6 (**a**, **c**) An 18-year-old patient with breast hypertrophy. (**b**, **d**) The same patient postoperatively 15 years after surgery using Sepúlveda's **L** technique

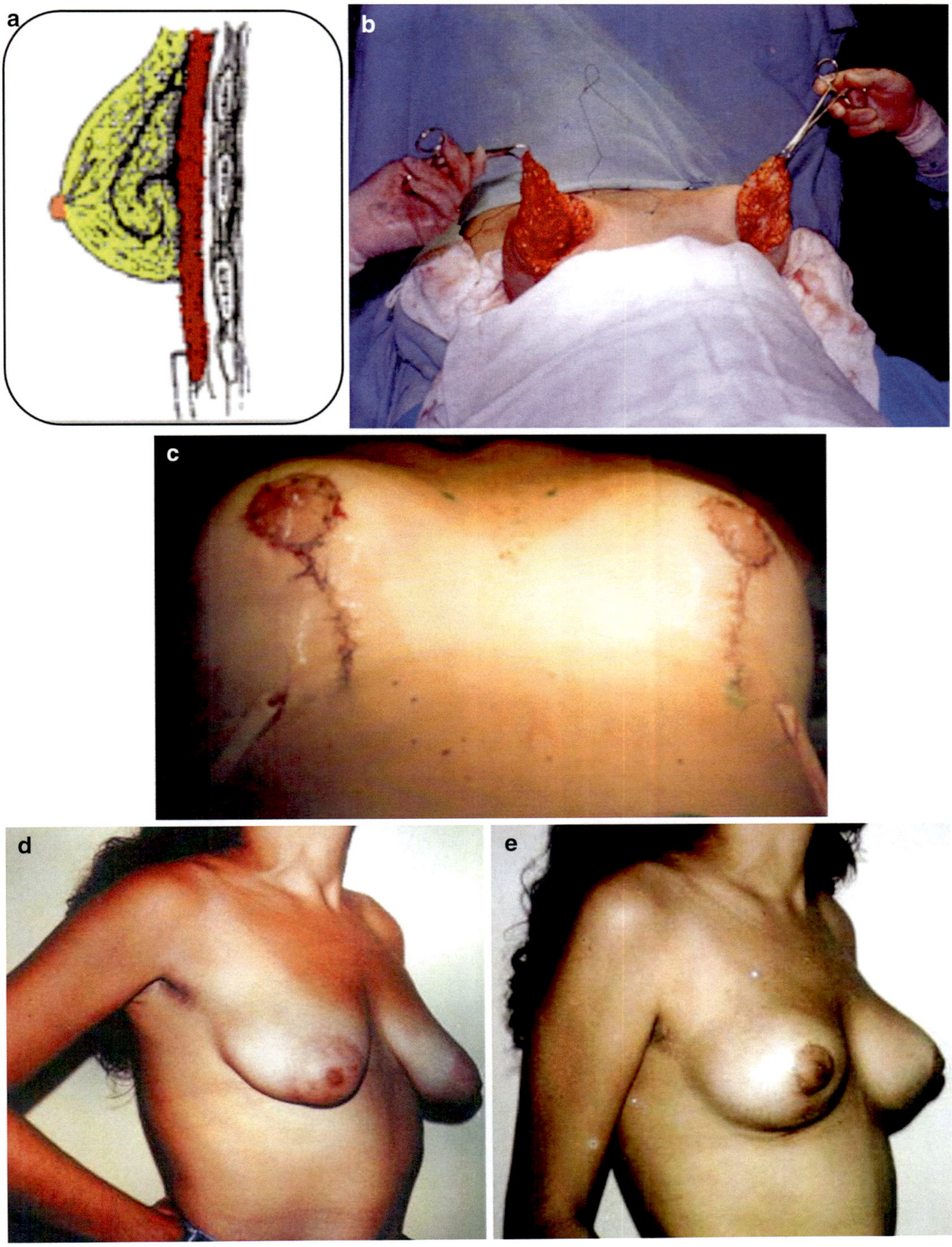

Fig. 27.7 (**a–c**) Fatty skin resection of the superior pedicle. (**d**) and (**f**) Preoperatively. (**e**) and (**g**) Six months postoperatively. (**h**) and (**j**) Preoperatively. (**i**) and (**k**) One year postoperatively. (**l**) Preoperatively. (**m**) Six years postoperatively. (**n–p**) In accordance with the degree of ptosis, the incision of the skin could end in a vertical incision in an L or small T shape. The sutures and the dressing are the same as in the old techniques (made in the past)

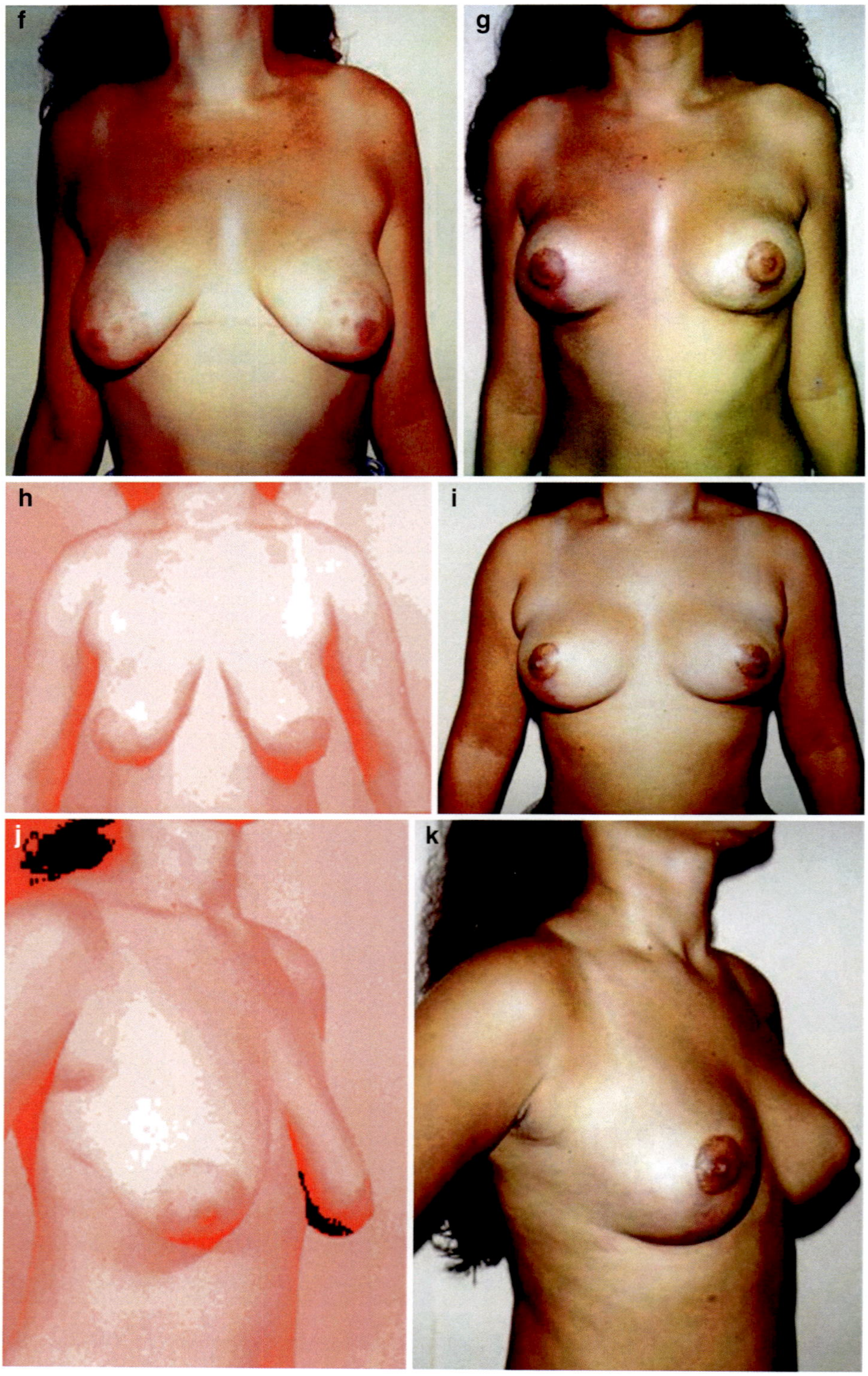

Fig. 27.7 (continued)

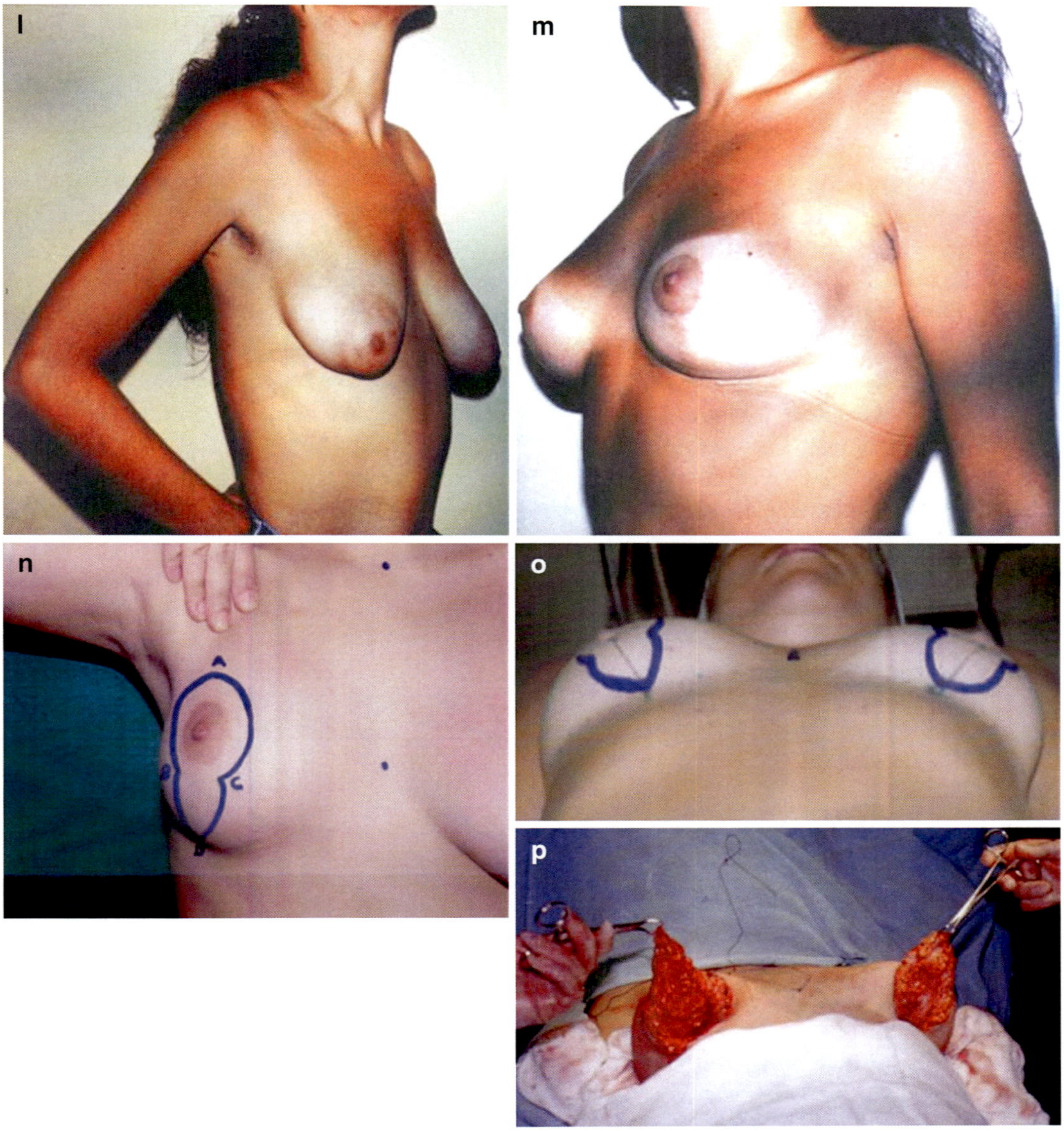

Fig. 27.7 (continued)

27.4 Complications

We have been using this technique for 34 years, operating on 1213 cases, and the rate of complications is lower than the previously used technique, with only 2% having a small amount of cutaneous damage on the suture line.

27.5 Discussion

Asymmetry of the breast was only observed in those who presented large asymmetry preoperatively, and in whom precise removal had not been done, cases observed by us, but did not constitute complaints by patients, who, on the contrary, showed satisfaction with the results obtained.

The patient satisfaction rate shows that 80% considered the results to be excellent, 15% good, and 5% satisfactory.

This study was carried out in patients operated on more than 2 years. The rate of satisfaction was observed in patients who had pregnancies or a weight gain above 10 kg, and who presented ptosis Converse (1964).

Conclusions

In juvenile patients with severe hypertrophy, moderate hypertrophy, and ptosis, we use the **L** technique, based on the Sepúlveda's technique (1981) with some modifications.

We have operated on 1213 patients using this technique. The complication rate shows that 2% of the cases had cutaneous damage because of the suture line, and there were hypertrophic scars in 3% of the cases, for which the patients were reoperated.

Because there is no horizontal incision toward the xiphoid cartilage, but a marking of the breast toward the mid-mammary line, the results are more lasting. We observed that **90%** of the patients found the results to be excellent, 7% good, and **3%** satisfactory (patients who presented hypertrophic scars). We consider that these results are a consequence of the final aspect of the breast, which resembles a prosthesis.

In studies relating to the satisfaction of the patients concerning the final results, the same standards were used, independent of the techniques carried out.

We strongly believe that the final aspect of the breast, which resembles a prosthesis, is because of our adapted techniques, such as from Sepúlveda's, Peixoto's, and Arié–Pitanguy's, with liposuction of the axillary and median portions.

References

Converse JM (1964) Reconstructive plastic surgery. W.B. Saunders, Philadelphia

Longacre JJ, De Stefano GA, Holmstrand K (1964) Breast reconstruction with local derma and fat pedicle flaps. Plast Reconstr Surg 24:563–576.

Pitanguy I (1971) Mastoplastias. Estudo Comparativo da Evolução Técnica em torno 1.196 Casos Pessoais. Rev Bras Cir 61:227

Pitanguy I (1984) Mamaplastia Redutora e Mastopexia—25 anos de experiência. Rev Bras Cir 74:265–288

Pitanguy I (1996) Hipertrofias Mamárias. Estudo Critico de Técnica Pessoal. Rev Bras Cir 5:263

Sepúlveda A (1981) Tratamento das Assimetrias Mamárias. Ver Bras Cirurgia 71:11–18.

28 Mammoplasty Planned Using the Divine Proportion and Assembled with Multiplanar Layers (Golden Ratio Mammoplasty)

Osvaldo Pereira

28.1 Introduction

The current techniques indicated to treat breast reduction, mastopexy with or without implant, are planned using the pinch test, prefabricated molds, and many empirical strategies. In addition, the remaining tissue is assembled to form the base of the cone. Many approaches use bidigital evaluation to plan the amount of vertical resection and to evaluate the ideal positioning of the nipple–areola complex (NAC): Arié (1957), Avelar (1994), Erol and Spira (1980), Franco and Rebelo (1977), Geogiade et al. (1979), Corine et al. (2014), Ribeiro (1989), Peixoto (1980), Perez-Macias (2004), Torres et al. (2005), Nahabedian et al. (2000), Erol and Spira (1980), Hugo and McClellan (1979), Hoopes and Maxwell (1979), among others.

The purpose of this study is to plan mastopexy and breast reduction according to the principle of the divine proportion, phi, associated with convergent multiplanar assembling of the new breast. The strategy is based on the constancy of the submammary fold, orientated over a V-shaped triangle with the 60° vertex at the umbilicus and each branch opening in the direction of the acromioclavicular joint. The divine proportion and its relationship with nature and the human body has been documented by Theodore (1914), Huntley (1970), and Hemenway (2005).

O. Pereira, M.D.
Clínica Jane Hospital Ilha,
Deputado Antonio Edu Vieira, Florianópolis,
SC 88040001, Brazil
e-mail: osvaldojpf@gmail.com

28.2 Method

The strategy has been prospectively investigated in 265 patients, encompassing $n = 530$ breasts. The mean age was 36 years. The follow-up ranged from 6 months to 3 years.

Technique: The principle of divine proportion orientates the creation of the new breast that is planned over a V-shaped 60° triangle with the vertex situated over the umbilicus, point u. It works as a point of fugue orientating the creation of the new breast. The two branches of the isosceles triangle open in an angle of 60° from point u, parallel to the mammary line, close to the acromioclavicular joint. P1, the key point of the strategy, is situated at the intersection of each branch of the V triangle with the submammary fold. It is marked using a compass with the patient in the orthostatic position. Using a compass, the distance measured in centimeters from P1 to the midline, point m, is transposed to the midsternal line cranially, determining point m′. According to the golden ratio, point P2, the apex of the new breast, is situated over each branch of the V-shaped triangle at the distance from P1 equal to (P1 → m) cm × phi = (P2 → m′) cm. Coincidently, the distance between P1 → P2 in centimeters measured with a compass is almost the same as that distance between P2 → m′ (Fig. 28.1).

J.M. Avelar (ed.), *Breast Surgery*, https://doi.org/10.1007/978-3-319-54115-0_28

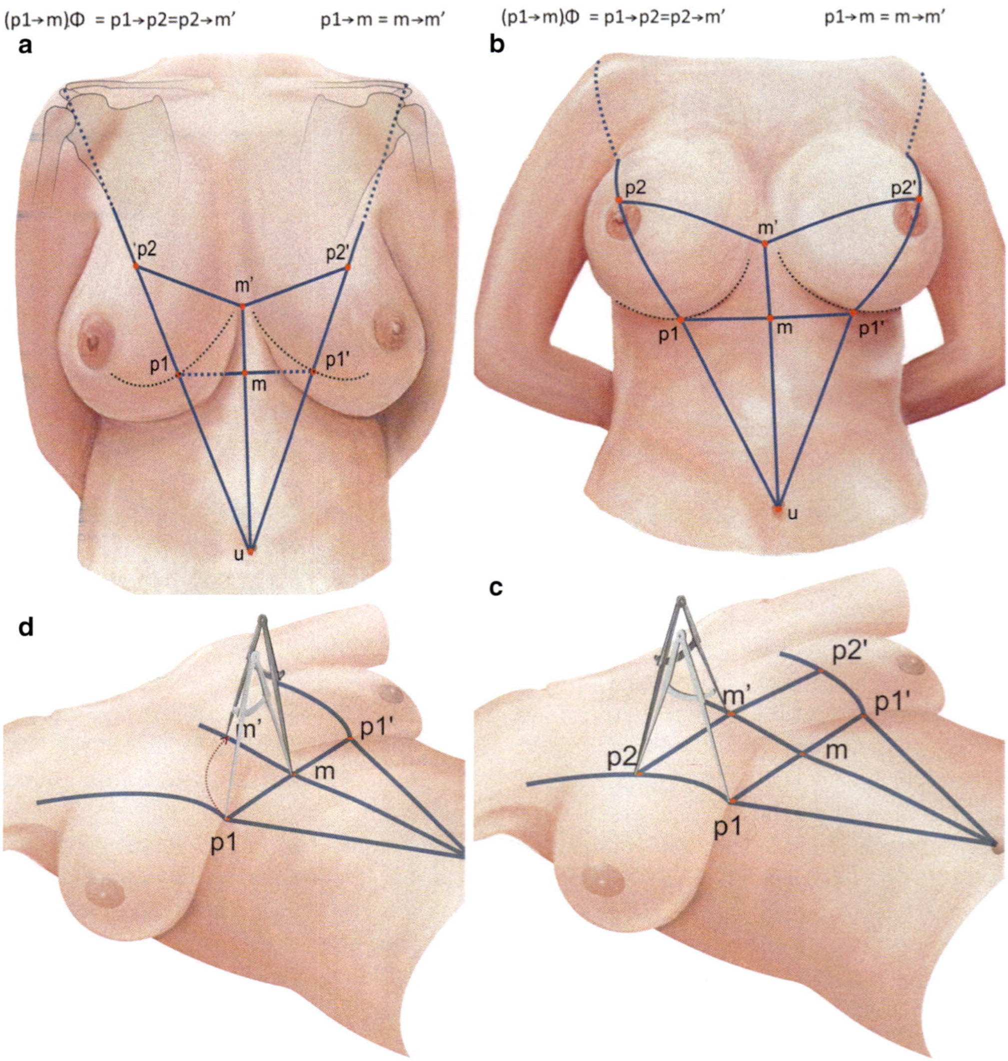

Fig. 28.1 (**a**) The golden ratio can be seen in a balanced breast. In the example, if P1 → m = 7.5 cm, then P1 → P2 = (P1 → m).phi = 7.5 cm × 1618 = 12.1 cm, which is the expected distance between them. When P1 → m = 7 cm, the projected P1 → P2 = m′ → P2 = 7. phi(1.618) = 11.3 cm. (**b**) Plan of the new breast. With the patient in a standing position, the sub-mammary fold is delineated. The 30° vertex of the compass? is positioned over the umbilicus, point u. The isosceles branches of the triangle run in the direction of the acromioclavicular joint. Its intersection with the submammary fold gives the origin of P1, the key point. P2, the superior border of the areola of the new breast, is situated over the axis of each triangle at a distance from P1 (P1 until m) × phi. The distance of P1 until m = m toward m′. (**c**) Planning the new breast with the patient in 30° dorso-flexion. The distance between point P1 to m is transferred to point m, the medial line, composing the triangle P1 → m → u → P1. The distance of P1 → m is transferred to m → m′. (**d**) P2 is situated over the branch of the triangle with the vertex at point u (umbilicus) at an angle of 60°. The distance P1 → P2 = m′ → P2 = P1 × phi(1.618). In the example, if P1 → m = 7; P1 → P2 = 7 × (1618) = 11.3 cm. Coincidently, most of the times m → m′ = one third of distance m′ → u

Pulling the breast upward with a hook at point P2, the same distance between P1 → P2 is transposed from that point downward marking the limit of the base of the cone and the amount of skin or hypertrophic tissue to be resected. For example, if the distance between point P1 until m = 7.5 cm, P2, the ideal position of the apex of the new breast, is situated at the distance: P1 → m (7.5 cm) × phi(1.618) = 12.1 cm from P1. That distance is equal (P2 → m′) in centimeters (Fig. 28.2). The final scar is converted into an inverted T. It can be converted into an L shape if the distance between the medial limit of the breast to be resected, point C (medial corner of the new cone of the breast after resection), until the sub-mammary fold, P1, is less than 2 cm.

The breast is assembled with multiplanar layers. The auxiliary pulls the external and medial quadrant in the direction of P1. Depending on the extent of tissue resection, usually four to eight retention sutures are used between the inner layers of the breast integument and the pectoral muscle (Fig. 28.3). The main layer is the suturing of the mammary inferior border with the submammary fascia of Scarpa along the submammary fold. Histological analysis carried out by Muntan et al. (2000) and the clinical use of this structure utilized by Lockwood (1999) reinforce its importance (Fig. 28.4). Usually six to eight adhesion sutures are used from lateral in the direction of P1 and two to three from the mammary sternal medial border, also in the direction of P1 (Fig. 28.5). In the same fashion, the dermal layer is sutured. The V branch of the triangle guides the objective amount of vertical resection along the axis P1 toward P2. The cone

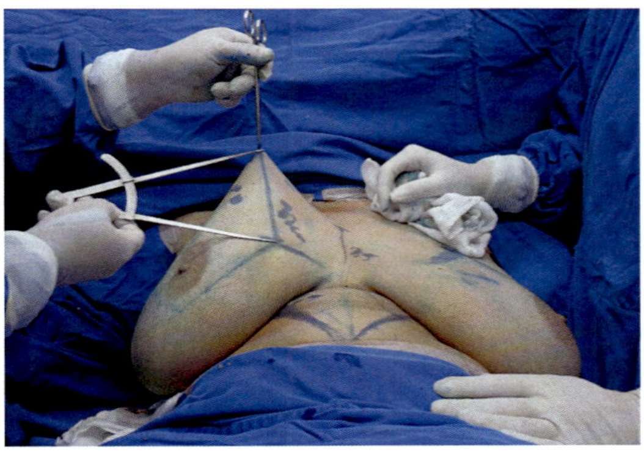

Fig. 28.2 The amount of the tissue resected is calculated pulling the breast with a hook at P2. In this case, P1 to m measured 7.5 cm. Then, the horizontal excess of the hypertrophic integument preserves 12.1 cm from P2 (7.5 cm × 1.618) of the new mammary cone

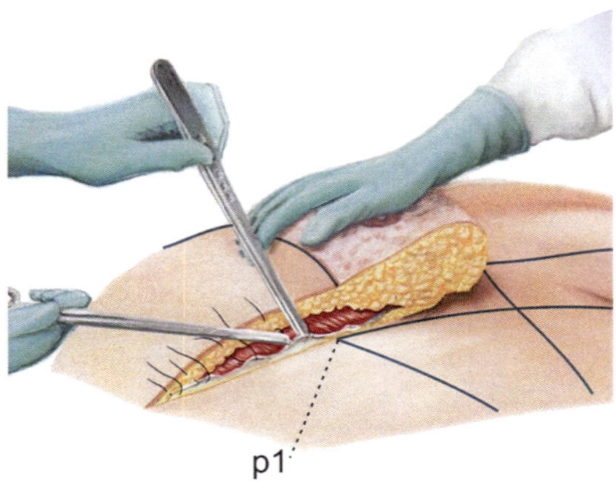

Fig. 28.4 The main layer is made between the breast integument to the fascia of Scarpa at the level of the submammary fold. It is a very strong layer. Finally, the suturing ends with running sutures of the subdermal and cuticular layers

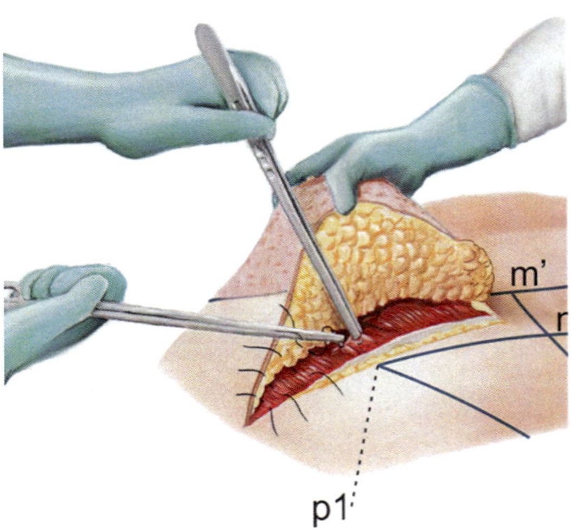

Fig. 28.3 Breast assembly is oriented by the axis of the umbilicus and the acromioclavicular joint. The integument is sutured in a multiplanar fashion with absorbable retention sutures over the pectoralis major muscle. The breast tissue is rotated from lateral to point P1

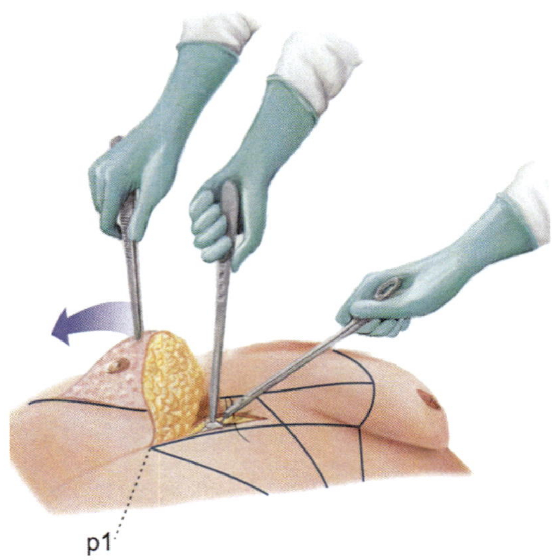

Fig. 28.5 Rotation of breast tissue from the sternum region to P1 in the same fashion indicated from the axillary region to P1 completes assembly. The vertical amount of skin is objectively evaluated and completed using Schwarzmann's maneuver

breast is molded temporarily with continuous sutures guided by the branches between P1 → P2 along the 60° triangle with a vertex at point u. The vertical skin excess is evaluated objectively. The epithelium is removed to complete Schwarzmann's maneuver. If necessary, the dermis around the NAC can be incised to help its transposition at P2. Lipoplasty under the areola eases its new positioning. Its inferior border to P1 is the same as P1 → m. However, considering that the gravity action from that distance is subtracted from 1 cm to result in a final transoperative proportion of the upper pole/lower pole of 55/45 (Fig. 28.6).

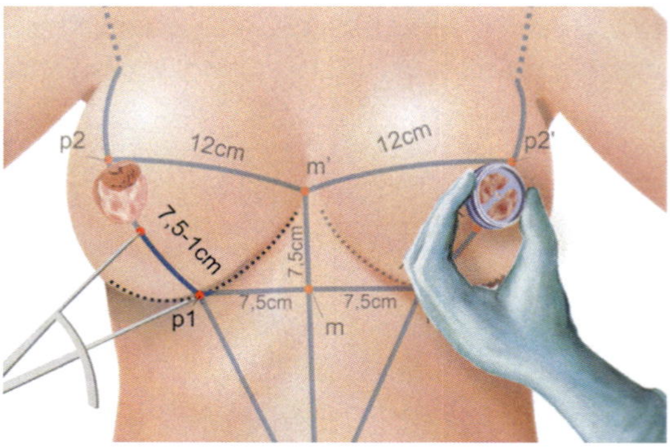

Fig. 28.6 The nipple–areolar complex (NAC) is positioned on the apex of the breast along the branch of the triangle that starts at the umbilicus. In general, the distance from P1 to the inferior border of the areola is the same: (P1 → m) – 1 cm. The reduction of (–1 cm) is to compensate for the action of gravity that will have an effect over time

28.3 Results

To have an objective analysis of the aesthetic result, the data were evaluated according to Strasser's (1999) grading. In this system, the flaws are classified according to five headings: malposition, distortion, asymmetry, contour deformity, and scarring. All the negative attributes of a result. The absence any of the flaws is a perfect result. Under this system, a perfect result obtains zero points. One to four points is classified as a good result, 5–14 as mediocre, and 15 or greater as a poor result.

Two hundred and twenty-one patients in our data scored good result (83%). Balance of the breasts was a constant in most of the cases of breast mastopexy and substantial reduction (Fig. 28.7).

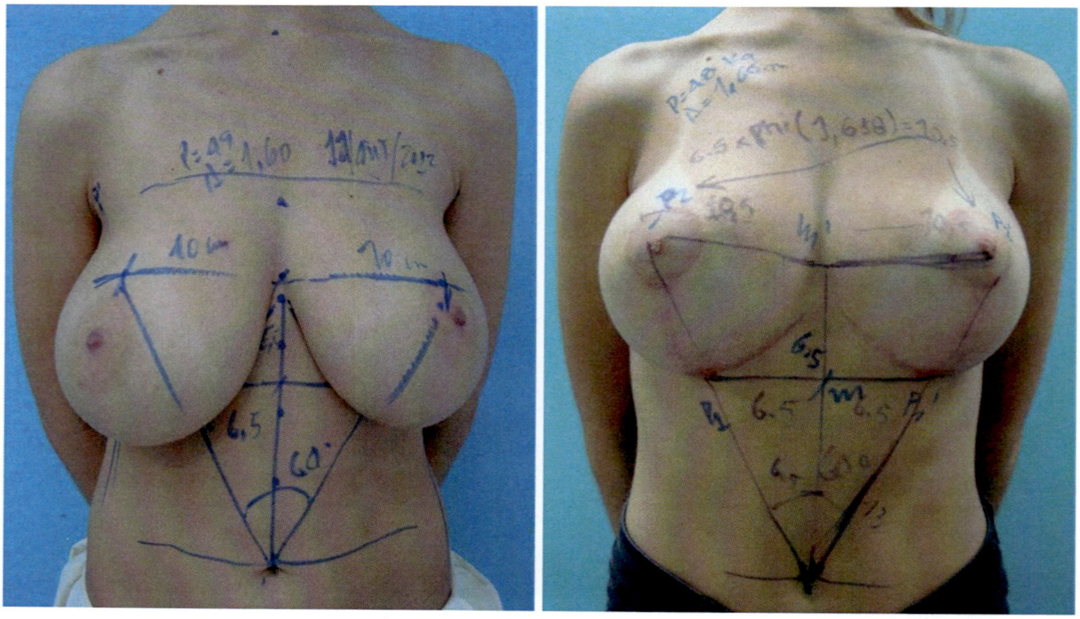

Fig. 28.7 Pre- and postoperative view of a 20-year-old woman, weight 48 kg, height 1.60 m, presenting breast asymmetry, ptosis, and grade 1 hypertrophy. P1 → m distance was 6.5 cm. The distance of between P1 to P2 (superior border of the areola) is 6.5 × phi(1.618) = 10.5 cm = m′→ P2. Resection of 290 g on the right side and 220 g on the left side. This case was grade 2 in Strasser'sclas- sification, in which the flaws are classified according to five headings: malposition = 0, distortion = 0, asymme- try = 0, contour deformity = 0, and scar = 2

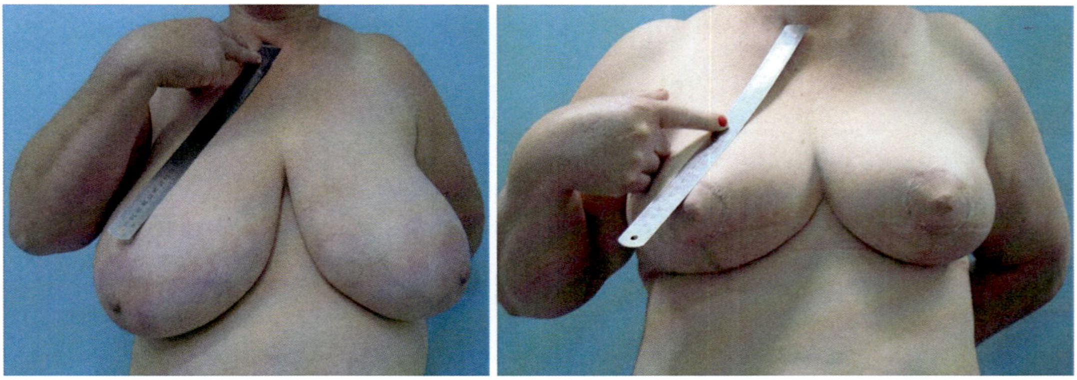

Fig. 28.8 Views pre- and 3 months postoperatively of a 52-year-old patient presenting grade 3 breast hypertrophy, weight = 102 kg, height = 1.74 m. On the right side 1183 g was resected and 1073 g on the left side. The golden ratio was based on: P1 → m = 9 cm; P1 → P2 = 14.1 cm. The distance between the clavicle and NAC of the right breast was more than 34 cm. Postoperatively, the distance was 24 cm

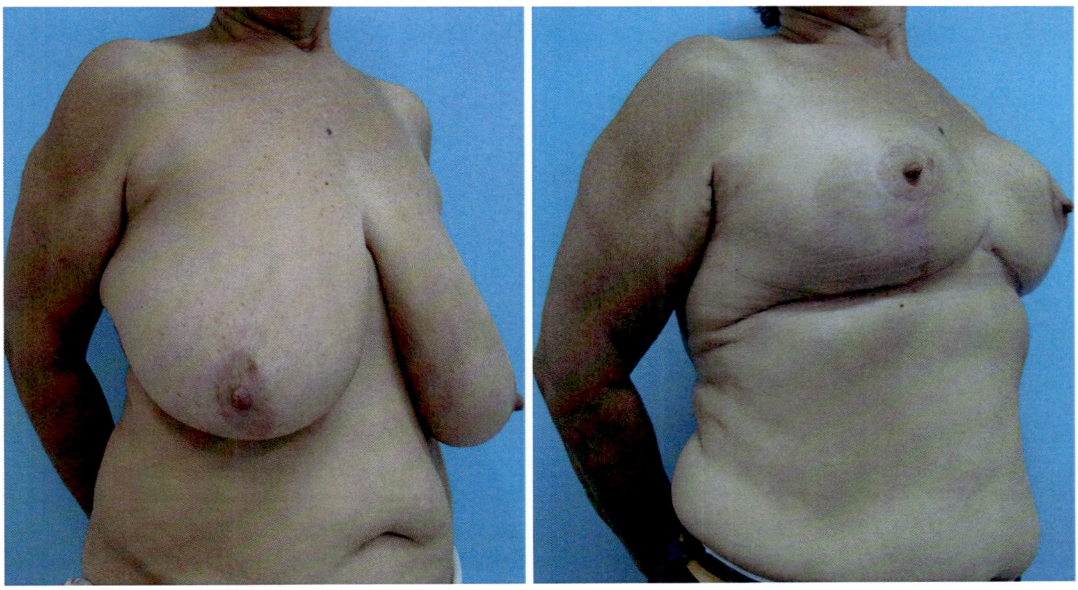

Fig. 28.9 A 58-year-old patient after breast reduction and significant ptosis. On the oblique view, we can see the NAC rotation proportioned by multi-planar layered assembly (compare with the black nevus position at the upper pole). The cutaneous laxity of the axillary region is also corrected using lateral and medial breast rotation in the direction of P1 associated with multi-planar layered assembly

Convergent mobilization of breast tissue to point P1 reduced axillary laxity and obtained satisfactory upper pole projection. Good scaring was noticed overall at the sub-mammary fold. Complications were few: delayed healing at the inverted T scar confluence in 19 patients (7%), asymmetry in 16 (6%), and partial nipple necrosis in 4 (1.5%). In large breasts in which the distance from the clavicle to the NAC was equal to or greater than 30 cm, the NAC was transposed to P2 attached to the upper pedicle (Figs. 28.8 and 28.9).

28.4 Discussion

The current mammoplasty techniques are planned using a pinch test, prefabricated molds, and sometimes complex empirical marking. This study evo-

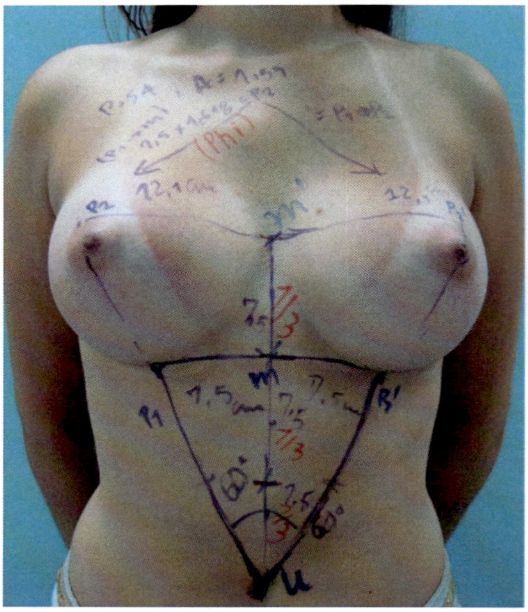

Fig. 28.10 A 19-year-old woman with an attractive breast, weight = 54 kg, height = 1.59 m. The divine proportion is noticeable when the mammary structure is reconfigured to a 60° V triangle with one vertex at the umbilicus (point u) and each isosceles branch opening to the articulation between the acromium and the clavicle. P1 → m, the distance from the intersection between the submammary fold and the branch of the triangle to the medial line reveals a closed relationship with the golden ratio. In the figure, P1 → m = 7.5 cm. P2, the superior border of the NAC is positioned at the distance: (P1 → m) × constant phi(1.618). If the distance P1 → m is 7.5 cm, P1 → P2 = 7.5 × phi = 12.1 cm = m′ → P2. The one third principle is present between m′ → m and m′ → u

cates the mathematical principles present in a balanced breast (Fig. 28.10). The new mammary cone is planned, taking into consideration the submammary fold, a constant structure that is the base of confection of a new breast. The method also embodies another objective parameter: a triangle with the apex, point u, situated at the umbilicus. Each branch opens 60° in the direction of the acromioclavicular joint parallel to the anatomical mammary line. P1, the key point of the strategy, is situated on the intersection of the submammary fold line and each branch of the V-shaped triangle. Each axis of the isosceles branch of this triangle orientates the creation of the new breast. An intrinsic proportion between the two geometric figures exists: the triangle and the cone of the breast. The anatomical NAC is divergent, because it is positioned over the curved rib arches (Fig. 28.11). Point

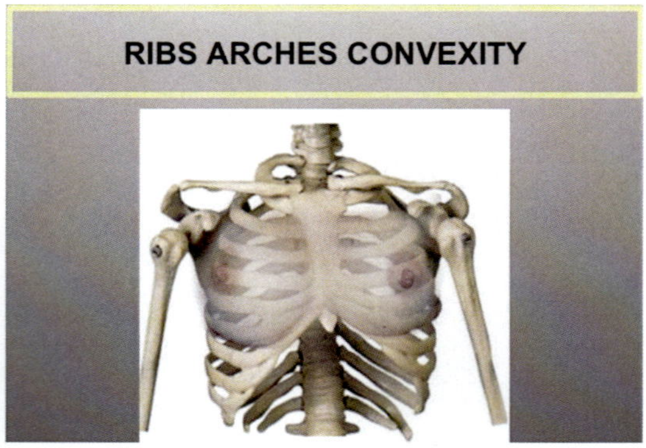

Fig. 28.11 Schematic drawing showing the divergence of the breast cone and the NAC because of the convexity of the costal arches of the ribs

P2 is vertically positioned at the distance of P1 to the point m—the intersection with the midsternal line—times the constant phi, 1.618. Horizontally, the distance is the same from that point to m′. It orientates the ideal point of the superior border of the NAC when measured with a compass from P1. This distance is the same as P2 − m′. The mathematical principle of the one third proportion is usually visualized between the P1 → P2 in centimeters until point u, the umbilicus, lying over the respective branch of the V-shaped figure, i.e., the distance between P1 → P2 is commonly is one third of P2 → u. This proportion is also recorded between the points m′ → u at the sternal midline, i.e., m′ → m is one third of the distance between m′−u.

In this way, we add precision to planning the apex cone. In contrast to many current techniques that use the pinch test to position the superior border of the areola, Pitanguy (1959) imagined the superior border of the areola, feeling the projection of the finger over the upper pole after touching the medium part of the breast integument at the submammary fold. Wise (1956) utilized prefabricated molds with their apex at a constant distance from the clavicle. Tebbetts (2014) considers the half size of the submammary fold to project the NAC and to evaluate the vertical and horizontal excess to be resected. Others consider the superior border of the NAC to be positioned at a distance of 19–20 cm from the clavicle. These strategies express the challenging difficulties in adding mathematical precision according to each biotype.

Multiplanar assembling connects many layers converging the skin envelope from an external

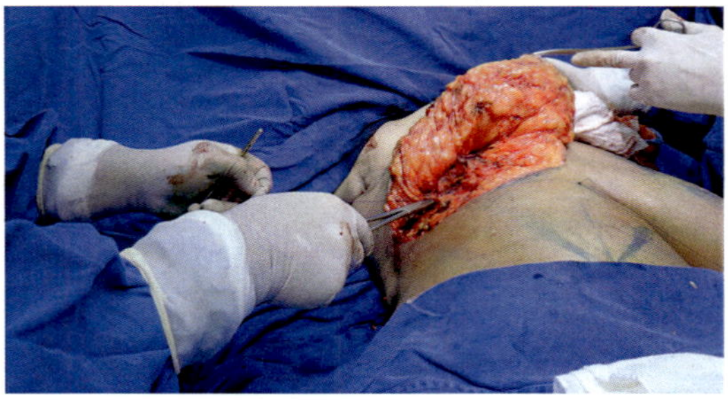

Fig. 28.12 Breast assembly with multiplanar layers, starting inside out, with multiple adhesion stitches approximating the breast tissue and the pectoralis major muscle

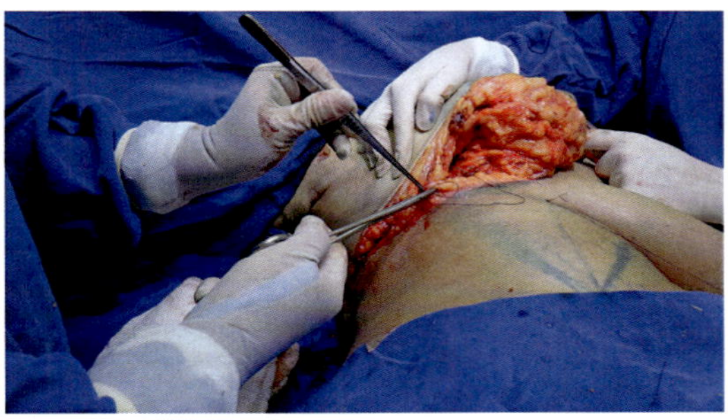

Fig. 28.13 Multiple sutures between the breast's remaining border and the fascia of Scarpa comprise the strongest layer. It helps to give projection to the upper pole and minimizes axillary flaccidity

and internal quadrant to the key point P1. The point u works as point of fugue with each branch in the direction of the acromioclavicular articulation. The new breast cone is assembled inside out with multiplanar layers, with that line, which works as a guide. The inner part of the tissue is sutured to the muscle fascia of the serratus muscle laterally and the pectoralis major muscle medially (Fig. 28.12). The second suture layer connects the breast tissue to the fascia of Scarpa along the line of the submammary fold. This layer is very strong (Fig. 28.13). It contributes to medial rotation, minimizes scar tension and dead space, and gives support to the upper pole. It works as a biological implant, presenting a similar effect to a mammary prosthesis at the end of the transoperative session. The multiplanar assembly is finished with dermal and subcuticular layers. It diverges from the breast tissue assembly, as most mammoplasty techniques do, because basically these approaches suture the points B and C referring to the remaining breast integument border after resection of the hypertrophy or mastopexy. It expands the muscle–glandular single retention suture to rotate the lateral quadrant, as indicated by Uebel (2013).

The convergent assembly helps to elevate the NAC with the upper pedicle, one of the most challenging tasks in larger hypertrophy or ptosis. It is transposed without difficulties because the lateral rotation in the direction to P1 transfers the ptotic NAC medially more easily. It works the same way as the techniques indicated for severe breast hypertrophy or ptosis with medial pedicle rotation utilized by Naufal et al. (2010) and Ariyan et al. (1989), or using the areola attached with an inferior pedicle, as demonstrated by Ariyan (1980). It contributes to avoiding amputation and the free graft of the NAC utilized in large breasts proposed by Thorek (1946) among others (Casas et al. 2001).

Centripetal rotation of breast tissue minimizes the axillary laxity, contributes to the transposition of the NAC, and adds volume to the upper pole of the breast. In this way, it works as an "autologous" implant at the end of the procedure (Fig. 28.14).

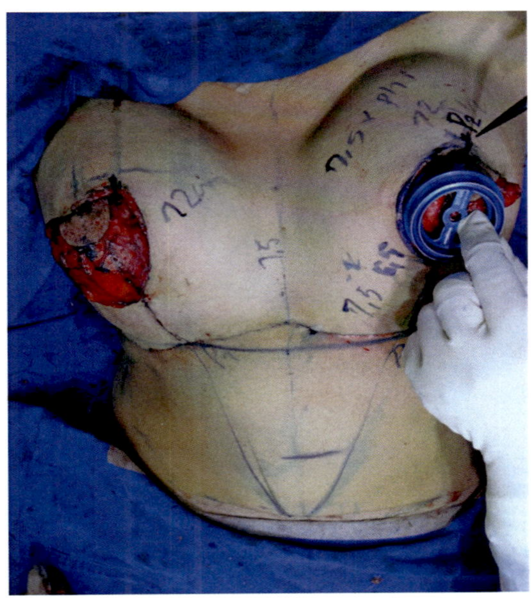

Fig. 28.14 Multiplanar layered assembly rotates the breast tissue from lateral to medial toward point P1 and from medial to P1. It helps NAC repositioning and gives fullness to the upper pole similar to an implant. The mammary cone is built over the branches of the 60° triangle that starts from the umbilicus in the direction of the acromioclavicular joint. The inferior border of the NAC is positioned at the distance between (P1 → m) − 1 cm, owing to the gravitational force. In this case, it was 7.5 − 1 cm = 6.5 cm. At the end of the surgery, the relation of the upper pole/lower pole is 55/45

Many contributions have been made to give bulk to the upper pole and prevent early breast ptosis. Inferior pedicle rotation to the upper pole is one of the most popular strategies (Ribeiro 2005, 1975; Castro 1983; Hall-Findlay 2002; Caldeira et al. 1999). Other techniques associate the inferior pedicle with a pectoral muscle belt described by Daniel (1994). Graf et al. (2003) indicated the same strategy associated with a vertical scar. In the past, we have supported the superior pedicle under the inferior third of the pectoralis major muscle, which works as a pocket (Pereira Filho 1995). Later, we proposed total coverage of the inferior pedicle by the pectoralis major muscle, which functioned as a biological implant. After oncological considerations, we stopped using that variation. Swanson (2011), investigating almost 100 mammoplasty reduction techniques using photometric analysis concluded that it is very difficult to maintain long-term upper pole fullness. He indicates a mammary prosthesis to achieve upper pole fullness and inferior convexity (Swanson 2015).

Nowadays there is a tendency of some surgeons to replace partially mammary tissue with implants as indicated by Saldanha et al. (2010). However, the presence of a synthetic product and its potential complications are relevant disadvantages. Also, it seems a paradox to replace part of the mammary integument in women who may become pregnant in the future, with a risk of damaging breastfeeding. We prefer to preserve breast tissue under the NAC and resect more tissue of the lateral quadrants to gain more projection under the upper pole. The strongest adhesion suture layer is made between the breast tissue and fascia of Scarpa. It rotates the medial and lateral quadrants to P1. Then, it contributes to the biological implant effect, as demonstrated in a preliminary letter (Fig. 28.15) (Pereira Filho et al. 2012).

The 60° V shape figure also orientates the inclination of the vertical scar and the position of the NAC. Usually, the inferior border of the areola is situated at 6–7.5 cm from P1. It follows the golden ratio, the distance between P1 and P2/phi. Taking into consideration the gravity action that contributes to natural mammary ptosis we deduct 1 cm from that measurement. Pursuing the ideal breast, the mammary shape ends at the transoperative view in a proportion of 55/45 (upper pole/lower pole). The gravity force over the mammary tissue changes that proportion to 45/55, which is considered more attractive according to a study by Mallucci and Brandford (2014).

Complications were few: minimal scar ulceration at the inverted T confluence in 19 patients (7%), asymmetry in 16 (6%), and partial nipple necrosis in 4 (1.5%).

After creation of the skin envelope, the scar usually ends in an inverted T. It can be reconfigured to an L shape, if the distance between the medial limit

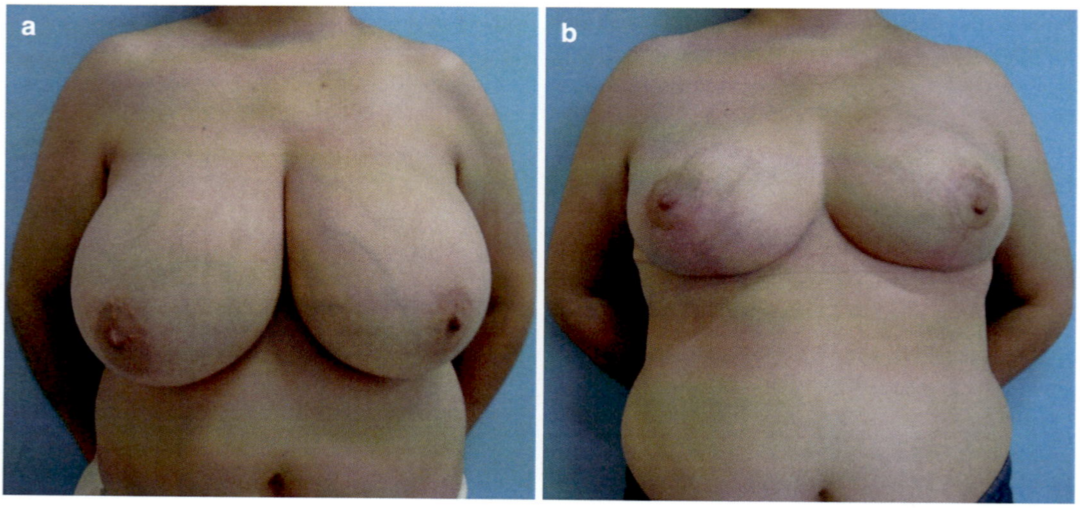

Fig. 28.15 A 34-year-old patient presenting a grade 3 hypertrophic breast, 1 year later after resection of 1060 g from the right side and 1015 g from the left side. This case scored 2 in Strasser's classification, i.e., malposition = 0, distortion = 0, asymmetry = 0, contour deformity = 0, and scar = 2

of the breast to be resected, point C (the medial corner of the new cone breast after resection), until the submammary fold, P1, is less than 2 cm (Fig. 28.16). It is an objective way of comparing current L-shaped scar mammoplasty approaches in which demarcation has been empirical, as used by Dufourmentel and Mouly (1961), or accurately addressed with more specific parameters as in Chiari Júnior (2002) and Bozola et al. (1982).

Precision in mammoplasty has been a challenging subject. The method we proposed defines quantified parameters for nipple position, and vertical horizontal skin resection that takes into consideration more than the breast width suggested by Tebbetts (2013). The golden ratio has been incorporated into the practice of Bozola et al. (2011) to help implant design preference. The study defines a comprehensive process guided by the universal principle of the divine proportion. In the assembly process, the breast cone is sculpted inside out, orientated by objective parameters. The technique preserves tissue under the NAC. It emphasizes tissue resection at the base and lateral quadrant, the area that is more susceptible to tumors. It contributes to upper pole projection using autologous tissue, reduces axillary laxity, and minimizes dead space. We have been investigating these principles since our first publication (Pereira Filho et al. 2012).

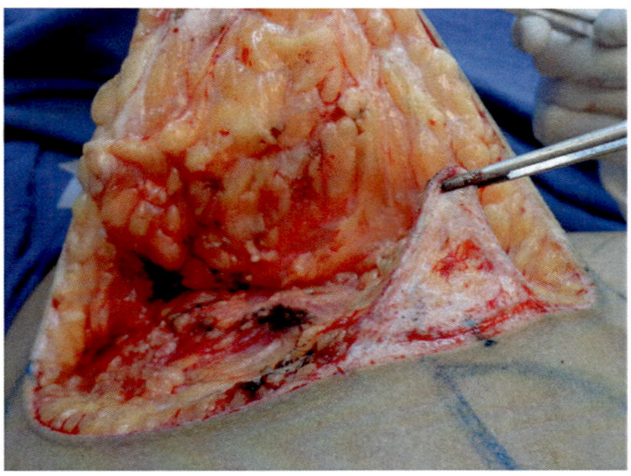

Fig. 28.16 A small triangle bridge with a base at P1 is preserved to minimize ulceration and delayed healing at the confluence of the vertical and horizontal scars

The complication rates are low. To minimize the most prevalent complication, scar ulceration at the inverted T, we now preserve a small triangle of tissue at the confluence of the vertical and horizontal scar (Fig. 28.17). This expands on the strategies advocated by Mahajan et al. (2006) that avoid tension at the confluence of the T scar, and the use of small darts indicated by Hoeflin (1992).

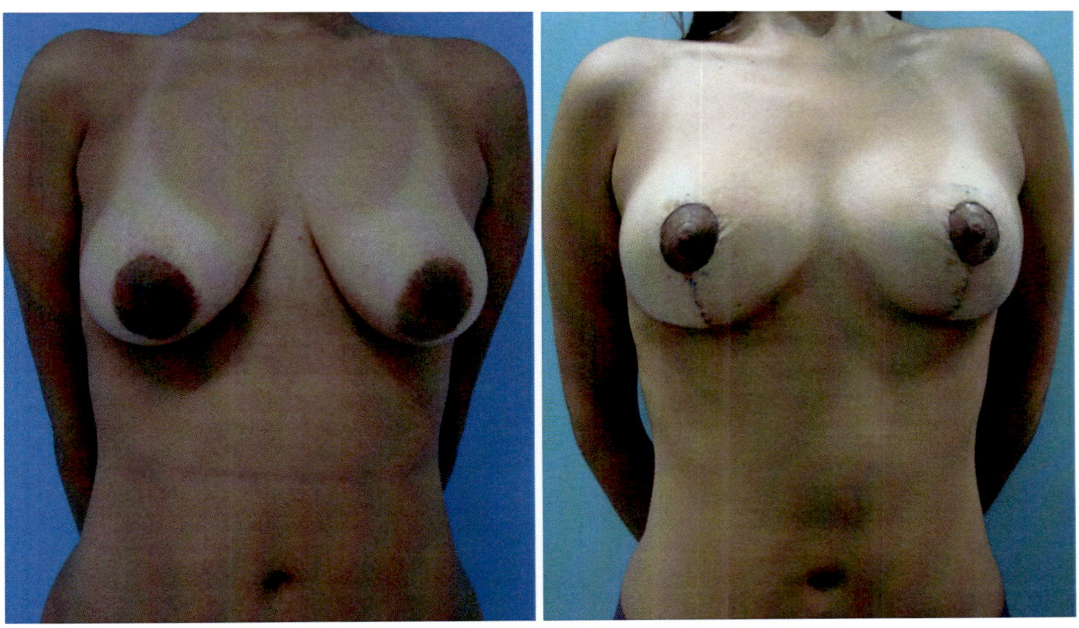

Fig. 28.17 A 31-year-old woman presenting moderate ptosis. The final L-shaped scar was possible because the distance of the cone breast to P1 was less than 2 cm

The approach proposed can then be considered for the armamentarium of plastic surgery in conjunction or associated with other methods described in mammoplasty.

Conclusion

Mammoplasties planned according to the golden ratio and assembled with multiplanar layers produce a proportionately balanced aesthetic breast, built over the V-shaped triangle with a 60° vertex at the umbilicus, guided by a constant submammary fold. The convergent assembly with multiplanar layer sutures using progressive multiple retention sutures provides rotation of the breast tissue and skin envelope guided by the branches of the triangle. As a consequence, it reduces the laxity at the axillary region, adds bulk to the upper pole, eases NAC elevation, contributes to a lower tension scar, and minimizes dead space (Fig. 28.18).

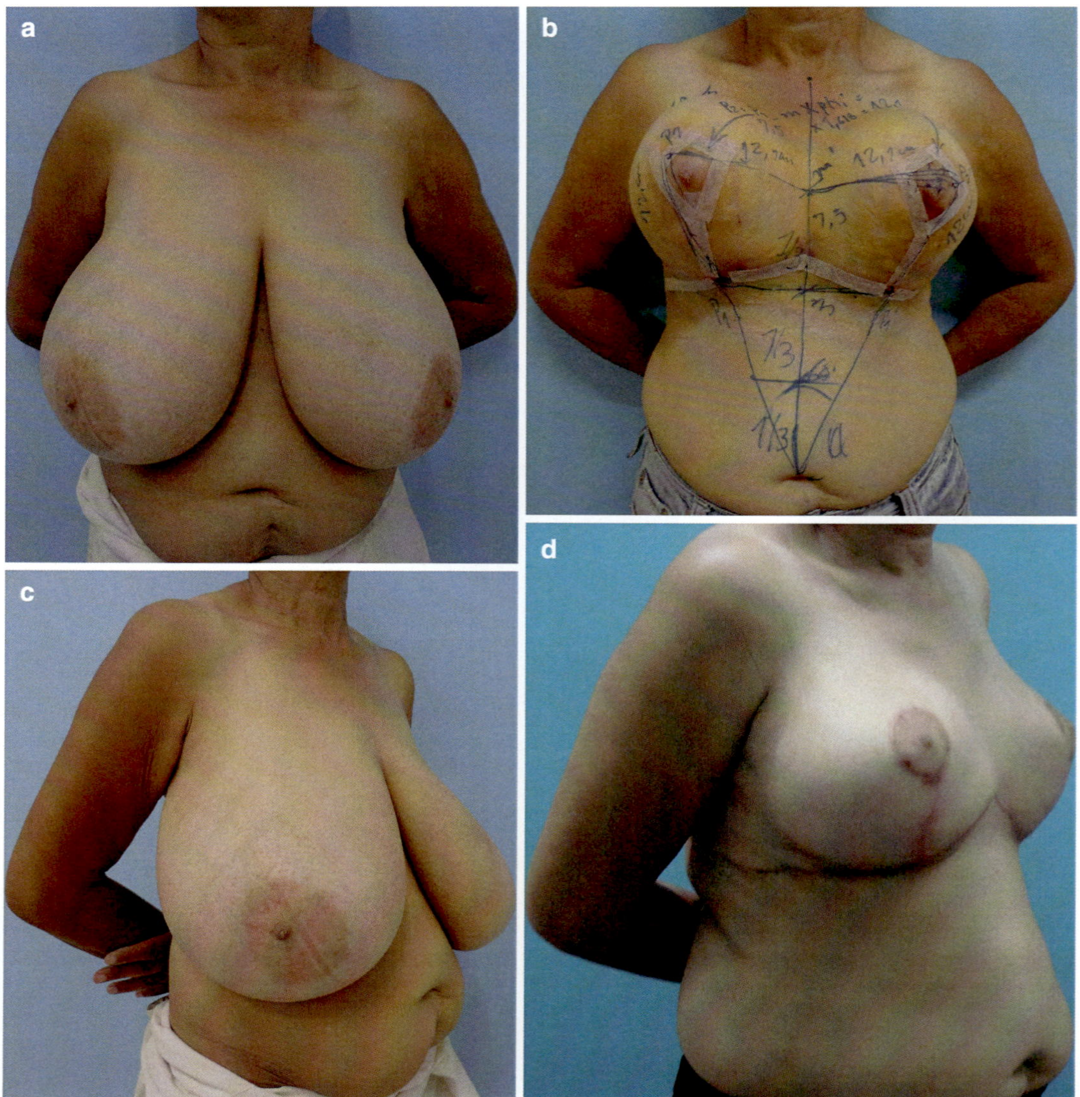

Fig. 28.18 (**a**) A 64-year-old patient presenting severe breast hypertrophy. (**b**) One week later after resection of 975 g from the right side, 1035 g from the left side, and breast lipoplasty of 1000 mL in volume. The distance from P1 to m was 7.5 cm. P1 → P2 = (P1 → m) × phi = 7.5 × 1618 = 12.1 cm. (**c**) Oblique view showing severe ptosis and axillary flaccidity. (**d**) Four months after mammoplasty using the approach discussed in the study. It was scored 2 according to Strasser's grading: malposition = 0, distortion = 0, asymmetry = 0, contour deformity = 0, and scar = 2

A low rate of complications was recorded. The approach adds precision to mastopexy and breast reduction and the principles are useful in planning breast augmentation.

Therefore, the technique should be considered in the arsenal of approaches indicated to correct mammoplasty.

References

Ariê G (1957) Nova Técnica em Mamaplastia. Rev Latinoam Cir Plast 3(28)

Ariyan S (1980) Reduction mammaplasty with the nipple-areola on a single, narrow, inferior pedicle. Ann Plast Surg 5(3):167–177

Ariyan S (1989).Finger RE, Vasquez B, Drew GS, Given KS Superomedial pedicle technique of reduction mammaplasty. Plast Reconstr Surg 83:471–478.

Avelar J (1994) Mamaplastia. Conduta Pessoal Simetria e Funcional Anais XXXI Congresso SBCP, Belo Horizonte, out, 1994

Bozzola A et al. (1982). Mamaplastia em L. Rev AMRIGS, Porto Alegre 26(3):207

Bozola AR, Longato FM, Bozola AP (2011) Análise geométrica da forma da beleza da mama e da forma da prótese na proporção phi: aplicação prática. Rev Bras Cir Plast 26(1):94–103

Caldeira AML, Lucas A, Grigalek G (1999) Mastoplasty: the triple-flap interposition technique. Aesthet Plast Surg 23:51–60

Casas L, Byun MY, Depoli PA (2001) Maximizing breast projection after free-nipple-graft reduction mammaplasty. Plast Reconstr Surg 107:955–960

Castro CC (1983) Redução mamária pela técnica do retalho dermoadiposo de pedículo inferior. Rev Bras Cir 73:47

Chiari Júnior A (2002) The L short-scar mammaplasty. Clin Plast Surg 29:401–409

Corine W, Megan V, Rohrich R (2014) Mastopexy and reduction mammoplasty pedicles and skin resection pattern. Plast Reconstr Surg Global Open 2(8):e202

Daniel MJ (1994) Mamaplastia com retalho de Músculo Peitoral. Arq Catarinense Med 23:121–122

Dufourmentel L, Mouly R (1961) Plastie Mammarie pour le Méthode Oblique. Ann Chir Plast 6:47

Erol O, Spira M (1980) A mastopexy technique for mild to moderate ptosis. Plast Reconstr Surg 65(5):603–609

Franco T, Rebelo C (1977) Cirurgia Estética. Livraria Atheneu, Rio de Janeiro

Geogiade NG, Serafin D, Reifkohl R et al (1979) Is there a reduction mammaplasty for "all seasons?". Plast Reconstr Surg 63(6):765

Graf R, de Araujo LRR, Rippel R, Neto LG, Pace DT, Biggs T (2003) Reduction mammaplasty and mastopexy using the vertical scar and thoracic wall flap technique. Aesthet Plast Surg 27:6–12

Hall-Findlay EJ (2002) Pedicles in vertical breast reduction and mastopexy. Clin Plast Surg 29:379–391

Hemenway P (2005) Divine proportion ϕ (phi) in art, nature, and science. Sterling, New York

Hoeflin SM (1992) Using skin dart to improve breast reduction and mastopexy scars. Plast Reconstr Surg 89(5):996

Hoopes JE, Maxwell GP (1979) Reduction mammaplasty: a technique to achieve the conical breast. Ann Plast Surg 3:106–113

Hugo NE, McClellan RM (1979) Reduction mammaplasty with a single superiorly-based pedicle. Plast Reconstr Surg 63:230–234

Huntley HE (1970) The divine proportion – a study in mathematical beauty, aesthetic claim. Dover, New York

Lockwood T (1999) Reduction mammaplasty and mastopexy with superficial fascial system suspension. Plast Reconstr Surg 103:1411–1420

Mahajan AL, Chapmann TW, McDiarmid J (2006) Preventing "T" junction dehiscence in mammaplasty. Plast Reconstr Surg 117:2100

Mallucci P, Brandford OA (2014) Population analysis of the perfect breast. A morphometric analysis. Plast Reconstr Surg 134:436–447

Muntan CD et al (2000) Inframmary fold: a histologic reappraisal. Plast Reconstr Surg 105(2):549–556

Nahabedian MY, McGibbon BM, Manson PN (2000) Medial pedicle reduction mammaplasty for severe mammary hypertrophy. Plast Reconstr Surg 105:896–904

Naufal RR, Pinheiro AS, Maciel PJ, Mélega JM (2010) Impacto da mamoplastia redutora com técnica do pedículo medial na redução dos sintomas dolorosos em pacientes com gigantomastia. Rev Bras Cir Plast 25(3 Suppl 1):55

Peixoto G (1980) Reduction mammaplasty: a personal technique. Plast Reconstr Surg 65:217–225

Pereira O, Bins-Ely J, Paulo E (2012) A retrospective photometric study of 82 published reports of mastopexy and breast reduction. Plast Reconstr Surg 130(6):890e–891e

Pereira Filho OJ (1995) Dynamic muscular support for mammaplasty. Transactions of the 11th congresso of the international confederation, Yokohama, Japan, p 397–398

Pereira Filho OJ, Bins Ely J, Lee KH (2012) Mamoplastia orientada pela proporção áurea(phi) associada à rafia interna com suturas progressivas. Rev Bras Cir Plást 27(3 Suppl 1):54

Perez-Macias JM (2004) Personal mastopexy technique for breast stabilization: update. Br J Plast Surg 57:178

Pitanguy I (1959) Breast hypertrophy. Trans. Intern. Soc. of Plast. Surgeons, 2nd Cong. London, E&S. Livingstone, Edinburgh, 1960

Ribeiro L (1975) A new technique for reduction mammaplasty. Plast Reconstr Surg 55:330–334

Ribeiro L (1989) Redução Mamária. In: Cirurgia Plástica da Mama. Medsi, Rio de Janeiro

Ribeiro L (2005) Pedículos em Mamaplastia. Atlas e Texto. Guanabara Koogan, Rio de Janeiro

Saldanha O et al (2010) Mamaplastia redutora com implante de silicone. Rev Bras Cir Plast 25(2):317–324

Strasser EJ (1999) An objective system for the evaluation of cosmetic surgical results. Plast Reconstr Surg 104:2282

Swanson E (2011) A retrospective photometric study of 82 published reports of mastopexy and breast reduction. Plast Reconstr Surg 128(6):1282–1301

Swanson E (2015) Ideal breast shape: women prefer convexity and upper pole fullness. Plast Reconstr Surg 135(3):641e–643e

Tebbetts JB (2013) A process for quantifying aesthetic and functional breast surgery: I. Quantifying optimal nipple position and vertical and horizontal skin excess for mastopexy and breast reduction. Plast Recontr Surg 132:1040

Tebbetts JB (2014) A process for quantifying aesthetic and functional breast surgery: I. Quantifying optimal nipple position and vertical and horizontal skin excess for mastopexy and breast. Plast Reconstr Surg 133:421e–422e

Theodore AC (1914) The curves of life. Dover, New York, pp 465–466

Thorek M (1946) Plastic reconstruction of the breast and free transplantation of the nipple. J Intern Coll Surg 9:194

Torres E, Salgado F et al. (2005). Breast pathology and reduction mammaplasty Pitanguy I. Plast Reconstr Surg 115:729–734.

Uebel CO (2013) Abdominoplastia e Mastopexia. In: Contorno Corporal e Lipoaspiração. Elsevier, pp 75–83

Wise RJ (1956) A preliminary report on a method of planning the mammaplasty. Plast Reconstr Surg 7:367–375

29 Vertical Mammaplasty: Vertical and Transverse Flaps through a Vertical Incision

Antonio Carlos Abramo

29.1 Introduction

Appropriate nipple–areola location with an adequate size, shape, and projection of the breast and a limited scar have guided the ideal result in reduction mammaplasty techniques (Xi et al. 2014). Moreover, the return of the sensitivity of the nipple–areola complex (NAC) is part of what is considered an ideal result in reduction mammaplasty. Return of the sensitivity of the NAC in reduction mammaplasty using a superior pedicle for the NAC is related to the amount of mammary tissue removed and elevation of the NAC (Abramo 1991).

Breast reduction with limited vertical incision has been indicated as an alternative in reducing mammaplasty. Vertical mammaplasty is achieved for young patients with moderate ptosis and moderate breast hypertrophy. Furthermore, it has also been indicated for patients over 50 years of age with severe ptosis and large breast hypertrophy (Beer et al. 2002). The fascial system within which the breast is enclosed provides a structural support to the breast, which is helpful in vertical mammaplasty. The thickness of the superficial layer of the breast reinforces the closure, not only at the junction of the NAC with the upper portion of the vertical scar, and along the vertical closure ensuring long-term stabilization of the mammary cone (Komya et al. 2015). Well-balanced breasts with an appropriate NAC location and a limited vertical scar have been widely described in reduction mammaplasty (Lassus 1996).

Arié (1957) reinforced the principles of vertical mammaplasty by performing a vertical spindle-shaped skin resection with a wide round dermal pedicle for the areola and resection of the mammary tissue along the vertical axis of the breast. Vertical triangular resection of the breast tissue has been also performed to reduce the breast volume in vertical mammaplasty (Flageul and Karcenty 2000).

Different models of vertical flaps with inferior pedicles have been reported as an additional element to increase the projection of the mammary cone (Ribeiro et al. 2002). In addition, several transverse supports to avoid downward displacement of the vertical flap with the inferior pedicle have also been reported. However, support of the vertical flap through a loop of the pectoralis major muscle can flatten the lower pole during the muscle contraction, through the pressure exerted by the muscle over the vertical flap (Graf and Biggs 2002).

A.C. Abramo, M.D., Ph.D.
Head Professor, Division of Plastic Surgery at General Hospital São Luiz Morumbi, Post Graduate Course in Aesthetic and Reconstructive Plastic Surgery of ACA-Institute of Assistance in Plastic Surgery of São Paulo, Rua Afonso de Freitas, 641 04006-052 São Paulo, SP, Brazil

J.M. Avelar (ed.), *Breast Surgery*, https://doi.org/10.1007/978-3-319-54115-0_29

Abramo et al. (2004) described two transverse flaps of mammary tissue with a pedicle at the distal end of the vertical pillars of the breast to enhance the lower pole and support the vertical flap, avoiding its long-term downward displacement. Some guidelines, such as marking the incisions, setting the NAC location, the amount of breast tissue resected, were followed to prevent later breast distortions after vertical mammaplasty.

Modification of the mosque-shaped areolar marking has been used to avoid NAC distortion after its transposition (Vogt et al. 2000). Liposuction in the lateral tail of the breast, without the need for skin resection, provided a suitable contour for the breast in vertical mammaplasty (Lejour 1994).

An adjustable vertical marking in conjunction with a vertical rectangular flap and two transverse triangular flaps of breast tissue are proposed here to achieve a long-term appropriate relationship among shape, projection, and volume of the breast with appropriate NAC location.

29.2 Method

29.2.1 Marking

Marking is carried out before surgery with the patient in a sitting position. A line is drawn from the nipple to the clavicle, 6–7 cm from the sternal notch. To avoid upward advancement of the NAC, point A is marked on the nipple–clavicular line 1–3 cm below the projection of the inframammary fold, establishing the superior limit of the new site of the areola. From point, a circle is outlined with a diameter ranging from 7 to 9 cm, allowing skin resection in accordance with the degree of breast hypertrophy and ptosis. The vertical diameter of the circle, represented by the line AD, is in continuity with the nipple–clavicular line, running through the NAC. From point D, the half-length of the vertical diameter is prolonged downward to the inframammary fold, defining point D_1 as the lower limit of the vertical incision. Point D1 is located on the inframammary fold or 1–2 cm above it, in accordance with the degree of breast ptosis or hypertrophy.

The transverse diameter of the circle, represented by the line BC, is displaced downward 1–2 cm along the vertical diameter, in accordance with the degree of breast hypertrophy or ptosis. Its intersection with the circumference of the circle determines points B1 and C1. The approach of points B1, A, and C1 defines the new size and location of the areola. From points B1 and C1 two curved lines with the concavity turned over the vertical diameter are drawn toward point D1. The degree of the concavity of the lines C_1D_1 and B_1D_1 is established by the amount of skin to be resected. Its length depends upon the degree of breast ptosis or hypertrophy.

Closure of the curved lines creates a vertical straight line ranging from 6 to 7 cm long. Marking is not strictly the same for both breasts; it depends on the degree of ptosis of each breast. A precise statement of the main points of the incisions marking may be accompanied by Figs. 29.1 and 29.2.

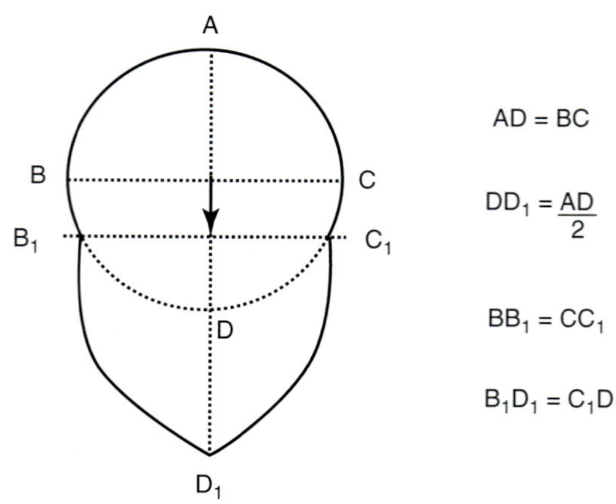

Fig. 29.1 Diagrammatic representation of the skin marking pattern

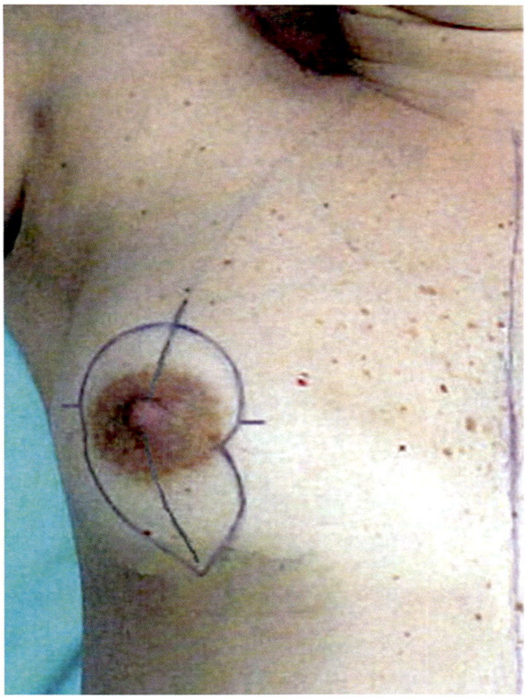

Fig. 29.2 Marking of the pattern on the breast skin

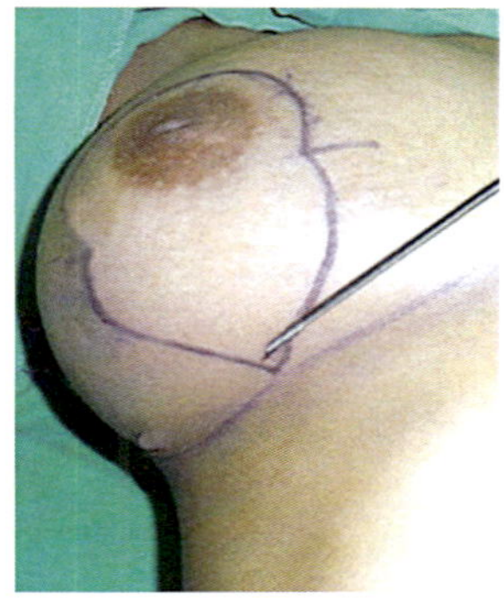

Fig. 29.3 Liposuction performed at the lateral tail of the breast

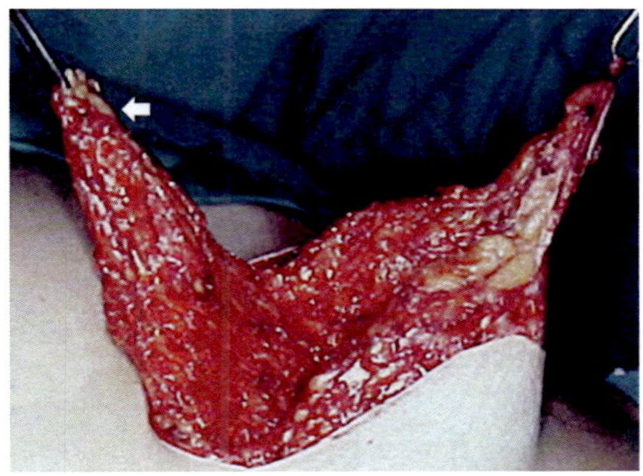

Fig. 29.4 The pedicle of the vertical flap is settled above the inferior limit of the vertical incision. The *arrow* shows the mammary tissue located beneath the areola added to the vertical flap

29.2.2 Operative Technique

Liposuction of the lateral tail of the breast is performed to avoid resection of skin and breast tissue at this level, adding a lateral horizontal lengthening to the vertical scar (Fig. 29.3). It is usually performed before the skin incisions. After incision around the skin marking provided by the pattern, the periareolar area is de-epithelialized and the skin inside the marking is resected. A vertical rectangular flap with inferior pedicle is dissected in the lower pole of the breast, 2 cm away from the skin incision, from the inferior limit of the vertical incision to the areola (Fig. 29.4). The pedicle of the vertical flap is 3 cm long and 5–7 cm wide supported over the fifth and sixth intercostal spaces. Its length is the same as the lower pole of the breast and is increased by the mammary tissue located beneath the areola (Fig. 29.4). The vertical flap is 5–7 cm wide and 3 cm thick for breast hypertrophy and the entire thickness of the lower pole for breast ptosis.

Resection of breast tissue is carried out only for breast hypertrophy, being performed transversely from the medial to the lateral portions of the breast, just above the pedicle of the vertical flap (Fig. 29.5). A vertical subglandular tunnel is dissected over the pectoral fascia toward the second intercostal space, to accommodate the vertical rectangular flap. The tip of the vertical flap is fixed on the pectoral fascia over the third rib and its lateral edges are fixed along the course of the subglandular tunnel (Fig. 29.6). A full-thickness

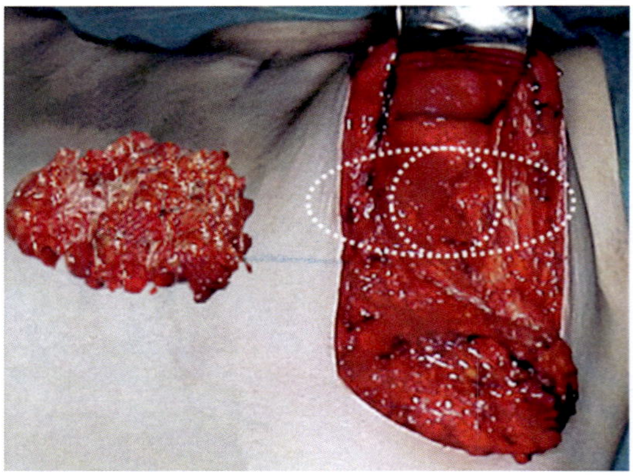

Fig. 29.5 Diagrammatic transverse resection of mammary tissue, performed just above the pedicle of the vertical flap. Amount of mammary tissue resected over the sternal area

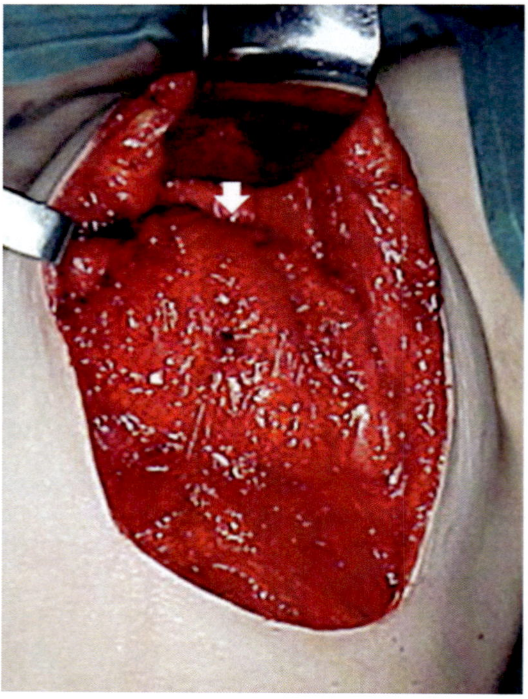

Fig. 29.6 The *arrow* indicates the vertical flap fixed in the pectoral fascia at the third rib

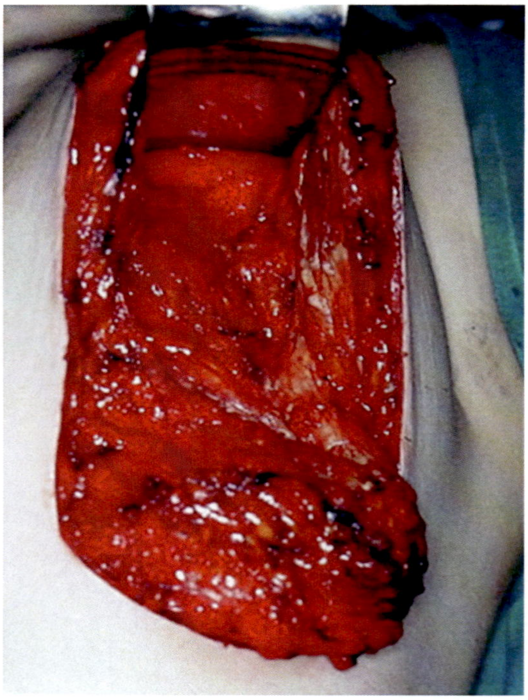

Fig. 29.7 Dissection of the medial triangular flap with pedicle supported on the lower half of the medial vertical pillar of the breast

incision is made in the vertical pillars of the breast, from the upper end at the areola to half of its length, and from the incision margin to the cut edge of the vertical pillar. Dissection of the vertical pillars creates two transverse triangular flaps with pedicles supported on the lower half of the pillars (Fig. 29.7). The length of the transverse flap corresponds to half the length of the vertical pillar and the thickness ranges according to the amount of breast tissue at the incision margin.

A subglandular tunnel is dissected at the inframammary fold on each side of the pedicle of the vertical rectangular flap to accommodate the end of the transverse triangular flap. Criss-crossing of the transverse triangular flaps is performed with the lateral triangular flap placed inferior to the medial one. The tips of the triangular flaps are anchored on the pectoralis fascia at the end of the subglandular tunnels, approaching the vertical pillars in the midline of the breast (Fig. 29.8). The triangular flaps are joined together, creating a transverse support sling for the vertical flap at the lower pole of the breast.

Closure of the vertical pillars is carried out in two layers, at the superficial layer of the superficial fascia of the breast and at the intradermal level. The two-layer closure provides better support for the reshaped breast changing the curve lines to a straight line (Fig. 29.9).

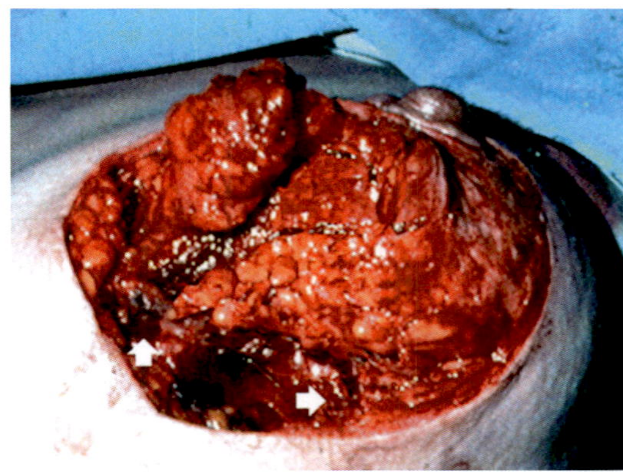

Fig. 29.8 The *vertical arrow* shows the tip of the lateral triangular flaps anchored on the pectoral fascia at the end of the medial transverse subglandular tunnel. The *horizontal arrow* indicates the subglandular transverse lateral tunnel

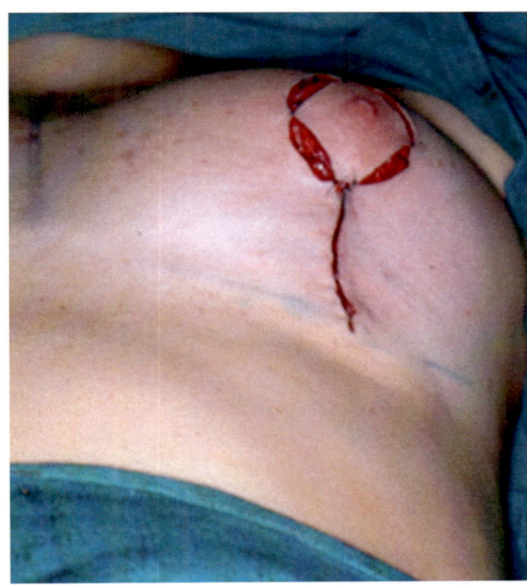

Fig. 29.9 Closure of the breast vertical pillars reinforces the breast projection. After closure, the curve lines of the patterns become a limited vertical straight line. Appropriate relationship among size, shape, projection, and location of the areola with a vertical scar on the right breast

29.2.3 Results

Breast elevation with a natural balance of shape, projection, volume, NAC location, and a limited vertical scar were achieved after mammaplasty, combining vertical and transverse flaps through a vertical incision. In addition, fullness of the upper pole was also achieved, ensuring the long-term balance of the breast. Figure 29.10 illustrates the long-term result.

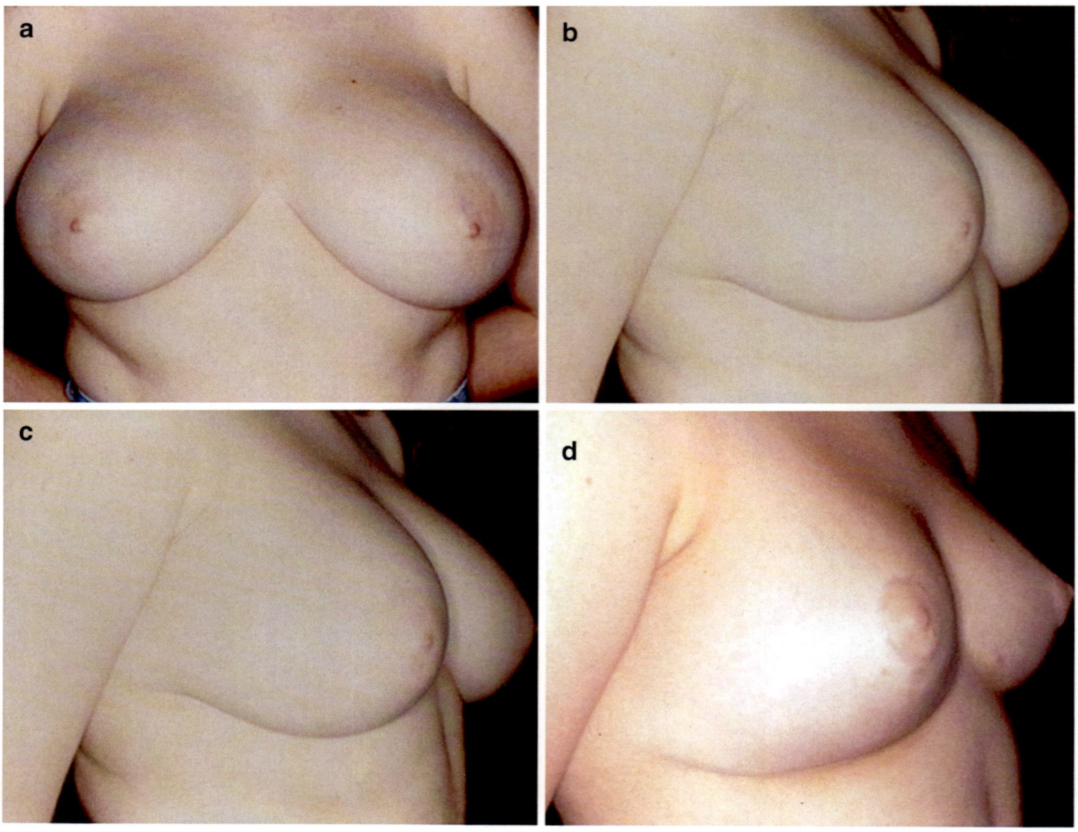

Fig. 29.10 (**a–c**) Breasts with moderate to large hypertrophy and moderate degree of ptosis without asymmetry. (**b–d**) Reduction mammaplasty combining vertical and triangular flaps with a vertical incision recovering the mammary cone. Two and a half years postoperatively

29.3 Case Report

Figure 29.11 shows a 47-year-old woman, who had undergone two pregnancies, and who had breast asymmetry. The degree of ptosis and hypertrophy in the right breast was moderate, whereas in the left breast, only mild ptosis without hypertrophy was observed. Point A was placed 1 cm below the projection of the inframammary fold on the breast skin. From point A a circle 9 cm in diameter was outlined around the NAC. Downward displacement of the transverse diameter along the vertical diameter of the circle was 2 cm. The length of each one of the lower

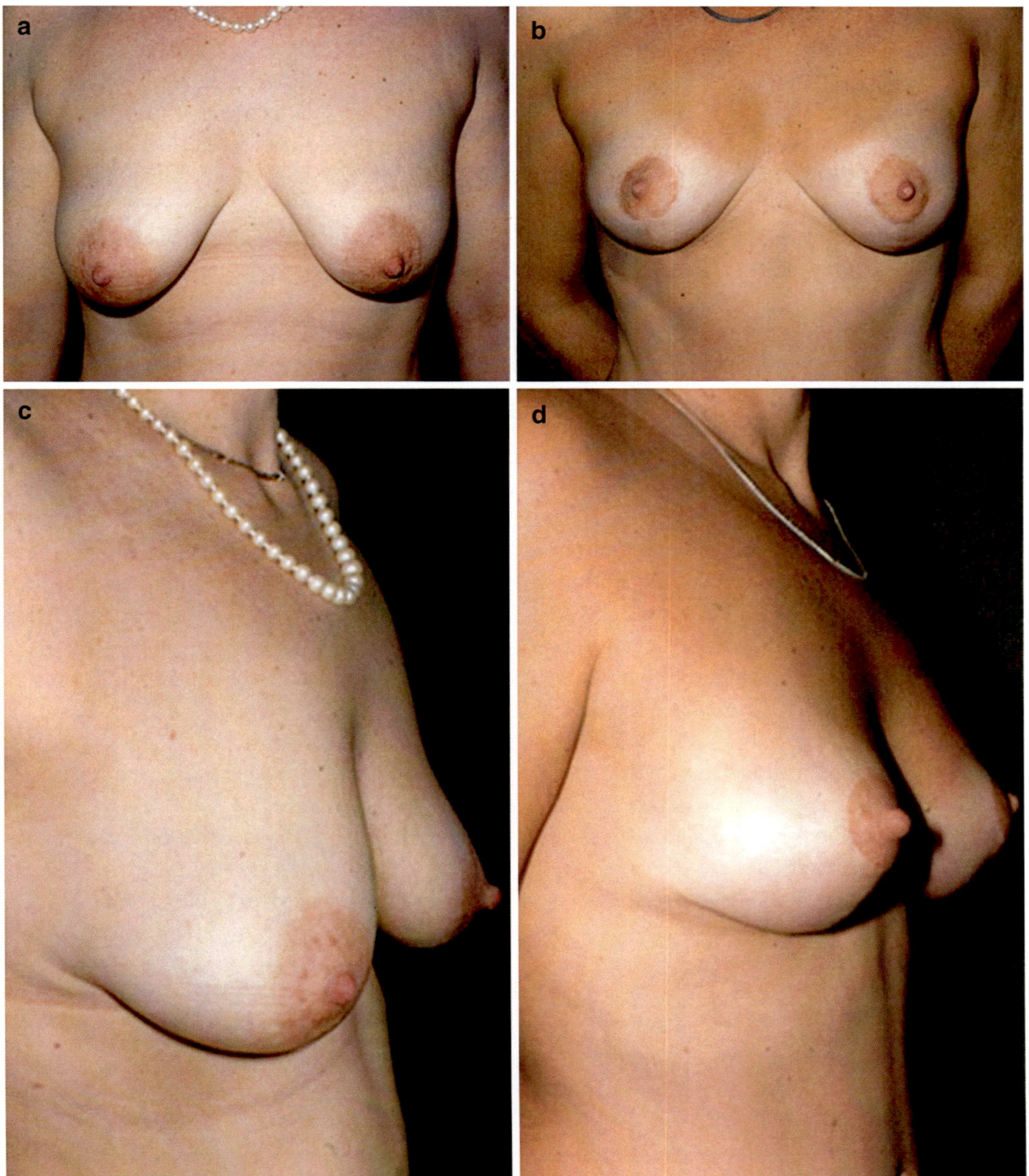

Fig. 29.11 (**a–c**) Breast asymmetry with a moderate degree of ptosis and hypertrophy in the right breast, and mild ptosis without hypertrophy in the left one. (**b–d**) Two years after the surgery, fullness of the upper pole remains

vertical curve lines created by the marking was 6 cm. The distance between them at the major concavity was 11 cm. Resection of mammary tissue in the right breast was 307 g and in the left one 212 g. Distinctive resection of mammary tissue was performed to adjust the breast asymmetry. A natural balance of size, shape, projection with proper elevation of the NAC, and a limited vertical scar at the lower pole of the breast was achieved combining vertical and transverse flaps through a vertical incision.

29.4 Complications

Despite the satisfactory performance achieved with vertical mammaplasty, some controversies have been reported. Critical evaluation of vertical mammaplasty has reported excessively long vertical scars, upward displacement of the areola, or poor long-term projection of the breast (Hidalgo 1999). In addition, larger reductions underneath the NAC may compromise the fullness of the upper pole (Aksu et al. 2015). Recurrence of breast ptosis can also occur after conventional vertical mammaplasty. However, it is unusual in mammaplasty combining vertical and transverse flaps through a vertical incision. Breast asymmetry after vertical mammaplasty can be caused either by recurrence of ptosis or by inadequate resection of mammary tissue. Skin dehiscence and necrosis, loss of sensitivity, and distortion of the NAC are complications that may occur in reduction mammaplasty, but were not found in mammaplasty combining vertical and transverse flaps through a vertical incision.

29.5 Discussion

Mammaplasty employing vertical and transverse flaps of mammary tissue through a vertical incision provided a natural contour for the breast, with well-balanced upper and lower poles, and appropriate location and sensibility of the NAC. According to Abramo and Viola (1993) maintenance of the upper pole of the breast attached to the pectoral muscle keeps safe the cutaneous branches of the third and fourth intercostal nerves, preserving the sensitivity of the NAC. The length of the vertical incision provided by the vertical marking created a limited vertical scar in the lower pole with no compromise of the inframammary fold.

Breast projection, shape and volume were obtained by the bulk of the vertical flap and the overlapping of the triangular flaps over the vertical flap. The criss-crossing of the triangular flaps also supports the vertical flap, ensuring long-term stabilization of the mammary cone. The continuity of the vertical diameter of the circle with the nipple–clavicular line provides a safe transposition of the NAC without distortion of the areola, as the nipple–clavicular line represents the course of the natural displacement of the areola (Abramo et al. 1999). The lower limit of the incision 1–2 cm above the inframammary fold enables easy accommodation of the skin at this level, holding the scar above the inframammary fold.

Variations in width and thickness of the vertical flap are helpful for appropriate breast projection, allowing for more removal of breast tissue in reducing mammaplasty and less in mastopexy, in this way adjusting the breast volume. The length of the vertical rectangular flap increased by adding the mammary tissue located underneath the areola, providing greater projection to the upper pole of the breast. In addition, the pedicle of the vertical flap placed 1–3 cm above the lower limit of the vertical incision allows the upward displacement of the flap, improving the upper pole fullness.

To ensure the long-term projection for the breast, the lateral edges of the vertical flap are fixed on the aponeurosis of the pectoralis major muscle, making its downward displacement more difficult. The transverse sling of mammary tissue created by the criss-crossing of the triangular flaps also supports the vertical flap into position with no pressure over the flap, avoiding its downward advancement, therefore enhancing the fullness of the upper pole. In addition, the criss-crossing of the triangular flaps also increases the amount of breast tissue at the lower pole, ensuring the long-term projection of the breast.

Conclusion

Mammaplasty combining vertical and transverse approaches projects the breast through the vertical flap and supports the mammary cone through the transverse sling achieved by the criss-crossing of the triangular flaps. The unequal direction of the vectors of the vertical and triangular flaps redistributes the tension exerted over the mammary cone, improving balanced shape, projection, and volume for the breast in the long term. Liposuction involving only the lateral tail of the breast improves the breast contour, reducing the bulge at the axillary area without the need for skin resection.

References

Abramo AC (1991) Pattern for reduction mammaplasty that uses a vertical dermal pedicle. Aesthetic Plast Surg 15:265–270

Abramo AC, Viola JC (1993) Avaliação da Sensibilidade do Complexo Aréolo-Mamilar (CAM) Após Mamaplastia Redutora. An Paul Med Cir 120(1):9

Abramo AC, Oliveira LMF, Milan R, Mateus S (1999) Evaluation of the nipple-areola complex sensibility after reduction mammaplasty by superior vertical dermal pedicle. Rev Bras Cir Plast 14(1):7–16

Abramo AC, Teixeira JC, Galindo A (2004) Mammaplasty combining vertical and transverse approaches through a vertical incision. Plast Reconstr Surg 113(2):508–516

Arié G (1957) Una nueva técnica de mastoplastia. Rev Latinoam Cir Plast 3:23–31

Beer GM, Morgenthaler W, Spicher I, Meyer VE (2002) Modifications in vertical scar breast reduction. Br J Plast Surg 54:341–347

Flageul G, Karcenty B (2000) À propos des plasties mammaires: la méthode verticale triangulaire on "Verticale triangulaire technique". Description, indications, rétrospective sur six ans. Ann Chir Plast Esthet 45:531–547

Graf R, Biggs TM (2002) In search of better shape in mastopexy and reduction mammaplasty. Plast Reconstr Surg 110:309–317

Hidalgo DA (1999) Update on vertical mammaplasty (discussion). Plast Reconstr Surg 104:2303

Komya T, Ito N, Imai R, Itoh M, Naito M, Matsubayashi J, Matsumura H (2015) Anatomy of the superficial layer of superficial fascia around the nipple-areola complex. Aesthetic Plast Surg 39:209–213

Lassus C (1996) A 30 years experience with vertical mammaplasty. Plast Reconstr Surg 97:373–380

Lejour M (1994) Vertical mammaplasty and liposuction of the breast. Plast Reconstr Surg 94:100–114

Öksüz S, Ülkür E, Peker F (2015) Superior pedicle reduction mammoplasty supported with inferior pedicle chest wall-based flap: refinements to the technique. Aesthetic Plast Surg 39:69–77

Ribeiro L, Accorsi Jr A, Buss A, Marçal-Pessoa M (2002) Creation and evolution of 30 years of the inferior pedicle in reduction mammaplasties. Plast Reconstr Surg 110:960–970

Vogt PM, Muhlberger T, Torres A, Peter FW, Steinau HU (2000) Method for intra-operative positioning of the nipple-areola complex in vertical scar reduction mammaplasty. Plast Reconstr Surg 105:2096–2099

Xi W, Perdanasari AT, Ong Y, Han S, Min P, Su W, Feng S, Pacchioni L, Zhang YX, Lazzeri D (2014) Objective breast volume, shape and surface area assessment: a systematic review of breast measurement methods. Aesthetic Plast Surg 38:1116–1120

Vertical Mammaplasty

30

Ruth Graf, Priscilla Balbinot, and Daniele Pace

30.1 Introduction

Breast surgery techniques have changed over the years with improved results. Recent efforts have been made to shorten scars and achieve a good breast shape in the long term. The aim of a mammaplasty/mastopexy procedure is to improve breast ptosis by lifting the breast including the gland and the nipple–areola complex (NAC), to correct breast ptosis and hypertrophy, remodel the breast parenchyma to provide a natural and firm aspect to the breast, reduce skin scars, and provide the patient with low rates of morbidity and complications.

Vertical mammaplasty is a technique with a many advantages and it produces stable results. Dartigues (1925) was the first author to describe a vertical scar technique used for mastopexy. Arié (1957) described a technique for reduction mammaplasty that resulted in a vertical scar, which did not gain popularity because the vertical scar often crossed the inframammary crease and extended onto the chest wall, leaving an unsightly scar. It was only in 1969 that Lassus renewed interest in vertical breast scar reduction by developing a technique using a superior dermoglandular pedicle for transposition of the NAC: a central excision en bloc of skin, fat, and gland; no undermining; and resulting in a vertical scar. In 1994, Lejour described a modification of Lassus' technique, beginning the breast reduction with liposuction to eliminate fat contributing to the breast volume. The skin surrounding the excised area was undermined and the superior dermoglandular pedicle was sutured to the pectoral fascia, joint pillars improved breast shape, and suturing the skin of the vertical wound above the inframammary crease. Lassus' and Lejour's techniques demonstrated positive outcomes when applied not only in mild and moderate cases of breast hypertrophy, but in severe cases as well (Lassus 1970; Lejour 1994).

A desirable long-term outcome is achieved with breast shape redefinition using internal tissue, not with skin sutures, avoiding excessive scar tension. As a consequence, over time the breast developed a phenomenon commonly referred to as a "weight-bridge," that is, a heavy lower pole and loss of projection in the upper pole of the breast. A loop of muscle flap is a suggested modification to reduce the weight-bridge phenomenon over time. Performing the chest wall-based flap technique under a sling of pectoralis major muscle permits maintenance of this

R. Graf, M.D., Ph.D. (✉)
Pietà Centro Médico, Hospital de Clínicas – Rua General Carneiro, 181, Alto da Glória, Rua Solimões, Curitiba, PR, Brazil
e-mail: ruthgraf@uol.com.br

P. Balbinot, M.D., M.Sc.
Federal University of Parana, Rua General Carneiro, 188 – Hospital de Clinicas, Curitiba, PR, Brazil
e-mail: pribalbinot@gmail.com

D. Pace, M.D., M.Sc.
Pietà Centro Médico, Rua Albino Silva, Curitiba, PR, Brazil
e-mail: danielepace@hotmail.com

J.M. Avelar (ed.), *Breast Surgery*, https://doi.org/10.1007/978-3-319-54115-0_30

redefinition, together with liposuction to the lateral breast area to better define the lateral fold.

The goals of a vertical scar technique associated with a chest wall-based flap and bipedicled pectoralis major muscle flap are: upper pole fullness with the patient in a supine position and maintenance of the breast position in the standing position, minimal breast descent providing a better aesthetic outcome in the long-term follow-up, a vertical scar that does not cross the new inframammary crease, and no flattening of the central position of the breast (NAC) area as such using the periareolar approach (Graf et al. 2003, 2016; Hall-Findlay and Shestak 2015).

30.2 Method

30.2.1 Technique

Skin markings are made with the patient in a standing position. Precise measurements must be taken using the inframammary fold (IMF), the NAC, and the suprasternal notch as key landmarks. The midline of the chest and IMF are marked. First, lines are drawn straight down the midline from the suprasternal notch to the xyphoid process, from a point 5 cm from the suprasternal notch at the clavicle to the NAC and then straight down to the areola. Setting the nipple height is extremely important. The position is determined by multiple factors. The distance from the sternal notch to the nipple should be within a range of 17–19 cm and it is influenced by height, breast, and body type. With a horizontal maneuver, the breast is moved medially and laterally and two points (B and C) are marked, using the vertical line inferior to the areola as a reference, which demonstrates the excess skin. Using these three points as a reference, a curved line is drawn around the areola in an oval shape, similar to the periareolar technique. The medial portion of this line is, on average, 9 cm from the midline, and the lateral portion is, on average, 12 cm from the anterior axillary line. The vertical incision ends 2 cm above the IMF. Point D is marked, 2–4 cm above the IMF. Points BD and CD are joined together in a curved line of approximately 5–7 cm (Fig. 30.1).

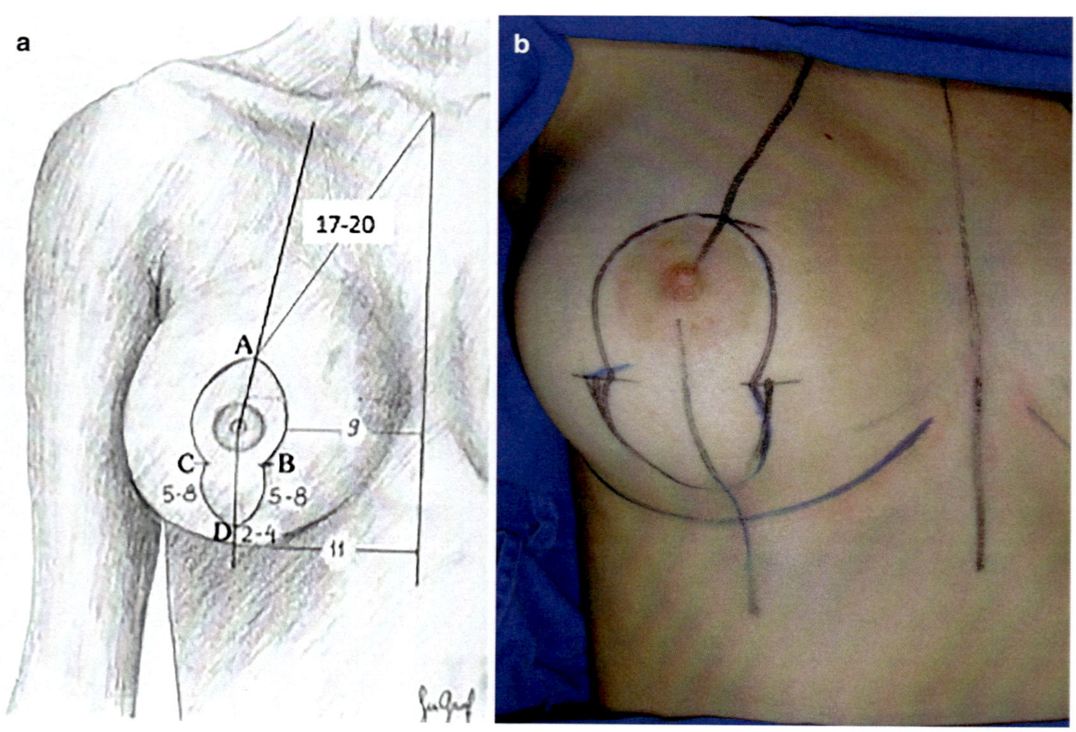

Fig. 30.1 (**a**, **b**) Preoperative skin markings and are of skin resection

30.2.2 Operative Procedure

The patient is placed supine on the operating table and, after induction with general or epidural anesthesia (local is possible) and prep and drape, the incision markings are infiltrated subdermally (except superior to the areola), with dilute epinephrine in saline solution (1:100,000) and then tattooing is performed as four cardinal points and more four points between these are made in the NAC (Fig. 30.2).

The surgery is initiated by marking the areola with a 42-mm areolotome. Surgery begins with de-epithelialization of the area previously described. The dermis is incised along the marked lines, up to 1.5–2 cm superior to points B and C, sparing the upper portion of the areola, which is the pedicle for the NAC (Fig. 30.3). Thereafter, dissection of breast tissue is initiated in the lower half area between the skin and the areola, parallel to lactiferous ducts, avoiding cutting them, toward the chest wall, reaching the pectoral fascia

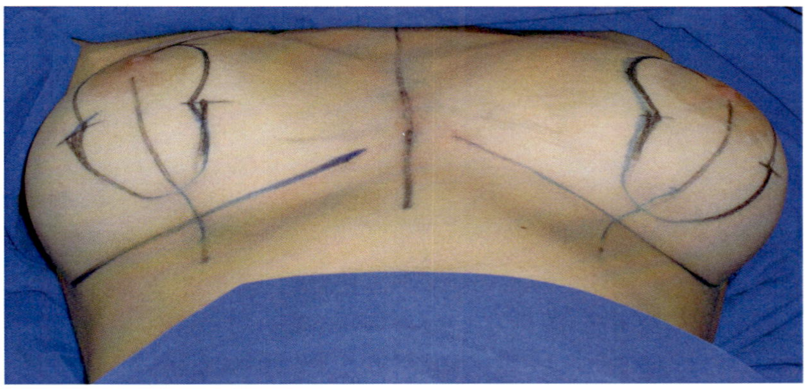

Fig. 30.2 Skin markings (operative table)

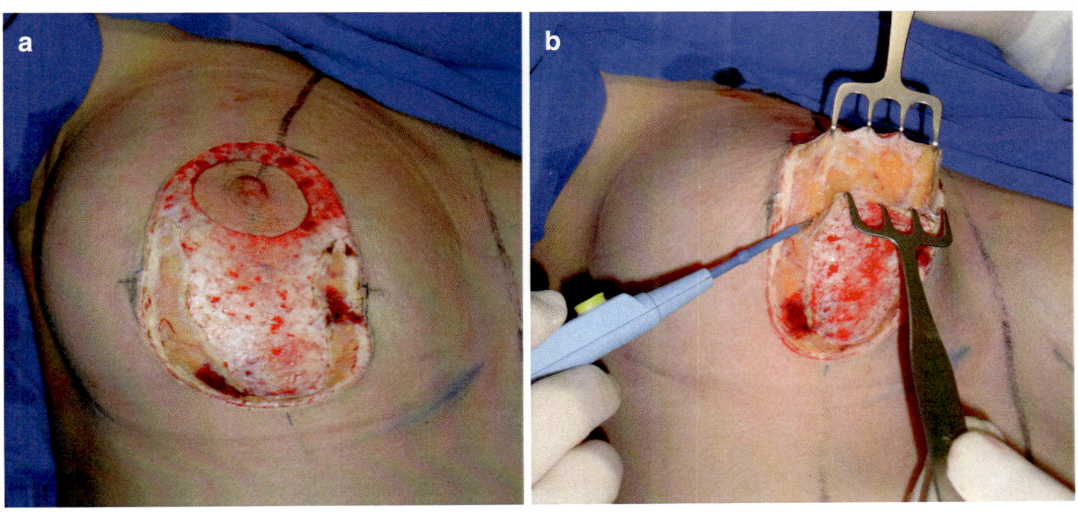

Fig. 30.3 (**a**) Chest wall-based flap creation. (**b**) Dermal incision

at the level of the fourth intercostal space. The incision is then made obliquely in the upper portion of the flap, leaving enough breast tissue on either side (future breast pillars) (Fig. 30.4).

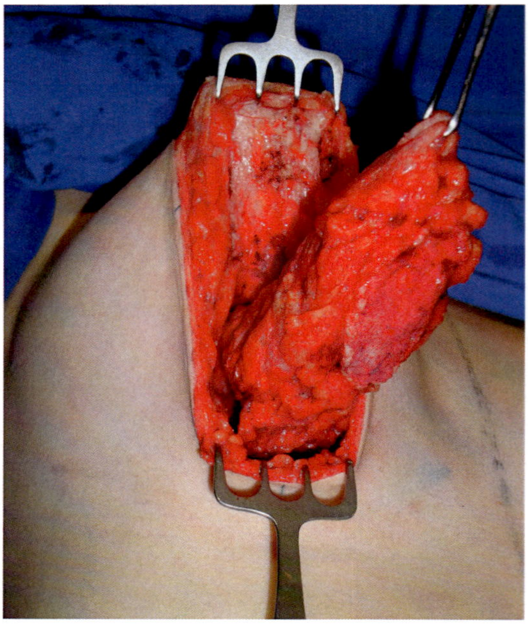

Fig. 30.4 Chest wall-based flap undermined

Breast tissue is undermined to the level of the second intercostal space, at the level of the pectoral fascia. The lower portion of the flap is dissected carefully down to the original inframammary crease leaving a 0.5–1 cm mastectomy flap, widening its base until the chest wall flap is formed, which will be based on the arteries of the fourth and fifth intercostal spaces, with the following approximate dimensions: 6–8 cm wide and 4 cm thick. Great care must be taken at this point not to undercut the flap (chest wall pedicle).

A strip of pectoral muscle approximately 8–10 cm long and 1.5–2 cm wide is marked with methylene blue, which is dissected just superior to the base of the chest wall flap, using no more than one-half of the muscle thickness, wide enough to accommodate the chest wall-based flap with no compression at all and the donor site is closed with 2-0 nylon. Its caudal or inferior line is at the cephalic end of the flap base. This loop is used to help hold the flap in position in the upper pole. The dermis of the chest wall-based flap is then sutured to the pectoral fascia with a running 2-0 nylon suture, starting laterally and finishing medially (Fig. 30.5) (Daniel 1995).

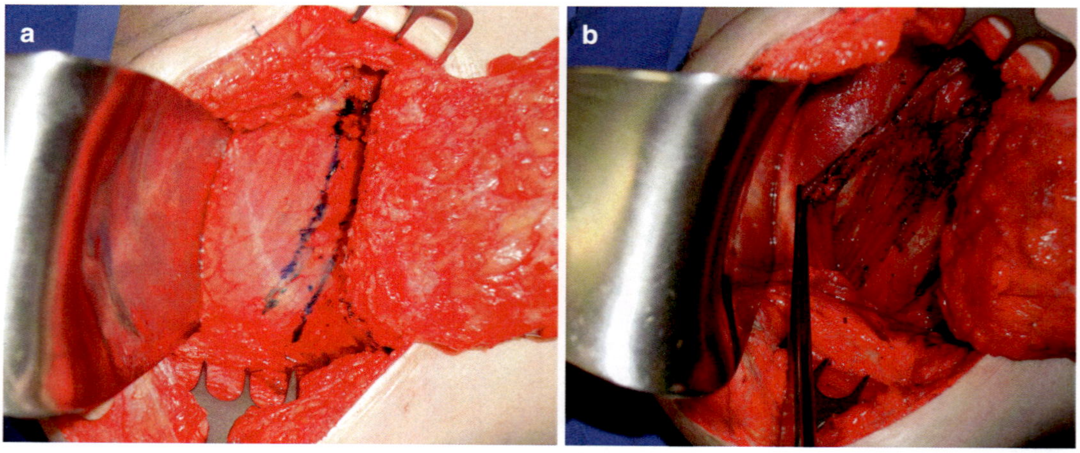

Fig. 30.5 (**a**, **b**) Pectoralis major loop is created just superior to the chest wall-based flap

The flap is now freely mobile and is based on vessels from the fifth and sixth intercostal spaces, as a perforator flap. The breast tissue is retracted upward and cephalic and dissected off the pectoral fascia up to the second intercostal space, creating a space in the upper pole of the breast into which the flap will be fixed (Fig. 30.6).

With the flap in the correct position and the breast suspended by the hook in the NAC, breast tissue excess is removed, if necessary. It is important to avoid resections from the medial column to avoid flattening of the medial breast. Breast tissue excess is removed just after the flap is sutured, to maintain the same size of the columns (Fig. 30.7). The upper breast flap of the gland

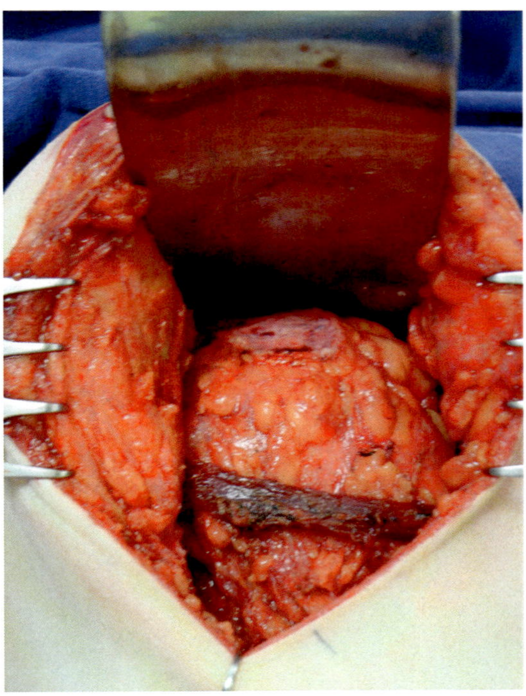

Fig. 30.6 Chest wall-based flap is sutured to the pectoral fascia at the second intercostal space

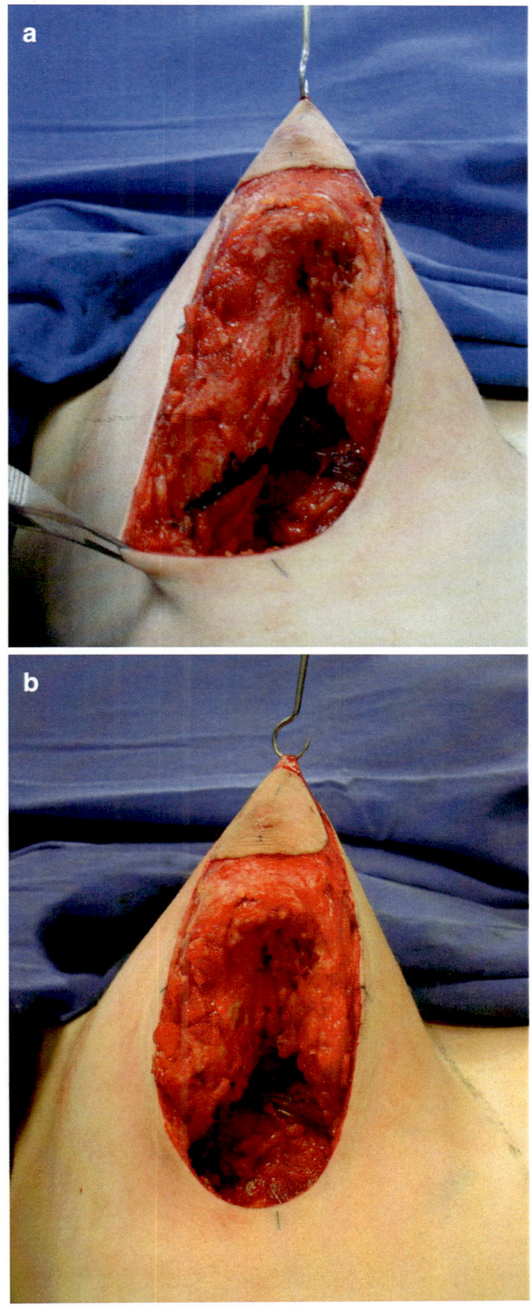

Fig. 30.7 (**a**, **b**) Breast tissue excess is removed just after the flap is sutured, to maintain the columns at the same size

(the superior part of breast tissue) is sutured to the muscle plane at the second intercostal space to lift the undermined breast tissue and improve upper pole projection (Fig. 30.8).

Closure starts with suturing of the columns with 2-0 nylon in several layers (Fig. 30.9). A round block suture is applied around the NAC to homogeneously distribute the periareolar skin and to reduce tension on the NAC. Eight cardinal points are marked in the periareolar skin and in the areola. The running suture is administered using 3-0 colorless nylon. Passing through the deep dermis of the outer skin and the areolar deep tissue, the suture takes a small amount of tissue between the markings in the areola, and large amounts right on the markings of the periareolar skin. Tensioning the suture reduces the periareolar circumference up to the desired diameter for the NAC (about 4.5 cm) (Fig. 30.10).

The deep dermis is sutured, placing together points B and C as the first suture and then the skin is sutured. Point D is fixated to the deep

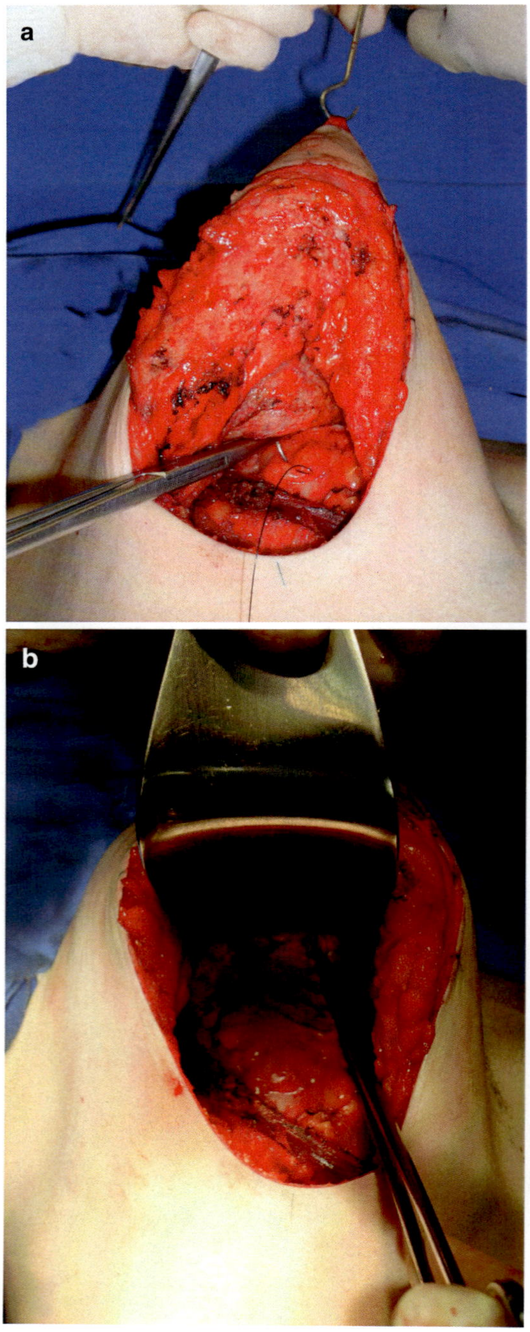

Fig. 30.8 (**a**, **b**) Superior part of the breast tissue is sutured to the chest wall base flap to lift the undermined breast tissue and improve upper pole projection

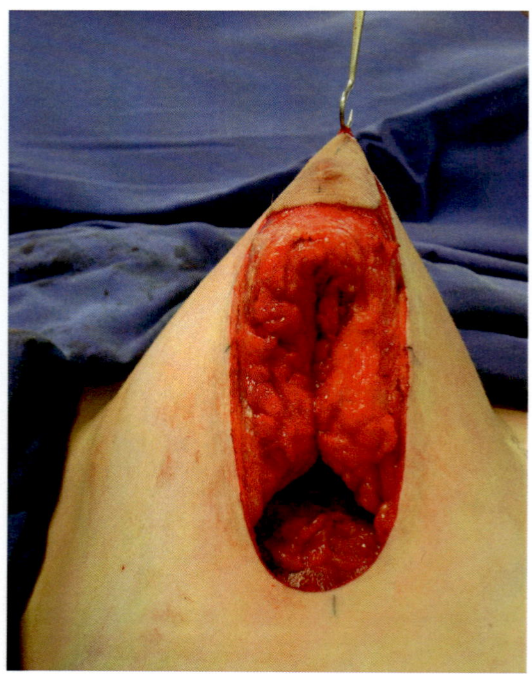

Fig. 30.9 Closure starts by suturing the columns with 2-0 nylon in several layers

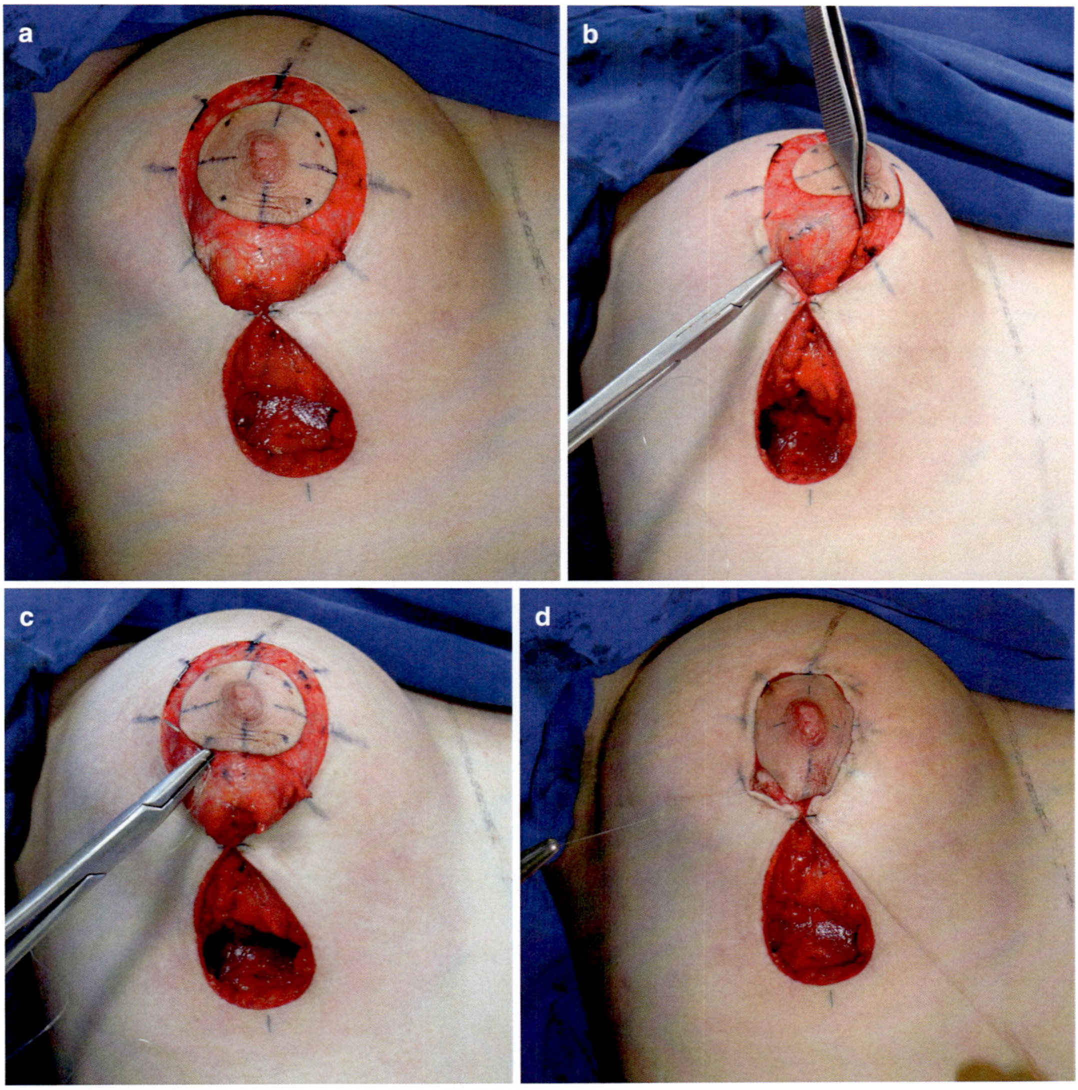

Fig. 30.10 (**a**) Eight cardinal points are marked in the periareolar skin and in the areola. (**b**) A running suture is made using a 3-0 colorless nylon and starts at the inferolateral part of the nipple–areola complex (NAC). (**c**) Passing through the deep dermis of the outer skin and the areolar deep tissue, the suture takes a small amount of tissue between the markings in the areola, and large amounts right on the markings of the periareolar skin. (**d**) Finished round block suture

plane so that the vertical suture is kept at the same level as the new inframammary crease (Fig. 30.11). Subcutaneous tissue is undermined from the glandular tissue to elevate the vertical scar and to enable suturing of the dermis to the columns superiorly (Fig. 30.12). A subcuticular suture with 4-0 Monocryl is applied to the vertical scar to shorten it. Starting from point D, vertical skin is closed with sutures of 3-0 Monocryl. Anchoring the deep dermis to the underlying columns, these sutures elevate the whole vertical component, placing point D at the level of the new IMF. Thus, the final vertical scar end ups at the level or slightly above the new inframammary crease. Final skin closure is carried out using a running intradermic suture of 4–0 Monocryl (Fig. 30.13). Drainage is not routinely used.

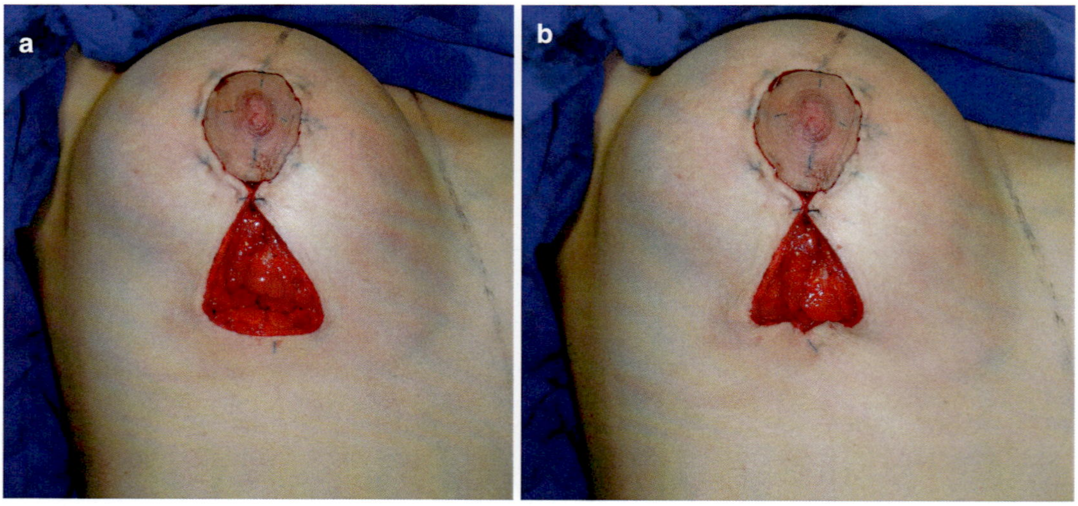

Fig. 30.11 (**a**, **b**) Vertical suture is kept at the same level as the new inframammary fold

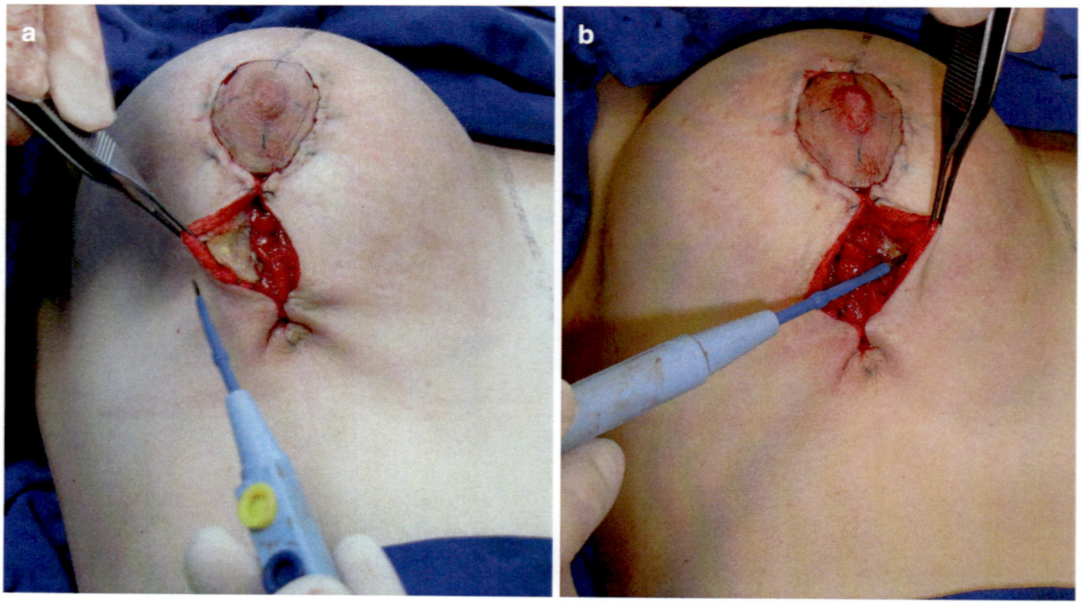

Fig. 30.12 (**a**, **b**) Subcutaneous tissue is undermined by the glandular tissue to elevate the vertical scar and to enable suturing of the dermis to the columns superiorly

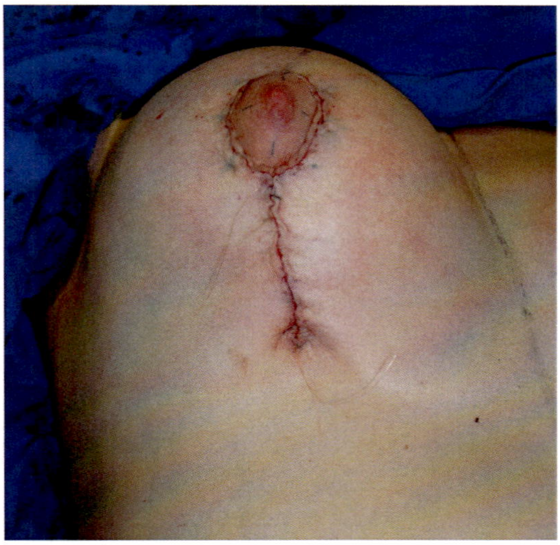

Fig. 30.13 Final suture

30.3 Discussion

Recently, working with the philosophy of the periareolar technique associated with the vertical scar technique, it has been possible to reduce the scar length, thus avoiding its elongation across the inframammary crease by compensating for skin excess around the areola. It was observed that in every single technique performed, after descent, the breast shape lost upper pole fullness. The inferior portion of the breast tissue can be used to fill in the upper pole or the areola to achieve a better shape. A mastopexy or reduction without an augmentation often lacks projection and desired volume and tends not to hold its shape over time (Cerqueira 1998; Chen et al. 2004).

In contrast to a breast reduction, it is a mistake to place the nipple too low because in this technique the bottoming-out effect is minimized. The shape of the skin to be excised is typically not perfectly round and concentric, but may be more oval and excentric to lift the nipple and not overly narrow the width of the breast, added by a vertical incision to elevate the lower pole. With this technique, we can achieve better breast projection and, the same time, reduce the breast base width (Fig. 30.14).

By employing the chest wall-based flap holding the muscle loop when performing, a predictable and safe result can be achieved, with a minimized risk. When suitable patient selection is made, long-term results can be achieved (Figs. 30.15, 30.16, and 30.17).

It is important to perform skin and areola tattooing at cardinal points before making the incision. In this way, proper parameters are maintained and suitable areolar spread is achieved at the end of the surgery. Round block suture with non-absorbable stitches (colorless nylon because Gore-Tex© is not available in Brazil) is applied, such as with Dennis Hammond's technique. Eight cardinal points guide the areolar spread and the suture takes greater amounts of tissue at the external border just in marked points and smaller amounts of tissue between the marked points on the areola. This suture helps to maintain long-lasting results and to prevent areolar enlargement. The round block suture starts and ends at the lateral lower part of the areola, always leaving the notch in the same spot. When the patient complains that she can feel the suture, after 1 year it is removed at the office under local anesthesia.

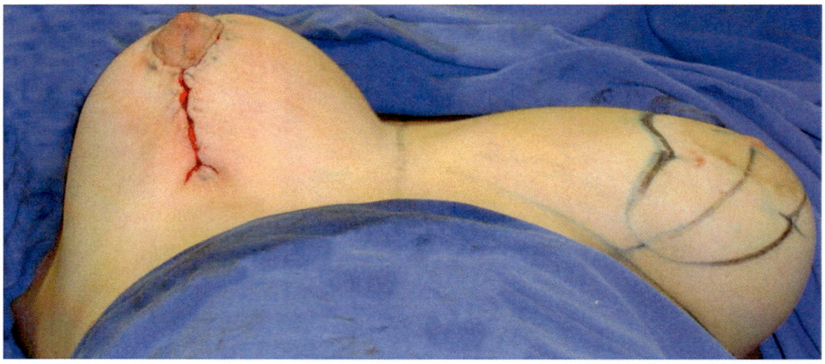

Fig. 30.14 Note the difference between the two breasts with regard to breast projection and base width

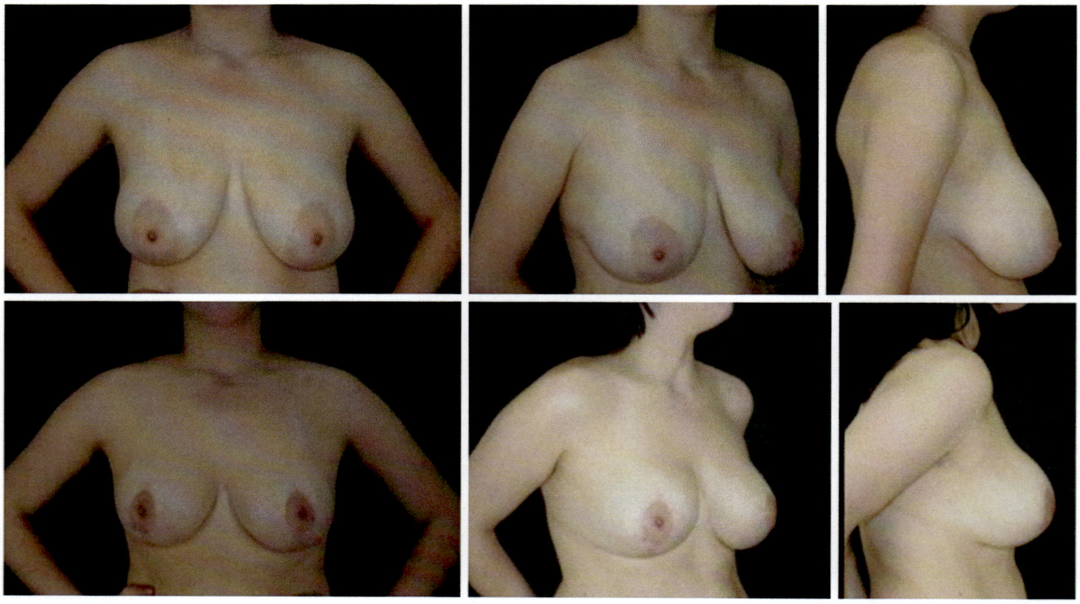

Fig. 30.15 One year postoperatively with a vertical technique and chest wall-based flap sustained by a pectoralis major loop

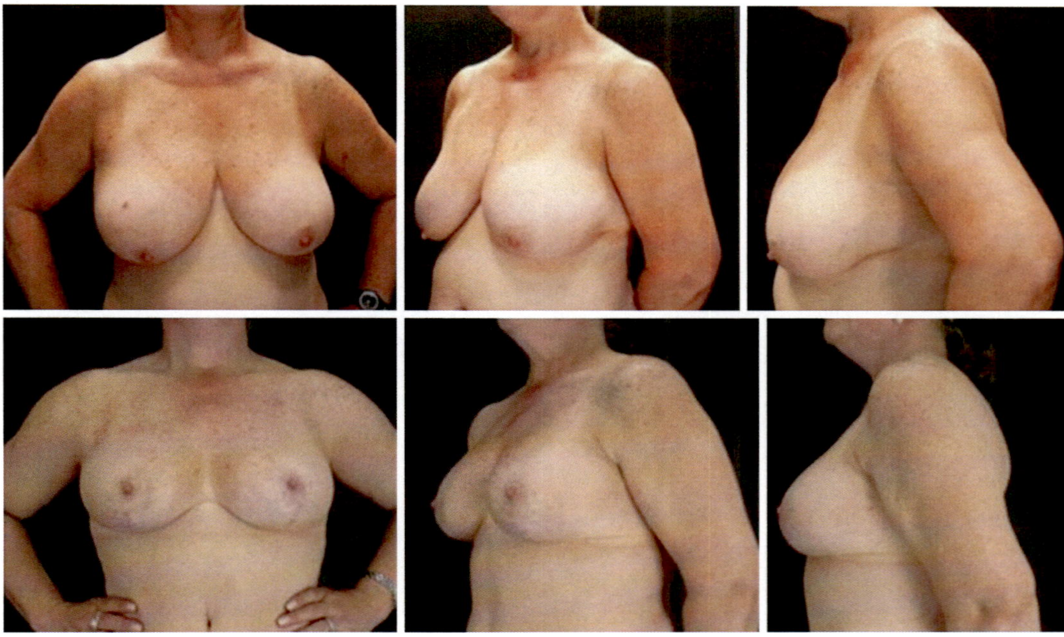

Fig. 30.16 Two years postoperatively using the same technique

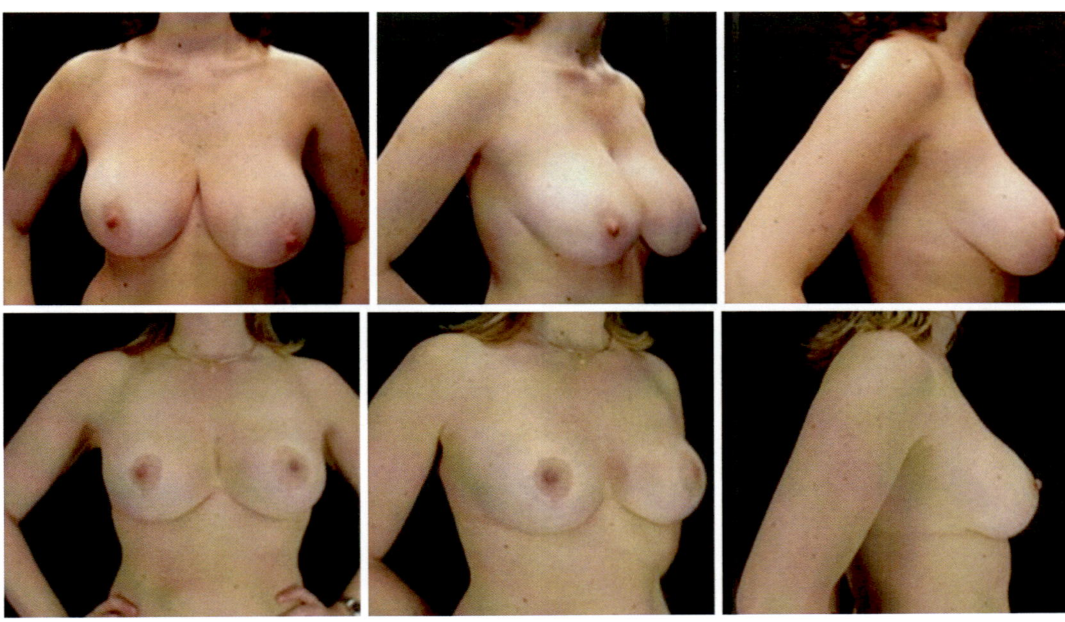

Fig. 30.17 Three years postoperatively using the same technique

30.4 Complications

The most common complication related to the chest wall-based flap is fat necrosis in the distal portion of the flap, which can be dealt with by surgical revision to remove this tissue. Superficial wound dehiscence and inferior skin and fat excess are minor complications and are avoided by using a suitable technique.

Seroma or hematoma is avoided with careful hemostasis during surgery. Other complications seen are wound-healing problems in the vertical scar owing to the wrinkles related to the shrinking of the scar.

Conclusions

The vertical mammaplasty method has a low rate of complications. Wound healing seems to be the main problem after mammaplasty, but major deformity is rarely encountered. Complications that necessitate a second operation are very rare. Patient satisfaction after vertical mammaplasty is usually very high. There is often a great benefit for the patient, both physically and psychologically.

References

Arie G (1957) Una nueva tecnica de mastoplastia. Rev Latinoam Cir Plast 3:23

Cerqueira AA (1998) Mammoplasty: breast fixation with dermoglandular mono upper pedicle under the pectoralis muscle. Aesthet Plast Surg 22:276–283

Chen CM, White C, Warren SM, Cole J, Isik FF (2004) Simplifying the vertical reduction mammaplasty. Plast Reconstr Surg 113(1):162–172

Daniel MJB (1995) Mammaplasty with pectoral muscle flap. Presented at 64th American annual scientific meeting, Montreal

Dartigues L (1925) Traitement chirurgical du prolapsus mammaire. Arch Franco-Belg Chir 28:13

Graf R, Reis de Araujo LR, Rippel R, Neto LG, Pace DT, Biggs T (2003) Reduction mammaplasty and mastopexy using the vertical scar and thoracic wall flap technique. Aesthet Plast Surg 27(1):6–12

Graf R, Tolazzi A, Balbinot P et al (2016) Influence of the pectoralis major muscle sling in chest wall-based flap suspension after vertical mammaplasty: ten-year follow-up. Aesthet Surg J 36(10):1113–1121

Hall-Findlay EJ, Shestak KC (2015) Breast reduction. Plast Reconstr Surg 136(4):531

Lassus C (1970) A technique for breast reduction. Int Surg 53:69

Lejour M (1994) Vertical mammaplasty and liposuction of the breast. Plast Reconstr Surg 94:100

Check for updates

31 Martire's Technique for "L" Mastoplasty

Lybio Martire Jr.

31.1 Introduction

During the 1970s and the beginning of the 1980s, there was a greater concern with regard to scar reduction in mastoplasty. Various new techniques resulted in L-shaped scars; some of them were derived from techniques that had already been used before, with inverted T-shaped scars, whereas others were based on new principles.

We had the opportunity to observe and accomplish some of these techniques but we developped our own technique with new principles.

Meanwhile, problems such as enlargement, length of lateral scars, and centralization of the cone were found. There were some critics of the complexity of this system during accomplishment or in relation to the oblique scars that were not L-shaped and scheduled surgeries that were supposed to result in L-shaped scar but actually resulted in an inverted T. In the congress, the question of X-shaped scars was discussed with the intention of reducing scars without damaging the shape.

All of this made us concerned about and look for a solution to this problem, and think about how to elaborate a new way of gaining favorable results that is easy to use, easy to understand without any doubts, that can also be used in any case of breast hypertrophy and all kinds of ptosis as universal procedures.

In 1985, we started to use the procedures and techniques described above and we presented for the first time in 1988 during "*Jornada Carioca de Cirurgia Estética*," when we talked about "*Cuidados e Táticas em mastoplastia em "L"*", presenting with the main objective to show the studies we had done and the tactics that we were using to avoid the problems mentioned previously.

We started presenting our new technique at scientific meetings, emphasizing the characteristic of being a "simple and objective technique" and a universal procedure that can be used in any treatment of all cases of hypertrophy and breast ptosis.

What made us elaborate on the technique was the conclusion that the most important philosophy in L-shaped mastoplasty is to obtain in a well-defined way what we call point L, which is the extremity of the lateral flap (see Fig. 31.6). The suitable definition of this point, which supports the principle of our technique, makes the lateral piece have an exact size to avoid strain on the scar and to position the cone correctly, and the possibility of obtaining an L-shaped scar in 90°, which is important to avoid enlargement.

L. Martire Jr, M.D.
University Department of Plastic Surgery, Surgical Technique and History of Medicine, Titular of Brazilian Society of Plastic Surgery, Titular of Federation Ibero Latinoamericana de Cirurgia Plástica y Reconstructiva, Titular of Brazilian College of Surgeons, Fellow of International College of Surgeons, Titular Founder of Brazilian Society of History of Medicine,
Endereço: R. Caravelas, 546, Vila Mariana, São Paulo, SP, Brazil
e-mail: LybioJunior@gmail.com

J.M. Avelar (ed.), *Breast Surgery*, https://doi.org/10.1007/978-3-319-54115-0_31

For the last 28 years, we have treated all degrees of mammary hypertrophy and ptosis with this procedure, obtaining 90° L-shaped scars with lateral extension and a pleasing shape.

31.2 Method

With the patient in a semi-sitting position draw a midline medially and after that two midclavicular lines passing the nipple and crossing the submammary sulcus with a distance depending on the size of the patient's thorax, which can vary from 10 to 12 cm. The fact that determines the distance is the midclavicular line being parallel to the midline medially (Fig. 31.1).

Delimit the classic point "A" from Pitanguy's (1978) technique, which is the projection of the submammary sulcus above the areola (Fig. 31.2b). In slightly accentuated ptosis, this point remains a little above the nipple–areola complex (NAC). This shape, called point A can be 1, 2, 3, 4 or more centimeters above the areola, depending on the degree of breast ptosis. The next step, in a horizontal line that crosses the nipple, is carried out by bidigital clamping of the breast to determine points B and C (Fig. 31.2c). The distance between them depends on the size of the breast or the degree of flaccidity; it could be 6, 7, 8, 10, 12 cm or more.

The distance between point B and the nipple is projected over the submammary sulcus. The intersection point of the submammary sulcus with the midclavicular line is called point E (Fig. 31.2a). The fourth part of this measure should be projected in the medium direction beyond the midclavicular line (Fig. 31.2a). The medium extremity of this line is called point F and the lateral extremity point D (Fig. 31.2a).

Once it is done, raise the breast with one of the hands and draw a diagonal line from the nipple to point D and another that crosses the first and runs from point B to point E. The intersection of these two diagonal lines determines the key point of the surgery, which is denominated point L (Fig. 31.2b). From this point, we put together points A, B, and C with arched lines. Point "B" through the line that is also arched is joined to point L, this one to point D, and point F to point C (Fig. 31.2c).

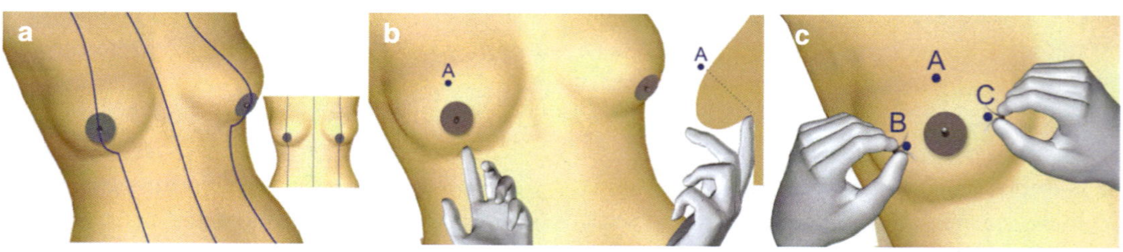

Fig. 31.1 Medial and midclavicular lines must be parallel and what determines the distance between them is the parallelism, which may vary, on average, between 9 and 12 cm, depending on the width of the thorax and delimitation of points A, B, and C from Pitanguy's technique

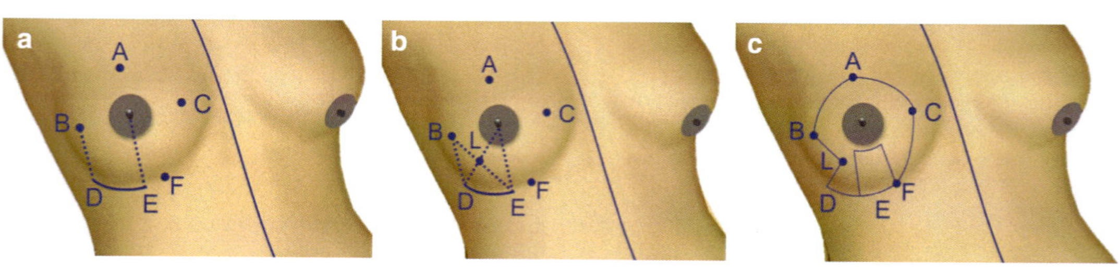

Fig. 31.2 (**a**) Delimitation of points D, E, and F. (**b**) Delimitation of point L, the key point of surgery. (**c**) Union of points A, B, C, and L, showing the end view of the marking and the introduction of the inferior pedicle flap

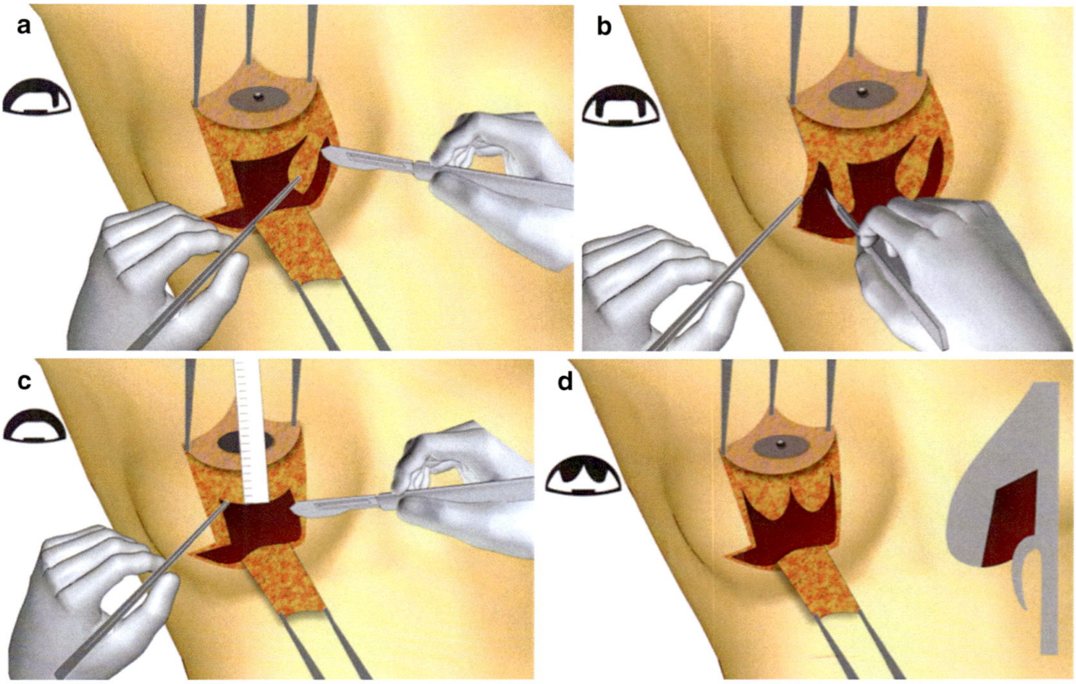

Fig. 31.3 Preparation of (**a**) the medial flap and (**b**) the lateral flap. (**c**, **d**) The tissue resection, if necessary, is carried out by removing the base of the breast

In our technique, we always use an inferior pedicle flap similar to that described by Ribeiro (Ribeiro and Backer 1973); it is point F on its medial border and point L the side limit, determining the width of the flap (Fig. 31.2c).

Schwarzmann's maneuver is performed, and extended to the flap with an inferior pedicle. This is made a thicker at its base and thinner at the extremity, leaving the skin totally free, being joined just at the breast muscle, where the irrigation comes from.

The lipectomy should encourage the emptying of the whole medial and lateral poles of the breast. The flaps of lateral and medial skin are about 1.5–2.0 cm thick along their entire length (Fig. 31.3a, b). If breast reduction is needed, we perform a lipectomy according to Peixoto's technique (Martire 1990): a resection of the entire base of the breast (Fig. 31.3c, d).

After resecting, the breast is divided into two pieces, creating two flaps, one lateral and the other medial, which will be crossed, always with the medial over the lateral (Fig. 31.4c, d).

Before crossing to build the breast, it is necessary to fix the inferior pedicle flap starting from the base to the extremity to avoid apex promotion of a submammary sulcus elevation. It means to avoid elevation or retraction of the submammary sulcus (Fig. 31.4b).

During the external mounting, point L is joined to point F" (Fig. 31.5a). Point B is sutured 1 cm below point C (Fig. 31.5b). From this step, a conventional suture can be made, with a tobacco pouch at the top of the cone to make it easier to position the new areole (Fig. 31.5). If it is necessary to take away excess tissue (in the case of extreme flaccidity), the resection process never should be performed in the lateral flap, only in the medial flap (Fig. 31.6). The areola is placed at the extreme part of the cone in this technique. There is no reason to be concerned about the distance between the areola and the submammary sulcus because the accommodation happens equally not raising the areole later (Fig. 31.6).

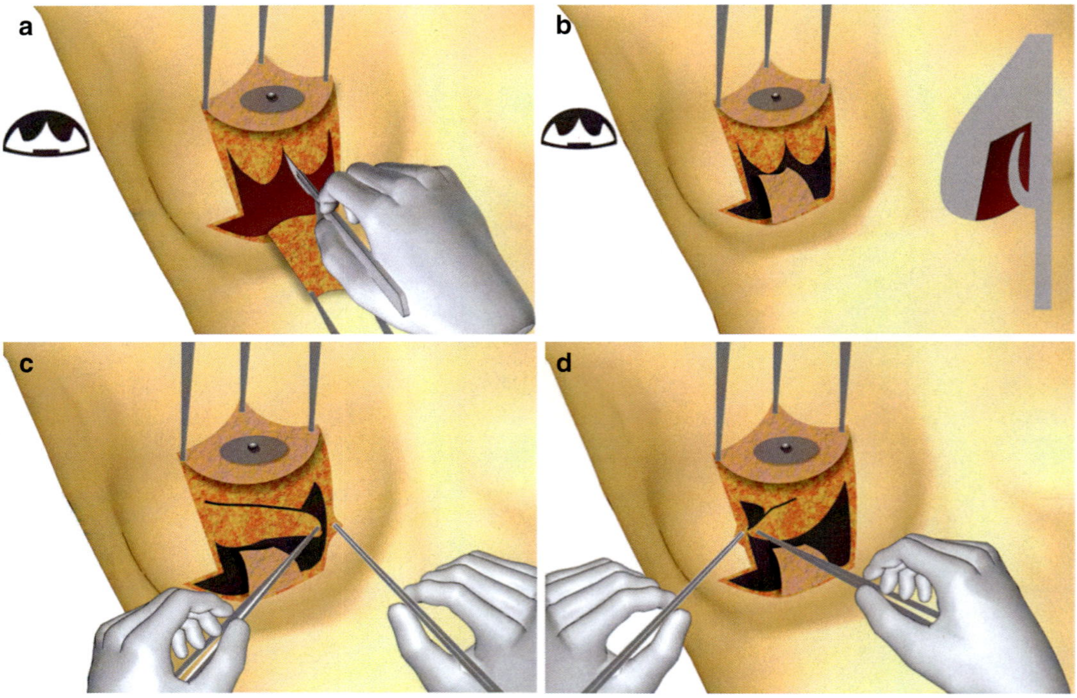

Fig. 31.4 (**a**) Splitting the breast tissue, (**b**) fixing the inferior pedicle flap, and crossing of the lateral and medial flaps, firstly been made by (**c**) fixing the lateral flap and over it, (**d**) setting the medial flap

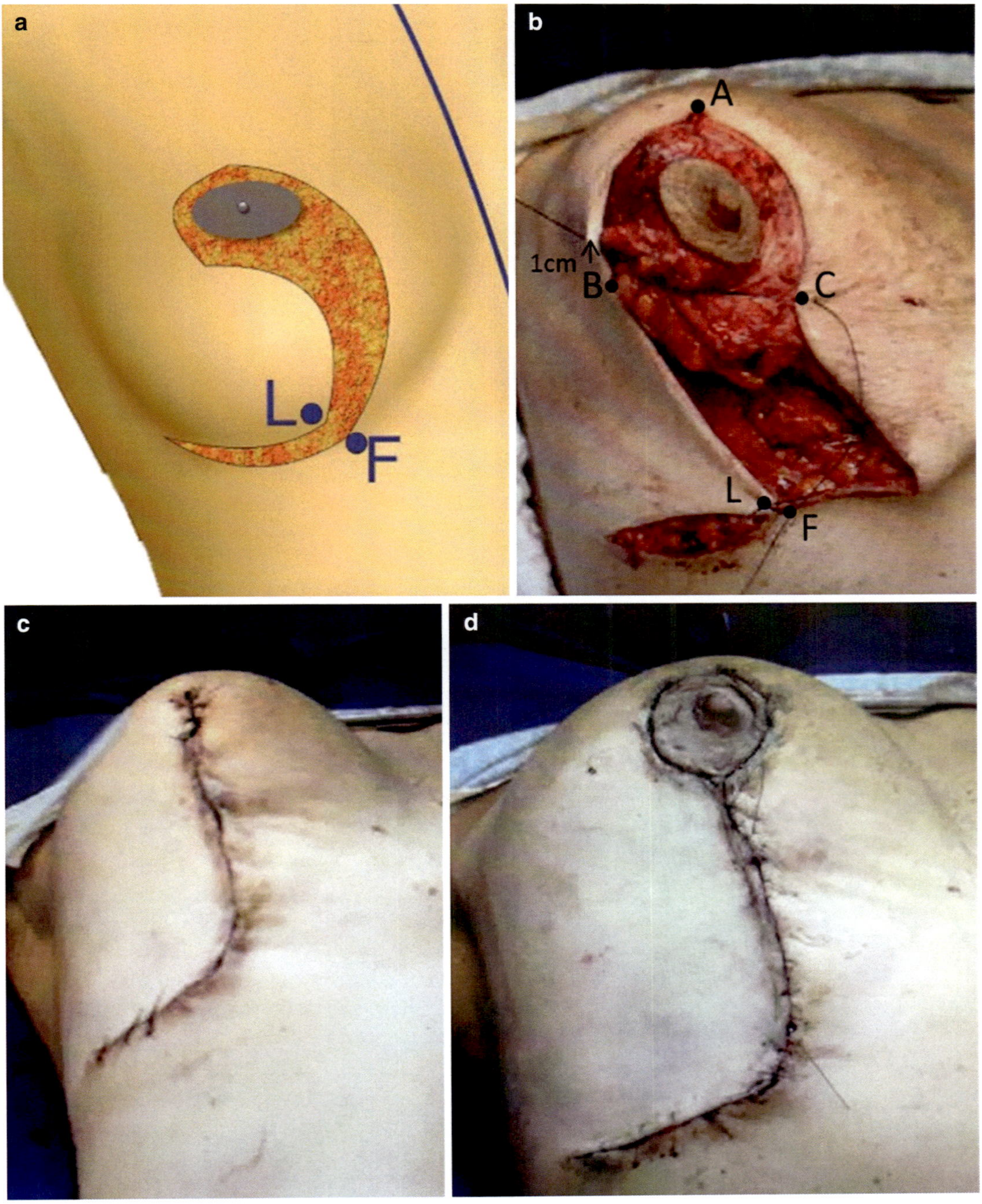

Fig. 31.5 Resection of the skin, if necessary, is carried out exclusively on the medial flap, never on the lateral flap. We can also observe how the areola is automatically positioned at the apex of the breast cone

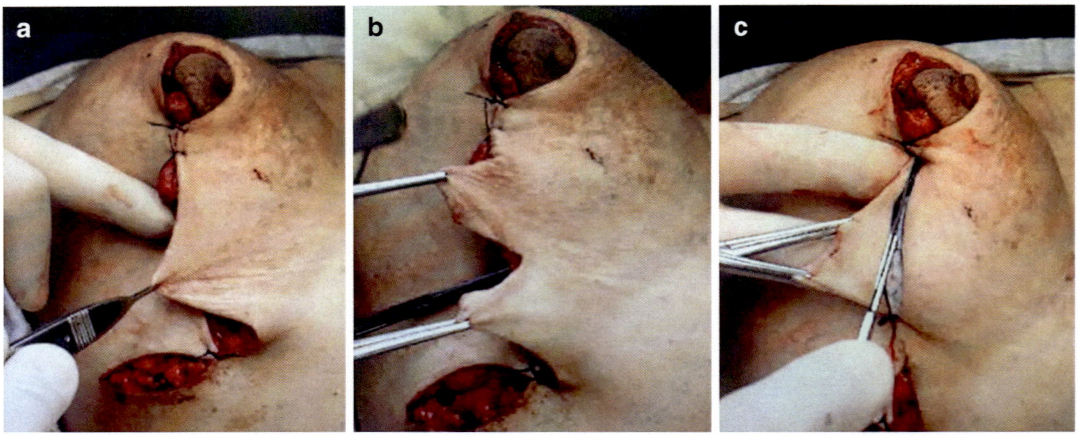

Fig. 31.6 Breast assembly phases showing the union of (**a**) points L and F, and (**b**) of points B and C (1 cm above point B). (**c**, **d**) It can be seen that the nipple–areola complex is not affected by drift and its distance to the mammary fold need not be measured. It is important that the areola be positioned at the apex of the breast cone

31.3 Discussion

The most important aspect of this technique is that it can be carried out in breasts of all sizes and with all degrees of ptosis or flaccidity, but also at any age, making it a universal procedure.

The small resulting scar is also a relevant factor and it appeals greatly to the patients.

Since we created this technique, all our mastoplasties have been carried out in this manner, with satisfactory results in our evaluation and with a 100% satisfaction rate in our patients.

It is also a straightforward procedure with 0 marking that is easy to understand and carry out, as we observe the precautions described in the method.

The long-term evaluation shows that the result remains satisfactory for many years with a pleasing shape and proper positioning of the breasts.

31.4 Complications

The incidence of complications is very low because the NAC does not suffer traction, positioning itself naturally, and the lateral and medial flaps of the breast are broad-based and therefore very well irrigated.

Thus, in all the time we have been performing this technique, that is, for 28 years, we have observed very few complications, which were restricted to partial suture dehiscence in the vertical scar (in two cases), partial necrosis of the lateral flap (in three cases), liponecrosis or liposclerosis with hardened nodule formation (in ten cases).

Conclusion

The procedure described here has been carried out by the author for 28 years and, according to the evidence observed in the results during this time, we conclude that it is excellent, considering that it is suitable for all shapes of breasts and that it is convenient, produces favorable results, has a low complication rate, and has durable results (Figs. 31.7, 31.8, 31.9, 31.10, 31.11, 31.12, 31.13, 31.14, 31.15, and 31.16).

Special Thanks Illustrations created by Prof. Dr. José Marcos dos Reis.

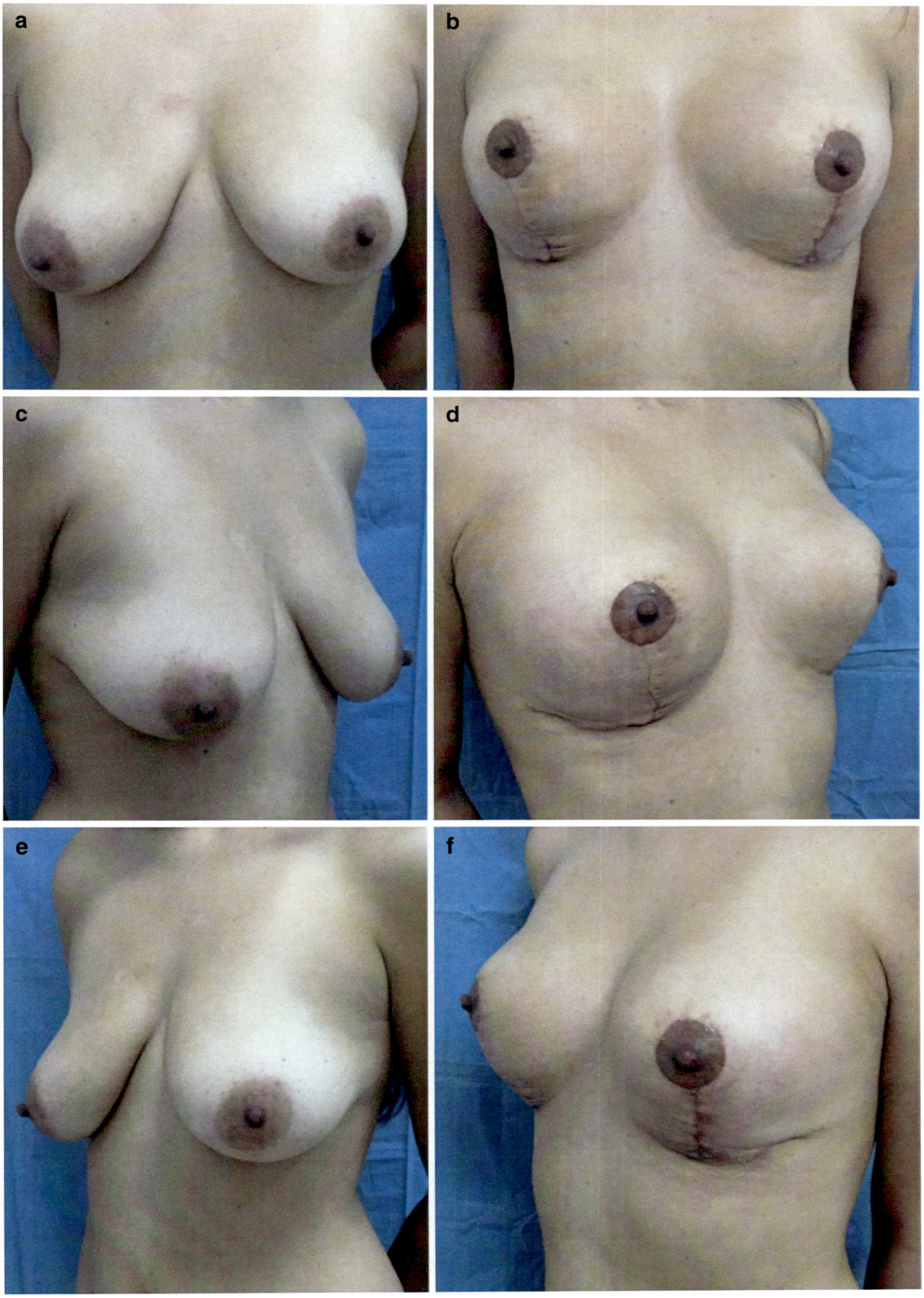

Fig. 31.7 A 30-year-old, pre- and 1 month postoperatively. (**a**, **b**) Frontal, (**c**, **d**) right side, (**e**, **f**) left side

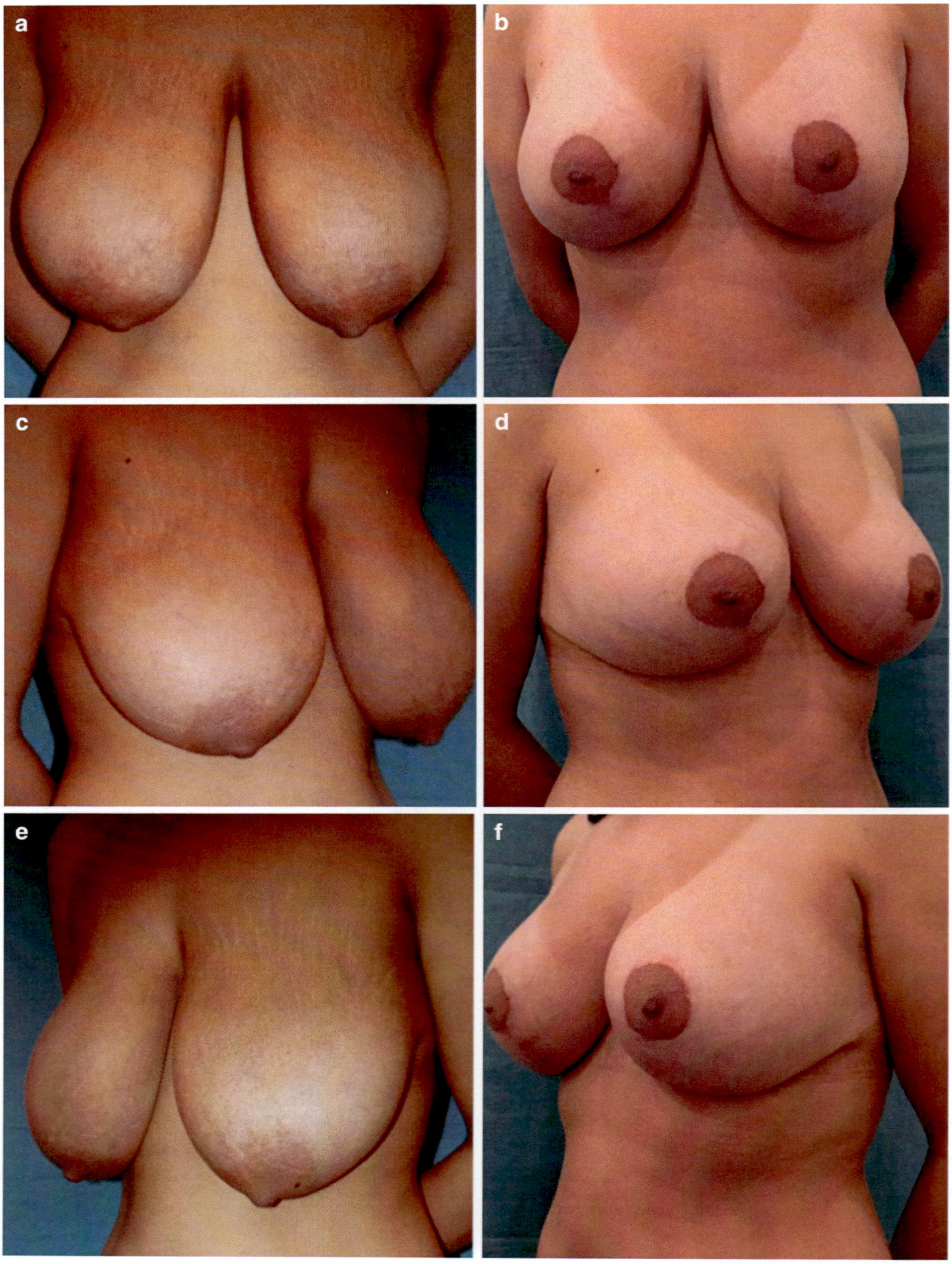

Fig. 31.8 A 29-year-old, pre- and 1 year postoperatively. (**a**, **b**) Frontal, (**c**, **d**) right side, (**e**, **f**) left side

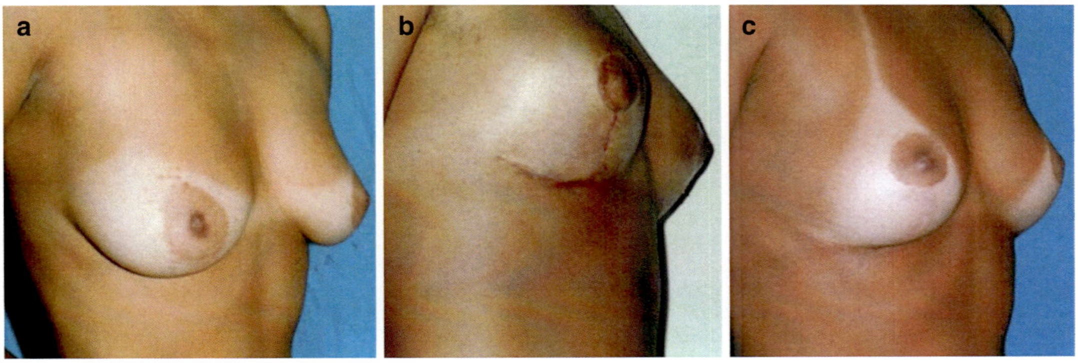

Fig. 31.9 A 28-year-old. (**a**) Pre-, (**b**) 1 month postoperatively, and (**c**) 1 year postoperatively

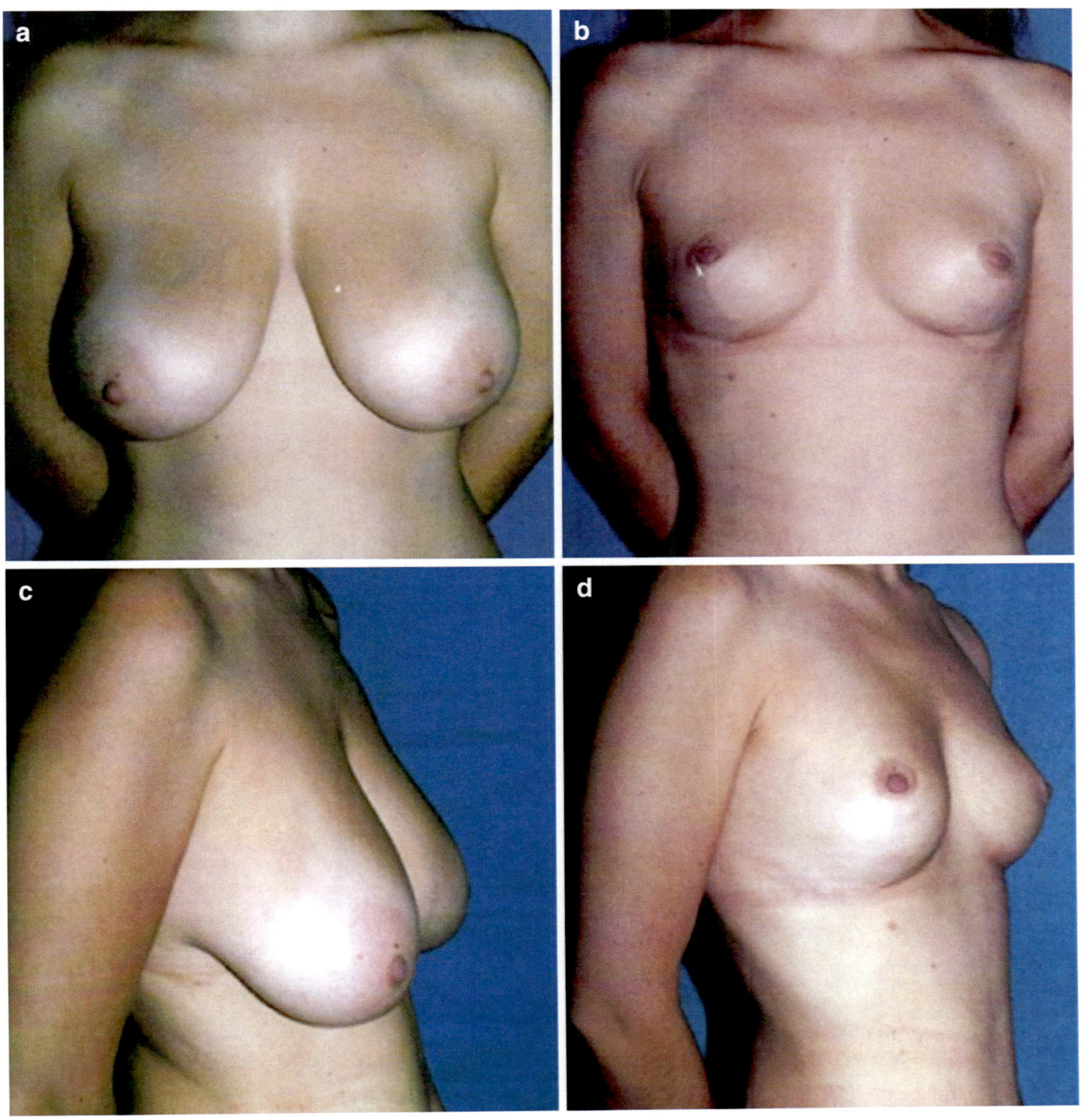

Fig. 31.10 A 31-ear-old, pre- and 2 years postoperatively. (**a**, **b**) Frontal, (**c**, **d**) right side

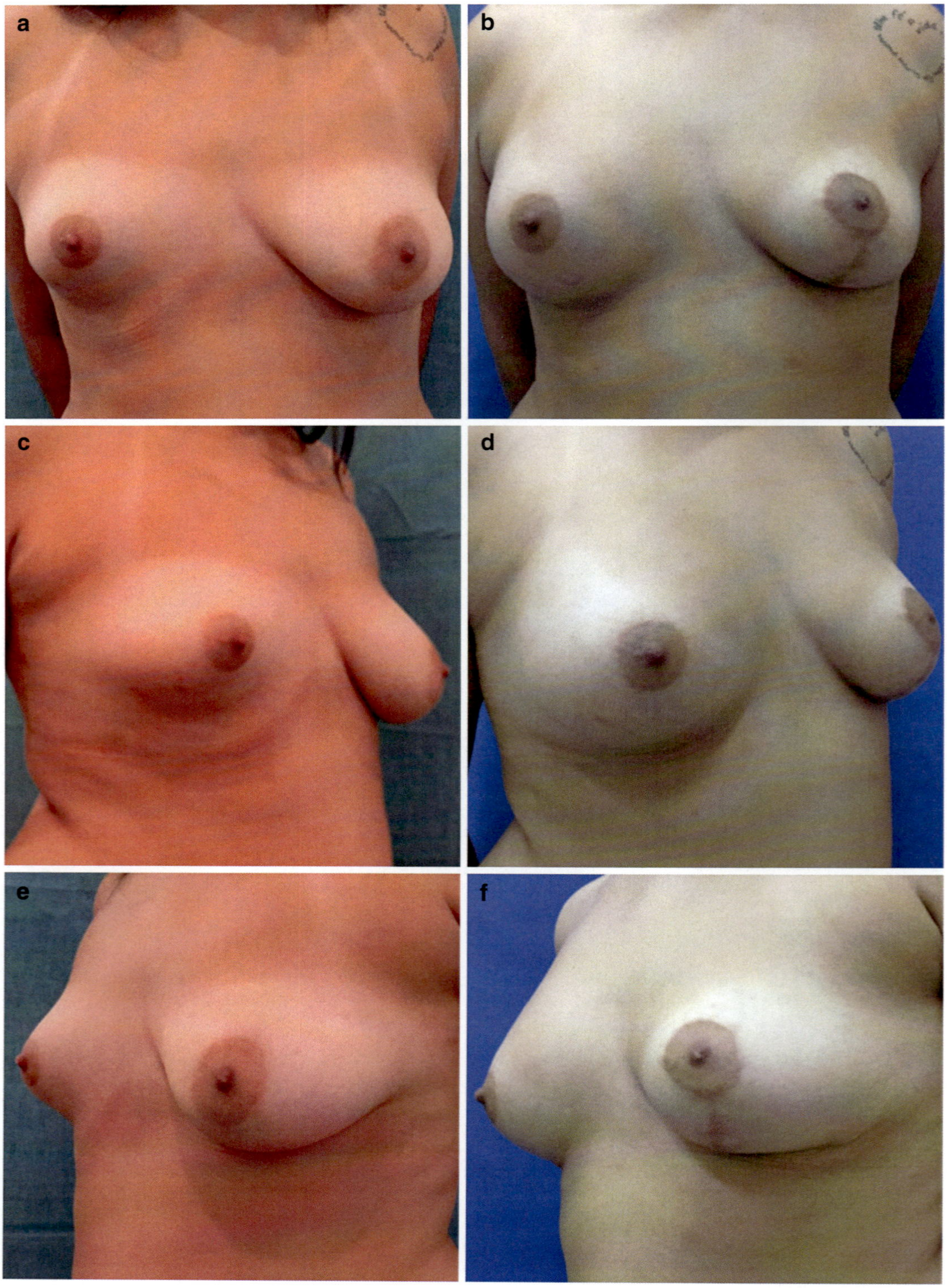

Fig. 31.11 A 24-year-old, pre- and 6 months postoperatively. The left breast was operated on using this technique; in the right breast, a silicone prosthesis of 350 cc was implanted. In this case, there was an even greater advantage, of course, in using a technique with less scarring and without the medial branch

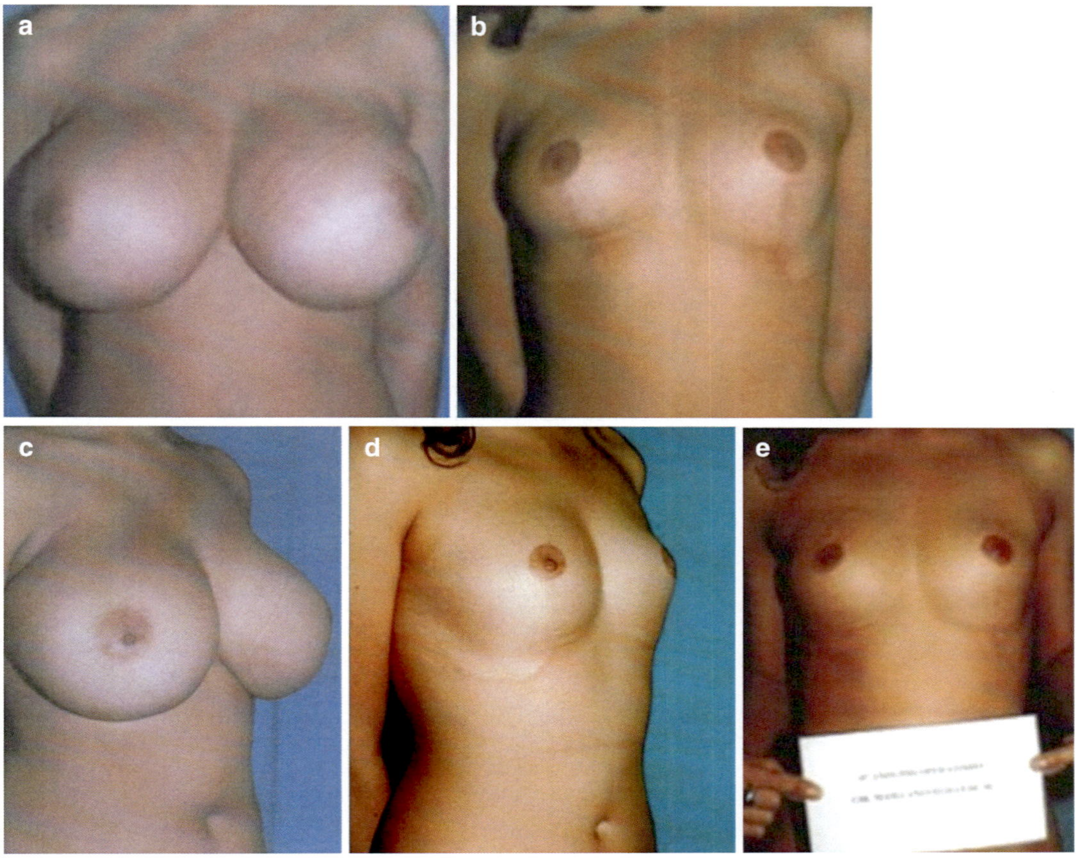

Fig. 31.12 A 19-year-old, with severe breast hypertrophy, (**a**, **b**, **c**, **d**) pre- and 1 year postoperatively and (**e**) 7 years postoperatively. In this case, the scar, in its entire extent, benefited the patient, who had symmastia (joined breasts)

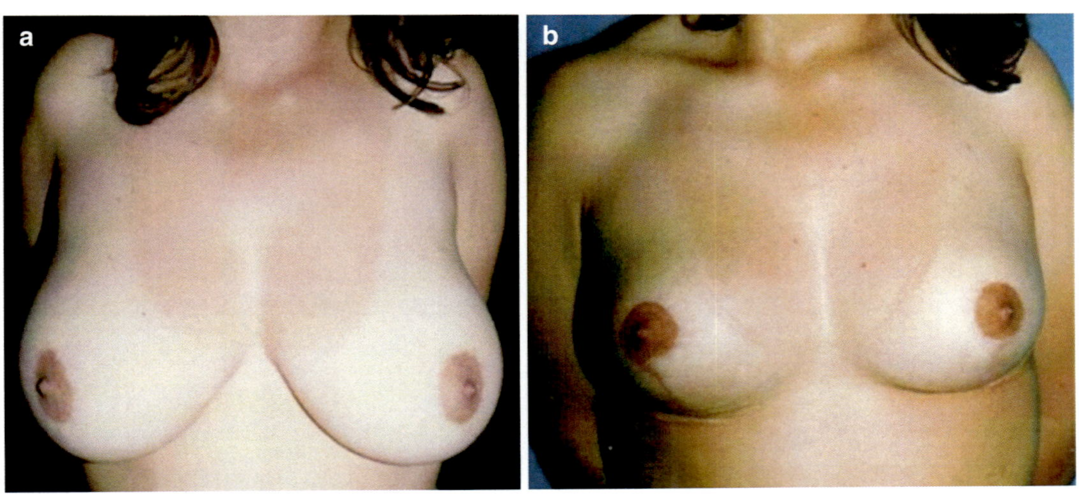

Fig. 31.13 A 17-year-old, (**a**) pre- and 4 months (**b**) postoperatively

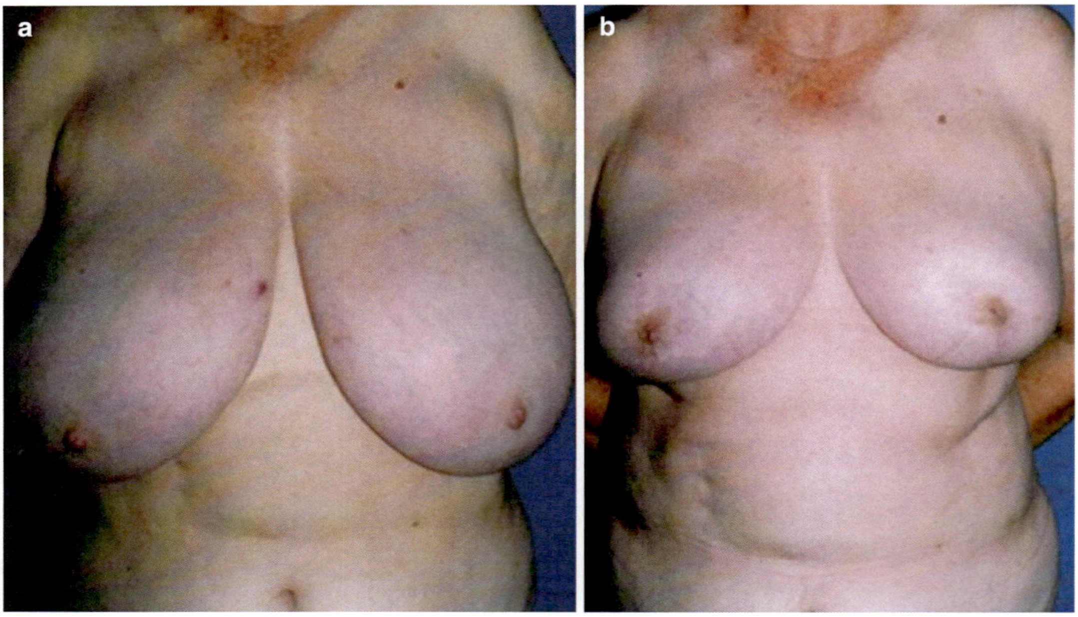

Fig. 31.14 A 70-ear-old, (**a**) preoperatively and (**b**) 2 years postoperatively

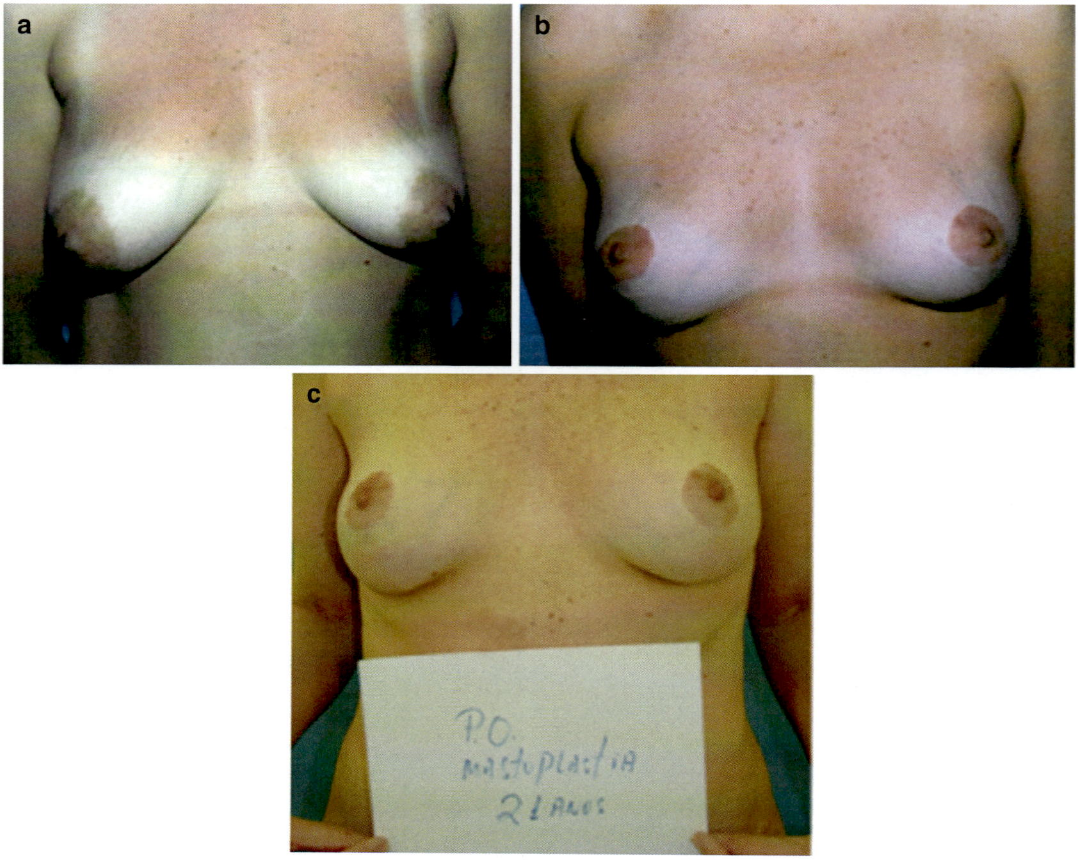

Fig. 31.15 A 26-year-old, (**a**) pre-operatively, (**b**) 1 year postoperatively, and (**c**) 21 years postoperatively

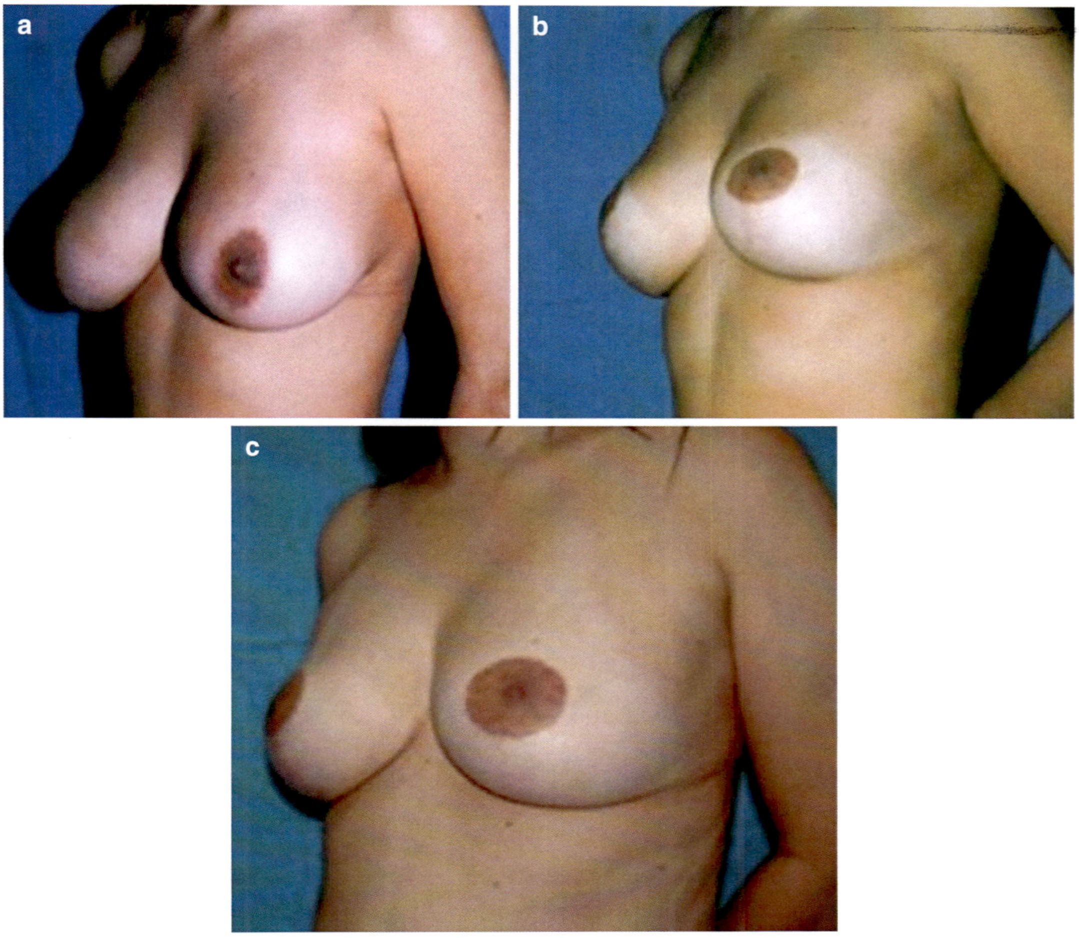

Fig. 31.16 A 24-year-old, (**a**) pre- and (**b**) 1 year postoperatively and (**c**) 22 years postoperatively

References

Lalardrie J (1974) Chirurgie Plastique Du Sein. Massonet Cie, Éditeurs, Paris

Marino H (1978) Plasticas Mamarias. Lopez LibrerosEditores, 2ª Ed. Buenos Aires

Martire L Jr (1988) Cuidados e Táticas em Mastoplastia em "L". 8ª Jornada Carioca de Cirurgia Estética, Rio de Janeiro

Martire L Jr (1990) Mastoplastia em "L" – Nossa Sistematização Simples e Objetiva. Annals of XXVII Congresso Brasileiro de Cirurgia Plástica

Martire L Jr (1994) Mastoplastia em "L" – Nossa Sistematização Simples e Objetiva. Annals of XXXI Congresso Brasileiro de Cirurgia Plástica

Martire L Jr (1997) Mastoplasty in "L" – personal technique. Annals of international congress on aesthetic plastic surgery

Peixoto G (1980) Reduction mammoplasty: a personal technique. Plast Reconstr Surg 65:217–226

Pitanguy I (1978) Mamaplastia. Guanabara Koogan, Rio de Janeiro

Ribeiro L, Backer C (1973) Mastoplastiascon pedículo de seguridad. Rev Esp Cir Plast 6:223–234

32 Breast Reduction with L Scar After 30 Years: Indications and Limitations

Antonio Roberto Bozola

32.1 Introduction

In this chapter, the author describes the limitations of and indications for the L mammoplasty technique after his 30-year experience of performing it. In 1990 (Bozola 1990a), he described the L mammoplasty technique, which leaves out the medial segment of the horizontal scar, and classified mammary hypertrophy in accordance with shape and volume. He proposed a new anatomical analysis of the breast based on three breast projections (Bozola 1990b; Bozola et al. 2011), He determined the resection marks of the excess skin according to the size of the ptosis and related how to provide a beautiful breast with suitable shape and volume in each case.

32.1.1 Anatomy of the Beautiful Shaped Breast and Classifications of Mammary Hypertrophy

If we consider the shape of the breast as being similar to an irregular cone that can be observed from three-dimensional points of view (frontal, lateral, and vertical), it is possible to determine:

(a) Frontal view – based on the breast implantation on the normal thorax comprising two horizontal lines: the lowest horizontal breast line (LHBL) that connects the inframammary sulcus where they meet the breast meridian line (point I), and the highest horizontal breast line (HHBL), which connects the highest point of the two anterior axillary folds. This results in an oval geometric figure that presents a smaller horizontal diameter than the vertical diameter in a ratio of 1:1.3 (Fig. 32.1). Figure 32.1 also shows its vertical axis ABCD (breast meridian) containing the golden ratio (Bozola et al. 2011), which means that the AD segment is to BD as the BD segment is to CD. If the ratio of the breast axis is 1:1.5 or it approximates 1:1.618, the result is a beautiful breast.

(b) Lateral view – inclining a golden triangle (which contains the phi ratio) over 18° (angle of Louis) in relation to the vertical axis of the body, this will also result in a beautiful breast (Fig. 32.2). From the profile, a normal and beautiful breast, with no ptosis, is located above the horizontal plane A (LHBL), which passes the inframammary sulcus and coincides with point I (the intersection of the breast meridian line with the inframammary sulcus). Another horizontal plane, M, crosses the apex of the mammary cone and divides the breast into two segments: superior and inferior. Where plane M crosses the breast meridian, point M is determined. In general, the nipple is found there (sometimes the nipple–areola complex (NAC) may be ectopic – outside of the apex of the cone). The ideal

A.R. Bozola, M.D.
Regent Cirurgia Plástica da Fac. de Medicina de São José do Rio Preto, São José do Rio Preto, SP, Brazil
e-mail: drbozola@gmail.com

J.M. Avelar (ed.), *Breast Surgery*, https://doi.org/10.1007/978-3-319-54115-0_32

measurement of the breast from the apex of the cone to point I (LHBL) is between 7 and 12 cm. The section of the breast above the apex of the cone to the HHBL measures 1.618 times the size of the inferior section.

(c) Vertical view – From the vertical point of view of the individual (when the patient looks at her breasts). A normal and beautiful/attractive breast is located between two vertical lines: the vertical lateral breast line (VLBL) and the

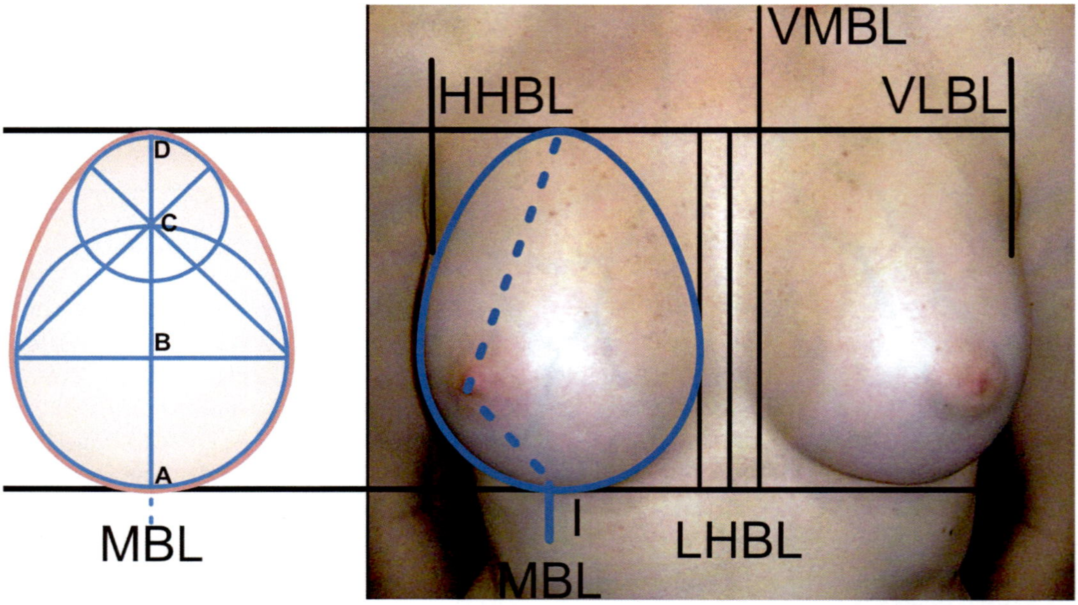

Fig. 32.1 In a frontal view: a perfect breast shape comprising the lowest horizontal breast line (LHBL) and highest horizontal breast line (HHBL) and the mammary meridian

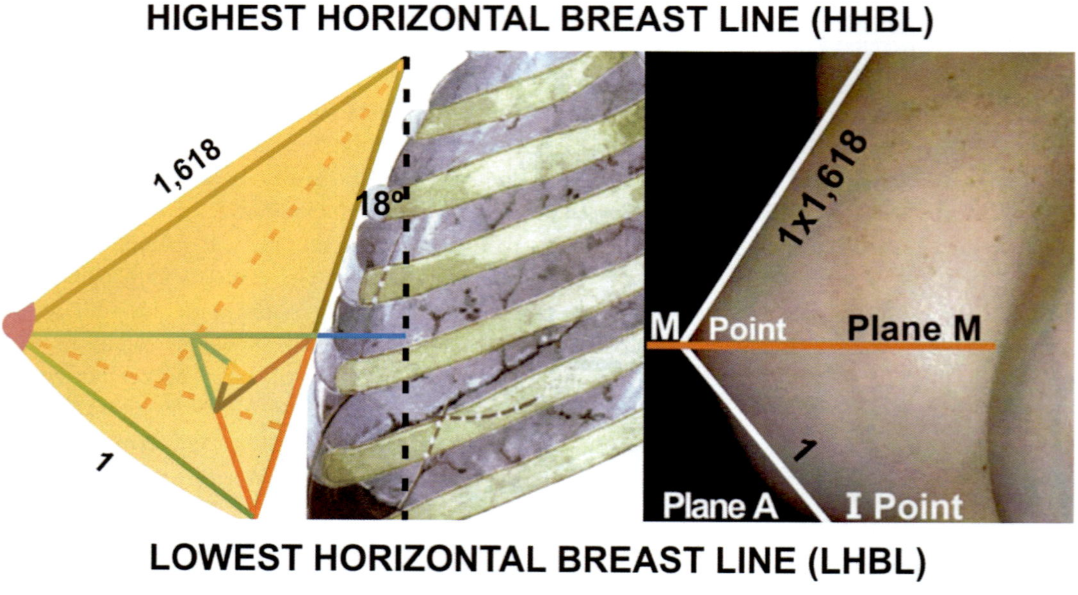

Fig. 32.2 In a lateral view: a perfect breast shape that is located above the LHBL line and that is similar to a golden triangle presenting an inclination of 18°

vertical medial breast line (VMBL) (Fig. 32.3). The former coincides with the anterior axillary line and the latter is situated 1–2 cm lateral to the middle line of the sternum bone. Applying a geometric analysis of the breast, it is possible to join the five golden triangles by their closest sides and by their apexes, forming a golden pentagon. If this pyramid pentagon is turned on its vertical axis, a golden cone is obtained. This presents a ratio of 1:1.618 between its height and base. If we curve its lines from the base and the apex, we obtain a figure that resembles a beautiful breast. The NAC must be on the apex of the cone.

In the author's opinion, the phi proportion can help plastic surgeons to provide beautiful breast shapes for their patients. The shape of the breast contains and molds its volume. Volume can be

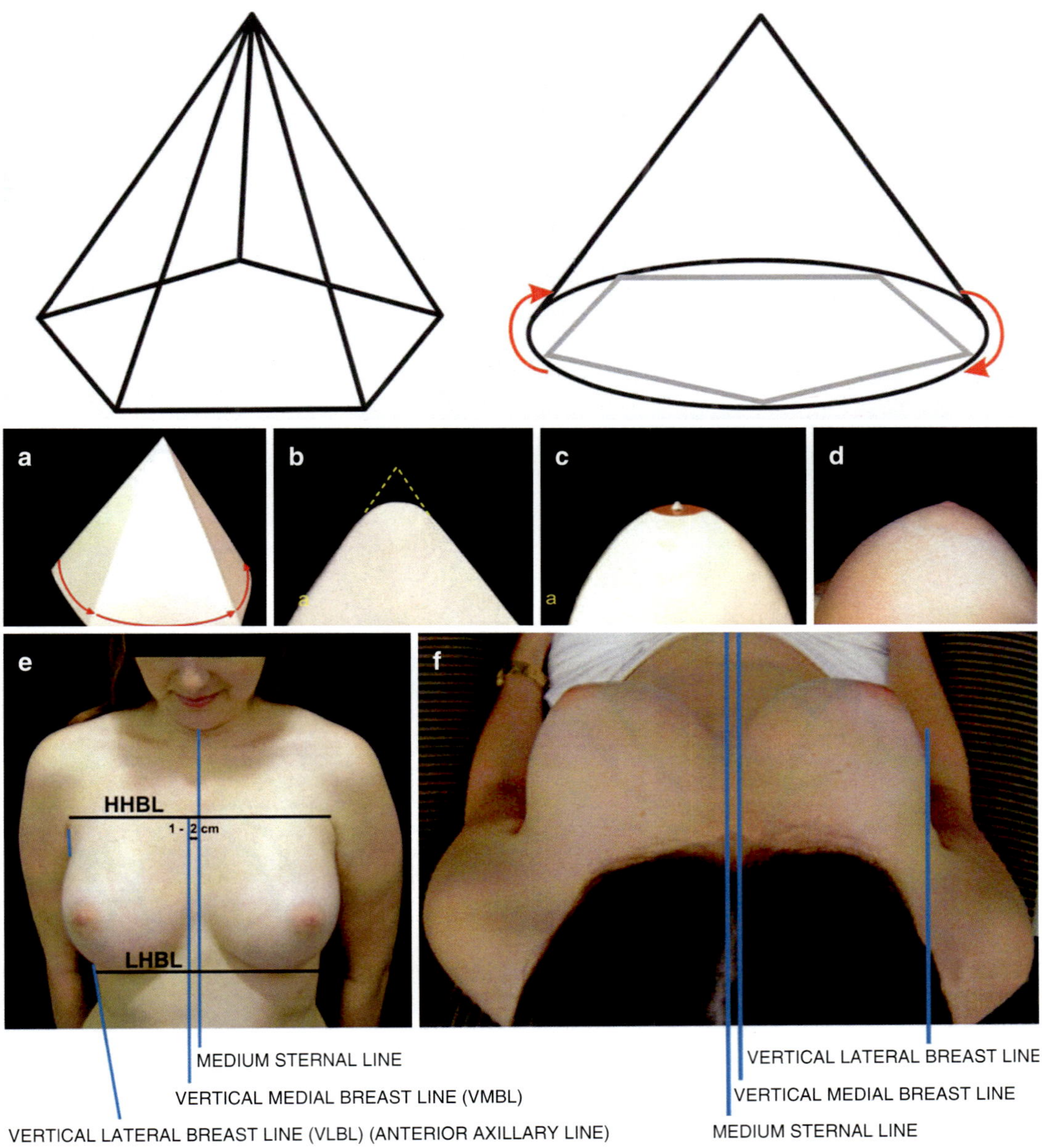

Fig. 32.3 (**a–d**) In a vertical view: a perfect breast shape constructed by joining the five golden triangles by their closest sides and by their apexes, forming a golden pentagon

changed over time because of different cultures, individual wishes, and fads. But a beautiful breast shape does not change. He also claims that phi must not be fixed as an exact measure, but rather be an indisputable reference.

32.1.2 Diagnosis of Breast Shapes and Volume Alterations

The diagnosis of the breast shapes and volume alterations can be determined in accordance with the metric changes of breast implantation on the thorax and their relationship with breast projection. It is possible to divide mammary hypertrophy into four groups (Fig. 32.4).

Group I (*GI*): the breast presents a normal base and projection. Its volume is adequate, but the shape is modified owing to ptosis. From the frontal view we can observe a reverse of the vertical and horizontal diameters. The superior section of the breast becomes empty and, from the lateral view, plane M can be observed below plane A.

Group II (*GII*): the breast presents a small projection and its base of implantation is wide. If it is beyond the VLBL and MVBL lines, symmastia and/or lateral axillary extension are caused.

Group III (*GIII*): the breast presents a large projection, but its base is minor/small and does not reach the VLBL and MVBL lines.

Group IV (GIV): the breast presents a large base and projection. We can combine GII and GIV, but those proportions can be found in GII, GIII, and GIV.

Ptosis: the breast presents a large volume and the elastic resistance of the skin is poor. In a frontal view, the point and plane M can be observed descending from plane A and point I into/toward the inframammary sulcus. These movements always take place gradually and over time (Fig. 32.5). The vertical diameter is reduced, and the horizontal diameter is widened. The upper pole of the breast becomes empty. The positions of points I are unalterable over time and they become points A when they are projected onto their breast meridians. It is the measurement between points A and M that indicates the skin surplus and how to execute the incisions and their skin extensions. Thus, the scars depend on the ptosis. If we have to

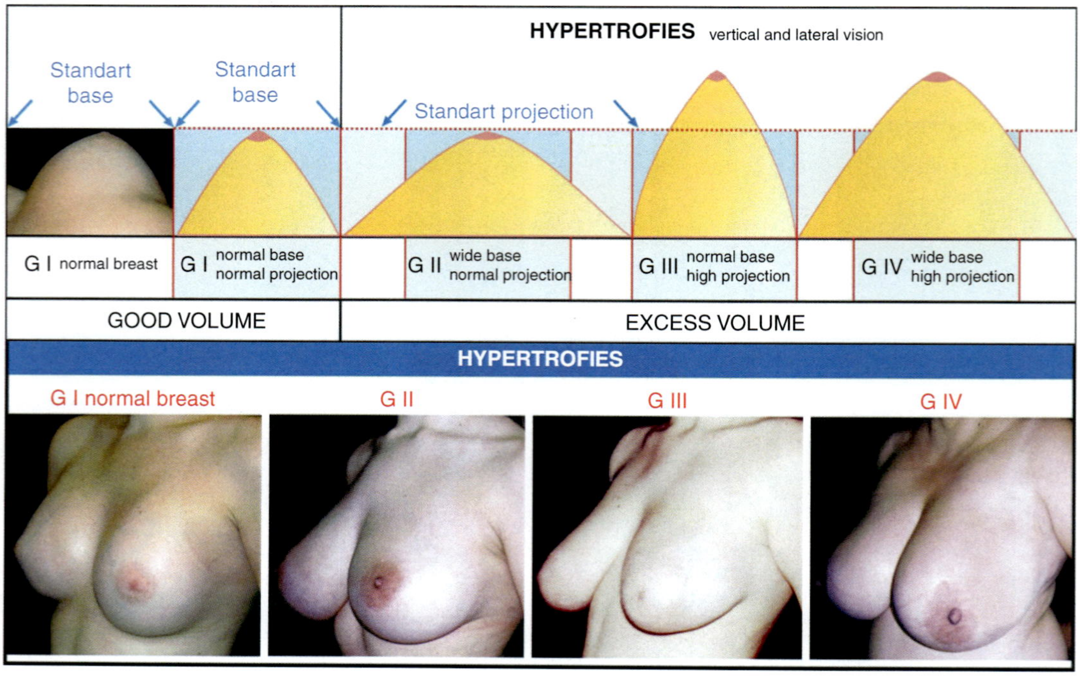

Fig. 32.4 Classifications of mammary hypertrophy according to the extent of the breast implantation on the normal thorax and their projections

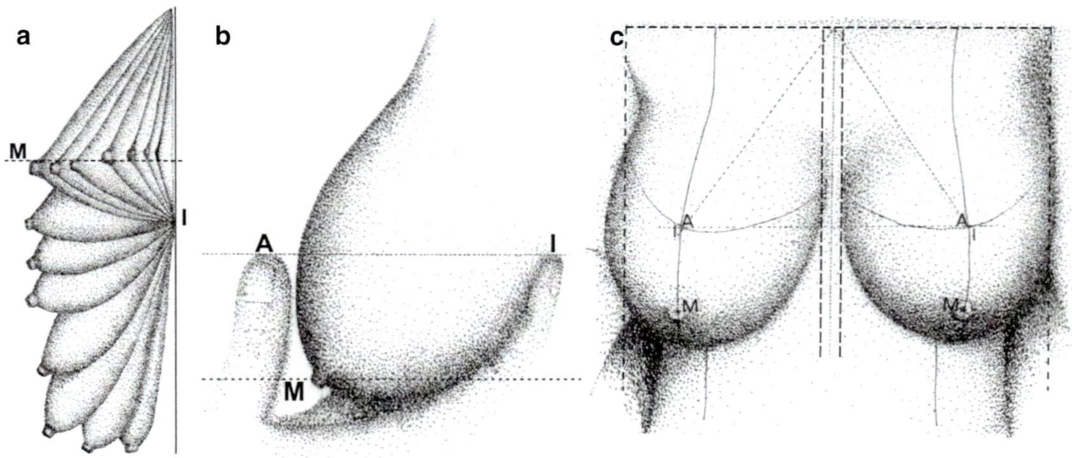

Fig. 32.5 (**a**) Schema of anteroposterior breast growth and its projections into the space that subjects it to gravitational forces, making it sag over time. (**b**) Point I when it is projected onto the breast determining point M. (**c**) A frontal view of the breast points already described

remove a small/minor volume, this means that we will obtain a small/minor scar. Points I and their corresponding points A (Pitanguy 1963) should be equidistant from the medial breast and external line. Points M are sometimes located in an ectopic position in ptosis cases.

There is a direct relationship between the A–M measurement and the final scar. With AM: 0–2 cm the alterations are in shape, volume, and NAC position, no ptosis, and it is possible to perform surgery resulting in a periareolar scar (Aboudib and Castro 1998; Andrews et al. 1975; Baran et al. 2001; Benelli 1990; Bozola 2009; Bustos 1992; Fayman et al. 2003; Goes 1996; Martins 1986; Ribeiro et al. 1998). With 3 cm, I had a final vertical scar (Ariê 1957; Bozola 1984; Ribeiro 1990) in those with an A–M measurement of 4–7 cm, an L scar (Bozola 1990a, b, 2011; Bozola 1984; Chiari 1992; Elbaz and Verheerke 1972; Horibe et al. 1956; Meyer and Kessehing 1975; Regnault 1974; Sepulveda 1981); and in those with A–M distances an inverted T scar (Lima 1979; Mckissock 1976; Peixoto 1980; Pitanguy 1963; Pontes 1973; Strombeck 1960). The T technique allows an extension of A–M value plus 2 cm, which reduces the horizontal scar by half, because of the skin compensations that are described later. The T technique provides an extension of only two times the A–M value plus 2 cm.

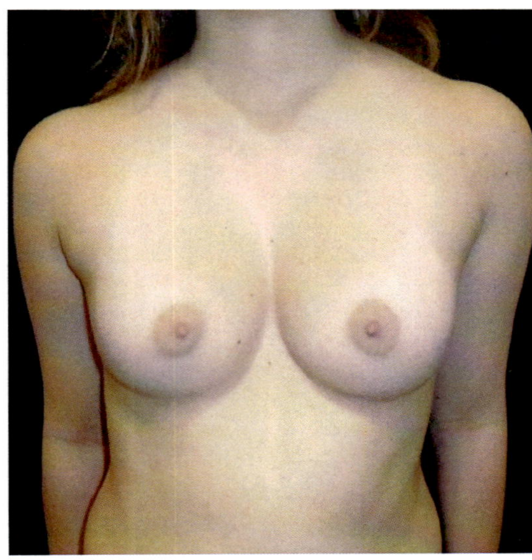

Fig. 32.6 Alteration of the thorax shape (pectus excavatum), which changes the breast bases of implantation and their projections

NAC: ectopic positions on the vertical and horizontal axes, diameter, shape, projection, and color must be individually analyzed.

Breast symmetry: diagnosing aesthetic diseases of the breast depends on their shape, volume, ptosis, NAC positions, axillary extension, pectoral pillars, anatomical thorax alterations, curvatures of the ribs, projection of the external bone (Fig. 32.6), musculature, and spinal pathological conditions.

32.2 Method

Skin markings: with the patient standing up to obtain the HHBL, LHBL, VMBL, VLBL, the mammary meridian, points I, A, and M, and the A–M measurement (Fig. 32.7). The, with the patient in a supine position, with arms at 90° relative to the thorax, the marks are made according to the A–M measurement. Place your flattened hand on the lateral breast side and push it until you can correct the breast meridian (Fig. 32.8a).

A superior semicircle with a radius A–M based on the pivot point M is drawn (Fig. 32.8a). From point I on the meridian of the breast, mark the A–M measurement upward. Based on the pivot point at its superior extremity, mark a quarter of the circle in the lower medial quadrant, also with the radius A–M, and join it to the medial end of the superior semicircle (Fig. 32.8b). From point I, the A–M measurement is transferred laterally on the submammary fold and the horizontal A–M is marked, elevating its extremity in the same proportion as the intended reduction in the diameter of the base of the breast (1–2 cm) (Fig. 32.8c). From the lateral extremity of this marking, up to point A, with a little upward traction of the skin, a line is marked where the curved oblique A–M is drawn. The oblique A–M is curved approximately 2 cm too (Fig. 32.9a).

The lateral superior semicircle is then joined to the inferior marking.

On the latero-superior quadrant, I draw a skin prevent triangle based on two equal arches that join each other at the bisector of the angle of the meridian and a horizontal line passing to M, height 1–2 cm, and give the surgeon a small amount of excess skin to aid in closure and to prevent tightness below the areola (Fig 32.9b).

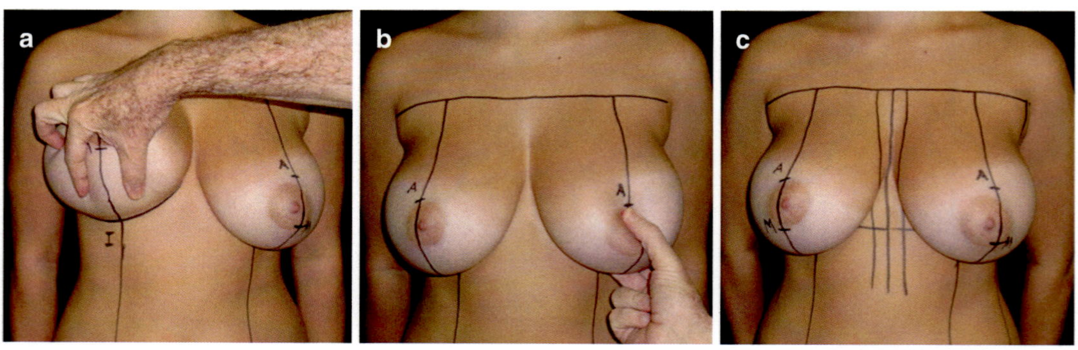

Fig. 32.7 (**a**) Point I. (**b**) Obtaining point A through a point I projection on the breast. (**c**) With the patient standing and presenting the large projection of point M on the breast ectopic cone comparing with the NAC and the mammary lines and points

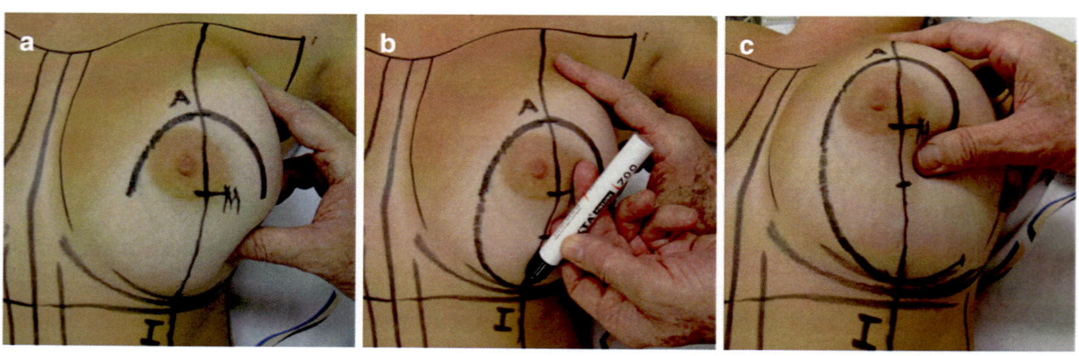

Fig. 32.8 (**a–c**) Marking out the skin resections based on the measurement of A–M. Please see the text

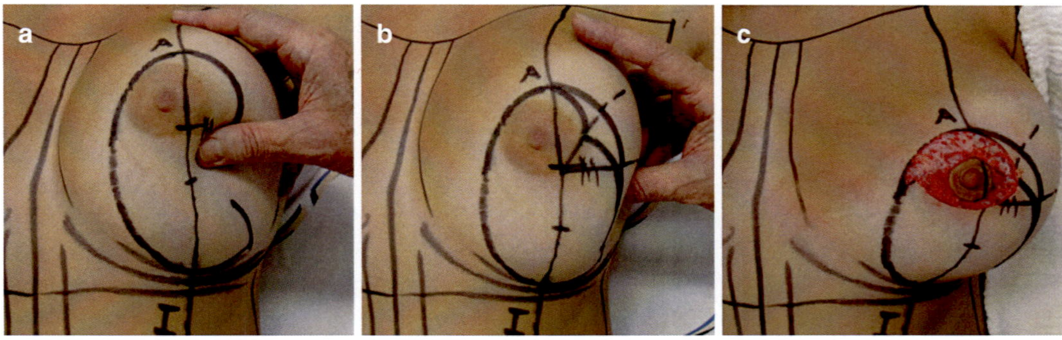

Fig. 32.9 (**a–c**) Skin resections already marked and superior de-epidermization

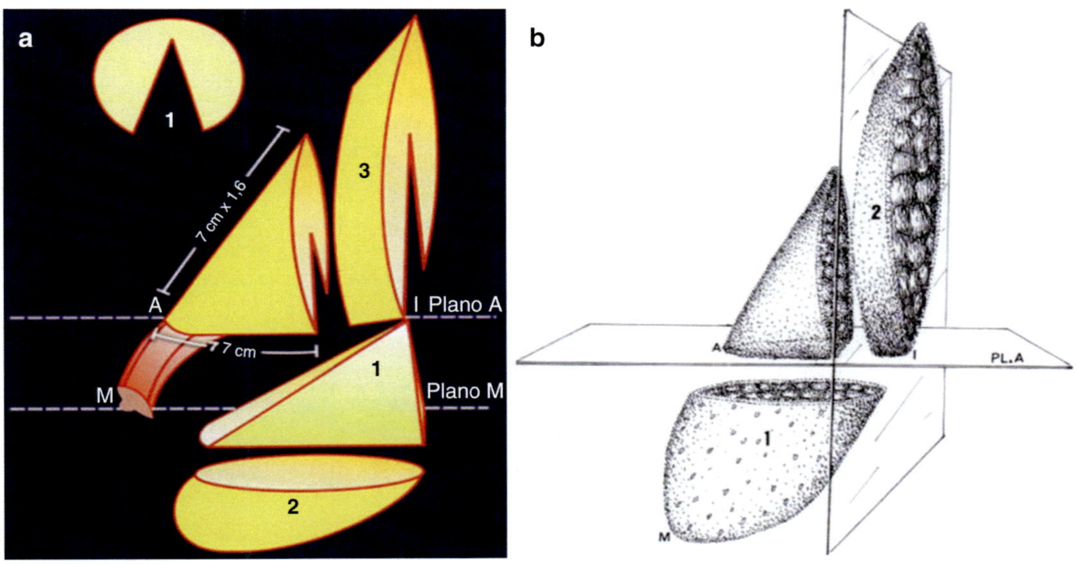

Fig. 32.10 (**a**, **b**) Schema of the breast tissue removal in group IV. *1* A breast reduction wedge in its latero-lateral diameter. *2* Ptosis of the breast volume. *3* A resection of the breast base to aim to reduce its projection, providing the remaining breast tissue with a suitable shape and a volume inside the mammary lines. The areolar pedicle is de-epidermized

32.2.1 Mammary Glandular Resection

The mammary gland resection and assembly is variable according to each group.

Group IV: to correct this type of breast, it is necessary to carry out a resection of the ptotic excess under plane A, and a resection of the vertical wedge to reduce the base (Figs. 32.10a and 32.11a), in addition to a resection of the base, in two parts, medial and lateral, reducing the height (Fig. 32.10). It is possible to reduce the projection with a resection and an inverted wedge under the NAC, easily elevating it. The lateral and medial parts are sutured to each other, except under the areola when the A–M measurement is much longer. The first and superior stitch the same as in GII.

All the time, think about the possibility of obtaining the shape, proportion, and volume described in Fig. 32.10.

It is important for the subcutaneous tissue in the whole the wound to be maintained at the same thickness as the subcutaneous tissue in the thorax.

During the resection of the breast tissue, this thickness must be left to avoid damage to the neurovascular supply to the skin and gland because this is embryologically ectodermic. The resection of the base of the mammary cone should follow the thoracic curvature so that the gland can be removed up to the axillary region. Resections of excess gland under plane A should accompany the skin mark parallel to point I. If this is done perpendicular to the thorax, it cuts the normal future cone, flattening its inferior pole. In all cases, it is important to leave a small flap of subcutaneous fat with an inferior pedicle and fixed naturally on the thorax, at point I, to avoid an empty appearance when the patient raises her arms (Fig. 32.11d) This is to rebuild the inferior aspect of the cone. When the patient has the upper pole emptied, a long and narrow flap is necessary to fill the breast, and increase the vertical diameter. The medial and lateral columns of the breast tissue must be sutured together to avoid dead spaces, except in the subareolar area, when the A–M measurement is longer.

Group III: The resection is performed in the base to reduce the height of the mammary cone with "amputation of the base" (Fig. 32.11b–c). It is possible to reduce a small excess of projection with an inverted wedge. In this case, it is not a good idea to suture the lateral and medial columns to reduce the projection.

Group II: After resection of the ptotic mammary gland under plane A, to correct the ptosis,

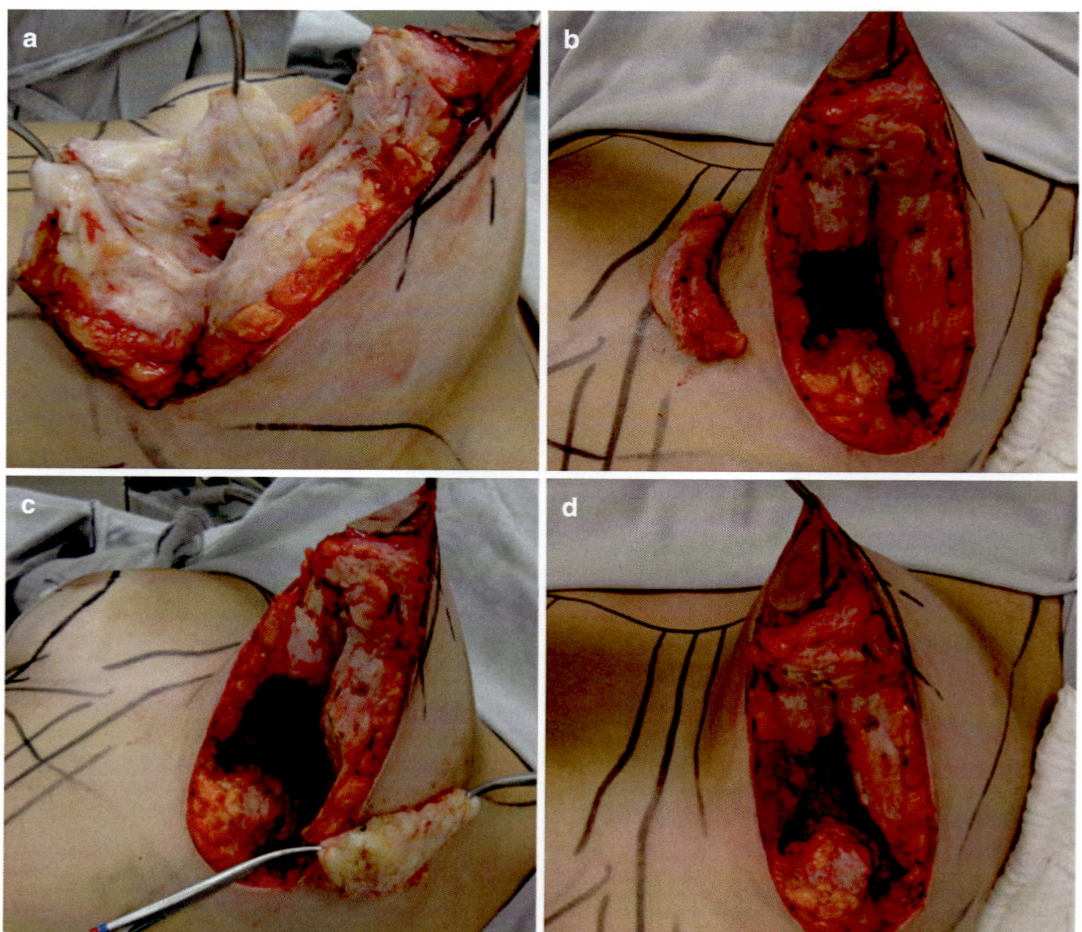

Fig. 32.11 (**a**) Ptosis and wedge resection as a whole (group IV), or leaving it entire or as part of it as an inferior pedicle (flap; group I). (**b**) Resection of the medial base (groups III and IV). (**c**) An inferior minor flap that is always left in groups II, III, and IV. (**d**) Resection of the lateral base (groups III and IV)

except for the NAC and its pedicle, a wedge is resected from near the apex to the base of the mammary gland to reduce its horizontal diameter and the lateral and medial glands are sutured to each other. The superior and first stitch fixes the aponeurosis of the pectoralis major muscle. The diameters are inverted. (Fig. 32.11a).

Group I: as there is no excess of mammary tissue, an axial flap is made of the mammary gland that is under plane A, except the NAC and its pedicle (Figs. 32.10a and 32.11a). The axial flap can be de-epithelialized or the skin can be completely removed. The remaining breast is freed from its insertion into the pectoralis major muscle, enough to slide the flap under the mammary gland and suture it vertically on the aponeurosis of the pectoralis major muscle (Ribeiro et al. 2002). Afterward, the lateral and medial glands are sutured together, or not, if the projection of the breast is to be reduced. In cases where there is an excess of axillary extension, part of the lateral flap is resected. With all these maneuvers, the inferior pole of the breast is emptied, the postero-anterior direction is increased, and the breast is filled. Again, the vertical diameter is longer than the horizontal diameter.

Suturing of the skin: pulling point A in a vertical and medial direction, the skin compensation is made to the lateral up to point I or 1 cm more medial than this with oblique A–M and horizontal A–M (Fig. 32.12a). Now, to adjust the difference between the great medial and the

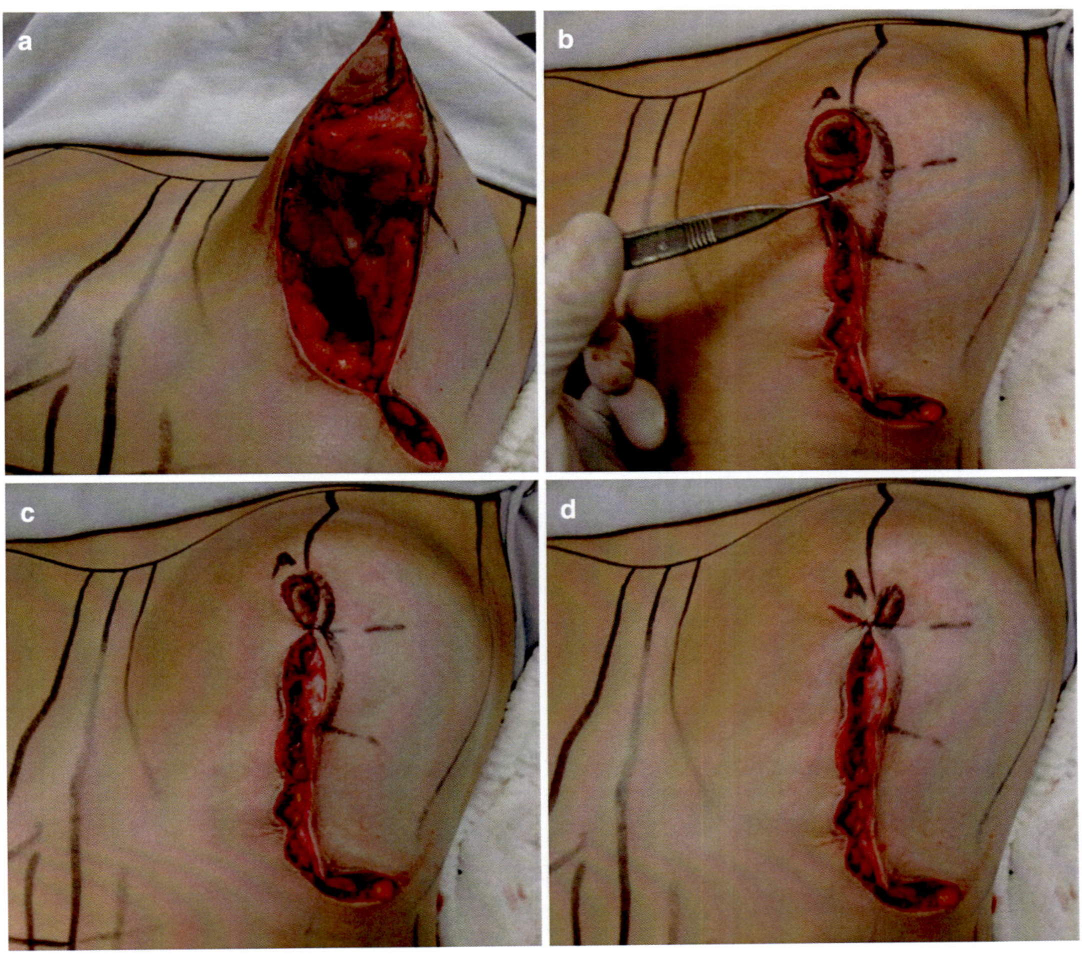

Fig. 32.12 (**a**) At the beginning of the suture from the lateral to the medial side. (**b**) The suturing of point I toward the areolar region with a semi-colon shape and a possibility of using or not using the skin security triangle. (**c**) The end of the vertical suture. (**d**) The end of the V–Y suture

short lateral surgical margins. At the beginning, it is necessary to execute the subcutaneous suture and then the skin suture. On the medial side, the needle should be inserted in a parallel incision line and, from the side, the needle should be inserted in a perpendicular direction. This suture is called a "semi-colon shap". What adjusts the slope naturally (Fig. 32.12b). To remove the tension to elevate the areola, an incision is made in the dermis in the lateral part of the areola. The tension on point A is released, and the lateral and medial sides are equally distributed and sutured to each other from the sulcus to the top, where a purse-string suture is inserted. The skin triangle in the supero-lateral quadrant is resected partial or totally or sutured under the areola to adjust the vertical suture (Fig. 32.12b), if the ptosis is small. If the ptosis is medium, it is not necessary to insert the purse-string suture as well; thus, I insert three stitches (v–y) around the skin excess at the extremity of the cone, or end in a vertical suture (Fig. 32.12c). After both, if the breast has considerable ptosis, the skin excess will exist mainly on the medial side; because of this, a purse-string suture is inserted (Fig. 32.13a). After both breasts are sutured, the new position of the NAC is marked in such a way that its superior margin is situated at the apex of the mammary gland (Fig. 32.13b). The purse-string suture is removed, or the three stitches, and the left and right sides of the circles are compared. The excess skin is removed, and the areola is sutured into the new position. If the diameter of the de-epithelialized area around the areola is more than twice its size, this is not good. Its suitable size measures one and a half times of the size of the areola.

During the suturing of the areola (Fig. 32.13c), there must be similar tension at the cardinal points, and there will be wrinkling of the skin, mainly on the medial side, when the A–M measurement is approximately 7 cm, which will disappear over a period of 60 days. When large wrinkles occur in patients with very elastic skin or an A–M measurement of more than 7 cm, the results are not good, and this is the only limiting factor in maintaining the final L scar. If this occurs, the skin excess is rotated downward to the medial submammary fold, where a resection is carried out with a final short inverted T scar, twice the size of an L scar.

Also, the limiting factor in obtaining a final L scar is not the volume, but the degree of ptosis, which is related to skin elasticity. For example, depending on the A–M measure, it is easier to obtain a final L scar in resections of 600 g than in

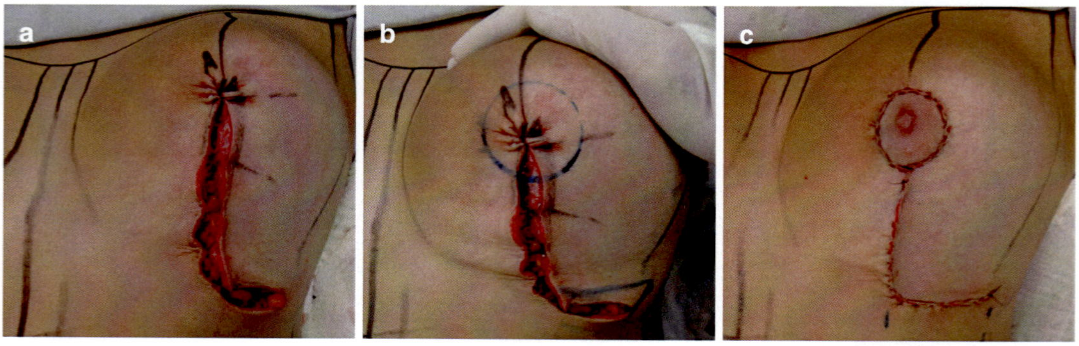

Fig. 32.13 (**a**) The end of the areolar bag to aim the circular compensation, based on the measurements of the excess skin. (**b**) Marking the location of the nipple–areola complex and correcting the position of the horizontal and lateral suture upward to the glandular edge, pushing the breast with the hand upwards. (**c**) The concluded sutures resulting in a horizontal scar that measures at most A–M +2 cm, and the vertical scar measures the same height of the new breast cone

those of 200 g. The excess skin that is removed by the purse-string suture corresponds to the skin resected in the medial part of the mammary fold in the inverted T technique.

Sometimes it is necessary to correct the horizontal scar, to put it up on the inferior glandular border, to compress the breast toward the upwards and remove a lateral skin triangle to compensate and increase it to 2 cm.

The suturing of the wound must begin from the sulcus and go up to the apex, and the breast tissue must have a rotation from lateral to medial, ending with a purse-string suture at the level of the areola, which allows more skin to be resected, resulting in a small scar.

Another important factor in the standardization of results is to leave the same size and volume of breast tissue columns in all patients, and the inferior pedicle flap if necessary, with the lateral one a little longer than the medial one, to follow the curvature of the thorax. Also, the standardization of volume that remains will give final symmetry, even in preoperatively asymmetrical breasts. Perfect unitary build-up of resections of the skin, an envelope suture with minimal tension, and a good areola position will provide good long-term results.

32.3 Results: Discussion and Conclusions

In the L technique, good and bad final results are proven only about 6 months after the surgery. They can be in relation to ptosis (Figs. 32.14 and 32.15), shape and final volume, breast asymmetries, and nipple diameter. If the technical maneuvers have not been correctly executed, the consequences will be apparent. When the sutures of the mammary cone are built from its upper mammary pole toward point I (in the superior-most position with the aponeurosis of the pectoralis muscle) the final shape results are good and durable. The irregularities of the confluence of the vertical and horizontal scars are reduced if A–M has a maximum value of 7 cm. The skin resection that leaves the ratio of content to container prevents residual ptosis and bad final scars. The NAC diameter can increase if skin tension exists around. The larger the volume removed, the greater the scarring. So, a minimum percentage of breast asymmetry should be permitted (Fig. 32.16).

The NAC sensibility presents in a normal state when the mammary gland detachments are reduced because it preserves the peripheral breast tissue of the thorax.

If it was possible to lift the NAC without tension, traction, or twisting, there was no necrosis of the NAC in this series of patients. Most of my patients were very happy with the final result in the immediate and late postoperative periods.

After undermining the resected glandular tissue slightly, the lymphedema is small too, and in the late follow-up period its regression reduces the volume by about 10–15%.

The L scar technique is executed through/with/for skin compensations as the breast apex towards its base, from the medial breast side to the lateral side, on the inframammary sulcus. It is indicated for any size of ptosis, but in cases of severe ptosis, it will extend beyond the VLBL and the scars will offer bad final results over time because of the movements of the patient's arms.

Throughout man's evolution, the limbic brain systems have been marked out with attractive features of what is visually beautiful. One mathematical proportion has been repeatedly referred to be contained in beautiful general forms up to the present day. Beautiful is an adjective that determines what the human vision can capture from shapes, volumes, proportions, outlines, lights, glows, shadows, colors, movements, and postures. Plastic surgeons must recognize why a breast is beautiful and how to correct their aesthetic changes (Atalay 2004; Bashour 2006; Eco 2004; Etcoff 1994, 1999; Gil and Médici Filho 2002; Langlois et al. 1987; Livio 2005; Marquardt 2010; Ono et al. 2007; Preston 1993; Ricketts 1982).

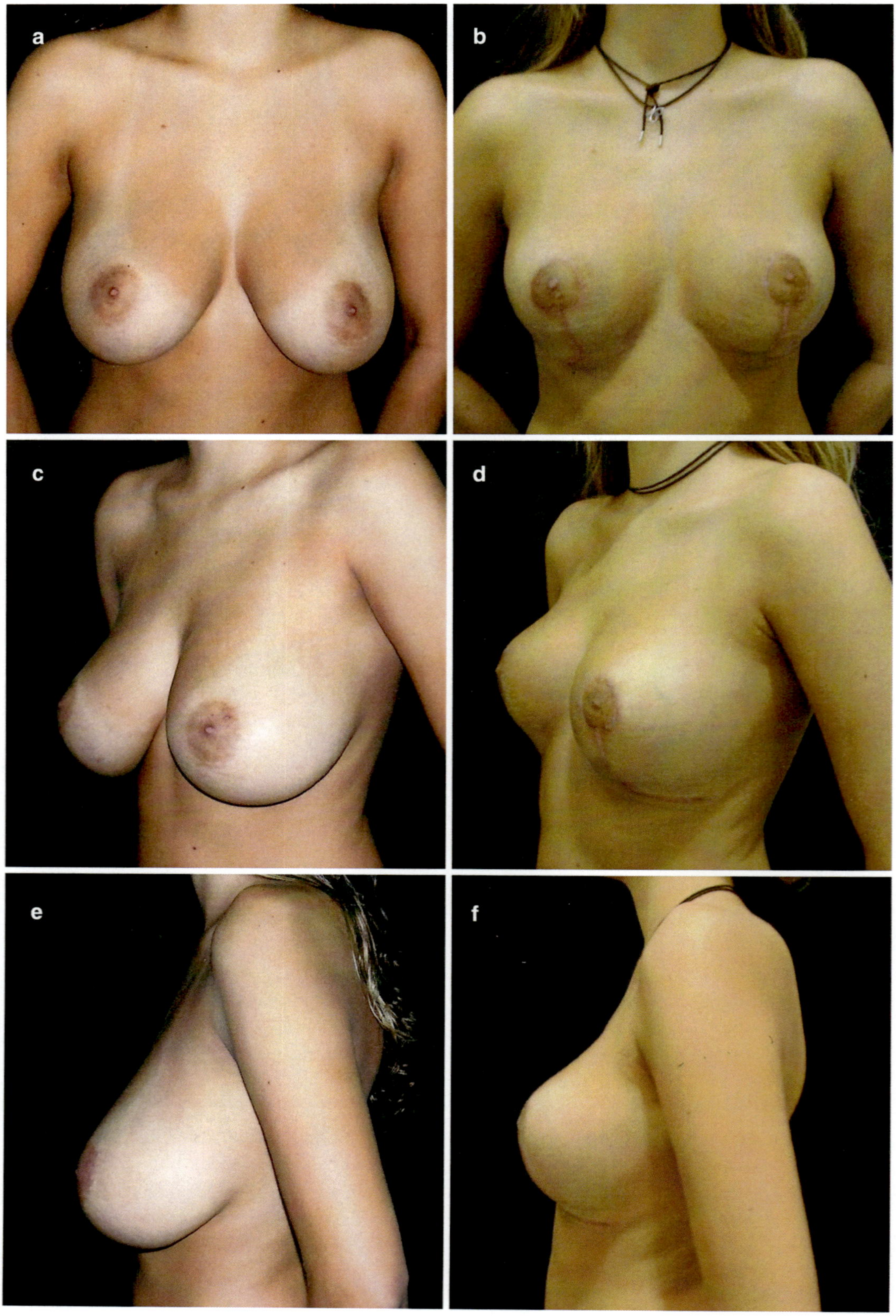

Fig. 32.14 (**a–f**) Pre- and postoperative pictures in a frontal, oblique and lateral view of a group IV mammoplasty presenting an L scar

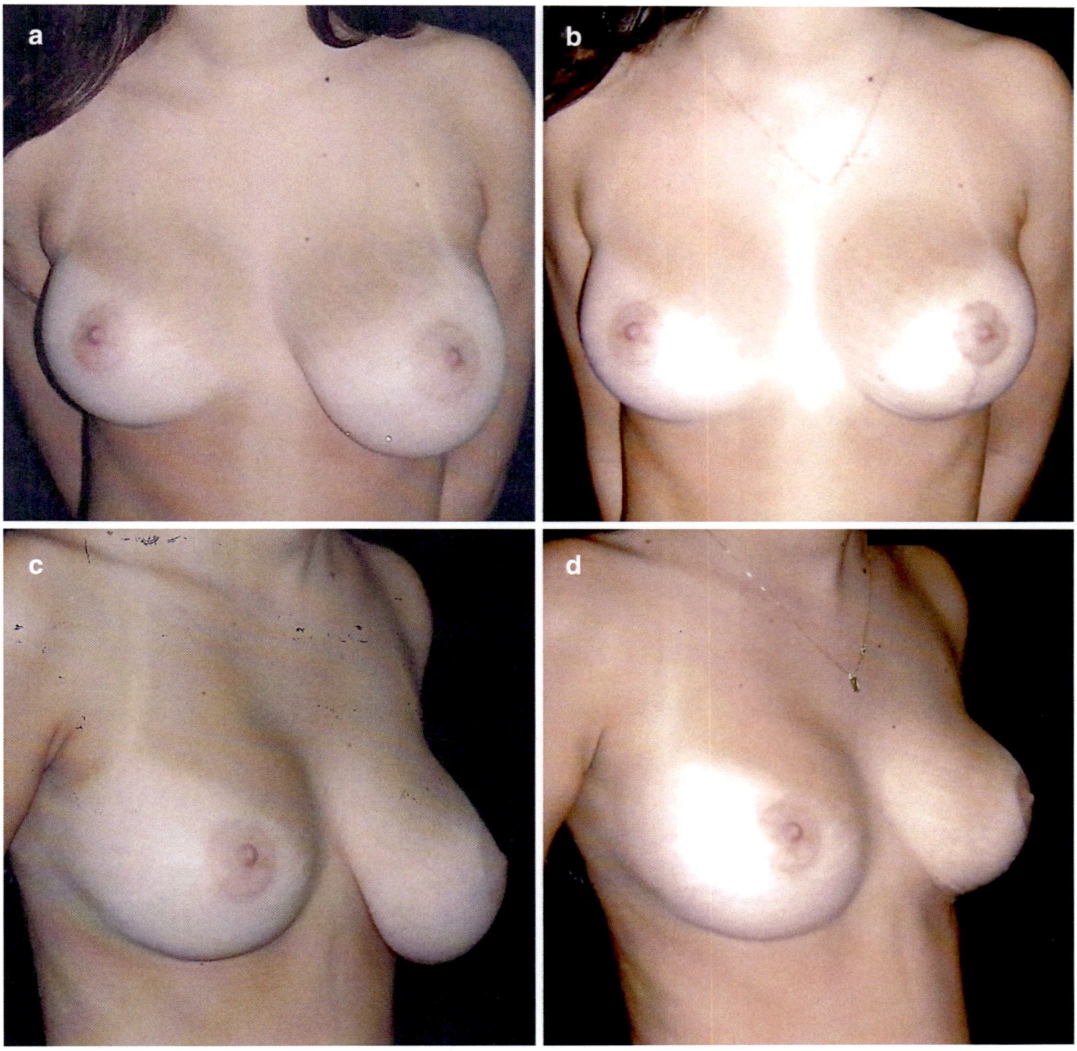

Fig. 32.15 (**a–h**) *Right* and *left* breast sides observed from a frontal, oblique, and lateral view, applying the concepts of the L scar technique just on the left breast, patterning form and volume of the right breast

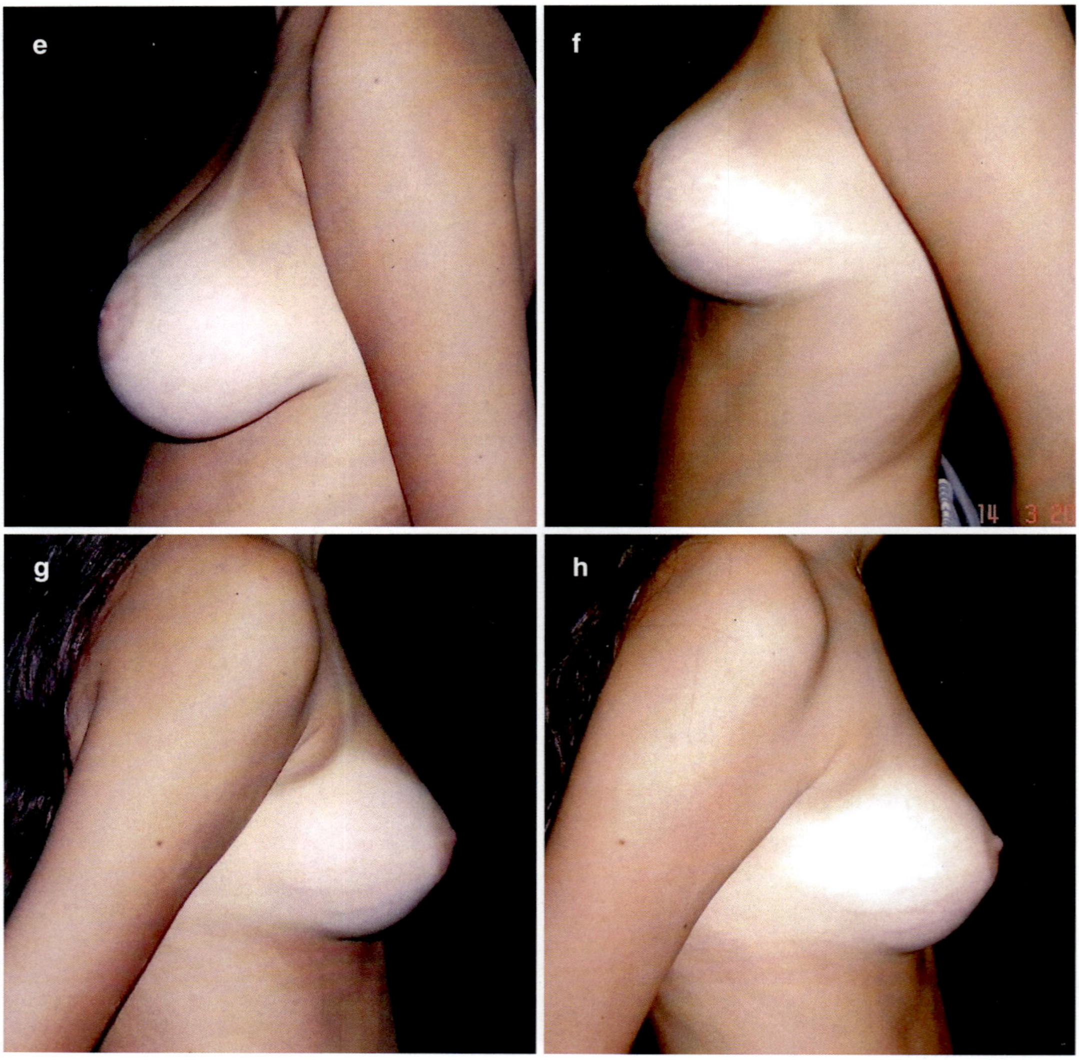

Fig. 32.15 (continued)

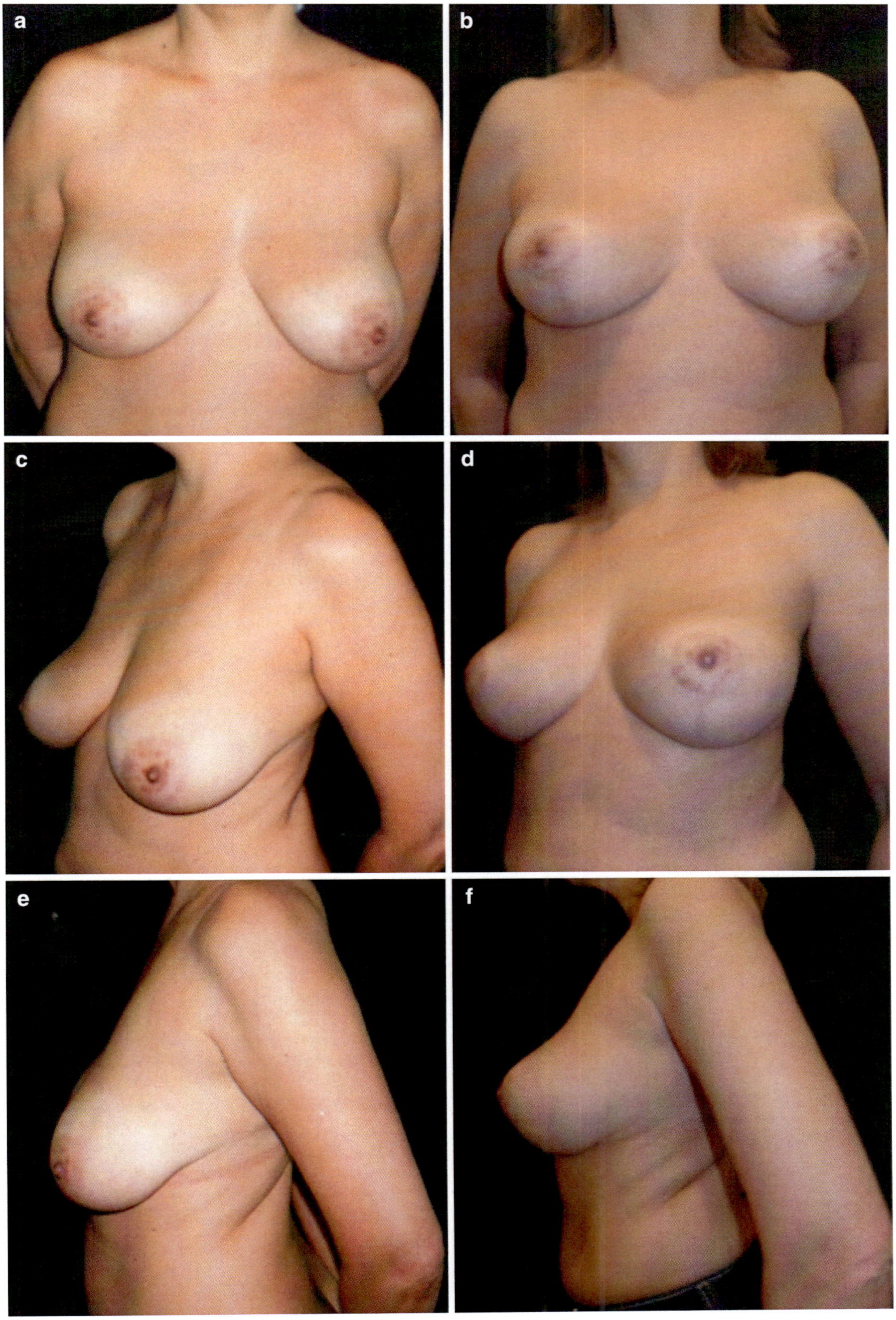

Fig. 32.16 a Pre and pos op of breast reduction Ppying the L scar technique.

References

Aboudib JH, Castro CC (1998) Mammaplasty utilizing the periareolar approach. Aesth Plast Surg 22:51–57
Andrews JM, Jshizuki MMA, Martins DMSF, Ramos RR (1975) An areolar approach to reduction mammaplasty. Br J Plast Surg 28:166
Ariê G (1957) Una nuevatecnica de mastoplastia. Rev Latinoam Cir Plast 3:23
Atalay B (2004) Math and the Mona Lisa, the art and science of Leonardo da Vinci. Harper Collins, New York
Baran CN, Peker F, Sensöz O, Baran NK (2001) Unsatisfactory results of periareolar mastopexy with or without augmentation and reduction mammaplasty: enlarged areola with flattened nipple. Aesth Plast Surg 25:286–289
Bashour M (2006) History and current concepts in the analysis of facial attractiveness. Plast Reconstr Surg 118(3):741–756
Benelli L (1990) A new periareolar mammaplasty: the "roundblock" technique. Aesth Plast Surg 14:93–100
Bozola AR (1984) Mamaplastia- Técnica de Ariê "Invertida"- Nota Prévia,in Anais da 1 Jornada Sul Brasileira de Cirurgia Plástica. ArtgrafLtda 157–160
Bozola AR (1990a) Reduction mammaplasty: preferred techniques. In: Goldwyn RM (ed) Reduction mammaplasty. Little Brown, Boston, pp 407–437
Bozola AR (1990b) Breast reduction with short L scar. Plast Livio Reconstr Surg 85(5):728–738
Bozola AR (2009) Periareolar breast reduction. Aesth Plast Surg 33:228–234
Bozola AR, Longato FM, Bozola AP (2011) Análise geométrica da forma da beleza da mama e da forma de prótese baseado na proporção Phi: aplicação prática. Rev Bras Cir Plást 26(1)
Bustos RA (1992) Periareolar mammaplasty with silicone supporting lamina. Plast Rec Surg 89(4):646–657
Chiari A Jr (1992) The L short-scar mammaplasty: a new approach. Plast Reconstr Surg 90:233
Dufourmentel C, Mouly R (1961) Plastic mammaire par la methode oblique. Ann Chir Plast 6:45
Eco U (2004) Storia della belleza. Bompiani, Milan
Elbaz JS, Verheerke G (1972) La cicatrice en L dans les plasties mammaires. Ann Chir Plast 17:283
Etcoff NL (1994) Psychology. Beauty and the beholder. Nature 368(6468):186–187
Fayman MS, Potgieter E, Becker PJ (2003) Outcome study: periareolar mammaplasty patients' perspective. Plast Reconstr Surg 111:676–684. (discussion 685–687)
Gil CTLA, Médici Filho E (2002) Estudo da proporção áurea na arquitetura craniofacial de indivíduos adultos com oclusão normal, a partir de telerradiografias axiais, frontais e laterais. Ortodontia 35(2):69–85
Goes JCS (1996) Periareolar mammaplasty: double skin techniquewith application of polyglactine or mixed mesh. Plast Reconstr Surg 97:959–968
Goldwyn RM (ed) (1976) Plastic and reconstructive surgery of the breast. Little Brown, Boston, pp 269–283
Horibe K, Spina V, Lodovici O (1956) Mamma plastia redutora: nuevo abordaje del metodo lateral-obliquo. Rev Latinoam Cir Plast 2:7
Langlois JH, Roggman LA, Casey RJ, Ritter JM, Rieser-Danner LA, Jenkins VY (1987) Infant preferences for attractive faces: rudiments of a stereotype? Dev Psychol 23(3):363–369
Lima JC (1979) Breast reduction: new method and refinements. Transactions of the 7th International Congress of Plastic Reconstrutive Surgery, São Paulo, pp 518–521
Livio M (2005) La proporción áurea, la historia de PHI, el numero más sorprendentedel mondo. Editorial Ariel, Barcelona
Marquardt SR (2010) Marquardt beauty analysis (web site). Accessed 15 March
Martins PDE (1986) Mamaplastia periareolar com transposição de retalhos. Rev Soc Bras Cir Plast 6:1–10
Mckissock PC (1976) Correction of macromastia by the bipedicle vertical dermal flap. In: Goldwyn RM (ed) Plastic and reconstrutive surgery of the breast. Litlle Brown, Boston, pp 215–229
Meyer R, Kessehing UR (1975) Reduction mammaplasty with an L-shaped suture line. Plast Reconstr Surg 55:139
Ono E, Walter-Porto COT, Medici-Filho E, Moraes LC, Moraes MEL, Castilho JCM (2007) Análise da proporção áurea em indivíduos dolico, braqui e mesofaciais, por meio de radiografias cefalométricas laterais. Rev Odontol Ciênc 22(56):154–159
Peixoto G (1980) Reduction mammaplasty: a personal technique. Plast Reconstr Surg 65:217
Pitanguy I (1963) Mammaplastias. Rev Latinoam Cir Plast 7:139
Pontes AA (1973) Technique of reduction mammaplasty. Br J Plast Surg 26:365
Preston JD (1993) The golden proportion revisited. J Esthet Dent 5(6):247–251
Regnault PCI (1974) Reduction mammaplasty by the "B" technique. Plast Reconstr Surg 53:19–24
Ribeiro L (1990) The Lozaenghe technique. In: Goldwyn RM (ed) Reduction mammaplasty. Little Brown, Boston
Ribeiro L, Canzi W, Buss A, Accorsi A (1998) Tuberous breast: a new approach. Plast Reconstr Surg 101:42–50. (discussion 51–52)
Ribeiro L et al (2002) Creation and evolution of 30 years of the inferior pedicle in reduction mammaplasties. Plast Reconstr Surg 110(3):960–970
Ricketts RM (1982) The biologic significance of the divine proportion and Fibonacci series. Am J Orthod 81(5):351–370
Sepulveda AA (1981) Tratamento das assimetrias mamárias. Rev Bras Cir 71(18):11
Strombeck JO (1960) Mammaplasty: report of a new technique based on the two pedicle procedure. Br J Plast Surg 13:79–91

Mastoplasty: The L Technique

33

Vilibaldo Cabral de Paulo

33.1 Introduction

From the aesthetic point of view, we believe that contemporary plastic surgery has reached perfection with regard to volume, shape, positioning of the breasts and the quality of the scars, thanks to the generous contributions of numerous techniques, among which we highlight, Arié's (1957), Strombeck's (1960/61), and Pitanguy's (1963). However, from a subjective point of view in daily contact with the patients, many patients are dissatisfied with the scars of the inverted T technique, especially with regard to the medial segment, despite the professing satisfaction with the overall result.

Facing this concern, plastic surgeons, especially those of the Brazilian School, were motivated to develop and improve surgical techniques and tactics to minimize the stigma of scars, which was already part of our daily work.

Authors such as Geraldo Peixoto in 1980 published a personal technique that reduced the size of the inverted T. Eulalio José Neiva 1984 proposed a pentagonal resection to reduce the horizontal line of the T. Yhelda de A. Felicio (1984) presented a technique with one areolar scar, and then other authors such as Ricardo Bustos (1985), Sampaio Goes (1989) and Pedro Martins (1989), contributed to the improvement of periareolar mastoplasty. Based on the techniques of Arié (1957) and Dufourmental and Mouly (1961), there was an increase in the number of techniques with lateral incisions such as that of Horibe (1976), and the J technique published in 1981 by Sepulveda. In Bozola (1992), Bozola published his L technique.

Inspired by the work of Bozola, we began to perform this technique in 1983, at first in patients with simple ptosis and small hypertrophy. Enthusiastic with regard to the good aesthetic results and the apparent acceptance of our patients, we were also encouraged to practice it in cases of medium and large hypertrophy; today, it is the technical procedure that has been almost exclusively adopted to treat different presentations of aesthetic breast deformities (Merriman 1984; Hakme et al. 1983).

33.2 Materials and Methods

After 33 years spent performing mastoplasty using the L technique in patients with small hypertrophy and ptosis, we gradually started to employ this technique in medium and large hypertrophy. The ages ranged between 12 and 68 years.

In isolated cases, we apply the same technique for sequelae correction as for other techniques to

Work done at the Clinic for Aesthetic Plastic Surgery and Reconstructive VILIBALDO CABRAL PAUL and University Hospital of the Federal University of Paraíba.

V.C. de Paulo, M.D.
Avenida Coremas, 172, João Pessoa, PB,
58013-430, Brazil
e-mail: vilibaldocabral@hotmail.com

J.M. Avelar (ed.), *Breast Surgery*, https://doi.org/10.1007/978-3-319-54115-0_33

reduce the medial segment of the T at the time of silicone prosthesis insertion when there was a need to correct mammary ptosis, offer better accommodation of the content and container, and give rise to a better aesthetic configuration.

In our assessment, we consider hypertrophy:

- Small: when the breasts fit comfortably into a brassiere of Brazilian size 42 or 44, or when it was necessary to resect up to 400 g of dermo-glandular tissue.
- Medium: when the breast fit into a size 46 brassiere, or when 400–800 g was resected.
- Large: when the breast fit into a for a brassiere above size 48, or there is resection of more than 800 g.

33.3 Surgical Technique

We proceeded to mark the skin of the cutaneous resection area (simple ptosis) or dermo-glandular (hypertrophy), calculating the excess through interdigital pinching of the lower pole of the breast, trying to model the future breast cone using this maneuver (see Fig. 33.2). At the apex of this cone or slightly below, point A of the future location of the nipple–areola complex (NAC) is marked. From there we go down with a curved line toward the medial pole meeting the midclavicular line with the inframammary crease, point B" always going above that point and proceeding toward the anterior axillary line, stopping before the skinfold limit of the submammary groove that originates from the interdigital clamping point D. Then we went down with another curved line by the lateral pole to a point C, which when approaching it from point B, these two curved lines form a perfect angle, with the points A and B as the vertices (see Fig. 33.3).

Starting from point C, we draw a line that can be straight or curved toward point D. The final alignment results in a shape resembling a comma viewed in the right breast and after resection and subsequent suturing in a U, viewed in the left breast (Figs. 33.1, 33.2 and 33.3).

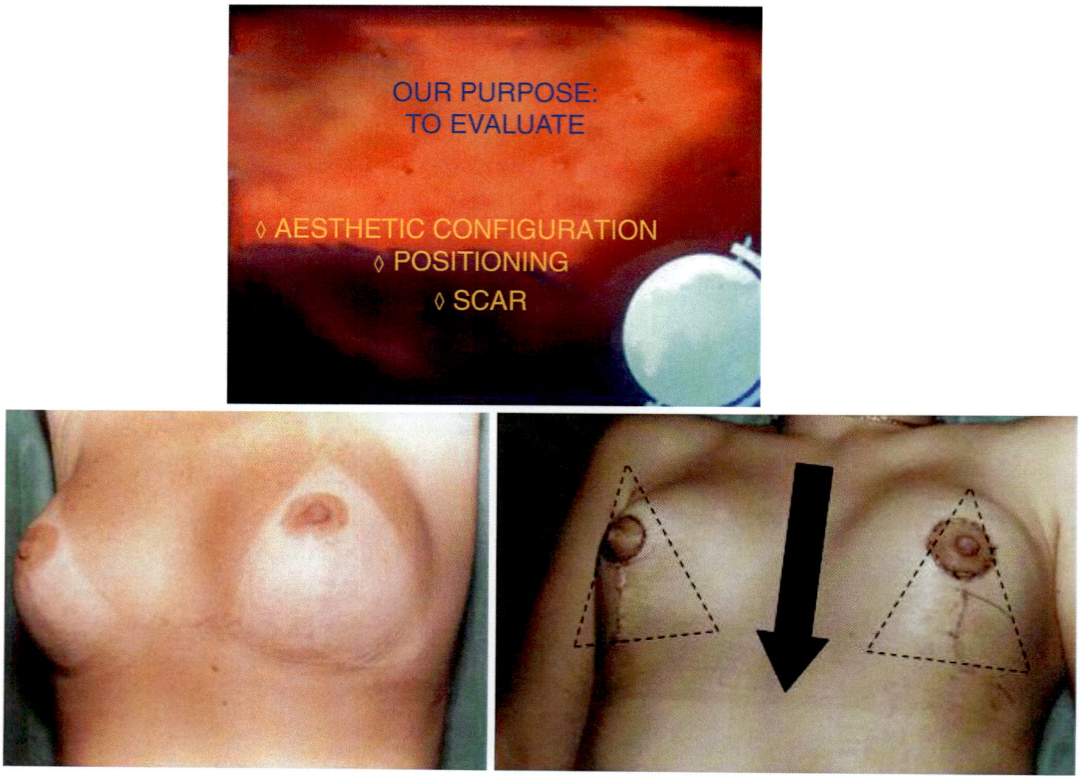

Fig. 33.1 Intermamario Canyon free of scars

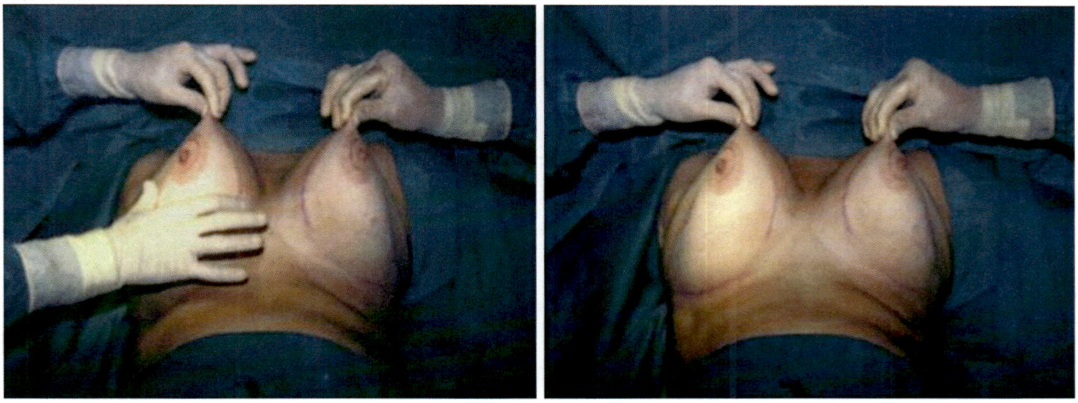

Fig. 33.2 Marking

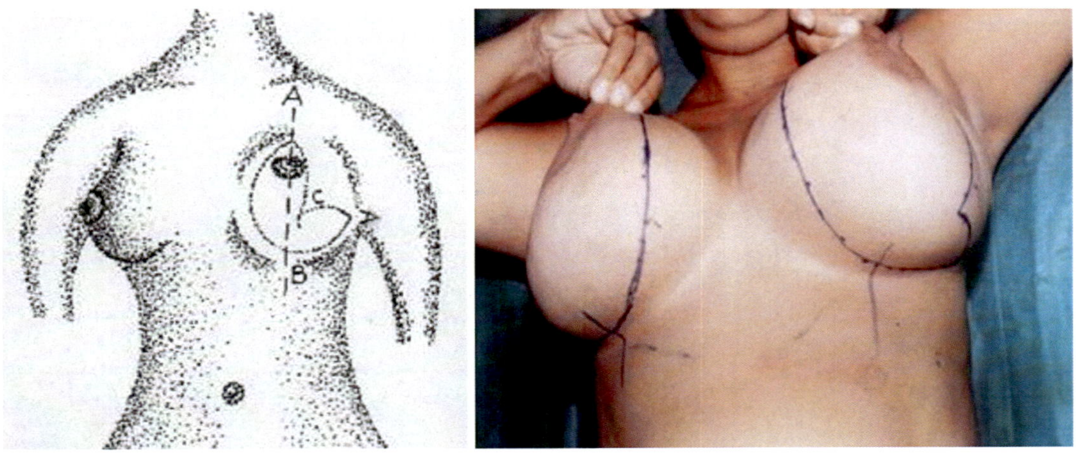

Fig. 33.3 Marking

We resect the excesses of atypical breast contents without following patterns standards, according to the need and the individuality of each case, the first withdrawal being only the necessary excess, either wedge-shaped or "watermelon cut" according to Arié, now as a keel shape, as Pitanguy advocated, and sometimes combining techniques such as those of Pitanguy and Peixoto to reduce the volume and height of the breast cone (in large hypertrophy).

The remaining breast content in the upper, medial, and lateral poles should be sufficient to allow the breast to be filled that favors the shape of a cone in height and diameter in perfect proportionality with the contour of the patient's torso.

In any resection technique, we are always careful to leave more content in the lateral pole, making a greater resection of the medial pole to avoid flattening of the lateral pole (Fig. 33.4). The structure is made of a breast approaching the lateral pole towards the medial pole, fixing them to one or more points with non-absorbable sutures (Mononylon 3–0), Transfixing the weight of the chest in a slightly higher position to compensate for future chest fall (as a "bridge"). The skin sutures are made with sparse intradermal points of absorbable suture (braided polyglycolic acid) and poliglecaprone thread in an intradermal continuous suture without removal. The areolas are sutured with nylon 5–0 at separate points. We do not use drains and the dressing of gauze pad and cotton and crepe bands is applied for 24 or 48 h placed in a brassiere (Figs. 33.5, 33.6, 33.7, 33.8, 33.9, 33.10, 33.11, 33.12, 33.13, 33.14, 33.15, 33.16., 33.17, 33.18, 33.19, 33.20, 33.21, 33.22 and 33.23).

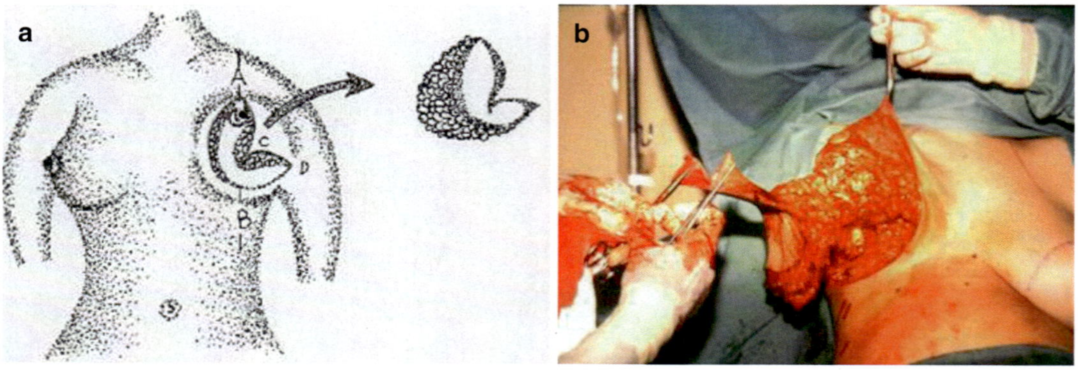

Fig. 33.4 (**a**, **b**) Surgical resection

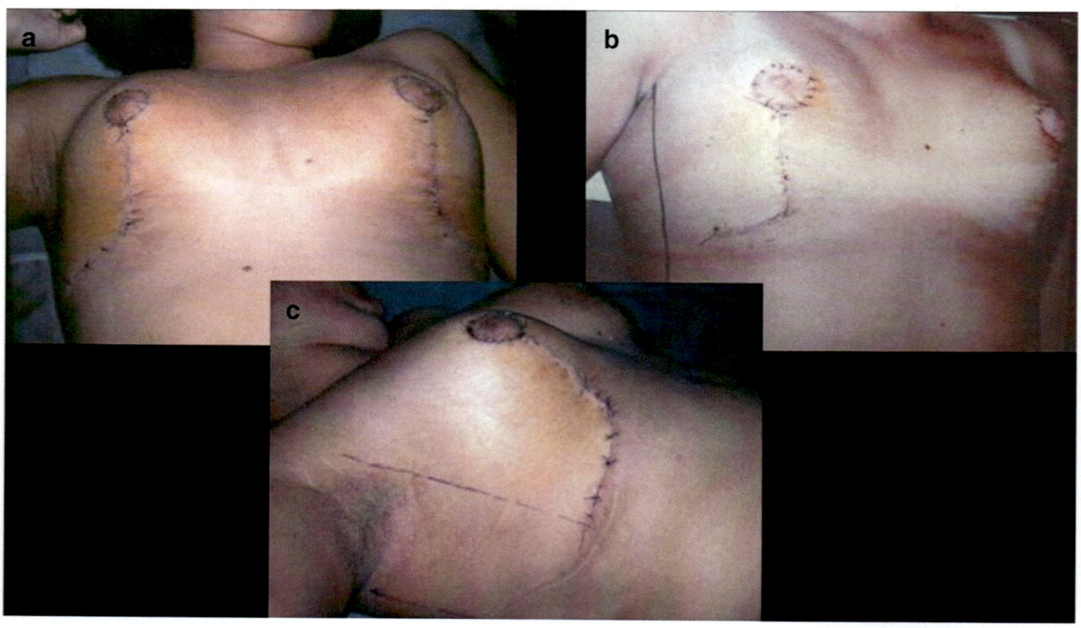

Fig. 33.5 Scars (**a**, **b**) and (**c**) - post operative

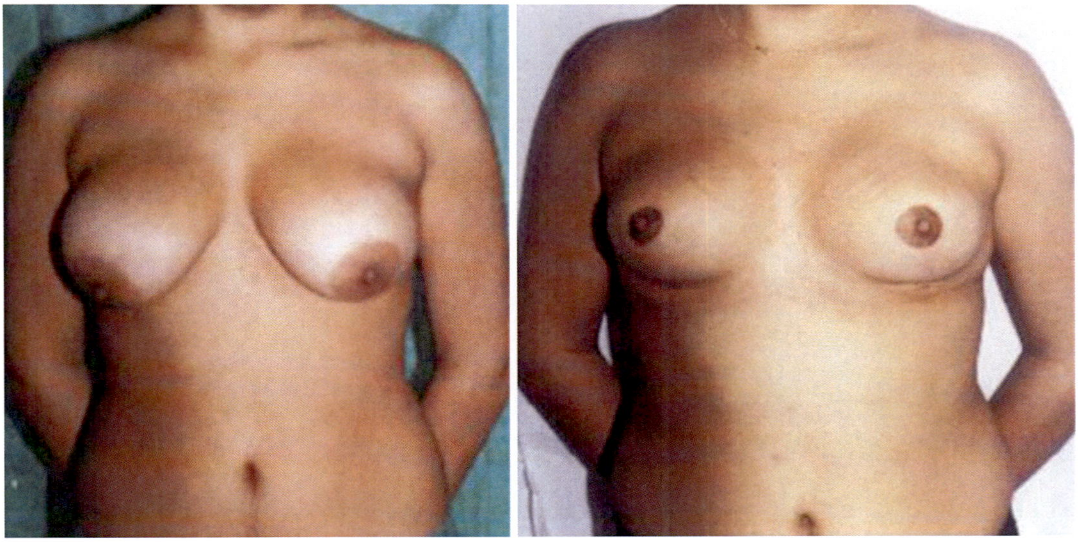

Fig. 33.6 Before and after small hypertrophy

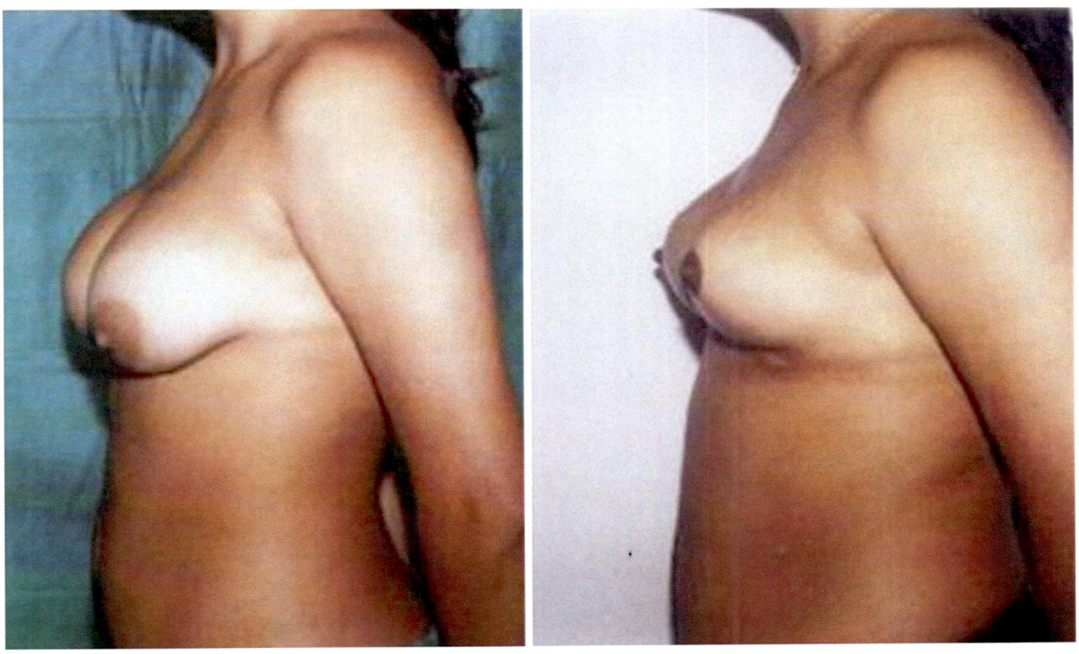

Fig. 33.7 Before and after small hypertrophy

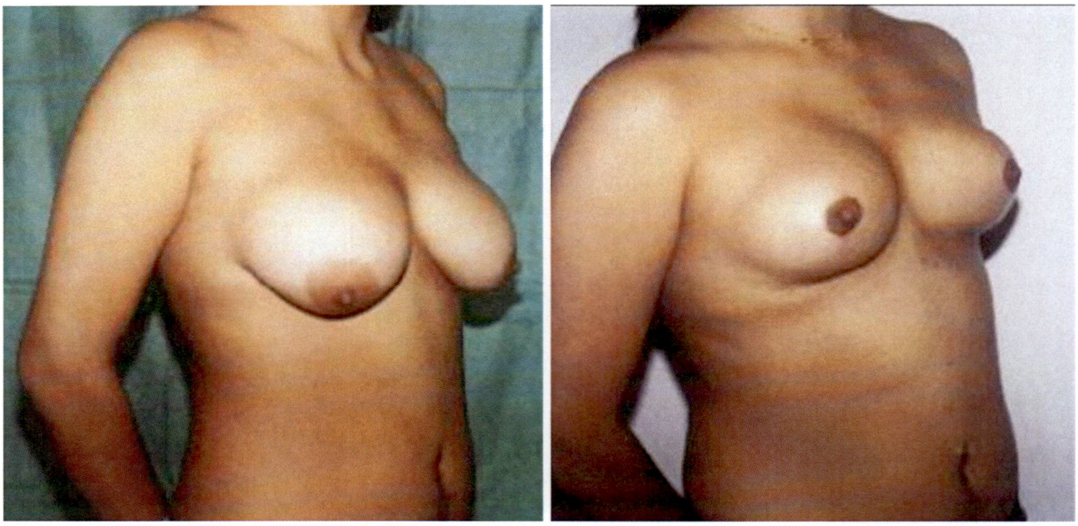

Fig. 33.8 Before and after small hypertrophy

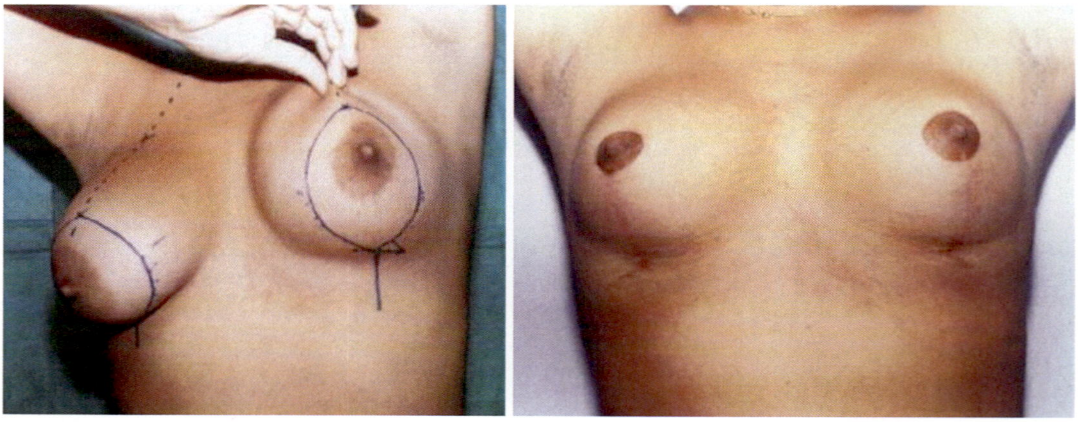

Fig. 33.9 Before and after small hypertrophy

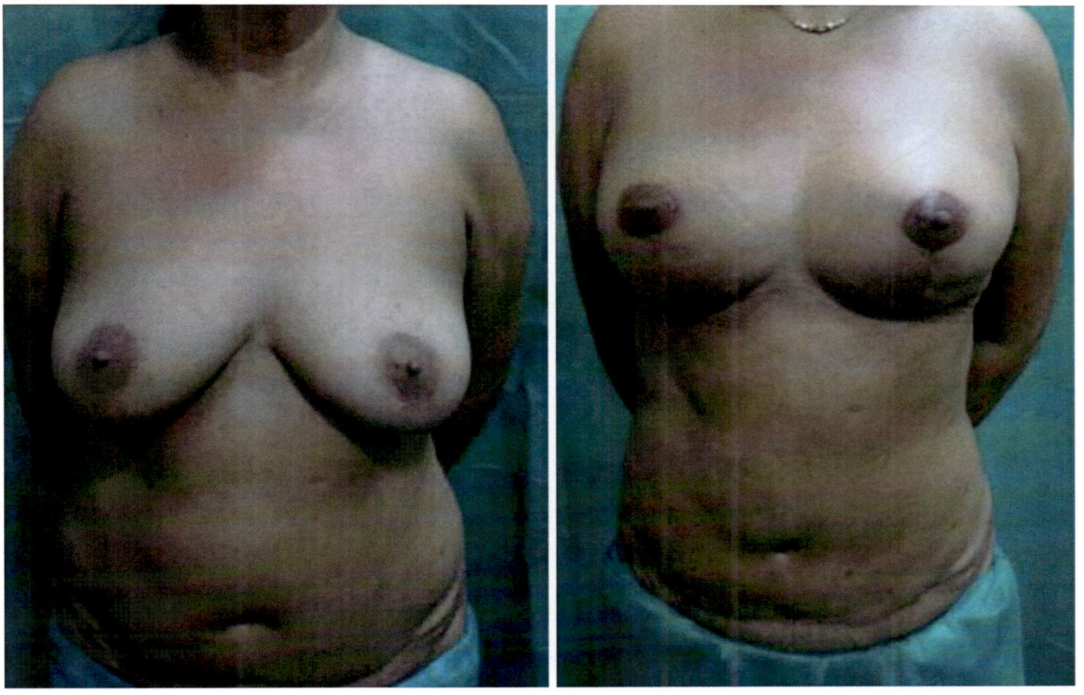

Fig. 33.10 Before and after small hypertrophy

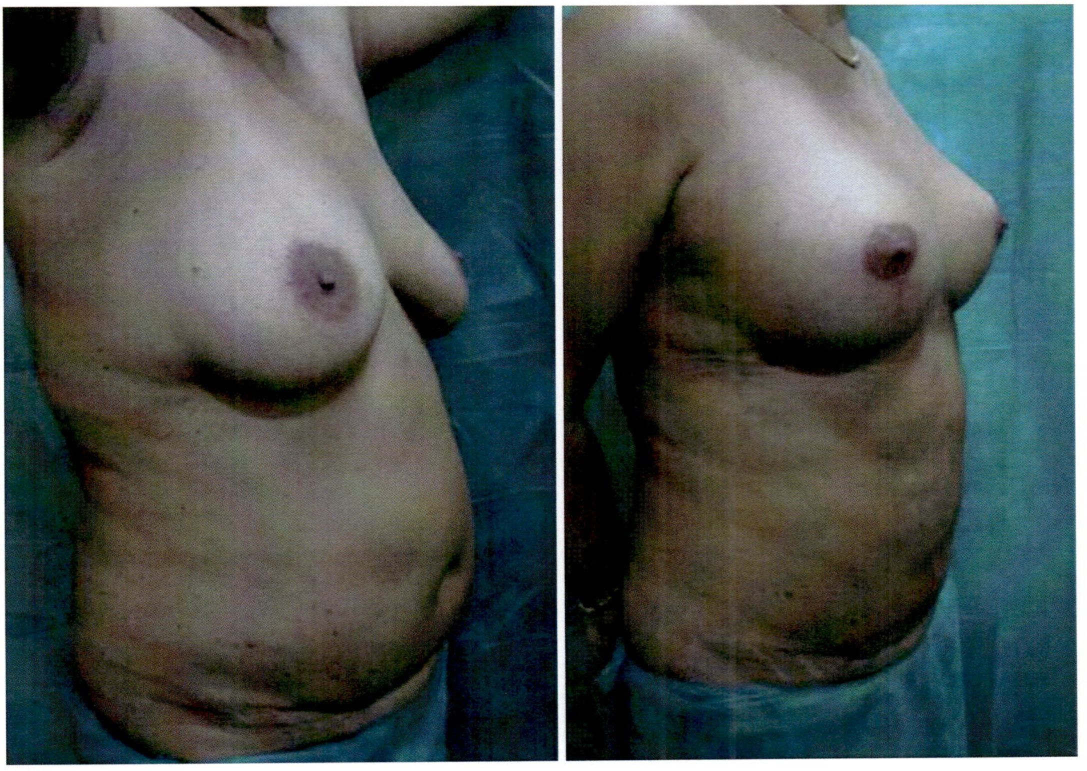

Fig. 33.11 Before and after small hypertrophy

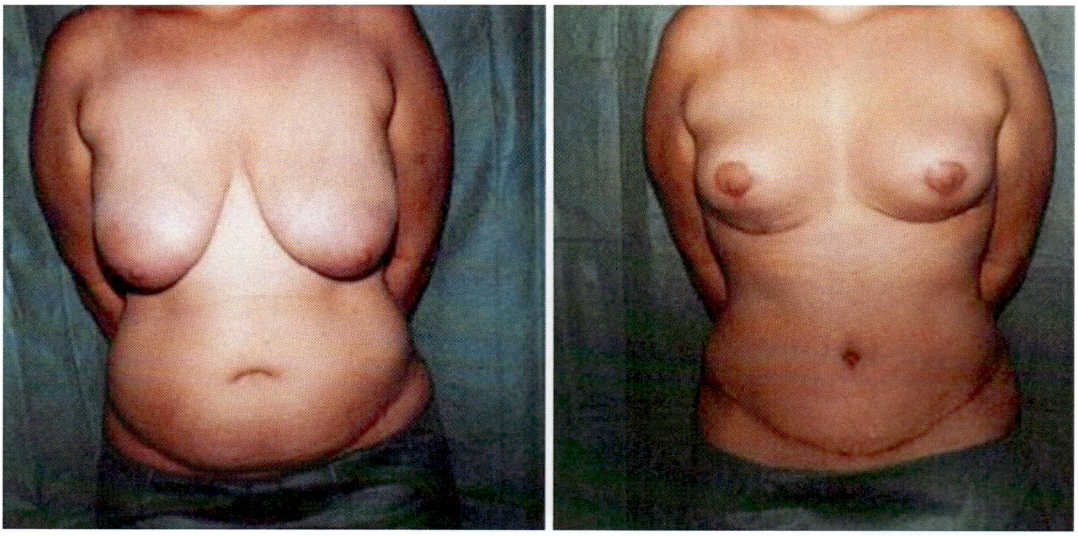

Fig. 33.12 Before and after medium hypertrophy

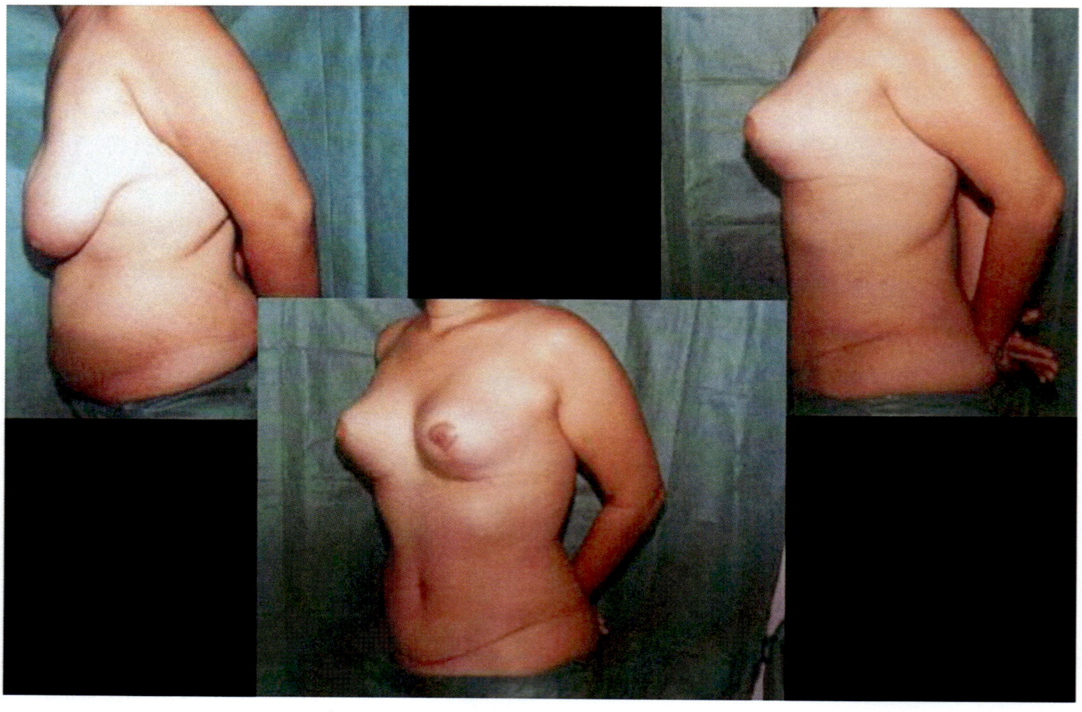

Fig. 33.13 Before and after medium hypertrophy

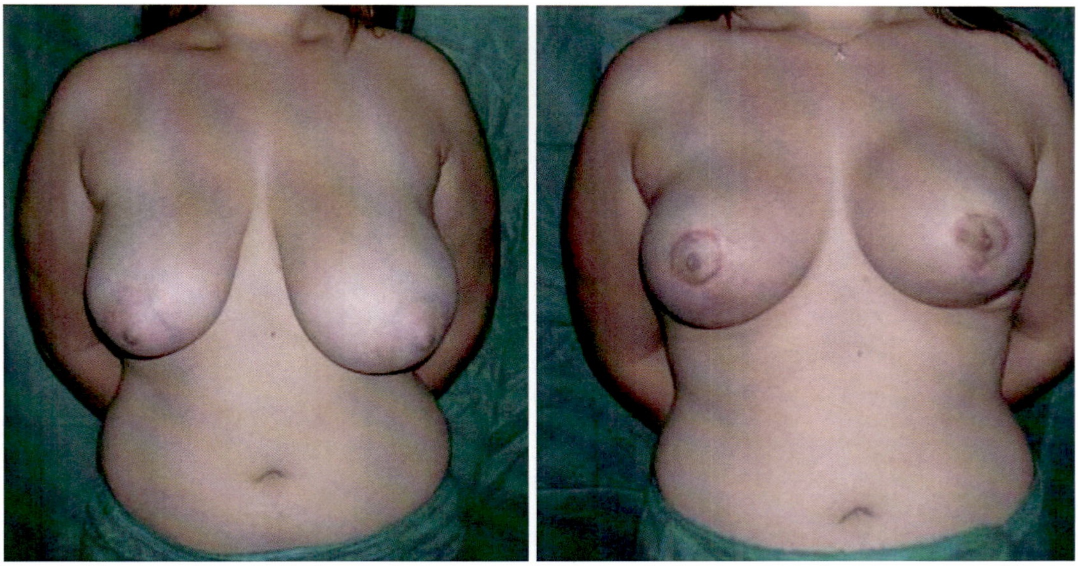

Fig. 33.14 Before and after medium hypertrophy

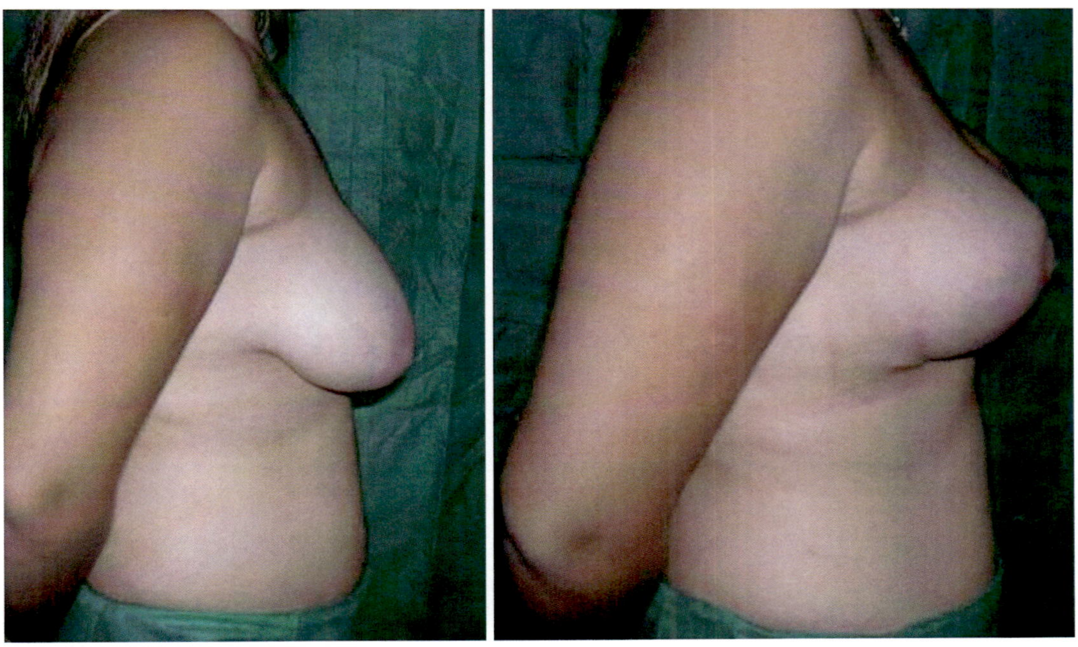

Fig. 33.15 Before and after medium hypertrophy

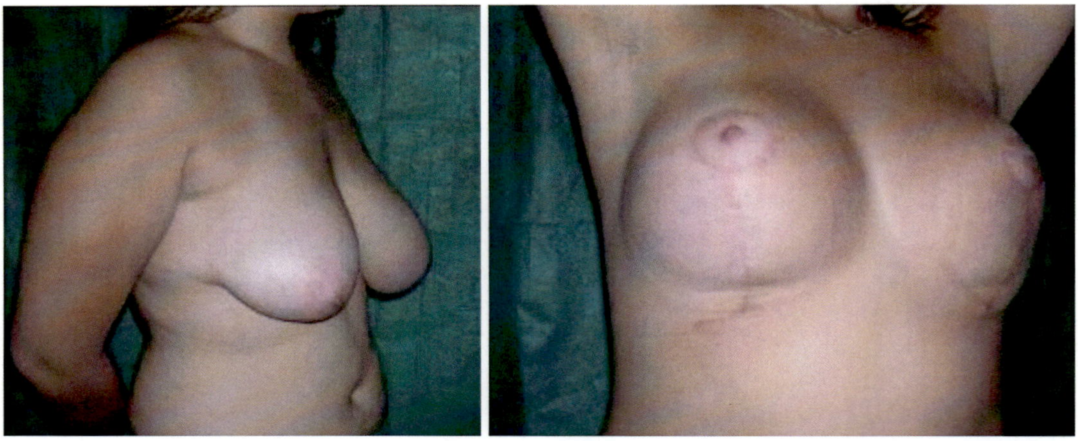

Fig. 33.16 Before and after medium hypertrophy

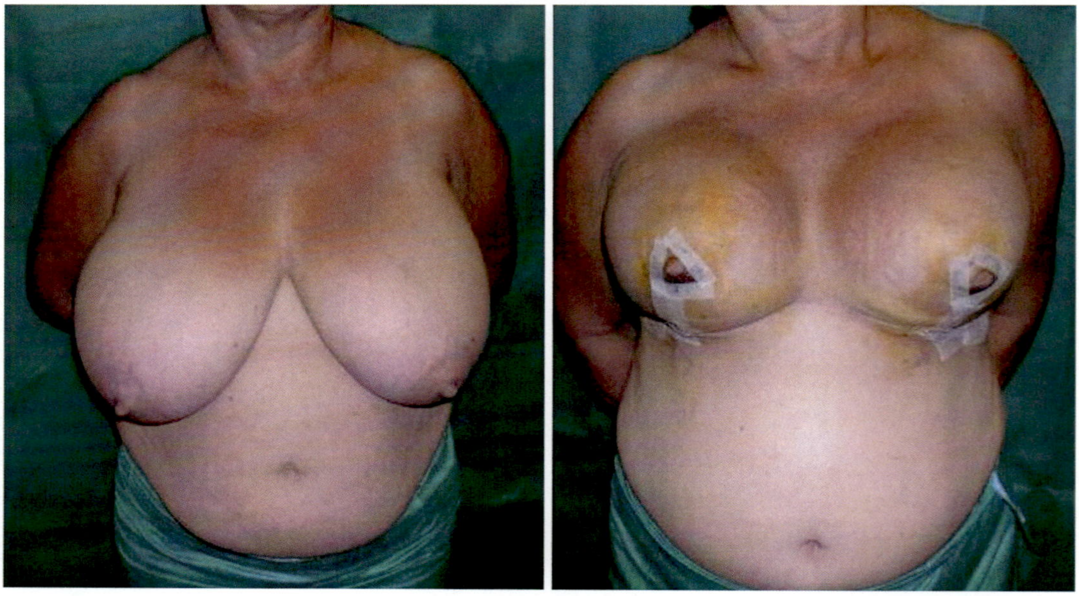

Fig. 33.17 Before and after large hypertrophy

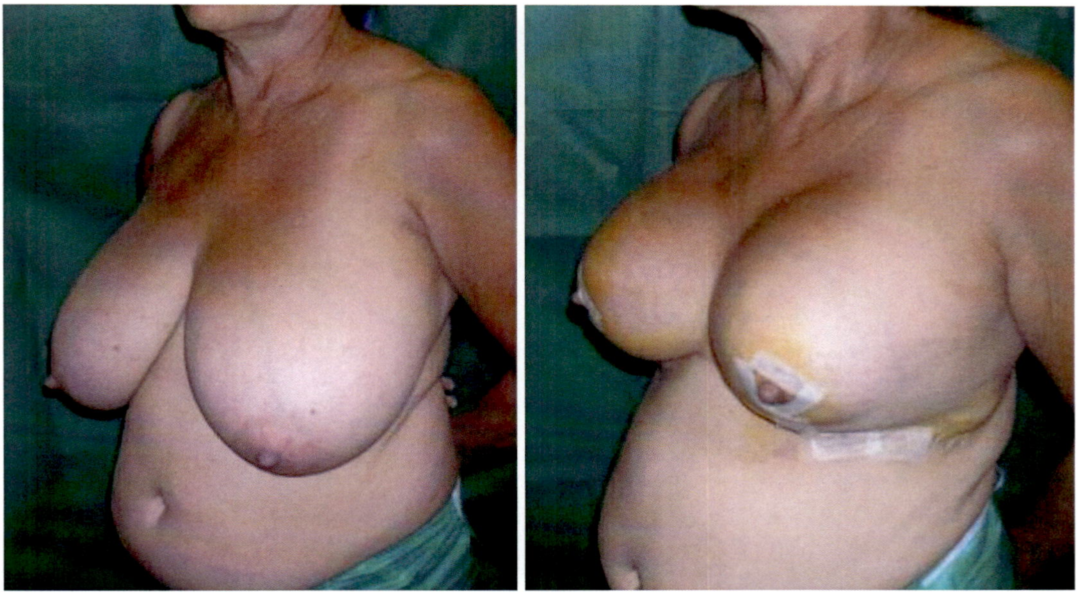

Fig. 33.18 Before and after large hypertrophy

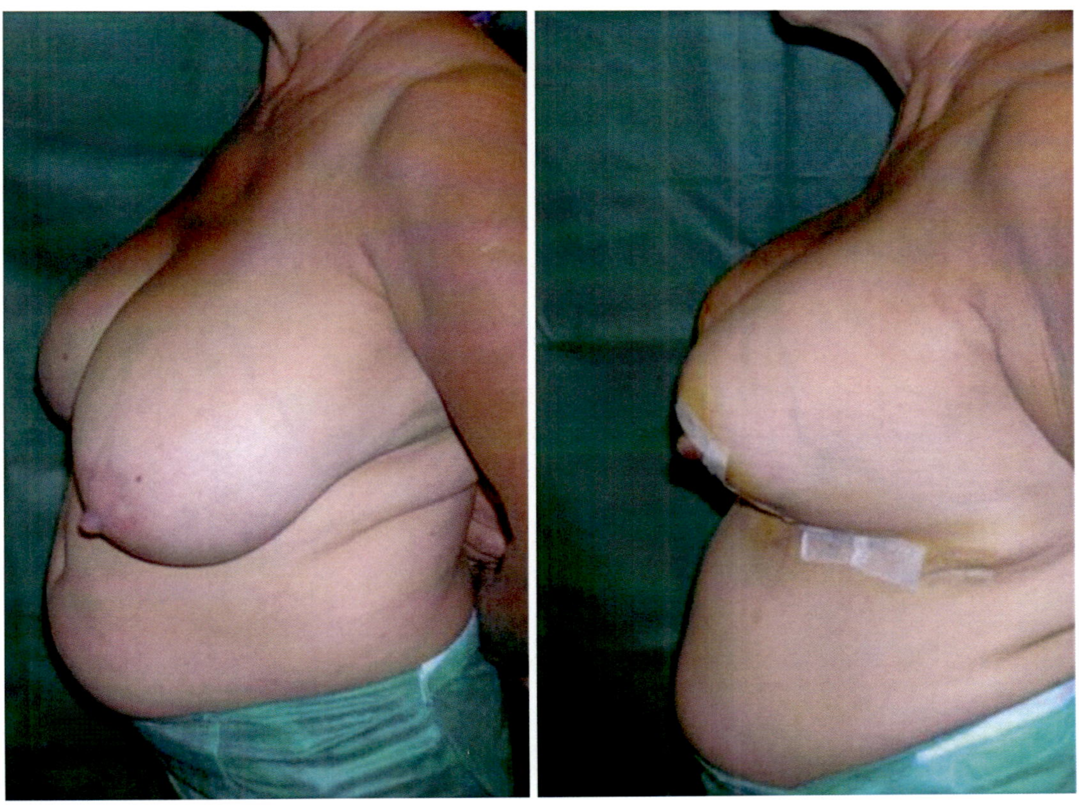

Fig. 33.19 Before and after large hypertrophy

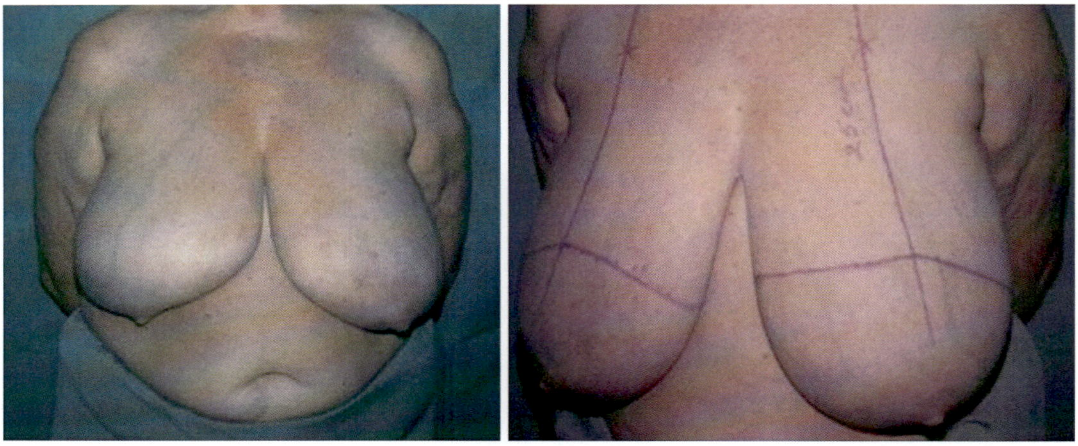

Fig. 33.20 Before and after large hypertrophy

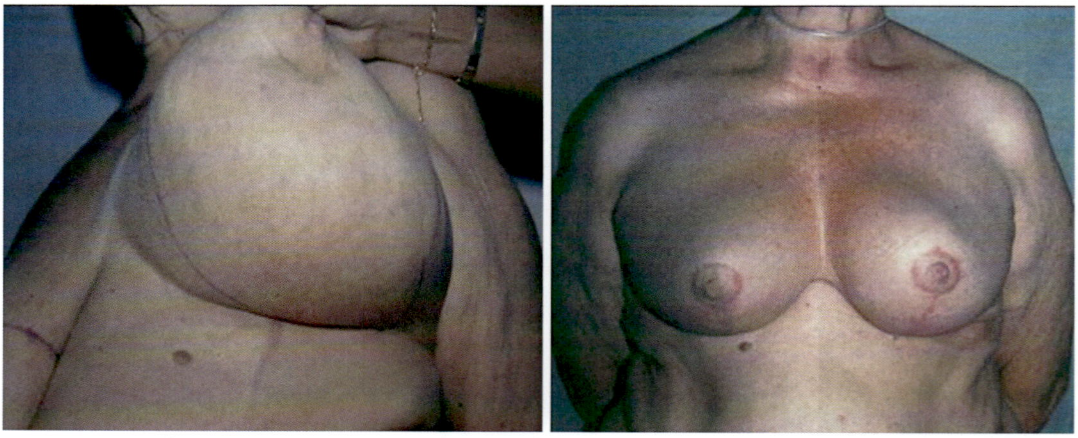

Fig. 33.21 Before and after large hypertrophy

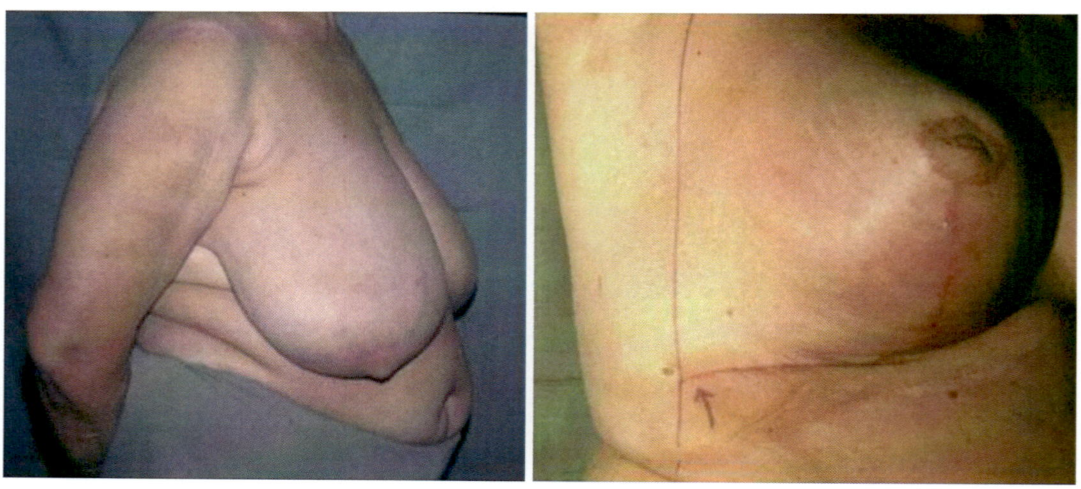

Fig. 33.22 Before and after large hypertrophy

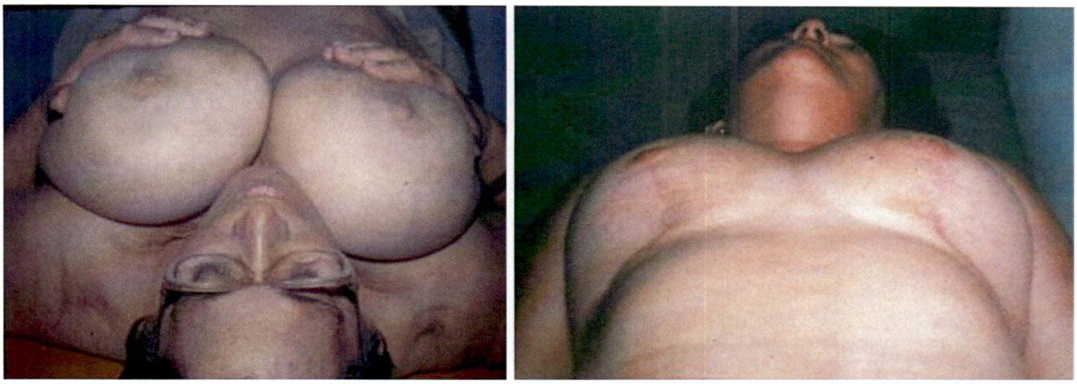

Fig. 33.23 Before and after large hypertrophy

33.4 Discussion

The L technique is a versatile procedure that can be performed easily and in a shorter surgical time, in patients with ptosis, small and medium hypertrophy, and, with skill and some tactical resources, in large hypertrophy.

At first, we noticed a certain flattening of the lateral pole, which was corrected when we came to resect more content of the medial pole, preserving sufficient breast tissue in the lateral pole, which when pulled and rotated medially, filled the space created, favoring the frame of the breast cone with effective filling of the upper pole, eliminating excess volume and allowing a graceful setting of the intermammary space. We usually call it INTERMEDIATE CANYON, which is very often required by patients who intend to display it at the neckline of their clothes.

After 33 years of working with this technique, we make 1600 g of reductions in each breast and never had difficulties with the elevation of the NAC, we do not feel the need to resort to the dermoglossous flap by Ribeiro (1975), or the interbreeding of flaps suggested by Sperli 1977 and Farid in 1983 with the intention of better filling the upper pole and providing better support.

More than 4000 patients were operated on using this technique and in a recent survey a sample of 100 patients found that a good aesthetic configuration was maintained, preserving the upper pole, with a small degree of ptosis, and inapparent scars. We only had one case of reoperation for ptosis correction at 6 years postoperatively, in a patient who became pregnant soon after surgery.

33.5 Complications

We had no severe complications, except in one case in which a subareolar hematoma caused suffering and complete necrosis of the areola and nipple, which had to be properly rebuilt. There were no complaints of loss of sensitivity. A few patients had hypertrophic scars and were treated with intracicatricial infiltration with corticosteroids. There were no cases of infection.

Conclusion

In our current routine, besides the Arié technique or the Arié–Pitanguy version for small ptosis, the L technique seems to be the best option for mastoplasties, because of both the objective aspects of aesthetic presentation that it offers, as in the fulfilment of the artistic sense of the surgeon and the great satisfaction of the patients that we have increasingly witnessed.

The resection of a greater volume of glandular content in the medial pole to be advanced to the lateral pole to fill the space, this allows the excess underarm extension to be corrected to sufficiently fill the upper pole and provide good fixation of the breast. It has been proven by 33 years of follow-up that these effects can be long-lasting.

References

Arié G (1957) The new Tactics of Mastoplastics. Lat Amer Cir Plast 3:23–28

Bozola AR, et al. (1992) Mastoplasty 1—personal contribution. Rev AMERIGS Porto Alegre 26(3):207–214

Bustos RA, Loureiro LEK, Thome CE (1985) Breast reduction of glandular retail trilobal inferior pedicle periareolar incision. In: XXII Cong transcript. Bras Cir Plast 44–489, Lawn—RS

Dufourmentel C, Mouly R (1961) Plastie mammaire par la methode oblique. Ann Chir Plast 6(1):45–48

Eulalio JN (1984) Breast reduction for pentagonal resection. In: The XXII Cong. Bras. Cir. Plast. 481/483. 1984, Rio de Janeiro, 82

Felicio de AY. (1984) Mamaplastia redutora com incisão periareolar. In: Anais da I Jornada Sul Brasileira de Cirurgia Plástica; Florianópolis. pp 307–311

Merriman Y (1984) Breast reduction with one areolar scar. Bras Cir Plast 481/483. Rio de Janeiro

Goes JCS (1989) Periareolar mammaplasty: double skin technique with mesh. Rev Soc Bras Cir Plast 13:9–13

Horibe K, Spina V, Lodovici O (1976) Breast reduction: Nueva Abordage delmetodo oblique side. Cir Plast Ib Lat Am II:7

Hakme F, Gomes BS, Muller P, ME S (1983) Technical L in ptosis Mmárias with making Retail Cruzado. Ver Bras Cir 73(2):37

Martins PDE (1989) Mastoplasty periareolar with patchwork transposition. In: Communication in Brazilian Congress. Cir. Plast., Blumenau—Santa Catarina

Pitanguy I (1963) Mammoplasty. Lat Am 7:139

Peixoto G (1980) Reduction mammaplasty the personal technique. Plast Reconst Surg 65:277

Ribeiro L (1975) A new technique for reduction mammaplasty. Plast Reconstr Surg 55(3):330–334

Strombeck J (1960) Mammaplasty: report of a new technique based on the two pedicle procedure. Br Plast Surg 13:79–90

Sperli A (1977) Mastoplasties Esthetic en las Ptosis. El boundary between el use them silicones y las mastopexies. In: 5th Cong. Arg. Cir. Aesthetics. Buenos Aires

34 Mastoplasty: Personal Technique with L Scar

Armando Chiari Jr.

34.1 Introduction

Breast reduction with an inverted T pattern has consistently resulted in a high degree of patient satisfaction in relation to shape and lasting results. However, the extensive incisions required have led plastic surgeons to seek short scar techniques. The elimination of the horizontal incisions certainly leads to more extensive vertical scars and to an excess of skin excess at the lower extremity of the scar. Especially in the cases of larger breasts, the elimination of the vertical incisions leads to areolar enlargement, scars of poor quality, and ptosis relapse.

The L short scar, or Chiari technique, seeks to maximize the utilization of the principle according to which the most important thing is what remains, not what is removed (Chiari 1992, 2001, 2002, 2013; Chiari and Grotting 2011). The resulting L scars are used for small, medium, and large reductions. The mini-l scars are used for mastopexies with the associated use of prosthesis. With reduced scars, this technique creates a good shape and good long-term results (see Figs. 34.7, 34.8, 34.9, 34.10 and 34.11), preserving breast sensitivity (Chiari 1992; Chiari et al. 2012) in a large series of patients.

This technique, which uses a superomedial transposition pedicle, an extensive undermining from the thoracic wall, and resects middle and inferior portions of the breast, is described.

A. Chiari Jr., M.D., Ph.D.
Department of Surgery, Medical School, Federal University of Minas Gerais, Rua Herculano de Freitas, Belo Horizonte, MG CEP 30441-039, Brazil
e-mail: chiari@chiari.com.br

34.2 Method

34.2.1 Preoperative Markings

The design of the skin that will remain is based on the design of the medial line *BC* and the more superiorly placed lateral line *B′C′* (Fig. 34.1). Markings are based on the midsternal line, the inframammary fold, and its projection on the anterior surface of the breast (point A), rather than on a predetermined pattern (Chiari 1992). Therefore, we delimit the amount of skin strictly necessary (Figs. 34.1 and see 34.3) for reshaping the medial (*line BC*) and the lateral (*line B′–C′*) portions of the breasts. After resection, these lines *BC* and *B′C′* are sutured together to form the vertical scar and a lateral dog ear (see Figs. 34.5 and 34.6).

With the patient in a standing position, the mid-mammary and midsternal lines are marked. Point A is marked on the projection of the submammary sulcus, on the mid-mammary line, and point A′ is marked 2 cm above it. Afterward, the patient is placed supine and all the following marks are made on a stretched skin (Chiari 1992, 2001, 2002, 2013; Chiari and Grotting 2011).

J.M. Avelar (ed.), *Breast Surgery*, https://doi.org/10.1007/978-3-319-54115-0_34

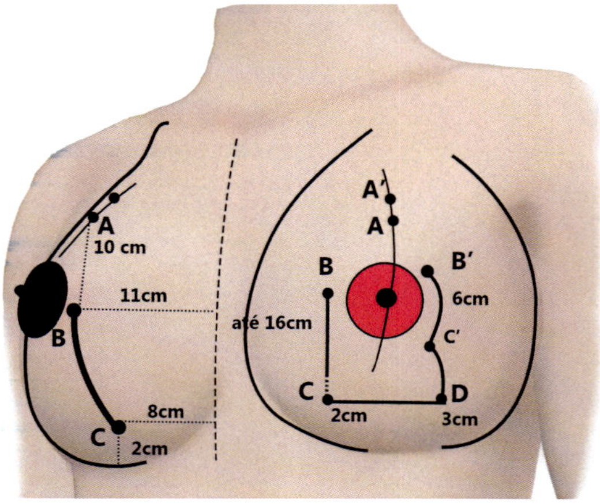

Fig. 34.1 Point A is the projection of the inframammary fold onto the anterior surface of the breast, with the patient standing. Point A′ is marked 2 cm above it. All the subsequent markings are made with the patient in a supine position, with the skin stretched. The main medial markings, line BC, refer to the midsternal line, to the inframammary sulcus, and to point A. The larger and more affected by ptosis the breast is, the longer line BC will be, and the closer point B′ should be from point A, with its lateral distance from the areola determined by trial and error. The formation of an adequate mammary cone is sought by uniting points B and B′ using bidigital maneuvers (Chiari 1992, 2001, 2002, 2013; Chiari and Grotting 2011).

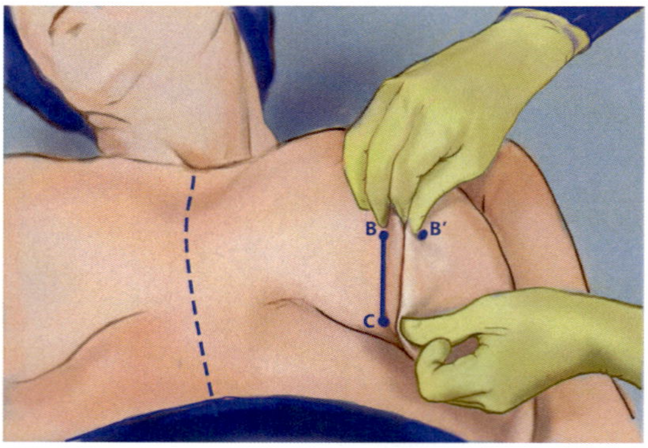

Fig. 34.2 Opposing point B to point B′ using bidigital maneuvers, we show the new breast cone, which must have good projection without tension

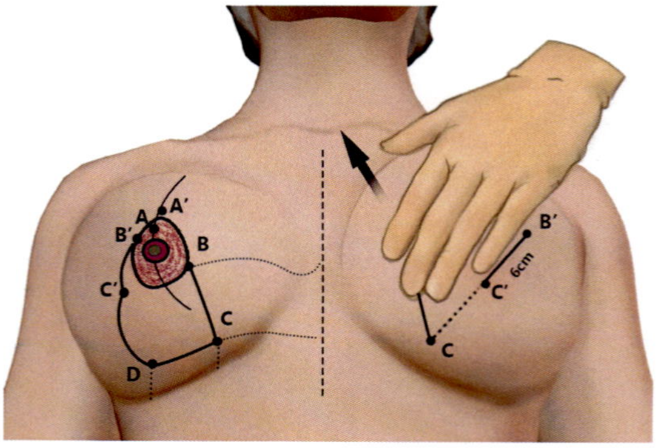

Fig. 34.3 Point B′ is marked between the nipple and point A. The larger and more affected by ptosis the breast is, the closer point B′ should be from point A. Line B′C′ has a length of 6.0 cm and is marked in the direction of point C, with the breast skin stretched in a superior and medial direction. The surgeon should check the adequacy of markings by bidigital maneuvers, bringing together the main lines BC and B′C′. Point C′ may have its position changed to a more lateral one, according to the surgeon's own feeling in relation to the quantity of skin that will remain

Point C is marked 8 cm from the midsternal line and 2 cm (for larger breasts) from the submammary sulcus (Fig. 34.1). Point B is marked 11 cm from the midsternal line and 10 cm from point A. The larger and more affected by ptosis the breast is, the longer line BC will be (Fig. 34.1). In bigger patients or in those whose chests are wider, the distance from points C and B to the midsternal line should increase from 8 and 11 cm to 9 and 12 cm or to 10 and 13 cm respectively.

Point B′ (Fig. 34.1) is marked between the nipple and point A, the larger and more affected by ptosis the breast is, the closer point B′ should be from point A (Fig. 34.1). The lateral distance from the areola is determined by trial and error: opposing point B to point B′ with bidigital maneuvers (Fig. 34.2) we show the new breast cone, which must have good projection without tension (Chiari 2002, 2013; Chiari and Grotting 2011). Point C′ is marked 6 cm from point B′, originating line B′C′C, with the breast skin stretched medially and upward (Fig. 34.3). The surgeon should check the adequacy of markings by bidigital maneuvers, bringing together the main lines BC and B′C′ (Fig. 34.2). Point C′ may have its position changed to a more lateral one, according to the surgeon's own feeling in relation to the quantity of skin that will remain.

Finally, point D is marked 3.0 cm from the inframammary sulcus (for larger breasts, Figs. 34.1 and 34.3), at the end of the skin fold that is formed by the union of lines BC and B′C′, by the use of bidigital maneuvers (Chiari 1992, 2001, 2002, 2013; Chiari and Grotting 2011). For patients whose breasts are smaller, the distances from points C and D to the inframammary sulcus are 1.0 cm and 1.5 cm respectively.

34.2.2 Surgical Technique

With the patients in a supine position, the skin bordered by points A, B, B′, and by a line extending 1.5 cm inferiorly, the new areola is de-epithelialized (Figs. 34.1 and 34.3), after marking the new areola within 4.3 cm. The skin is incised along line CD and the adipose capsule is dissected 1.0 cm caudally. This dissection is extended slantwise upward until above the inferior border of the pectoralis major muscle, preserving the mammary tissue adhered to the muscle fascia – enough to avoid retractions on line CD.

Then, the breast is extensively undermined at the level just above the pectoralis major muscle fascia up to the superior border of the breast. This undermining is prolonged medially and laterally, up to two resistant fascial structures. Laterally, this fascial structure is surgically isolated by using a blunt detacher. The chest anterolateral wall skin is detached about 6 cm horizontally, from the end of the incisions that originated the lateral branch of the L scar. The detachment should go beyond the anterior axillary line. From that point, the skin detachment is vertically turned aside, toward the corresponding axilla, about 7 cm (Chiari et al. 2012). The structure, isolated in that way, was called the lateral neurovascular pedicle of the breast (Chiari 1992) and contains blood vessels and the anterior divisions of the lateral cutaneous branches of the third, fourth, and fifth intercostal nerves (Chiari 1992; Chiari et al. 2012; Sarhadi et al. 1996; Würinger et al. 1998; McCulley and Rousseau 1999), which are important for nipple–areola sensitivity. In all techniques, incisions, resections, and detachments at the level of the anterior axillary line and beyond it involve a higher risk for lesions to this pedicle (Benelli 1990; Chiari 1992; Chiari et al. 2012; Sarhadi et al. 1996; Würinger et al. 1998; McCulley and Rousseau 1999).

The patients are placed in a semi-sitting position for the parenchymal resection. The breasts are pulled upward, from point A (Figs. 34.4 and 34.5). Mammary resection starts through an incision made along line C′D, which continues vertically toward the chest. The glandular incisions along lines BC and B′C′ converge at 60° to the thoracic wall (Fig. 34.4; Chiari 1992, 2001, 2002, 2013;

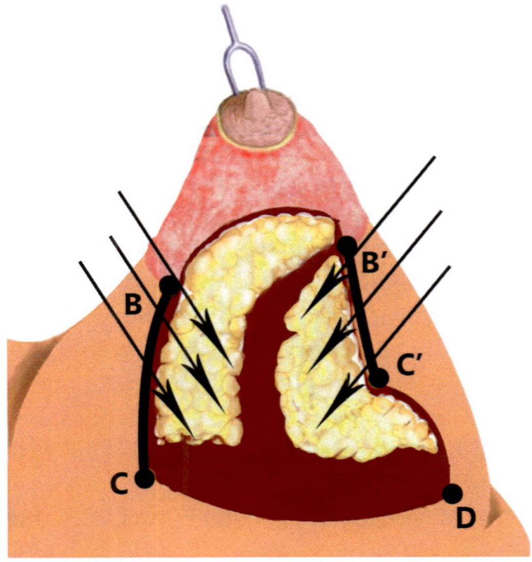

Fig. 34.4 Incisions from lines BC and B′C′ converge in the mammary tissue at 60° toward the chest (Chiari 1992, 2001, 2002, 2013; Chiari and Grotting 2011). An incision or a resection of the necessary mammary tissue is made in the superior pole, (Chiari 1992, 2001, 2002, 2013; Chiari and Grotting 2011) between the areola and point B′

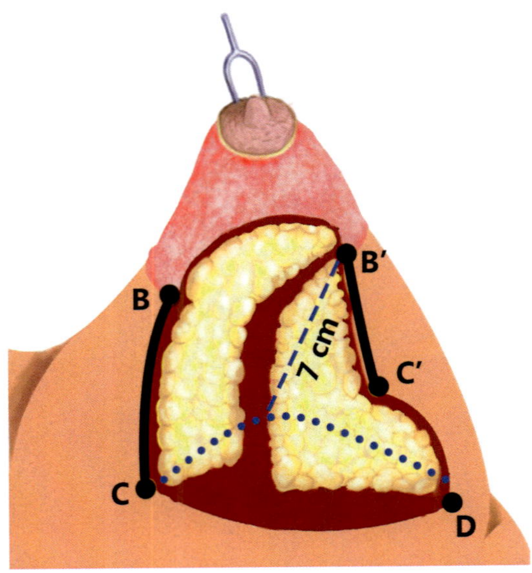

Fig. 34.5 Left breast with the main oblique incisions made in the mammary tissue. The bases of the pillars formed (*horizontal blue lines*) are resected, making them 7 cm in height

Chiari and Grotting 2011), retaining a portion of glandular tissue in the upper pole and beneath the nipple–areola complex (NAC) and inferiorly two pillars of mammary tissue, which, when brought together, provide the bulk of the breast. In breasts with a firm parenchyma, an incision or a resection of the necessary mammary tissue is made in the superior pole (Chiari 1992, 2001, 2002, 2013; Chiari and Grotting 2011), between the areola and point B′ (Figs. 34.4 and 34.5). The bases of the pillars formed are resected, making them an average of 7 cm high (Fig. 34.5). When performing this maneuver, good care should be taken to preserve the lateral neurovascular pedicle of the breast (Chiari 1992; Chiari et al. 2012; Sarhadi et al. 1996; Würinger et al. 1998; McCulley and Rousseau 1999).

After careful hemostasis and beginning at the bases, the medial and lateral pillar bases are sutured together, in addition to lines BC and B′C′, forming the vertical stem of the L scar (Figs. 34.5 and 34.6). When it comes to large breasts with elastic skin, the lateral line B′C′, which is 6 cm long, is sutured to the much longer line BC (Fig. 34.1); the compensation folds that result from this skin compensation disappear around the third postoperative month (Chiari 2013).

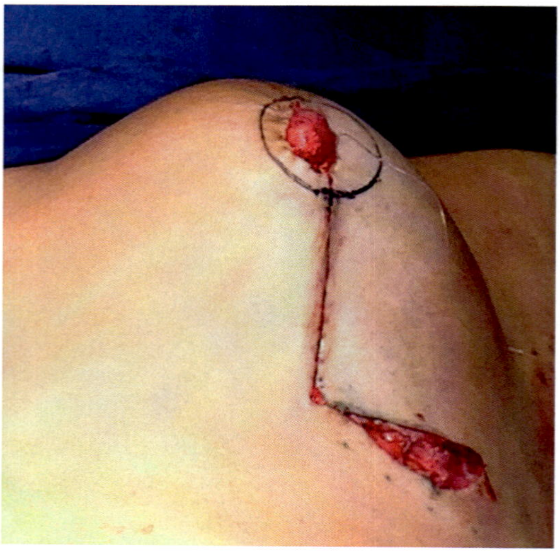

Fig. 34.6 The medial line BC was sutured to the lateral line B′C′, originating the vertical stem of the L-shaped scar. A temporary skin compensation pouch is made using more medial skin (Chiari 1992, 2001, 2002, 2013; Chiari and Grotting 2011) to achieve a well-projected mammary cone top, without tension. The new areolar position is marked within 3.6 cm and de-epithelialized with the vertex at one point between A and A′, according to the surgeon's own feeling in relation to the quantity of skin that will remain

A temporary skin compensation pouch is made using more medial skin, (Chiari 1992, 2001, 2002, 2013; Chiari and Grotting 2011) to achieve a well-projected mammary cone top, without tension (Fig. 34.6). The new position of the areola is marked within 3.6 cm and de-epithelialized, with the vertex in one point between A and A′, according to the surgeon's own feeling in relation to the quantity of skin that will remain (Fig. 34.6).

The amount of periareolar skin removed is small, being much bigger in the middle and inferior parts of the breast (Chiari 1992, 2001, 2002, 2013; Chiari and Grotting 2011). A continuous circular intradermal suture (Benelli 1990; Chiari 2002, 2013; Chiari and Grotting 2011) is applied with colorless 4–0 Monocryl®, fixed within 4.3 cm, to prevent areolar enlargement and to rotate the skin that remains at the top of the mammary cone from medial to lateral. In some cases with more tension at the top, I still use colorless 4–0 Mononylon® (Chiari 2013). The areola is placed within the limits of the four cardinal points.

At the superior margin of the lateral skin fold, it is necessary to resect a skin compensation triangle to raise and adjust the lower edge of the L-shaped horizontal scar to the new sulcus (Fig. 34.6) (Chiari 1992, 2013).

34.3 Discussion

In 200 women examined, the average length of the chest width was 32 cm. Dividing this distance by 4, resulted in 8 cm, which is the distance of point C from the midsternal line, near the submammary sulcus. At this level, in a frontal view, because the thorax is curved in the lateral portions, 8 cm seems to place point C (and along with it the vertical stem of the L-shaped scar and the areola) a little lateral to the middle of each hemithorax. This position is important for eliminating the medial surplus skin resected in the classic inverted T techniques and at the same time, for positioning the breasts more laterally and not straight ahead (Chiari 1992).

Points C and C′ are united at the level of the submammary sulcus (Figs. 34.1, 34.3, and 34.6) and points B and B′ are united at the level of the new areola (Figs. 34.1, 34.3, and 34.6). At this point, the breast must be designed with more skin (11 cm and not 8 cm) to project the breast from the thorax (Chiari 1992).

Line B′C′ is traced on distended skin with a length of 6.0 cm (Figs. 34.1 and 34.3). With the breast remodeled and without skin distention, the vertical stem of the L-shaped scar (originated by the union and compensation of lines BC and B′C′) will have an average length of 5.0 cm (Fig. 34.6). Therefore, we delimit the amount of skin that is strictly necessary (Figs. 34.1, 34.3 and 34.6) to reshape the medial (line BC) portion of the breasts (Chiari 1992, 2001, 2002, 2013; Chiari and Grotting 2011).

Since 1988 I have operated on 1,476 patients aged 13–68 years. The technique has attained a good shape and projection, with patients having a considerable degree of skin elasticity, even in patients with large hypertrophy (over 600 g) and severe ptosis (Figs. 34.7, 34.8, 34.9, 34.10 and 34.11). It is possible for patients with insufficient skin elasticity and those with severe ptosis to achieve a good result if we draw line BC no longer than 8.0 cm. The resulting surplus skin in the inferomedial pole is removed by resection of a medial dog ear that is only de-epithelialized. The resultant scar has an L-T shape, always smaller than a classic inverted T scar (Chiari 1992, 2002; Chiari and Grotting 2011).

Especially in the cases of larger breasts, the elimination of the horizontal incisions in the

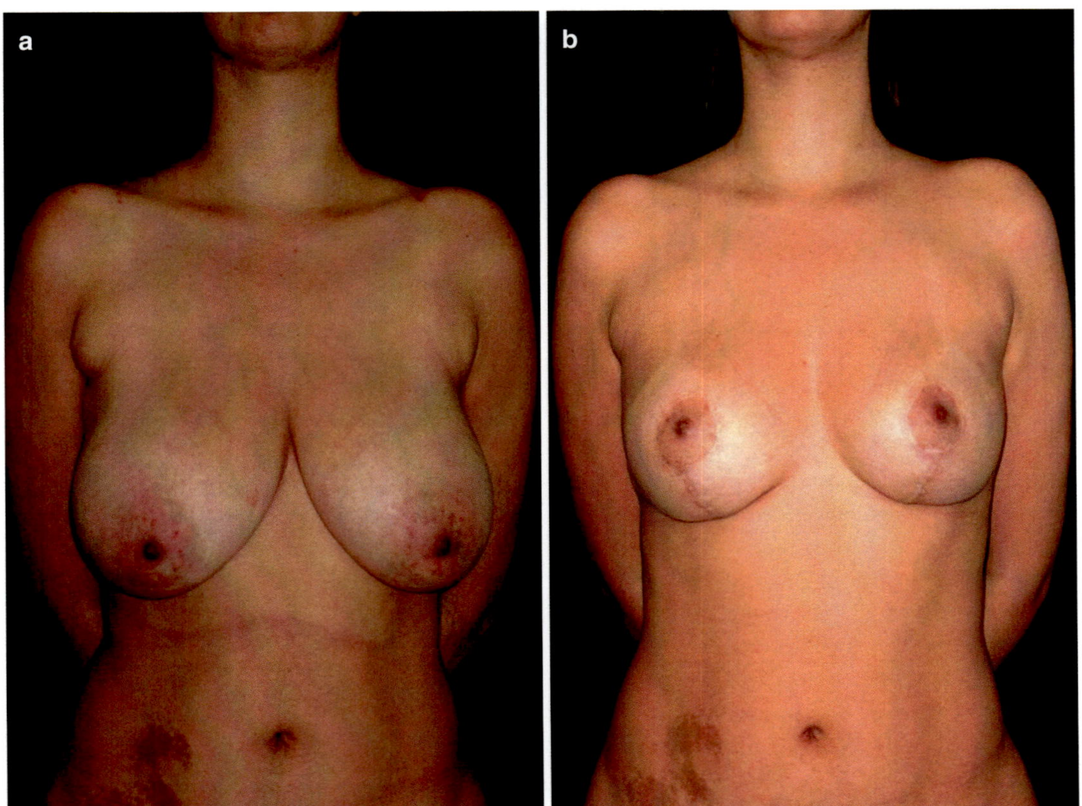

Fig. 34.7 A 27-year-old patient, before (*left*) and 6 months after (*right*) resection of 600 g from the right breast and 630 g from the left breast, with the resulting L-shaped scars

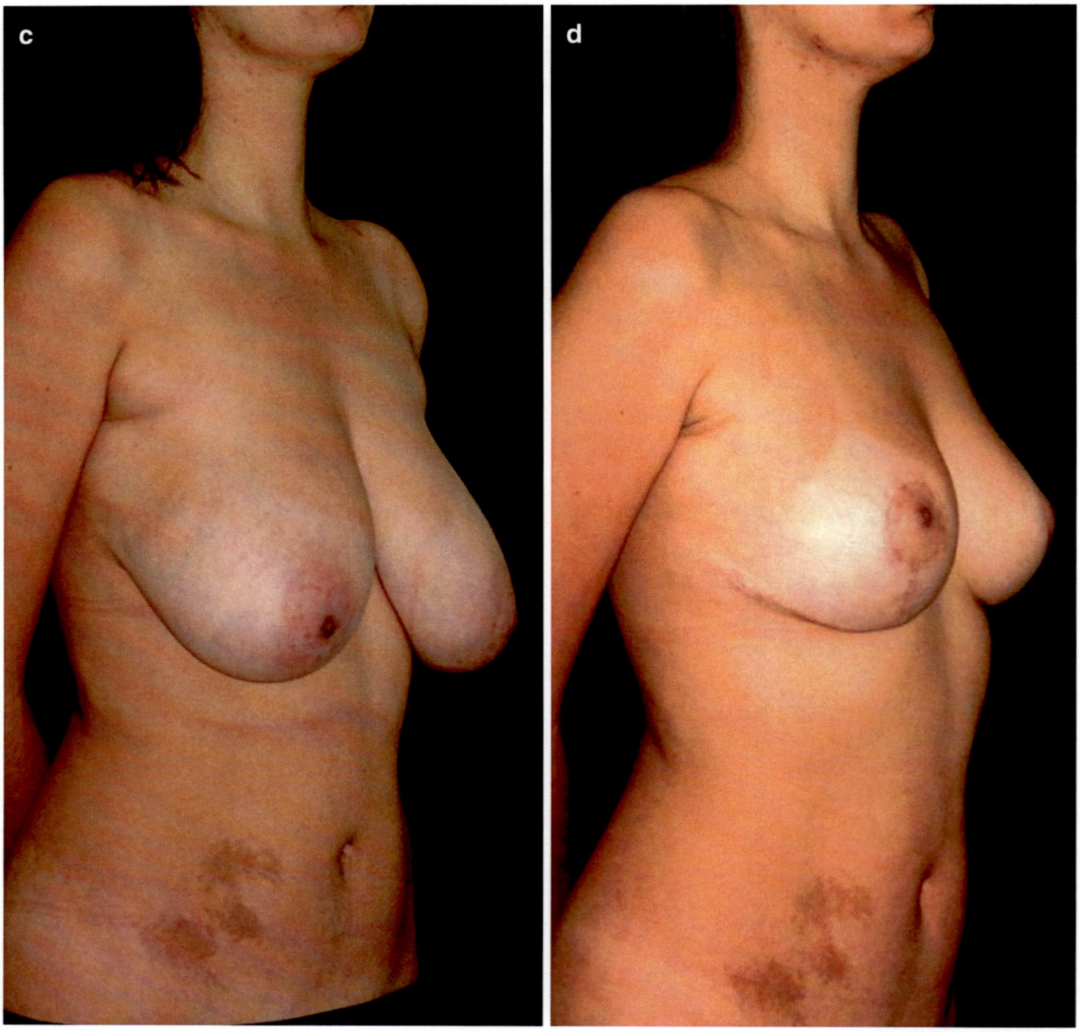

Fig. 34.7 (continued)

vertical scar techniques can lead to more extensive vertical scars, excessive curvature of the inferior poles, and to excess skin in the lower extremity of the scar. In Brazil, large parts of the body are exposed all year round and I think that we cannot ask the patient to wait for skin accommodation or a better shape. In my opinion, surgeons must do their best to obtain a good shape and an excellent projection in the operating room.

Between 1999 and 2003, the vertical and the mini-L variants of the technique were emphasized (Figs. 34.9 and 34.11) and shown in two publications by Chiari (2001, 2002). In some patients with fatter mammary content, poor skin elasticity, and more severe ptosis, there was apparently good accommodation of the skin in the operating room, but time and gravity caused a curvature of the inferior poles, with ptosis relapse and areolar enlargement. Routine indication for a suture in a periareolar pouch (Benelli 1990) with colorless 4–0 Mononylon® minimized, but did not solve the problem (Chiari 2013). Nowadays, the markings of the variants with mini-L and vertical scars (Chiari 2001, 2002) are indicated, especially for mastopexies with the associated use of prosthesis.

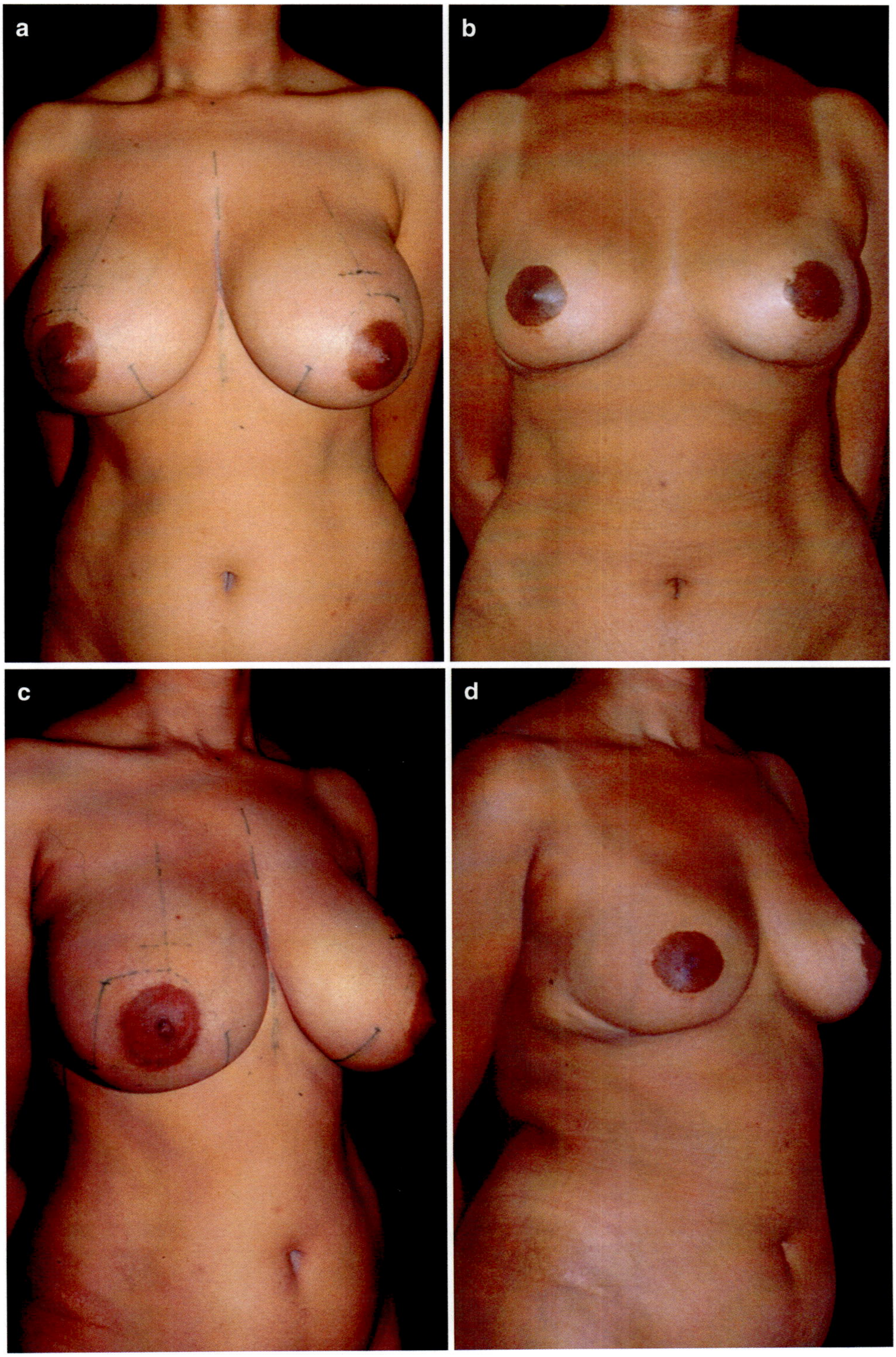

Fig. 34.8 A 22-year-old patient, before (*left*) and 5.5 years after (*right*) resection of 560 g from the left breast and 590 g from the right breast, with the resulting L-shaped scars

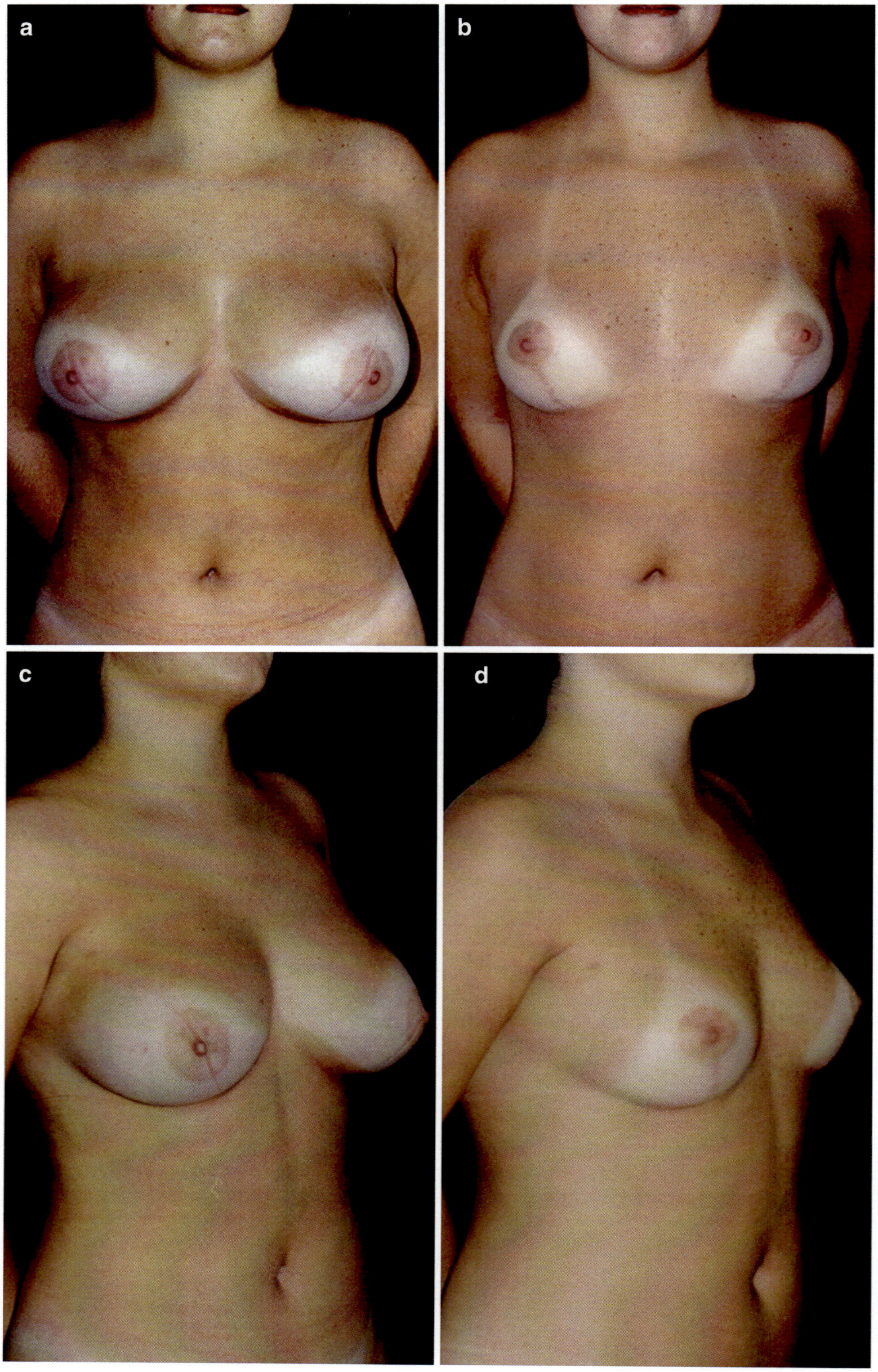

Fig. 34.9 A 21-year-old patient, before (*left*) and 12 months after (*right*) resection of 210 g from the right breast and 240 g from the left breast, with the resulting mini-L-shaped scars

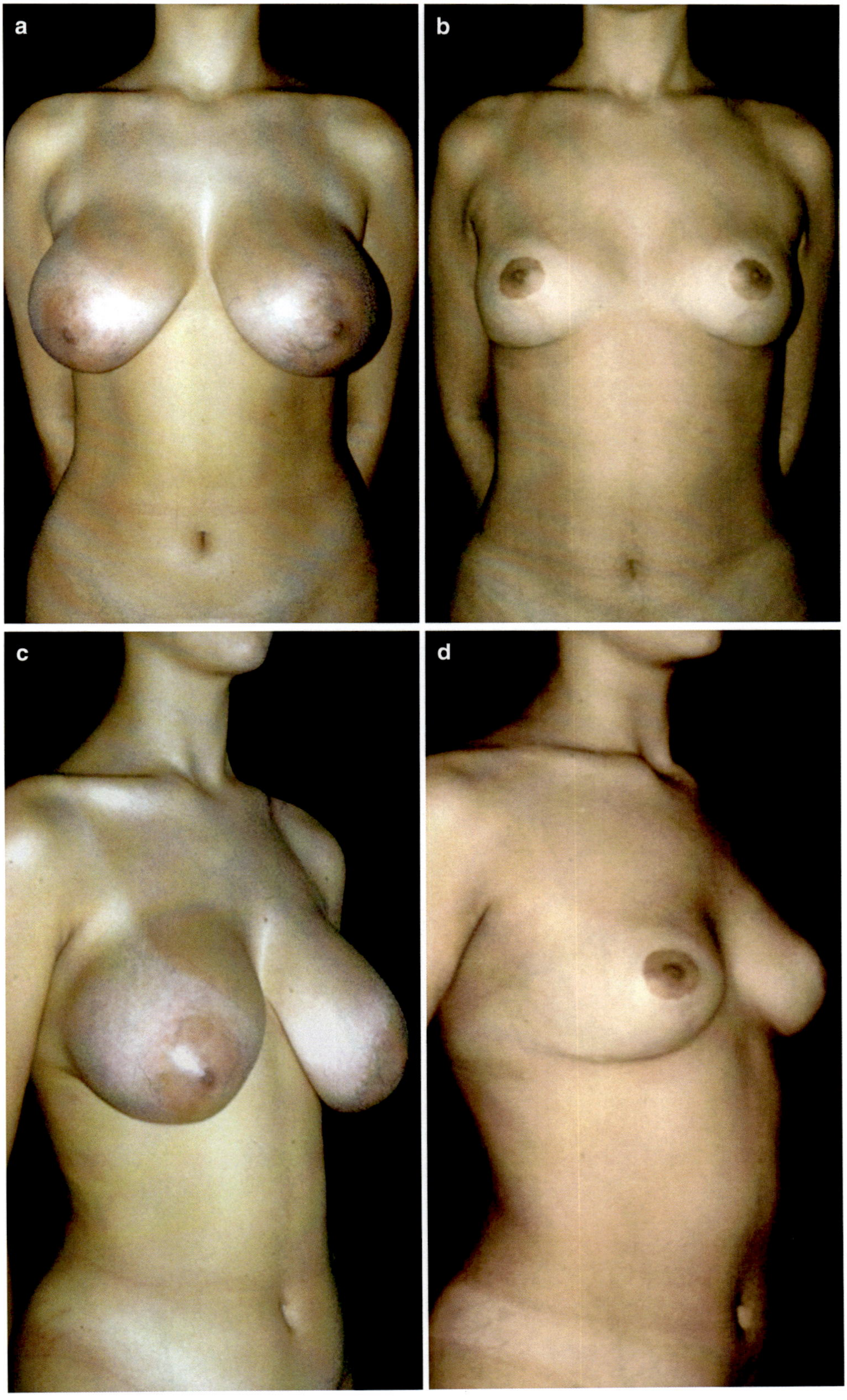

Fig. 34.10 A 23-year-old patient, before (*left*) and 3 years after (*right*) resection of 610 g from the left breast and 480 g from the right breast, with the resulting L-shaped scars

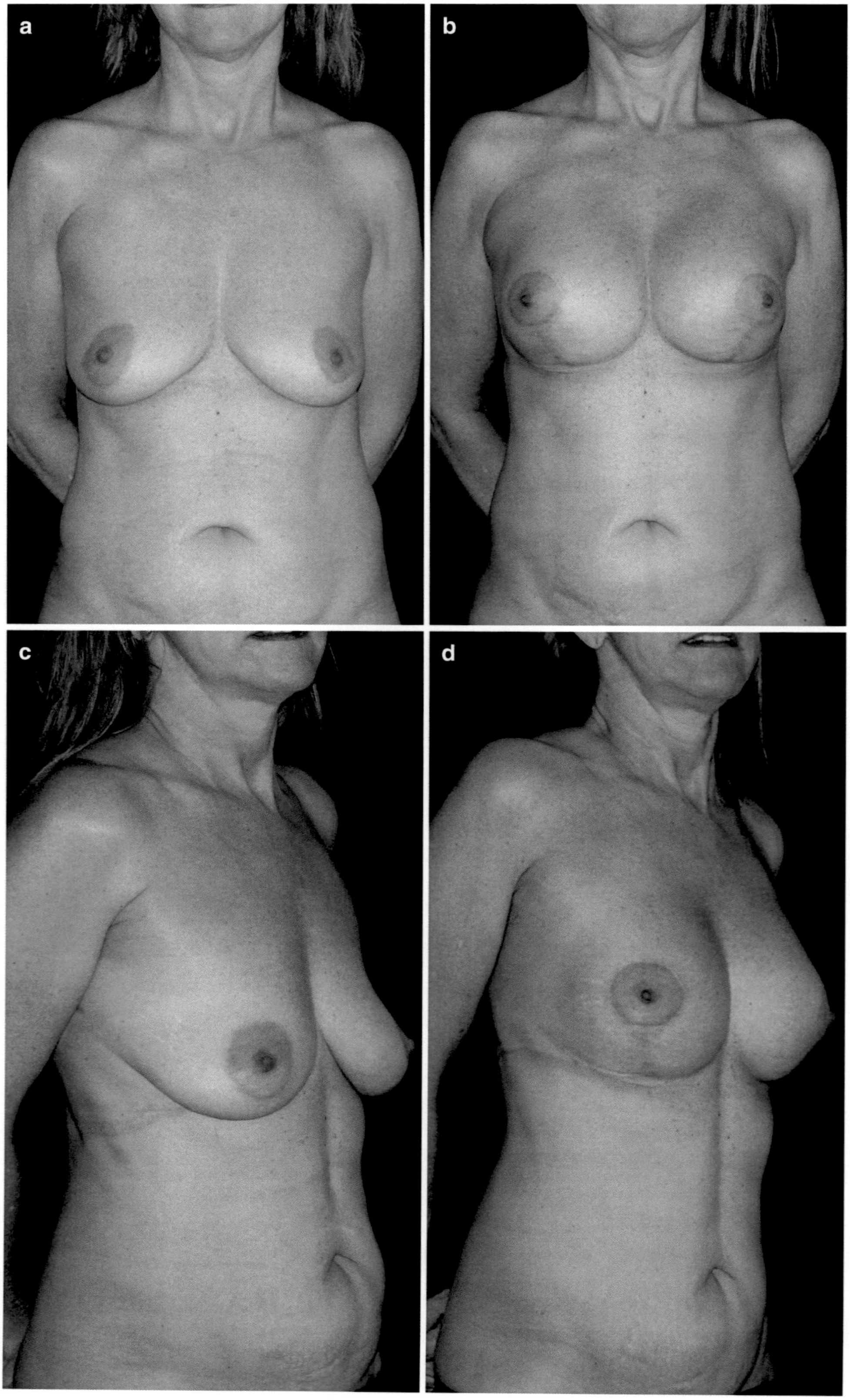

Fig. 34.11 A 53-year-old patient, before (*left*) and 2 years after (*right*) resection of 61 g from the left breast and 46 g from the right breast, associated with the use of 220 cc silicone implants and the resulting mini-L-shaped scars

34.4 Complications

Areolar enlargement, bad periareolar scars, and early ptosis relapse are avoided by resection of a small amount of skin at the top of the mammary cone.

Sensitivity of the NAC has been consistently retained by maneuvers adopted to preserve the lateral neurovascular pedicle of the breast (Chiari 1992; Chiari et al. 2012; Würinger et al. 1998).

No hematomas developed because I ensure that good hemostasis is carried out.

Small sloughing of the areola may rarely occur and is treated conservatively with daily dressings with good lubrication and carboxytherapy.

Most patients that could be followed up breast-fed their babies, but with a smaller amount of milk; the success rate of postoperative breast feeding is unknown.

Conclusions

By marking the skin that will remain, the Chiari or L short scar mammaplasty makes it possible to carry out large resections in the middle and inferior parts of breasts, rendering removal of excessive amounts of periareolar skin unnecessary. As a result, the scars are short, with elimination of the medial limb, a shortened lateral limb, an undistorted areola, and with adequate length of the vertical stem of the L, without surplus skin in the inferior pole of the breast.

This technique creates a good shape and long-term results, preserving breast sensitivity, in a large series of patients, including large-breasted ones.

References

Benelli L (1990) A new periareolar mammaplasty: the "round block" technique. Aesthetic Plast Surg 14:93–100

Chiari A Jr (1992) The L short-scar mammaplasty: a new approach. Plast Reconstr Surg 90:233–246

Chiari A Jr (2001) The L short-scar mammaplasty: 12 years later. Plast Reconstr Surg 108:489–495

Chiari A Jr (2002) The L short-scar mammoplasty. Clin Plast Surg 29:401–409

Chiari A Jr (2013) The L short-scar mammaplasty. In: Neligan PC (ed) Plastic surgery, vol 5, 3rd edn. Elsevier Saunders, New York, pp 206–215

Chiari A Jr, Grotting J (2011) The L short-scar mammaplasty. In: Spear SL (ed) Surgery of the breast. principles and art, 3rd edn. Lippincott WillIams & Wilkins, Philadelphia, pp 1128–1143

Chiari A Jr, Nunes TA, Grotting J, Cotta FB, Gomes RCB (2012) Breast sensitivity before and after the L short-scar mammaplasty. Aesthetic Plast Surg 36: 105–114

McCulley SJ, Rousseau TE (1999) A modified Chiari L short-scar mammoplasty—the technique and results. Br J Plast Surg 52:112–117

Sarhadi NS et al (1996) An anatomical study of the nerve supply of the breast, including the nipple and areola. Br J Plast Surg 49:156–164

Würinger E, Mader N, Posch E, Holle J (1998) Nerve and vessel supplying ligamentous suspension of the mammary gland. Plast Reconstr Surg 101:1486–1493

35 Inferior Pedicle to Improve Mastoplasty

Marcelo Paulo Vaccari Mazzetti,
Ryane Schmidt Brock, and Rayssa Sauaia

35.1 Introduction

The new era of breast reduction or mastoplasty was introduced by Pitanguy's technique and principles in the last century. Before him, several other authors have described methods trying to find an efficient and safe surgical method of reducing and uplifting breast hypertrophy (Pitanguy 1959, 1967; Lexer 1912; Kausch 1916; Avelar 1993).

Pitanguy achieved this goal with his principles and technique, which are known all over the world. We used to follow Pitanguy's surgical principles associated with an inferior pedicle flap with de-epithelialized dermis, subcutaneous, and mammary tissue.

The technique of an inferior pedicle was perfected in the second half of the past century by Sinder (1970, 1974) and later by Ribeiro and Backer (1973) and Ribeiro et al. (2002). Many authors contributed to the development of this technique, presenting important contributions several years later (Graf et al. 2000; Rohrich 2006).

Our long-term postoperative results demonstrated new breast ptosis with loss of superior breast projection, especially in large and moderate sized breasts. The gravitational force and human posture led to an initial loss of result. Motivated to avoid this problem, we adopted this technique 10 years ago (Fig. 35.1).

With the acquired experience, we noticed that the superior pedicle is very versatile, not only for remodeling, but also to maintain a long-lasting result, increase the mammary upper or superolateral pole, elevate the superior abdominal wall and it is also useful for compensating for breast glandular loss in lateral columns after tumor resection, nodular or cystic excision and over-resection during mammoplasty (Avelar 1980). It can also be useful for patients after gastroplasty and severe weight loss.

The ptosed tissue can be transformed into an authentic autogenous "mammary implant" and it can be positioned to increase antero-posterior breast projection and the medial breast pole.

M.P.V. Mazzetti, M.D., M.Sc. (✉) • R.S. Brock, M.D., M.Sc. • R. Sauaia, M.D.
Defeitos da Face Studies and Research Center, Department of Plastic Surgery, Ceci Avenue, 475, São Paulo, SP 04065000, Brazil
e-mail: dr.marcelovaccari@gmail.com

J.M. Avelar (ed.), *Breast Surgery*, https://doi.org/10.1007/978-3-319-54115-0_35

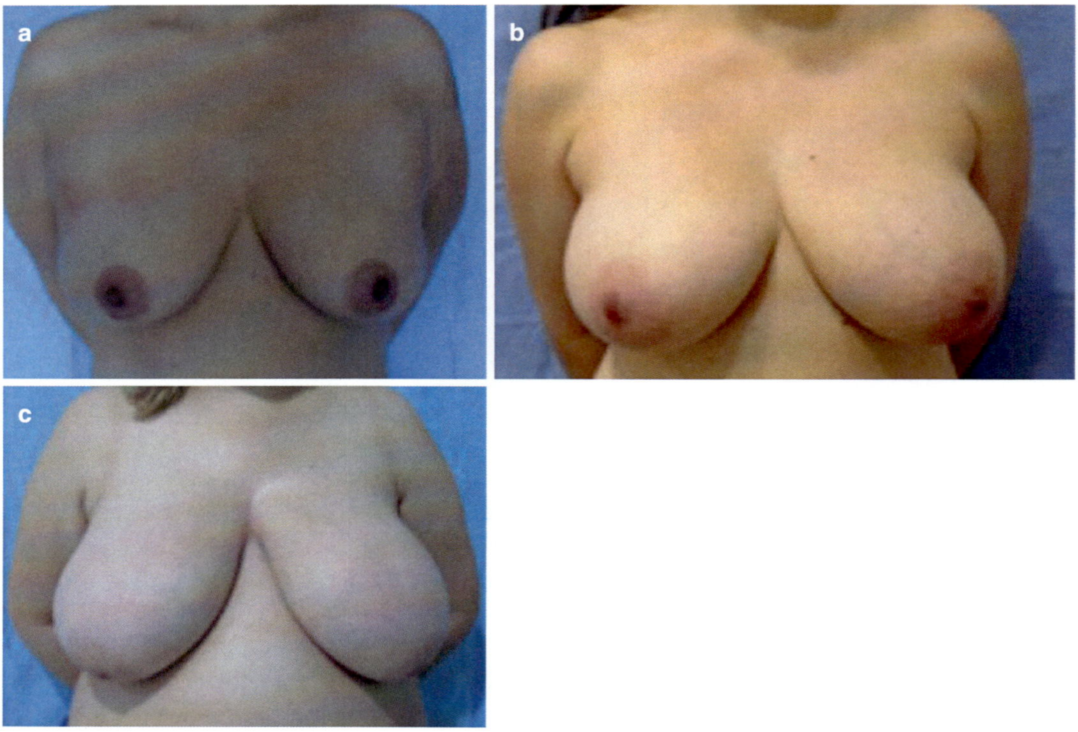

Fig. 35.1 Different types of breast ptosis and grades of hypertrophy. All these patients were subjected to the inferior pedicle technique: (**a**) and (**b**) had no glandular resection and (**c**) had a reduction in volume

35.2 Methods

35.2.1 Surgical Principles

We follow Pitanguy's principles and the technique involving an inferior pedicle, with personal modifications, such as:

1. The surgical marking must be made according the surgeon's creativity and customized for each patient.
2. Determining Pitanguy's point A is key and the first point of reference for other demarcation points.
3. The resection of the mammary gland, when necessary, is performed as a "keel" incision in the median line.
4. Creation of two mammary columns on each side of the mammary gland, which are essential after creation of the inferior pedicle and/or gland resection.
5. Creation of the "third pedicle" on the upper pole of the breast, which provides adequate vascular support to the remaining mammary gland after creation of the inferior pedicle and/or gland resection.
6. Creation of the inferior pedicle.
7. Fixation of the inferior pedicle to an anterior portion of the second costal arch.
8. The remaining mammary gland maintains anatomical communication with the galactophorous ducts and nipple.
9. The two mammary columns are sutured between each other and over the inferior pedicle, including it in the inferior sutures.
10. No "dead space" is present after the suturing of the inferior pedicle and mammary columns.
11. No cutaneous undermining.

35.2.2 Surgical Markings

During the preoperative period, all patients are photographed and marked according to Pitanguy's technique in an orthostatic position. The marking consists of the definition of points A, B, and C and then a continuous line extended below from B and C to the mammary fold to determine the inferior pedicle (Figs. 35.2 and 35.3) (Pitanguy 1967).

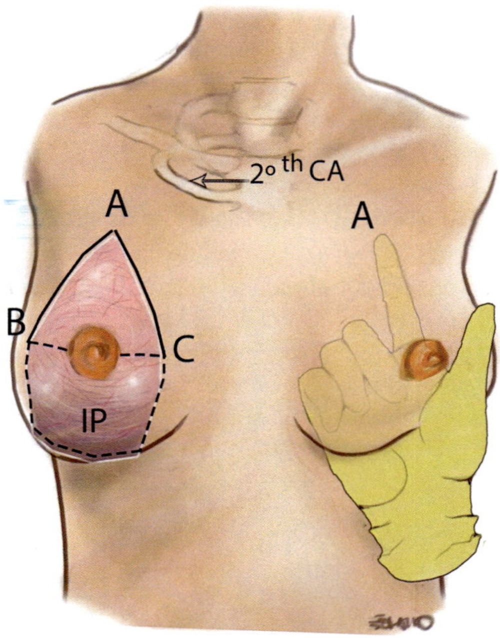

Fig. 35.2 Drawing demonstrating the marking points "A", "B" and "C" and straigth lines down to inframammary fold to delimited the inferior pedicle. Marking A point with finger projection of the inframammary fold and the projection of the second costal arch (2th CA), where the inferior pedicle will be attached

Point A: the upper point, the superior areolar edge should correspond to the projection of the inframammary fold and it must be at the line drawn 4–5 cm from the midline at the clavicular projection point passing by the nipple.

Points B and C are the lateral and medial points that establish the amount of skin to be resected and the length of the vertical scar. It is defined using the "pinch test."

Distance BC corresponds to the width of the inferior pedicle, and the lengthening corresponds to the distance of the new inferior areolar border. The thickness must be between 2 and 4 cm.

Below points B and C, a vertical line to the inferior mammary fold is marked that should be the projection of the flap with the inferior pedicle. According to each breast, surgical marking of the flap must be made, taking into consideration all anatomical aspects, in addition to the shape and size.

35.2.3 Surgical Technique

The surgery is done using general anesthesia associated with local infiltration with lidocaine and epinephrine solution 1:200.000 U, only in the incision lines and to undermine the glandular area in the fascial plane.

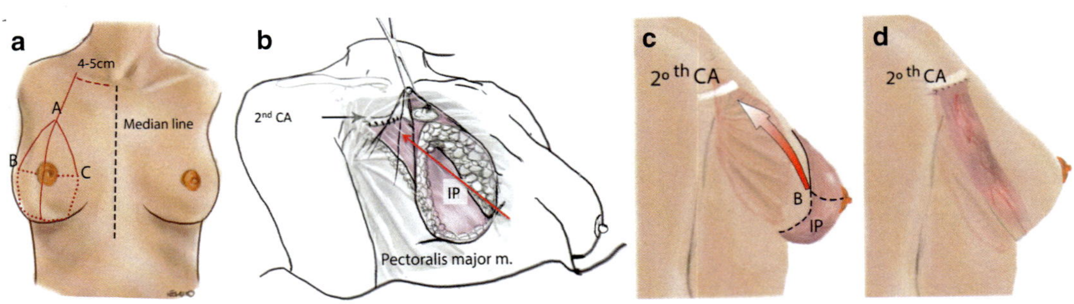

Fig. 35.3 Drawing demonstrating the marking points "A", "B" and "C" (**b**) Oblique view of the inferior pedicle (IP) and its movement up to second costal arch (2nd CA) (*red arrow*). (**c**) Lateral view of inferior pedicle disection. (**d**) Upper pole breast projection caused by the inferior pedicle attached in the second costal arch (2th CA)

The skin area inside the lines is de-epithelialized preserving the dermis and neural ending.

The inferior pedicle is marked and dissected perpendicular to the chest wall, up to the muscular plane. It must have a minimum thickness of 2 cm. The operation is performed under general anesthesia after meticulous surgical marking. Cutaneous incisions are made to create the inferior flap with the inferior pedicle. The flap is then de-epithelialized and sutured to the osteocartilaginous structures. The central area of the mammary gland is excised (Fig. 35.4).

A fascial subglandular plane is dissected up to the second cartilaginous costal arches, where the upper extremity of the inferior pedicle is fixed in the osteocartilaginous structure using a Mononylon 2–0 suture.

At this moment, when asymmetry or glandular hypertrophy is presented, the glandular tissue is resected at the lateral and medial columns, leaving at least 1 cm thickness (minimal resection). If necessary, a second resection is carried out at the median glandular tissue under the nipple–areolar complex (NAC; major resection).

The lateral and medial columns are sutured to each other and with the inframammary fold at same time with the dermal basis of the pedicle. The lateral "dog ear" is now marked and resected and the inferior fold is defined and sutured.

Finally, the NAC is marked and repositioned. Usually, the NAC is positioned between 6 and 8 cm from the inferior mammary fold in a vertical median breast line. The final aspect immediately after surgery shows a good result with inverted T-shaped incisions (Fig. 35.5). From the lateral view, a later result shows a well-balanced breast with inconspicuous scars (Fig. 35.6).

For secondary mammaplasty, the same procedure may be employed, as the inferior flap is sutured in an upward position to give more projection to the breast. This flap is even a good procedure for the treatment of very flabby breasts with severe ptosis to improve the superior pole of the breast. So far, in cases of gigantomastia with very fatty tissue, the flap with inferior pedicle is a useful procedure for achieving greater breast projection (Fig. 35.7).

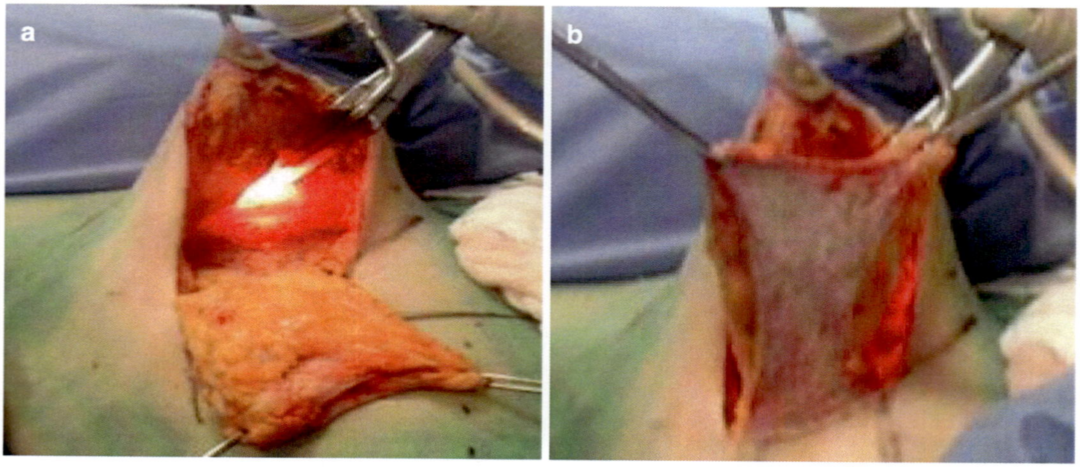

Fig. 35.4 Intraoperatively, with (**a**) an inferior pedicle flap dissection with 3-cm thickness. (**b**) Inferior pedicle elevated with dermis maintenance to preserve neurovascular endings and give support to adequate fixation in the osteocartilaginous structure of the second costal arch

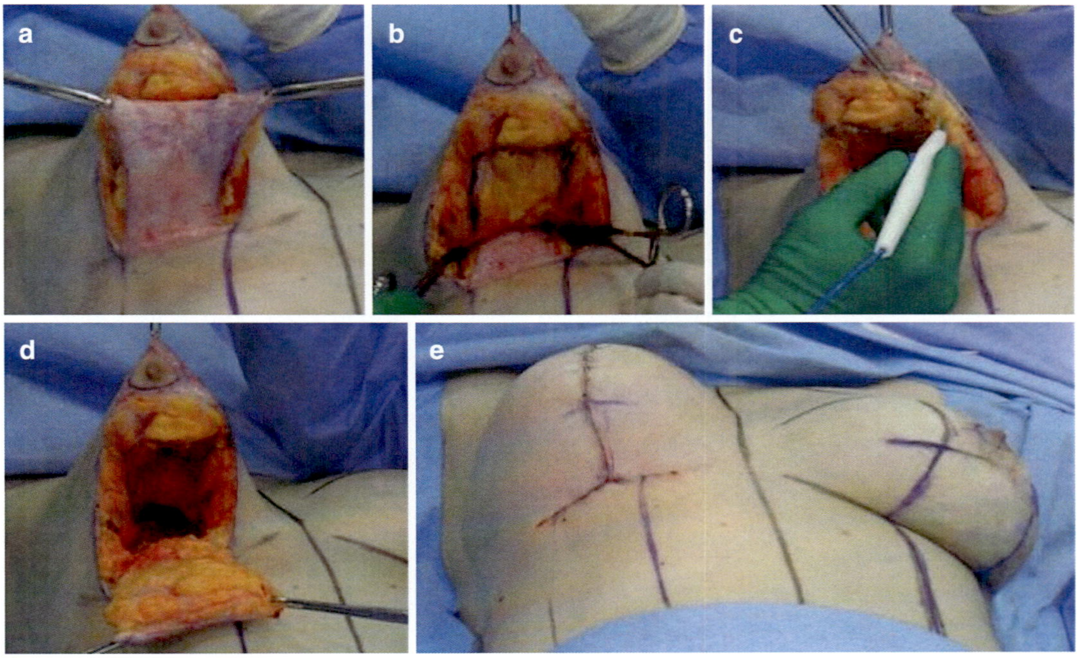

Fig. 35.5 Technical procedure sequence. (**a**) De-epithelialized inferior pedicle elevated. (**b**) Positioning the inferior pedicle where it is fixed in the osteocartilaginous structure and breast resection marking. (**c**) Resection of the median glandular tissue. (**d**) Breast central tissue resected with the three results of Pitanguy's pedicles. (**e**) Right breast at final closure without nipple exposure and left breast with previous marking

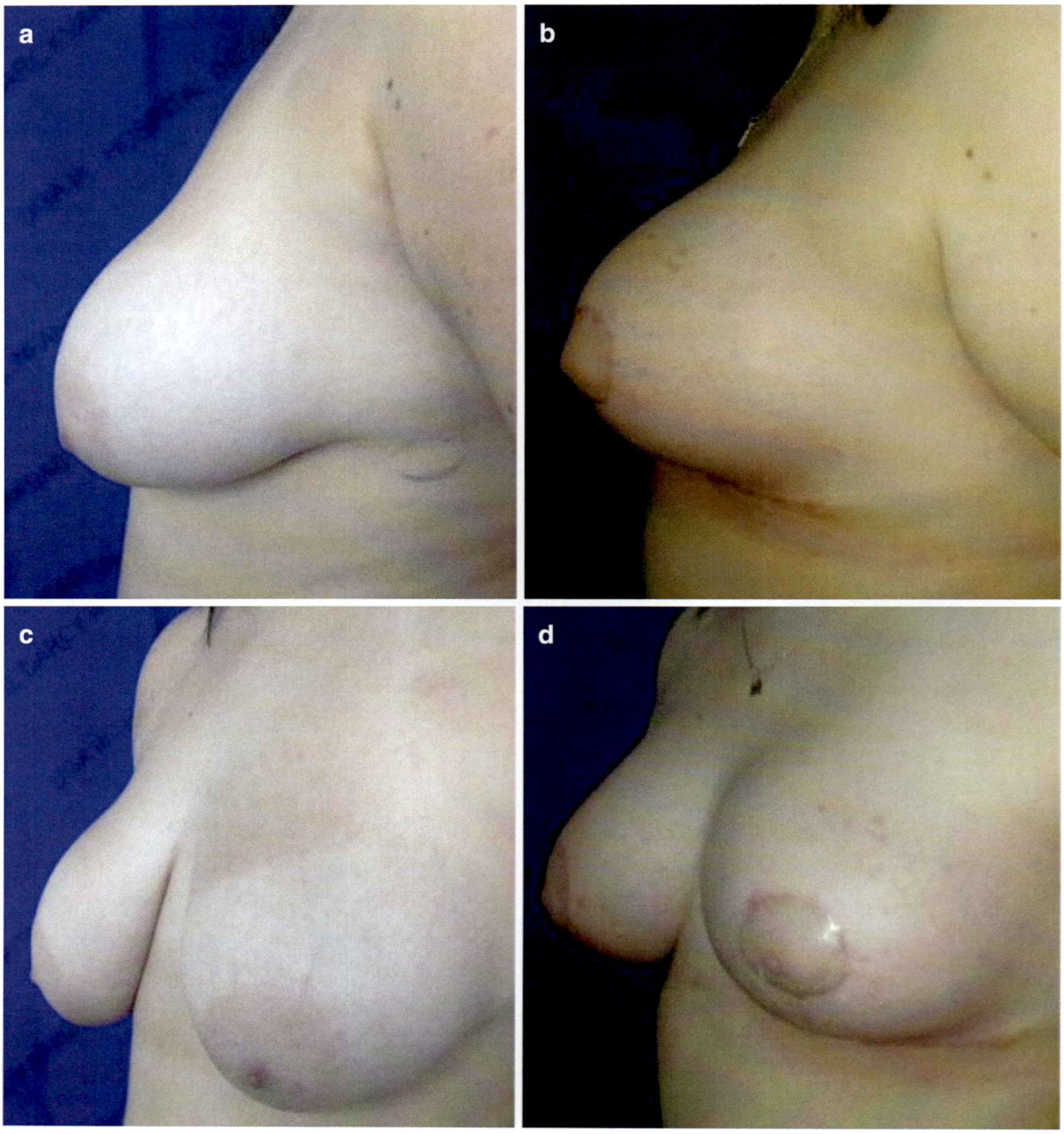

Fig. 35.6 (**a**) Preoperative lateral view of mammary ptosis. (**b**) Lateral view 30 days postoperatively without glandular resection. (**c**) Oblique preoperative view and (**d**) 1 month postoperatively of mammoplasty with an inferior pedicle

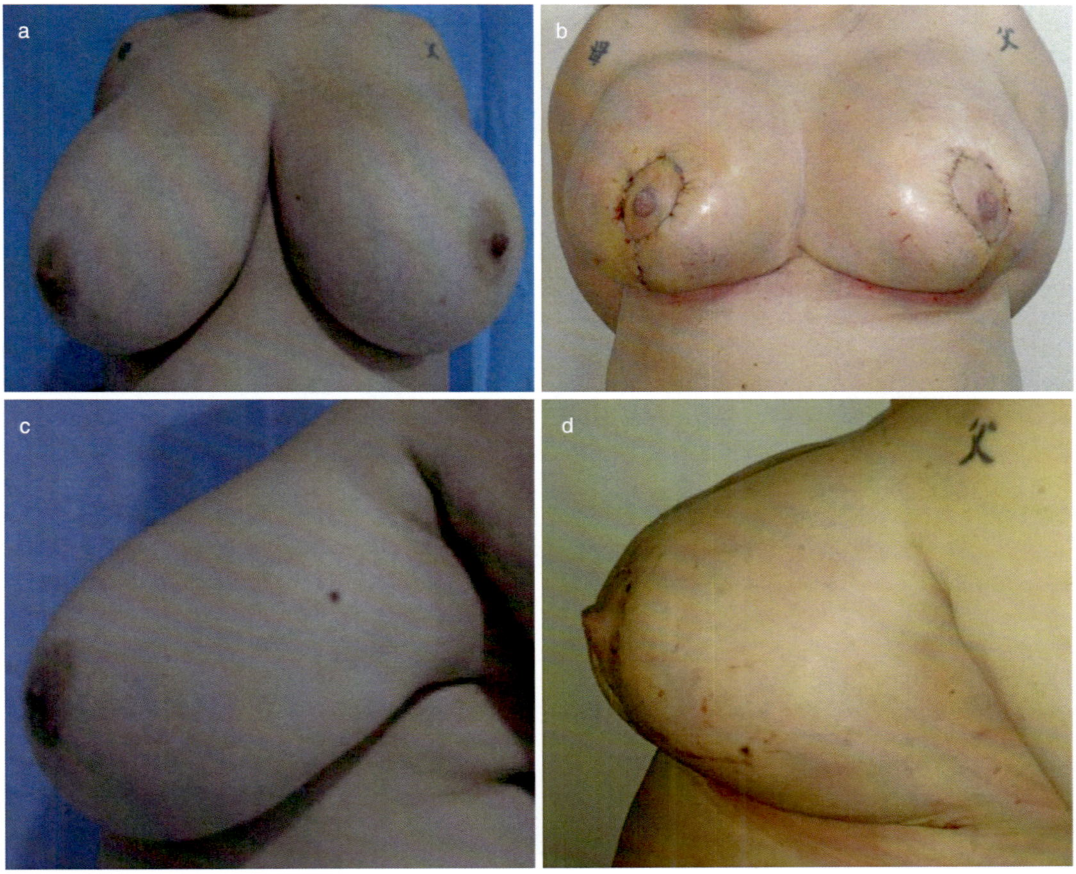

Fig. 35.7 Patient with gigantomastia subjected to mammoplasty with an inferior pedicle and a resection of 2100 g on the right side and 2310 g on the left side. (**a**) Preoperative frontal view. (**b**) Frontal view 10 days postoperatively. (**c**) Preoperative lateral view and (**d**) 10 days postoperatively

35.3 Discussion

Mammoplasty is one of the most common procedures performed by plastic surgeons today (ASPS 2013). The breast surgery is indicated for breast hypertrophy, ptotic and asymmetric breasts, glandular over-resection after tumor resection or severe weight loss after gastroplasty. Some authors used similar techniques to correct ptosis after implant removal (Ribeiro 1975; Avelar 1993; Rohrich 2006; Graf and Biggs 2002; Hönig et al. 2010).

In Brazil, until the end of the past century, women desired small breasts; however, this beauty pattern changed to larger breasts and Brazilian plastic surgeons received at their private practice a large number of patients with the single desire to elevate the breast without volumetric reduction.

To achieve these kind of results, we started to use their own local tissue to remodel the breast. The ptosed tissue is fixed on the osteocartilaginous skeleton of the chest.

The technique described follows Pitanguy's principles of marking with a superior vascular pedicle; however, it has modifications to improve long-lasting results with a well-vascularized inferior pedicle.

The inferior pedicle is an autologous tissue transfer of the volume of the ptotic glandular tissue to a posterior volume (Hönig et al. 2010; Hammond et al. 2015).

Initially, the inferior pedicle was located in the inferior portion of the breast; however, some authors changed the inferior pedicle position and in some cases put it under the muscle, whereas others fixed the pedicle in the muscular fascia. We believe the fixation in an osteocartilaginous structure permits better superior traction and better upper breast pole projection, other fixation points are made for adequate positioning of the inferior pedicle (Lexer 1912; Strömbeck 1960; Graf and Biggs 2002).

Another important technical detail is to create the inferior pedicle with the patient lying down without any traction of the breast by the medical assistant. The surgeon must hold the "entire" breast in his/her hand and avoid any positional interference during pedicle creation. The incisions must be done in a vertical line, avoiding oblique incisions. The oblique incisions could be dangerous to the mammary columns, decrease vascular supply to the nipple, decrease the contact of the galactophorous ducts, and deform the harmonious shape of the new breast.

Starting at the new inferior areolar border allows an increase in the lengthening of the inferior pedicle, with a resulting better projection of the superior breast pole. In our point of view, the more glandular tissue fixed, the more reduced the chances of mammary ptosis in the post-operative period.

The versatility of this pedicle is wide: if the surgeon needs during the surgery to fill an anatomical area in the breast it could be used. If the surgeon needs reduce the size of the breast the pedicle could be smaller or eliminated.

In some cases of a superior abdomen sagging, which is occasionally present after a liposuction procedure in this area or is a natural characteristic of the woman, the use of an inferior pedicle with superior traction results in a good option to solve the problem and in other cases the abdominal tissue could be used to improve mammary volume. This option is very useful for fixing three problems during same procedure: eliminate a sagging superior abdomen, increase the size of the breasts without implants, and correct mammary ptosis. The patient must be advised that this will be not a simple mammoplasty, but a complex procedure, with an increased risk of complications and care during the postoperative period (Figs. 35.8, 35.9, and 35.10).

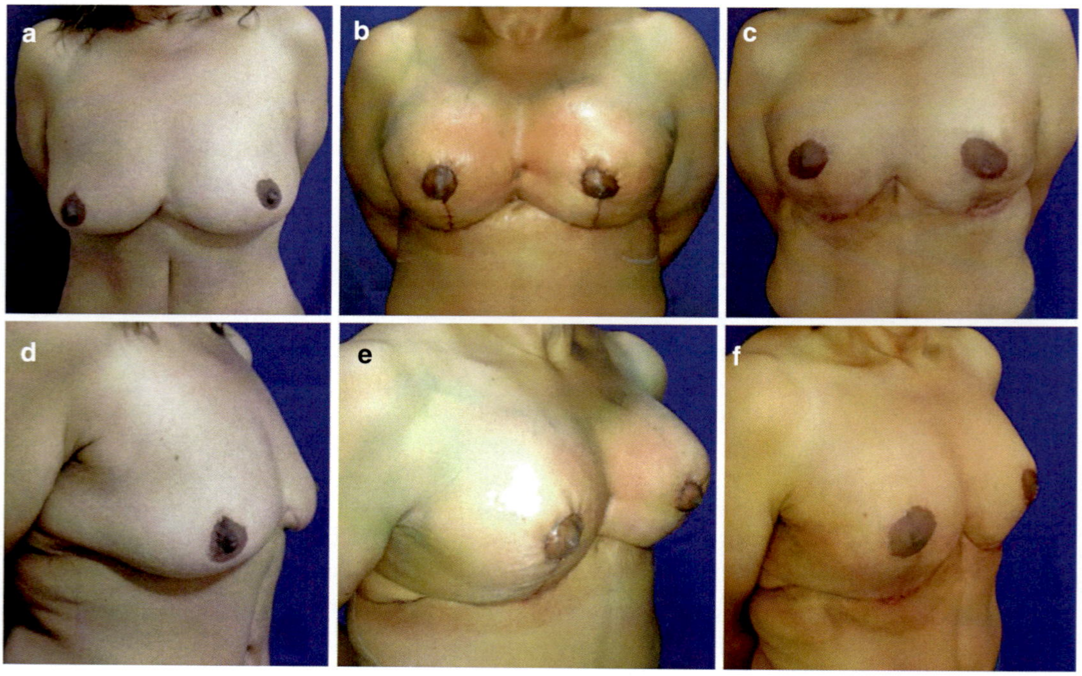

Fig. 35.8 Patient subjected to an extended inferior pedicle (EIP) to the superior abdomen and elevation. (**a**) Preoperative frontal view, with a deep fold in the superior abdomen medium line with sagging skin. (**b**) 1 week after mammoplasty with EIP, with the skin marks for reconstruction of the intermammary fold. (**c**) Frontal view 60 days postoperatively, the intermammary fold skin marks have disappeared. (**d**) Oblique preoperative view. (**e**) 1 week postoperatively. (**f**) Oblique view 60 days postoperatively of mammoplasty with treatment of medium fold superior sagging abdomen and adequate projection of the breast without prosthesis

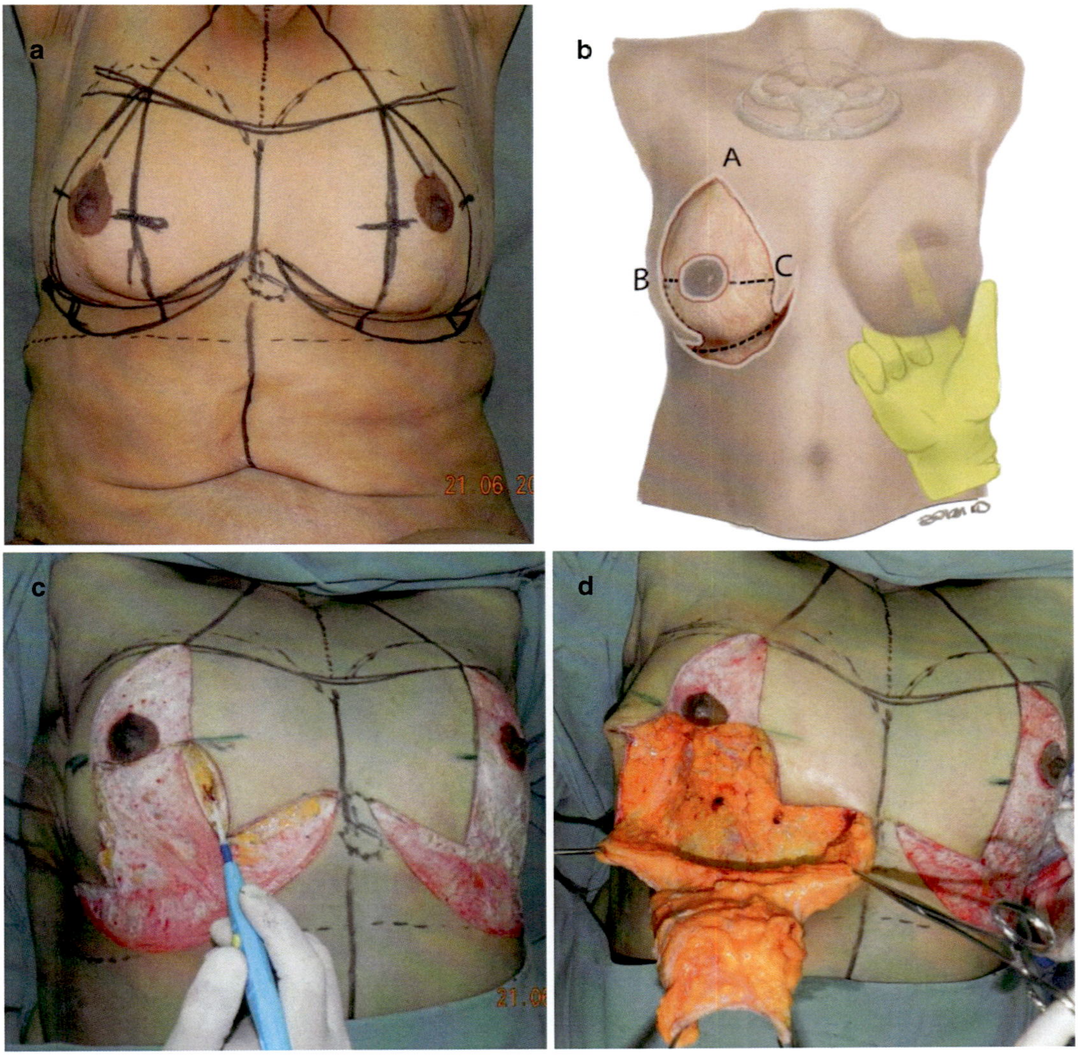

Fig. 35.9 Patient subjected to extended inferior pedicle (EIP) to the superior abdomen and elevation, (**a**) Preoperative frontal view, with a deep fold in the superior abdomen medium line with sagging skin and surgical markings. (**b**) Drawing with the EIP markings. (**c**) Creation of the EIP with electrocautery. (**d**) Extended displacement under the superior sagging abdomen for treatment of medium fold and increased volume of the new breast without silicon prosthesis

A reasonable number of patients search us with the desire for implants. Often they tell us: "I'd like to have a mammary implant to pull up my breasts," but when we asked about the size of their breasts, they answer: "It's ok, I like the size of my breasts, but they are saggy and droop." This is a perfect and common situation for using the inferior pedicle technique and avoid mammary implants. Satisfaction that they do not have to have for implants is the most common patient reaction. Actually, this is the most common procedure in our breast surgery practice, sometimes associated with lipoinjection (Chap. 50; Fig. 35.11).

Patients undergoing the inferior pedicle technique with an inverted T scar frequently experience bottoming out (Rohrich 2006). For this reason, our choice is to use the inferior pedicle technique to avoid this long-lasting result.

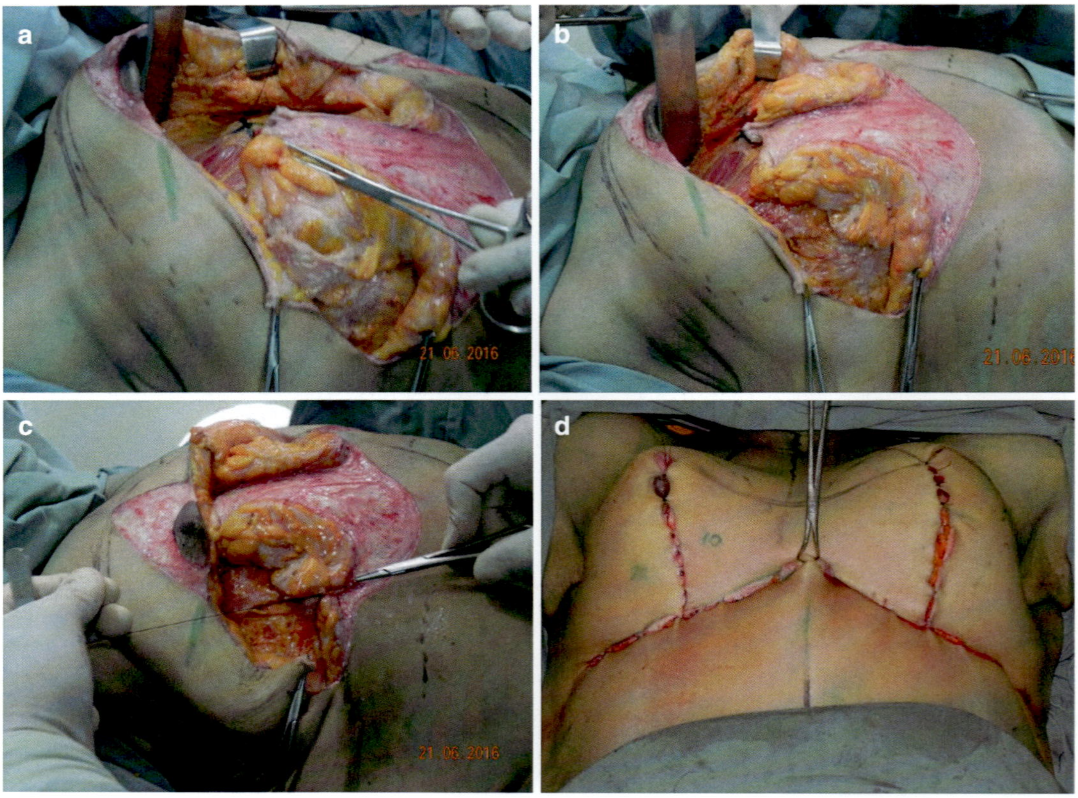

Fig. 35.10 Intraoperative steps of EIP with (**a**) upper traction to the second costal arch (green X indicated by the *red arrow*). (**b**) Fixation of EIP in the second costal arch. (**c**) Complementary fixation of EIP in the pectoral fascia. (**d**) Structured breasts without exposure of nipples and elevation of the central part of the superior abdomen

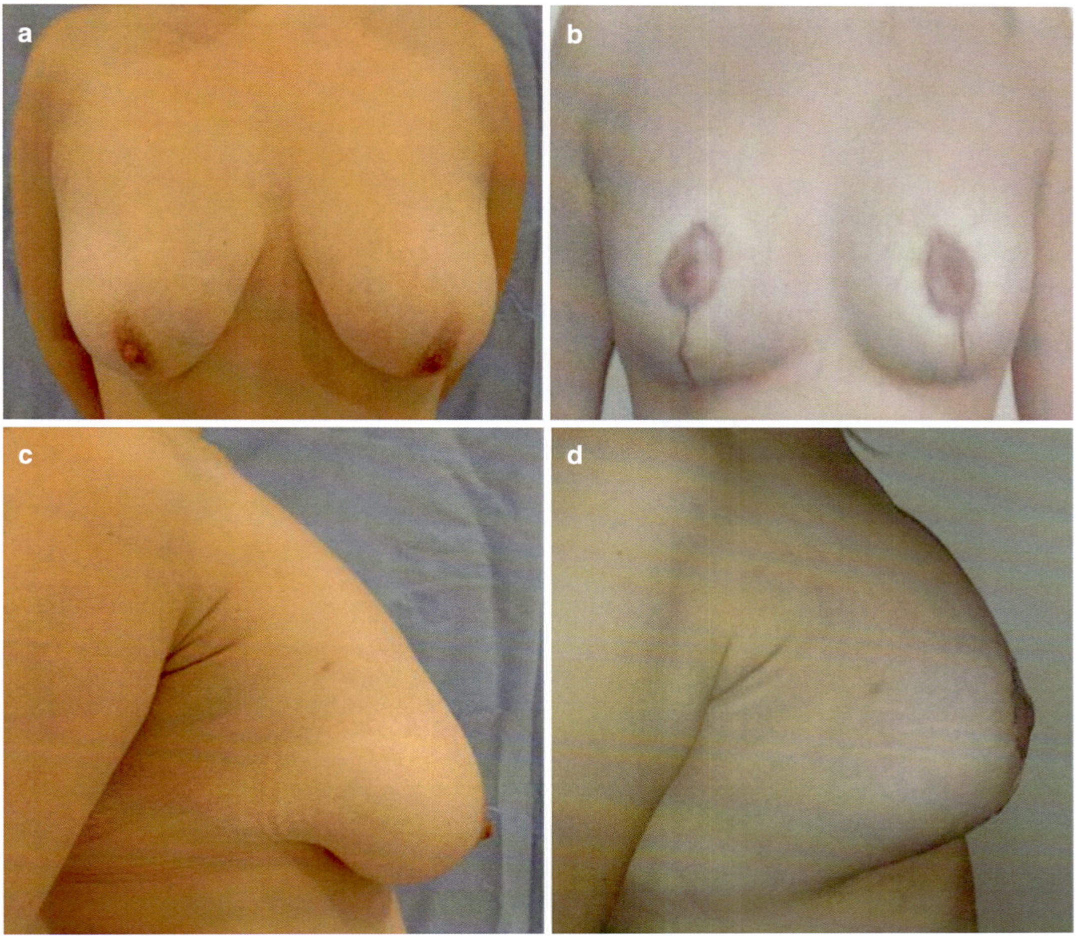

Fig. 35.11 Surgical result of the combined inferior pedicle technique with major pectoral muscle lipoinjection. (**a**) Frontal preoperative view of a patient with ptosis. (**b**) Frontal postoperative view of 3 months after surgery. (**c**) Lateral view of preoperative and (**d**) 3 months postoperatively of mammoplasty with an inferior pedicle, demonstrating improved projection of the upper pole of the breast

35.4 Complications

The bottoming out consequence, the most common after use of the inverted T technique, was not observed in our patients' postoperative results. However, in some cases, we observed the NAC directed upward and some cases had a high inferior pole with a long vertical measurement (Rohrich 2006).

Conclusion

The technique of auto breast augmentation using an inferior pedicle-based flap demonstrated long-lasting results, with better anteroposterior projection, a better superomedial pole and better ptosis correction.

Acknowledgement The authors have no conflicts of interest.

The study had no financial support.

References

American Society of Plastic Surgeons (ASPS) (2013) http://www.plasticsurgery.org/Documents/news-resources/statistics/2013-statistics/plastic-surgery-statistics-full-report-2013.pdf

Avelar JM (1980) Dermoadiposeglandular flap with superior pedicle on mastopexy (Retalho dermoadiposeglandular com pediculo superior nas mastopexia). In: Brazilian symposium on breast surgery, sponsored by Brazilian society of plastic surgery—Regional of São Paulo, August, São Paulo

Avelar JM (1993) Reduction mastoplasty under local anesthesia (Mastoplastia redutora sob anestesia local). In: Juarez M. Avelar (ed) Loco-regional anesthesia on aesthetic surgery—(Anestesia Loco-regional em cirurgia estética). Editora Hipócrates, São Paulo, 29:244–60

Graf R, Biggs TM (2002) In search of better shape in mastopexy and reduction mammoplasty. Plast Reconstr Surg 110(1):309–317

Graf R, Biggs TM, Steely RL (2000) Breast shape: a technique for better upper pole fullness. Aesthetic Plast Surg 24:348–352

Hammond DC, O'Connor EA, Knoll GM (2015) The short-scar periareolar inferior pedicle reduction technique in severe mammary hypertrophy. Plast Reconstr Surg 135(1):34–40

Hönig JF, Frey HP, Hasse FM, Hasselberg J (2010) Inferior pedicle autoaugmentation mastopexy after breast implant removal. Aesthetic Plast Surg; 34:447–454.

Kausch W (1916) Die Operationen der mammahypertrophie. Zentralbl F Chir 43:713–716

Lexer E (1912) Hypertrophie bei der mammae. Munch Med Wochenschr 59:2702

Pitanguy I (1959) Breast hypertrophy. In: Walace AB (ed) Transaction of the international society of plastic surgeons, Second Congress, London. Livingstone, Edinburg, p 509–517

Pitanguy I (1967) Surgical correction of breast hypertrophy. Br J Plast Surg 20:78

Ribeiro L (1975) A new technique for reduction mammaplasty. Plast Reconstr Surg 55:330–334

Ribeiro L, Backer E (1973) Mastoplastia com pedículo de seguridade. Rev Esp Cir Plast 16:223

Ribeiro L, Accorsi A Jr, Buss A, Marcal-Pessoa M (2002) Creation and evaluation of 30 years of the inferior pedicle in reduction mammaplasties. Plast Reconstr Surg 110:960–970

Rohrich RJ, Gosman AA, Brown SA, Reisch J (2006) Mastopexy preferences: a survey of board-certified plastic surgeons. Plast Reconstr Surg 118(7):1631–1638

Sinder R (1970) Thesis presented and approved for associated-professor at the former National School of Medicine (Faculdade Nacional de Medicina), current Federal University of Rio de Janeiro (UFRJ), with subject on mammoplasty

Sinder R (1974) The use of dermo-adipose flap in abdominoplasty and mammoplasty—personal technique (Uso de retalho dermo-adiposo em plásticas de mamas e de abdome—técnicas pessoais). In: XI Cong Bras Cirurgia Plástica, Belo Horizonte-MG

Strombeck JG (1960) Mammaplasty report of a new technique based on two pedicle procedure. Br J Plast Surg 13:79–90

36 Endoscopic Breast Reduction and Lifting

Marco Aurélio Faria Correa

36.1 Introduction

New concepts regarding skin elasticity were introduced into the field of plastic surgery by way of innovative techniques of liposuction and periareolar breast reduction (Avelar and Illouz 1986; Peixoto 1980; Ribeiro 1989). These new concepts, which concern the capacity of the skin to retract, allowed the author to investigate the feasibility of applying endoscopic methods to subcutaneous tissue to avoid skin resection. The author began by modifying the mini-abdominoplasty technique and techniques for breast reduction and mastopexy—endoscopy was also used as an aid for flap harvesting and placement of tissue expanders—and to develop promising research regarding axillary inguinal lymph nodes dissections (Faria-Correa 1992).

Video endoscopic methods have been used in different surgical fields such as gynecology, orthopedics, and general surgery, where many advantages have been shown. There is less tissue trauma, lower rate of infection, and minimal scarring.

Laparoscopic procedures used pressurized CO_2 gas to create a space between the laparoscope and the tissue to allow visualization. In the subcutaneous tissue, however, pressured gas is not recommended because of the risk of embolism. To circumvent this risk, the author developed the "subcutaneous tomoscope," which is an instrument that transfers into a transparent capsule the space needed for illumination and visualization. The optical cavity functions much the same way as a scuba diving mask does while serving as a blunt dissector because of its wedge-shaped capsule (Faria-Correa 1992). Specially designed retractors were developed to increase the necessary working space in addition to instruments such as special needle holders and needles Fig. 36.1). All of these instruments were designed to work through minimal incisions.

With video endoscopy, delicate processes can be performed through minimal incisions that can be made at strategically placed and remote sites avoiding visible scars. This is an important goal in the field of aesthetic surgery where scars are undesirable and may sometimes compromise the final aesthetic result.

M.A. Faria Correa, M.D.
Dr. Marco Faria Correa Plastic Surgery Pte Ltd,
38 Irrawaddy Road, Singapore 329563, Singapore
e-mail: drmarco@drmarco.com

J.M. Avelar (ed.), *Breast Surgery*, https://doi.org/10.1007/978-3-319-54115-0_36

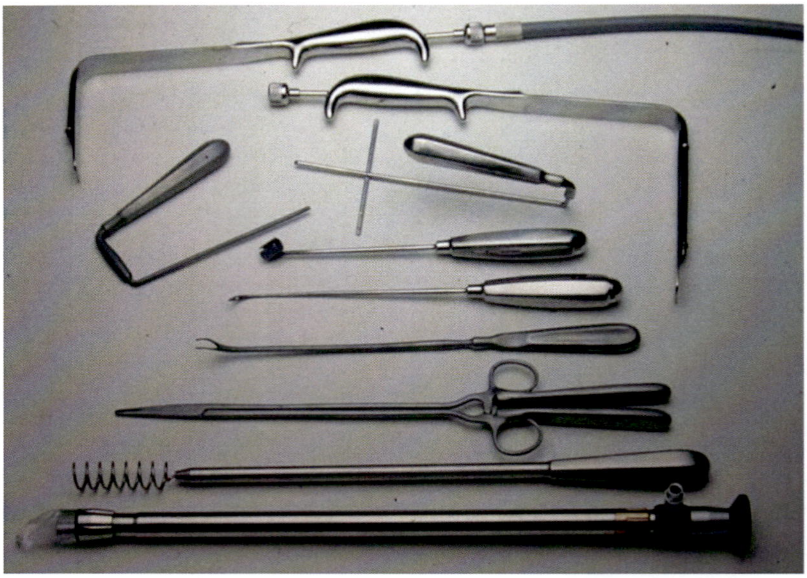

Fig. 36.1 Set of instruments developed by the author from top to bottom: light source retractors; single and cross puncture elevators; transcutaneous suture set guide, a modified Reverdin needle, and a fondue fork; a modified needle holder; "screw-suture"; "subcutaneous tomoscope"

36.2 Materials and Methods

Endoscopic versions of mastopexy and breast reduction were first performed in November 1992. Since then, the endoscopic technique has been used to treat 196 patients. The patients ranged in age from 14 to 58 years. They presented with first- or second-degree ptosis with or without hypertrophy. Patients were selected on the basis of having good skin elasticity without significant excess skin. Breastfeeding and striae were not considered contraindications as long as the patient maintained good skin elasticity. Premature moderate ptosis recurrence was observed when the endoscopic technique was applied to patients presenting with skin flaccidity. An important application for this technique is in patients with a small degree of breast asymmetry, particularly in young patients. The larger breast can be reduced with no visible scar or loss of sensation to match the smaller, unoperated breast.

36.2.1 Technique

The traditional video endoscopic system and the subcutaneous tomoscope, associated with endoscopic instruments, were used to create an optical space. Thus, monitor control could be used without CO_2 distension. Some instruments were modified and new ones were developed, creating a set of instruments that facilitate this procedure. Regular laparoscopic forceps and scissors connected to electrocautery were used.

36.2.2 Positioning of the Patient and the Team

Proper positioning of both the patient and the surgical team is important for facilitating this procedure. The monitor is placed over the patient's head and the anesthesiologist stays beside the patient's head. The surgeon works beside the patient. The surgical table must be adequate to allow change in the patient's positioning from supine to sitting.

36.2.3 Planning

In planning the mammoplasty, the breast must be observed as a three-dimensional structure (Figs. 36.2, 36.3 and 36.4). Working endoscopically and considering the three-dimensional breast volume as a cone, looking upward, the bottom of the cone can be seen (Fig. 36.5). The goal is to work on the base of the glandular cone. The first step is to plan the undermining of an enlarged

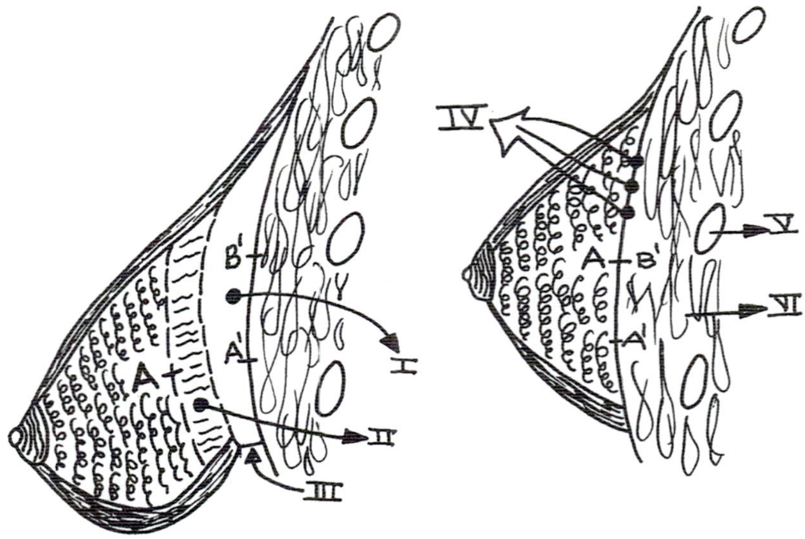

Fig. 36.2 Video-endoscopic breast reduction and mastopexy technique: A and A'—level point; B′—*upper position*; I—retromammary pocket; II—tissue resection area; III—submammary sulcus incision; IV—sutures to fix the gland in its new position at the pectoral fascia; V—ribs; VI—muscle

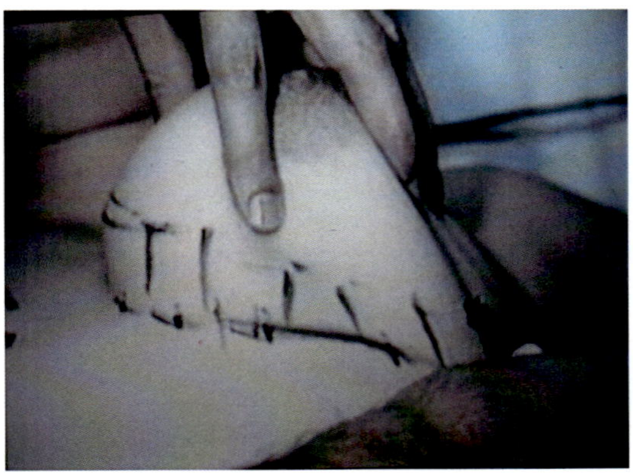

Fig. 36.3 Marking shows externally the breast tissue to be resected from the base of the glandular cone

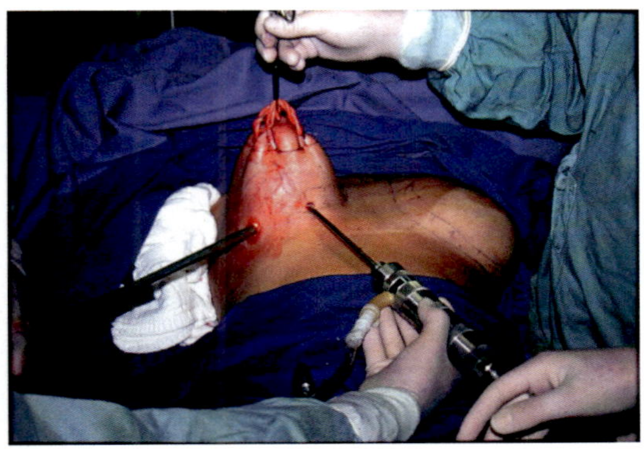

Fig. 36.5 Transoperative view showing two small incisions (2 cm) at the submammary sulcus, through which the shaver and scope are introduced. Transcutaneous lifting sutures are used to maintain the optical cavity

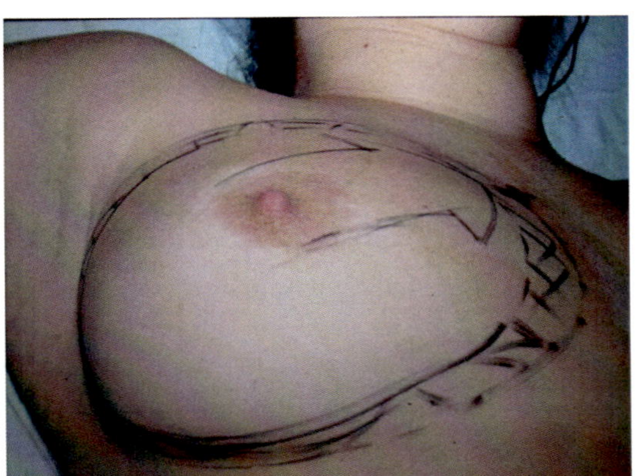

Fig. 36.4 *Arrow* shows the direction of the mastopexy toward upper-medial

area between the breast and the pectoralis fascia, thus creating a retromammary pocket. Both gland advancement (mastopexy) and breast tissue reduction are planned to proceed from the bottom of the cone. If only mastopexy is needed, the incisions are marked at the inframammary fold. If breast reduction is intended, the incisions must be placed a little above the fold.

36.2.4 Anesthesia and Infiltration

General, epidural or local anesthesia can be used. To reduce bleeding, the process is begun by infiltration of epinephrine/saline solution (1:500,000).

This is infiltrated at the base of the breast in the area to be undermined and inside the breast tissue.

36.2.5 Incisions

One or two incisions (1–2 cm) are made in the submammary sulcus. If necessary, a third incision can be made at the axilla to help tissue resection or suture placement.

Traditional open surgery is carried out in three dimensions; however, when working exclusively with a monitor view, the third dimension is lost. This can be improved by simultaneously working through two different ports, such that we "triangulate" to a focal point. This provides us with a depth-of-field feeling in the operative area. The best performance is achieved with a triangulation of approximately 30–45° (Fig. 36.5).

36.2.6 Dissection

A retromammary pocket is created between the breast and the pectoralis fascia (Fig. 36.2). This undermining must be wide enough to allow the advancement of the ptotic gland from the lower lateral to the upper medial position on the chest wall. This also provides an ample area of internal scarring between the chest wall and the deep part of the breast tissue. This ample retromammary pocket is created with the aid of the tomoscope by blunt dissection under endoscopic control. The dissection area is similar to that where breast implants are placed. The bleeding is controlled endoscopically by the use of laparoscopic forceps connected to the electrocautery maneuvering them under monitor view. The dissection of the retromammary pocket is completed by using laparoscopic scissors connected to the electrocautery. The use of pressured gases to create and maintain the work space is avoided. The optical cavity can be provided with the aid of specially designed, long and thin elevators and retractors that are introduced through the work ports. An external lift can be used by placing sutures through the anterior portion of the cone of the breast (Fig. 36.5).

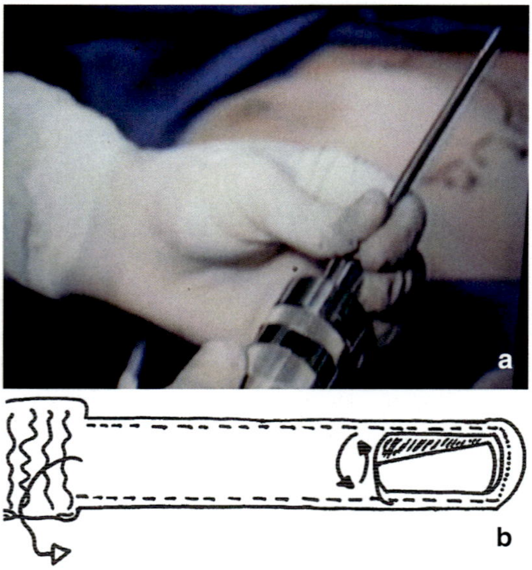

Fig. 36.6 (**a**) Shaver—a video-arthroscopic instrument, originally employed to resect the meniscus and debride the fibrotic tissue inside the knee, here used to carry out breast reduction. (**b**) Shaver instrument cannula. There are two cannulas, one rolling inside the other, a punching aspirator

36.2.7 Breast Tissue Resection

The tissue resection is performed at the base of the gland under endoscopic control, preserving the anterior cone and glandular ducts. A video arthroscopic shaver can be used to reduce the breast. The shaver works as a punching aspirator. There are two cannulas, one rolling inside the other (Fig. 36.6); both are equipped with windows through which the breast tissue is aspirated and resected. Some breast glands may be too rigid; therefore, its tissue cannot be resected by this punching aspirator. Thus, the procedure is performed by the use of a knife, scissors, electrocautery or laser. This type of breast is the one that is seen on mammography presenting with a large amount of white fibrous tissue.

By resecting only the base of the breast cone, the functions and sensation are preserved. This is a physiological mammoplasty. The axillary pole and bottom of the mammary cone are resected. There is no resection of even small amounts at the upper pole of the gland. Working endoscopically, the internal breast volume can be felt externally by hand palpation. By properly planning the tissue resection, the breast is modeled and sculptured into its new shape.

36.2.8 Breast Lifting Fixation

After obtaining adequate hemostasis, the next step is to lift and fix the gland into its new position (Fig. 36.7). Sutures are used to position the mammary gland and fix it to the pectoralis fascia. Suturing can be performed with laparoscopic needle holders. As many sutures as needed are placed to help in positioning the breast so that it is held in place during the maturation of the internal cicatrix, which ultimately fixes the breast permanently in position. Patients with good skin quality are good candidates for this procedure and gain an aesthetic advantage with the repositioning of the gland, as this recreates an upper pole to the breast.

36.2.9 Dressings and Postoperative Care

Suction drains are used during the first 12 h and then removed. A Micropore tape dressing (Fig. 36.8) helps to reposition the gland in its new site. This dressing is maintained for 20 days for a long-term support. Continuous use of a supporting bra is recommended for at least 3 months thereafter and as long as possible throughout the patient's life.

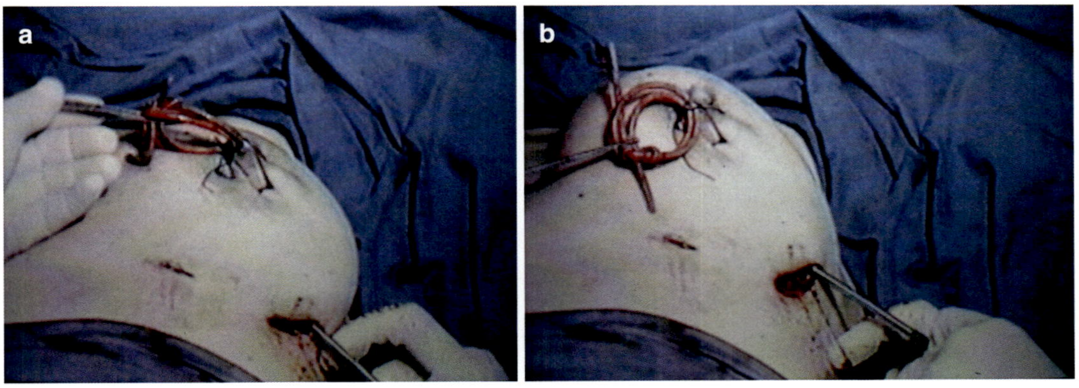

Fig. 36.7 (**a**, **b**) Grasping and testing the correct position for placing the sutures

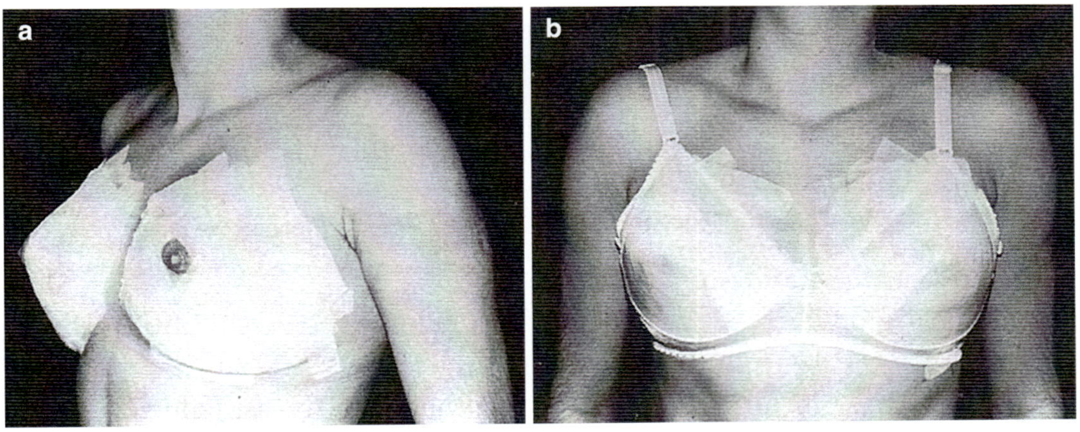

Fig. 36.8 (**a**, **b**) Micropore modulator dressing and drainage

36.2.10 Complications

Among the 196 cases, five cases of hematoma were observed in patients in whom no drains were used and 22 patients had early ptosis recurrence in 22 patients because of poor skin elasticity.

36.3 Discussion

The endoscopic breast reduction and mastopexy techniques preserve breast function and sensation with minimal scars (Figs. 36.9 and 36.10) (Faria-Correa 1993, 1994a, b, 1995a, b, c, d, 1994c, d, e; Faria-Correa 2000). An important goal is to treat

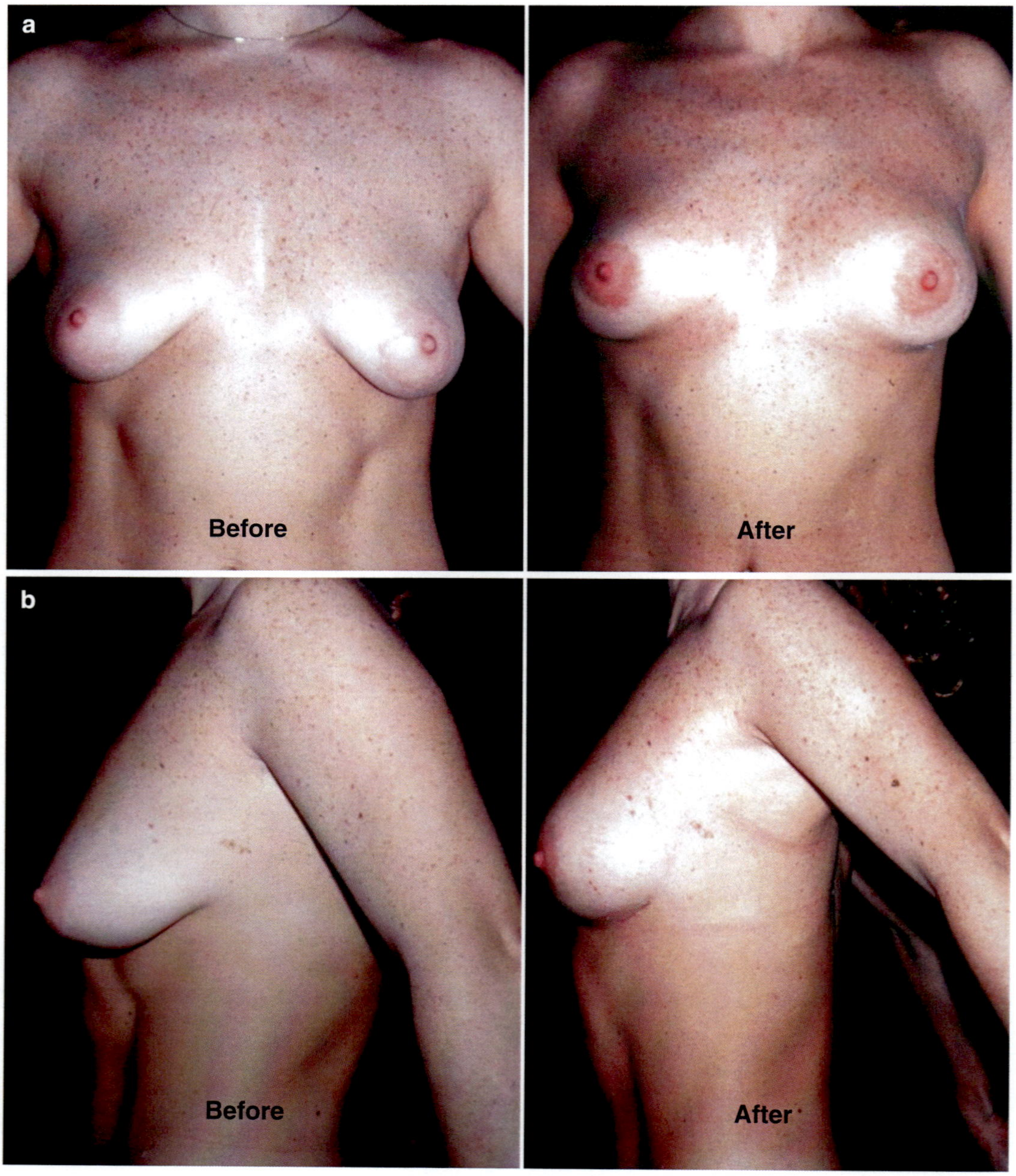

Fig. 36.9 (**a**) Preoperative view of a 32-year-old patient, who had breastfed two children, presenting with breast ptosis, a moderate amount of striae, and a moderate degree of flabbiness. (**b**) Eight months after endoscopic breast lift

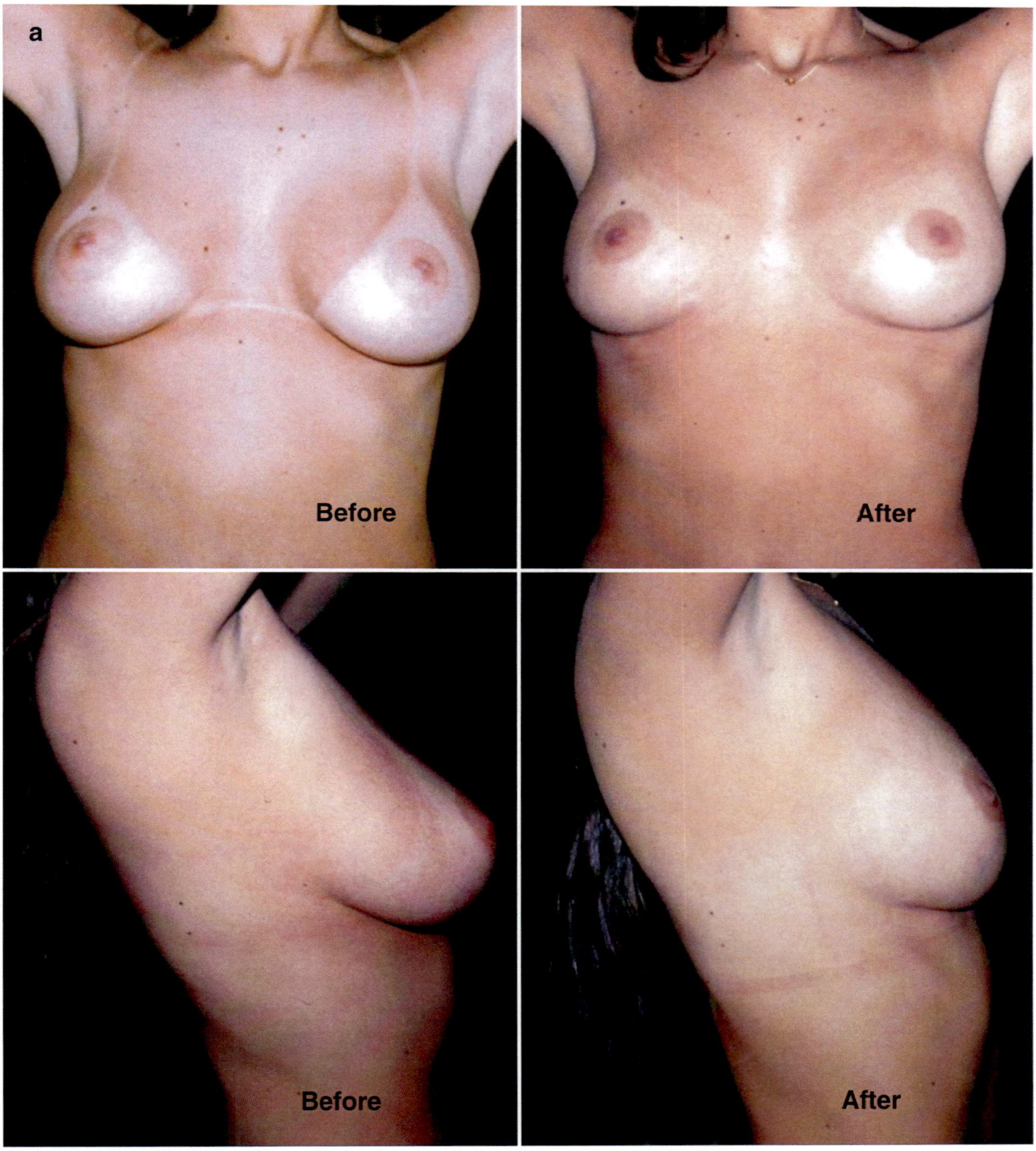

Fig. 36.10 (**a**) Preoperative view of a 20-year-old patient with good skin elasticity, breast hypertrophy, ptosis, but no striae. (**b**) Two years after video-endoscopic breast reduction and lift (120 g from each breast), showing a nice upper pole, good skin retraction, no damage to function or sensation, and no visible scars

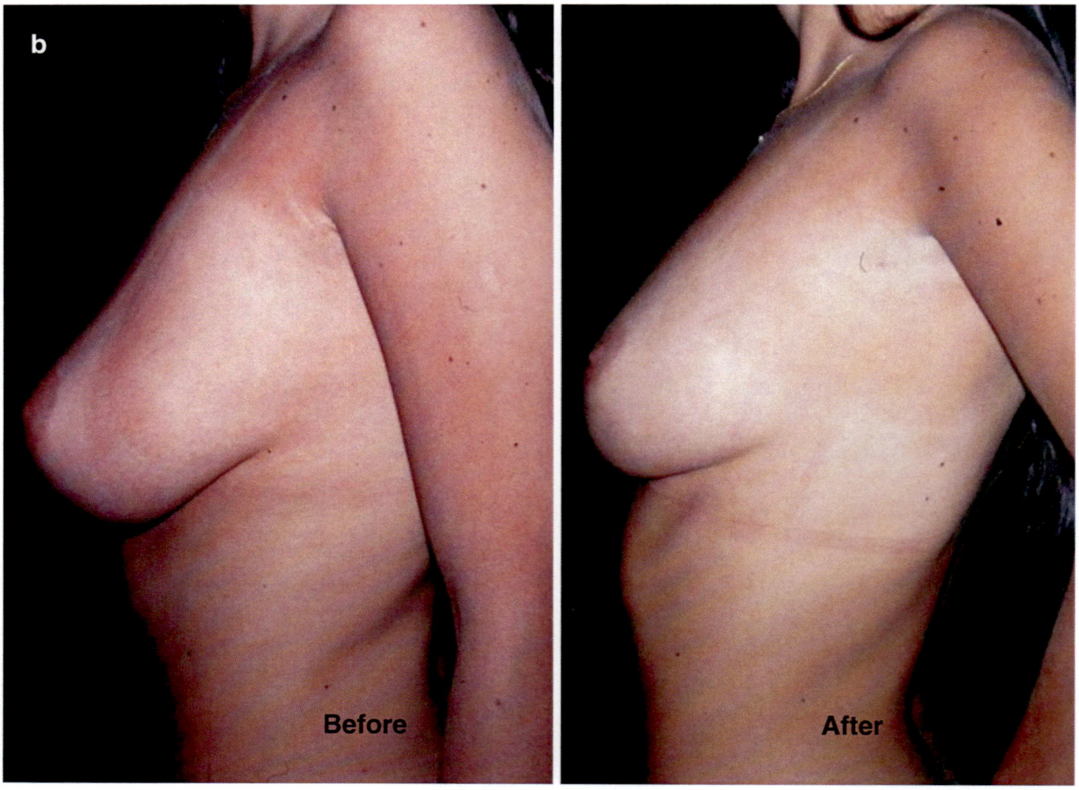

Fig. 36.10 (continued)

mammary asymmetry without using prostheses or adding long scars to the breast as opposed to the traditional procedures.

The breast is an anatomical structure that grows perpendicularly from the chest. The effects of gravity pull the breast down whether the patient is old or young, or operated on or not. The maintenance of a long-term good result depends not only on the technique used by the author, but also on the skin elasticity for retraction. Successful long-term follow-up relies on breast weight and precautions taken by the patient, such as the use of a steadfast modulator bra especially during the practice of sports.

In patients whose skin does not have the capacity to retract, the results are transitory as in usual mastopexies. Nevertheless, characteristic of this minimally invasive technique that have been attracting patients' interest is the lack of visible scars and the maintenance of sensitivity and function.

Conclusions

The results of 23 years' follow-up in 196 patients permit us to recommend its use in first-degree ptosis and breast reductions in younger patients. The technical procedure presented shows its utmost effectiveness and best aesthetic results in young patients who present with a small amount of hypertrophy or asymmetry, but with good skin elasticity and who do not have significant excess skin. The author believes that the use of these endoscopic techniques is a new trend in plastic surgery when properly applied.

References

Avelar JM, Illouz YG (1986) Lipoaspiração. Hipocrates 3:320

Faria-Correa MA (1992) Videoendoscopy in plastic surgery: brief communication—a videocirurgia na cururgia plastica. Rev Soc Bras de Cir Plastica Est Reconstr 7:80–81

Faria-Correa MA (1993) Mamoplastia videoendoscopica e abdominoplastia videoendoscopica (subcutaneoscopica). In: Tournieux AAB (ed) Atualizacao em Cirurgia Plastica Estetica. Santa Isabel Livraria e Editora, Sao Paulo, pp 411–418

Faria-Correa MA (1994a) Mamoplastia por endoscopia. Rev Cirurg Plas Ibero Latino-Americana 20:121–127

Faria-Correa MA (1994b) Mamoplastia Videodndoscopica. Arquivos Catarinenses Med 23:116–118

Faria-Correa MA (1994c) Mammoplastia por endoscopia. J Cirurg Plast Ibero-Latino-Americana 20(2):121–127

Faria-Correa MA (1994d) Mammoplastia videoendoscopica. Rev Soc Bras Med Estet 4:33–36

Faria-Correa MA (1994e) Endoscopic mammoplasty. In: Transactions of the 7th Asian congress of plastic and reconstructive surgery, Bangkok, Holistic

Faria-Correa MA (1995a) Endoscopic abdominoplasty, mastopexy, and breast reduction. Clin Surg 22(4):723–745

Faria-Correa MA (1995b) Breast lift and reduction. Endosc Plast Surg:194–202

Faria-Correa MA (1995c) Endoscopic mammoplasty. World J Plast Surg 1:118–119

Faria-Correa MA (1995d) Videoendoscopic subcutaneous techniques for aesthetic and reconstructive plastic surgery. Plast Reconstr Surg 96(2):446–453

Faria-Correa MA (2000) Reducao e pexia mamaria por videoendoscopia. In: Saltz R (ed) Cirugia da Mama-Esttica e Reconstructiva de Ricardo Ribeiro. Livaria e Editora Revinter, Sao Paulo, pp 319–327

Peixoto G (1980) Reduction mammoplasty. A personal technique. Plast Reconstr Surg 65(2):217–226

Ribeiro L (1989) Circurgia Plastica da Mama. Medsi, Rio de Janeiro

37 Mammoplasty Using a Periareolar Approach

Jose Horacio Aboudib
and Fernando Serra-Guimarães

37.1 Introduction

Reduction mammoplasty is one of the most frequently requested forms of breast plastic surgery (International Society of Aesthetic Plastic Surgery 2015; Hammond and Kim 2016).

For decades, it has evolved technically; however, a greater impulse occurred in the late 1950s and 1960s with the incorporation of contributions from Arié, Strombeck, and Pitanguy (Strombeck 1960; Pitanguy 1960) to existing techniques. Since then, mammoplasty has become a common operation with regard to obtaining breasts with adequate shape and projection, and a low incidence of complications.

After obtaining breasts with a suitable shape and size, there was concern about obtaining breasts with reduced scarring. During the 1980s, Peixoto (1989) touched plastic surgeons presenting a technique that resulted in smaller scars based on skin retraction properties. This added to the contributions of Bustos (1992) Goes (1989), Goes (1996), Benelli (1993), and others, and led to improvement of the technique, which proposed breast reduction through a periareolar incision restricting the scar to the area of transition from the skin pigmentation of the areola to the breast skin.

A review of the historical evolution of periareolar breast reduction shows that it was first described in 1916 by Kausch (1976), who performed circular resections near the areola. In 1928, Noel (1928) proposed lifting the breast with skin resection in the upper periareolar region in a half moon shape two or three times to take the areola to the desired position. In some cases, the scar was completed around the areola to accommodate the skin surplus. In 1969, Hinderer (1969) proposed correcting mild ptosis using a double periareolar incision. In 1970, Souza (1970) proposed that skin retraction property would allow glandular resection using the periareolar technique, skin ressection, reaching a perfect balance between the breast volume and skin coverage. In this technique, the breast parenchyma would provide support through its attachment to the pectoralis major muscle at the level of the second rib.

In the 1990s, Benelli (1993) revised the technique and concluded that the lack of support of the skin resulted in an early breast ptosis, in addition to the centrifugal pull of the periareolar incision leading to enlargement of the areolar diameter. Based on this, he presented a new technique, periareolar mastoplasty, performing permanent cerclage, which he called "round block," and inferior pole-crossing mastopexy.

J.H. Aboudib, M.D., Ph.D. (✉)
Plastic Surgery, Pedro Ernesto University Hospital, Rio de Janeiro State University, Estrada da Gávea, RJ 22610001, Brazil
e-mail: jhaboudib@gmail.com

F. Serra-Guimarães, M.D., Ph.D.
Plastic Surgery, Pedro Ernesto University Hospital, Rio de Janeiro State University, Rua de Paranhos Antunes, RJ 10010601, Brazil

J.M. Avelar (ed.), *Breast Surgery*, https://doi.org/10.1007/978-3-319-54115-0_37

The evolution of the described techniques brought progressive improvement of results. Aboudib JH, Cadoso de Castro C, Coelho RS, Cupello AM (1991). Therefore, reduction mammaplasty with a periareolar approach incorporated important contributions that became a progressively safer and more effective, providing more satisfactory and lasting results (Hammond and Kim 2016).

37.2 Method

37.2.1 Marking

The procedure begins with the marking of the incisions in the breast with the patient in a standing position, before anesthesia.

The entire circumference of the breast is defined, which is the limit for infiltration and cutaneous detachment. The midclavicular point is determined, and from this a line is drawn through the nipple to the inframammary groove. At this line, we mark the projection of the inframammary fold: this is called point A′. This point represents the new position of the nipple. A point is marked 2 cm above A′, called point A, which is the future location of the upper edge of the nipple–areola complex (NAC; Fig. 37.1).

Starting from the inframammary fold toward the NAC, at a variable distance of 4–7 cm, point B is marked, which corresponds to future lower edge of the areola. Medial and lateral to the nipples, depending on the existing skin excess, points C (future medial border of the areola) and D (future lateral border of the areola) are defined. Point C is approximately 7–10 cm from the sternum bone and point D 8–12 cm of the anterior axillary line. The union of these points A, B, C, and D creates an oval figure, which is the amount of skin to be resected.

37.2.2 Operation

The surgery is performed under local anesthesia and sedation. Anesthetic infiltration is held in the plane between the subcutaneous tissue and the mammary gland throughout the length of the breast and between the gland and the pectoralis major muscle. The anesthetic solution is composed of 0.05% bupivacaine and adrenaline (1/400,000) for a total of approximately 150 mL for each breast.

Patients are operated on in the supine position. During the resection of excess breast parenchyma and superior rotation of the flaps, the back is raised to 45°. The arms remain at a 90° angle with the trunk.

After marking the new size of the areola (usually between 3.5 and 4 cm) with methylene blue, we began the incision over this marking followed by detachment of the skin with a blade to the circle joining points A, B, C, and D, without concern with regard to preserving the dermis. An incision is made along the circle A–B–C–D and the skin between this marking and areola is then resected (Fig. 37.2).

Using scissors, we dissected the dermis and fat tissue that are separate from the mammary parenchyma (Fig. 37.3) In the upper pole of the

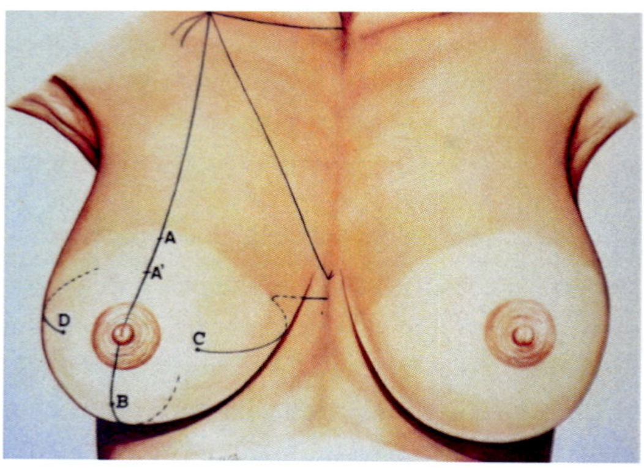

Fig. 37.1 Marking the new position of the nipple–areola complex (NAC). The union of A, B, C and D represents the amount of skin removed

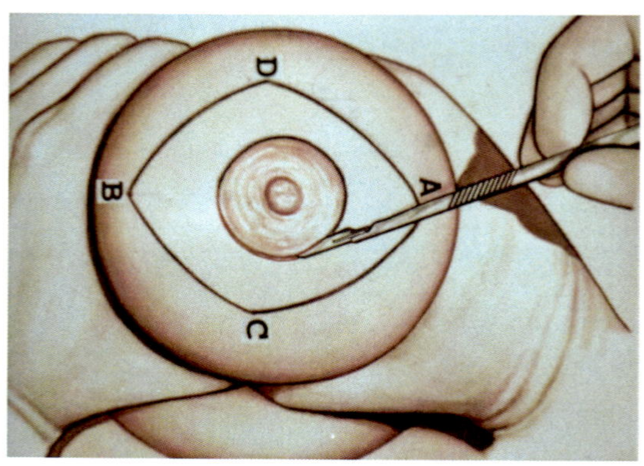

Fig. 37.2 Incision in the NAC and in the lines AC/CB/BD/AD, with removal of the skin

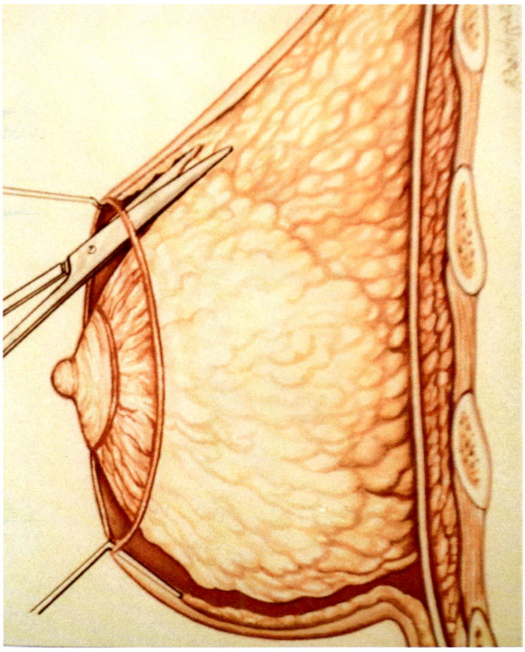

Fig. 37.3 Subcutaneous detachment performed around the circumference of the breast, in the plane between the subcutaneous tissue and the breast parenchyma

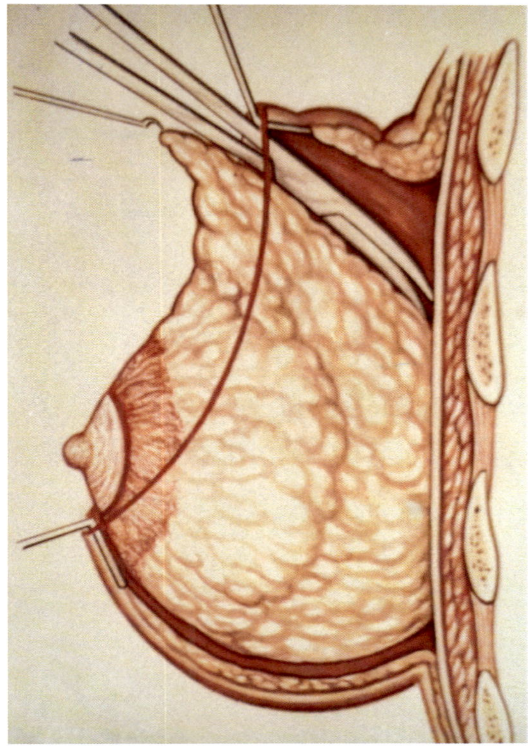

Fig. 37.4 Detachment of the upper glandular parenchyma of the aponeurosis of the pectoralis major muscle

breast, to follow the displacement accompanying the deep part of the glandular tissue, a greater amount of subcutaneous tissue adhered to the skin, so that in this region, the flap (especially at the base) is thicker than in the other quadrants. The glandular parenchyma remains connected only to the muscular plane, and is vascularized by the perforating branches.

Then, the upper pole of the breast is dissected from the pectoralis major muscle (Fig. 37.4). This is an avascular plane and can be dissected by divulsion. The detachment limit is the projection of the upper edge of the areola (Fig. 37.5).

Thus, we prepared the entire upper pole, which will be resected. The breast tissue is pulled upward with the use of two forceps (Fig. 37.6). The tissue to be resected corresponds to the breast tissue above the semicircle, which is determined by a compass at a distance of 7–8 cm from the nipple (Fig. 37.7). This is the usual distance from the upper base of the breast to the nipple. Above this semicircle, all breast tissue is resected. This step is critical for the proper fitting of the breast.

After this resection (Fig. 37.8), a V shape is determined, whose opening is defined from the maximum limit of the upper rotation of the side pole and medial pole toward the middle line (Fig. 37.9).

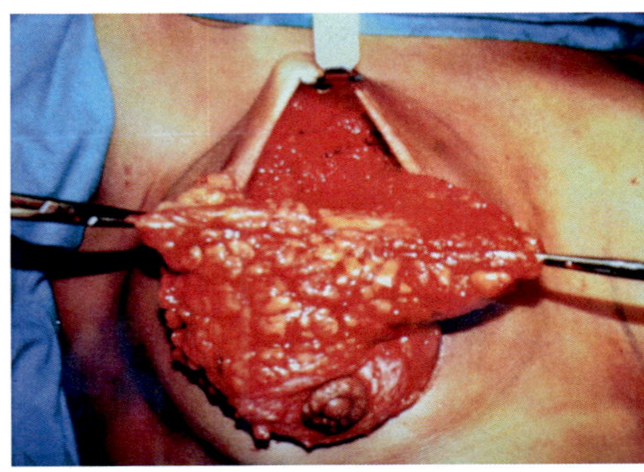

Fig. 37.5 Glandular detachment concluded

This resection is usually higher in the side pole, which has a higher rotation. After resection, the medial and lateral flaps are rotated superiorly to the midline (Fig. 37.10) to ensure reduction of the base and anterior breast projection (Fig. 37.11). The lateral and medial flaps are sutured to the pectoralis

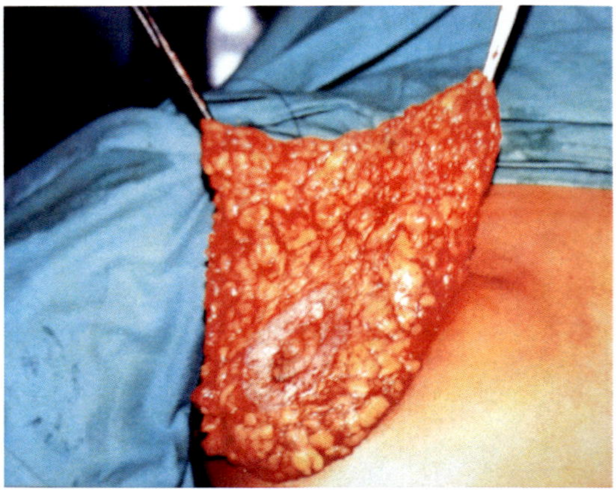

Fig. 37.6 Breast parenchyma prepared for resection

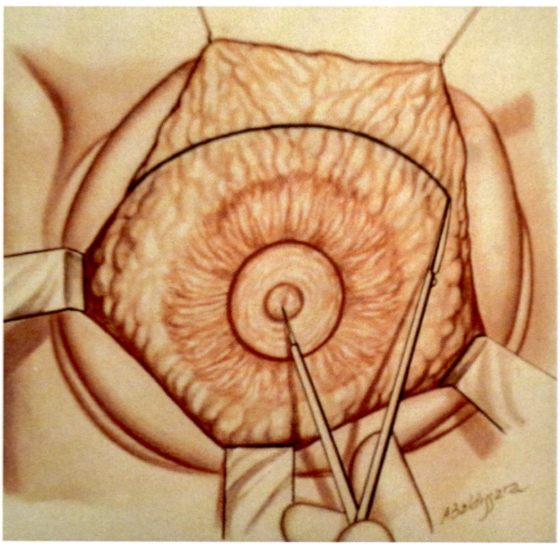

Fig. 37.7 Marked semicircle with concavity downward and 8 cm from the nipple

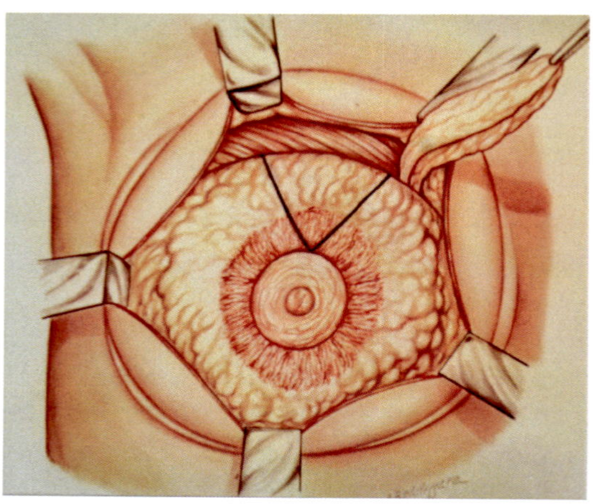

Fig. 37.8 Resection of the upper pole of the mammary gland above the marked semicircular line and demarcation of the wedge to be resected

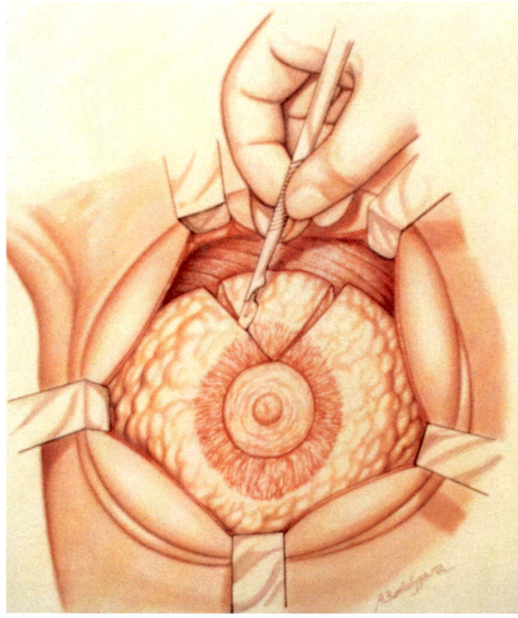

Fig. 37.9 V-shaped resection of the upper breast pole

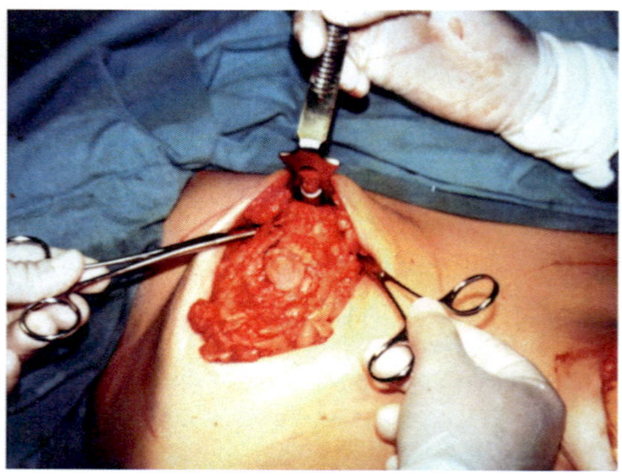

Fig. 37.10 Flaps being translated superiorly and fixed in the upper pole

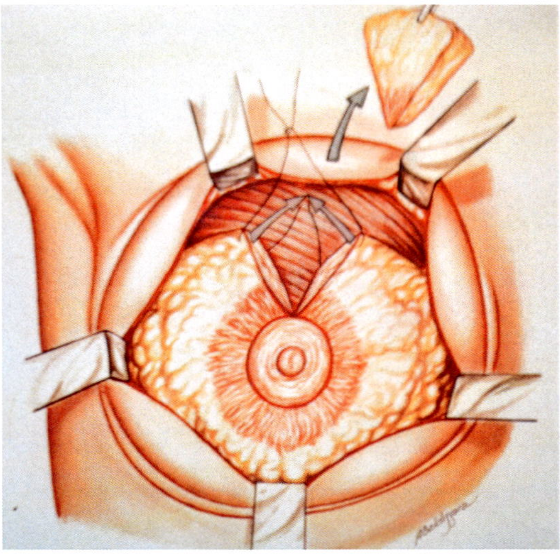

Fig. 37.11 Suture of the flaps in the midline after V-shaped resection and upward rotation

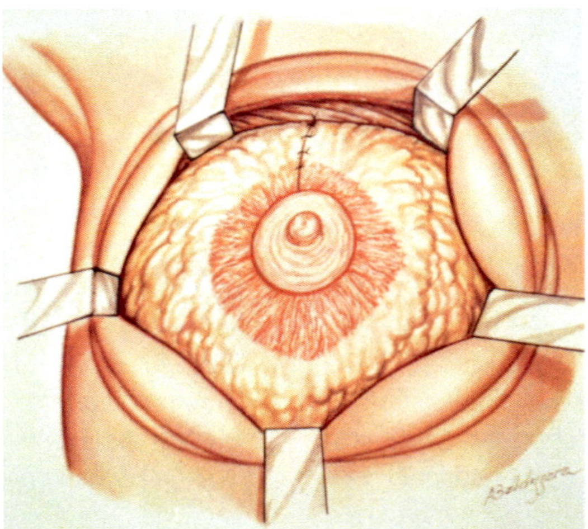

Fig. 37.12 Sutured flaps in the upper pole

major muscle and to one another in the midline superiorly (Fig. 37.12) using Mononylon 3–0 wires.

Once the upper anchorage has been successfully completed, the entire base of the breast (Fig. 37.13) is sutured to the muscle layer, narrowing the redundant tissue to gain greater anterior projection of the breast, which is often overcorrected at the end of surgery (Fig. 37.14) to oppose the counteracting force that will be exerted by the skin.

We then performed circular intradermal suturing with Mononylon 3–0 wire (Fig. 37.15),

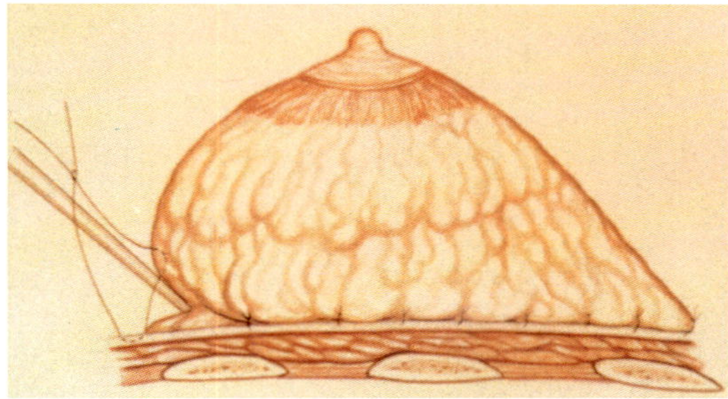

Fig. 37.13 The base of the breast is sutured to the aponeurosis of the pectoralis major muscle to achieve greater projection of the breast

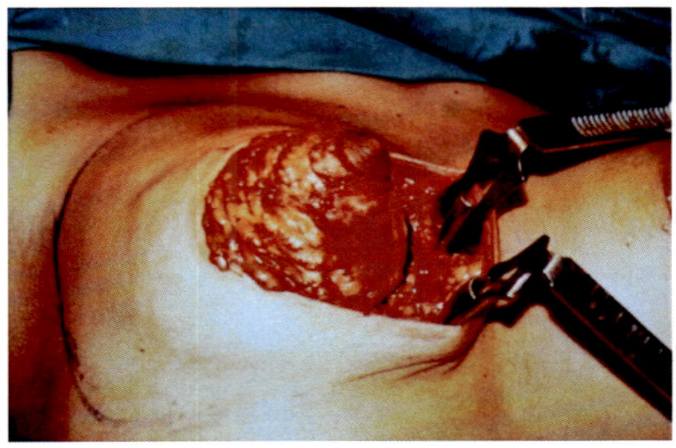

Fig. 37.14 Projected cone-shaped breast parenchyma

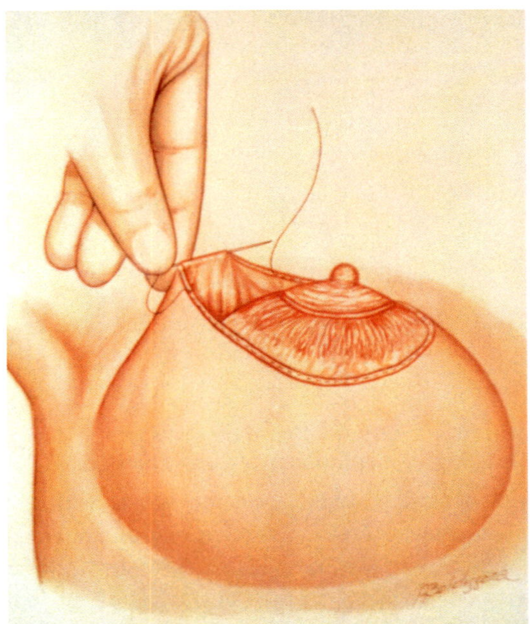

Fig. 37.15 Circular intradermal suturing with Mononylon 3–0

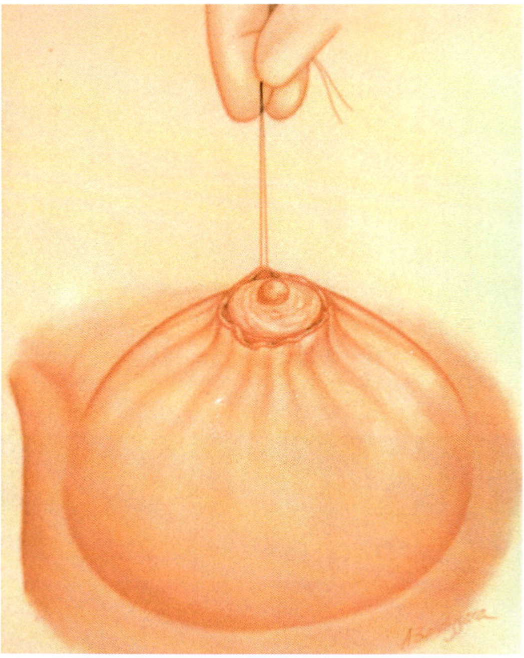

Fig. 37.16 Tensioned circular suture, approximating the skin edges to the outer limits of the NAC

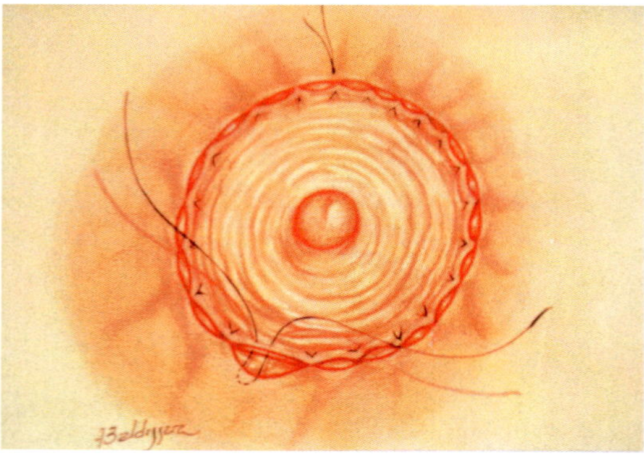

Fig. 37.17 5-0 mononylon "U" stiches areolar suture

which, when pulled to the predetermined size of the areola (Fig. 37.16), contains the tension that would be exerted on the suture with the consequent increase in the areolar diameter.

Suturing of the skin is performed with U-shaped stitches (Figs. 37.17 and 37.18), all around the areola. At the end of the surgery, the breast has a conical shape, with the scar limited to the areola (Fig. 37.19).

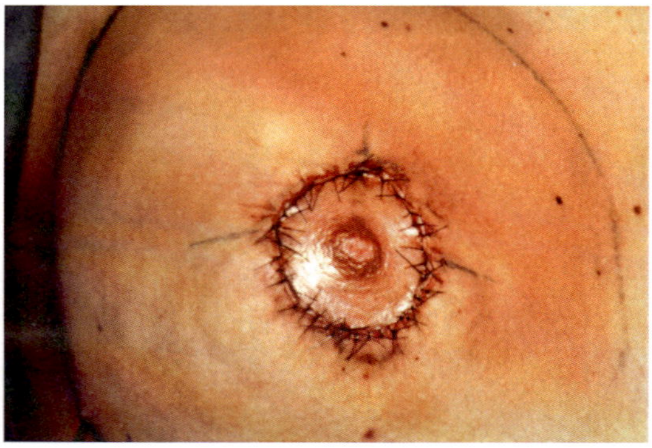

Fig. 37.18 Suture final aspect

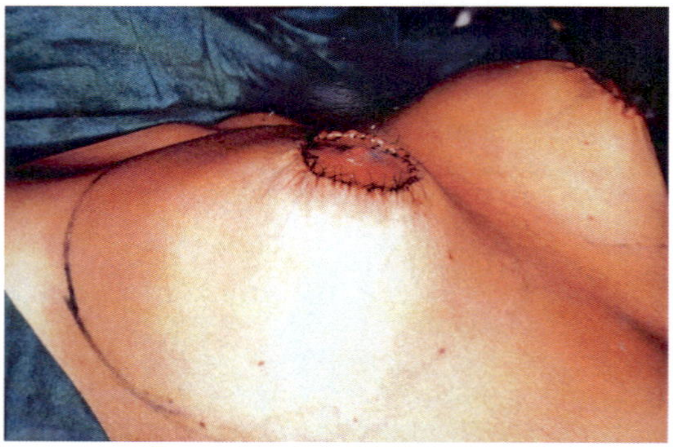

Fig. 37.19 Immediate postoperative

We use aspirative drain and slightly compressive occlusive dressing with gauze and cotton wool. Drain and dressing are removed after 24 h. The stitches are removed between the 7th and 15th postoperative day. The circular intradermic suture is not removed.

This technique applies to breast ptosis with mild and moderate hypertrophy, due to the limit for skin resection. The age of patients undergoing periareolar mammaplasty is predominantly less than 25 years. The breast resection usually ranges between 100 and 400 g and cutaneous resection between 4 and 14 cm.

37.3 Discussion

The development of mammaplasty was initially marked by techniques that sought to achieve good shape and projection of the breasts and

Table 37.1 Complications

Complication	Skin necrosis	Epidermolysis	Areola sensibility change	Dehiscence	Seroma	Total
Percentage	2	2	6	6	2	18

resulted in large scars, as the Strombeck and Pitanguy techniques (Strombeck 1960; Pitanguy 1960). Later there was a demand for techniques for breast reduction with progressively smaller scars like "L", vertical, and finally periareolar scars. Initially the periareolar technique failed due to skin necrosis secondary to large subcutaneous detachments. Knowledge of the importance of preserving the subdermal vascular plexus and the standardization of this dissection assured an adequate skin vascularization eliminating large necrosis (Hammond 2016).

Complications such as increased areola diameter and early ptosis were corrected with the application of periareolar suture round block and adjustments in parenchymal resections, respectively. In the technique presented here the upper pole "V" resection associated with the fixation of the breast muscle plane ensures good projection of the breast and stable results in the medium and long term.

It is common to observe wrinkling of the skin around the areola due to excess skin in relation to the size of the nipple areola complex. This wrinkling usually disappears between 2 and 5 months postoperatively. In cases of large resections patients are warned of the possible need for scar revision, after the sixth month postoperatively.

The age of the operated patients, with a predominance of patients under 25 years old is justified in better skin elasticity and lower skin excess at this age. Currently the authors restrict the indication of this technique to patients with good skin elasticity, which usually occurs under 25 years old.

The main reason for performing reoperations was the appearance of the scar. Concern about the scar was in fact the reason for the development of techniques that result in smaller scars. Studies evaluating other techniques also prove to be the scar the main focus of criticism by the patients.

37.4 Complications

The study of complications of periareolar approach shows a total complication rate of 18%. (Table 37.1)

The reoperation rate after 72 months of follow-up is 46% and the principal cause was the periareolar scar. Revisions in the scar on an outpatient basis were performed in 46% of patients and reoperation for residual sagging applying the scar "inverted T at 6%. These events were considered complications. Two percent of patients require reoperation due to small skin necrosis. The dissection must be subcutaneous, with preservation of the subdermal vascular plexus. Superficial dissections are more susceptible to skin necrosis.

When asked about satisfaction with the surgery, 86% of patients reported being satisfied or very satisfied, somewhat satisfied, and 8% 6% were dissatisfied. These numbers are close to those observed in patients undergoing breast reduction with inverted "T" scar (Aboudib-Cadoso de Castro et al. 1991).

Conclusion

The periareolar approach has a high level of satisfaction by the patients. The main indication is young patients with small to moderate breast hypertrophy and good skin elasticity. However, the skin periareolar resection presents high scar revision index.

References

Aboudib JH, Cadoso de Castro C, Coelho RS, Cupello AM (1991) Analysis of late results in postpregnancy mammoplasty. Ann Plast Surg 26:111–116

Benelli LA (1993) A new periareola mammaplasty: the "round block" technique. Aesthetic Plast Surg 14:93–100

Bustos RA (1992) Periareolar mammaplasty with sikicone supporting lamina. Plast Reconstr Surg 89(4):646–657

Goes JCS (1989) Periareolar mammaplasty double skin technique. Rev Bras Cir Plast 4(23):55–63

Goes JCS (1996) Periareolar mammaplasty double skin technique with application of polyglactine or mixed mesh. Plast Reconstr Surg 97:959

Hammond DC, Kim K (2016) The short scar periareolar inferior pedicle reduction mammaplasty: management of complications. Clin Plast Surg 43(2):365–372. Epub 2016 Feb 5

Hinderer V Primera experiencia con una nueva técnica de mastoplastia para petosis ligera. VI Reunión Nacional de la Soc. Española de Cir. Plástica y Reconstructiva. Madri, Nov 1969

International Society of Aesthetic Plastic Surgery. ISAPS global statistics 2015. http://www.isaps.org/Media/Default/global-statistics/2015%20ISAPS%20Results.pdf. Accessed 12 May 2016

Kausch M, Zarem, Harvey A.M.D. (1976) Plastic and Reconstructive Surgery of the Breast: R. M. Goldwyn (ed.), 565 pages, Boston, Little, Brown & Company, 1976.

Noel A (1928) Lopez-Martinez. La chirurgie esthétique; nouveaux procédés chirurgicaux de correction du prolapsus mammaire. Le Concours Méd:41

Pitanguy I (1960) Breast hipertrophy. In: Transactions of international society of plastic surgeons, 2nd congress, London, 1959, Livingstone, Edinburgh, LTDA

Souza AM (1970) Mastoplastia por incisão periareolar superior. ARS Curandi. 28:80–82

Strombeck JO (1960) Mammaplasty—report of a new technique based on the two pedicle provedure. Br J Plast Surg 13:79

Peixoto G (1989) Reduction mammaplasty. In: Ribeiro L (ed) Cirurgia Plástica da mama. MEDSI, Rio de Janeiro, pp 113–127

38 Critical Analyses on the Periareolar Approach to Mastoplasty

João Francisco Vale Pereira and William Seidel

38.1 Introduction

Many techniques with only incision around the areola have been developed to minimalize scarring in mammaplasties. We use a periareolar mammoplasty approach as the first choice in all our mammaplasties, both reduction mastopexy or breast increase with prosthesis. We started with techniques described by other authors, and over time we began to use the technique with characteristics modified from standard techniques. For some postoperative characteristics observed at the time, the side approach is used in most cases, for reasons explained below; however we believe that it is formally indicated for breasts with mild ptosis and breasts with tuberous features with greatly enlarged areola, constricted base, mild ptosis where the goal is to reduce the diameter of the areola, improve breast contour, and projection, with or without the use of an implant.

J.F. Vale Pereira, M.D.
Clinica Vale Pereira, Av. Osvaldo Rodrugues Cabral, 88015-710 Florianópolis, SC, Brazil
e-mail: xanicovallepereira@gmail.com

W. Seidel, M.D. (✉)
VIVVA Clinica, Rua Padre Roma sala 409, 88010-090 Florianópolis, SC, Brazil
e-mail: wseidel.plastica@gmail.com

38.1.1 History

The development of modern plastic surgery in the late nineteenth century and throughout the twentieth century brought innumerable mammoplasty techniques. Initial reports of mammoplasty with periareolar scarring ranged from Kausch (1916), Biesenberger (1931), Arié (1957), Strömbeck (1960), Pitanguy (1961), Andrews (1975), Peixoto (1983), Benelli (1990), Góes (1990), Bustos (1992), and Vale Pereira (1993). It is noteworthy that in the late 1980s and early 1990s we performed this technique often, which led us to participate as speakers at the XXVII Brazilian Congress of Plastic Surgery in Rio de Janeiro from 11 to 16 November 1990 on the periareolar breast lift technique, and also at *VII Corso Internazionale didactic—operative Chirurgia Estetica* 1990, held in Rome 29–30 April. We then published an article in the *Rivista Italiana de Chirurgia Plástica* as *Mamoplastica Periareolare* in 1993. It is also important to discuss here the preference for breast volume of Brazilian women, which in past decades was often a question of breast reduction throughout the exponential growth period of breast enlargement with silicone implants until today, when the preference is for a smaller breast volume and demand is for mastopexy, either with or without silicone implants.

J.M. Avelar (ed.), *Breast Surgery*, https://doi.org/10.1007/978-3-319-54115-0_38

38.2 Method

Through case studies and personal experience, we show why the primary indication was not for periareolar breast lift in all cases, particularly in reducing mammoplasty to treat severe ptosis, but this approach is only indicated for selected cases, which will be shown below.

We carried out a review of our cases using photographic files of patients operated on in our clinic over the years, correlating with them with those of established colleagues and their experiences with this mammoplasty approach.

38.3 Discussion

Bustos (1992), one of the pioneers in modern periareolar breast lift, showed his approach through the report of his 5-year experience with the technique, including 485 cases operated on between July 1985 and December 1989. Such cases included moderate ptosis, severe hypertrophy and/or a combination of the two. Resection of the excess breast tissue was carried out, but much of the gland was preserved, which provided the chance to maintain functionality, and the fact that the skin envelope was not violated, diminishing the chances of skin necrosis. It was performed using a silicone blade to help shape the breast and prevent ptosis, which had no interference to touch or imaging tests.

In our technique, periareolar mastoplasty by Vale Pereira (1993), which greatly relied on Bustos et al.'s technique, a design was made, point A, 18 cm from the ipsilateral midclavicular point and 6 cm from the inframammary fold, was made. The area of skin was decorticated between those points in a circular fashion while maintaining a symmetrical diameter (Fig. 38.1),

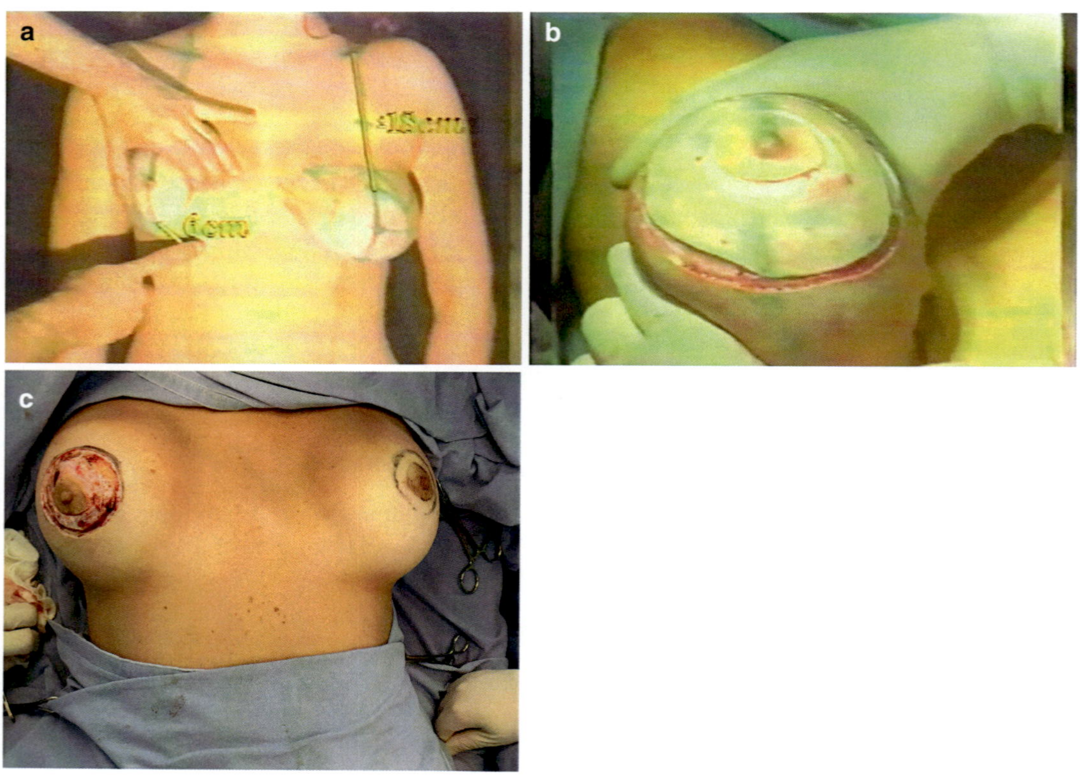

Fig. 38.1 (**a**) Marking points – 18 cm from the ipsilateral midclavicular point, and 6 cm from the mammary fold (picture of old technique). (**b**) Area of skin was decorticated between those points in a circular fashion while maintaining a symmetrical diameter (picture of old technique). (**c**) Circular area of skin decorticated (picture from recent patient)

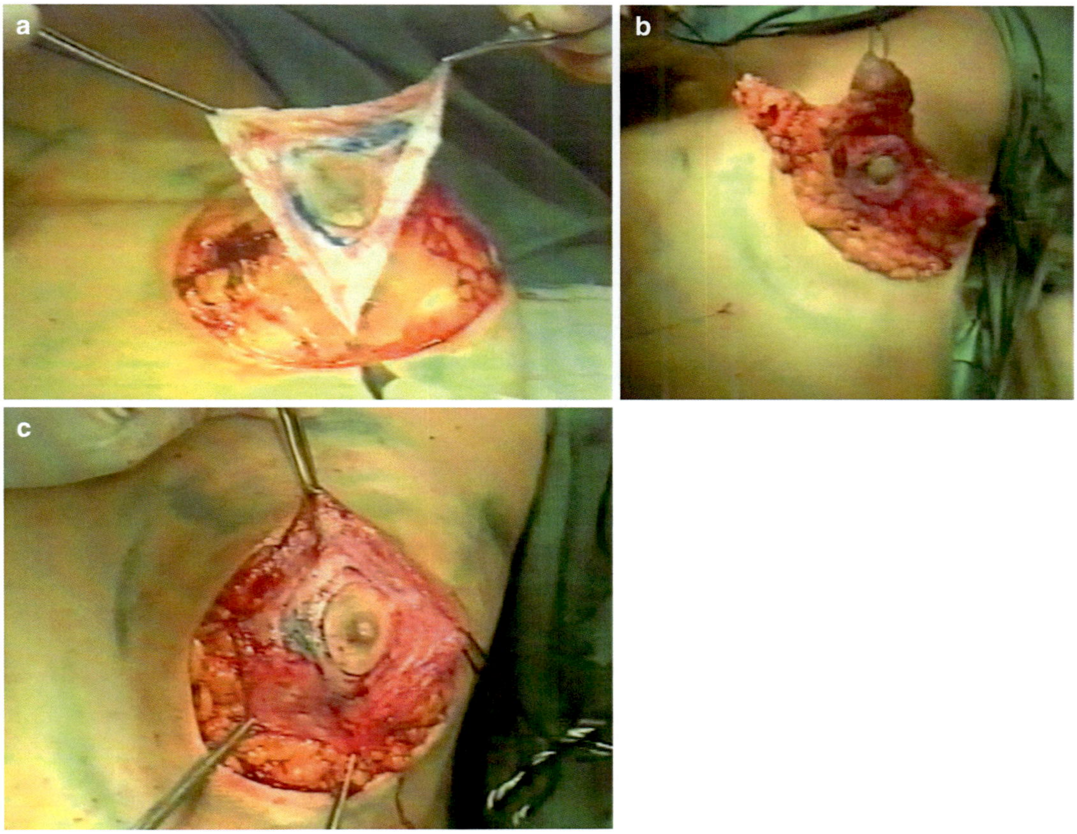

Fig. 38.2 Steps of periareolar mammoplasty. (**a**) Dermis flap to cover cone breast. (**b**) Three triangular flaps. (**c**) Recovered breast cone

preserving a flap of the dermis, which served as a cover for the mammary cone afterward. After an incision, we performed periareolar detachment of the skin followed by resection of the glandular tissue through a demarcated triangle. Three triangles in the upper pole were preserved, two were resected plus a resection or imbrication in the lower pole, as reduction and correction of ptosis were required. Then the breast was closed to form the cone of the mammary gland after covering with the dermal flap (Fig. 38.2). An important technical detail was that three or more circular suture layers were made in a teardrop shape involving the whole breast cone and a fixed circular suture was performed around the entire breast cone at the pectoralis major muscle on the upper pole (Fig. 38.3), to obtain the gland suspension effect and avoid early ptosis. This technique has been widely used by us and presented at congresses and conferences (Fig. 38.4).

Benelli (1990) introduced the concept of periareolar breast lift using a device called "round block." A circular suture is performed after large detachment and subsequent removal of skin as needed for correction of hypertrophy or breast ptosis, a technique that is used widely.

Góes et al. (2004) in his work performed periareolar mastopexy or breast reduction using polyglactin polyester mesh to obtain a controlled conical shape of the breast, as a skin envelope alone does not prevent early ptosis or extension of the areola. Therefore, he used a mesh device to prevent ptosis and enlargement of the areola.

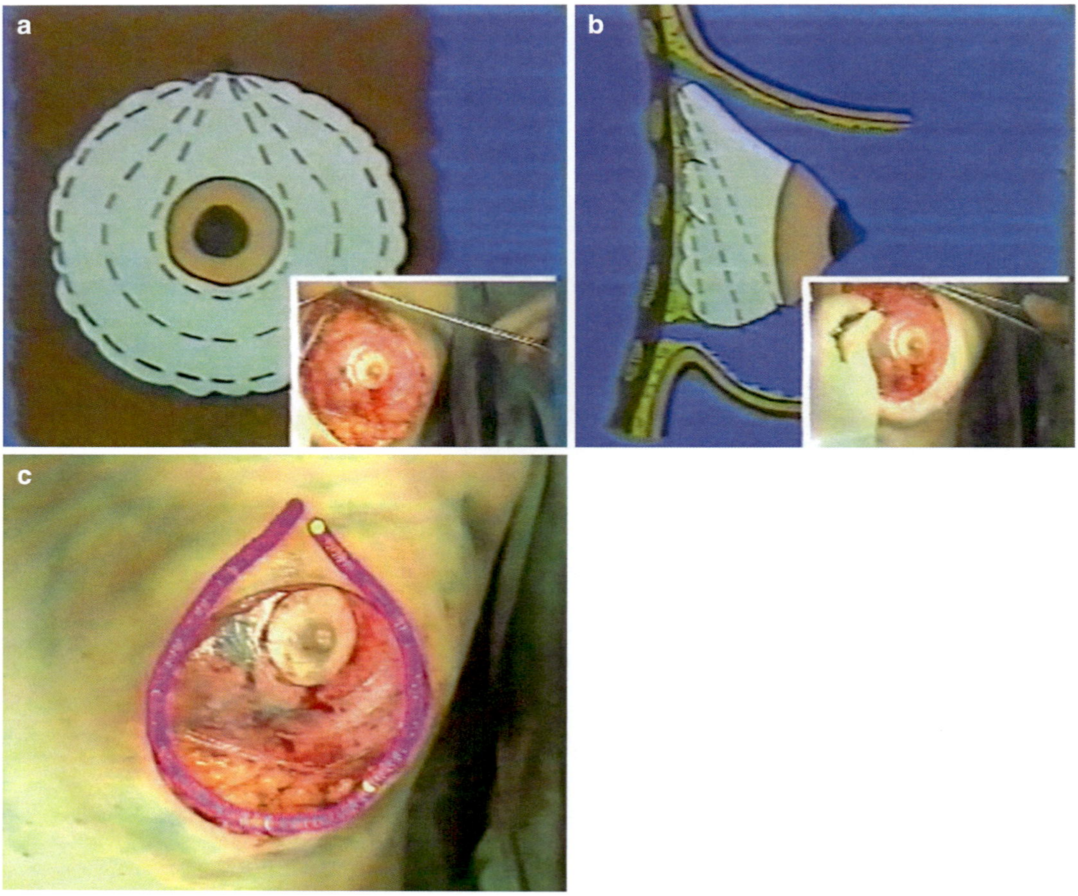

Fig. 38.3 Suture in teardrop shape. (**a**) Schematic drawing of front view suture in a teardrop shape. (**b**) Lateral view. (**c**) Marking the teardrop shape

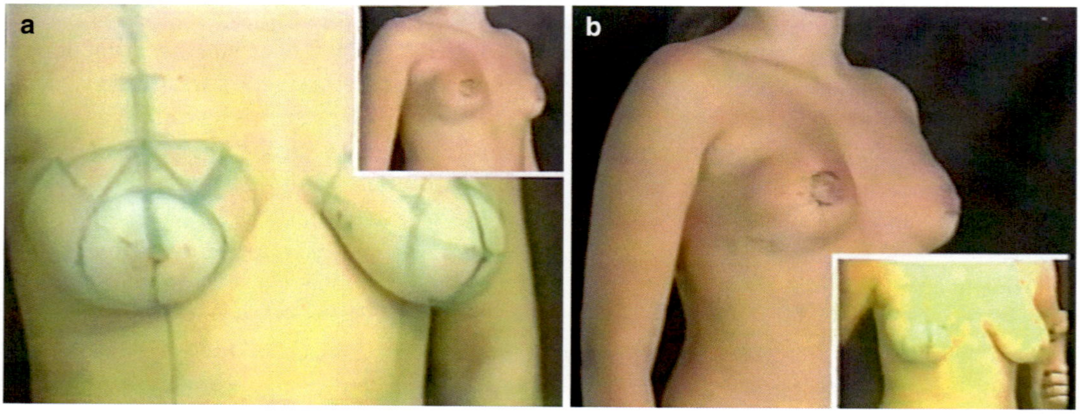

Fig. 38.4 (**a**) Preoperative and (**b**) postoperative views of a periareolar mammoplasty in a 17-year-old patient

38.4 Complications

Enlargement of the areola, loss of nipple projection, and flatness of the whole breast are the most frequent consequences of periareolar mammoplasty (Baran et al. 2001). Although initially use of surgical resources in the immediate postoperative period is to try to prevent complications by using suitable sutures, during the later postoperative period enlargement, loss of projection, and recurrence of ptosis may be observed (Fig. 38.5) (Baran et al. 2001). We believe that the consolidated statement for a periareolar approach in a breast is that it is most effective in breasts with tuberous characteristics: increased areolar diameter in that one of the surgical goals is to reduce the diameter of the areola, a high mammary fold and constricted base also often associated with pseudo-herniation of the breast tissue by the areola, and in cases of pseudoptosis or ptosis grade I according to Renault (1976). In these cases, it is still our first-choice approach. For a reduction in breast volume, we believe that a technique with a vertical component and often associated with a horizontal scar as needed, provides a more satisfactory result for breast reduction, better design of the breast, with a more harmonious contour and prevention of the enlargement of the areola after surgery for better distribution of the tension between all sutures.

It is important to make some criticism of these impressive works, first on the use of a silicone blade, which in some cases when we used it resulted in fibrosis and postoperative discomfort and had to be removed. Moreover, in cases of large ptosis and hypertrophy, recurrence and poor prognosis of the periareolar scar were experienced. We use round block suture in borderline cases if the periareolar approach is indicated, to try to "get rid" of a vertical scar. It allows greater removal of skin and prevents enlargement of the areola after surgery. This lock when there is a very large surplus of skin and the consequent resection of this skin, making a very large diameter for a circular suture, forming skin folds (Fig. 38.6). However we observed that although the immediate postoperative period has the appearance of closure being irregular, the evolution is favorable, in some cases we make use of retinoic acid in these skin irregularities, which assists in the retraction of the skin. We believe that this cutaneous fold aspect does not contraindicate the use of the technique.

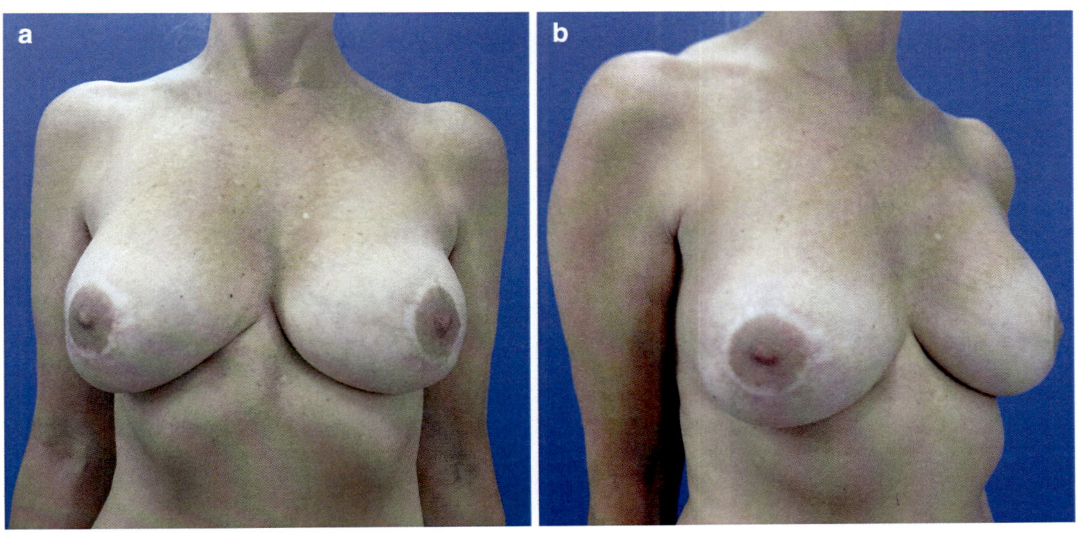

Fig. 38.5 Bad result of periareolar mammoplasty, 1 year postoperatively, enlargement of the areola and breast ptosis

Thus, by observing early ptosis, even though the technique could be performed successfully, we do not perform this routine approach in cases of breast reduction and mastopexy without the use of implants in cases of significant ptosis or hypermastia.

38.4.1 Current Surgical Technique

In indicated cases, pseudoptosis treatment or discrete breast ptosis with discrete cutaneous surplus is associated with the use of silicone gel breast implants. This is a description of our current technique for mild ptosis correction via periareolar mastopexy with use of a polyurethane-covered silicone gel implant: the marking is performed preoperatively, highlighting the whole breast area to be removed, and the area to be incised, which may be circular or semicircular, in which case only insertion is performed without removal of the skin implant. All patients were operated on in our clinic Vale Pereira—Florianópolis SC, the preferred anesthesia technique is epidural anesthesia under the supervision of the clinic. The solution to be infiltrated is 250 mL 0.9% physiological saline and 1 mL adrenaline. The incision is made with a scalpel on the skin and below the gland planned with the help of electrocautery. Sometimes it is necessary to perform resection of retro-areolar glandular breast tissue. Molds are used for testing and the choosing of the polyurethane implant. Closure is carried out using glandular planned Mononylon 3–0 by separate points in the subdermal layer and Mononylon 4–0 wire in a continuous intradermal suture. When large amounts of skin are removed, a suture is held in a "round block" with Mononylon 2–0 (Fig. 38.7; Table 38.1).

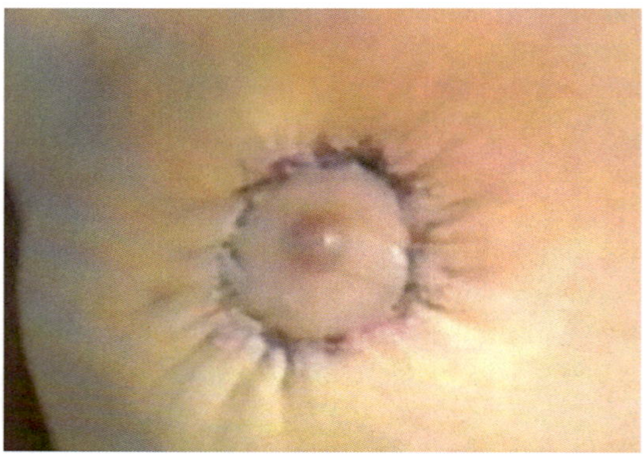

Fig. 38.6 Folded aspect of skin in round block suture

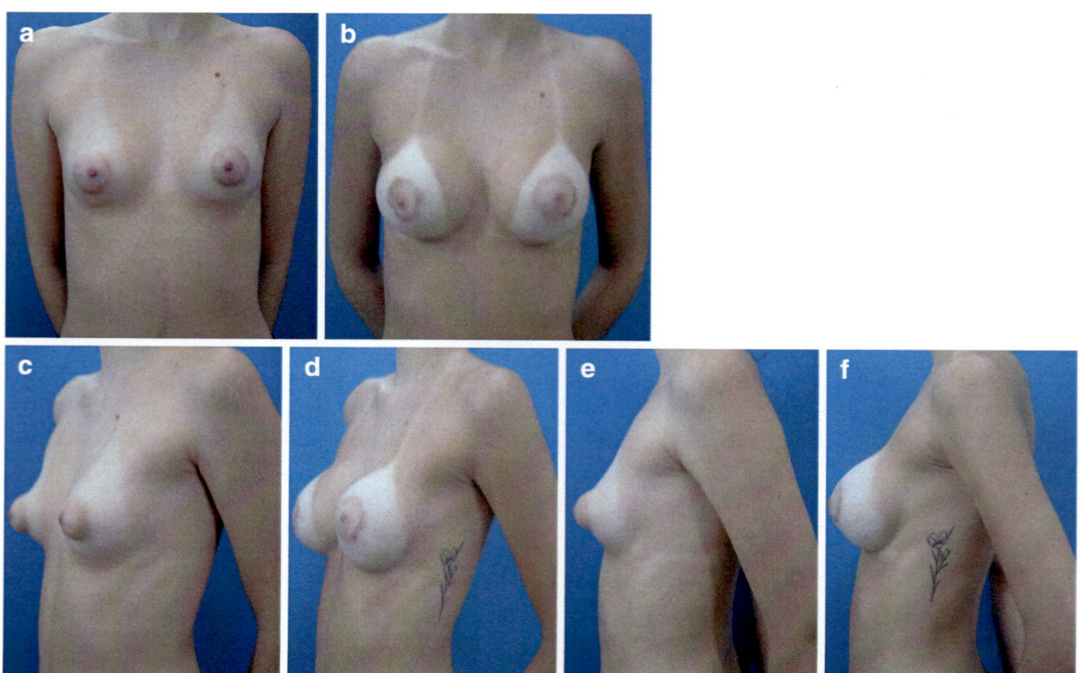

Fig. 38.7 (**a**, **c**, **e**) Preoperative views of a 20-year-old patient with tuberous breasts. (**b**, **d**, **f**) One year postoperatively in periareolar mammoplasty with breast implants (current technique)

Table 38.1 Criteria for indication of periareolar approach to mastoplasty

Periareolar mammoplasty: personal approach João Francisco Vale Pereira	
Indication for use of this technique:	Indications for which we failed to accomplish a solution:
1—Mild breast ptosis, Renault grade I pseudoptosis[a]	1—Severe hypertrophy
2—Tuberous breasts: enlarged areola, constricted base, high groove	2—Severe ptosis
3—Enlarged areola in nontuberous breasts with mild ptosis	3—Significant association between ptosis and hypertrophy[b]

[a]Generally where this technique is indicated, we make use of polyurethane-covered silicone gel implants (and less postoperative ptosis and capsular contracture are observed)
[b]In cases discouraging the exclusive use of the periareolar approach, we demonstrated a preference for a technique to present a vertical component, often a horizontal incision, and therefore scarring

Conclusion

Taking into account our experience over the years with postoperative follow-up in the clinic of patients operated on using the periareolar technique, we can conclude the indications for this technique are much reduced, as it fails to perform reducing mammaplasties in cases of large ptosis and breast hypertrophy because of the high rate of recurrence and rates of reoperations due to enlargement of the areola, complaints about scarring, and especially the recurrence of ptosis. It is often necessary to associate a vertical and horizontal incision to make the correction scar. We also note that the use of a silicone mesh or screen or Mononylon suspension sutures (teardrop shape) do not provide lasting results or replace the skin removed at the lower pole of the breast, with vertical and horizontal scarring. Today, we believe that the indication for periareolar mammoplasty is considered for cases of tuberous breasts with enlarged areola, mild ptosis, ptosis and pseudoptosis grade I according to Renault's classification, and in most cases it is associated with the use of polyurethane-covered silicone gel implants.

References

Arié G (1957) Nova Técnica em Momoplastia. Revista Latino Americana de Cirurgia Plástica 3:28

Baran CN, Peker F, Ortak T, Şensöz Ö, Baran NK (2001) Unsatisfactory results of periareolar mastopexy with or without augmentation and reduction mammoplasty: enlarged areola with flattened nipple. Aesth Plast Surg 25:286–289

Benelli L (1990) A new periareolar mammaplasty: the "round block" technique. Aesth Plast Surg 14(2):93–100

Biesenberger H (1931) Deformitäten und Kosmetische Operationen der Weibblichen Brust. Viena Mauddrich

Bustos RA (1992) Periareolar mamaplasty with silicone sheeting. Plast Reconstr Surg 89(4):646–657

Góes JCS, Landecker A, Lyra EC, Henríquez LJ, Góes RS, Godoy PM (2004) The application of mesh support in periareolar breast surgery: clinical and mammographic evaluation. Aesth Plast Surg 28:268–274

Peixoto G (1983) Reduction Mammaplasty: Conceptual Evolution. Transo f the VIII Cong Inter of Plast Surg Montreal 543:544

Pitanguy I (1961) Mammaplastias: Esudo de 245 Casos consecutivos e Apresentação da técnica pessoal. Rev Bras Cir 42:201

Regnault P (1976) Breast ptosis. Definition and treatment. Clin Plast Surg 3(2):193–203

Strombeck JD (1968) Reduction Mammaplasty in Plastic Surgery. A Concise Guide to Clinical Pratice. Ed. By Grabb WC, And Smith JW. Boston: Little Brown and Co.

Vale Pereira JF (1993) Mastoplastica Periareolare. Rivista Italiana di Chirurgia Plastica

Tuberous Breast

39

Ricardo Cavalcanti Ribeiro,
Luis Emilio Fuentes López, and Sergio Romay

39.1 Introduction

The formation of the mammary gland begins before sexual differentiation. The development of the mammary ridge or milk line, which is a surface spread of embryonic ventral ectoderm, extending from the axilla to the inguinal bilaterally, begins by the fifth week of embryonic life. The mammary crest, from which usually develops a single pair of mammary glands, disappears in human embryos at around the seventh week, persisting in only a small portion of the pectoral region. This involution of the milk crest is characteristic of the human species.

Subsequently, there is invagination of the local ectoderm that will form the primary breast bud, which will give rise to 15 or 20 secondary branches. At first, these sprouts, consisting of ectodermal cells, are massive and branch out into the middle of the mesenchyme. In the third trimester of pregnancy, the ducts become tunneled, with a light appearance in their interior, open out into the mammary pits, which rise and form the nipple. The ramifications of the ducts end in a blind bottom, constituting lobular duct units or cellular terminals.

Breast engorgement and secretion of colostrum, due to hormonal stimulation from the mother through the placenta, occurs in approximately 80% of infants of both sexes. There is spontaneous regression of this phenomenon around the third or fourth week after birth, with the gradual elimination of hormones by the conceptus.

Until the onset of puberty, the female breasts usually remain underdeveloped, starting development with ovarian stimulation that begins in this period. From then on, the development is glandular, together with the fat and connective tissue. During pregnancy, the development of the mammary glands is completed.

Russo and Russo describe the development of the breasts, especially in their early years, to make the biological phenomena that govern the mammary epithelium comprehensible:

Nulliparous breasts consist of type I lobes, also called virgin lobes, because they are present before menarche. This type is the most undifferentiated. The lobes are formed of clusters of 6–11 ductules per lobe.

Type II lobes are formed from the first; they have a more complex morphology and are formed by a larger number of ductular structures per lobe.

Type III are characterized by having an average of 80 ductules or wells per lobe. They are often found in women on hormone therapy and during pregnancy.

Head of Division of Plastic and Reconstructive Surgery of Universidade Federal do Estado of the Rio de Janeiro (UNIRIO)

R.C. Ribeiro, M.D., Ph.D. (✉)
Division of Plastic Surgery of Casa de Portugal, Brazilian Society of Plastic Surgery, Carlos Chagas Institute, Rio de Janeiro, RJ, Brazil
e-mail: rribeiro@centroin.com.br

L.E.F. López, M.D. • S. Romay, M.D.
Division of Plastic and Reconstructive Surgery, Carlos Chagas Institute, Rio de Janeiro, RJ, Brazil

J.M. Avelar (ed.), *Breast Surgery*, https://doi.org/10.1007/978-3-319-54115-0_39

Type IV lobes are considered the ultimate expression of development and differentiation. They are found during pregnancy and lactation, and furthermore, are not noticed in nulliparous women in the post-puberty period. This differentiation diminishes the possibility of breast cancer—a pregnancy to term before the age of 24, according to those authors, reduces the relative risk (RR) of breast cancer development fourfold.

Changes in breast morphology can be divided according to the time they are diagnosed into congenital and development; and from the pathophysiological point of view and functional morphology. But many of these morphological changes can coexist with functional problems; thus, the authors consider the first classification more appropriate.

39.2 Tuberous Breasts

The concept of tuberous breasts has been studied as a change in breast morphology since the last century, although Longacre (1954) and Goulian (1971) had studied this breast alteration and proposed its treatment with the use of a dermoadipose pedicle to enlarge the breast base. It was only in 1976 that Rees and Aston described it as a "tuberous breast" for the first time. Several authors actively participated in search techniques for the correction of this abnormality and so far, innovative techniques have been published with satisfactory results (Jurado 1976; Pitanguy 1984; Ribeiro et al. 2002; Rohrich et al. 2002; Robbins 1977; Wallace et al. 1998).

Given that breasts identify a woman's femininity and that their function is not limited to breastfeeding and raising children, and as they play a key role in sexual development and social acceptance, we can consider it important that the changes they reach are harmonious in appearance or they can otherwise cause unwanted psychological conduct with falling levels of self-esteem and stress of neurotic or bipolar disorders that could generate a progressive and destructive dissatisfaction with a woman's personal development.

39.3 Definition

The term "tuberous breast" is used to define a syndrome consisting of a hypoplastic alteration of the breast, where there is a base of insufficient diameter for the glandular content, accompanied by a pseudo-herniation of the same through the areola, with a deficit of skin wrap and a poorly positioned inframammary crease, which is usually located above the desired location; thus giving the tubular appearance that identifies it.

This entity is not recognized as a medical condition or actual disease but, apparently, has a strong association with other types of deformities, as elaborated in an article published by DeLuca-Pytell et al. This was a review of the incidence of tuberous breasts in 375 patients undergoing mammoplasty who only sometimes presented mammary asymmetry. It was performed through a retrospective preoperative analysis, and presented interesting results, for example, that 80.1% of patients who underwent mammoplasty had mammary asymmetry, and of the patients with asymmetry, 80.8% had some type of tuberous breast, compared with only about 7% of patients with symmetrical breasts. This strong association can provide the etiology, which remains unknown, and the development of optimal techniques for treatment (Figs. 39.1, 39.2, 39.3, 39.4, 39.5, 39.6, 39.7, 39.8, 39.9, and 39.10).

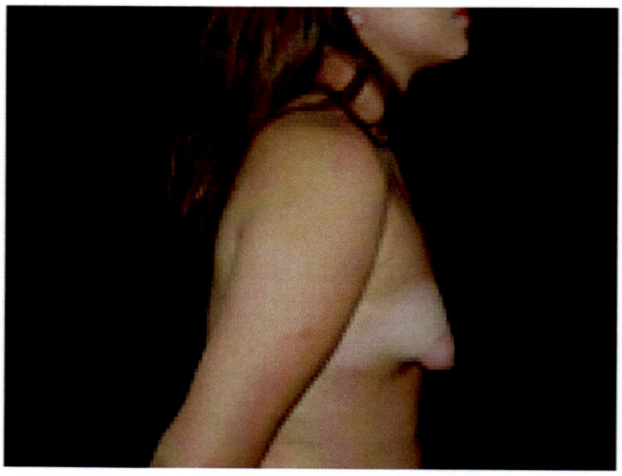

Fig. 39.1 Right side of a female patient with tuberous breast

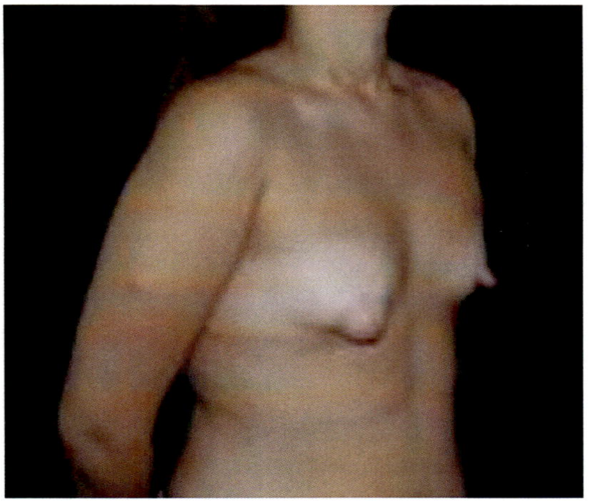

Fig. 39.2 Same patient on oblique view showing severe hypoplasia of left breast

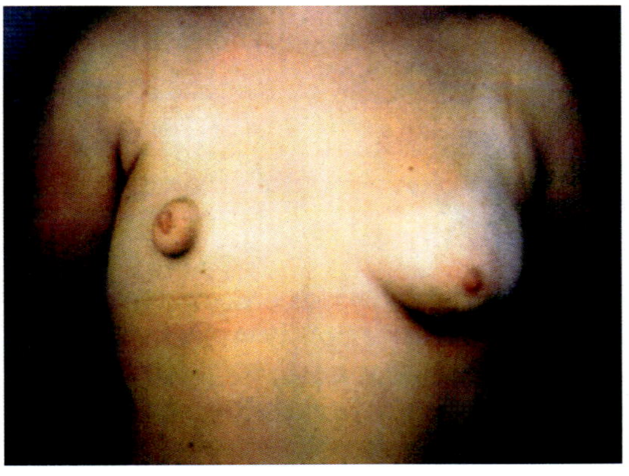

Fig. 39.3 A female patient with severe asymmetric breast: hypoplasia on right side and tuberous on left

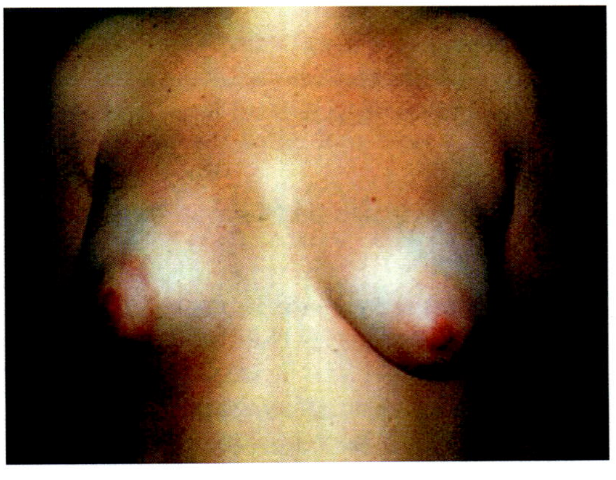

Fig. 39.4 Tuberous breast with asymmetry

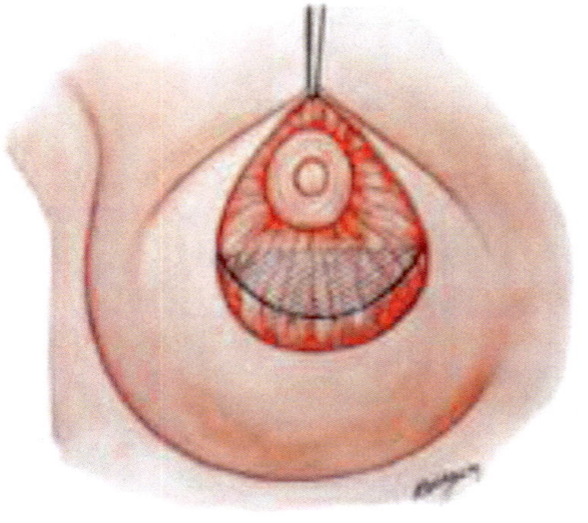

Fig. 39.5 Drawing shows the technique for correction of tuberous breast: deepithelized periareolar area with demarcation of a curved incision below the nipple-areolar region

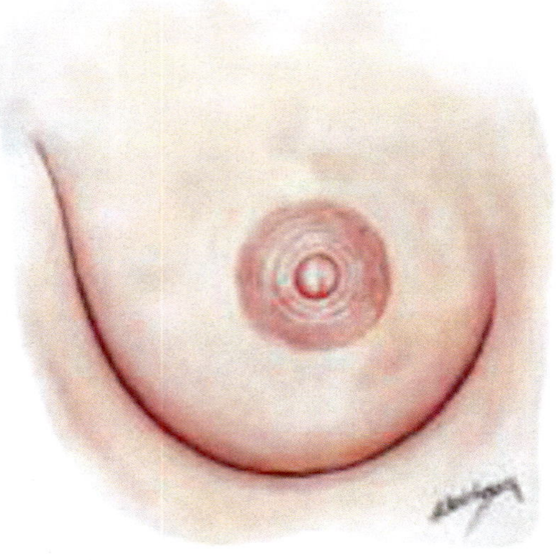

Fig. 39.6 Drawing shows the final aspect after correction of tuberous breast throught periareolar incision

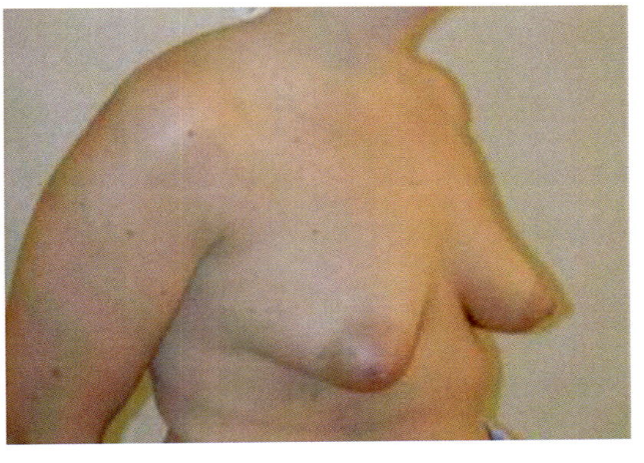

Fig. 39.7 Preoperative photo of a patient on oblique view showing bilateral teberous breast

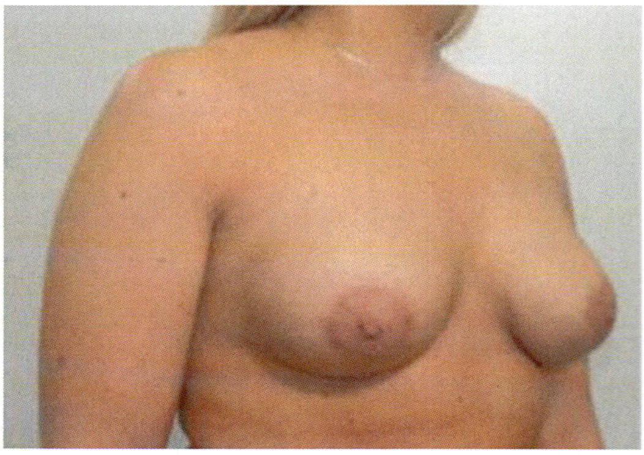

Fig. 39.8 Same patient after correction of tuberous breast

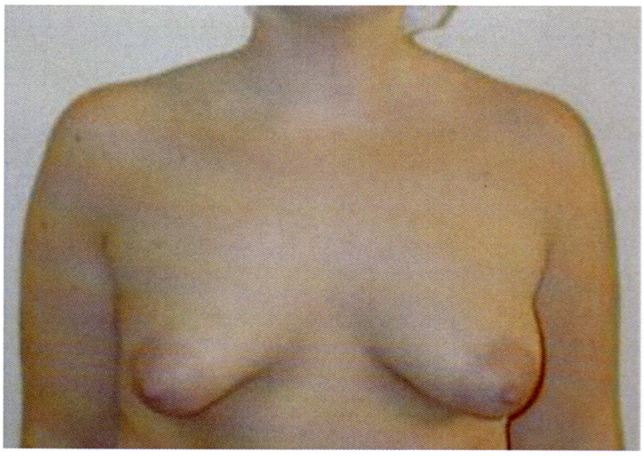

Fig. 39.9 Preoperative of the same patient in frontal view with bilateral tuberous breasts

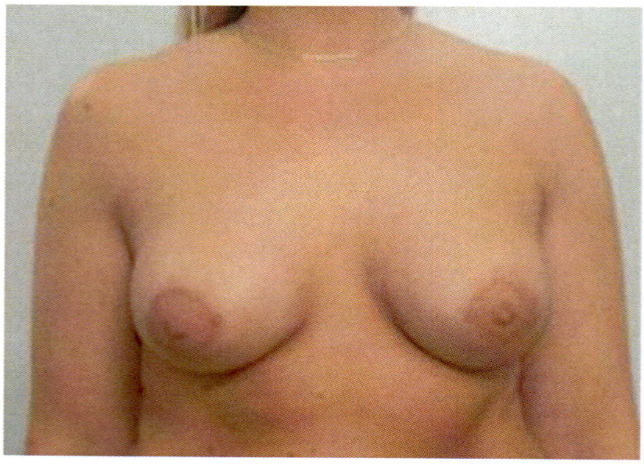

Fig. 39.10 Post operative photo of the same patient

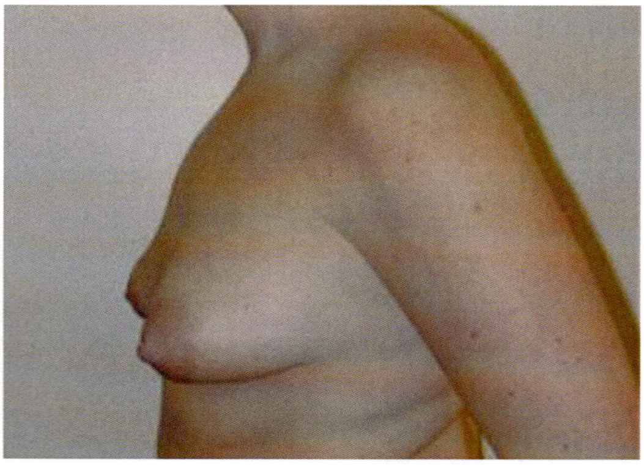

Fig. 39.11 Left side of the same patient showing ptotic and tuberous breasts

39.4 Classification

Morphologically, various proposals for tuberous breast classification have been described, one of which was advocated by Meara et al. (2000), most frequently used today. However, in the same year, Von Heimburg presented a more refined version of this classification, which we consider adequate for academic purposes and is useful in comparing the postoperative results of procedures performed by different surgeons using different techniques to define the degree of correction of the defect (Fig. 39.11).

39.5 General Aspects

Clinical findings

Tuberous or tubular breasts are characterized as:

- Deficiency of glandular tissue plus elongation
- Enlargement and swelling of the NAC—constriction/herniation
- Narrow base—absence or poor lower pole
- Association with other congenital breast diseases

– Classification of tuberous breasts. (Source: Plastic and Reconstructive Surgery 2005 Dec; 116 (7): 1894–99.)

Type I: hypoplasia of the inferomedial quadrant of the breast.
Type II: hypoplasia of the inferomedial and inferolateral quadrants (lower pole of the breast).
Type III: hypoplasia of the lower breast pole with skin deficiencies in the subareolar region.
Type IV: severe mammary constriction with a very narrow base.

Discussion
Surgical technique
Surgical treatment

Single stage or several stages

Expanders: reconstruction of the breast with an expander behind the pectoralis major muscle, to distend the skin, thus acquiring enough volume to change the expander for a final mammary implant.
Permanent implants
Glandular mobilization resections
Glandular flaps (Lyacir Ribeiro)

After the recognition of tuberous breasts, Bass et al., in 1978, reported his technique, emphasizing the existing pseudo-herniation in the NAC. Toranto described a correction in two surgical stages and Williams had a known specific treatment for this entity. However, good results have only been achieved as of 1993 by Teimouriam and Adham, whose technique consisted of two incisions (areolar and submammary) and the use of an implant.

Dinner, also, in 1987, and Eliot, in 1998, used submammary groove flaps for treating tuberous breasts, and later Versaci, in 1991 and 1994, suggested the use of tissue expanders and repair at various surgical stages. Muti, in turn, began to combine the use of glandular flaps with the inclusion of implants through a periareolar incision with or without the vertical scar as a complement.

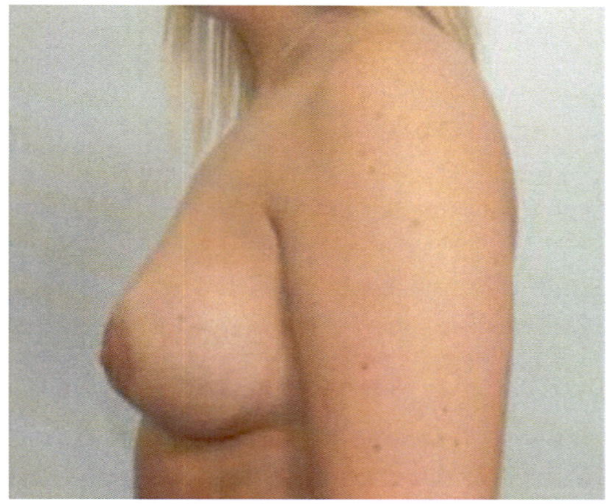

Fig. 39.12 Left side of the same patient after operation

Liacyr Ribeiro published several articles proposing a technique based on dividing the breast into two hemispheres (upper and lower). The lower segment is folded onto itself, creating the lower pole of the breast. At the same time, the areal constriction is released. This surgery may be performed with or without implants. We describe this surgical sequence in Fig. 39.12.

39.5.1 Association Between Tuberous + Poland Syndrome (Type 1)

39.5.1.1 Surgical Sequence

With the patient in a semi-seated position, a new areola is designed with an areola cutter 4–5 cm in diameter and the periareolar excess is marked. Then, the new inframammary crease is marked, usually positioned 1.5–2 cm below the original crease. Next, the periareolar region is denuded with subsequent breast division into two flaps, an upper areola—the pedicle and other inferior pedicle releasing carefully medial and lateral extensions of the upper flap. The flaps should be carefully handled, especially the lower, to avoid prejudicing the intercostal perforating vessels that nourish the flaps.

The lateral and medial portions of the inferior pedicle wither, and it is ready to be inverted upon itself to create the lower pole of the breast and the bottom of the fascia of the pectoralis major muscle is secured with non-absorbable suture. This inferior pedicle receives its vascularization from the fourth, fifth, and sixth intercostal arteries. The superior part, with the release of the constricted ring of skin, slips naturally onto the pedicle, forming the base of the breast to be enlarged.

The areola's final suture is made with continuous round block wired non-absorbable nylon 2-0 stitches. In certain situations, it may be necessary to suture points with interrupted 5-0 nylon 6-0 or other yarns may be used according to the surgeon's preference.

It is considered important to fix the breast with hypoallergenic tape for a period of approximately 15 days for modeling purposes.

39.5.2 Morphological Changes of the Breast and Thoracic Wall

Conclusions

The tuberous breast can constitute a therapeutic confrontation. Understanding the classification and having the knowledge of the above-mentioned techniques aid plastic surgeons in the surgical treatment of tuberous breasts. Expanders, implants, and pedicle flaps are excellent tools when operating on this type of syndrome. These techniques provide excellent aesthetic results, with both physician and patient satisfaction.

References

Jurado J (1976) Plásticas mamárias de redução baseadas em retalho dérmico vertical monopediculado. Anais XII Congresso Brasilei- ro de Cirurgia Plástica, vol 29

Pitanguy I (1984) Mamoplastia reductora con retallo superior em hipertrofia mamaria. Rev Bras Cir 74:265–284

Ribeiro L, Accorsi A Jr, Buss A, Marcal-Pessoa M (2002) Creation and evolution of 30 years of the inferior pedicle in reduction mammaplasties. Plast Reconstr Surg 110(3):960–970

Robbins TH (1977) A reduction mammaplasty with the areolanipple based on an inferior dermal pedicle. Plast Reconstr Surg 59(1):64–67

Rohrich RJ, Gosman AA, Brown SA, Tonadapu P, Foster B (2004) Current preferences for breast reduction techniques: a survey of board-certified plastic surgeons 2002. Plast Reconstr Surg 114(7):1724–1736

Wallace WH, Thompson WO, Smith RA, Barraza KR, Davidson SF, Thompson JT II. (1998) Reduction mammaplasty using the inferior pedicle technique. Ann Plast Surg 40(3):235–240

40 Body Contouring Surgery: Combined Breast Surgery in Lipoabdominoplasty

Célio Ferreira Leão, Gheisa Moura Leão, Mário Junqueira Souza, Tiago Almeida Vale, Giovani Araujo Godinho Filho, and Célio Coelho Neto Leão

40.1 Introduction

Considering the progress that has taken place in the fields of technology and in the measures used in patient safety in plastic surgery, it has become possible to incorporate mastopexy, or breast augmentation, into body contouring lipoabdominoplasty, with a trained team, during the same surgery, as long as it does not exceed the 5 h limit.

The development of this surgical process, published here, began with the work done by the author of this chapter presented at the XXXVII Brazilian Congress of Plastic Surgery (XXXVII Congresso Brasileiro de Cirurgia Plástica) (Leão 2000). A central subcutaneous tunnel is created from the umbilicus up to the xiphoid process, allowing rectus abdominis muscle plicature. Clinical observation has shown that the lateral abdominal flaps remain attached to the aponeurosis through subcutaneous adhesions found after liposuction. This flap adhesion is similar to that observed when applying the Baroudi and Ferreira knots maneuver (1998). It is necessary to clarify that the evolution of this surgical technique into the combined breast lipoabdominoplasty described

C.F. Leão, M.D. (✉)
Faculdade de Medicina da Universidade Federal de Goiás (School of Medicine of the Federal University of Goiás), Goiânia, GO, Brazil

Escola de Medicina da Pontifícia Universidade Católica de Goiás (School of Medicine of the Pontifical Catholic University of Goiás), Goiânia, GO, Brazil

Serviço de Cirurgia Plástica da Santa Casa de Misericórdia de Goiânia (Plastic Surgery Service of the Santa Casa de Misericórdia Hospital of Goiânia), MEC/SBCP, Goiânia, GO, Brazil

Sociedade Brasileira de Cirurgia Plástica (Brazilian Society of Plastic Surgery), São Paulo, SP, Brazil
e-mail: celioleao1@hotmail.com

G.M. Leão, M.D.
Escola de Medicina da Pontifícia Universidade Católica de Goiás (School of Medicine of the Pontifical Catholic University of Goiás), Goiânia, GO, Brazil

Serviço de Cirurgia Plástica da Santa Casa de Misericórdia de Goiânia (Plastic Surgery Service of the Santa Casa de Misericórdia Hospital of Goiânia), MEC/SBCP, Goiânia, GO, Brazil

Sociedade Brasileira de Cirurgia Plástica (Brazilian Society of Plastic Surgery), São Paulo, SP, Brazil

Clínica de Cirurgia Plástica—Allure (Allure Plastic Surgery Clinic), Goiânia, GO, Brazil

M.J. Souza, M.D. • T.A. Vale, M.D.
G.A. Godinho Filho, M.D.
Serviço de Cirurgia Plástica da Santa Casa de Misericórdia de Goiânia (Plastic Surgery Service of the Santa Casa de Misericórdia Hospital of Goiânia), MEC/SBCP, Goiânia, GO, Brazil

C.C.N. Leão, M.D.
UNIG—Hospital da Plástica (UNIG—Hospital of Plastic Surgery), Rio de Janeiro, RJ, Brazil

J.M. Avelar (ed.), *Breast Surgery*, https://doi.org/10.1007/978-3-319-54115-0_40

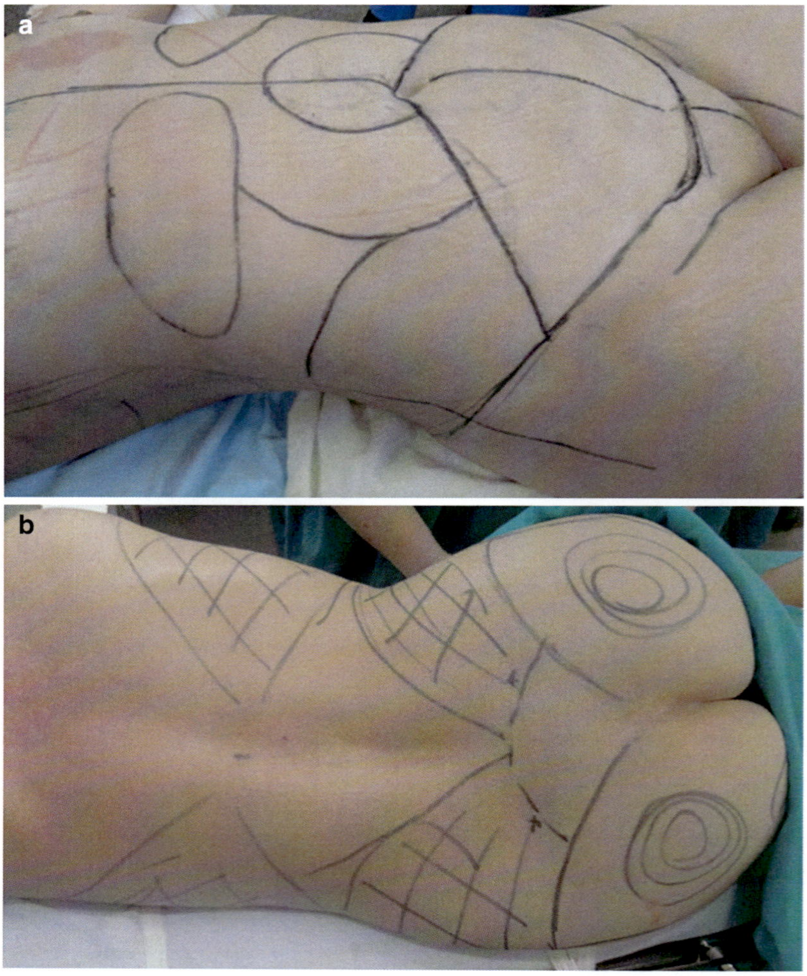

Fig. 40.1 (**a**, **b**) Front and back design of liposuction and lipoabdominoplasty

here, was only possible because of the advent of Illouz liposuction (1980) and the definite association between liposuction and classical abdominoplasty (Fig. 40.1) (Avelar 2000).

Since then, we have included breast implants and fat grafting of the buttocks, complementing the body contouring surgery (Fig. 40.2).

We have devised a new plication, from the fascia of Scarpa to the aponeurosis of the abdominal musculature, now closing the surgical tunnel previously described (see Fig. 40.6). The goal of this suture is to markedly improve the body contouring surgery, providing a new silhouette by sliding not only the abdominal flap, but also the entire thoracic–dorsal–flank–abdominal flap, as if we restitched a new garment over a thinner body (see Fig. 40.7).

This view of the body characterizes a new perspective, as it is now seen in its entirety instead of in its segmented form. This has resulted in a new insight into body contouring and the surgical process.

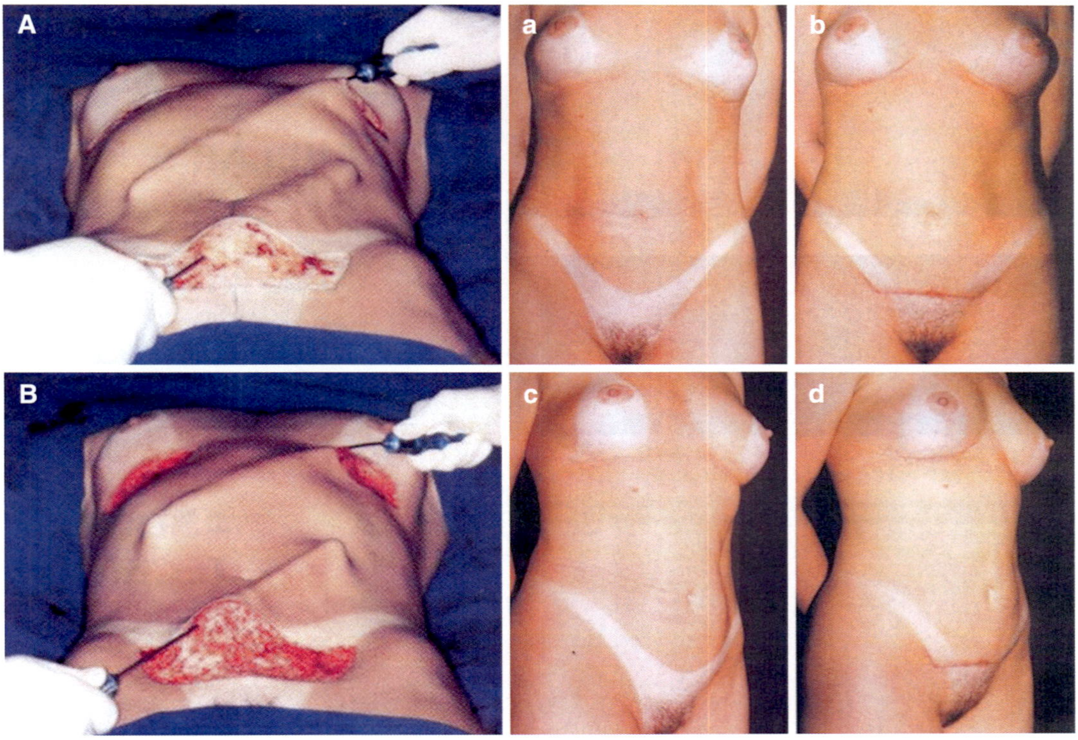

Fig. 40.2 (**a**, **b**) Definitive liposuction combined with abdominoplasty. (**c**, **d**) Postoperative Avelar's technique, front and oblique

40.2 Method

In the period from 2000 to 2010, a total of 606 surgeries were conducted; in a second period, from 2010 to 2015, 163 were conducted, totaling 769 procedures in female patients, with an average age of 30 years (Fig. 40.3).

40.2.1 Surgical Technique

40.2.1.1 Tumescent Liposuction

- The patient should be positioned in a ventral decubitus position for the beginning of the procedure (Fig. 40.4b).
- First, the saline solution is infused (1,000 mL/3 capsules of adrenaline in a proportion of 1/0.33 Ml); infiltration is done with a 4-mmcannula around the back. The liposuction of the back and flank is initiated using vibroliposuction, a procedure that sets the liposuctioned fat aside in a sterile flask.
- The total amount of fat to be taken should not exceed 5–7% of the body weight. The buttocks fat graft is carried out with the fat obtained from these areas until the desired volume is reached, varying from 250 mL to 600 mL of the supernatant fat.
- This procedure should take 40 to 60 min.
- The patient is put into the dorsal decubitus position (Fig. 40.4a).
- The saline solution is infused (1,000 mL/3 capsules of adrenaline in a proportion of 1/0.33 mL); the infiltration is performed with

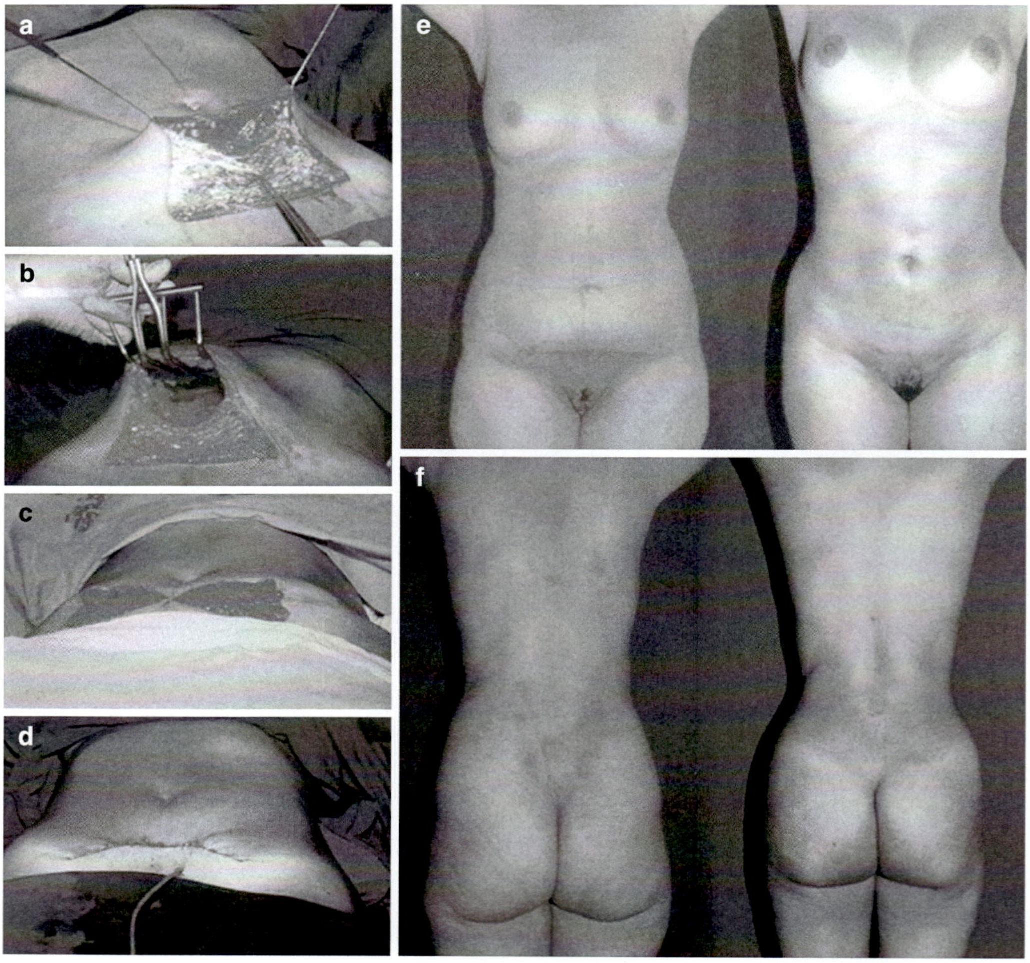

Fig. 40.3 (**a–d**) Leão's technique. Xipho-umbilical tunnel creation for the rectus abdominis muscle plicature. (**e**, **f**) Pre- and postoperative liposuction and fat grafting of the buttocks

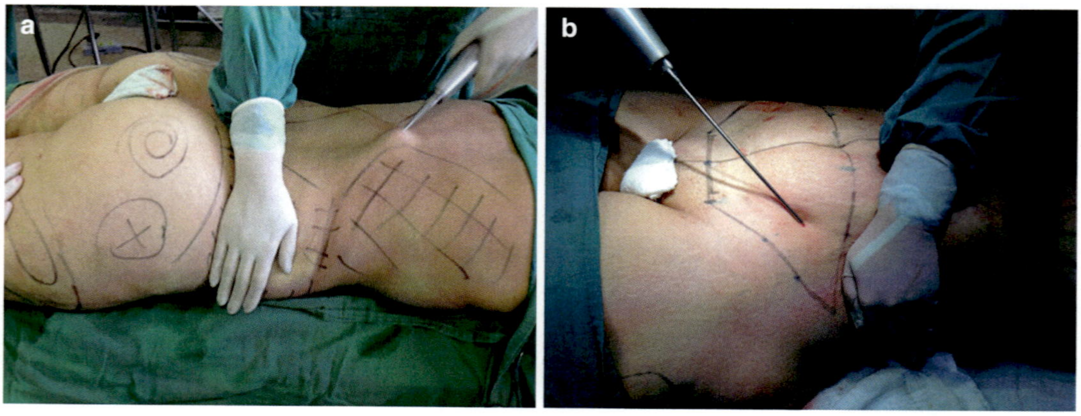

Fig. 40.4 (**a**) Dorsal decubitus: vibroliposuction of the back, chest, and flanks. (**b**) Ventral decubitus: abdominal and flank vibroliposuction, connection with the dorsal area making a liposuctioned flap pattern in a roll shape

a cannula of 4 mm in the entire abdomen. After infiltration, the vibroliposuction device is used to carry out liposuction of the entire abdominal flap.

- Then, another surgeon begins the breast surgery design.
- The liposuction of the abdominal area connects to the dorsal area, making a unique subcutaneous thinner flap pattern in a roll shape.

40.2.1.2 Breast Implant

- The inframammary approach is used in 80% of the patients; in 20%, other approaches are used, with implants ranging from 280 cc to 350 cc on average (Fig. 40.5b).
- For mastopexy, the Pitanguy (1971) outline should be used as a primary reference, begin the opening of the breast vertically, separating the mammary tissue and placing the implant (200 cc to 260 cc), using a subfascial plane to ensure better support for the breast and the mammary implant. Once the implant inclusion is done, review the outline and set point A, which will be the new position of the nipple–areola complex (NAC), leaving from 16 cm to 17 cm between the hemi-clavicular line and the areola, whose diameter varies from 3.8 cm to 4.2 cm. Afterward, the excess skin to be removed is defined. Internal stitching with Nylon 3-0 is carried out, subdermal and intradermal with Monocryl 4-0 in the vertical and horizontal scar tissue (Fig. 40.5a).

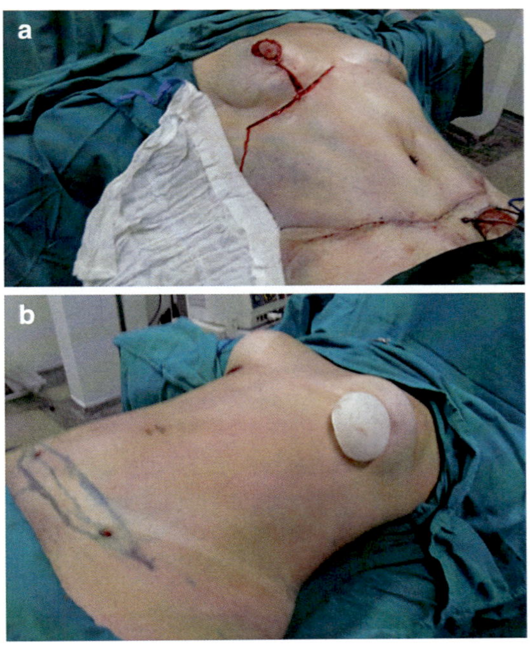

Fig. 40.5 (**a**, **b**) Preoperatively, mammary or inclusion of implant performed at the same time as the lipoabdominoplasty

40.2.1.3 Abdomen

- Once liposuction of the abdomen is concluded, the Callia (1965) outline is performed.
- After displacement of the abdominal flap, infraumbilically, circumvent the umbilical scar tissue, maintaining its vascularization and keeping a distance of 4–5 cm from the Alba line or the abdominal average.
- After the hemostasis review, perform the plication of the rectus abdominis muscles, using Nylon 0-0 or braided surgical thread 3-0. The suturing maybe continuous or separate.
- Then, fixation of the umbilical scar tissue to the northern, southern, eastern, and western points with Nylon 3-0.
- After the conclusion of the plication of the rectus abdominis, correcting its diastasis, a continuous running suture is made between the fascia of Scarpa and the aponeurosis of the rectus abdominis muscles, thus closing the dermal tunnel previously opened from the xiphoid appendix to the pubis (Fig. 40.6).
- Observe that, as the suture is being made, the thoracic flank abdominal flap slides over the abdomen as if it were covering this body segment again and as a whole, giving a new aesthetic to the body contouring surgery.
- At this moment, already with the new umbilical scar tissue defined at its new flap point, begin the closing by planes (Fig. 40.7).

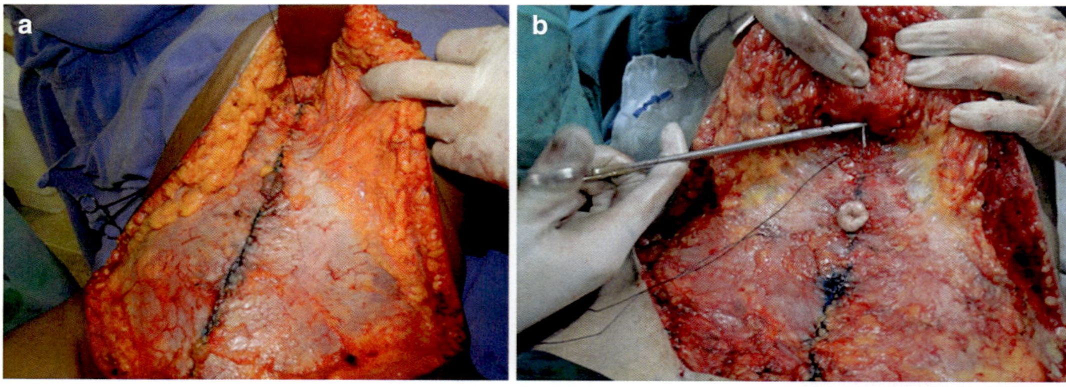

Fig. 40.6 (**a**, **b**) Beginning of the plication of the fascia of Scarpa at the level of the xiphoid appendix

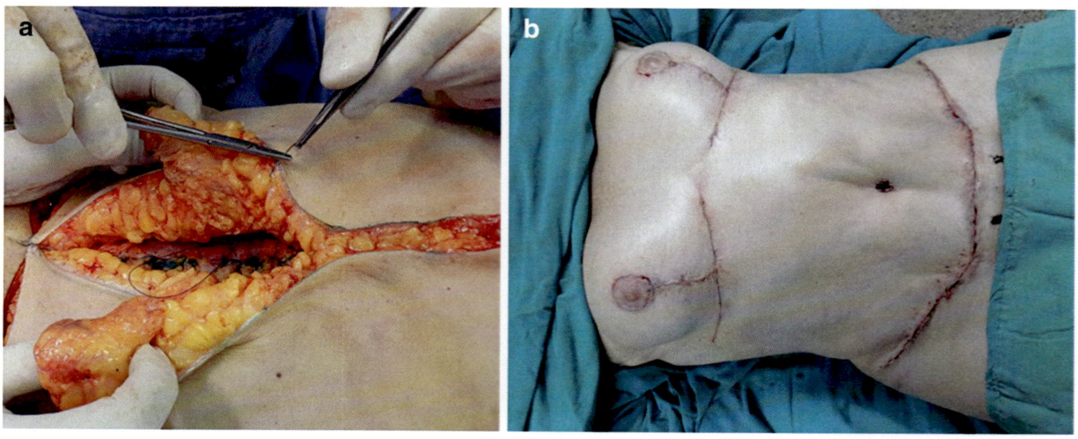

Fig. 40.7 (**a**) Detail of the suture of the fascia of Scarpa passing the aponeurosis in a continuous running semicolon suture. (**b**) Immediate postoperative image of the breast surgery combined with lipoabdominoplasty performed within the same surgery of an average of 5 h

40.2.2 The Fascia of Scarpa

It is believed that the fascia of Scarpa is a phylogenetic remainder of the piloerector muscle of birds. As it is interspersed in the adipose tissue, it is divided into superficial and deep (areolar and lamellar layers). It is composed of connective tissue of varying thickness, reaching millimeters in obese individuals and in certain parts of the body. It plays a relevant role in the maintenance of the form and esthetic of the individual. In surgical terms, it can show itself thick enough to ensure adequate anchorage of the point in determined suture lines, besides being mandatory to avoid its retraction and the formation of unaesthetic scar tissue.

The vascularization of the abdominal infraumbilical Scarpa follows abdominal vascularization, with emphasis on the deep system composed mainly of perforator veins coming from the deep epigastric arteries, both superior and inferior, and extensive anastomotic networks.

In this area, lymphatic drainage occurs via two systems: a superficial one and a deep one, each distributed in adipose and deep tissue.

The premise of the conservation of the fascia of Scarpa results from this fact and, consequently, from the preservation of the deep lymphatic system, confirmed in subsequent studies, which showed a smaller rate of seromas when surgeries were performed in such a way.

Under these conditions, it is worth highlighting that the duration of surgery is the same as for a body contouring lipoabdominoplasty (Figs. 40.8, 40.9, 40.10, 40.11, 40.12, 40.13, 40.14, 40.15, 40.16, 40.17, 40.18, 40.19, and 40.20).

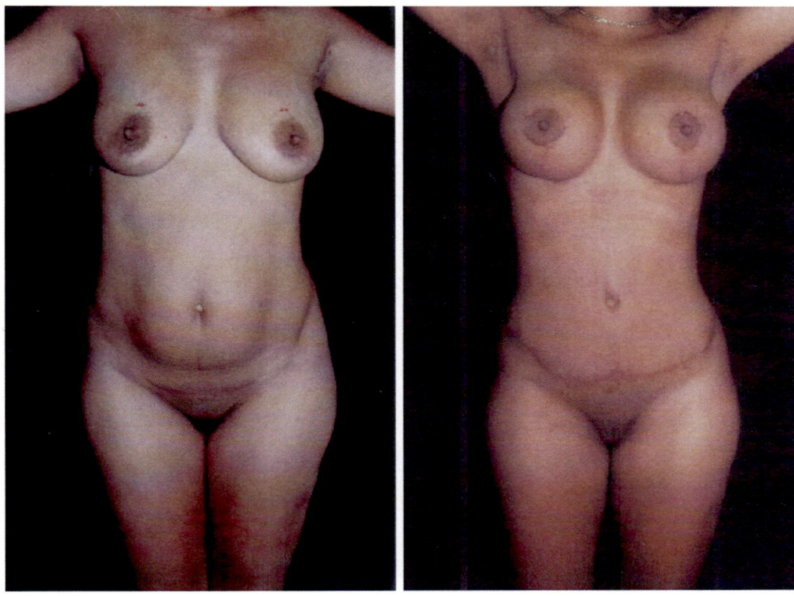

Fig. 40.8 Front view: lipoabdominoplasty and implant inclusion (pre- and postoperatively)

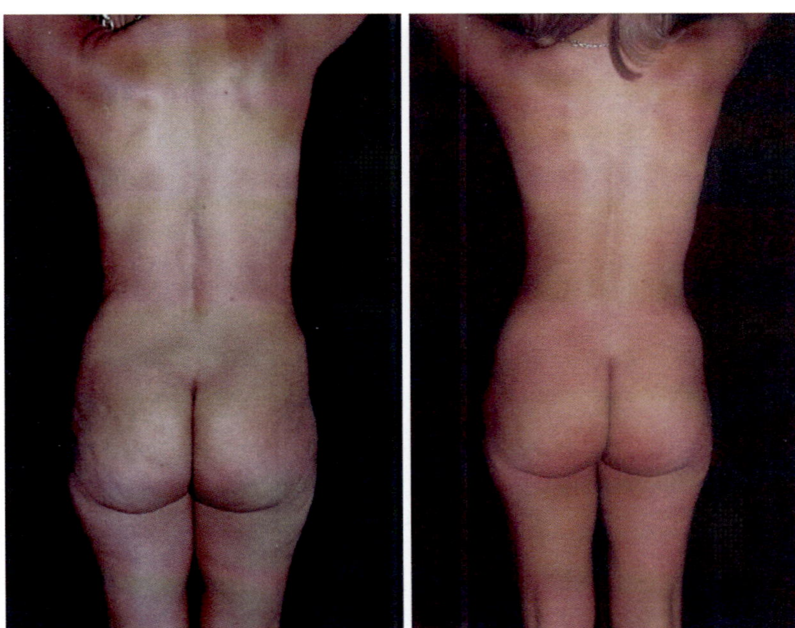

Fig. 40.9 Back view: vibroliposuction with fat grafting of the buttocks (pre- and postoperatively)

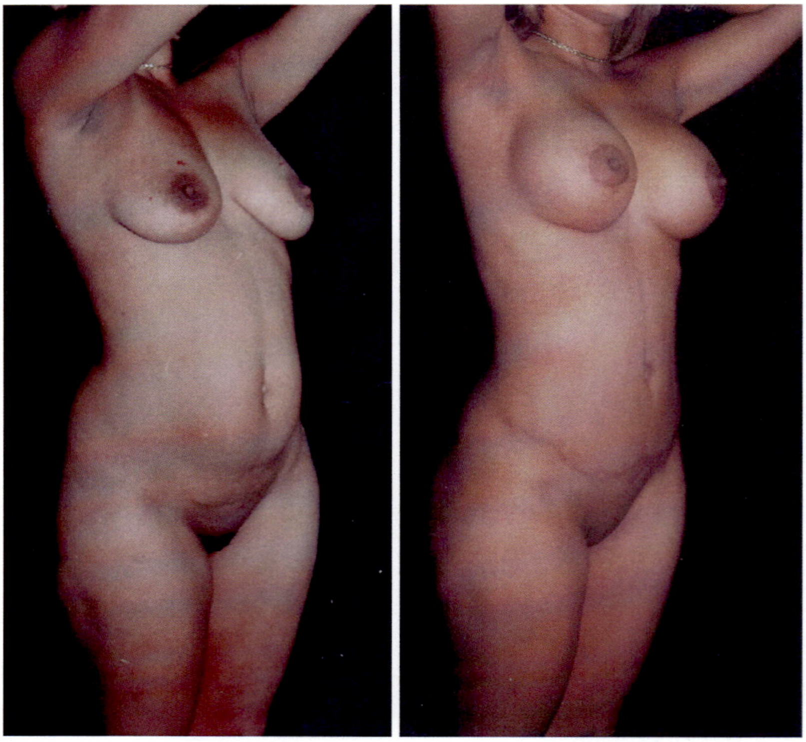

Fig. 40.10 Oblique view: vibroliposuction, breast implant, fat grafting of the buttocks (pre- and postoperatively)

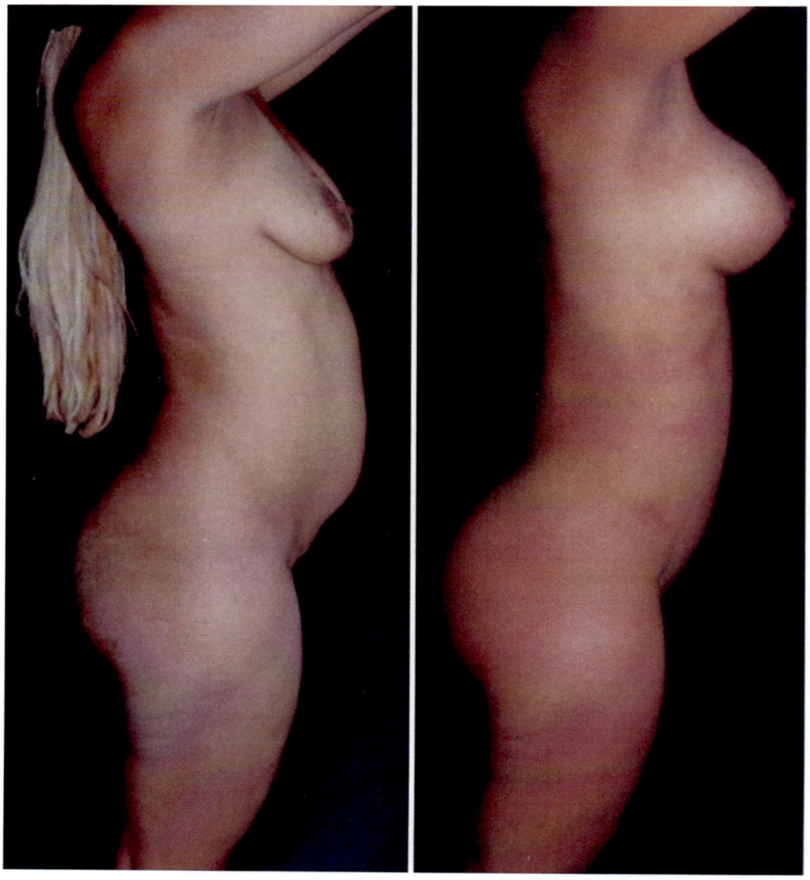

Fig. 40.11 Side view: vibroliposuction, breast implant, fat grafting of the buttocks (pre- and postoperatively)

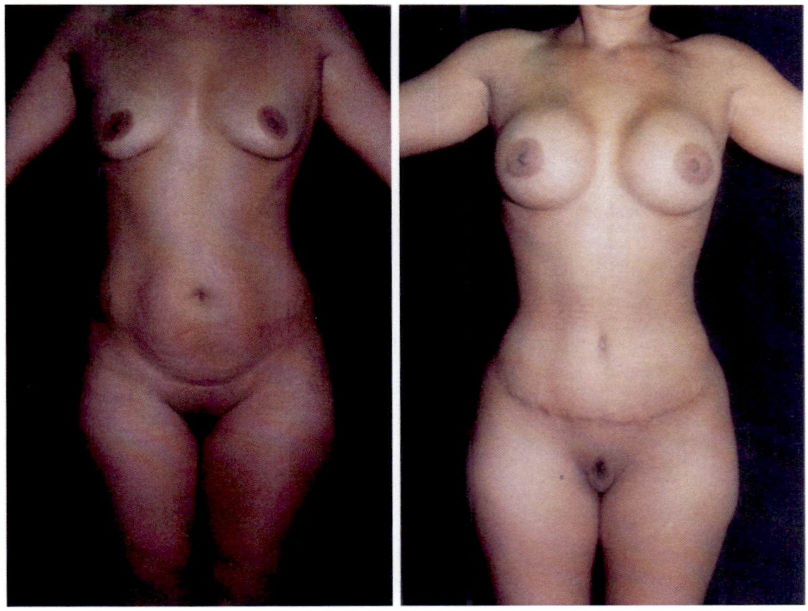

Fig. 40.12 Front view: vibroliposuction, abdomen, and breast implant (pre- and postoperatively)

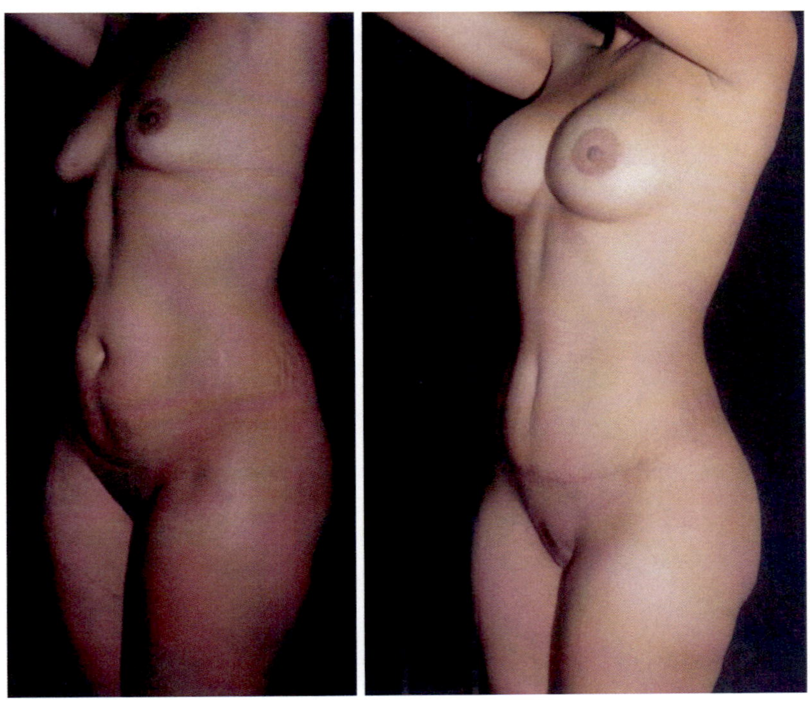

Fig. 40.13 Oblique view: vibroliposuction, abdomen, chest, and back (pre- and postoperatively)

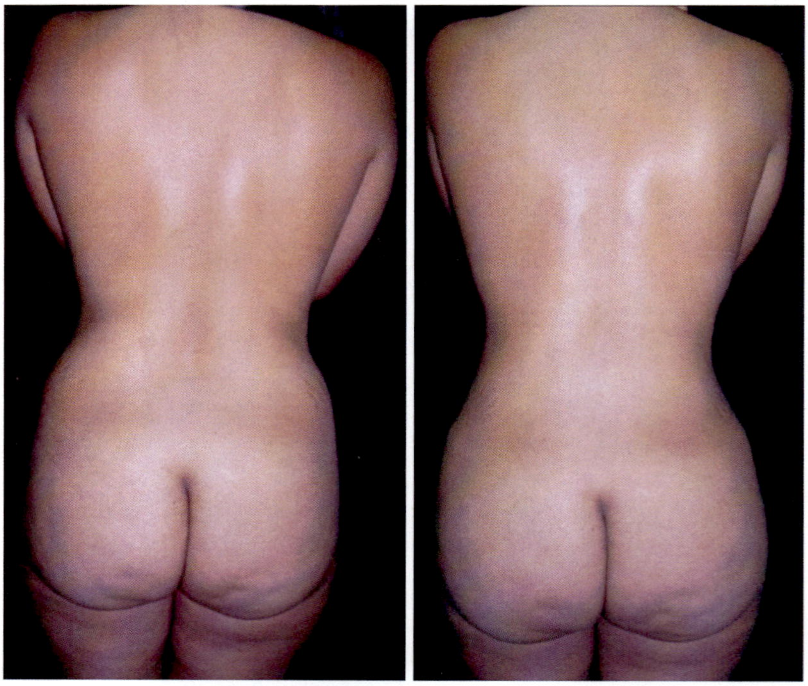

Fig. 40.14 Back view: back and flank vibroliposuction. Fat grafting of the buttocks (pre- and postoperatively)

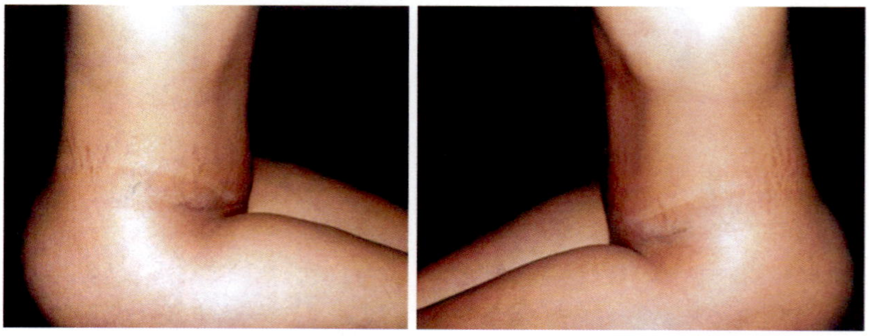

Fig. 40.15 Seated view: abdomen, back, and fat grafting of the buttocks (postoperatively)

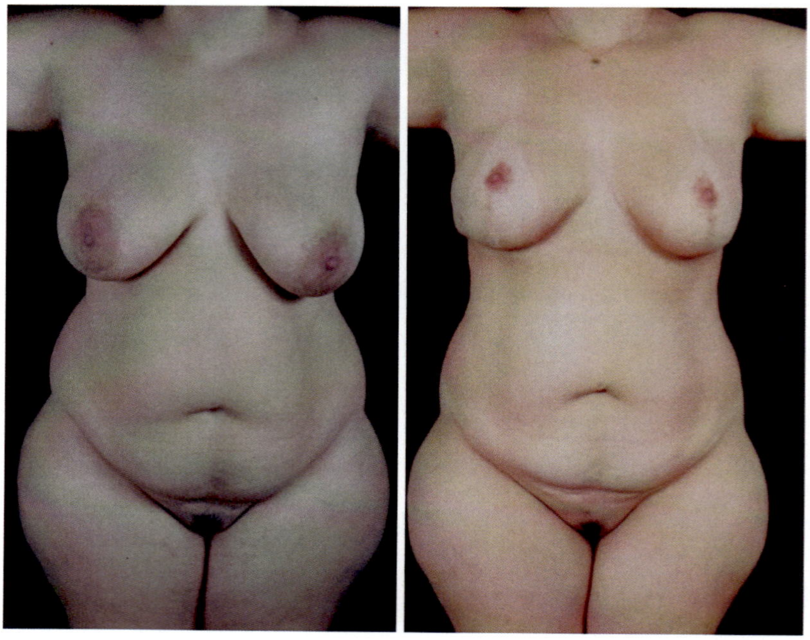

Fig. 40.16 Front view: non-aesthetic outcome because of the patient being overweight (pre- and postoperatively)

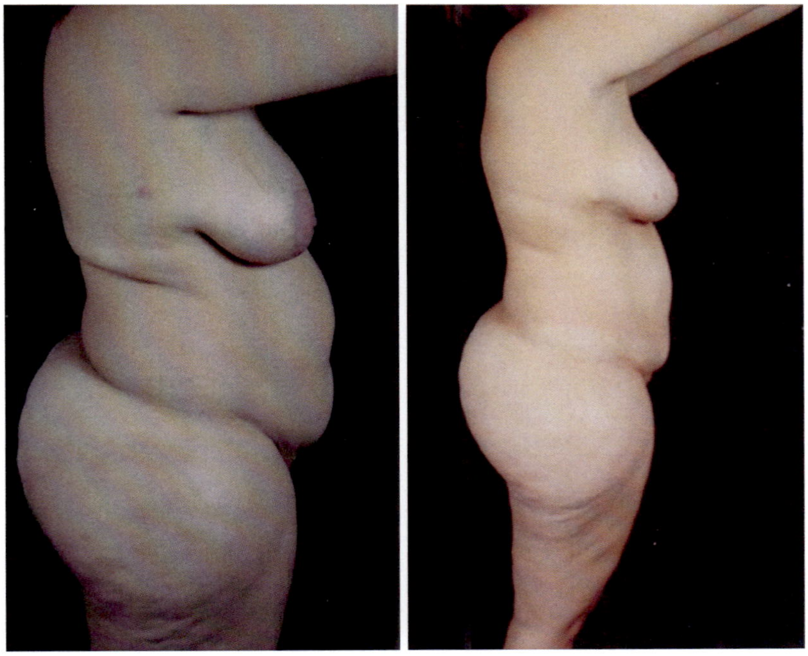

Fig. 40.17 Side view: non-aesthetic outcome because of the patient being overweight (pre- and postoperatively)

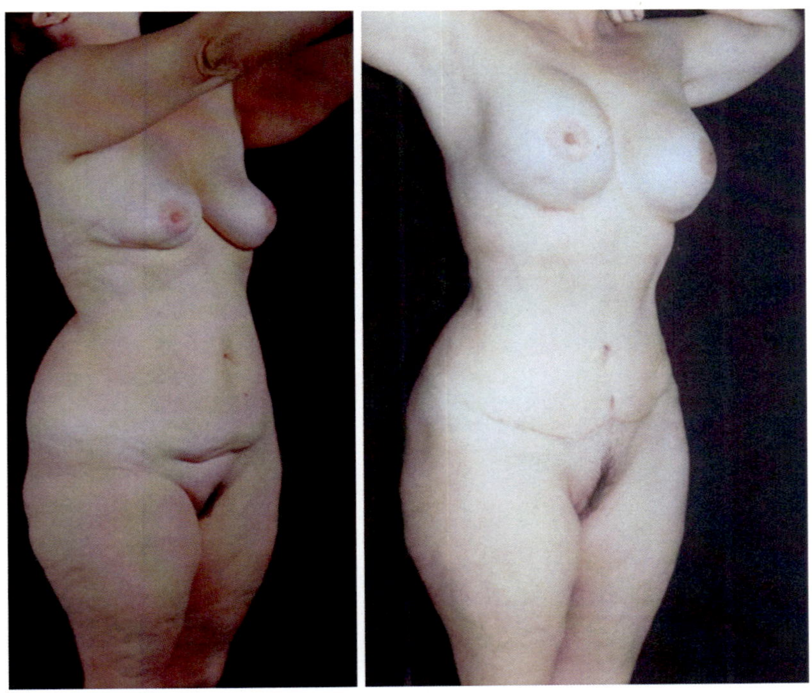

Fig. 40.18 Oblique view: lipoabdominoplasty with breast implant included with a non-aesthetic outcome (pre- and postoperatively)

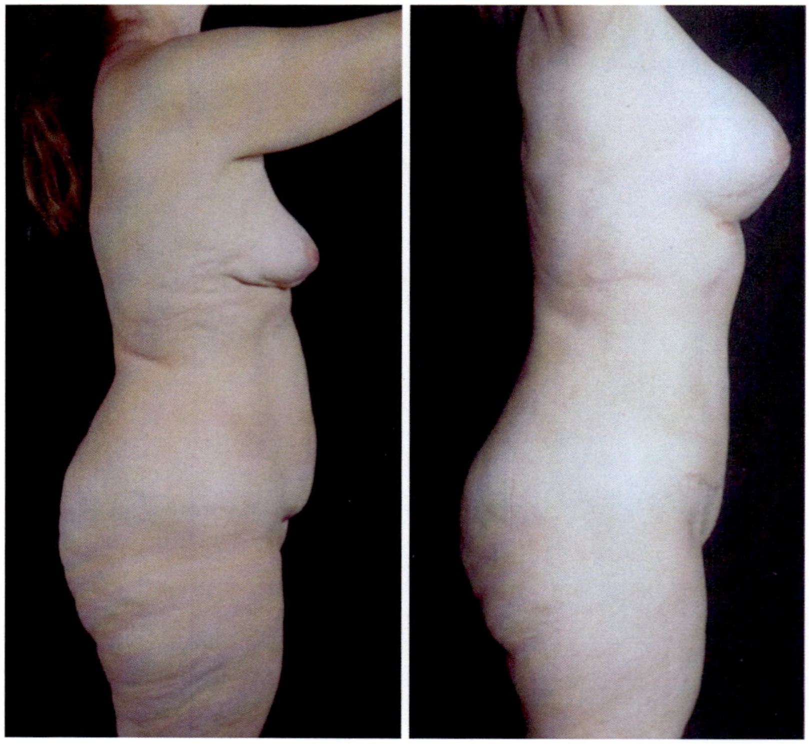

Fig. 40.19 Side view: lipoabdominoplasty with breast implant included with a non-aesthetic outcome (pre- and postoperatively)

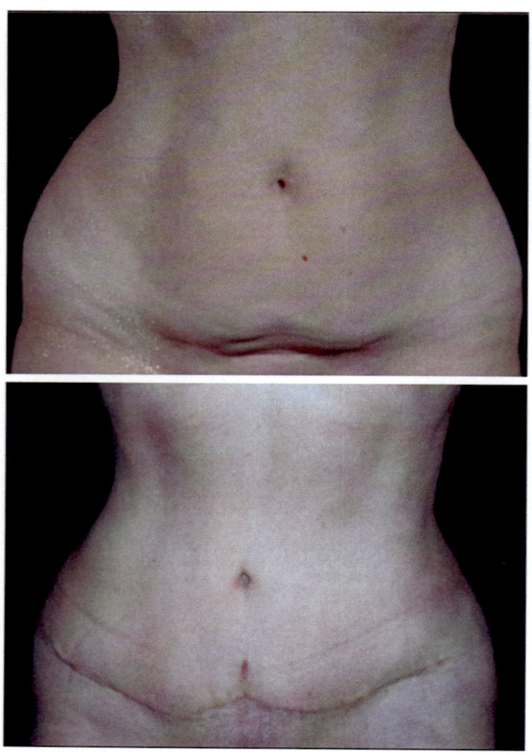

Fig. 40.20 Front view: lipoabdominoplasty in a patient with poor skin elasticity (pre- and post-postoperatively)

40.2.2.1 Patient Safety and Selection

World literature tells us that two thirds of the complications and adversities in surgical procedures can be avoided and that, approximately, one third progress to death or leave permanent sequelae that must be avoided at all costs in our specialty because of their consequences. Hence, it is necessary to follow the patient safety protocol of the World Health Organization (WHO) (Ferraz 2009):

- Qualified surgical team, duly trained to work in harmony
- Trained anesthesiology team with experience in plastic surgery
- Safe place to perform the procedures
- Use of pneumatic compression device in the lower limbs throughout the surgery and until 24 h after the procedure
- Stimulation of early walking
- Use of elastic support stockings, of medium compression, for 10 days
- Prescription of enoxaparin (40 mg) subcutaneously, for 10 days.

40.2.3 Patient Selection

- BMI less than 30
- Comorbidity scanning
- Mandatory preoperative examinations are performed by a cardiologist and an anesthesiologist.

40.3 Discussion

The progress of surgical techniques and the increase in safety regarding the surgical procedure allowed the patient to be seen as an entity and not in a segmented way, as used to be the case.

Thus, body contouring surgery is today a reality and, in many cases, can be achieved in a single surgery. This fact not only brings surgical benefits, but also ensures a shorter recovery time for the patient, which, according to the dynamics required by modern times, is imperative.

The viability of the combined breast lipoabdominoplasty, or the breast surgery within lipoabdominoplasty, depends on the absolute security of the patient. When carried out in this way, the procedure has an effect on this patient, a great body contouring result.

40.4 Complications

Adequate selection of the patients based on mandatory preoperative examinations by a cardiologist and an anesthesiologist, comorbidity scanning, and BMI around 30 are factors that considerably lessen the number of complications. In our study carried out during the period 2010–2015, a total of 163 patients were operated upon without any severe complications, such as deep vein thrombosis, thromboembolic prophylaxis, permanent sequelae or death. Epidermolysis, minor necrosis, hypertrophic scars, and complaints about the umbilical aesthetics were registered.

40.4.1 Cases

Six months preoperatively and post-operatively.

Conclusion

Our long-term experience has been accompanied by constant updating regarding advances in medicine and technology, especially concerning the benefits that the plastic surgery brings to the patient. Combined breast lipoabdominoplasty shortens the surgical times and maintains the quality of the postoperative results both in the short and in the long term, with a low index of complications. All surgeries performed have been progressing well, it is also important to notice. During these 15 years, we have not verified any severe complications, such as thrombosis or pulmonary embolism, or severe cases of infection, as we have been conducting the selection of patients according to criteria, with a surgical team of recognized expertise and a high degree of proficiency, that works in harmony and synchronicity.

Annexes

The intention of this chapter is to bring not only the author's experience but also his dedication to plastic surgery along these years.

References

Avelar J (1999) Uma nova técnica de abdominoplastia: sistema vascular fechado de retalho subdérmico dobrado sobre si mesmo combinado com lipoaspiração. Rev Bras Cir 88/89(1\6):3–20

Avelar JM (2000) Abdominoplasty: a new technique without undermining and fat layer removal. Arq Catarin Med 29:147–149

Babcock W (1916) The correction of the obese and relaxed abdominal wall with special reference to the use of buried silver chain. Am J Obstet 74:596–611

Barcudi R, Ferreira CA (1998) Seroma: how to avoid it and how to treat it. Aesthet Surg J 18(6):439–441

Bozola AR, Psilakis JM (1988) Abdominoplasty: a new concept and classification for treatment. Plast Reconstr Surg 82(6):983–993

Brasil. Ministério da Saúde (2014) Documento de Referência para o Programa nacional de Segurança do paciente. Fundação Oswaldo Cruz e Agência Nacional de Vigilância Sanitária. Secretaria de Atenção à Saúde. Programa Nacional de Segurança do Paciente. Coleção institucional do Ministério da Saúde, ed. 1.ª, edição—2014—1500 exemplares, Brasília, p 42

Callia W (1965) Contribuição para o estudo da correção do abdômen em pêndulo e globono – técnica original (Tese de Doutorado). Faculdade de Medicina da USP, São Paulo

Illouz YG (1980) Une nouvelle techinique pour lês lipodystrophies localisées. Rev Chir Esth Franc 6:9–14

Jaimovich CA, Mazzarone F, Parra JFN, Pitnaguy I (1999) Semiologia da parede abdominal: seu valor no planejamento da abdominoplastia. Rev Soc Bras Cir Plast 14(3):21–50

Kelly HA (1910) Excision of the fat abdominal wall lipectomy. Surg Gynecol Obstet 10:229

Leão CF (2000a) Abdominoplastia: Uma nova abordagem. In: Anais do XXXVII Congresso Brasileiro de Cirurgia Plástica, Porto Alegre, RS, 12–15 nov

Leão CF (2000b) Curso de Abdominoplastia. Chair man: AR Bozola: In: Anais do XXXVII Congresso Brasileiro de Cirurgia Plástica, Porto Alegre, RS, 12–15 nov

Leão CF (2010) Lipodorsoabdominoplastia: 10 anos de experiência. Rev Bras Cir Plast 25(4):688–694

Leão CF (2014) A Dorsolipoabdominoplastia, abordagem circunferencial para melhorar resultados, como faço. XXI Encontro Associação dos ex-alunos do professor Pitanguy

Pitanguy I (1971) Surgical reduction of the abdomen, things and buttocks. Surg Clin North Am 51(2):479–489

Sinder R (1975) Plastic surgery of the abdomen: técnica pessoal de abdominoplastia, com prévio descolamento de retalho supra-umbilical e uso de retalho dermoadiposo. In: VI Congresso f Plastic and Reconstructive Surgery, Ago 25, Paris, France

Thorek M (1942) Plastic surgery of the breast and abdominal wall. Charles Thomas, Springfield

Secondary Mastoplasty for Repair of Unfavorable Results

41

Juarez M. Avelar

41.1 Introduction

Reduction mammaplasty is one of the more frequently performed procedures by plastic surgeons. Few patients come for revision procedures and even fewer present for a secondary or repeated reduction mammaplasty. This study defines the secondary reduction mammaplasty as performing an additional or repeated reduction of the breast size.

Reduction mastoplasty is a meticulous procedure demanding constant effort from plastic surgeons to improve surgical results (Avelar 1993). So far, a significant number of patients operated on elsewhere present unaesthetic surgical results that require a secondary operation for the repair of surgical problems. Most of the patients in whom I have performed a secondary operation complain about the unaesthetic appearance of the breasts, with moderate or severe asymmetry and malpositioning of the nipple–areola complex (NAC) (Avelar 1989). The first reference to secondary mammoplasty is reported by Maliniac (1959) in a useful description concerning unsatisfactory results after mammaplasty, with a wide description concerning all aspects of the surgery. Also, Myr and Myr (1968) published an important study regarding the cause of unsatisfactory results after mammoplasty. The most frequent complaint of patients he found was similar to what I have seen, which is related to the position of the NAC combined with ptosis of the mammary tissue. Some years later, Herman et al. (1975) described scar revision after reduction mastoplasty, which I have not seen among my patients.

So far, unsatisfactory results have been mentioned by Serletti et al. (1992), Davis et al. (1995), Boschert et al. (1996). Lejour (1997) proposed vertical mammaplasty as secondary surgery after other techniques. A series of 16 patients was reported by Hudson and Skoll (1999),as eight underwent a repeated or secondary reduction mammoplasty with a pedicled NAC and eight patients had inferior wedge excision. Also, Hoffman (1986) reported on the correction of breast asymmetry with recurrent abnormalities following reduction mammaplasty. Unaesthetic scars, malpositioning of the NAC, and an ungraceful shape of the breasts are some of the current problems that may occur after reduction mastoplasty operations.

Because the breasts are important organs for good harmony with the body contour, when unexpected situations occur, patients demand a new operation. Scar revision, repositioning of the NAC, and remodeling of the breasts to achieve a good balance between them are the most frequent

J.M. Avelar
Brazilian Institute of Surgery Plastic and Reconstructive, Alameda Gabriel Monteiro da Silva, 01442000 São Paulo, SP, Brazil
e-mail: juarezavelar@bol.com.br; institutodaorelha@uol.com.br; clinica-avelar@uol.com.br

J.M. Avelar (ed.), *Breast Surgery*, https://doi.org/10.1007/978-3-319-54115-0_41

disfigurements after mastoplasty operation, but I have not performed secondary or repeated reduction mastoplasty.

So far, procedures of mastopexy associated with augmentation mastoplasty are even more difficult as the combined complications of both operations may occur. It should only be performed after careful consideration of alternative options, including breast augmentation only, mastopexy only, or a two-stage procedure, which is not a topic for discussion here.

41.2 Method

41.2.1 Surgical Evaluation

During consultation, the surgeon must talk and listen to patients calmly to understand their complaints about unsatisfactory results. One fundamental question should be asked: the date of the last operation she underwent on her breasts. It is advisable to wait at least 1 year after the last procedure, as scar tissue formation is still in development during that period of maturation. The decision of a secondary operation must be taken after physical and psychological evaluation, as she is already frustrated and may undergo a reparatory procedure (Avelar 1990; Avelar and Gameiro 1990). There are some aspects that must be carefully evaluated: scars, location, and position of the NAC, symmetry of the breasts, harmony with the chest, and other considerations. The position, location, and size of the scars are the first stage when considering the breasts.

In the case of an unaesthetic location of the NAC, since they are the most important reference points of beauty of the breasts, patients complain a great deal about them. When primary mastoplasty was performed with the patient in a supine position on the operating table, it is quite difficult to achieve the correct location of the NAC, as the surgeon does not have enough anatomical references. In other hands, when mastoplasty is performed with the patient in a semi-sitting position, it is easy to mark the new location of the NAC, as the breasts are in a normal position. Therefore, to repair such an acquired abnormality is a constant challenge because of the malpositioned NAC, which is the most frequent one.

41.2.2 Surgical Planning

After meticulous evaluation, the surgeon may have enough information for surgical planning. If the breasts are still large, a secondary reduction mastoplasty may be performed. Nevertheless, if the scars are not well placed it is mandatory to plan the new operation for scar revision. So far, if the NACs are in the wrong location it is necessary to plan to achieve a good balance between them in future breasts. Such deformities are quite frequent when the previous operation has been done with the patient in a supine position on the operating table. When Pitanguy (1959, 1961); Pitanguy and Garcia (1972) introduced new concepts on reduction mastoplasty the semi-sitting position of the patient on the operating table improved the aesthetic results very much, as the submammary sulcus is well identified for the correct orientation of surgery. In fact, when the surgeon performs mastoplasty with the patient in a supine position, the final scars are in an adverse location, as the submammary creases are not respected during the operation.

To perform a secondary mastoplasty, it is necessary to achieve a good balance of the NAC with the breasts, as in all patients I have treated, there has been an excess of mammary gland in the lower segment of the breast and the NAC is located too high. Thus, it is necessary to transpose the glandular tissue from down upward. My preference is to create a dermal–adipose–glandular flap with a superior pedicle to rotate from down upward to repair the upper segment of the breasts, with consequent reduction of the lower one.

41.2.3 Surgical Demarcation

41.2.3.1 Pre-demarcation

Once the new mastoplasty is planned my preference is to do pre-marking 1 day before the

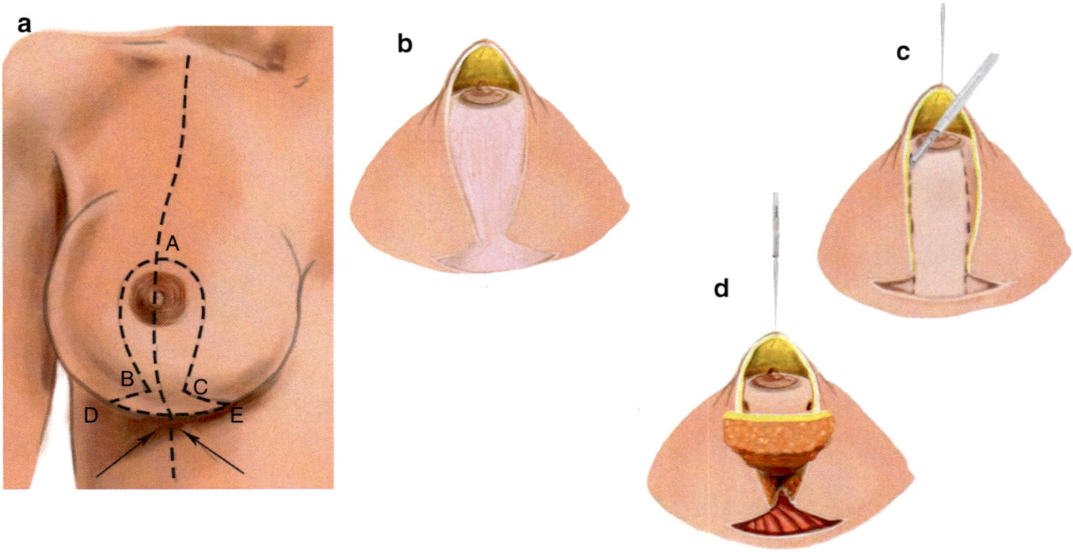

Fig. 41.1 Sequential drawings to demonstrate the creation of the dermal–adipose–glandular flap. (**a**) Surgical marking of the midclavicular line and skin incisions for mastopexy; Pitanguy's point A is a fundamental reference and points B, C, D, and E demarcate the area for skin excision. (**b**) The superficial layer of the skin was resected according to the markings. (**c**) Two parallel incisions are made from the nipple to the submammary sulcus. (**d**) The flap is raised and projected forward

operation at my clinic, when another evaluation is made. The first step is to determine Pitanguy's point A (Fig. 41.1a).

Afterward, the sternal notch is marked and a point is drawn 7 cm from it, on the midclavicular point. A line is drawn obliquely downward passing the nipple. When the nipple–areola regions are in an ectopic position, the surgeon's creativity must orientate the adequate location of the future areas (Fig. 41.1a).

41.2.4 Surgical Technique

41.2.4.1 Anesthesia

With the patient in operating room, the anesthesia is performed by intravenous sedation under the care of the anesthesiologist and the operating table is placed in a semi-sitting position. Local infiltration is employed.

41.2.4.2 Anesthetic Infiltration

After adequate surgical marking, according to each case, the anesthetic infiltration is carried out subcutaneously following the lines on the skin. My anesthetic solution is lidocaine (2%) 40 mL, distilled water 160 mL, adrenaline (1/1000) 1 mL, for a total solution of 201 mL.

With the use of this volume of infiltration it is possible to infiltrate both breasts. It is important to mention that the mammary tissue should not be infiltrated, but only at the base and at the subcutaneous level underneath the marking (Avelar and Catunda 1985; Avelar 1993).

41.2.4.3 Skin Incisions

The cutaneous incisions are made according to each patient, since the deformities were adequately evaluated and the operation is planned. There is no standard technique, as each patient presents peculiar surgical scars that must be incised to achieve aesthetic results.

41.2.4.4 Creation of the Dermal–Adipose–Glandular Flap

In all my patients who underwent repair of the breasts secondary to previous mastoplasty, I created a dermal–adipose–glandular flap with a superior pedicle to carry out adequate transposition from the lower segment to the superior one.

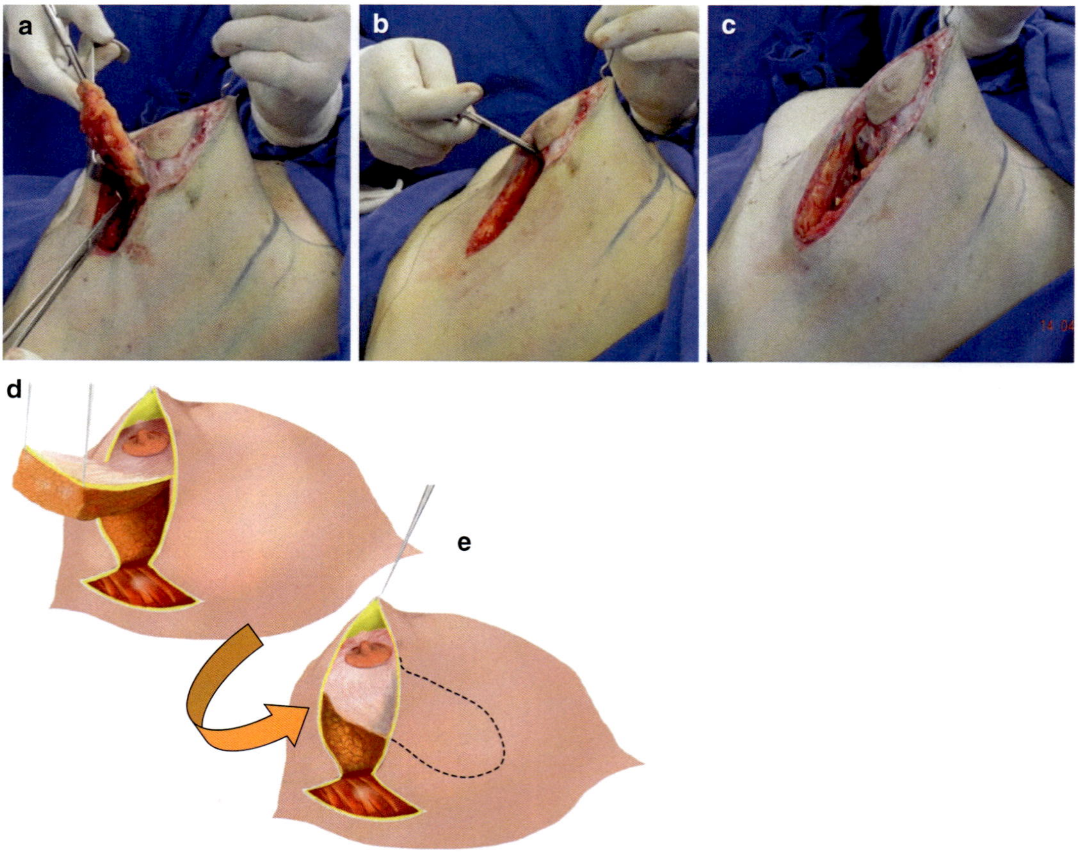

Fig. 41.2 Rotation of the dermal–adipose–glandular flap with a superior pedicle from down to backward, to be sutured to the aponeurosis of the pectoralis major. Peroperative photos (**a**), (**b**), and (**c**) show that the flap is already raised and rotated backward. Drawings (**d**) and (**e**) show the movement indicated by the *arrow*

After de-epithelialization the dermis, subcutaneous layer, and glandular tissue are cut by two parallel incisions. The flap is pulled forward and the base of the breast is undermined all over the mammary area (Fig. 41.1b–d). In the next step, the flap is rotated back and upward and sutured to the mammary tissue (Fig. 41.2). The donor area is then sutured. Patients who underwent this procedure present a great improvement to the breast by reducing the inferior segment and filling the superior one (Figs. 41.3, 41.4, 41.5). When the breasts present more mammary tissue, the flap is long

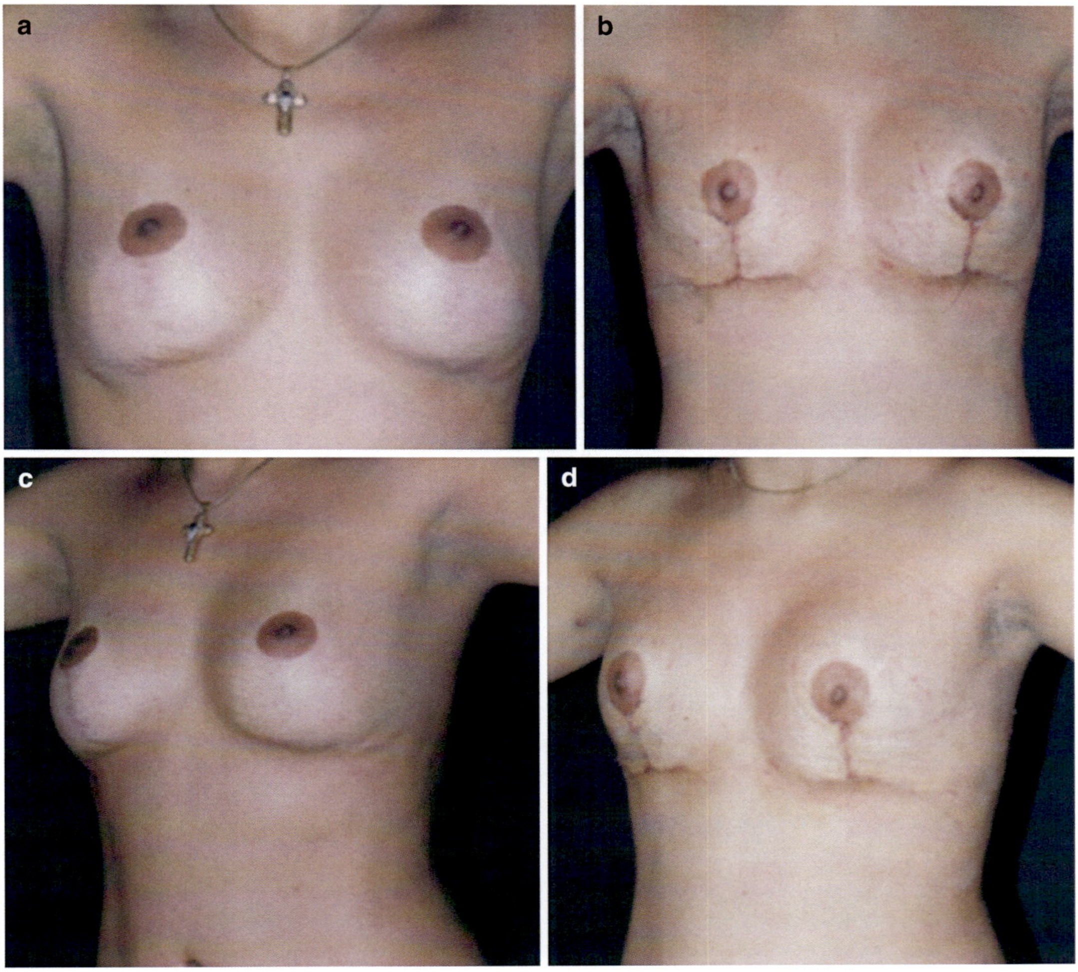

Fig. 41.3 Repair of an unaesthetic surgical result after mastoplasty carried out elsewhere. Photos (**a**) and (**c**) before repair of the nipple–areolar regions show a very high location; photos (**b**) and (**d**) after surgical repair

enough to be sutured to the aponeurosis of the pectoralis major (Figs. 41.6 and 41.7). There are cases in which it is necessary to combine cutaneous expansion with rotation of the dermal–adipose–glandular flap to obtain adequate skin covering on the superior segment of the breast (Fig. 41.8). This can even be combined with upper lipoabdominoplasty for the repair of the severe deformities of the breast due to fibrotic tissue secondary to previous operations (Fig. 41.9).

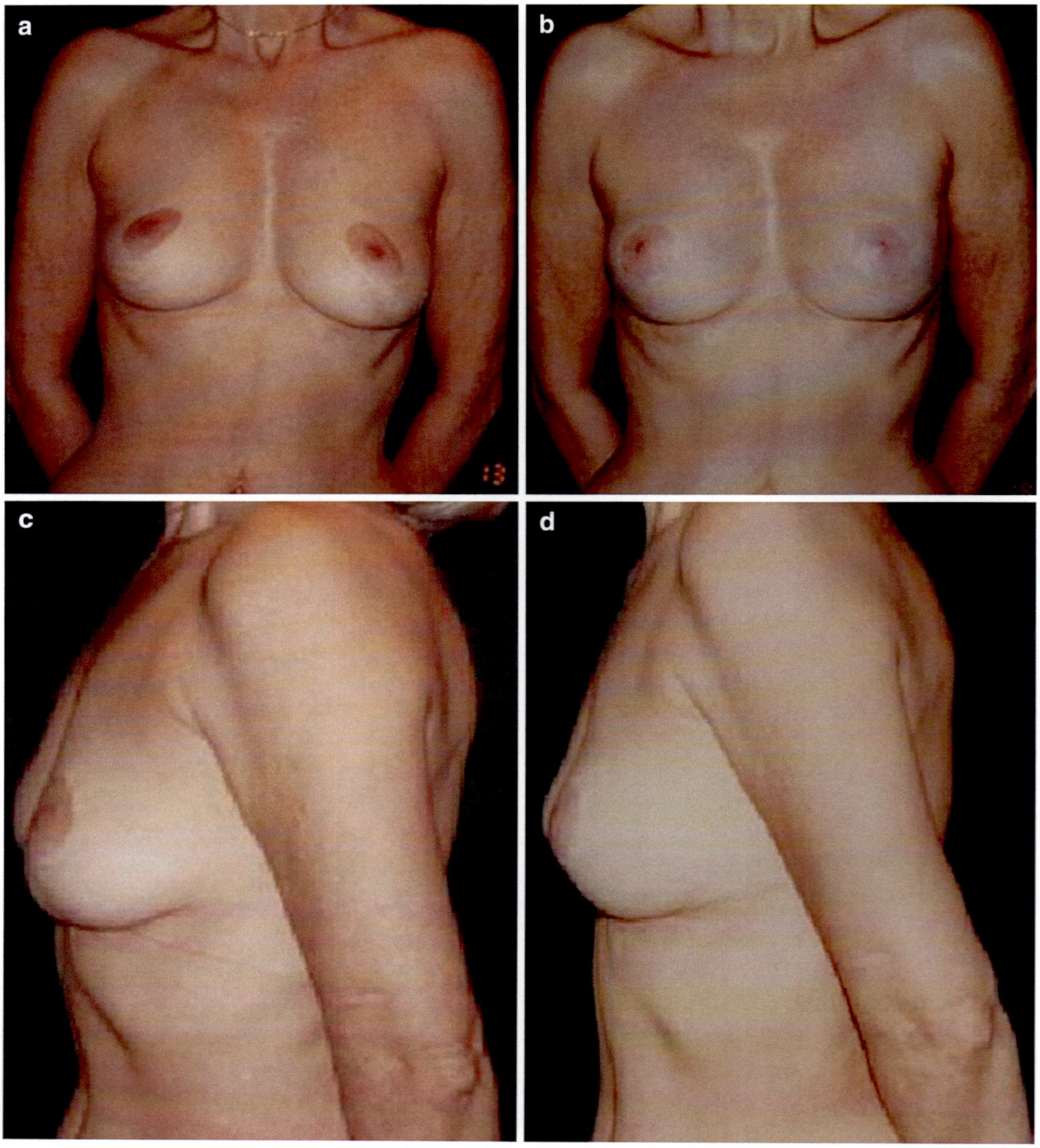

Fig. 41.4 Repair of an unaesthetic surgical result after mastoplasty carried out elsewhere. Photos (**a**) and (**c**) before repair of the nipple–areolar regions show a very high location; photos (**b**) and (**d**) after surgical repair

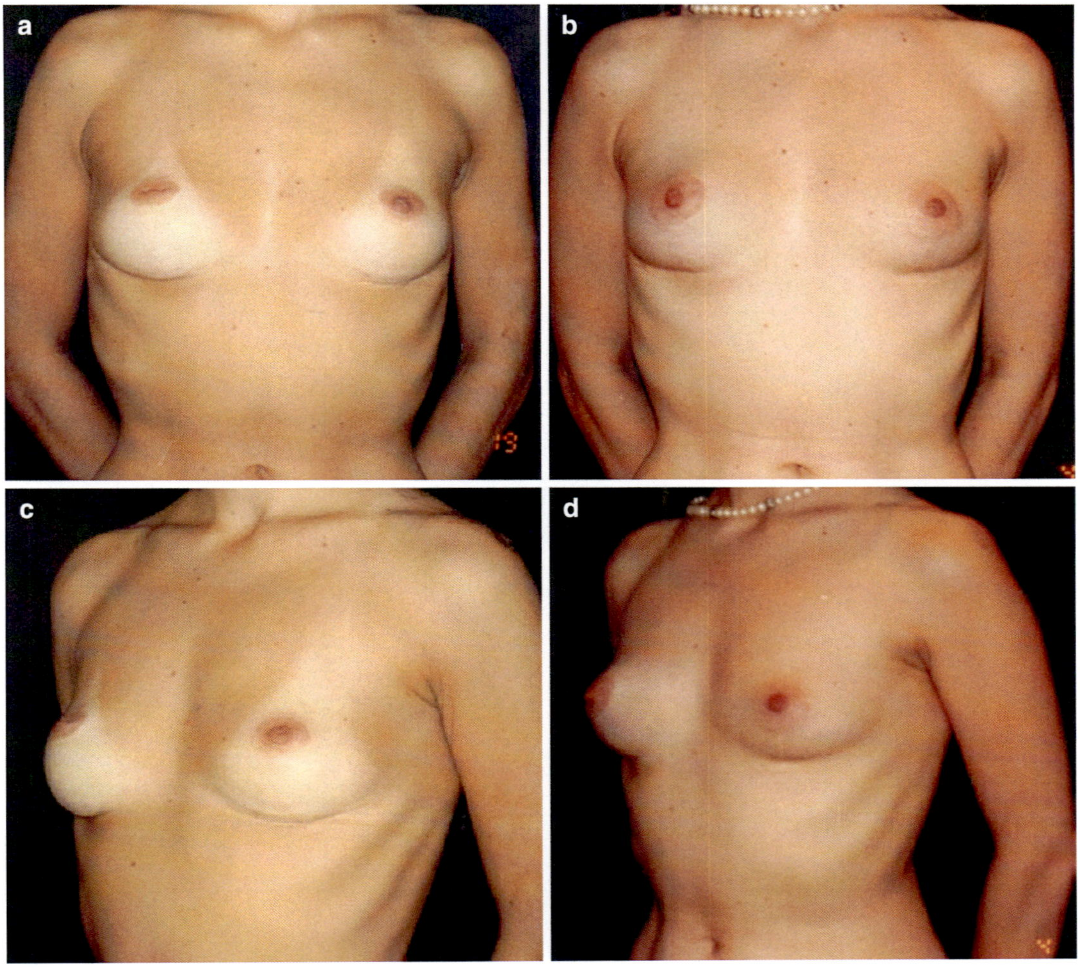

Fig. 41.5 Correction of an unaesthetic surgical result after mastoplasty operated elsewhere. Photos (**a**), (**c**) before repair of the nipple–areolar regions show very a high location; photos (**b**), (**d**) after surgical repair. The patient refused implants

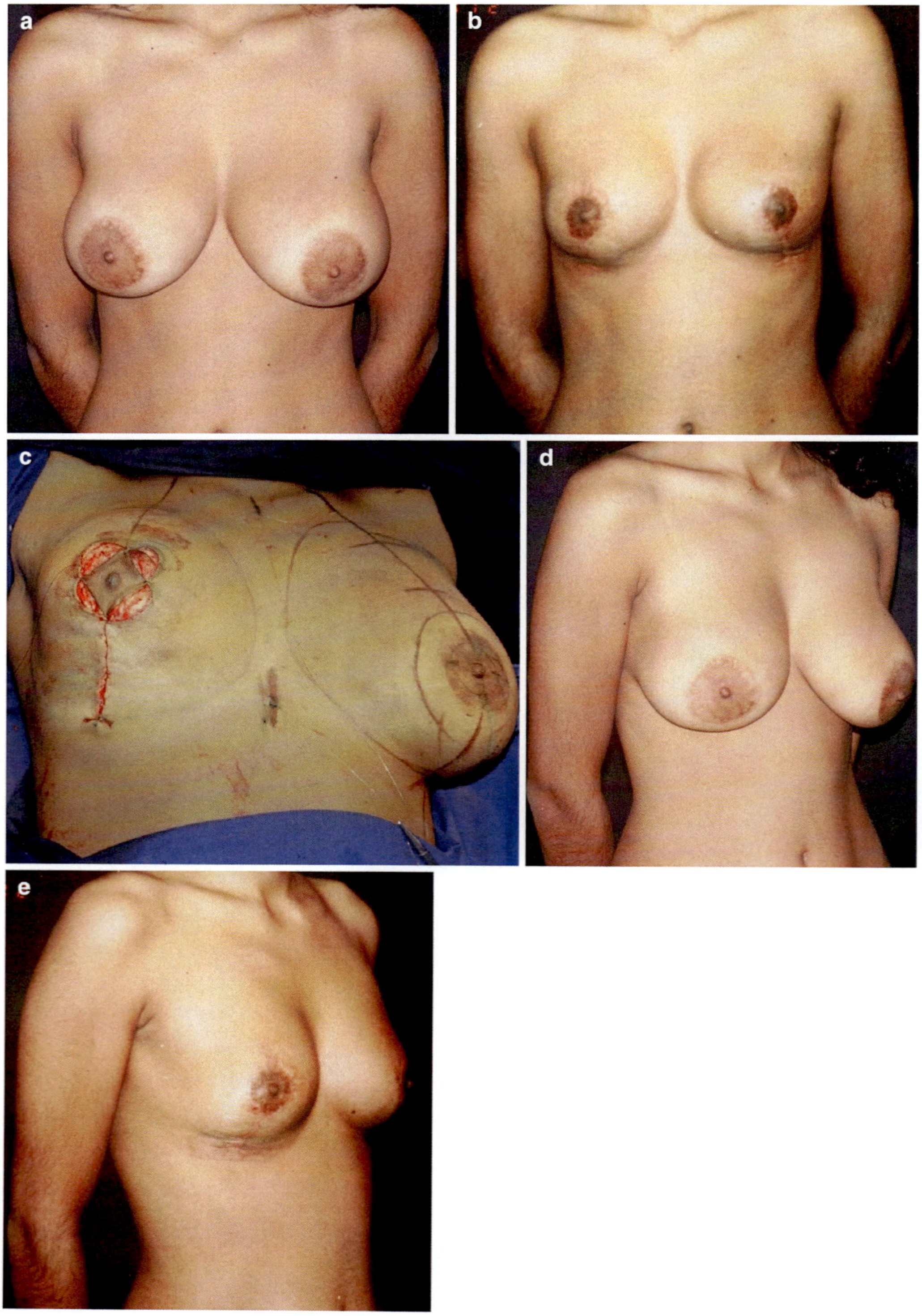

Fig. 41.6 A 33-year old patient presented an unaesthetic and asymmetrical surgical result of the breasts after periareolar mastoplasty carried out elsewhere. In photo (**a**) in the frontal view, the scars around the areola are visible. (**b**) After repair, she presents another scar around the areola and another one on the vertical. (**c**) Peroperative photo shows that the right breast has been repaired, with the nipple–areola in an adequate location. (**d**) Oblique view photo before repair. (**e**) After surgical reparation following the described procedure creation and rotation of the dermal–adipose–glandular flap

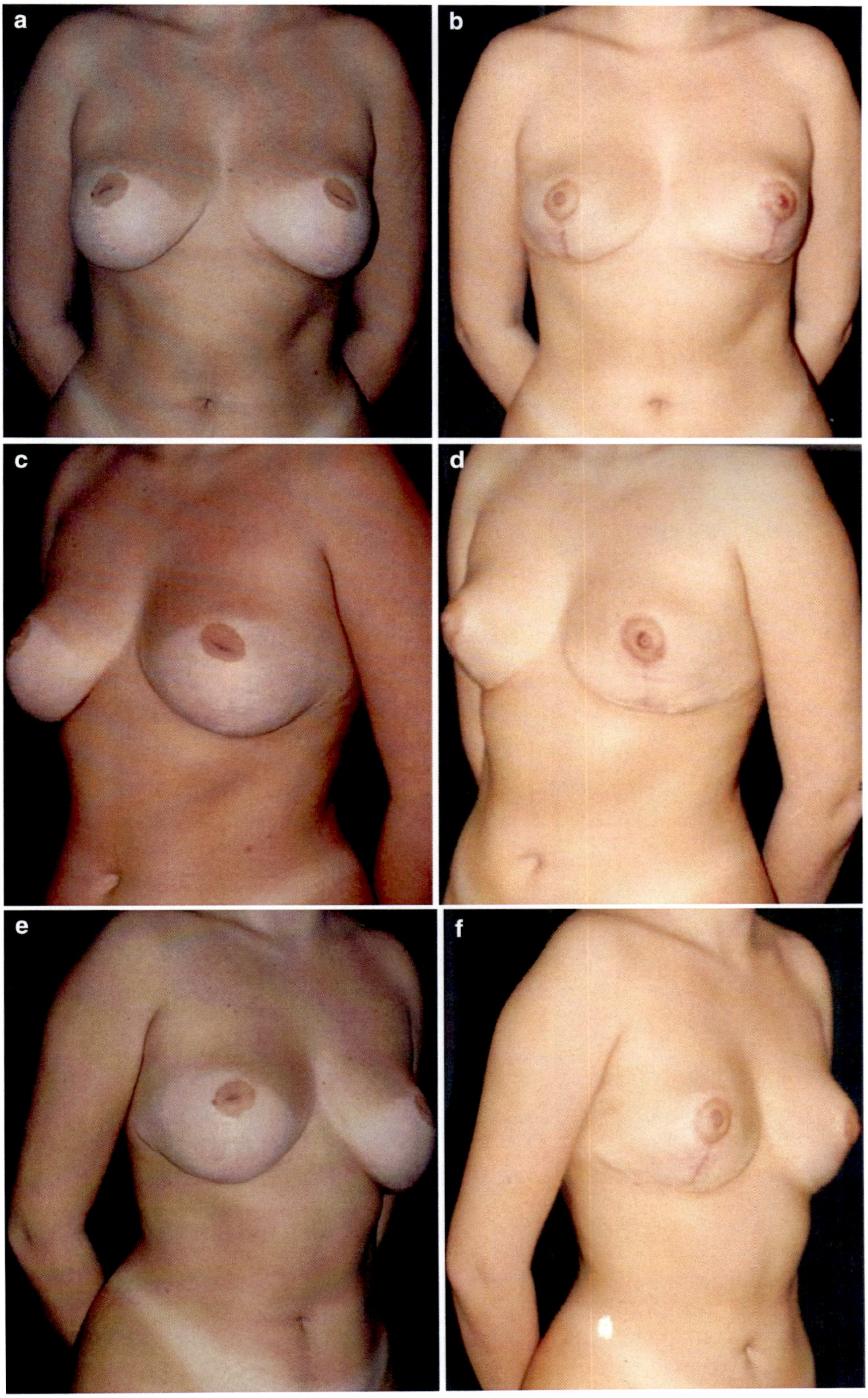

Fig. 41.7 A 35-year-old patient presented an unaesthetic surgical result after mastoplasty carried out elsewhere. Photos (**a**), (**c**), (**e**) before repair of the lower segment of the breasts is too low and the nipple–areolar regions show a very high location; photos (**b**), (**d**), (**f**) after surgical repair following the technique described

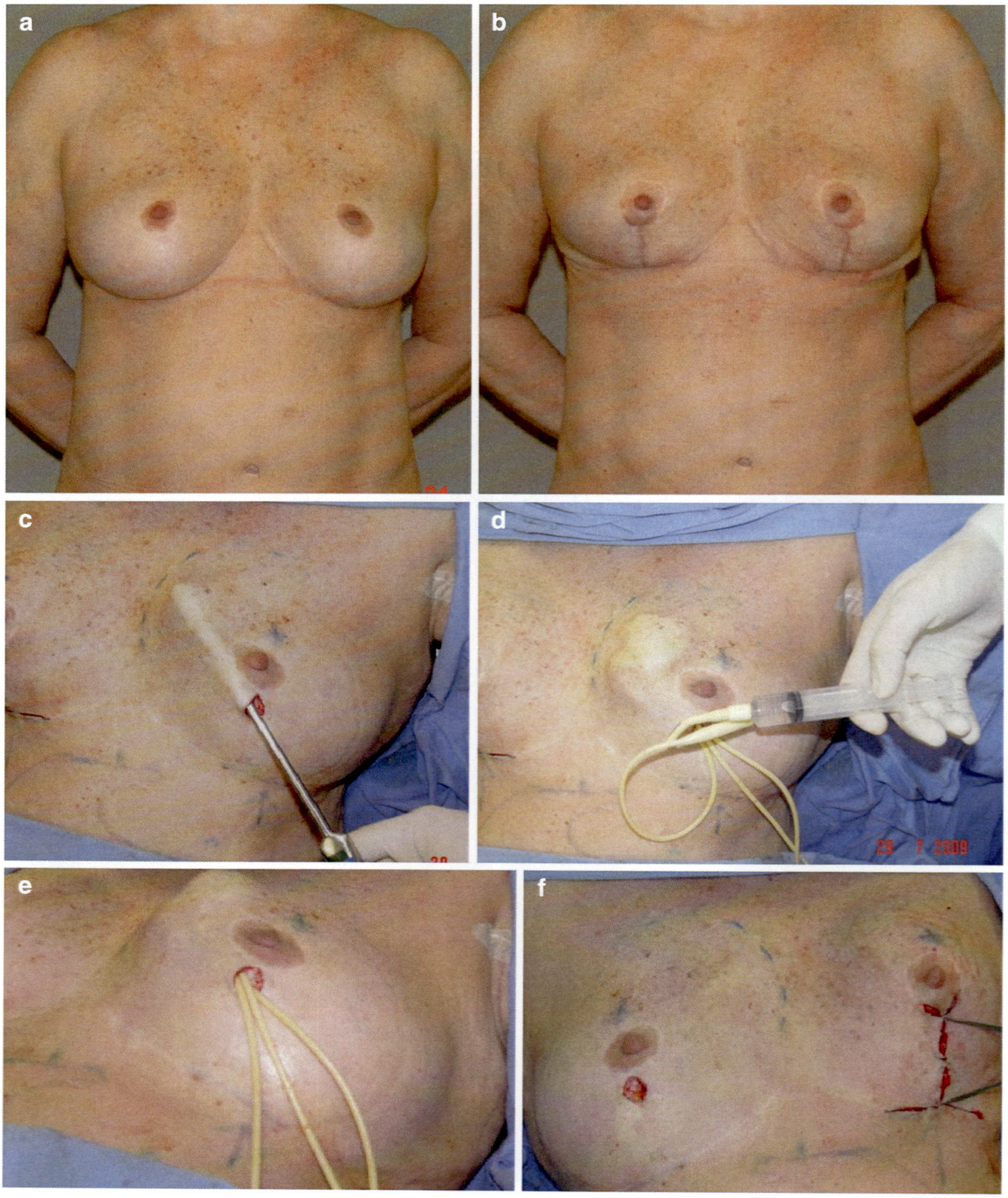

Fig. 41.8 Correction of an unaesthetic surgical result after two mastoplasty operations performed elsewhere. Photo (**a**) in frontal view before repair of the nipple–areolar regions show asymmetry and a very high location; photo (**b**) after surgical repair. (**c**) Peroperative photo showing tunnelization using a thin cannula underneath the skin on the left breast; photos (**d**) and (**e**) during surgery using a balloon to expand the skin on the upper pole of the left breast. (**f**) Peroperative photo shows that the right breast is already repaired; (**g**) both breasts were repaired; photos (**h**) and (**j**) before repaired; photos (**i**) and (**k**) show the final result on an oblique view and profile

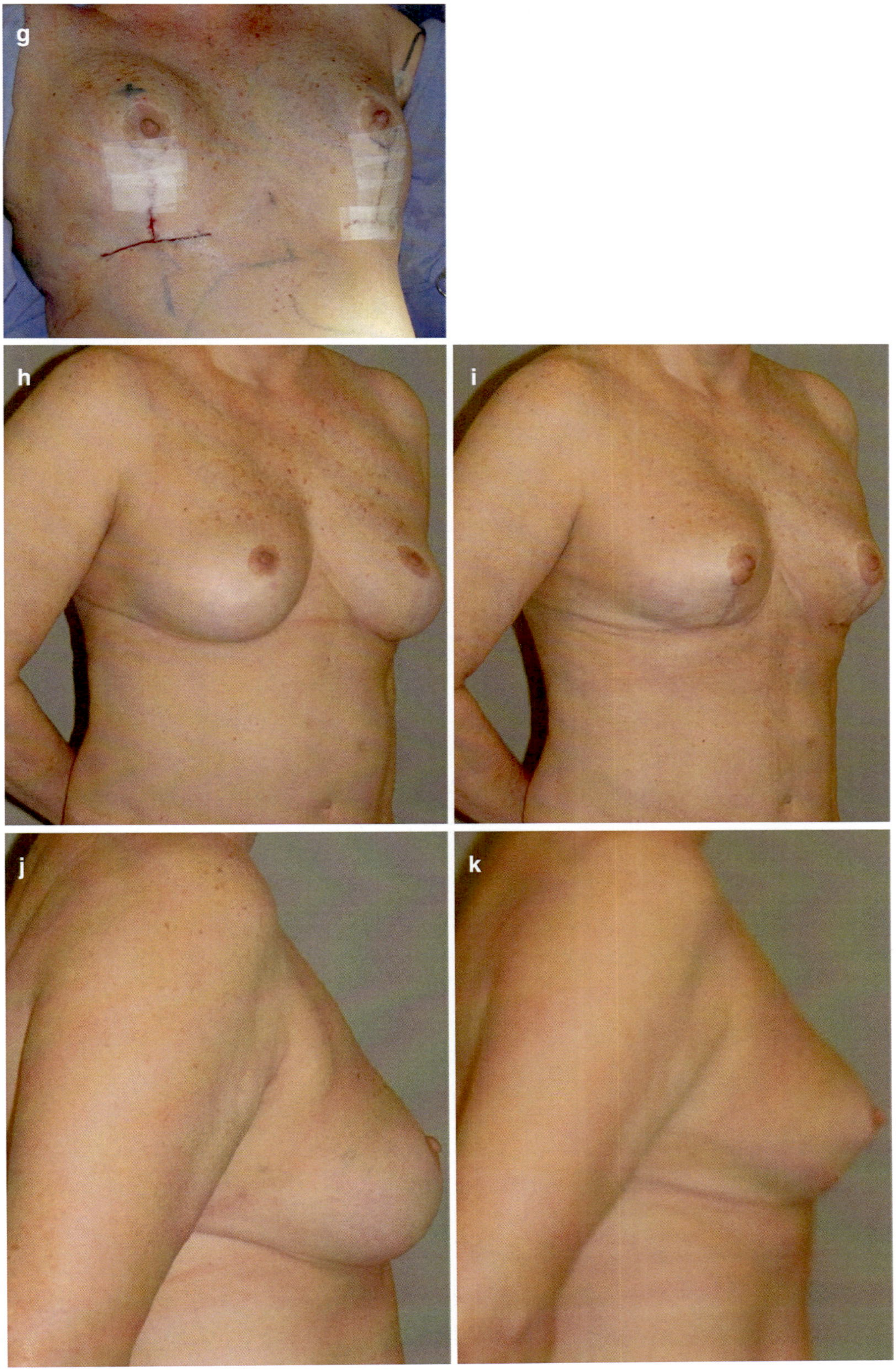

Fig. 41.8 (continued)

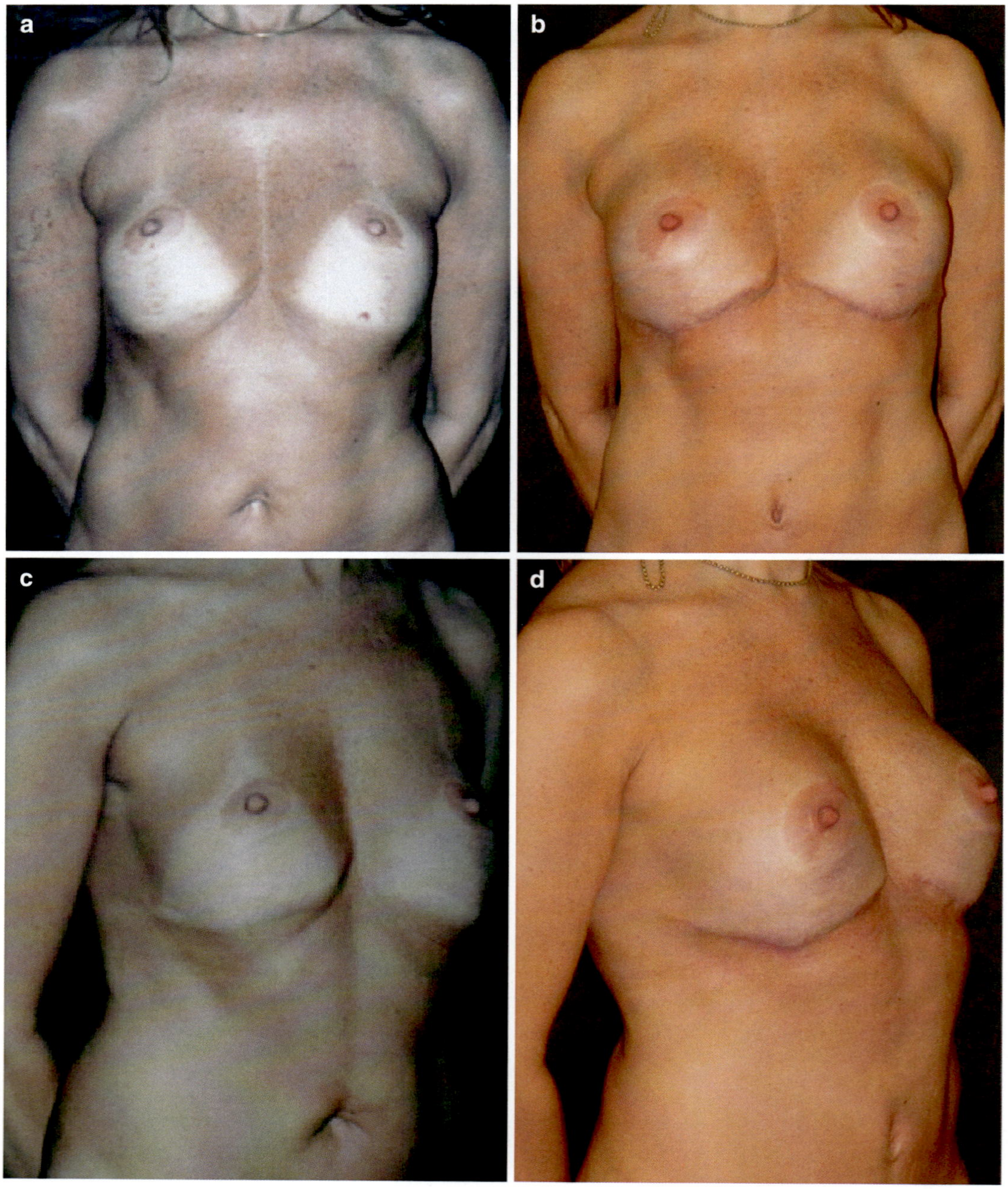

Fig. 41.9 A 35-year-old patient presenting an unfavorable aesthetic surgical result after mastoplasty. She had undergone two operations elsewhere. Photos (**a**) and (**c**) before repair of the nipple–areolar regions, which are located too high; photos (**b**) and (**d**) after surgical repair of the breast in combination with upper lipoabdominoplasty

41.3 Discussion

The most important concept for performing secondary mastoplasty as the basic support for the repair of unsatisfactory results is adequate surgical evaluation. Therefore, careful analysis of both breasts is a mandatory step before surgical planning. The decision to perform the procedure should be taken once there is a good understanding between surgeon and patient, as she is already frustrated after failure of the primary operation. She should be cautioned about the potential risks and possible adverse outcomes due to the peculiarity of each deformity. The surgeon must evaluate the presence of scars, the position of the NAC, and symmetry of the breasts, in addition to all the unaesthetic aspects of the previous operations. If a patient has already undergone more than one surgery, it means that she is twice as deeply frustrated and upset with regard to the breast operation (Fig. 41.9).

The most frequent situation is the unaesthetic position of the NAC that is located too high. Such problems may occur especially when the primary operation was performed with the patient in a supine position on the operating table during surgery.

The cutaneous–adipose–glandular flap is a useful procedure as it replaces the depression on the upper pole of the breast where it is missing the mammary gland. In fact, in most patients, the upper pole of the breast is flat, which the patient's main complaint.

41.4 Complications

The most feared situation when repairing a secondary mastoplasty is an unsuccessful result, as the patient is already frustrated because of the previous operations. To avoid such an unpleasant surgical result, it is necessary to analyze carefully all aspects of the secondary mastoplasty before planning the operation.

Some minor complications may occur: unaesthetic scars after the operation due to malpositioning of the previous ones and an imbalance of the NAC due to severe distortion before surgery. Bleeding during and after operation is rare, as the presence of scar tissue avoids such a situation. The scars around the areola may be irregular because of tension on the new region.

Conclusions

Secondary mastoplasty provides the surgeon with all the tools necessary to manage the unaesthetic issues of a woman's breast in a single operation: the size, shape, symmetry, and position of the NAC. This procedure must also take into consideration the patient's suffering due to previous operations and that she may expect too much from the surgical result. The surgeon should evaluate all deformities of the breasts in addition to his or her capacity and knowledge concerning the structure of the tissues. These opposing forces may result in difficulty obtaining the desired breast shape and in the risk of complications, such as delayed healing, infection, or unaesthetic scars.

References

Avelar JM (1989) Breast asymmetry (Assimetria mamária). In: Avelar JM (ed) Plastic surgery in infancy (Cirurgia plástica na infância), vol 2. Editora Hipocrates, São Paulo, pp 413–418

Avelar JM (1990) Fundamental principles in mastoplasty (Princípios fundamentales en las mastoplastias). In: Avelar JM, Malbec EF (eds) Historia. ciência 1 arte en cirugía estética, Ed. Hipócrates, São Paulo, pp 530–549

Avelar JM (1993) Reduction mastoplasty under local anesthesia. (Mastoplastia redutora sob anestesia local) In: Juarez M (ed) Loco-regional anesthesia on aesthetic surgery—(Anestesia loco-regional em cirurgia estética), vol 29. Avelar—Editora Hipócrates, São Paulo, pp 244–260

Avelar JM & Catunda MM (1985) Local anesthesia in body contour surgery. (Anestesia local na cirurgia do contorno corporal)—Anais do XII Congresso Brasileiro de Cirurgia Plástica, Gramado, RS, Novembro/1985: 415–416

Avelar JM & Gameiro CA (1990) New concepts in mastoplasty (Nuevos conceptos en la mastoplastia). In: Avelar JM, Malbec EF (eds) Historia, ciência y Arte en cirugía estética, Ed. Hipócrates, São Paulo, pp 550–559

Boschert MT, Barone CM, Puckett CL (1996) Outcome analysis of reduction mammaplasty. Plast Reconstr Surg; 98: 451–4.

Davis GM, Ringler SL, Short K, et al. (1995) Reduction mammaplasty: long term efficacy, morbidity, and patient satisfaction. Plast Reconstr Surg; 96: 1106–10.

Herman S, Hoffman S, Kahn S (1975) Revisional surgery after reduction mammaplasty. Plast Reconstr Surg 55(4):422–427

Hoffman S (1986) Recurrent abnormalities following reduction mammaplasty and correction of breast asymmetry. Plast Reconstr Surg 78:55–62

Hudson DA, Skoll PJ (1999) Repeat reduction mammaplasty. Plast Reconstr Surg 104:401–408

Lejour M (1997) Vertical mammaplasty as secondary surgery after other techniques. Aesthet Plast Surg; 21: 403–407.

Maliniac JW (1959) Harmful fallacies in mammaplasty. Persona communication. Abstract, International Congress of Plastic Surgery, London

Myr Y, Myr L (1968) Reduction mammaplasty. Plast Reconstr Surg 41(4):352–355

Pitanguy, I. (1959) Breast hypertrophy. In: Wallace AB (ed) Transactions of the International Society of Plastic Surgeons, Second Congress, Edinburgh, E. & S. Livingstone, p 509

Pitanguy I (1961) An eclectic approach to breast problems [Aproximação eclética ao problema das mamaplastias]. Rev Bras Cir 41:179–196

Pitanguy I, Garcia LC (1972) Aspectos importantes de técnica pessoal em mamaplastia. Bol Soc Cir Plast Reconstr Córdoba 4:7

Serletti JM, Reading G, Cladwell E, Wray RC (1992) Long term patient's satisfaction following reduction mammoplasty. Ann Plas Surg 28:363–5

42 Complications from Treatment with Mammoplasty

Ricardo Cavalcanti Ribeiro,
Pedro Felipe Suárez Cruz, and Flávio Rezende

42.1 Introduction

Reconstructive or aesthetic mammoplasty has played an important role in the evolution of the plastic surgery, and is nowadays the number one procedure for this specialty, surpassing procedures such as liposuction and others. The application of an appropriate surgical technique and the implementation of high quality materials are of utmost importance, to reduce the complications that may be present.

With the emergence of new, less aggressive surgical techniques and better quality materials, the spread of complications has decreased over time, facilitating the procedure and satisfactory results, both for the patient and for the doctor.

Many risk factors have been associated with complications in mammoplasty, which is why it is very important to know about and prevent them, and to take action to reduce the incidence of these complications. In Table 42.1, we cite the risk factors that have a major impact on these procedures.

Table 42.1 The principal factors that increase the risk of complications in mammoplasty

Clinical factors	Breast local factors	Factors related to the surgical procedure
Smoking	Size of hypertrophy	Surgical technique used
Hypertension	Commitment to skin by infectious process	Surgeon's lack of experience
Diabetes mellitus	Previous surgery	
Disorders of coagulation	Previous radiotherapy	

Source: Cirurgia Plástica Fundamentos e Arte. Volume IV; Mélega

Head of Division of Plastic and Reconstructive Surgery of Universidade Federal do Estado of the Rio de Janeiro (UNIRIO)

R.C. Ribeiro, M.D., Ph.D. (✉)
Division of Plastic and Reconstructive Surgery of Casa de Portugal, Brazilian Society of Plastic Surgery, Carlos Chagas Institute, Rio de Janeiro, RJ, Brazil
e-mail: rribeiro@centroin.com.br

P.F.S. Cruz, M.D.
Division of Plastic and Reconstructive Surgery, Carlos Chagas Institute, Rio de Janeiro, RJ, Brazil

F. Rezende, M.D.
Plastic and Reconstructive Surgery, Universidad Federal del Estado de Río de Janeiro, Brazilian Society of Plastic Surgery, Rio de Janeiro, RJ, Brazil

J.M. Avelar (ed.), *Breast Surgery*, https://doi.org/10.1007/978-3-319-54115-0_42

42.2 Methods

Through the use of electronic searches such as MEDLINE, PUBMED, SCIELO, and the written literature, a review of the literature from the 1990s through to 2016, using keywords such as (Complications in Mammoplasty, Complications in Mastopexy, Risk Factors in Mammoplasty, Complications in Reduction Mammoplasty, Seroma in Mammoplasty, Hematoma in Mammoplasty, Capsular Contracture, Implant Rupture, Breast Implant Rippling, Infection in Breast Surgery).

42.3 Discussion

42.3.1 Complications in Breast Aesthetic Procedures

The aesthetic approach to the breast has a significant relationship with reconstructive surgery, currently presenting a low incidence of around 1–10%, considering the large number of surgeries performed today.

Many of these complications occur in all procedures, which we discuss below (Baker 1975; Bender and Beck 1995).

Hematoma is usually displayed immediately and is associated with the bleeding of the surgical field. Clinically, the patient refers to discomfort in the thoracic region related to pain and local burning. In the physical examination, an edema may be found, associated with hardening and ecchymosis. To prevent such a complication, it is important to obtain a precise anamnesis with the aim of identifying risk factors inherent to the patient and to the use of any medication that predisposes to increased bleeding. Once the complication has shown up, the next steps are established, which could vary from simple needle aspiration to immediate intervention to carrying out hemostasis and drainage of the hematoma, thereby preventing the suffering of the adjacent tissues and reducing the risk of infection (Fig. 42.1).

Seroma is considered a very frequent complication of these procedures, which does not mean that it is easily resolved. It occurs because of the lymphatic damage that is part of the procedure. Clinically, it can go unnoticed; the patient may merely refer to serohematic secretion from the suture line. Discomfort or pain may occur in the case of large collections Brown et al. (1997). Seroma can be prevented through the careful dissection of tissues, the conscious use of electrocautery, and the use of vacuum drainage. Treatment methods consist in the periodic drainage of the seroma from the spontaneous form or by puncture.

Infection is associated with multiple causes; among the most common are the bad practices of

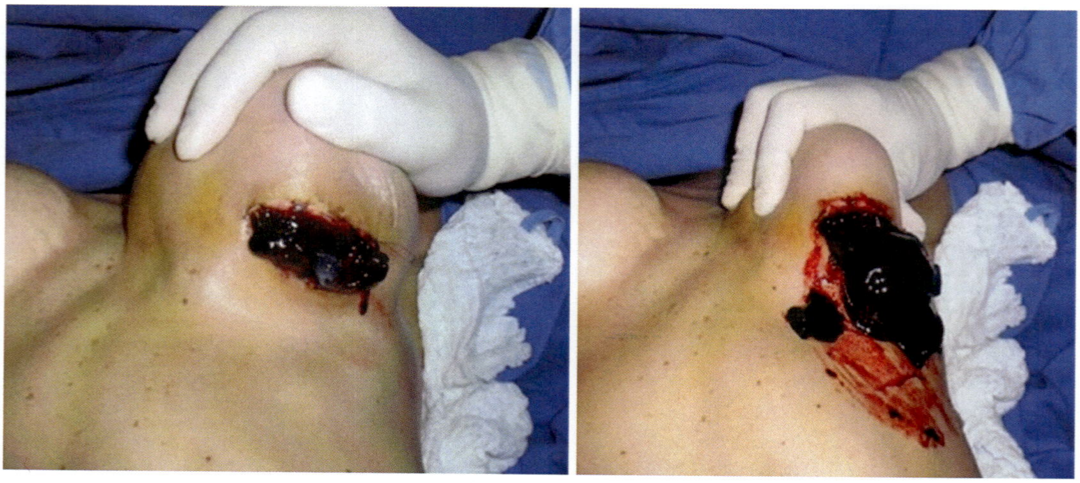

Fig. 42.1 A 23-year-old patient with a history of breast augmentation with implants, who referred in her second postoperative week to pain and increased breast volume. The revision was performed at a surgical center, where a large hematoma on the left breast is drained

asepsis and antisepsis and clinical conditions inherent to each patient. It clinically manifests with pain together with hardening and hyperemia in the region of the breast, with occasional purulent secretion and systemic fever-like symptoms. The microorganisms most frequently related to this process are *Staphylococcus aureus* and *Streptococcus* (Chen et al. 1991; Courtiss and Goldwyn 1976). Prevention is by use of a suitable surgical technique with appropriate sterile material, cleaning of the surgical field, and use of prophylactic antibiotics in the anesthetic induction. Treatment requires the use of broad-spectrum antibiotics, local care, and periodic evaluation of the patient.

Wound dehiscence occurs more frequently in the distal part of the skin flap. It is related to the excessive tension on the edges of the wound, thin skin, changes in skin perfusion correlated with smoking, infection, diabetic angiopathy, hypoproteinemia, chronic use of corticosteroids, and treatment with radiotherapy, etc Dos Santos et al. (2008). Treatment requires regular monitoring of the patient, resection of devitalized tissue, and closing the wound by first intention healing. For large losses, the use of skin grafts or skin flaps is necessary for resolution (Fig. 42.2).

Unsatisfactory scar or hypertrophic/keloid: Complication that is linked to the use of inadequate surgical techniques, involves excessive tension on the suture line, improper handling of tissues, material of low quality, and problems inherent to each patient Dos Santos et al. (2008).

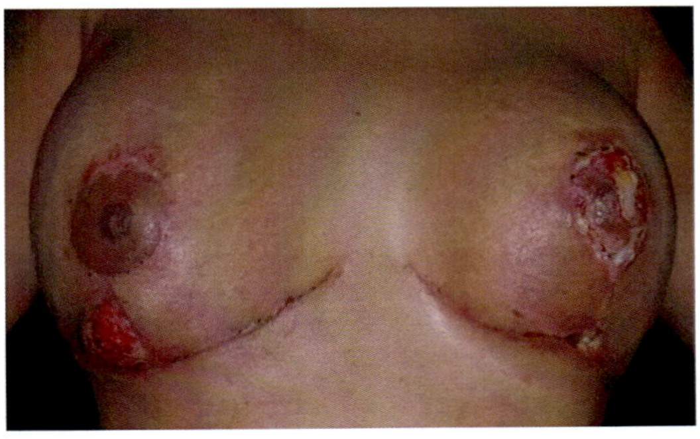

Fig. 42.2 A 30-year-old patient, postoperative day 25 after mastopexy with implants. There is evidence of wound dehiscence in the right inframammary region and left periareolar region

Thanks to local treatment with corticoids, pressure therapy, and beta therapy, significant improvements are achieved in the appearance of the scar, leaving second surgery to revise the scar as a last resort.

Next, we present the most prevalent complications in each procedure.

42.3.1.1 Mastopexy

The objective of this procedure is the correction of breast ptosis. For a better approach, the knowledge of the grades of ptosis is indispensable, taking into account the different classifications currently used.

The proper selection of patients is essential for obtaining satisfactory results, considering the degree of breast ptosis, the patient's age, skin quality, and the patient's expectations as a starting point.

A procedure that usually mobilizes the dermoglandular flap, which may create intense lipolysis, probably progressing to fat necrosis.

Necrosis of the Nipple—Areola complex: Slightly frequent complication. As associated risk factors include the development of very thin flaps, closure of the wound under tension, the use of postoperative dressing with too much compression and infection Filipe Volpe et al. (2012). Treatment depends on the degree of commitment, ranging from small local debridement up to the need to use grafts or flaps for defect coverage (Fig. 42.3).

Recurrence of breast ptosis: Patients who lose a large amount of weight have an important deficit of fatty tissue, a significant loss of breast-bearing capacity, and subsequent ptosis. The recurrence of the breast ptosis has been linked to surgical techniques that do not restore the anatomy of the breast, especially ligaments of suspension. Currently, several studies have been conducted to avoid this complication. Significant results have been found with the use of materials such as mesh that reinforce the sustainability of the breast and allow proper maintenance of the shape and position of this area for a longer period of time Gabriel et al. (1997).

Deformity of the breast: This correlates with the type of surgical technique used. It is clearly

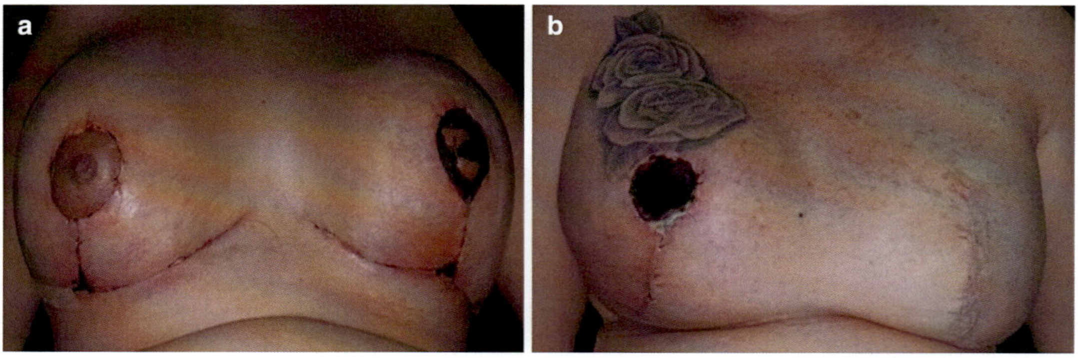

Fig. 42.3 Patient 10 days postoperatively after mastopexy with implants, who presented partial necrosis of the nipple–areola complex. (**a**) Patient on day 12 postoperatively after breast reconstruction with a *latissimus dorsi* flap, (**b**) presenting total necrosis of the nipple–areola complex

demonstrated in the inverted T mastopexy, in which the breast has a more flattened aspect. In the oblique technique, the breast acquires a more pointed form. The correction is performed through the surgical intervention.

Asymmetry of the Nipple—Areola complex: The surgical planning is of great importance to avoid a change in the location of the nipple–areola complex (NAC), requiring previous marking of the patient to obtain a satisfactory result.

42.3.1.2 Reduction Mammoplasty

The purpose of this procedure is the decrease in the content and breast container, for physical and psychosocial reasons referred to by the patient. From the physical point of view, there are negative effects such as pain in the neck and back region, the feeling of increased weight, maceration, irritation and infection in the inframammary region, pressure from the use of a brassiere, generating discomfort in the patient. Psychosocially, breasts with large volumes can result in frustration and shame in younger women, hampering sports and social activities.

Breast reduction is considered a significant procedure given that it includes dissections and extensive resections, which increase the number of complications, varying from environment to 10% Gabrielli et al. (2001).

Nipple—Areola Complex Epidermolysis: The involvement of the NAC is associated with ischemia by excess tension or venous congestion that leads to an alteration in the perfusion, partial or total loss of this segment. It is important to highlight that the excessive stress relief can be reversed over a 6 h period, thus avoiding this complication. In partial losses, scar revision may be necessary months after surgery. Total losses require entire reconstruction of the complex with diverse techniques in addition to the possibility of a tattoo that mimics this segment.

Alterations of the sensitivity: Relatively frequent complication related to the amount of breast tissue removed. It tends to occur with more intensity 6 months postoperatively, with a gradual recovery of sensation, as was reported by Courtis and Goldwyn (1976) in their studies. In some patients, hypoesthesia of the NAC may occur for up to 2 years Handel and Yegiyants (2016).

Unsatisfactory scars or hypertrophic/keloid: It is known that techniques employing vertical scars tend the lengthen the scar, rather than inducing scar hypertrophy. Horizontal scars present a greater tendency toward hypertrophy; thus, it is recommended to locate them in the mammary sulcus, where there will be less tension and they will be better camouflaged. Crossing of the halfway line that is associated with the appearance of keloid scar should always be avoided. For the initial treatment of the hypertrophic scar, the intralesional infiltration of corticoids is recommended 3 months postoperatively.

42.3.1.3 Augmentation Mammoplasty

Augmentation mammoplasty is considered to be one of the most frequently performed procedures in plastic surgery. Currently, satisfactory results have been obtained, allied with less aggressive surgical techniques, a better surgical set of instruments, and better quality implants, making this a simple technique.

Displacement of the implants: A major incidence of displacement appears in implants with a retromuscular location, related to the easy dissection of the areolar connective tissue, when the muscle exercises pressure during mobilization or sports. Patients with an implant in a retroglandular location present less or no displacement, owing to the more careful dissection that accommodates the implant appropriately Hölmich Lisbet et al. (2005).

Rippling: It is a frequent complication in patients who undergo breast augmentation with implants, presenting a great challenge to the plastic surgeon. Wrinkles on the skin are presented by a crease in the surface layer of the implant, associated with inadequate coverage, because of the failure of soft tissues and increased consistency in the surface layer of the implant. The ripples of the implant are more obvious in the upper pole of the breast at the cleavage line or in the lateral region. There is an increased incidence with the use of implants filled with saline solution compared with gel implants Laurence (2014). It is critical to inform the patient of the possible occurrence of this complication, before performing breast augmentation. The initial treatment of these patients is expectant. Currently, many of these patients are treated by small amounts of fat grafting in the superficial part of the soft tissue to minimize any possible complications that this procedure could present, and achieving satisfactory cosmetic results. Processes with difficult resolution require removal of the implant with a change in its position (Fig. 42.4).

Capsular Contracture: Considered one of the most common late complications in this type of procedure. It is known that all mammary implants suffer some grade of capsule formation associated with a natural reaction of the organism in response to a foreign body. Diverse causes have been related to the appearance of an anomalous capsule, but the exact etiology is still unknown. Clinically, the capsular contraction can vary from a simple appearance of the implant, to an excessive pain that forces the removal or exchange of the implant after the execution of capsulectomy vs capsulotomy Pittet et al. (2005). For a better

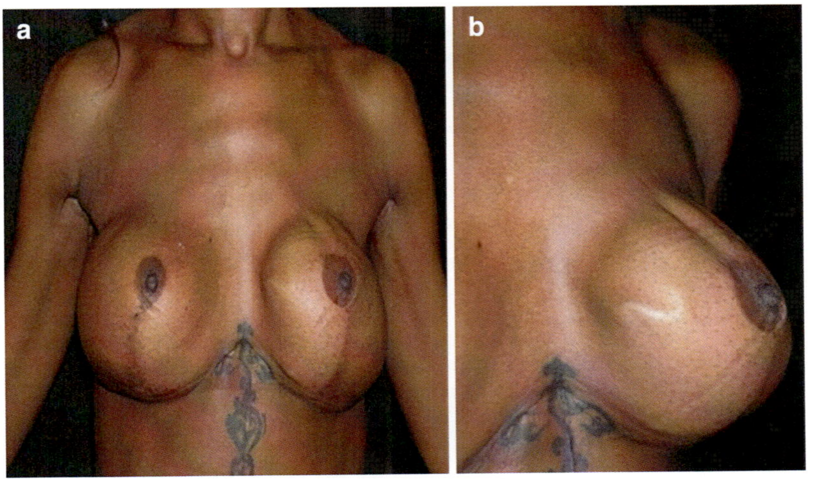

Fig. 42.4 Patient 2 years postoperatively after mastopexy with implants. A superficial position of the implants associated with the presence of rippling is observed

Table 42.2 Classification of capsular contracture

Grade I	Breast absolutely natural.
Grade II	Minimal contracture. Slight firmness of the breast.
Grade III	Moderate contracture. Breast firmer, a little painful.
Grade IV	Severe contracture. Breast very firm, painful.

Baker's Source (Plastic And Reconstructive Surgery Journal. 1995; 1119–23)

understanding, it is important to remember the classification, presented by Baker in the 1970s, which we show in Table 42.2 together with the main characteristics Raquel and de Moraes (2009).

Treatment of this complication is diverse. Patients with capsular contracture of the first grade can be treated in an expectant way, giving greater importance to the periodic evaluation. Capsular contracture of the second degree requires clinical intervention, through the use of ultrasound associated with manual and microcurrent lymphatic drainage, succeeding in regression of the process at an early stage in many cases. Patients with more severe cases (grades III and IV) are recommended to change their breast implant, repositioning the new implant with a preference for the submuscular plane associated with capsulectomy or capsulotomy and clinical treatment. At present, implants of better quality and a rough surface are those made of polyurethane or silicone, decreasing the incidence of capsular contracture.

Implant Rupture: Breast implants may have two types of rupture. First, in intracapsular rupture, the composition of the implant is contained by the fibrous capsule already formed, thus preventing movement. This type of rupture accounts for 80–90% of this complication. In extracapsular rupture, which represents 10–20% of all cases, the content of the implant is free in the breast cavity. As a diagnostic tool, we manage magnetic resonance imaging, which, together with the clinical findings of the patient, provide more accurate information on the detection of this complication.

Rupture may be observed with a high frequency in implants that contain saline solution. Clinical accounts by the patient such as a sudden loss of the size of the breast are usually associated with a trauma. This type of material does not present reabsorption on the part of the adjacent tissue, for which it requires extraction of the same and new placement of the implant. New-generation materials that contain cohesive gel do not present a risk of major rupture for the patient because the material does not split, and it is not even re-absorbed by the organism, which facilitates its extraction. In the therapeutic approach for these patients, we recommend removal of the breast implant with or without replacement, depending on the patient's desire and the surgeon's decision (Ricardo and Saltz 2012; Srinivasaiah et al. 2014; Tark et al. 2005).

Stretch Marks: Also known as striae distensae or skin rupture, stretch marks are related to a rapid stretching of the skin of the breast region, by the application of tension in a fast and sustained way that avoids progressive expansion. Factors favoring the appearance of stretch marks in patients with breast augmentation include the use of oral contraceptives, nulliparity, being overweight, a personal history of stretch marks, and patients of a young age van (Deventer et al. 2012; Vitug and Newman 2007).

Conclusion

Breast surgery is considered one of the most popular procedures performed in plastic surgery. Knowledge of different surgical techniques, the materials used, and the factors that increase the risk of complications are important for obtaining favorable postoperative outcomes. The recognition and early approach toward these complications prevent the development of sequelae that generate a negative impact on patient satisfaction.

References

Baker Jr JL (1975) Classification of spherical contractures. Presented at the aesthetic breast ymposium. Scottsdale, Arizona

Bender H, Beck L (1995) Complicações nas cirurgías da mama. In: Complicações intra e pós-operatorias em ginecología, pp 136–162

Brown SL, Silverman BG, Berg WA (1997) Rupture of silicone-gel breast implants: causes, sequelae, and diagnosis. Lancet 350(9090):1531–1537

Chen J, Gutkin Z, Bawnik J (1991) Postoperative infections in breast surgery. J Hosp Infect 17:61–65

Courtiss EH, Goldwyn RM (1976) Breast sensation before and after plastic surgery. Plast Reconstr Surg 58(1):1–13

Dos Santos M, Ricardo Frota B, Adolfo Ribeiro C, Motoka E, Aulus de Mendonça A (2008) Prevention and treatment of capsular contracture after mammary prosthesis implantation. Rev Bras Cir Plast 23(2)

Filipe Volpe B, Arthur Volpe B, Antonio Roberto B (2012) Striae distensae after breast augmentation. Aesthet Plast Surg 36(4):894–900

Gabriel SE, Woods JE, O'Fallon M, Beard CM, Kurland LT, Melton LJ (1997) Complications leading to surgery after breast implantation. N Engl J Med 336(10):677–682

Gabrielli F, Potenza C, Puddu P, Sera F, Masini C, Abeni D (2001) Suture materials and other factors associated with tissue reactivity, infection, and wound dehiscence among plastic surgery outpatients. Plast Reconstr Surg 107(1):38–45

Handel N, Yegiyants S (2016) Managing necrosis of the nipple areolar complex following reduction mammaplasty and mastopexy. Clin Plastic Surg 43:415–423

Hölmich Lisbet R, Fryzek Jon P, Kim Breiting Vibeke B, Anna Krag C, McLaughlin JK (2005) The diagnosis of silicone breast-implant rupture: clinical findings compared with findings at magnetic resonance imaging. Ann Plast Surg 54(6):583–589

Laurence GN (2014) Breast implant rippling and palpability. In: Mugea TT, Shiffman MA (eds) Aesthetic surgery of the breast. Springer, Berlin Heidelberg, pp 557–561

Pittet B, Montandon D, Pitte D (2005) Infection in breast implants. Lancet Infect Dis 5(2):94–106

Raquel Cristina Tancsik C, de Moraes AM (2009) Striae Distensae: physiopathology. Surg Cosmet Derm 1(3):137–140

Ricardo CR, Saltz R (2012) Cirurgia Da Mama. Estética & Reconstrutora, Segunda edicao: Complicacoes na Cirurgia de Mama, pp 361–370

Srinivasaiah N, Iwuchukwu OC, Stanley PR, Hart NB, Platt AJ, Drew PJ (2014) Risk factors for complications following breast reduction: results from a randomized control trial. Breast J 20(3):274–278

Tark KC, Jeong HS, Roh TS, Choi JW (2005) Analysis of 30 breast implant rupture cases. Aesthet Plast Surg 29(6):460–469

van Deventer PV, Graewe FR, Wuringer E (2012) Improving the longevity and results of mastopexy and breast reduction procedures: reconstructing an internal breast support system with biocompatible mesh to replace the supporting function of the ligamentous suspension. Aesthet Plast Surg 36:578–589

Vitug AF, Newman LA (2007) Complications in breast surgery. Surg Clin N Am 87:431–451

Part III

Aesthetic Reparation of Breast and Chest Wall Deformities

Asymmetrical Breasts: A Challenge for Aesthetic Repair

43

Juarez M. Avelar

43.1 Introduction

From birth until puberty, the breasts are latent. During puberty, a great physical change occurs in the female body caused by hormonal metabolic alterations when the breasts start to develop and assume an enormous importance in a woman's life. Also, abnormal development may occur in males during puberty and in adults caused by the action of hormonal disturbances, named gynecomastia, which is not the subject of this chapter.

From puberty, female breasts are an important symbol of femininity and they are responsible for significant expression in body contouring and in the sexual sphere. They have an even greater emphasis in adolescence when young girls begin a new part of their lives. Of the numerous changes in body structure during puberty, breast development is a new world with multiple functions. Any change in the aesthetic constitution can modify the body's silhouette, causing image disharmony and imbalance. In addition, the lactation function compromises the breast frame with regard to breast asymmetry.

As far as the presence of breasts in the female body have tremendous value and symbolism for the existence, asymmetries can attract more attention, leading to a search for surgical solution in adulthood or adolescence. Asymmetries with concomitant hypertrophy focus on women aged from childhood and puberty. In contrast, many congenital diseases confer an aesthetic imbalance to the anterior chest wall, causing serious disorder in the intimate well-being of the woman.

43.2 Classification: Congenital and Acquired

The incidence of mammary asymmetry among my patients is very high, and I may consider it quite unusual for a woman to have perfectly symmetrical breasts. Such an observation is so important that some abnormal evolution of breasts after mastoplasty may be due to structural asymmetry of the tissues (Avelar 1989, 1993). If a patient does not complain about that, it is adequate for the surgeon to show her before surgery. During consultation, I always ask my patients about any asymmetry and it is quite rare for someone respond to my question. However, during physical examination when she is in a standing position in front of two parallel mirrors in my examination room they quite often present some sort of abnormality.

Maliniac (1950) classified breast asymmetries into four categories:

1. Asymmetry with bilateral hypertrophy
2. Hypertrophy on one side and amastia or hypomastia on the other

J.M. Avelar, M.D.
Brazilian Institute of Plastic and Reconstructive Surgery, Sao Paulo, SP 01442-000, Brazil
e-mail: juarezavelar@bol.com.br

J.M. Avelar (ed.), *Breast Surgery*, https://doi.org/10.1007/978-3-319-54115-0_43

3. Hypertrophy on one side and the other a normal size
4. Amastia or hypomastia on one side and the other normal breast

So far, Juri (1989) has presented a brief classification of asymmetrical breasts of only three grades. Other authors have referred to this, such as Broadbent and Woolf (1978), Karim et al. (2009), Jales (2004), Sepúlveda (1981), with some reports concerning the asymmetry of the breasts and proposed specific classifications. As such abnormalities are quite frequent and are of great importance in plastic surgery, I proposed a classification according to the origin (Avelar 1989), which is helpful for surgical correction. Below, I present a classification into two major groups: congenital and acquired

A. Congenital

(a) Without chest deformity
  1. Bilateral hypertrophy (Fig. 43.1)
  2. Hypertrophy of one breast and normal size of the other (Fig. 43.2)
  3. Hypertrophy of one breast and hypomastia of the other (Figs. 43.3 and 43.4)
  4. Hypertrophy of one breast and ptosis of the other (Figs. 43.5 and 43.6)
  5. Bilateral hypomastia (Fig. 43.7)
  6. Hypomastia of one breast and normal size of the other (Fig. 43.8)
  7. Asymmetrical breasts with bilateral ptosis (Fig. 43.9)

(b) With chest deformity
  1. Bilateral hypertrophy
  2. Hypertrophy and normal size
  3. Hypertrophy and hypomastia
  4. Bilateral hypomastia
  5. Hypomastia and normal size

Illustrative photos of asymmetrical breast with chest deformities are shown in Chap. 45

(c) Without nipple deformity
  1. Atelia and normal size
  2. Amastia and normal size
  3. Amastia and hypomastia
  4. Polythelia
  5. Polymastia (Fig. 43.10)

(d) With nipple deformity
  1. Atelia and normal size
  2. Amastia and normal size
  3. Amastia and hypomastia
  4. Polythelia
  5. Polymastia

B. Acquired

1. Traumatic
   (a) Burns (Fig. 43.11)
   (b) Human bite (Fig. 43.12)
2. Iatrogenic
   (a) After mastectomy for resection of breast cancer (Fig. 43.13)
   (b) Secondary to augmentation mastoplasty
   (c) Secondary to reduction mastoplasty

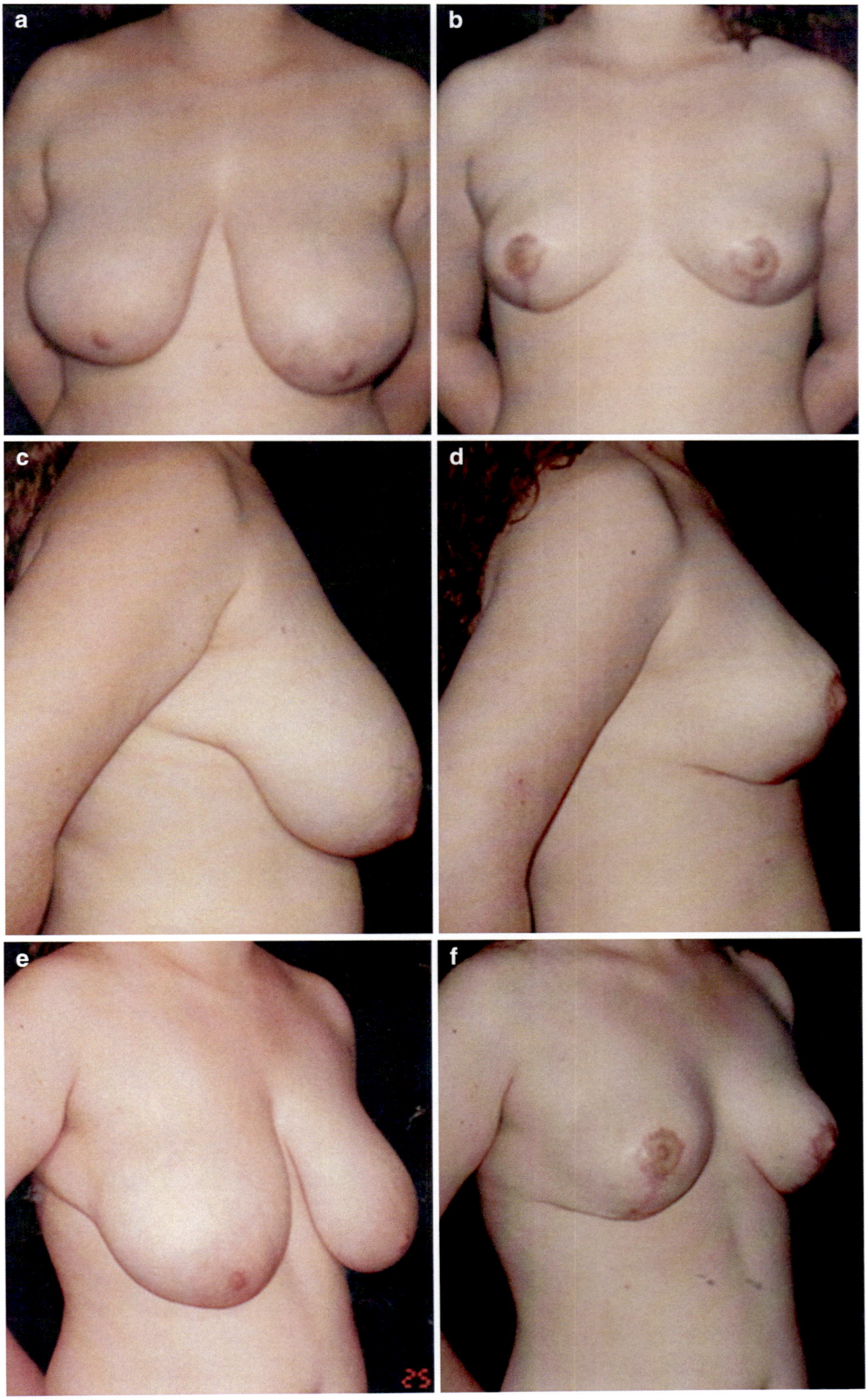

Fig. 43.1 A 29-year-old patient with large hypertrophic breasts with evident asymmetry. (**a**, **c**, **e**) Preoperatively. (**b**, **d**, **f**) After reduction mastoplasty using my approach, with small scars on the submammary folds

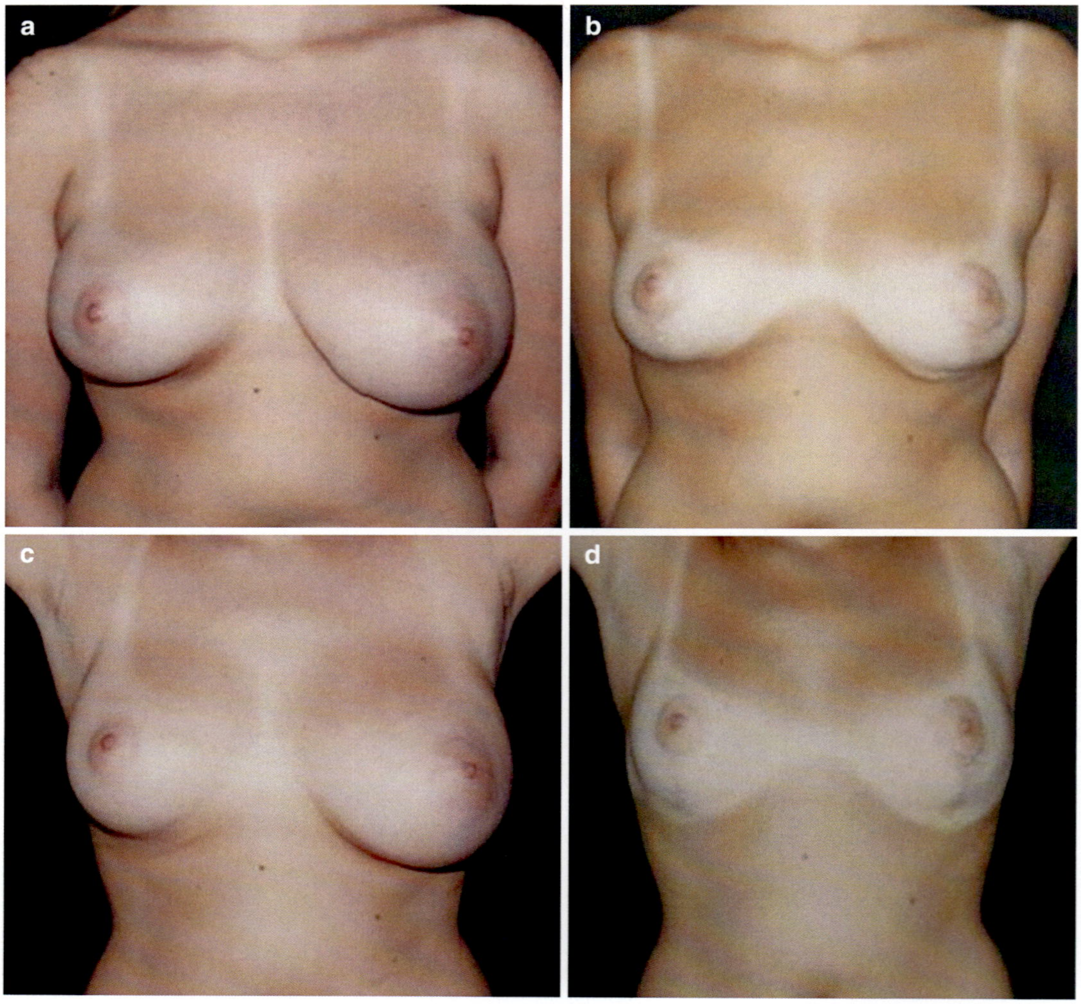

Fig. 43.2 Asymmetrical breasts: hypertrophic with ptosis on the left side and ptosis on the right side. (**a**) Before surgery. (**b**) After reduction mastoplasty on the left side with resection of 200 g and mastopexy on the right side. (**c**) Before surgery with arms up. (**d**) After surgery

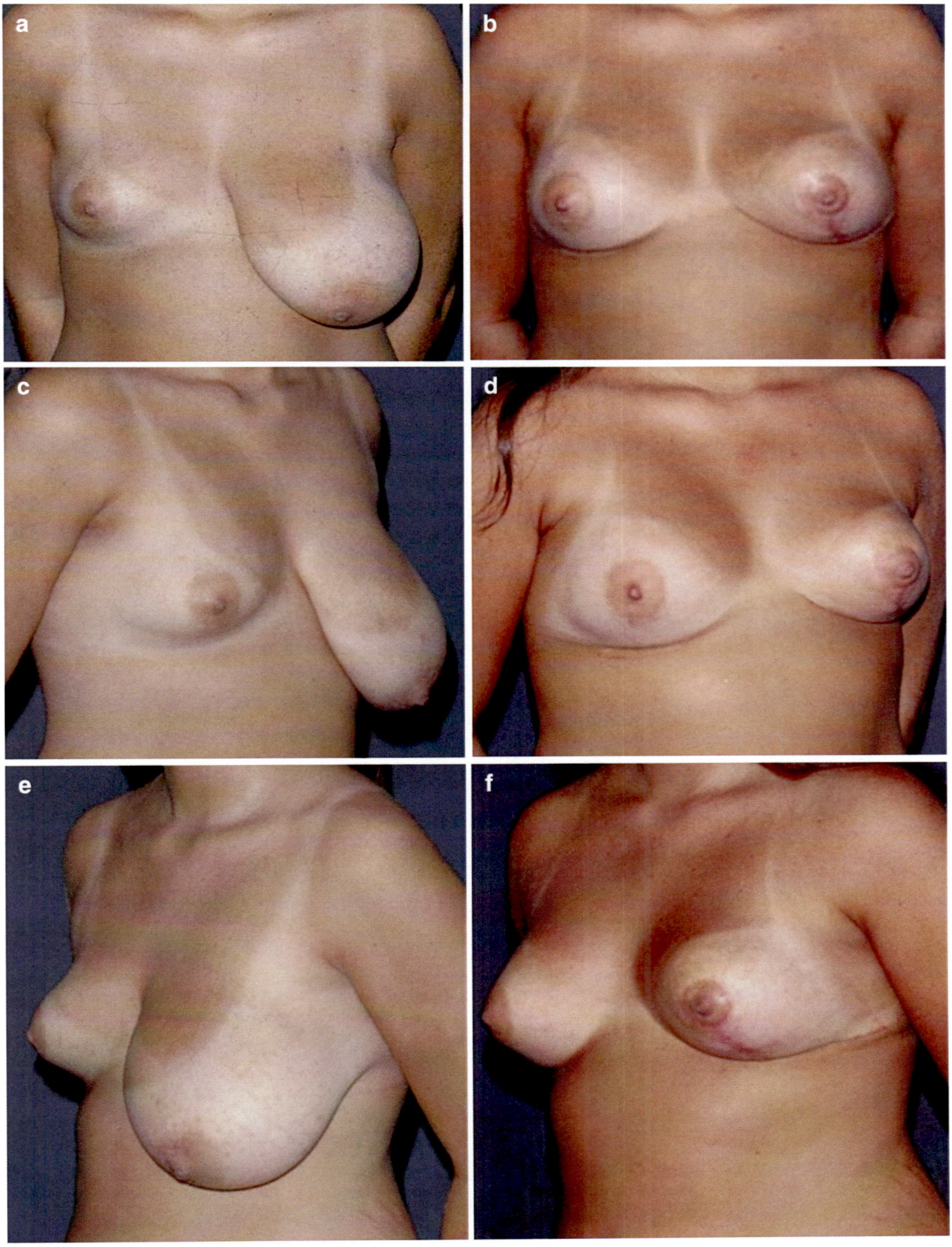

Fig. 43.3 Breast asymmetry in a 19-year-old girl: hypertrophic on the left side and hypomastia of the right breast. (**a**) Preoperative frontal view. (**b**) Postoperative view. 500 g was removed on the left side and 180 mL was implanted on the right side. (**c**) Preoperative oblique view on the right side. (**d**) Postoperatively. (**e**) Preoperative left view. (**f**) Postoperative left view

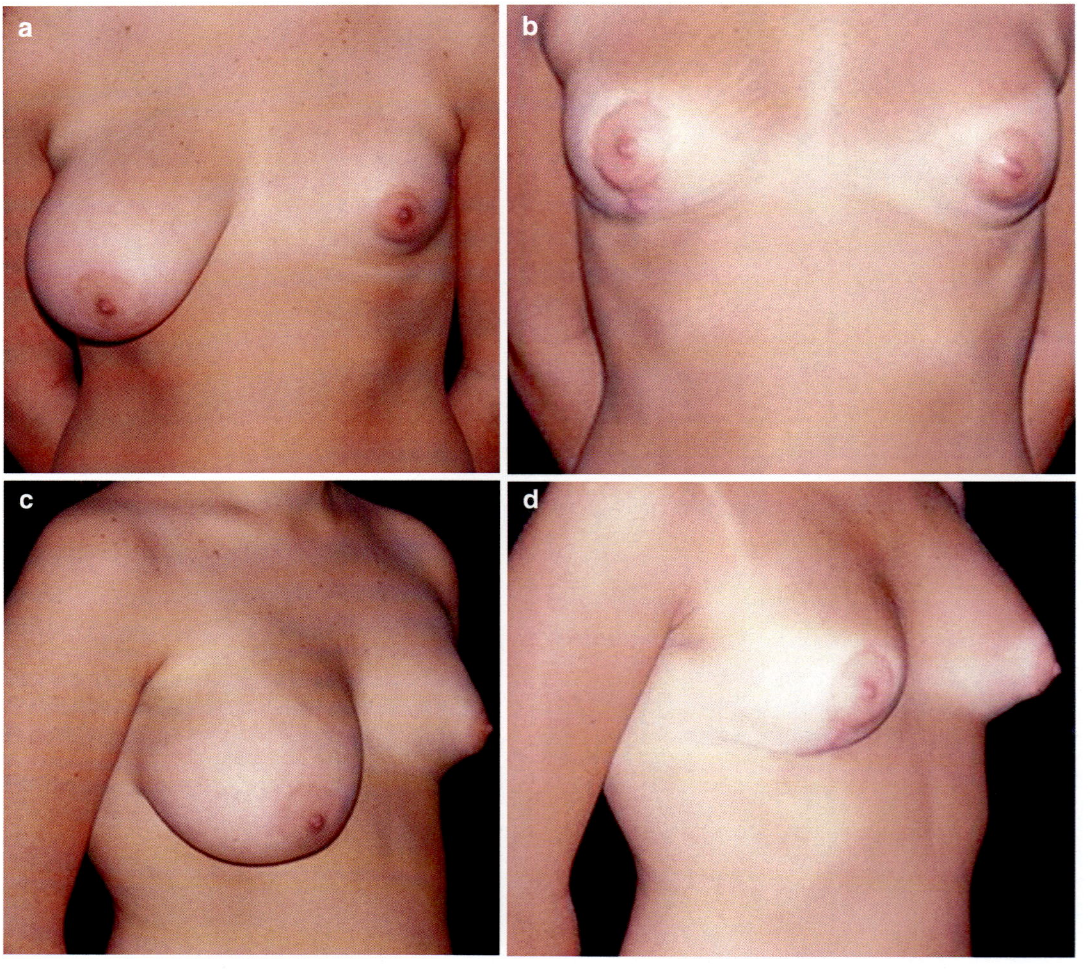

Fig. 43.4 Asymmetrical breasts: hypertrophic with ptosis on the right side and hypomastia on the left side. (**a**) Before surgery. (**b**) After reduction mastoplasty on the right side and implant of 160 mL on the left side. (**c**) Before surgery right view. (**d**) After surgery

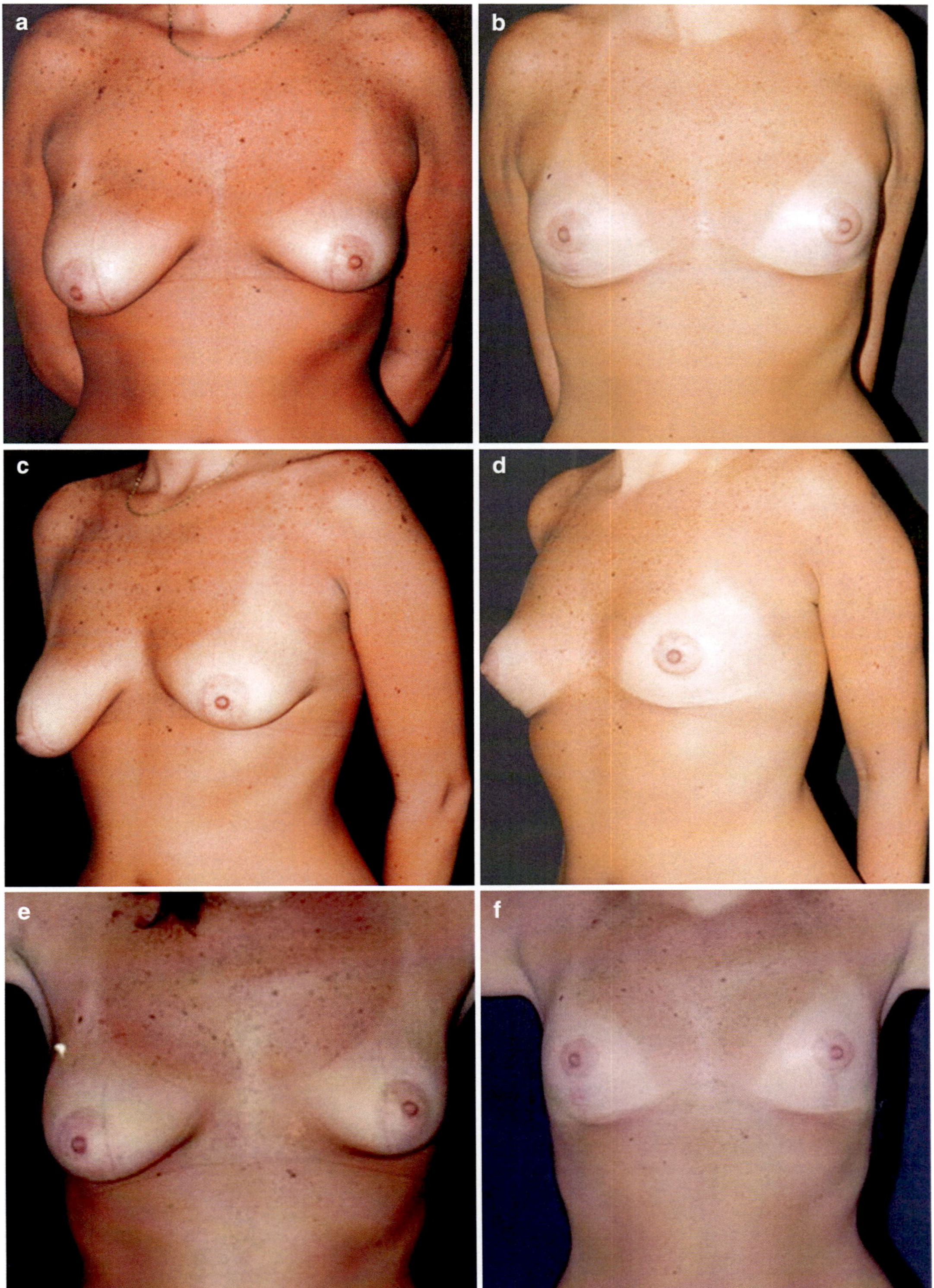

Fig. 43.5 Asymmetrical breasts: hypertrophic with ptosis on the right side and ptosis on the left side. (**a**) Before surgery. (**b**) After reduction mastoplasty with removal of 150 mg on the right side and mastopexy on the left side. (**c**) Before surgery left view. (**d**) After surgery. (**e**) Before surgery front view with arms up. (**f**) After reduction mastoplasty on the right side and mastopexy on the left side

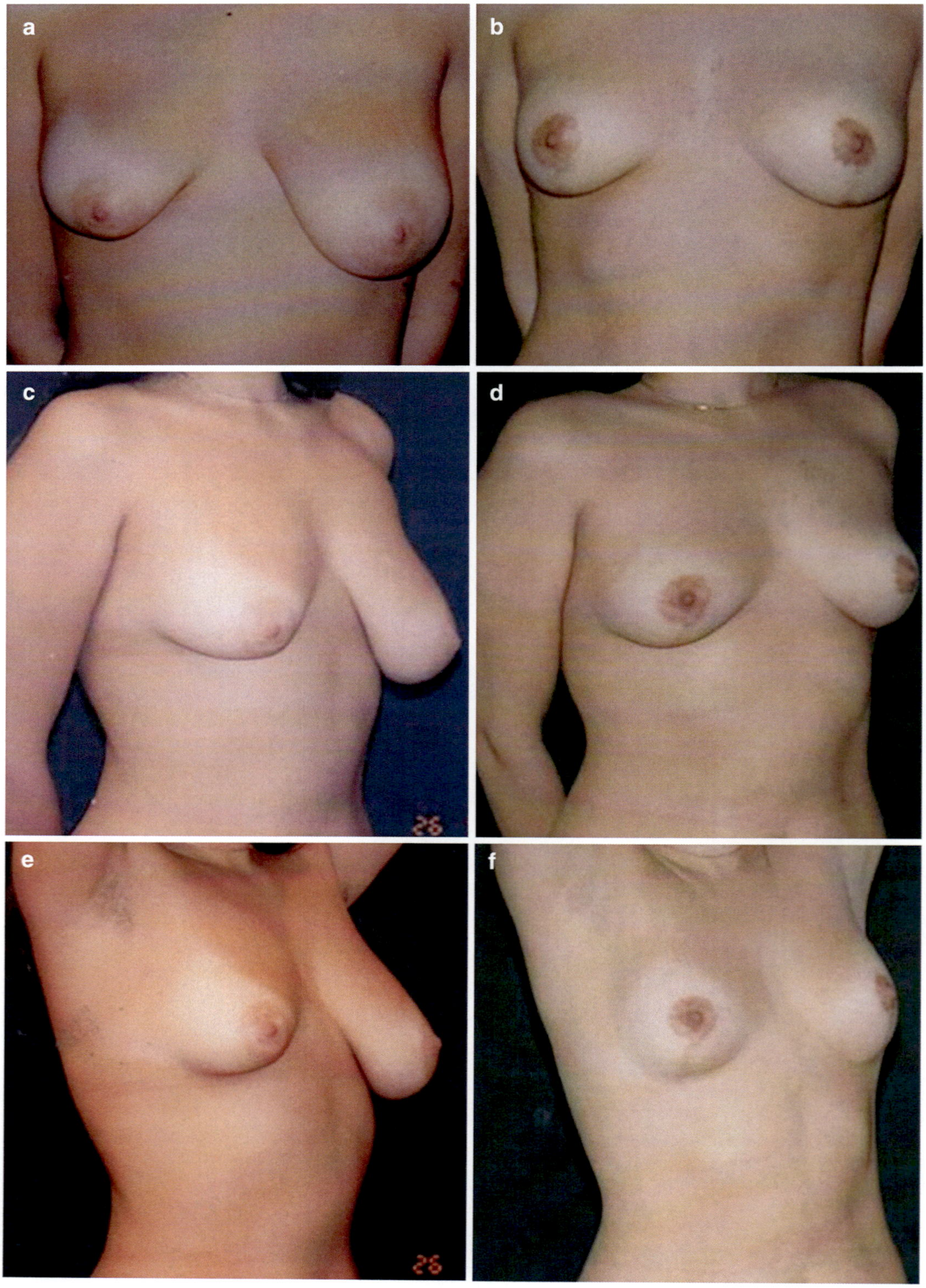

Fig. 43.6 Asymmetrical breasts: hypertrophic with ptosis on the left side and ptosis on the right side. (**a**, **c**) Before surgery. (**b**, **d**) After reduction mastoplasty on the left side and mastopexy on the right side. (**e**) Before surgery oblique view on the right side with arms up. (**f**) After reduction mastoplasty on the right side and mastopexy on the left side

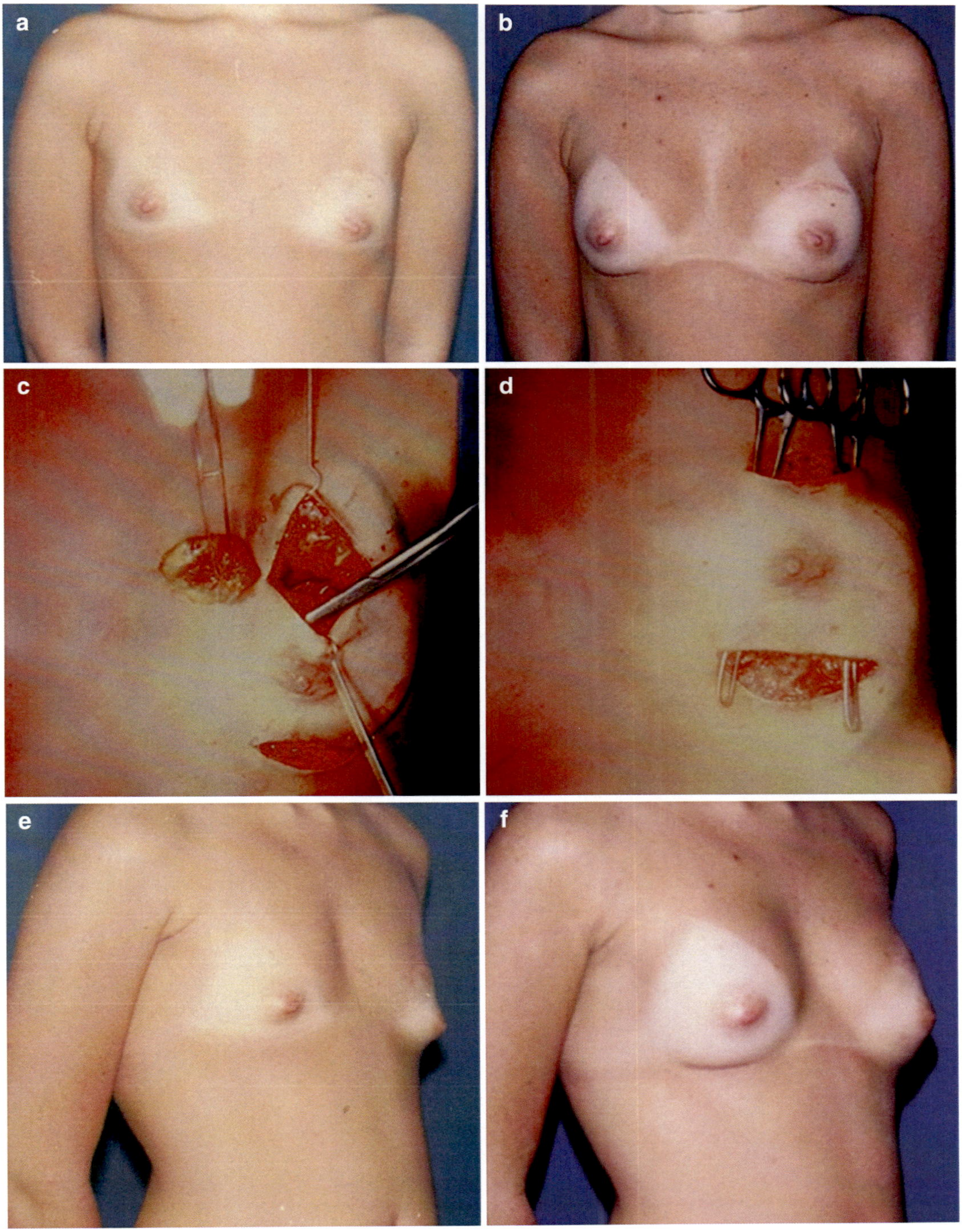

Fig. 43.7 Bilateral hypomastia with congenital ptotic breast on the left side. (**a**) Preoperative photo of a 17-year-old girl with a surgical scar above the nipple–areolar complex (NAC) on the left side due to a previous operation performed elsewhere as an attempt at correction of asymmetry. (**b**) After implantation of a 180-mL prosthesis with elevation of the left breast through the same scar. (**c**) Peroperative photo showing resection of a segment of skin and adipose tissue to lift the nipple on the left side. (**d**) After dissection of the panniculus with two forceps passing from top to bottom on the future submammary fold. (**e**) Preoperative photo oblique view on the right side showing the asymmetry of the nipple–areola regions. (**f**) After prosthesis implantation with correction of the ptotic NAC on the left side

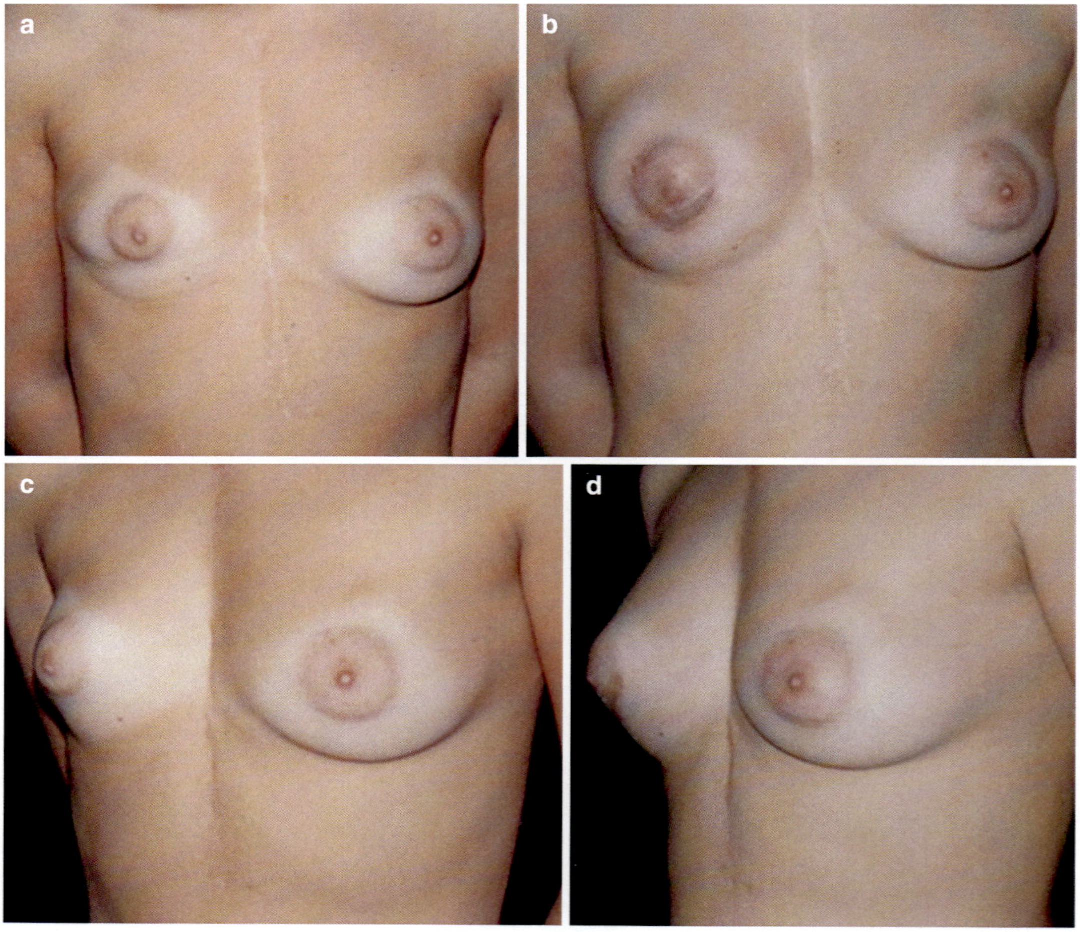

Fig. 43.8 Asymmetrical breasts: hypomastia on the right side with congenital abnormal breast development with a constricted breast, and a normal size on the left side. (**a**) Before surgery frontal view. (**b**) After implantation of a 180-mL prosthesis on the right side. (**c**) Before surgery left view. (**d**) After surgery

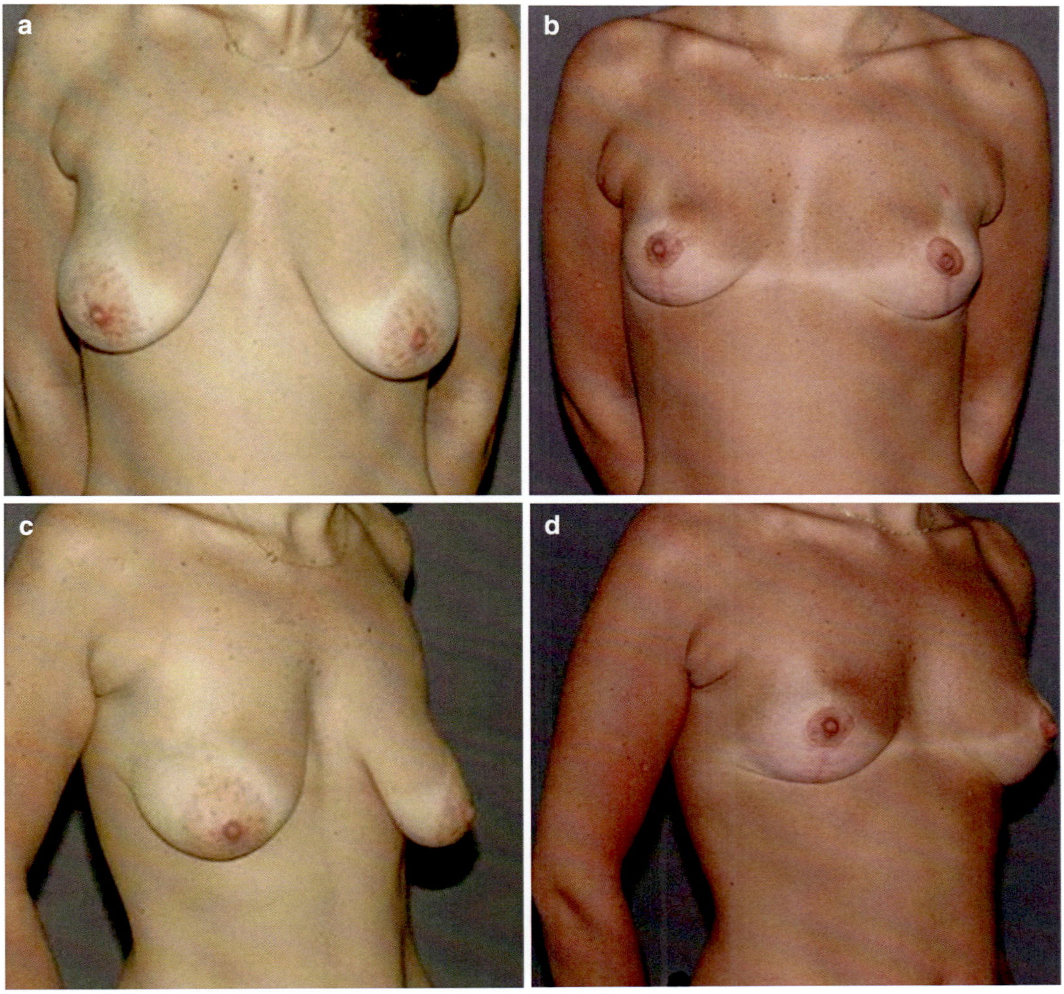

Fig. 43.9 Asymmetrical breasts with severe bilateral ptosis and flaccidity. (**a**, **c**) Before surgery. (**b**, **d**) After bilateral mastopexy with removal of 90 mg from the right side and 150 mg from the left side

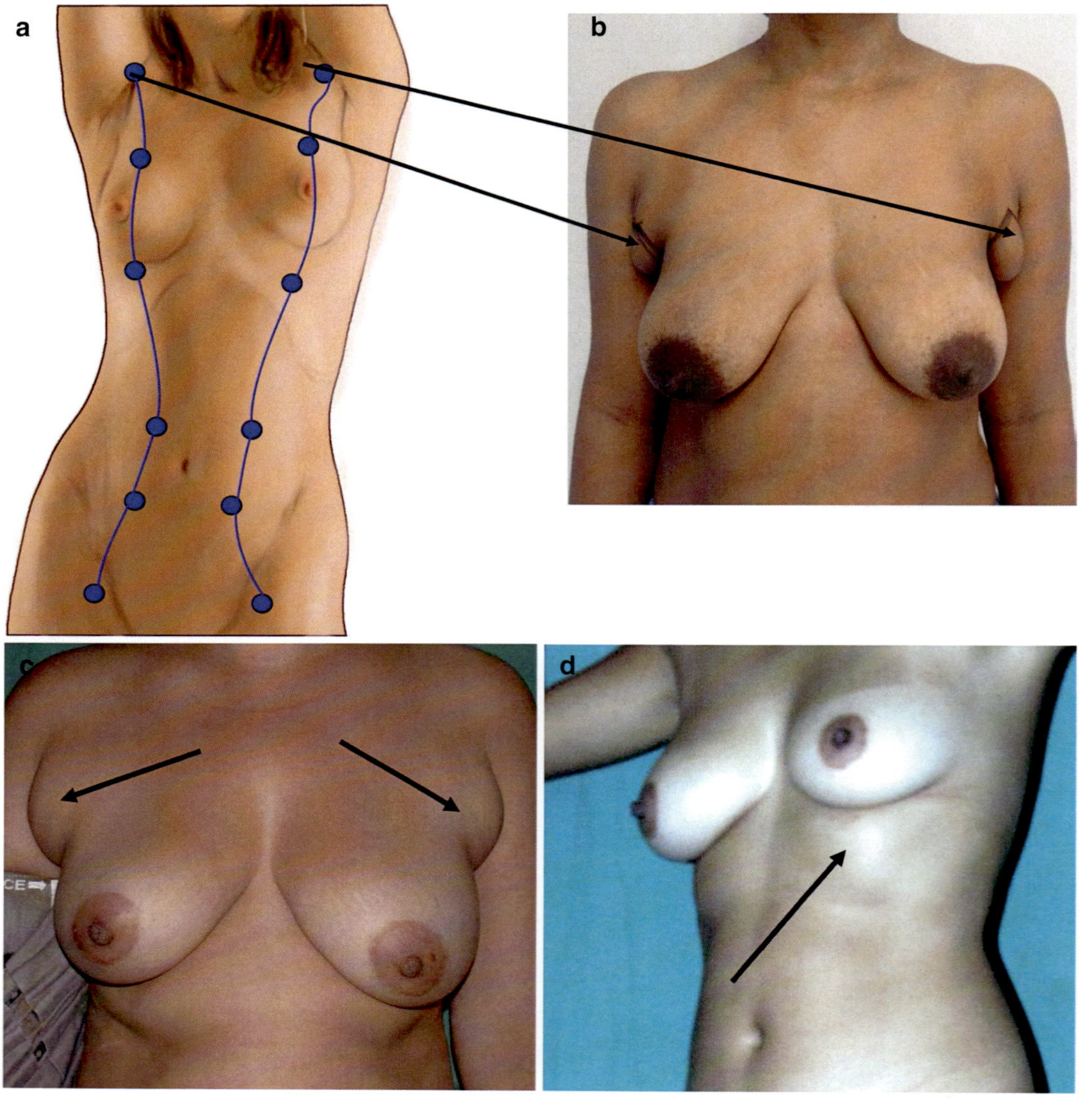

Fig. 43.10 Polymastia. (**a**) Diagram to demonstrate the location of the milk line where polymastia and polythelia may appear in women and men. (**b**) A patient presenting bilateral axillary polymastia. This photo is Dr Ricardo Cavalcanti's patient. Reproduced with kind permission

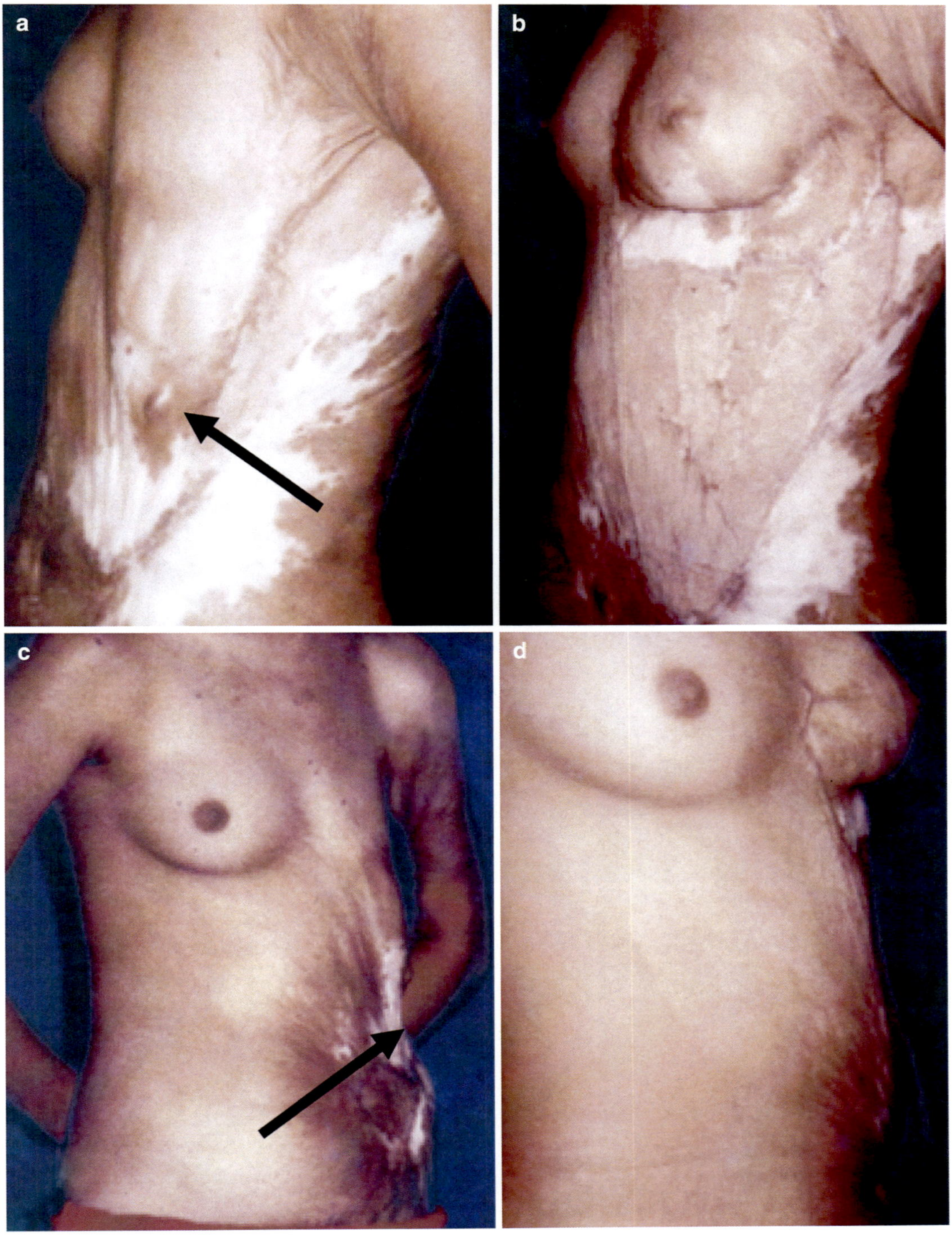

Fig. 43.11 Severely asymmetrical breast caused by burns. (**a**, **c**) A 17-year-old girl presenting complex and unaesthetic deformities of the left breast with retraction by scar tissue formation after burns. The *arrows* indicate the position of the NAC on the abdominal wall. (**b**, **d**) The final result after skin graft on the abdominal wall and remodeling of the breast by advancement of a cutaneous flap with repositioning of the NAC

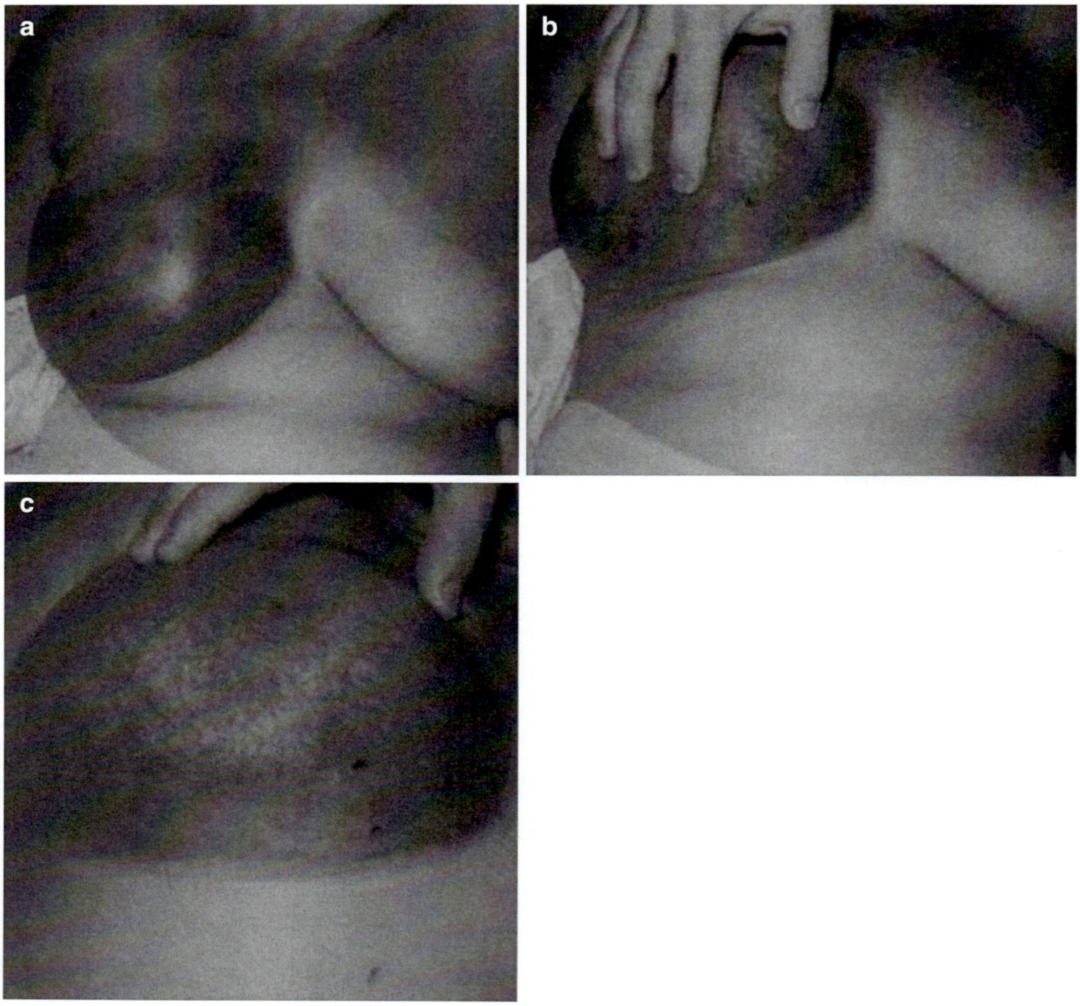

Fig. 43.12 Traumatic asymmetrical breast caused by severe hematoma formation due to a human bite on the right breast. (**a**) Front view with arms up showing a large hematoma on the right breast. (**b**) The breast is pulled up showing the limit of the hematoma on the submammary fold. (**c**) Close-up showing the breast with the nipple–areola region

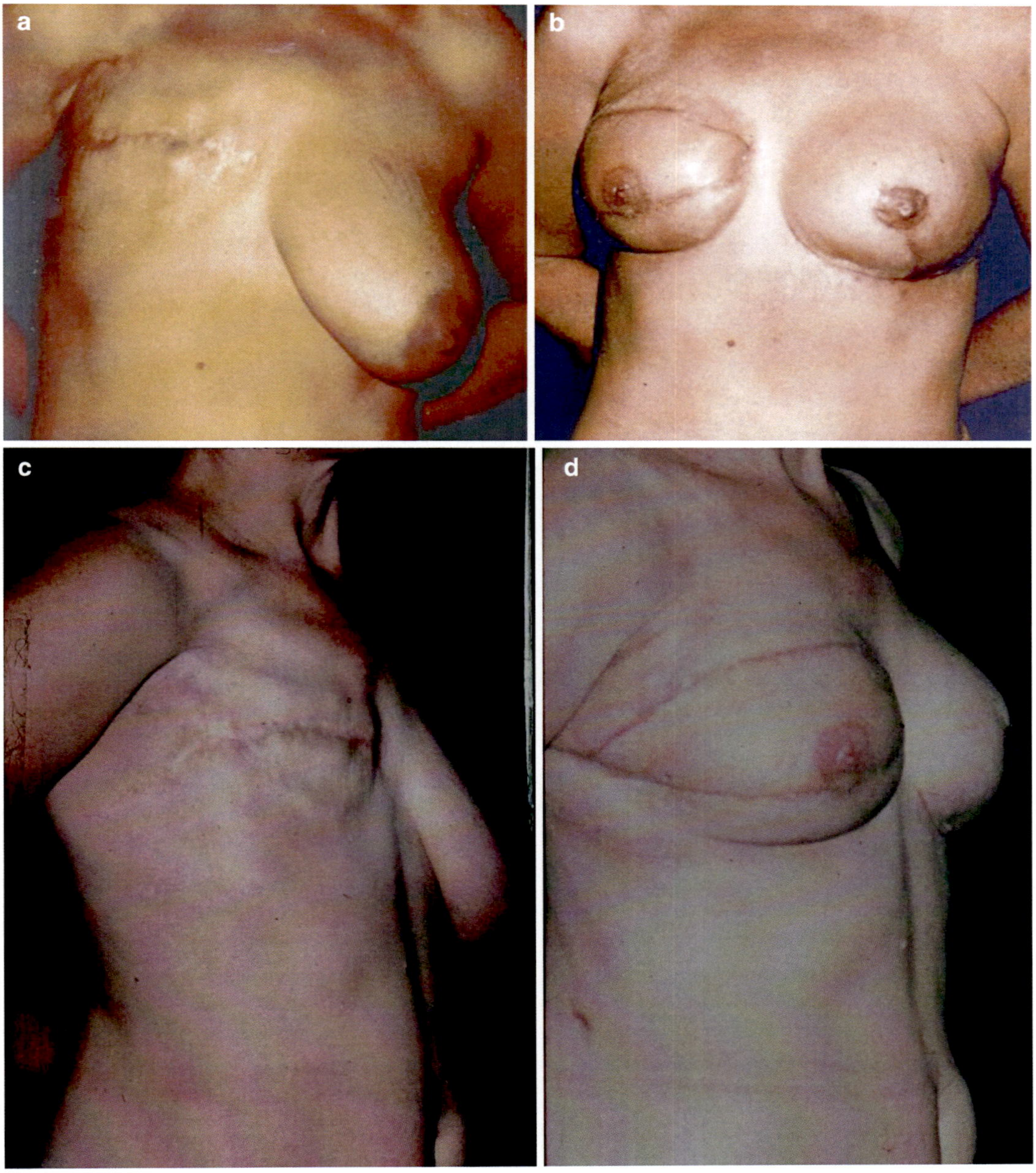

Fig. 43.13 A 54-year-old woman showing asymmetrical breasts due to radical mastectomy on the right side. (**a**) Frontal view showing the imbalance of the chest. (**b**) The same patient after reconstructions of the right breast with rotation of the latissimus dorsi muscle combined with silicone prosthesis implantation and reduction mastoplasty, with removal of 350 g from the left side. (**c**) Right side view before surgery. (**d**) After reconstruction of the right breast and reduction mastoplasty on the left side

43.3 Method

Aesthetic surgery for repair of asymmetrical breasts is even more complex than aesthetic mastoplasty, as it is mandatory to achieve a good balance between the two breasts.

43.3.1 Surgical Planning

I learned from Prof Pitanguy et al. (1973, 1977) that surgical planning is a basic step before performing any plastic surgery. However, when a patient presents with evident asymmetry between the two breasts, surgical planning is even more important, as sometimes two opposing operations must be performed. If one breast presents hypertrophy on one side and hypomastia on the other, we are obliged to plan reduction mastoplasty on one breast and augmentation mastoplasty using a silicone implant on the other. Nevertheless, quite often, surgical planning is much more complex, as bilateral hypertrophic breasts with severe asymmetry may involve a wide variety of deformities that require specific procedures to achieve aesthetic bilateral harmony.

43.4 Surgical Marking: Pre-Marking

It is my routine to carry out pre-marking at my clinic one day before the operation. I have found this useful, as it is another opportunity to see my patient once more to observe her abnormalities and to make some temporary marks on her breast and chest. Also, blood tests, clinical evaluation, and other pre-operative examinations required during the consultation can be carried out. At this time, some reference points are drawn on both breasts. In the case of mammary hypertrophy on one side, it is mandatory to landmark the reference points for reduction mastoplasty. According to the abnormality on the opposite breast adequate pre-markings are made.

The next day, when the patient is in operating room, the final surgical markings are made according to the deformity of both breasts.

43.5 Surgical Treatment

The correction of deformities of the breast requires surgery after proper clinical evaluation and meticulous surgical planning and marking as well. It is not the purpose of this chapter to describe the surgical techniques, as they are presented in detail in other chapters of this book. The reader can find descriptions that contain the approaches according to the deformity of the breasts to achieve harmony between them and the chest.

Asymmetry with breast hypertrophy on both sides requires bilateral reduction mastoplasty (Fig. 43.1). When a patient presents hypertrophy of only one breast, unilateral reduction mastoplasty is performed (Fig. 43.2). However, the most complex deformities are when patients present hypomastia of one breast and hypertrophy of the other. The surgical planning must be carried out with reduction mammaplasty on one side and breast augmentation on the opposite breast (Figs. 43.3 and 43.4). Both patients said that since the age of 10 years they had had hyperdevelopment of the breast on one side and underdevelopment of the other breast. The main purpose of operation is to correct the severe imbalance of the body contour, which can bring severe physical and psychological repercussions.

So far, some patients may present hypertrophy with ptosis of one breast and ptosis of the other breast (Figs. 43.5 and 43.6). Nevertheless, the asymmetry is even more complex when patients present bilateral hypomastia with congenital deformity of one breast, which requires breast augmentation combined with repair of the ptosis of the NAC (Fig. 43.7). Even, when a patient presents hypomastia on only one side, it is mandatory to perform unilateral augmentation mastoplasty with a silicone implant (Fig. 43.8).

The most frequent asymmetry of the breasts is ptosis associated with flaccidity, which requires bilateral mastopexy with removal of some of the mammary tissue to achieve a good balance of the two breasts (Fig. 43.9).

There are other congenital deformities that become evident only during puberty, when the breasts start to develop, as may occur when patients present polymastia or polythelia (Fig. 43.10). Patients complain about these abnormalities, but usually they are not aware of them unless they present monthly alterations related to menstruation.

Acquired asymmetry of the breasts is a special field in which patients with normal organs may damage them by several causes bringing imbalance to the body contour with physical and psychological repercussions. Deformities of the breast caused by burns to the chest are very common, when accidents occur in infancy or during adolescence. As the mammary glands originate and develop from the dermis they may be damaged when the trauma occurs to the chest wall. So far, it is advisable to be very careful when a child presents with burns on chest near the NAC. During puberty, when physical development includes significant alterations, the growing breast may show some asymmetry, which requires repair or reconstruction (Fig. 43.11). As I have many patients with ear deformities caused by burns, quite often some women present with associated abnormalities of the breasts. Other traumas may also damage the breast partially or totally. Human or animal bites are quite unusual causes, but when they occur, they may bring severe consequences (Fig. 43.12).

Nowadays, breast cancer is a great problem, which is more and more frequent. When unilateral or bilateral mastectomy is performed severe deformities can occur, which is a very wide field. Neither the pathological conditions nor the treatment are not with the scope of this chapter, but Fig. 43.12demonstrates the imbalance of the body contour caused by mastectomy. Therefore, in this chapter the problem is limited to including an example of the cause of asymmetrical breasts.

43.6 Discussion

The breasts are very important organs in women's intimate sphere and they have an even greater emphasis in adolescence when young girls begin a new part of their lives. The theme "breast asymmetry" has the greatest importance in the study of the pathological conditions of aesthetic breast surgery. Although it is recommended to delay surgical treatment until after puberty, quite often the problem originated at birth or during childhood (Figs. 43.3, 43.4, 43.7, and 43.8). The asymmetry does not only concern the volume of the mammary gland, but also the skin structures and nipple–areola regions. A broad classification of breast deformities is presented, addressing the diverse pathological conditions, emphasizing the appropriate age for surgery. Each patient must be treated according to the particular deformity of each breast. For this reason, clinical evaluation and surgical planning are very important steps to carry out before the operation.

Although breast asymmetry is not frequently described in the literature, but it represents a severe problem for patients. Most patients looking for a mastoplasty procedure present with some sort of asymmetry of the breasts, which may be solved during surgery. Maybe they do not complain about it before mastoplasty, but any asymmetry after the operation may cause dissatisfaction. For this reason, adequate evaluation is very important during consultation when surgery is planned, and during surgical marking.

43.7 Complications

As the operation is performed to repair asymmetrical breasts, the most feared complication is not achieving perfect bilateral harmony between the two sides because of the anatomical mammary structures of each breast. When the operation performed on one side is a reduction mastoplasty and on the other it is silicone prosthesis implantation, it is quite difficult to achieve a high level of bilateral symmetry. Even when mastopexy is performed on both sides, when patients have asymmetry, it is a constant challenge to achieve perfect symmetry.

As I have many patients with several kinds of asymmetry, it is mandatory to inform to each patient with regard to the limits of the operation and be specific in the written informed consent.

Conclusions

From birth until puberty the breasts are latent. From this period on, female breasts are an important symbol of femininity and they represent significant expression, not only in the physical aspects, but also from a psychological point of view, body contouring, and in the sexual sphere. When a young girl presents with asymmetric nipples or breasts, it is necessary to inform the mother about the indication for surgical correction. Each deformity may be treated according to the specific problem. The most frequent abnormality is bilateral hypertrophy with asymmetry. Therefore, surgical planning and surgical marking are essential to achieving good results with a good balance between the two breasts.

References

Avelar JM (1989) Breast asymmetry (Assimetria mamária). In: Avelar JM (ed) Plastic surgery in infancy (Cirurgia Plástica na Infância), vol 2. São Paulo, Editora Hipocrates, pp 413–418

Avelar JM (1993) Reduction mastoplasty under local anesthesia (Mastoplastia redutora sob anestesia local). In: Avelar JM (ed) Loco-regional anesthesia on aesthetic surgery—(Anestesia Loco-regional em cirurgia estética), vol 29. São Paulo, Editora Hipócrates, pp 244–260

Broadbent TR, Woolf RM (1978) Unsatisfactory results in augmentation mammaplasty—chest and breast asymmetry. Aesth Plast Surg 2(3):251–269. http://link.springer.com/article/10.1007/BF01577958

Karim KE-L, Ashraf Maher F, Ahmed Mabrouk AW, Abd-Al-Aziz Hanafy A-A-A (2009) A management-based classification for breast asymmetries. Egypt J Plast Reconstr Surg 33(1):95–100. http://www.esprs.org/Content/Journals/331_16.pdf

Jales RM (2004) Anatomia ultrassonográfica da mama. Faculdade de ciências médicas. http://www.fcm.unicamp.br/drpixel/pt-br/metodos-de-imagem/anatomia-ultrassonogr%C3%A1fica-da-mama

Juri J (1989) Mammary asymmetry: A brief classification. Buenos Aries Argentina. Aesthet Plast Surg 13(1):47–53. http://link.springer.com/article/10.1007/BF01570325#page-1

Maliniac JW (1950) Asymmetrical breast deformities. Am Surg 1934:734

Pitanguy I, Carreirão SE, Garcia LC (1973) Amastia unilateral. Rev Bras Cir 63(3/4):85–89

Pitanguy I, Viana GP, Daher M, Batti RB (1977) Mama extranumerária. Rev Bras Cir 67(7/8):273–278

Sepúlveda A (1981) Breast asymmetry—surgical treatment (Tratamento das assimetrias mamarias). Rev Bras Cir 71(1):11–18

44 Poland's Syndrome

Ricardo Cavalcanti Ribeiro,
Johana Buitrago Valderrama,
and Maria Gabriela Moreira Mangles

44.1 Introduction

In the nineteenth century, Poland (1841) published the first description of a congenital deficiency of the pectoralis major muscle (PMM) associated with brachysyndactyly Poland (1841). Later, Clarkson (1962) used the term Poland's syndactyly Clarkson (1962) and Baudinne et al. (1967) finally branded it Poland's syndrome Baudinne et al. (1967). Poland syndrome's is a sporadic, congenital, unilateral absence of the sternocostal head of the PMM that can occur with other ipsilateral chest wall and limb derangements. The deformity can also be complex with an ipsilateral absence of the ribs, axillary webbing, and foreshortening of the hemithorax Cooper and Johnson (1990).

Head of Division of Plastic and Reconstructive Surgery of Universidade Federal do Estado of the Rio de Janeiro (UNIRIO)

R.C. Ribeiro, M.D. Ph.D. (✉)
Brazilian Society of Plastic Surgery,
São Paula, SP, Brazil

Carlos Chagas Institute, Rio de Janeiro, PR, Brazil
e-mail: rribeiro@centroin.com.br

J.B. Valderrama, M.D.
Division of Plastic and Reconstructive Surgery of Casa de Portugal, Rio de Janeiro, RJ, Brazil

M.G. Moreira Mangles, M.D.
Division of Plastic and Reconstructive Surgery of Centro Policlinico Valencia, Valencia, Venezuela
e-mail: gabbymangles@gmail.com

Several studies have suggested a genetic factor or, even more likely, extrinsic factors between the sixth and the eighth week of pregnancy, may interfere with PMM migration and the separation of the digits that occurs during this period. The recent vascular hypothesis for the etiology of the Poland sequence implies that hypoplasia of the ipsilateral subclavian artery might be the origin of this birth anomaly Fedorov and Rozanova (2002) and Mace et al. (1972).

44.2 Discussion

44.2.1 Main Alterations Associated with Poland's Syndrome

- *Muscles*: the absence of the pectoralis minor muscle, absence of the clavicular and sternal segments of the PMM, hypoplasia of the serratus anterior, latissimus dorsi, deltoid, and infra- and supraspinatus muscles Psillakis and Altmann (1987).
- *Mammary glands*: areolar abnormalities, mammary absence or hypoplasia Hedge and Shokeir (1982), Goldberg and Mazzei (1977).
- *Thorax*: pulmonary herniation, hypoplasia of the ribs or deformities of the he Mace et al. (1972) mithorax depending on severity Hurwitz et al. (1994).
- *Ipsilateral superior limb*: skeletal hypoplasia affecting the hands Datta and Kingston (1994), forearms, upper arms and scapula; syndactyly, symbrachydactyly, polydactyly, brachysyndactyly, and axillary constrictions Mace et al. (1972).

J.M. Avelar (ed.), *Breast Surgery*, https://doi.org/10.1007/978-3-319-54115-0_44

Other abnormalities have been related to Poland's syndrome, these include dextrocardia, kidney hypoplasia Hedge and Shokeir (1982) and Shamberger et al. (1989), neurofibromatosis Alembik and Stoll (1994), myasthenia gravis, peroneal atrophy, microcephaly, craniofacial dysplasia, and Möbius syndrome Fedorov and Rozanova (2002) and Psillakis and Altmann (1987). There have also been reports of associated coagulation disturbances, psoriasis, systemic lupus erythematosus, Baselow–Graves' disease Reardon et al. (1990) and Ramos Niembro and Lom (1996), leukemia, and non-Hodgkin's lymphoma. Not all of these components are necessarily present, but the full syndrome consists of an assortment of these abnormalities David and Winter (1985).

44.2.2 Types of Poland's Syndrome

There are two major variations of Poland's syndrome: the simple (mild) form and the complex (severe) form. The type is based on the anatomy of the chest wall, because the severity of the hand deformity did not correlate directly with that of the chest wall Cavalcanti et al. (2007).

44.3 Simple Form

This most common form is characterized by the absence of the large, fan-shaped sternocostal head of the PMM. This renders the ipsilateral axillary fold deficient, a cosmetic feature that is usually mentioned by the patient. The clavicular head is present as a thin triangular bundle that attaches the humerus to the inferomedial third of the clavicle. Although the ribs and other musculoskeletal components also seem to be present, the breast and nipple–areola complex (NAC) are smaller and displaced somewhat toward the axilla. Because the pectoralis minor cannot be reliably tested, its presence cannot ordinarily be confirmed by physical examination. However, if the lengths of the clavicle, humerus, ulna, and phalanges are measured, they are usually found to be smaller on the affected side (Fig. 44.1).

44.4 Complex Form

The complex form, as in Poland's subject, is characterized by the absence of the sternocostal head of the PMM; rib and sternal aberrations; muscular displacements; and often a relatively severe brachysyndactyly. The clavicular head may be diminutive and the entire ipsilateral hemithorax and upper extremity components are notably smaller, even without measurement. An axillary web may be seen and seems to contain muscle tissue because some patients (or electrocautery during surgery) can cause it to contract. The serratus anterior may be absent, causing a winged scapula, even if the latissimus muscle is present. Other muscles may be deficient or displaced, as noted by Poland. The sternal body (gladiolus) and xiphoid process may be short and bifid, and the sternocostal cartilages on the affected side may be rotated and coalesced into a vertical bar. The insertion of the ipsilateral rectus abdominis muscle may be high, as if drawn up by

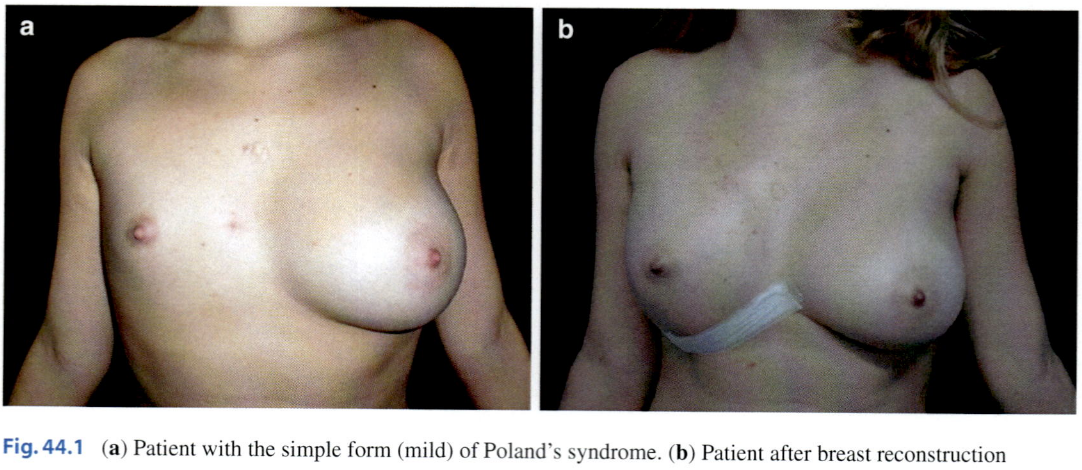

Fig. 44.1 (**a**) Patient with the simple form (mild) of Poland's syndrome. (**b**) Patient after breast reconstruction

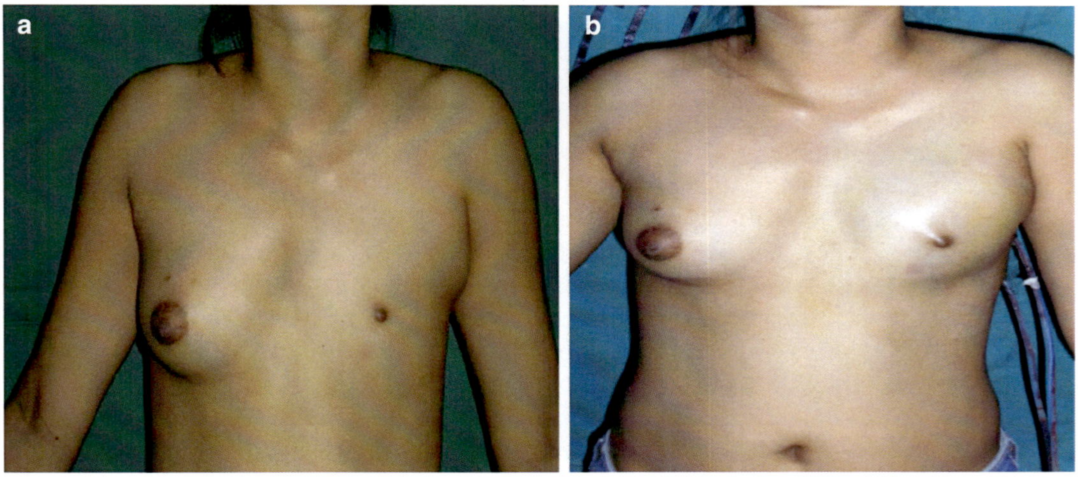

Fig. 44.2 (**a**) Patient with complex (severe) form of Poland's syndrome. (**b**) Patient after breast reconstruction

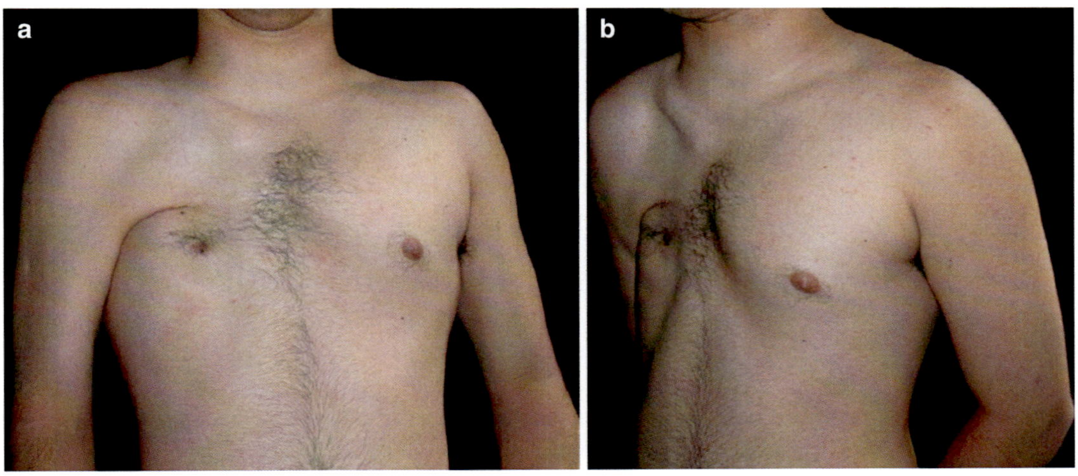

Fig. 44.3 Patient with complex (severe) form of Poland's syndrome

the shortened sternum and ribs; the clavicle is short; and the scapula is small, rotated, and resides higher than on the affected side. The anterior bodies of ribs 2–5 are thin and short, and their cartilages are often missing superolaterally. The latter are replaced by a tough pleurofascial membrane that can be seen to move with respiration (Figs. 44.2 and 44.3).

44.5 Radiological Staging

Imaging techniques play a fundamental role in the detection, location, and characterization of chest wall disorders, many of which have characteristic radiological appearances that allow definitive diagnosis. Sternal deformities can be visualized with X-rays and their severity quantified using computed tomography (CT) scans Jeung et al. (1999), which clearly show many abnormalities Wright et al. (1992). For chest wall disorders, the chest X-ray remains the basic imaging study for evaluating pathological conditions. Chest X-rays generally show hyperlucency on the affected side that mimics a radical mastectomy Hurwitz et al. (1994) and Wright et al. (1992). A mammogram is useful in showing breast asymmetry or the absence of the PMM. Poland's syndrome has been diagnosed in 1 out of 19,000 mammograms

Fokin and Robicsek (2002), according to Perez Aznar et al. (1996) failure to show the PMM on a mammogram is most often due to errors in positioning. Ultrasound also plays a complementary role in diagnosing thoracic pathological conditions Perez Aznar et al. (1996).

The advent of cross-sectional imaging techniques such as CT and magnetic resonance imaging (MRI) has enabled the precise localization of chest wall lesions and, in some cases, definitive diagnoses Jeung et al (1999). MRI shows better tissue contrast, but is less useful than CT in the study of pathological bone conditions. CT also depicts more clearly the absence of the PMM and allows better appreciation of nearby associated musculoskeletal anomalies, such as mediastinal widening Cavalcanti et al. (2007). CT and MRI together define, with precision, the muscular abnormalities, making these tools useful in the presurgical period. Hurwitz et al. (1994) justify the use of three-dimensional (3D) CT, among available imaging studies, for the planning of surgical procedures to ensure the best possible reconstruction Hurwitz et al. (1994). This imaging technique can offer an accurate representation of tissue deficits and asymmetry, thus helping in decisions regarding the transposition of muscular flaps and reconstructive techniques Reardon et al. (1990).

- *First degree (mild type)*: mammary asymmetry due to hypomastia or amastia and areolar asymmetry with or without partial absence of the PMM; no other musculoskeletal alterations are observed; other congenital alterations may or may not be present.
- *Second degree (severe type)*: hypomastia or amastia, areolar asymmetry, total absence of the PMM, and alterations of the ipsilateral muscle group and/or bones of the chest; ipsilateral superior limb alteration and other congenital alterations may or may not be present.
- *Third degree (extremely severe type)*: amastia, areolar asymmetry, major ipsilateral musculoskeletal chest alterations such as total absence of the PMM, the pectoralis minor muscle, the serratus anterior muscle; possible lung herniation; widened opening of the mediastinum; ipsilateral superior limb alteration; other congenital alterations may or may not be present Cavalcanti et al. (2009).

44.5.1 Surgical Technique

An algorithm for the planning of the surgical treatment is proposed based on the clinical and radiographic Poland's syndrome (CRPS) classification Cavalcanti et al. (2009). Corrections may include breast implants, customized breast implants, tissue expanders, local flaps, latissimus dorsi flaps, the Ravitch procedure, and contralateral symmetrization procedures such as mammary reductions or augmentations. Patients with second- and third-degree Poland's syndrome should be treated by a multidisciplinary team involving thoracic and orthopedic specialists (Table 44.1).

Table 44.1 Clinical and radiographic Poland's syndrome classification

Degree of presentation	Mammary alterations	Musculoskeletal chest alterations	Ipsilateral superior limb alterations	Other congenital alterations
First degree (mild type)	Amastia	None or partial	None	May be present
	Hypomastia or	Absence of pectoralis		
	areolar asymmetry	major muscle		
Second degree (severe type)	Hypomastia or amastia	Total absence of pectoralis major	No or small alterations	May be present
	Areolar asymmetry	Different alterations of the muscles and/or bones of the ipsilateral chest		
Third degree (extremely severe type)	Amastia	Different manifestations	Present	May be present
	Areolar asymmetry			

Table 44.2 Suggested surgical approach for each degree of presentation in the clinical and radiographic Poland's syndrome classification

Degree of presentation	Suggested surgical approach
First	• Breast implant
	• Contralateral mammary reduction or augmentation (symmetrization procedure when needed)
Second	• Tissue expander
	• Regional local flap
	• Breast implants or customized breast implant
	• Symmetrization procedure
Third	• Tissue expander
	• Customized breast implant when needed
	• Breast implants
	• Latissimus dorsi flap or another flap, such as the TRAM flap or free flap
	• Symmetrization procedure

TRAM transverse rectus abdominis myocutaneous

- *First degree (mild type)*: breast implants or customized breast implants and contralateral mammary reduction or augmentation when needed (symmetrization procedure).
- *Second degree (severe type)*: tissue expander when needed; regional local flap; breast implants or customized breast implants; and symmetrization procedure.
- *Third degree (extremely severe type)*: tissue expander; latissimus dorsi flap, or other flap such as a free flap or transverse rectus abdominis myocutaneous flap; breast implants or customized breast implants as needed; or other surgeries such as the Ravitch procedure and contralateral symmetrization procedure (Table 44.2.) Cavalcanti et al. (2009).

References

Alembik Y, Stoll C (1994) A boy with neurofibromatosis 1 and Poland anomaly. *Genet Couns* 5:167–170.

Baudinne P, Bovy GL, Wasterlain A (1967) A case of Poland's syndrome (in French). Acta Paediatr Belg 32:407–410

Bouwes Bavinck JN, Waver DD (1986) Subclavian artery supply disruption sequence. Hypothesis of a vascular etiology for Poland, Klippel-Feil and Möbius anomalies. Am J Med Genet 29:903–906

Cavalcanti Ribeiro R, Novaes W, España Quintero L, Moreira Mangles MG, Ibañez O'Kamell A, Quintella Gurgel G (2007) Mediastinal alterations in patients with Poland's 17 syndrome. Annals of 14th International Congress of International Confederation for Plastic, Reconstructive and Aesthetic Surgery, P/REC 57, June. Berlin, in German

Cavalcanti Ribeiro R, Saltz R, Moreira Mangles MG, Koch H. (2009) Clinical and Radiographic Poland Syndrome Classification: A proposal. Aesthetic surgery journal / the American Society for Aesthetic Plastic surgery 29(6):494–504.

Clarkson JH, Harley OJ, Kirkpatrick JJ (2006) Alfred Poland's syndrome: a tidy little controversy. J Plast Reconstr Aesthet Surg;59:1006–1008.

Clarkson P (1962) Poland's syndactyly. Guys Hosp Rep 111:335–346

Cooper RA, Johnson MS (1990) Mammographic depiction of Poland's syndrome. Br J Radiol. 63:302–303.

Datta D, Kingston E (1994) Myoelectric prostheses in management of Poland's Syndrome. Report of two cases. J Hand Surg Br;19B(5):659–61

David TJ, Winter RM (1985) Familial absence of the pectoralis major, serratus anterior, and latissimus dorsi muscles. J Med Genet;22:390–2.

Fedorov L, Rozanova LS (2002) State of the hemostasis system in Poland's syndrome. Vestn Khir Im I I Grek 161(4):29–32

Fokin AA, Robicsek F (2002) Poland's syndrome revisited. Ann Thorac Surg 74:2218–2225

Fraser FC, Ronen GM, O'Leary E (1989) Pectoralis major defect and Poland sequence in second cousins: extension of the Poland sequence spectrum. Am J Med Genet 33:468–470

Froriep R (1839) Observation of a case of absence of the breast (in German). Notizen aus dem Gebiete der Natur- und Heilkunde 10:9–14

Fryns JP, de Smet L (1994) On association of Poland anomaly and primary microcephaly. Clin Dysmorphol 3:347–350

Goldberg M, Mazzei R (1977) Poland syndrome: a concept of pathogenesis based on limb bud embryology. Birth Defects 13:103–115

Hedge HR, Shokeir MHK (1982) Posterior shoulder girdle abnormalities with absence of pectoralis major muscle. Am J Med Genet 13:285–293

Hurwitz DJ, Stofman G, Curtin H (1994) Three-dimensional imaging of Poland's syndrome. Plast Recontr Surg 94:719–723

Jeung MY, Gangi A, Gasser B et al (1999) Imaging of chest wall disorders. RadioGraphics 19:617–637

Mace JW, Kaplan JM, Schanberger JE, Gotlin RW (1972) Poland's syndrome: report of seven cases and review of the literature. Clin Pediatr 11:98–100

Mathes SJ, Seyfer AE, Miranda EP (2006) Congenital anomalies of the chest wall. In: Mathes SJ, Hentz VR, eds. Plastic surgery. vol 6, Trunk and lower extremities. Philadelphia: Saunders Elsevier;485–509.

Merlob P, Schonfeld A, Ovadia Y, Reisner SH (1989) Real-time echo-doppler scanner in the evaluation of patients with Poland sequence. Eur J Obstet Gynecol Reprod Biol 32:103

Perez Aznar JM, Urbano J, Garcia Laborda E, Quevedo Moreno P, Ferrer Vergara L (1996) Breast and pectoralis muscle hypoplasia. A mild degree of Poland's syndrome. Acta Radiol 37(5):759–762

Poland A (1841) Deficiency of the pectoral muscles. Guys Hosp Rep 6:191–193

Power D (1930) Alfred Poland (1822–1872). In: Power D (ed) Pharr's lives of the Fellows of the Royal College of Surgeons of England, vol II. John Wright, Bristol, p 184

Psillakis JM, Altmann EB (1987) Cirurgia craniomaxilofacial: osteotomias estéticas da face. Rio de Janeiro: Medsi, pp 317–23.

Ramos Niembro F, Lom OH (1996) Síndrome de Poland y autoinmunidad. Rev Mex Reumatol 11(3):92–96

Reardon W, Temple IK, Jones B et al (1990) Frontonasal dyplasia or craniofrontonasal dyplasia and the Poland anomaly? Clin Gen 38:233–236

Shamberger RC, Welch KJ, Upton J (1989) Surgical treatment of thoracic deformity in Poland's syndrome. J Pediatr Surg 24:760–765

Smith DW (1982) Recognizable patterns of human malformations. Genetic, embryologic and clinical aspects. WB Saunders, Philadelphia

Wright AR, Milner L, Bainbridge C, Wilsdon J (1992) MR and CT in the assessment of Poland syndrome. J Comput Assist Tomogr 16(3):442–447

45 Asymmetrical Breasts Associated with Chest Deformities

Juarez M. Avelar

45.1 Introduction

In addition to breast-feeding, the breasts are important organs for body contouring in women. Abnormalities of the breast, especially in combination with chest deformities, modify the body's silhouette, causing disharmony and imbalance of the image.

Although in males the breasts are not developed, I have several male patients with congenital abnormalities presenting chest deformities that cause complex unaesthetic imbalance and asymmetry of the body contours (Fig. 45.1).

To discuss this theme in this book is of enormous significance because of the interconnection

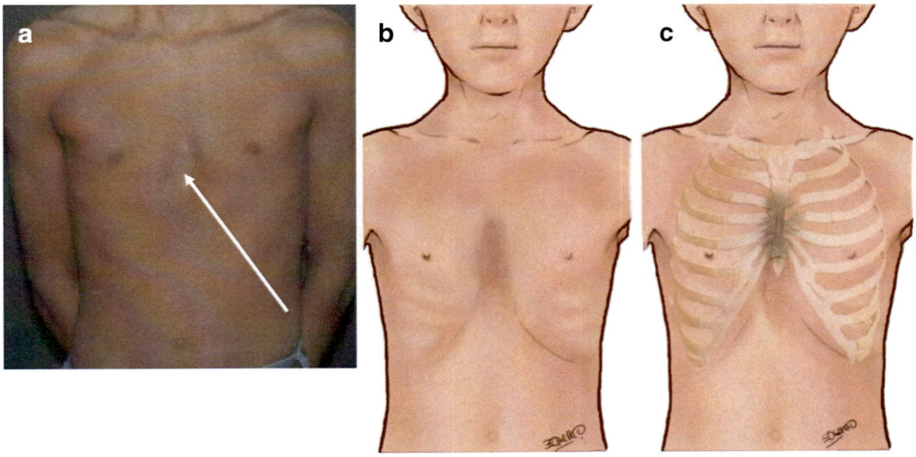

Fig. 45.1 Pectus excavatum. (**a**) A 7-year-old boy with congenital depression in the sternal region. (**b**, **c**) Drawings show the chest deformity in the sternal region

J.M. Avelar
Brazilian Scientific Institute of Plastic and Reconstructive Surgery, Alameda Gabriel Monteiro da Silva, São Paulo, SP 01442000, Brazil
e-mail: juarezavelar@bol.com.br; institutodaorelha@uol.com.br; clinica-avelar@uol.com.br

J.M. Avelar (ed.), *Breast Surgery*, https://doi.org/10.1007/978-3-319-54115-0_45

with various medical specialties and other areas of human knowledge.

Any deformity or even absence of the breasts from the female body have tremendous repercussions for the well-being of women, which require more attention and especially a harder search for a surgical solution in adulthood or adolescence. However, the problem is beginning to arouse interest and concern before puberty owing to disharmony of the body. Asymmetries with concomitant hypertrophy focus on women aged upward from childhood and puberty. In contrast, many congenital diseases confer an unaesthetic imbalance to the anterior chest wall, causing serious disorder in the intimate well-being of women and men as well.

45.2 Classification

As I used to have a large number of patients presenting complex deformities of the chest associated with abnormalities of the breasts and auricles, my previous classification was published (Avelar 1989). Nowadays, as there are more deformities of the chest among my patients, it is useful to include some other abnormalities in my previous classification so as to propose adequate surgical treatment. There are other classifications proposed by other authors with useful information concerning surgical repair (Coelho et al. 1988; Cavalcanti Ribeiro et al. 2007; De Souza Pinto et al. 1997). It is useful to mention the classification suggested by Cavalcanti Ribeiro et al. (2007) in three degrees for carrying out surgical planning.

Deformities of the chest may be classified into two major groups, acquired and congenital:

I. Acquired
   Traumatic
   Burns
   Iatrogenic (Ayer 1981)
   a. Post-cancer surgery
I. Acquired deformities of the chest are important topics, but are not described in this chapter
II. Congenital
   A. Deformities of the chest
      a. Pectus carinatum (Coelho et al. 2003)
         a1. Pectus carinatum superior
         a2. Pectus carinatum inferior (chicken breast, pigeon breast)
         a3. Pectus carinatum lateral
      b. Pectus excavatum
         b1. Chest deformities associated with breast abnormalities (Fig. 45.2)

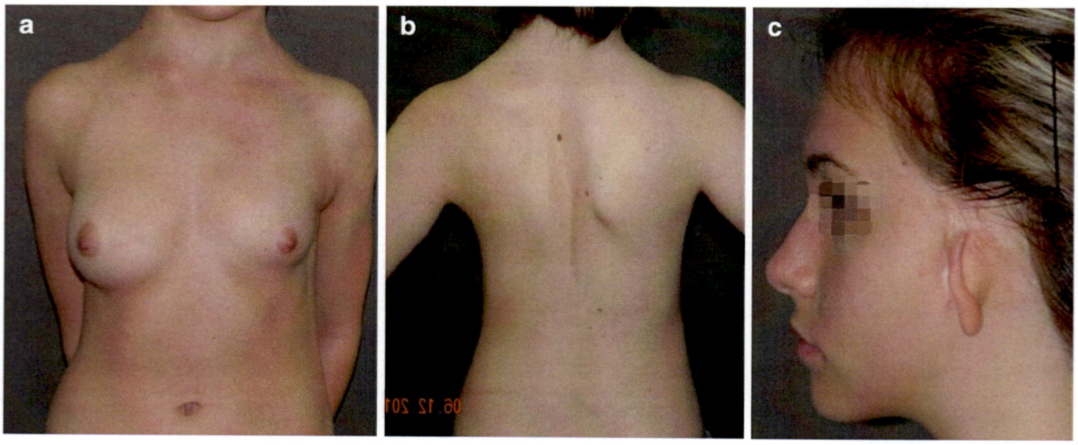

Fig. 45.2 A 17-year-old female patient with dysgenesis of the ear presenting asymmetrical breast and chest in addition to congenital torticollis. (**a**) Frontal view. (**b**) Back view, deviation of the column with asymmetry can be seen. (**c**) Lateral view of the face on the left side, the congenital deformity of the auricle can be seen

b2. Chest deformities associated with nipple–areola abnormalities (Fig. 45.3)

b3. Chest deformities without breast or nipple–areola abnormalities (Fig. 45.4)

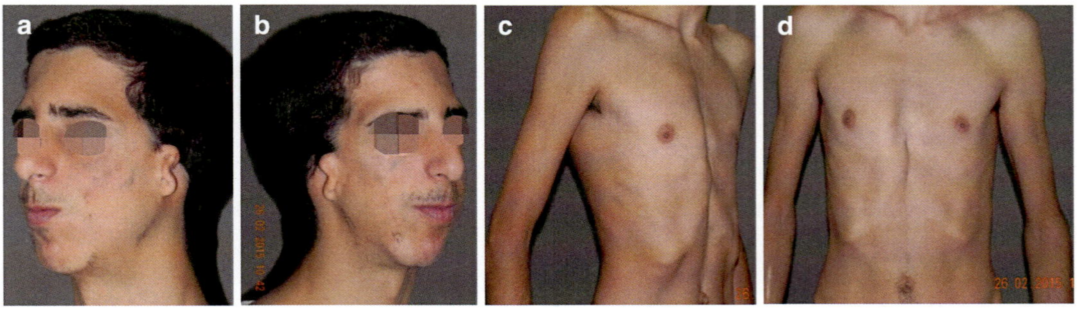

Fig. 45.3 A 20-year-old male patient with bilateral microtia associated with severe deformities of the chest. (**a**, **b**) Oblique view of the face showing bilateral microtia. (**c**, **d**) Oblique and frontal views showing severe and complex deformities of the chest

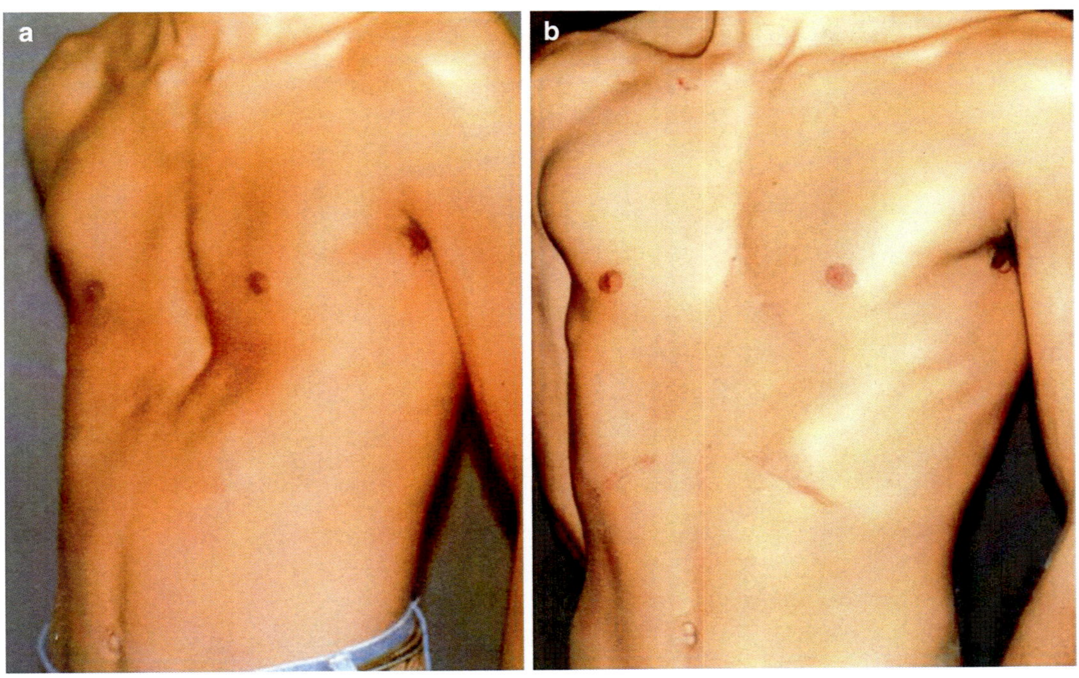

Fig. 45.4 Oblique view of a male patient presenting pectus excavatum. (**a**) Preoperative photo. (**b**) Postoperative photo after silicone implantation with a special prosthesis combined with resection of cartilage on the rib margin. (**c**) Preoperative photo of the same patient, frontal view showing the chest deformity. (**d**) Postoperative photo after silicone implantation combined with resection of cartilage on the rib margin. (**e**) Photo of the same patient with a model of the future implant. (**f**) Photo with preliminary prosthesis, which will be manufactured

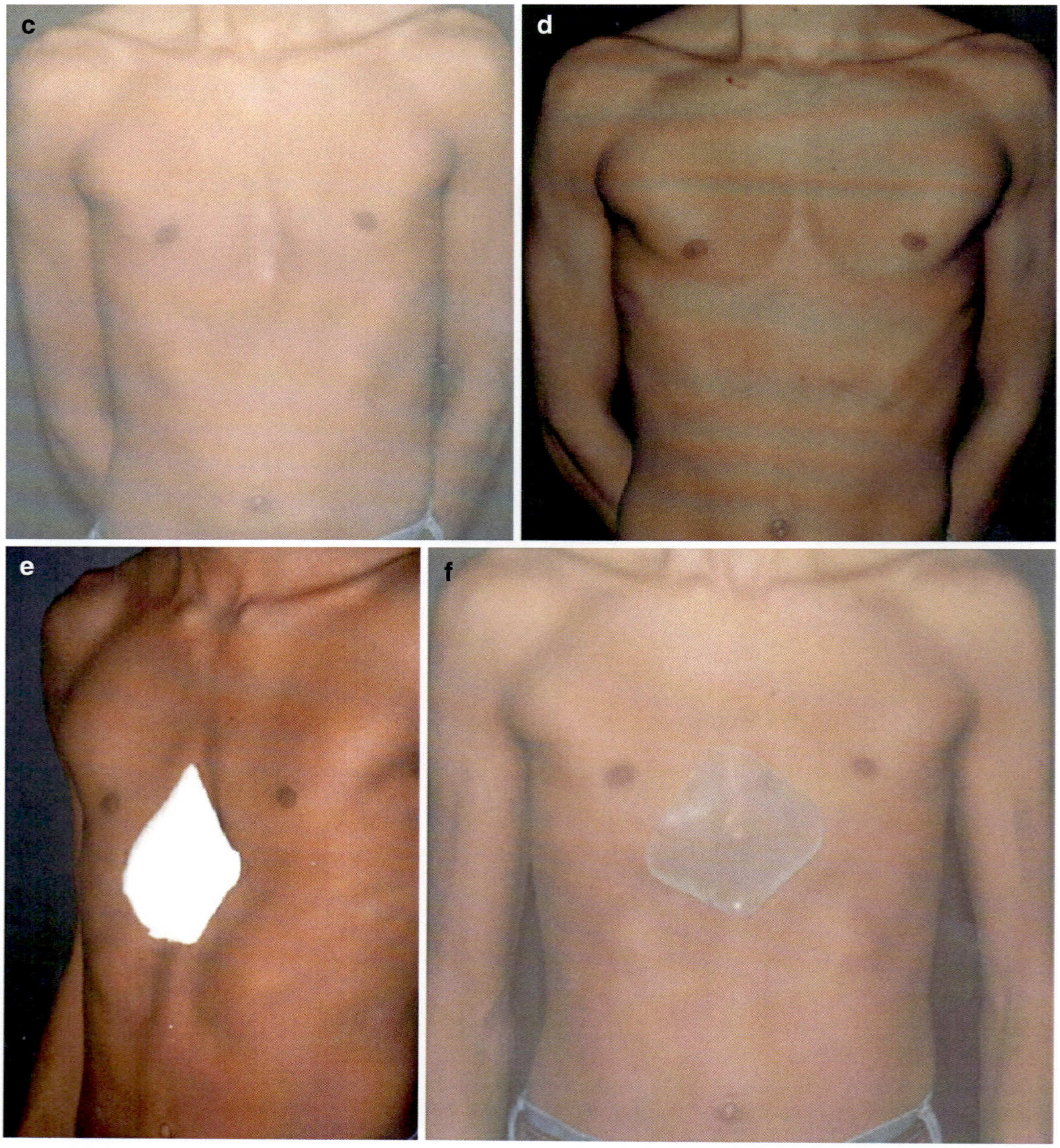

Fig. 45.4 (continued)

B. Deformities of the column associated with chest anomalies
   a. Deformities of the upper segment of the column (Fig. 45.5)
   b. Deformities of the medial segment of the column (Fig. 45.6)
   c. Deformities of the lower segment of the column (Fig. 45.7)
   d. Deformities of the upper, medial, and upper segments of the column (Fig. 45.8)

II. Congenital
   A. Deformities of the chest

It is useful to mention that patients with pectus carinatum present a lateral position of the nipple–areola regions in all three groups. Embryological development of the chest is projected forward and consequently the nipple–areola regions are located on the lateral sides of the chest.

a1. Pectus carinatum superior

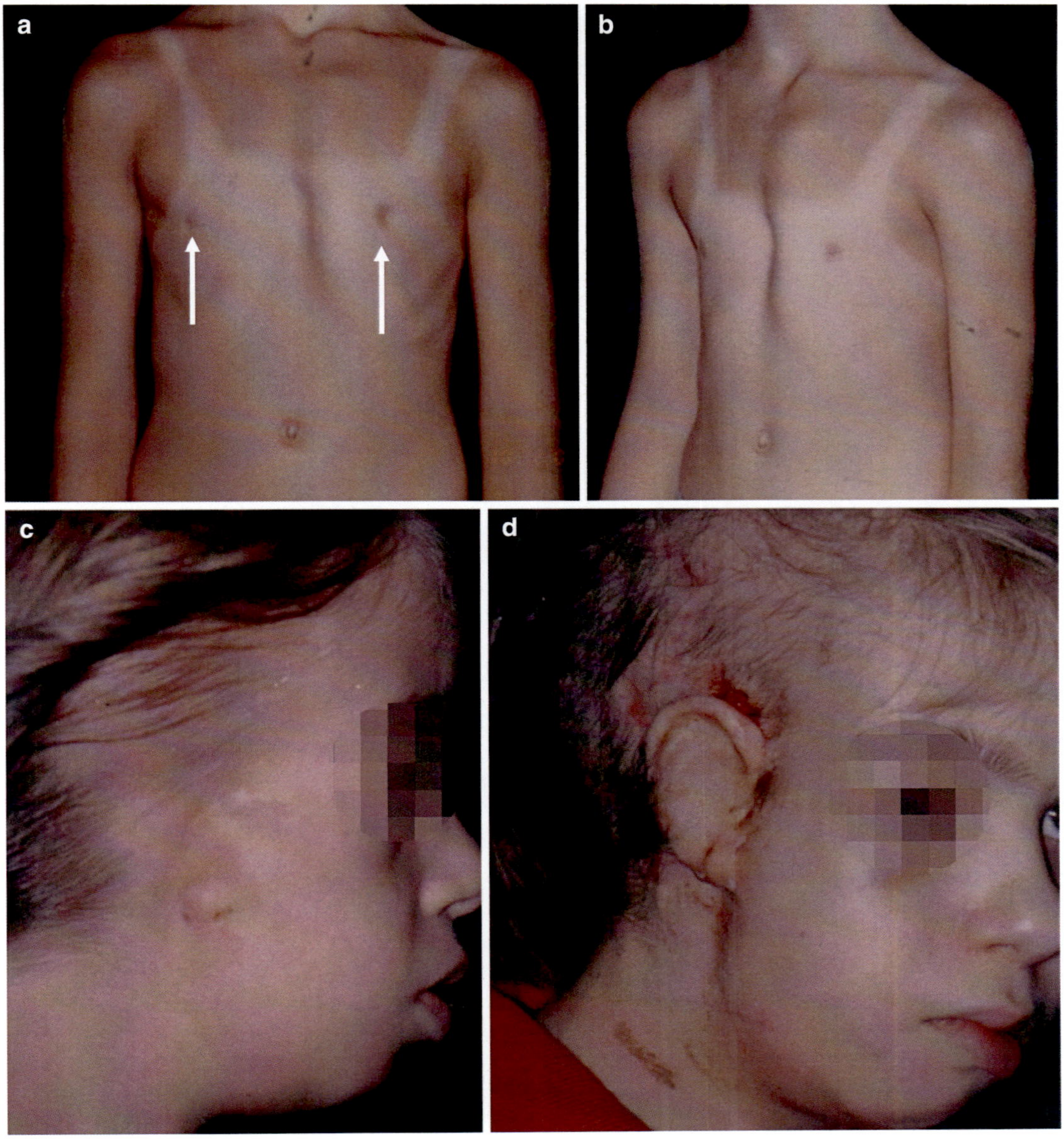

Fig. 45.5 A 9-year-old boy with anotia on the right side in association with severe deformity on both sides of the chest and pectus excavatum and asymmetry of the nipple–areola regions. (**a**) Frontal view with *arrows* indicating asymmetric nipple–areolar regions. (**b**) Oblique view. (**c**) Profile view of the right side of the face with anotia. (**d**) After ear reconstruction

a2. Pectus carinatum inferior (chicken breast, pigeon breast)
a3. Pectus carinatum lateral

On the other hand, in all patients presenting with pectus excavatum, the nipple–areola areas are located more medially, close to the sternal region (Fig. 45.5). Such an observation occurs in female and male patients with pectus carinatum and pectus excavatum.

B. Deformities of the vertebral column associated with chest anomalies

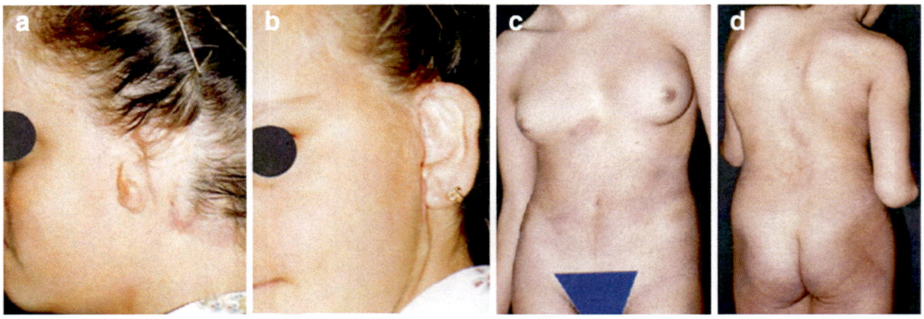

Fig. 45.6 A 16-year-old female patient with agenesis of the left ear presenting asymmetrical breast and chest. (**a**) Lateral view of the left side. (**b**) After ear reconstruction. (**c**) Frontal view, deviation of the whole body can be seen. (**d**) Back view, severe asymmetry of the torso and the column can be seen

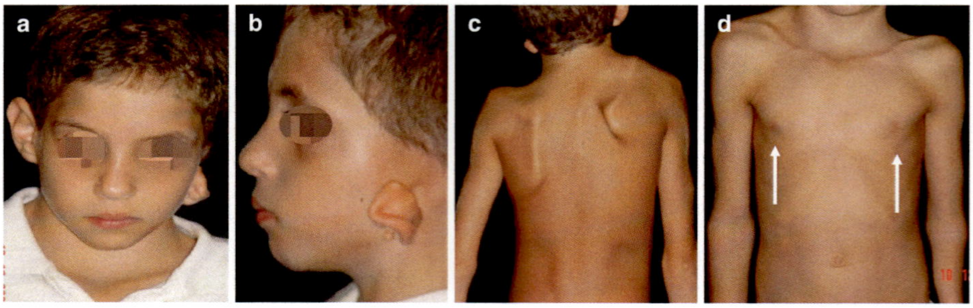

Fig. 45.7 A 7-year-old boy presenting complex associated anomalies of the left auricle with deformities of the torso. (**a**) Frontal view with asymmetrical auricles. (**b**) Profile view with severe anomalies of the left ear. (**c**) Posterior view showing severe deformities of the torso with asymmetry of the scapular bones and congenital torticollis. (**d**) Frontal view showing severe deformities of the neck and asymmetrical nipple–areola regions indicated by *arrows*

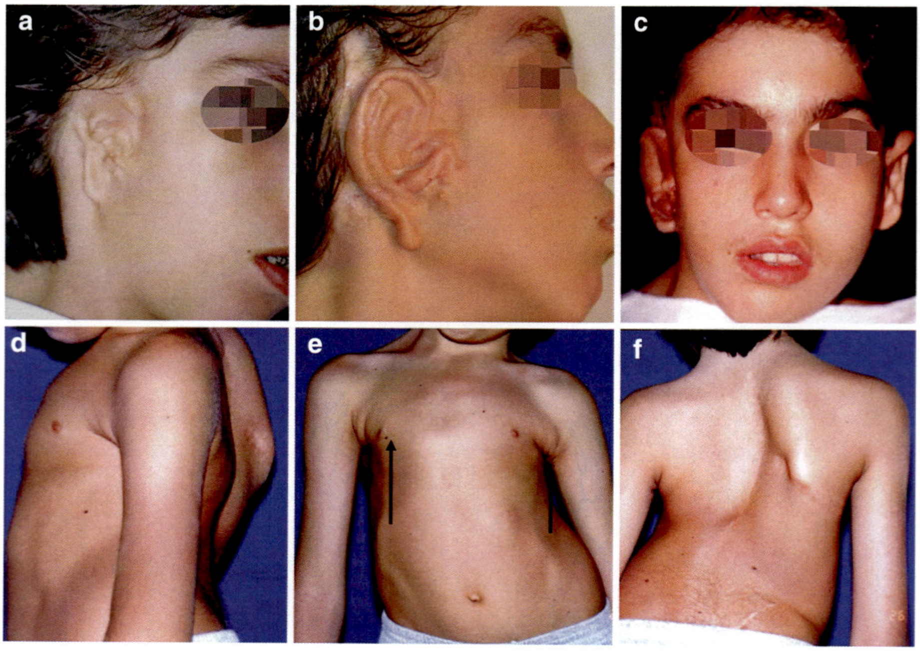

Fig. 45.8 A 11-year old boy presenting complex associated anomalies of auricle and torso and chest. (**a**) Profile view with microtia on right side; (**b**) after ear reconstruction; (**c**) frontal view with well balance of the reconstructed ear on right side with the left one; (**d**) profile view of left side of the torso; (**e**) frontal view of the chest with asymmetric nipple-areolar regions indicated by *arrows*; (**f**) posterior vie of the torso with asymmetry of the column and scapular bones as well

Patients classified in this group present with severe deformities of the vertebral column, with complex alterations of the anatomy that require an orthopedic approach. Some of my patients used to wear a special orthopedic apparatus to provide minimal conditions for the protection of the column (Fig. 45.6). Therefore, its treatment outside the scope of this chapter.

45.3 Method

45.3.1 Deformities of the Chest

The purpose of this chapter is to discuss only the surgical correction of the deformities of the chest that may be associated with breast abnormalities. The treatment is a complex procedure that must be performed according to the patient's complaints, following accurate surgical planning. Repair of breasts, breast asymmetry, and other deformities are described in other chapters of this book, and are thus not mentioned here.

45.3.2 Surgical Planning

According to the deformity of the chest, surgical planning must be carried out before the operation. I am not used to performing such repairs, as chest and heart surgeons are accustomed to it because abnormalities of the heart and lung are frequently associated.

45.3.3 Pectus Excavatum

Deformities of the chest classified as pectus excavatum in addition to pectus carinatum may be repaired by osteotomy of the ribs, as described by Coelho and Guimarães (2007). I am used to performing repair of the chest using silicone implants.

45.3.4 Surgical Demarcation

I am not used to performing osteotomy for the repair of such deformities, as my preference is to employ a special silicone implant. As each patient presents a specific deformity, it is necessary to prepare a unique implant for repair. Once the operation is scheduled, it is necessary to make a special model of the deformity. The deformity is marked on the chest the with patient supine on the examination table and the shape and size of the implant is delimited (Fig. 45.4). The special model is then prepared on the chest of the patient and is the basic instruction for the fabrication of the prosthesis. The new implant is created and sterilized and comes in a special packet matching the model in size, shape, and thickness (Fig. 45.4).

45.3.4.1 Pre-Marking

Pre-marking is carried out 1 day before the operation in my clinic with the patient in a standing position in front of two vertical mirrors. In this way, the patient can see all pre-markings and the location of the future scars so that she can sign the informed consent. Afterward, some more photos are taking showing all markings.

45.3.5 Surgical Technique

The operation is performed at the hospital under general anesthesia. As pre-marking has been done 1 day earlier, the full marking is completed following the key points already landmarked. Two incisions are marked on the projection of the rib margins as they quite often present excessive projection and it is necessary to remove some of the cartilage (Fig. 45.9).

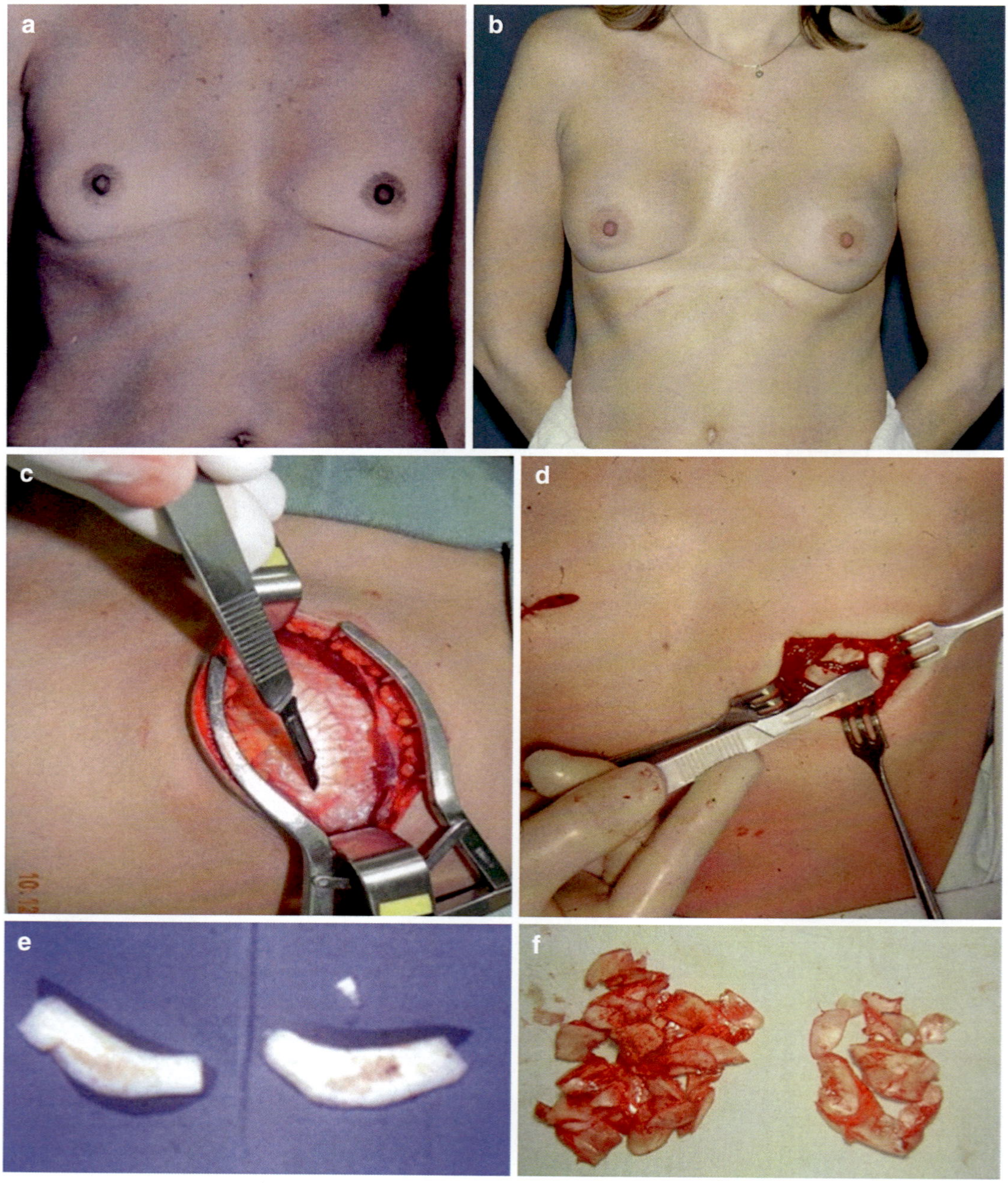

Fig. 45.9 Patient with pectus excavatum, combined with hypomastia and excessive projection of the rib margin. The surgical planning was to perform breast augmentation with a regular silicone implant, inclusion of a special implant for repair of pectus excavatum combined with resection of the cartilage of the rib margin. (**a**) Before surgery. (**b**) After all surgical procedures. Resection of the cartilage of the rib margin. (**c, d**) Preoperative photos showing resection of the rib margin on both sides. (**e**) Two pieces of cartilage removed from the rib margin. (**f**) Multiple small pieces of cartilage resected from a patient to achieve a good balance of the chest. Peroperative photos showing resection of the cartilage on the rib margin and implantation of a special prosthesis to repair the sternal deformity. (**g**) Two incisions were made on the rib margin on both sides. (**h**) Special prosthesis is being introduced through one incision to repair the sternal deformity. (**i**) Final aspect after resection of cartilage on the rib margin on both sides and the implant was introduced. (**j**) Preoperative photo of the same female patient, oblique view showing deep deformity in the sternal region, hypomastia. (**k**) After augmentation mastoplasty using a standard silicone implant. The model of the new prosthesis can be seen. (**l**) Final result after augmentation mastoplasty, resection of the cartilage of the rib margin and implantation of the special prosthesis to repair the external depression of pectus excavatum

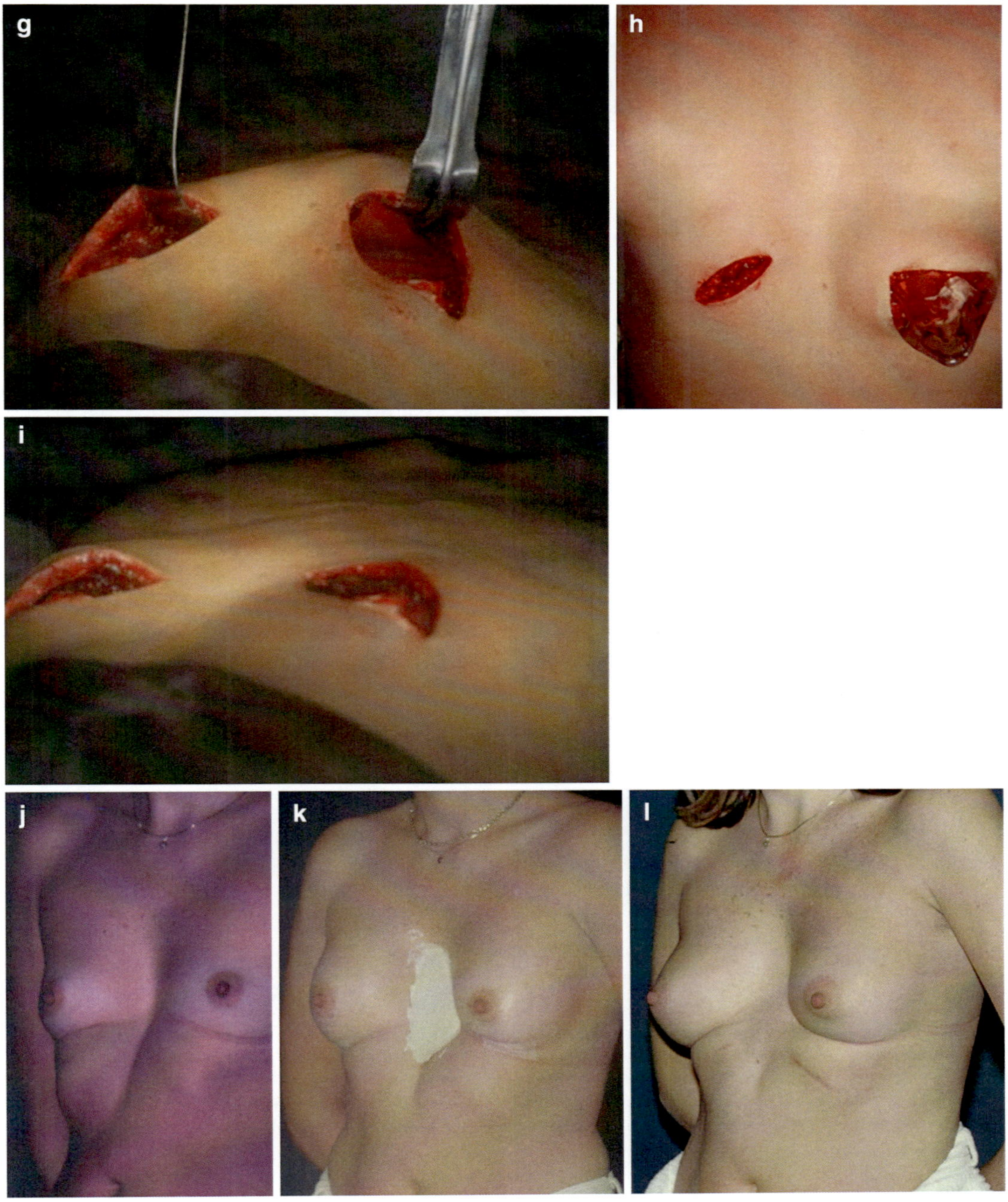

Fig. 45.9 (continued)

45.3.5.1 Anesthetic infiltration

After marking, anesthetic infiltration is carried out following the landmarks of the skin on the subcutaneous tissue underneath the incisions and all over the sternal area. My anesthetic solution consists of: lidocaine (2%) 40 mL, distilled water 160 mL, adrenaline (1/1,000) 1 mL, total solution 201 mL.

This amount of anesthetic volume is enough to infiltrate the sternal area and the projection of the rib margin.

45.3.5.2 Cutaneous Incisions are Made Following Marking

When a patient presents excessive projection of the rib margin it is necessary to remove some of the cartilage to achieve a good balance with the chest (Fig. 45.9a–f). Panniculus undermining from the cutaneous incision is done on the sternal area to create a wide pocket.

45.3.5.3 Prosthesis Inclusion

The special implant is then introduced through the cutaneous incision (Fig. 45.9g–i) to insert into the depression of the sternal region.

45.3.5.4 Suturing of the Wound is Performed from Deep Up to the Skin

The final result shows a good balance between breast and chest (Fig. 45.9j–l).

When a patient presents deformities of the chest associated with the breast, as may occur in Poland's syndrome, surgical corrections may be performed in a single operation (Fig. 45.10a, b). As there are deformities on the anterior aspect of the chest, transposition of the latissimus dorsi muscle may be carried out by rotation from the posterior aspect of the torso to the anterior side of the chest (Fig. 45.10c–f). The rotation of the latissimus dorsi muscle makes a movement similar to a pendulum to fill the upper part of the chest. As hypomastia may be associated with chest deformities, it is useful to include the silicone breast implant at the same time (Fig. 45.10g–j).

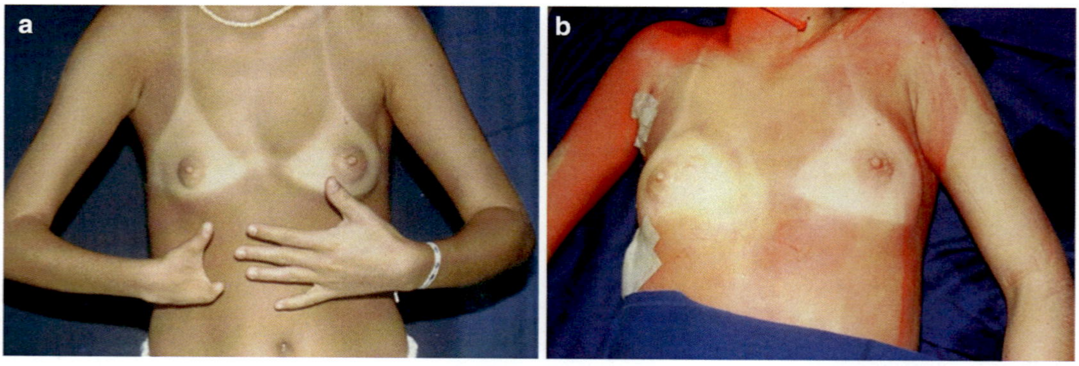

Fig. 45.10 A 17-year-old girl with Poland's syndrome with asymmetrical breasts and nipple–areola regions with dysgenesis of the right hand. (**a**) Frontal view of the chest with asymmetry before surgery. (**b**) Same patient after repair of the right side of the chest with rotation of the latissimus dorsi muscle combined with a silicone implant. (**c**) The *arrows* indicate two cutaneous incisions in the axillary region and the medial axillary line on the right side. (**d**) The latissimus dorsi muscle is already dissected and lying on the skin on the lateral side of the chest. (**e**) The *arrow* indicates the rotation arch of the muscle. (**f**) The muscle is already rotated and sutured to fill the upper segment of the anterior side of the chest combined with silicone implant for augmentation of the right breast. (**g**) Preoperative photo, oblique view, showing severe deformities of the right side of the chest. (**h**) Postoperative photo after repair of the deformities. (**i**) Preoperative photo, frontal view. (**j**) Same patient after the surgery described

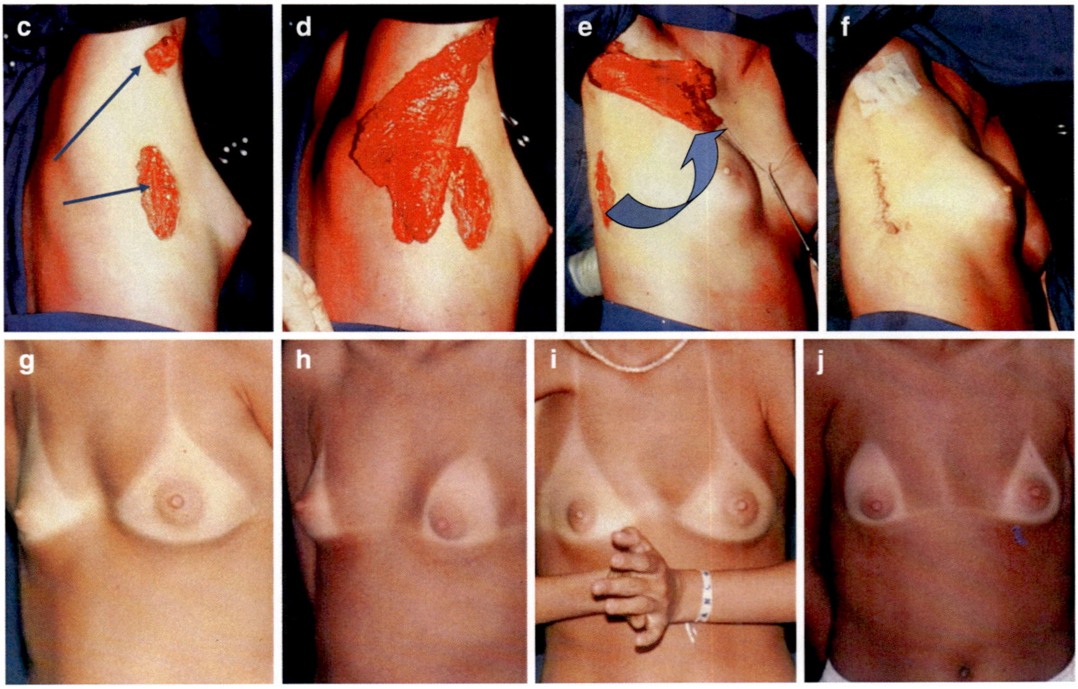

Fig. 45.10 (continued)

45.4 Discussion

Deformities of the chest and breast as well are severe problems in women as they bring complex unaesthetic alterations and imbalance to their intimate well-being. Correction of the breast must be carried out in adult life after physical development. It is advisable to first perform aesthetic surgery on the breast followed by repair of the chest deformities (Fig. 45.11). Pectus carinatum may be treated by osteotomy of the rib bones to reduce the projection of the sternal bone. Pectus excavatum may also be corrected by osteotomy of the rib bones, as described by heart and chest surgeons. Nevertheless, my preference is to perform inclusion of a silicone implant that has been specially fabricated for the patient, making a bespoke model for each one (Fig. 45.9) .

Once the model is prepared, the implant is manufactured, and sent in suitable condition for the operation.

I have also performed individualized implantations in male patients for the repair of severe pectus excavatum (Fig. 45.4). Again, special model is made in advance so that a unique implant can be created for each patient.

The operation is performed in hospital under general anesthesia. To avoid any scarring on the skin of the sternal region, which will cover the prosthesis, I make a cutaneous incision on the lateral border of the rib margin (Fig. 45.9). Cutaneous undermining must be carried out as deep as possible at the level of

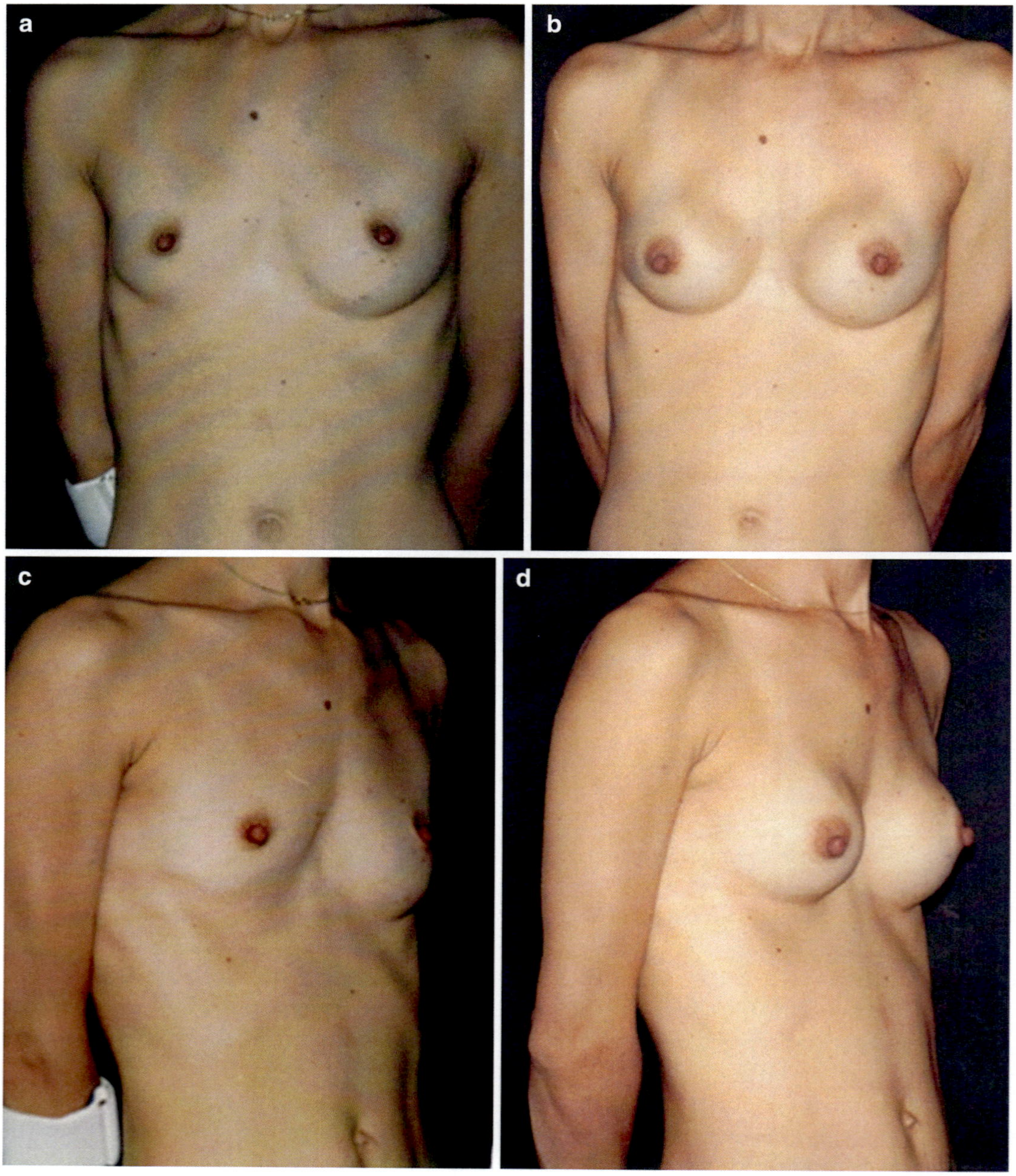

Fig. 45.11 Severe chest deformity associated with hypomastia and asymmetrical breasts. (**a**, **c**) Before surgery. (**b**, **d**) After bilateral augmentation mastoplasty with an implant of 155 mL on the left side and 220 mL on the right side to try to achieve a good balance of the breasts and chest. (**e**, **g**) Before surgery, oblique view on the left side and profile view on the right. (**f**, **h**) After mastoplasty with a mammary implant to try to achieve a good balance of the breasts and chest

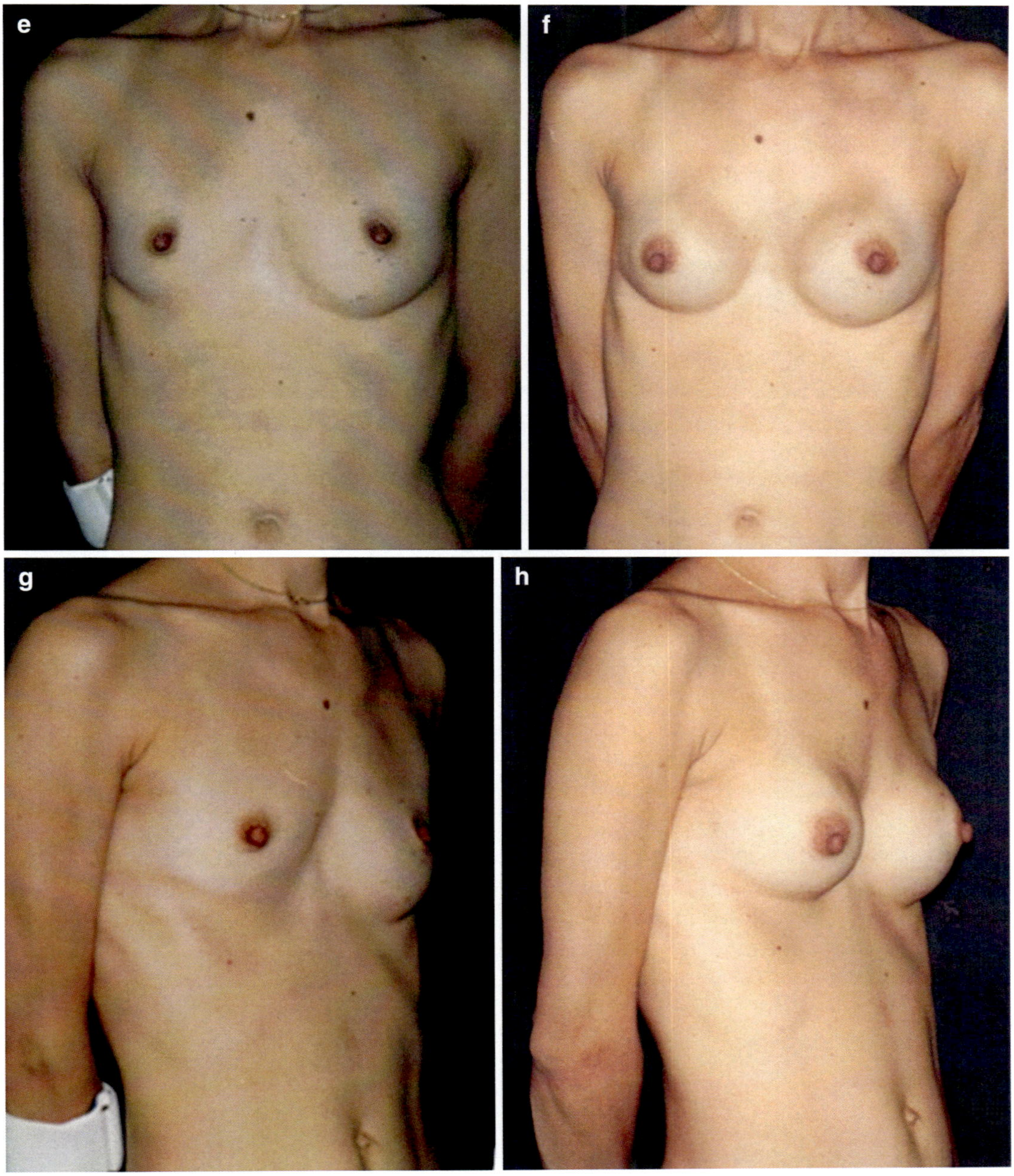

Fig. 45.11 (continued)

the periosteum of the sternal bone, where a pocket is created. Afterward, careful hemostasis must be performed. Following the operation, the special implant is then introduced through the cutaneous incision and it must be well placed on the sternal bone. I do not use any drainage after surgery.

45.5 Complications

The operation must be performed with great care regarding all steps of the operation. I have not experienced seroma formation, hematoma or infection, which may occur after silicone implantation. If the implant is too large, it may mar the surgical result. For this reason, it is mandatory to carry out adequate surgical planning.

Conclusions

Deformities of the chest with or without anomalies of the breasts may bring unaesthetic imbalance to the body contour. They may occur in both females and males. Although they are congenital anomalies with severe repercussions for the patients' well-being, the operation should only be performed in adulthood after complete physical development. Chest deformities such as pectus excavatum may be repaired by implantation of a special prosthesis through cutaneous incisions on the projection of the costal rib. However, pectus carinatum may be treated by osteotomy of rib cartilages. Asymmetrical breasts associated with deformity of the chest may be treated in the same operation or in two surgical stages.

References

Avelar JM (1989) Breast asymmetry. (Assimetria mamária). In: Cirurgia Plástica na Infância. Avelar J (Ed.). São Paulo: Ed. Hipocrates, pp. 413–423

Ayer E (1981) Breast asymmetry following thoracic surgery in childhood. Aest PlastSurg 5(2):169–172

Cavalcanti Ribeiro R, Novaes W, España Quintero L, Moreira Mangles MG, et al. (2007). Mediastinal alterations in patients with Poland's 17 syndrome. Annals of 14th International Congress of International Confederation for Plastic, Reconstructive and Aesthetic Surgery, P/REC 57, June. Berlin, Germany.

Coelho MS, Batlen LC, Guzzi A, Tozzo A (1988) Pectus excavatum/carinatum—Surgical results of the treatment (pectus excavatum/carinatum resultados do tratamento cirúrgico). Rev Bras Ortop 23:120–124

Coelho MS, Stori WS, Pizarro LDV, Zanin SA, Gonçalves JL, Bergonse NN (2003) Pectus excavatum/pectus carinatum: surgical treatment (pectus excavatum/pectus carinatum: tratamento cirúrgico). Rev Col Bras Cir 30(4):249–261

Coelho, MS, Guimarães PSF (2007) Pectus excavatum: terapeutic approach. (Pectus excavatum: abordagem terapêutica)—ARTIGO DE REVISÃO. Rev. Col. Bras. Cir 34(6):412–427 ISSN 0100-6991. doi: 10.1590/S0100-69912007000600011

De Souza Pinto EB, Queiroz Filho W, Erazo IP, MAS A, Wong LJ, Muniz AC (1997) Pectus excavatum: aesthetic surgical correction. (Pectus excavatum: correção cirúrgica estética). Rev Soc Bras Cir Plast 12(1):68–74

Check for updates

46 Aesthetic Approach to Breast Reconstruction

Ricardo Cavalcanti Ribeiro, Rawlson de Thuin, Isabel Vieira de Figueiredo-e-Silva, and Manuel Torreira Rios

46.1 Introduction

Alternatives to more conservative treatments have been developed since the beginnings of breast surgery. Multidisciplinary planning with oncologists, mastologists, and other specialists ensure a promising outcome in the approach toward breast reconstruction. As in any other form of reconstruction surgery, the surgeon should always keep in the mind the need to preserve the fullest extent of the area being operated, without ceasing to be effective in the treatment of the disease and without causing harm to the patient. The psychological and emotional factors play a huge role in patients undergoing reconstruction surgery. We should consider the patient as a whole and not just the treatment. It is not enough just to consider the type of surgery we will choose and the result we need to achieve without taking into consideration the psychological state of the patient. Otherwise, we may be able to achieve an excellent result, but the patient may not agree because she did not understand the surgery's limitations. To deal with expectations is very difficult, even more so, in an altered emotional state.

Techniques such as skin-sparing mastectomies, where the skin is preserved in patients undergoing mastectomies followed by immediate reconstructive surgery help to maintain the natural contour of the breast, allowing a better aesthetic result. The modified round block technique allows for scarless breast-conserving surgery. The knowledge of various breast reconstruction techniques and appropriately knowing which one to apply in each patient saves additional time in the surgery room and minimizes risks.

46.2 History

The need for a more aesthetic approach in breast reconstruction surgeries emerged in the 1990s when the concern with body image had increased worldwide. In countries like Brazil, where people care enough about their bodies and where breast cancer is most prevalent in the female population, the need for more aesthetic results has gained strength since then. Many patients

Head of Division of Plastic and Reconstructive Surgery of Universidade Federal do Estado of the Rio de Janeiro (UNIRIO)

R.C. Ribeiro, M.D., Ph.D. (✉)
Division of Plastic and Reconstructive Surgery of Casa de Portugal, Brazilian Society of Plastic Surgery, Carlos Chagas Institute, Rio de Janeiro, RJ, Brazil
e-mail: rribeiro@centroin.com.br

R. de Thuin, M.D.
Brazilian Society of Plastic Surgery, Carlos Chagas Institute, International Society of Aesthetic Plastic Surgery, Rio de Janeiro, RJ, Brazil

I.V. de Figueiredo-e-Silva, M.D.
Brazilian Society of Plastic Surgery, Carlos Chagas Institute, The American Society of Plastic Surgeons, Rio de Janeiro, RJ, Brazil

M.T. Rios, M.D.
Division of Plastic and Reconstructive Surgery, Carlos Chagas Institute, Rio de Janeiro, RJ, Brazil

J.M. Avelar (ed.), *Breast Surgery*, https://doi.org/10.1007/978-3-319-54115-0_46

were disappointed with the results achieved, which led Dr Audretsch, from Germany, to develop a surgical approach that came to be called oncoplastic surgery. Oncoplastic surgery is the technical convergence of oncological (ablative) and aesthetic breast surgery, which attempt to adequately remove end-stage breast cancer while retaining or producing a breast shape and appearance that closely approximates a normal breast. Early diagnosis and appropriate treatment helped to reduce the mortality rate and the expansion rate of tumors. Worldwide, countries have adopted oncoplastic ideology to find a halfway point between the oncological resection and aesthetic results (Cordeiro et al. 2004).

46.3 Methods

Analyzing the advantages and disadvantages of various approaches with the patients and other specialists, we conclude that performing an integrated surgery with the mastologist is crucial to having a better oncological and aesthetic outcome. In addition, the plastic surgeon should be updated and know the latest surgical techniques and their proper indications. Local and regional flaps, expanders, implants, lipofilling, nipple–areola reconstructions and pedicle flap-based reconstructions are all tools now available to plastic surgeons (Bostwick et al. 1978).

There are three main groups when categorizing reconstructive procedures and knowing them will help to improve outcomes. The patient groups are:

1. Immediate breast reconstruction
2. Mastectomy post-relapse associated with immediate breast reconstruction
3. Delayed breast reconstruction

Regarding group 1, the most convenient type of tumor treated with this procedure is the intraductal carcinoma using nipple-sparing or skin-sparing techniques occurring immediately after resecting the tumor. This group usually has a better outcome overall in quality and results (Neligan et al. 2013).

In group 2, patients have already been treated, but had some type of relapse and do not need treatment with radiotherapy (Jung et al. 2012).

Group 3 involves patients who temporarily cannot undergo any type of surgery. Reasons include the condition of the breast post-mastectomy, the biology of the tumor, the clinical state of the patient not allowing it, or the patient simply refusing to have surgery at that moment (Huemer et al. 2007).

46.4 Techniques

46.4.1 Local and Regional Flaps

Local and regional flaps are mainly used in reconstructive surgeries where a reasonable amount of breast tissue and skin is left after the mastologist has achieved resection of the tumor. Used in small or medium-sized breasts, this technique usually has better scarring outcomes and less visible scars, and includes glandular flaps in addition to dermoglandular flaps. The plastic surgeon usually looks for the most vascular donor site of a flap or flaps (more than one can be used to improve breast volume) and the ideal place is usually located infra-areolar or in the lateral part of the breast. Breast symmetry and CAP preservation should be a priority given the possibility. The latissimus dorsi, rhomboid flap, and thoracodorsal flap are some of those most commonly used (Bostwick et al. 1978). Regional flaps such as the transverse rectus abdominis myocutaneous (TRAM) flap is another excellent technique that has been well accepted and tolerated by patients undergoing breast reconstruction. Used in women needing large breast reconstruction, this procedure maintains the donor tissue connected to the original site to retain its blood supply, helping to format the breast mound (Figs. 46.1 and 46.2).

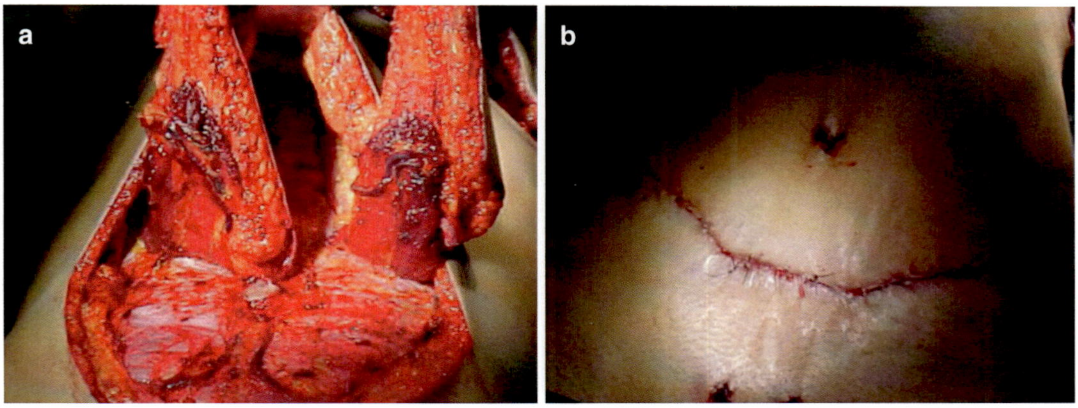

Fig. 46.1 (**a**) Bilateral elevation of the transverse rectus abdominis myocutaneous (TRAM) flap, where we observe a good arterial supply. (**b**) Donor site closed mimicking an abdominoplasty scar

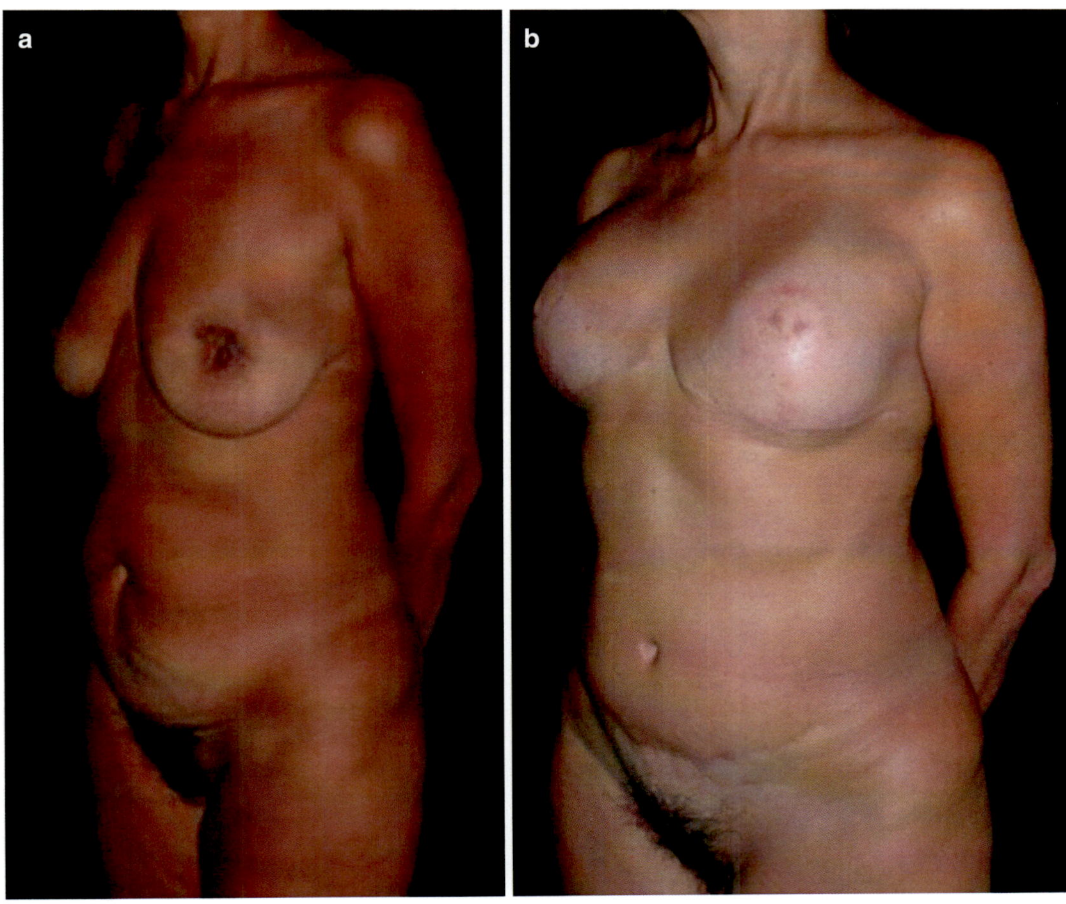

Fig. 46.2 (**a**) Profile of skin-sparing mastectomy with pedicled TRAM reconstruction (preoperatively). (**b**) Profile of skin-sparing mastectomy with TRAM (1 year postoperatively) and texturized implant 225 mL

46.4.2 Expanders and Implants

Reconstructing a breast with expanders and implants is easier and simpler than other techniques, such as skin flap reconstructions. We can use temporary implants (tissue expanders) or permanent tissue expanders (Becker implants) (Figs. 46.3 and 46.4). Both are placed under the pectoralis major muscle at the same time as the mastectomy. If we use a temporary implant, once the desired breast size is achieved, the expander is removed and a permanent implant is placed. With permanent expanders, we can achieve different results regarding volume and a safer reconstruction without the use of skin flaps.

The advantages of both types are the shorter hospitalizations and recovery time needed. The surgical risks are reduced too, but there are also

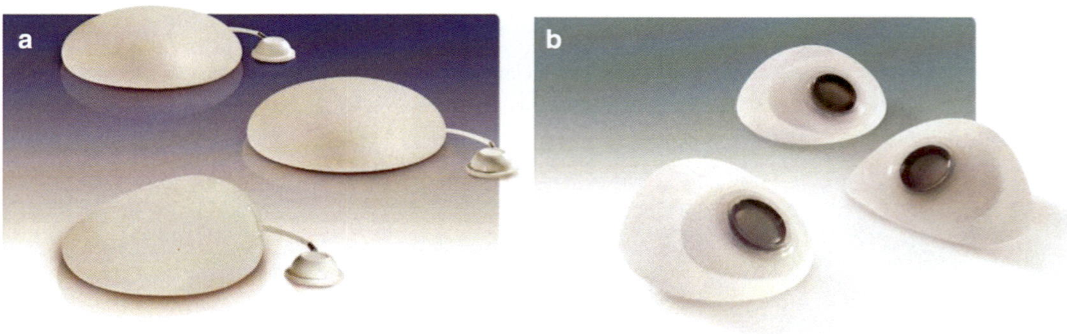

Fig. 46.3 (**a**, **b**) Becker expanders, both round and anatomic shape

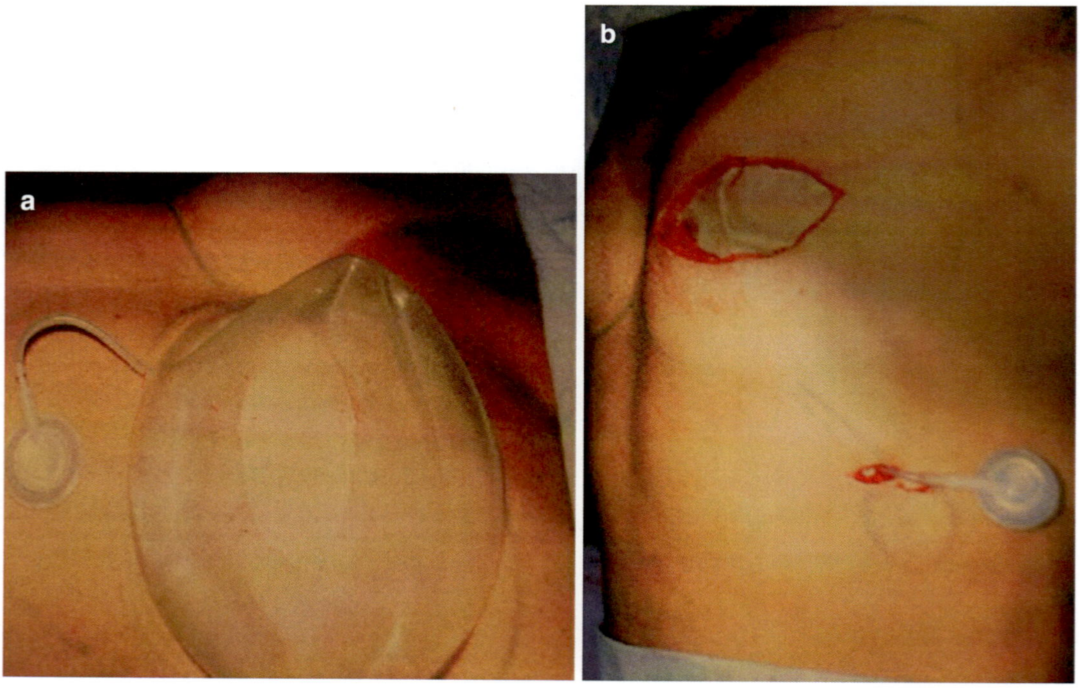

Fig. 46.4 (**a**) Round expander implant with remote valve. (**b**) Once the implant is placed the valve is situated at a certain distance

potential complications, such as ruptures, rippling, leakage, implant hardening, displacement, and wrinkling; the same as with breast augmentation surgeries. Implants are widely used to rebuild breasts as less surgery is required, involving just one body area, the chest; however, more than one procedure may be required to achieve the final result. Different implant fillers include saline, silicone gel, and combined saline–silicone.

Breast reconstruction with expanders and implants is mainly used when there is a small breast volume, but sufficient skin tissue as in skin-sparing mastectomies.

46.4.3 Round Block Technique

In cases of tumors, this technique produces very discreet scarring and a normal breast contour. In any peripheral extension and close to the nipple–areola complex (NAC) but without compromising it, it is possible to utilize this technique, which allows wide visualization of the oncological area being treated and gives a great opportunity for reassembly of the surgical space being treated, with obvious positive aesthetic repercussions (Benelli 1990).

The initial design corresponds to an area of approximately 1 cm in a circular periareolar form; next, the compromised oncological mammary area is resected with safe margins free from neoplasia and followed by the synthesis of the deep planes with absorbable sutures and closing of subcutaneous tissue the same way, approaching the cutaneous tissue around the NAC causing it to rise (Fig. 46.5). This may cause areolar asymmetry that results in future symmetrization of the contralateral NAC, in the same surgery or second seeing the final result after adjunctive radiation, which is considered the ideal scenario in terms of oncological safety and cosmetic results.

The NAC is a very important component of the breast and its final aesthetic result is crucial to patients diagnosed with breast cancer.

Despite its advantages, this technique is not for every patient. It is more suitable for patients with small to medium breasts and adequate areolar size. Restricted surgical exposure and difficulty in the skin dissection are commonly observed in patients with a small areola and inexperienced mastologists.

The marking on the patient is designed with the patient in a vertical position. If the areola is large but without mammary ptosis a semicircular incision is indicated. There is no need for additional markings in these cases. The incision is made exactly on the meeting point between the areola and surrounding skin. If the areola is small or has a slight ptosis a complete circumareolar epidermic decortication can be made. In these cases, the following markings should be made: point A, 19–21 cm from the midclavicular line and 10–12 cm from the sternal line. The ideal diameter of the NAC of 25–30 mm peripherally is designed as a complete epidermic ring and will be resected to reduce the excess tissue. The medial limit of the resection coincides with 10–12 cm from the sternal line and the same distance is kept for the lateral limit.

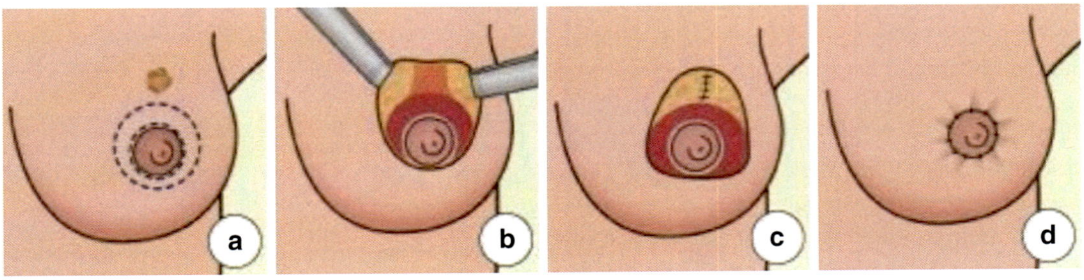

Fig. 46.5 (**a–d**) Round block incision marking followed by excision of the tumor, de-epithelialization and approximation of the NAC to its new position

46.5 Radiation Therapy

Radiation therapy is often indicated in breast cancer patients. After conservative treatment, the patient often needs to receive this treatment to prevent the tumor from growing again in the operated breast. Some studies suggest that patients with a life expectancy of less than 5 years and over 70 years of age may not prescind adjunctive radiotherapy. Patients over 70 years old, with a tumor size less than 2 cm and zero compromise of the lymphatic nodes within the armpit region and with positive estrogen receptors, may not need radiotherapy, even after preservation treatment of the breast because local recurrence in these situations is low when treated with a drug called tamoxifen sold under the name Nolvadex. The consensual recommendation for radiotherapy after radical mastectomy or mastectomy with reconstruction are the following situations: armpit area positive with four or more lymph nodes affected, Advanced tumors stage pT3 or pT4 with 1–3 lymph nodes affected, initial tumors pT1 or pT2 with 1–3 lymph nodes affected. The oncological approach post-mastectomies must be multidisciplinary and knowing the effects radiotherapy will have in the early stages and in the late in the esthetic results (Cordeiro et al. 2004).

46.6 Discussion

To succeed in breast reconstruction surgery, we need full integration between the plastic surgeon and the mastologist. To achieve success, the mastologist must fully understand the steps that are going to be taken to obtain the final result. The reconstruction can be immediate or not, depending on the type of breast cancer. The plastic surgeon must inform what type of breast volume he hopes to achieve, if the patient has cutaneous deficits how will he improve such defects, how will he deal with anatomical depressions, NAC reconstructions, and whether or not various surgeries will be needed to have an outstanding result. With these details taken into consideration, the incisions made on a breast with a tumor by the mastologist can be greatly modified now that he has a better understanding of the procedure trying to be accomplished.

46.7 Complications

When dealing with breast reconstruction complications such as asymmetry, necrosis of donor flaps, fibrosis, and infections can be experienced. Radiation therapy can be a key issue in a final aesthetic result in breast reconstruction, seeing that it may cause secondary surgeries to correct deformities caused by the radiation.

Conclusions

The knowledge of having several operating techniques is of great benefit when trying to achieve a greater percentage of breast conservation. The numerous options help to individualize patient treatment and care achieving more favorable results.

References

Benelli L (1990) A new periareolar mammaplasty the "Round Block" technique. Aesthet Plast Surg 14:93–100

Bostwick J III, Vasconez LO et al (1978) Breast reconstruction after a radical mastectomy. Plast Reconstr Surg 61(5):682–693

Cordeiro PG, Pusic AL, Disa JJ et al (2004) Irradiation after immediate tissue expander/implant breast reconstruction: outcomes, complications, aesthetic results, and satisfaction among 156 patients. Plast Reconstr Surg 113(3):877–881

Huemer GM, Schrenk P, Moser F, Wagner E, Wayand W (2007) Oncoplastic techniques allow breast-conserving treatment in centrally located breast cancers. Plast Reconstr Surg 120(2):390–398

Jung DY, Jeong WL, Young KC et al (2012) Surgical techniques for personalized oncoplastic surgery in breast cancer patients with small to moderate sized breast. J Breast Cancer 15(1):1–6

Neligan PC, Losken A (2013) Reconstructive surgery of the breast. The oncoplastic approach to partial breast reconstruction. Neligan Plast Surg 11:295–313

Aesthetic Repair of Nipple and Areolar Abnormalities

47

Helio Paoliello Jr. and Ricardo Paoliello

47.1 Introduction

The nipple areola complex (NAC) is an essential structure of the mammary anatomy. Patients with nipple or areola loss due to neoplasm, excisions, trauma or congenital absence, still suffer emotional distress, even after breast and NAC reconstruction. Other NAC conditions that require intervention are congenital and acquired or growth-related (athelia, polythelia, and amastia), post-traumatic, burn injuries, deformities, and breast surgery complications, such as breast reduction (Farhadi et al. 2006). In the case of neoplasms, a reconstructed breast brings significant psychosocial benefits to the patients (Fig. 47.1).

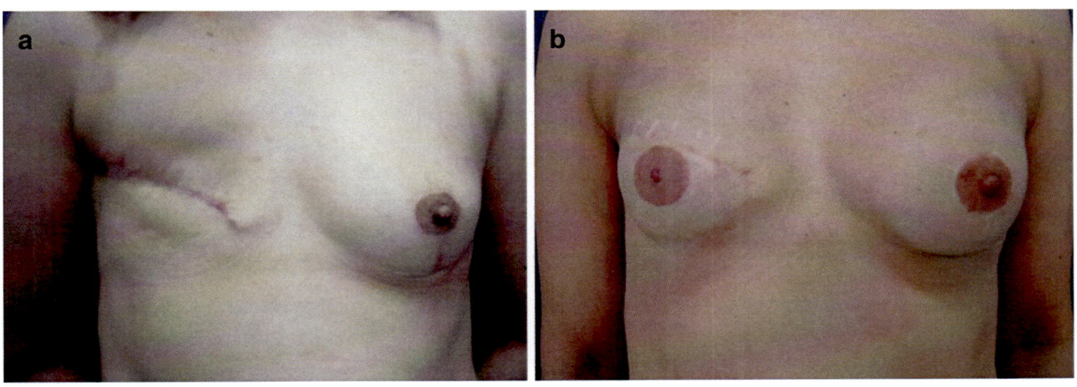

Fig. 47.1 Patient after (**a**) full mastectomy of the right breast and (**b**) after reconstruction of the breast and nipple–areola complex (NAC), via an areolar graft from the other breast and tattoo

H. Paoliello Jr. (✉) • R. Paoliello
Plastic Surgery Discipline, Faculdade de Medicina de Marília (FAMEMA), 1409, 7 de Setembro Street, Marília, SP 17502-020, Brazil
e-mail: heliopaoliellojr@yahoo.com.br; drricardopaoliello@gmail.com

J.M. Avelar (ed.), *Breast Surgery*, https://doi.org/10.1007/978-3-319-54115-0_47

Nipple reconstruction can be carried out at any moment after the conclusion of the mammary cone; however, if there is a need to symmetrize the other breast or administer radiotherapy, the surgeon must wait for the ideal time to perform it. The NAC reconstruction represents an important stage to the patient, from an aesthetic point of view (Ferreira et al. 1995).

Studies show that NAC reconstruction is highly related to the patient's general satisfaction and the acceptance of the patient's own body (Evans et al. 2005). Thus, the conclusion of the breast reconstruction through the creation of a NAC very similar to that of the opposite breast with regard to size, shape, projection, and position contributes greatly to the final result of the reconstruction.

The NAC, besides bringing harmony to the whole breast, has the primordial function of feeding, through the ejection of milk via the galactophorous ducts, and participates in female sexual pleasure through sensorial stimulus. These properties must be preserved when correcting hypertrophy and nipple inversion, and areolar hypertrophy, and will be compromised during surgery for the treatment of mammary tumors.

47.2 Method

We carried out a descriptive study based on a literature review and demonstration of techniques developed and implemented in Serviço de Cirurgia Plástica da Faculdade de Medicina de Marília, São Paulo, Brazil (FAMEMA).

47.3 Discussion

Ideally, the NAC is located at the most prominent point of the breast cone. The average size of the areola is 40 mm (between 35 and 45 mm) and the nipple is an average of 13 mm in diameter and 9 mm in height (Neligan 2013). However, we emphasize that the ideal size is the one that brings satisfaction to the patient, fulfilling her request and desire.

The areolar texture can be smooth or rough, depending on the location and number of Montgomery glands. There is a large variation in color, shape, size, and projection of the NAC, according to ethnic factors or as a result of aging, hormonal level variation (pregnancy and menopause), and weight change (Adams 1949).

47.3.1 Pathological Conditions of the Nipple

The diversity of nipple dimensions in the population makes it difficult to define hypo- and hypertrophy of this structure (Chang 2007). Thus, the perception of the patient and the proportion of the NAC in relation to the breast are key in the diagnosis. A higher incidence of nipple hypertrophy in people of Asian ethnic groups and of African descent has been observed (Fanous et al. 2009). Also, there is a classification of uni- or bilateral nipple inversion, in addition to specific treatment for a better result (Han and Hong 1999).

47.3.2 Nipple Hypotrophy

Of all the anatomical conditions of the nipple, hypotrophy is the one that contributes least to personal dissatisfaction. Puerile nipple in a breast with a proper shape and with an areola of a smaller diameter areola is common and well accepted by the female population. During pregnancy, hormone stimulation prepares this nipple for breastfeeding, changing the volume of the nipples (Lewis 1973). Eventually, after lactation, nipples may undergo atrophy at their base, leading to deformity and distal ptosis, similar to an acrochordon (Fig. 47.2), the correction of which is similar to that for hypertrophy: de-epithelialization of the atrophied area and burying it in the breast cone.

If nipple hypotrophy is the reason for the dissatisfaction, Table 47.1 describes ways to correct it.

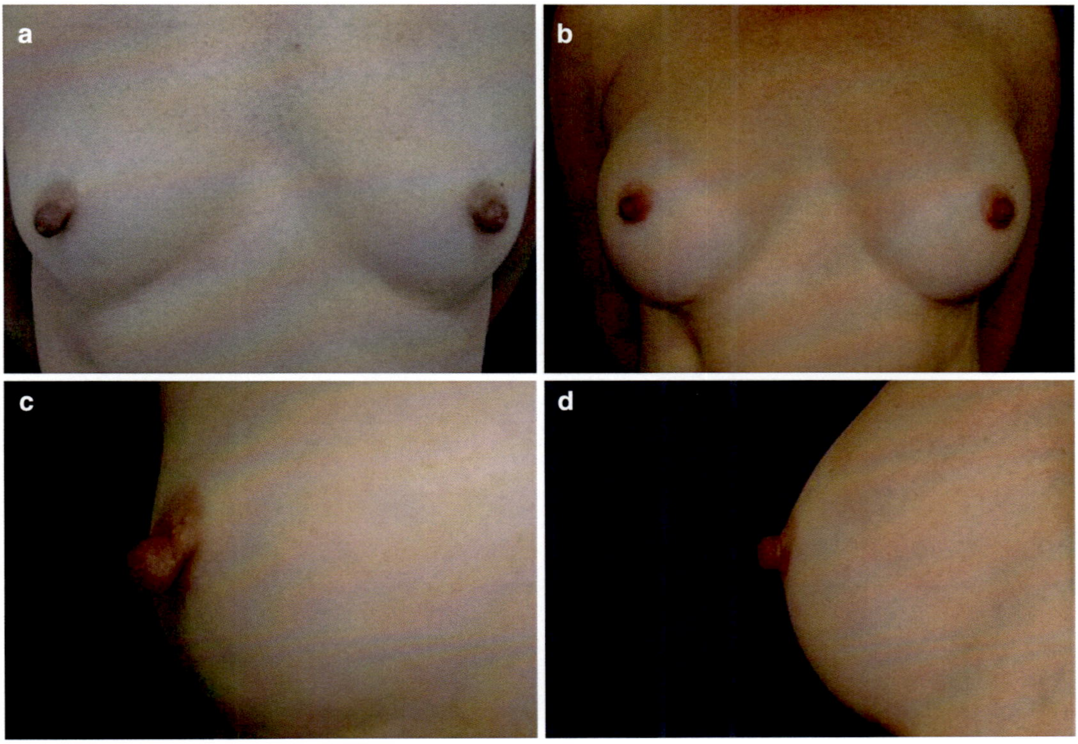

Fig. 47.2 Patient showing hypotrophy of the nipple base, (**a**, **c**) after lactation and (**b**, **d**) after surgical correction

Table 47.1 Various types of nipple reconstruction

Examples of techniques	
Local flap	Central based flaps
	Subdermal pedicle flap
	Double subdermal pedicle flap
	Pull-out/purse-string flap
Flaps with autologous graft augmentation	Cartilage graft
	Fat graft
Composite nipple graft	N/A
Flaps with allograft	AlloDerm™
Augmentation	Silicone gel
	Hyaluronic acid
	Calcium hydroxylapatite
	Artificial bone substance
	Polytetrafluoroethylene (PTFE)

47.3.3 Hypertrophy of the Nipple

More common among Asians and those of African descent (Fanous et al. 2009), hypertrophy of the nipple can cause discomfort and inhibition when projected under garments, mainly in tropical countries, because of the use of light clothing. Although facilitating breastfeeding, the demand for nipple reduction surgery in plastic surgery clinics has increased.

Use of the technique described by Pitanguy (Pitanguy and Macareno 1975; Pitanguy 1978) is widespread. In this technique, the nipple is divided horizontally into two parts, with excision of the lower portion and bending of the upper portion caudally, then suturing of the edges (Fig. 47.3).

Several other techniques with the same purpose are described in the literature: Lewis (1973), Sperli (1974), Regnault (1975), Vecchione (1979), Ferreira et al. (1995), Lai and Wu (1996), Lai et al. (1998), Chang (2007), Fanous et al. (2009).

Because of the simplicity and versatility, we adopted the technique with ring-shaped incisions (Fanous et al. 2009; Lewis 1973; Regnault 1975; Lai and Wu 1996). A circle is marked at the base of the nipple, and the height is varied according to the reduction desired. The second marking is performed

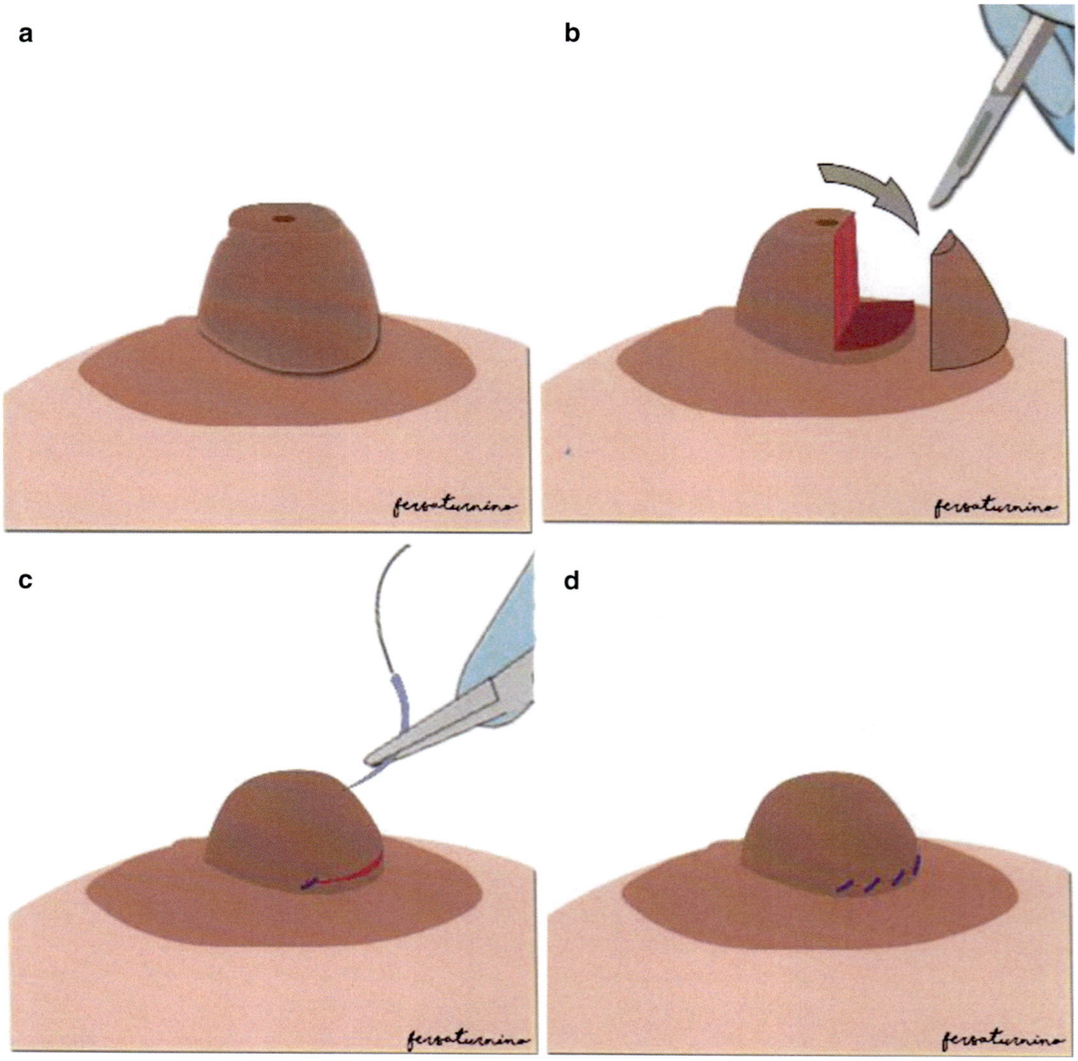

Fig. 47.3 Pitanguy's technique for nipple hypertrophy. (**a**) Hypertrophic nipple. (**b**) Horizontal incision dividing the nipple into two parts. (**c**) Caudal mobilization of the superior portion, folding in on itself. (**d**) Suturing of the edges and the final result

by setting a cylinder. A thin layer of skin in the area between the two incisions is then removed, the edges of which are approximated with non-absorbable, monofilament 5.0 or 6.0, burying the de-epithelialized segment. When the diameter of the papilla is excessive, a wedge of the papilla is

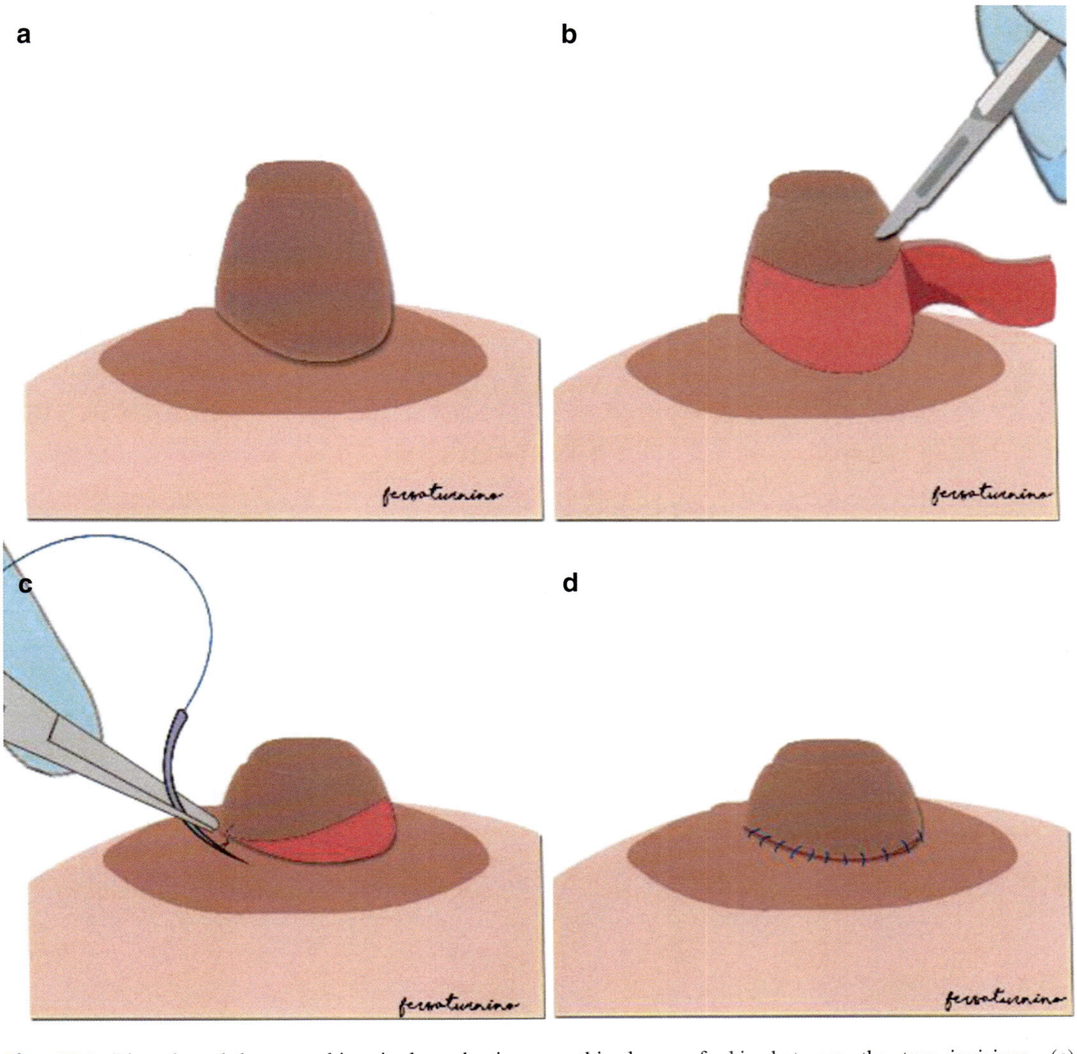

Fig. 47.4 Ring-shaped hypertrophic nipple reduction technique. (**a**) Hypertrophic nipple. (**b**) Incision at the base of the nipple; the distal incision varies according to the patient's desire for reduction, following a resection of a thin layer of skin between the two incisions. (**c**) Approximation of edges with a non-absorbable suture. (**d**) Final result

removed in its caudal part and the edges are sutured to close the wound area, following the same pattern of reduction in height. These techniques are aimed at saving the main milk duct (Figs. 47.4 and 47.5). The association between nipple reduction and silicone breast implants is quite common (Fig. 47.6).

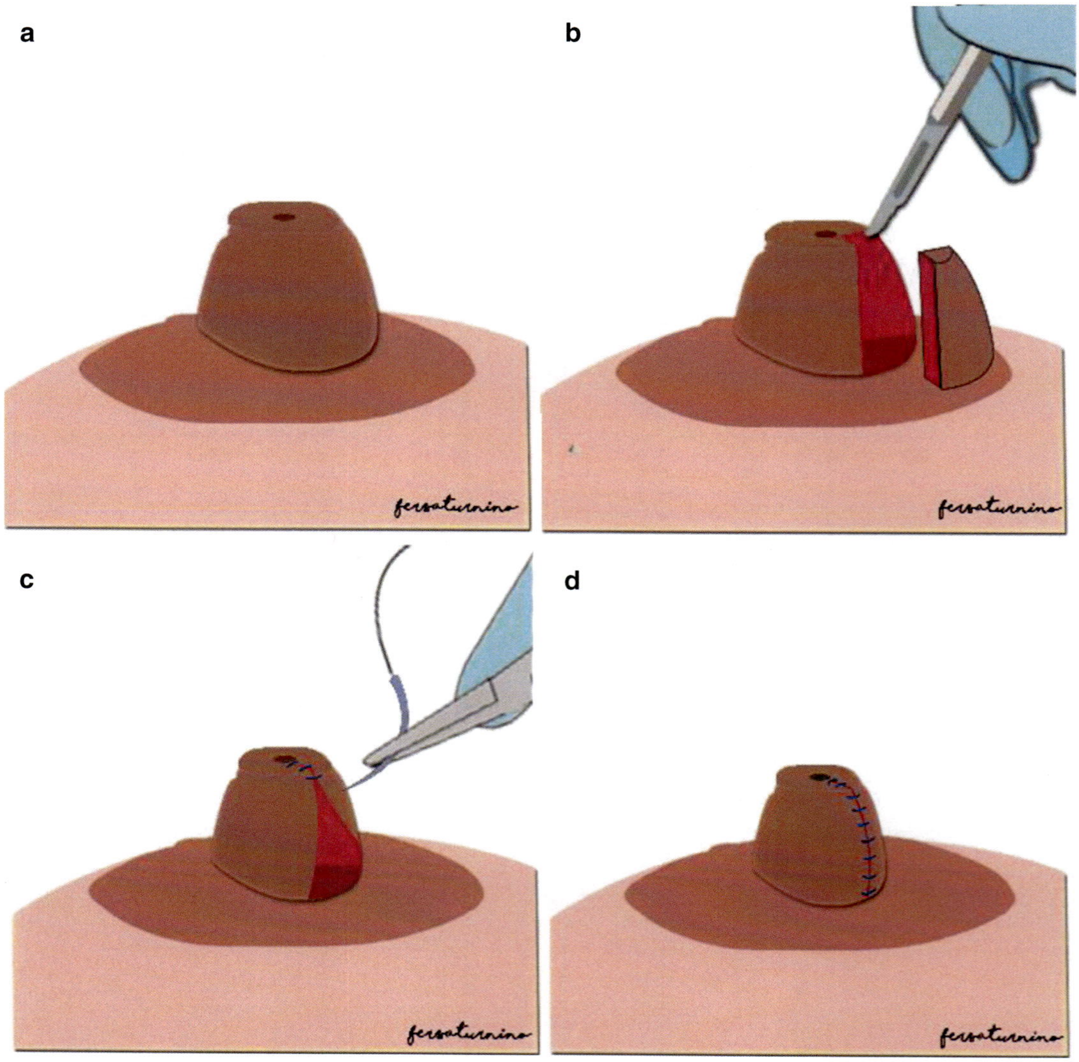

Fig. 47.5 Reduction technique for nipple volumetric hypertrophy. (**a**) Hypertrophied nipple. (**b**) Wedge resection of its caudal portion without reaching the main milk duct. (**c**) Approximation of edges with non-absorbable sutures. (**d**) Final result

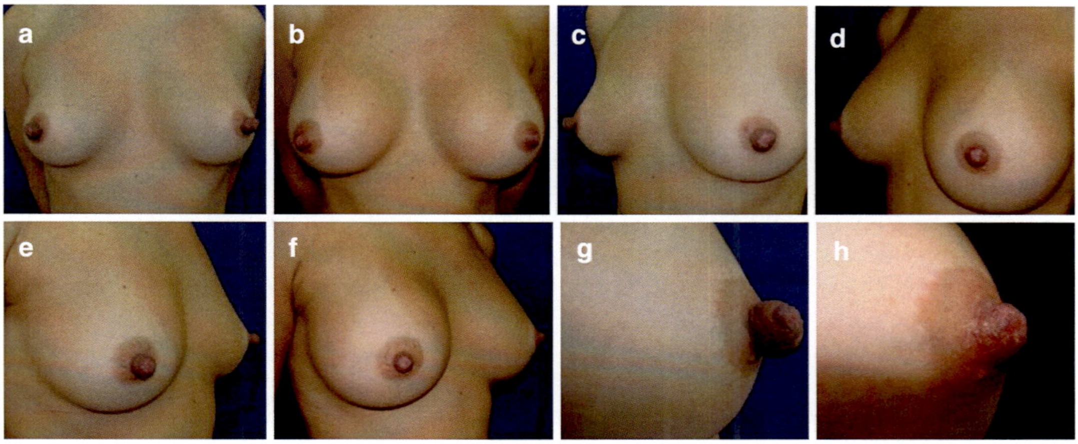

Fig. 47.6 Hypertrophic nipple. (**a**, **c**, **e**, **g**) After surgical correction with regard to height and diameter, using the techniques described in Figs. 47.4 and 47.5. (**b**, **d**, **f**, **h**) Submuscular silicone breast implants

47.3.4 Inverted Nipple

The inverted nipple diagnosis is made when the nipple is located in a plane below the areolar level, mainly due to fibrosis and an insufficient bulk of soft tissue in the nipple. This condition may be accompanied by the inflammatory and infectious processes of these structures, and endangers lactation and patients' self-esteem (Chang 2007).

In 1999, Han and Hong (1999) classified nipple inversion into three grades:

- Grade I: the inverted nipple can be easily pulled out manually and maintains its projection well without traction. Gentle digital pressure around the areola or gently pinching the skin causes the nipple to pop back out. It is believed to have minimal or no fibrosis.
- Grade II: the inverted nipple can be pulled out manually, but not as easily as in grade I. The nipple has difficulty maintaining its position and tends to retract. There may be a moderate degree of fibrosis.
- Grade III: the nipple is severely inverted and retracted. It is very difficult to pull out these nipples manually. Despite applications of pressure to the nipple to force it to protrude, it promptly retracts. The fibrosis is noticeable.

Several techniques have been described for the correction of this condition (Few et al. 1999), among them, those by Pitanguy and Macareno (1975) and by Pereira Filho et al. (2001). The technique we use consists of an infra-nipple semicircular incision encompassing 60% of the nipple circumference performed in the transition between the nipple and areola and the nipple pulled vertically using a simple hook. With blade 11, an "inverted cone," with its apex, the infra- and juxta-nipple, is incised, taking care not to completely incise the cranial pedicle, and a glandular flap is designed. Using the same blade, any remaining bands tethering the nipple down are released. After hemostasis, the resulting dead space is sutured with absorbable poliglecaprone 3–0 stitches from deep to the surface; thus, the flap obtained migrates anteriorly, adding bulk to the nipple. Skin is sutured using non-absorbable monofilament 6–0 suture. Dressing is carried out using interposing gauze, with a central circular hole, between the wound and a transparent plastic device (distal part of a syringe cut to the desired length), to which the nipple is anchored using non-absorbable monofilament 3–0 suture, allowing perfusion checks. The dressing is removed on the 5th day after surgery and the skin stitches after 10 days (Figs. 47.7 and 47.8).

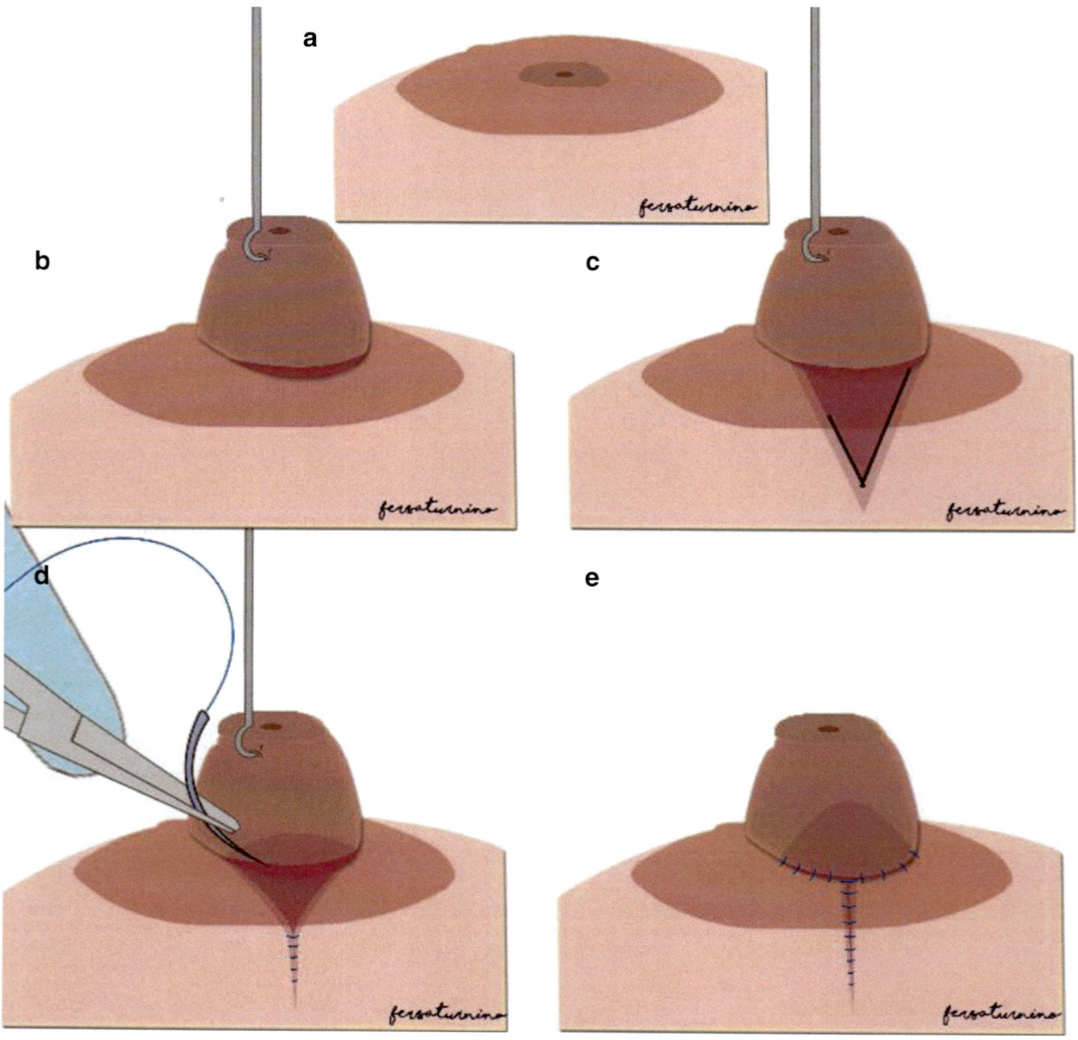

Fig. 47.7 Technique to treat inverted nipple. (**a**) Inverted nipple. (**b**) Nipple pulled vertically using a simple hook, followed by a 60% diameter semicircular infra-nipple incision between the nipple and areola. (**c**) Two to three centimeters deep "inverted cone" incision, maintaining a cranial pedicle glandular flap. (**d**) Dead space stitches using absorbable suture, from deep to the surface. (**e**) Skin stitches with non-absorbable suture and final result

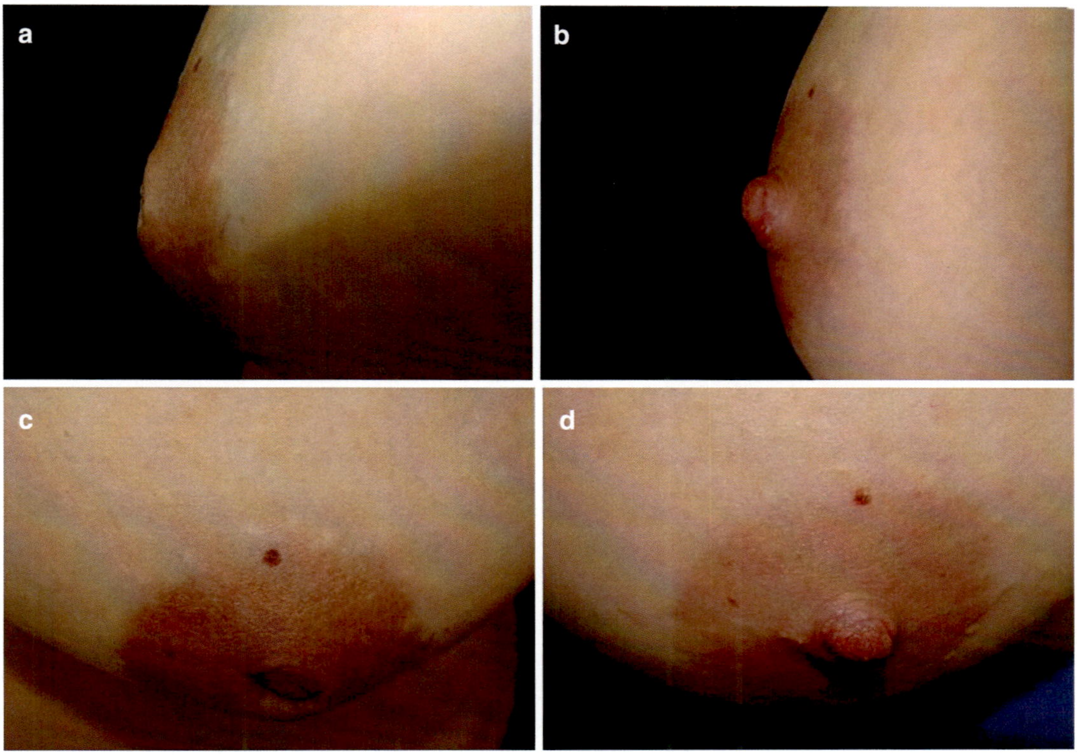

Fig. 47.8 (**a**, **c**) Inverted nipple. (**b**, **d**)After the surgical technique described in Fig. 47.6

47.3.5 Nipple Congenital or Post-traumatic Absence

When there is agenesis of the nipple, or its loss because of trauma, burn injury or mastectomy, several correction techniques have been described. The most frequently used are the skate flap technique (Fig. 47.9), described by (Farhadi et al. 2006); the star flap technique described by (Sisti et al. 2016); Di Lamartine et al. (2013), and the contralateral nipple graft, which is Pitanguy's technique (Fig. 47.10) (Pitanguy and Macareno 1975).

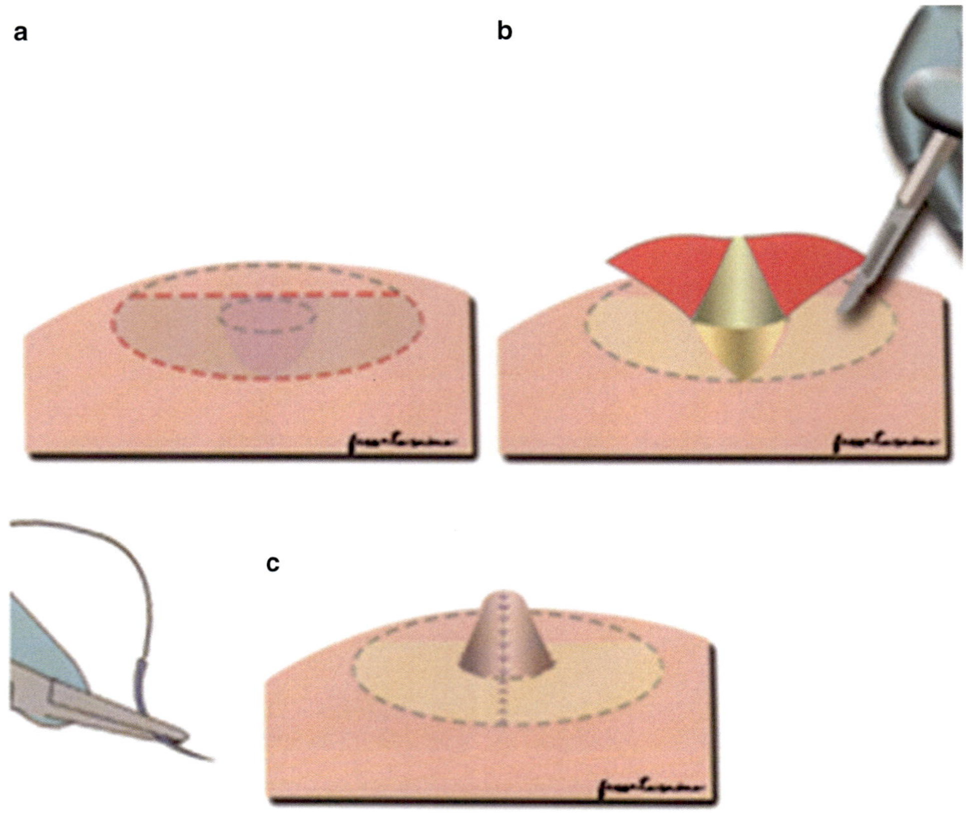

Fig. 47.9 Skate flap, for congenital or post-traumatic nipple correction. (**a**) Markings; the *gray dotted line* represents the future nipple and future areola; *red dotted line*, incision sites (transareolar incision is juxta-neonipple); *gray area*, superficial dissection; *purple area*, central deep dissection, which adds bulk to the neonipple. (**b**) After incisions and dissections. Medially migrated flaps, apex sutured at the lower point of the neonipple. (**c**) Final result, subcutaneous approximation and skin suture

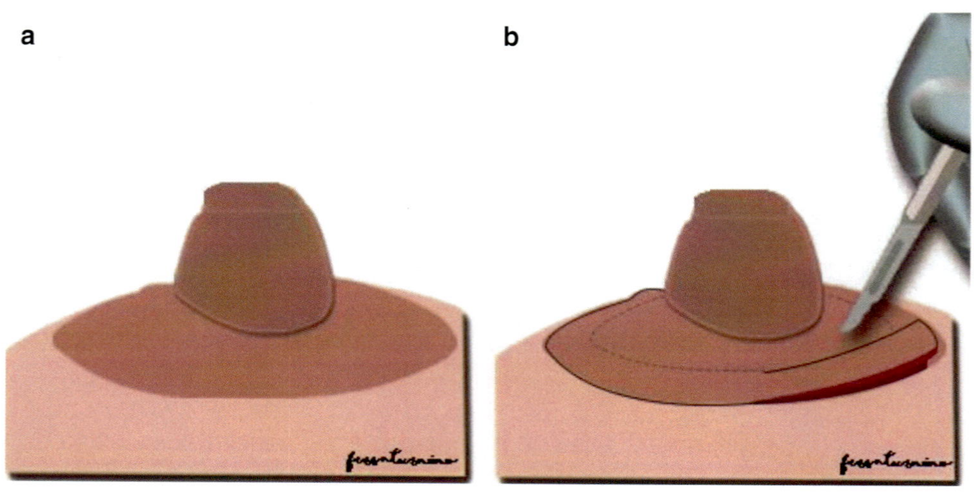

Fig. 47.10 Pitanguy's technique, areolar reconstruction with contralateral areolar skin graft. (**a**) Donor NAC. (**b**) Ring-shaped partial skin graft resection. Suturing is performed approximating the areola and the nearby skin. (**c**) The flap is incised in strips and sutured using non-absorbable spiral shaped sutures, until the exposed dermis is fully covered. (**d**) Final result

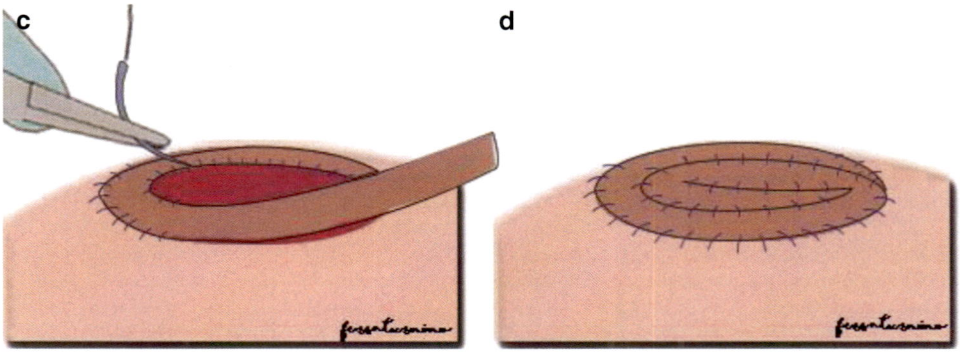

Fig. 47.10 (continued)

47.3.6 Areolar Deformities

Quite common, mainly after pregnancy or weight gain, areolar widening and hypertrophy are simple to correct and may be performed in association with a mastoplasty or circular peripheral resection of the widened areola (Benelli 1988).

Techniques for areolar reconstruction are contralateral partial areolar skin graft (Lewis 1973; Regnault 1975; Few et al. 1999; Wexler and Oneal 1973), partial skin graft from the medial proximal thigh or vaginal mucosa (Adams 1949; Schwartz 1976) or from the oral mucosa (Spina 1950).

Nowadays, tattooing or micropigmentation has been widely used (Riot et al. 2015). Ultraviolet light exposure has also been described as an attempt to increase graft pigmentation, without permanent results. Pigmentation provision and control results compared with contralateral NAC are rarely achieved (Farhadi et al. 2006; Elliott and Hartrampf 1990).

Although artistic tattoos have been known for millennia, their medical application has only recently been recognized (Riot et al. 2015). At the beginning, areolar micropigmentation was performed as a complement to a skin graft, as the latter lost its pigmentation; however, in the 1990's, Elliott and Hartrampf (1990) began using this technique as an isolated procedure for areolar creation. Tattooing or micropigmentation may also be used to correct shape, size, and reconstructed NAC location abnormalities (Saad 2001). It is an outpatient procedure, simple and low-cost, with no morbidity to donor sites and a low rate of complications, such as allergies and infections (Elliott and Hartrampf 1990). Retouching can be performed, as pigmentation decreases over time. The results are satisfactory.

47.4 Complications

Complications related to assistance for NAC reconstruction or correction include dyschromia, hyposensitivity, infections, and necrosis (Regnault 1975). For inverted nipple, partial or complete recurrence may occur (Han and Hong 1999).

Conclusion

Nipple–areola complex deformities are responsible for several degrees of psychosocial distress for patients. These deformities and their treatment should be widely known by plastic surgeons so that they can carry out treatment to correct or ameliorate these conditions.

References

Adams WM (1949) Labial transplant for correction of loss of the nipple. Plast Reconstr Surg 4:295

Benelli L (1988) Technique de plastie mammaire le round block. Rev Fr Chir Esth 13(50):7–11

Chang YC (2007) Aesthetic surgery for hypertrophic nipple: a simple technique. Rev Soc Bras Cir Plást 22(1):30–33

Di Lamartine J, Cintra Junior R, Daher JC, Cammarota MC, Galdino J, Pedroso DB, Cintra RH (2013) Nipple-areola reconstruction using the double opposing flap technique. Rev Bras Cir Plást 28(2):233–240

Elliott LF, Hartrampf CR Jr (1990) Breast reconstruction: progress in the past decade. World J Surg 14(6):763–775
Evans KK, Rasko Y, Lenert J et al (2005) The use of calcium hydroxylapatite for nipple projection after failed nipple-areolar reconstruction: early results. Ann Plast Surg 55:252-259;discussion 29
Fanous N, Tawile C, Fanous A (2009) Nipple reduction—an adjunct to augmentation mammoplasty. Can J Plast Surg 17(3):81–88
Farhadi J, Maksvytyte GK, Schaefer DJ, Pierer G, Scheufler O (2006) Reconstruction of the nipple-areola complex: an update. J Plast Reconstr Aesthet Surg 59(1):40–53
Ferreira LM, Neto MS, Okamoto RH, Andrews J d M (1995) Surgical correction of nipple hypertrophy. Plast Reconstr Surg 95:753–754
Few JW, Marcus JR, Casas LA et al (1999) Long-term predictable nipple projection following reconstruction. Plast Reconstr Surg 104:1321–1324
Han S, Hong YG (1999) The inverted nipple: its grading and surgical correction. Plast Reconstr Surg 104(2):389–395
Lai Y, Wu C (1996) Nipple reduction with a modified circumcision technique. Br J Plast Surg 49:307–309
Lai YL, Weng CJ, Samuel Noordhoft M (1998) Areolar reduction with inner doughnut incision. Plast Reconstr Surg 101:1695–1699
Lewis JR Jr (1973) Atlas of aesthetic plastic surgery. In: Cap 10: Breasts, 1st edn. Little, Brown and Company, Boston, p 231
Neligan PC (2013) Plastic surgery. In: Pate KM, Nahabedian MY (eds) Cap 22, Nipple aréola complex reconstruction, vol 5, 3rd edn. Elsevier, Philadelphia, p 500
Pereira Filho OJ, Bins-Ely J, Granemann AS et al (2001) Closed inverted nipple treatment through a microincision procedure. Plast Reconstr Surg 108:1000–1005
Pitanguy I (1978) Mamaplastia. Guanabara Koogan, Rio de Janeiro
Pitanguy I, Macareno A (1975) Reconstrução de aréola e mamilo. Rev Bras Cir 65(9/10):237–244
Regnault P (1975) Nipple hypertrophy. A physiology reduction by circumcision. Clin Plast Surg 2:391–396
Riot S, Devinck F, Aljudaibi N, Duquennoy-Martinot V, Guerreschi P (2015) Tatouage de la plaque aréolo-mammelonnaire en reconstruction mammaire: note technique. Ann Chir Plast Esthet 61:141–144
Saad JF (2001) Reconstrução do complexo aréolo-papilar com retalho em fechadura associado à pigmentação com tatuagem [dissertação de mestrado]. Universidade de São Paulo, Faculdade de Medicina, São Paulo, p 102
Schwartz AW (1976) Reconstruction of the nipple and areola. Br J Plast Surg 29:230–233
Sisti A, Grimaldi L, Tassinari J, Cuomo R, Fortezza L, Bocchiott MA, Roviello F, D'Aniello C, Nisi G (2016) Nipple-areola complex reconstruction techniques: a literature review. EJSO 42:441–465
Sperli AE (1974) Cosmetic reduction of the nipple with functional preservation. Br J Plast Surg 27:42–43
Spina V (1950) Neo-areoplasty with labial transplant: symmetrical correction of shape and volume of breast. Plast Reconstr Surg 6:400
Vecchione TR (1979) The reduction of the hypertrophic nipple. Aesthet Plast Surg 3:343–345
Wexler MR, Oneal RM (1973) Areola sharing to reconstruct the absent nipple. Plast Reconstr Surg 51:115

Part IV

Mastopexy and Breast Augmentation

Perspectives of Lipotransfer for Breast Augmentation

48

Alberto M.L. Caldeira, Walter Marrou Pautrat, and Miluska Bromley Cueva

48.1 Introduction

Fat transfer has become one of the most popular aesthetic and reconstructive procedures of the last decade. Originally intended as an autologous filler, as described by Neuber in 1893 when he used fat transfer to fill a depressed scar, over time we have witnessed the many properties it holds and how promising this technique has been shown to be with regard to tissue regeneration and modulation (Billings and May 1989; Chung et al. 2014).

For many surgeons, the initial enthusiasm of fat grafting was quickly abandoned because of reports involving the unpredictability of lasting results, mainly as a cause of fat reabsorption and poor recipient retention rates. As we show throughout this chapter, fat itself was not the problem, but our lack of understanding regarding the physiology of aspirated fat is what was really limiting the results of these autologous transfers. One notable surgeon who made improvements in the field during the mid1990s was Sydney Coleman, who standardized the technique to make it reproducible and have predictable results (Pu et al. 2015). He stated that fat should be transferred in small quantities to the recipient tissues and deposited in multilayered tunnels using a retrograde technique, so that most of the injected adipocytes would be in close contact with well-vascularized tissues, increasing the survival rate of the fat transferred. It was imperative not to inject fat as a bolus, because it would form lakes of transferred adipose tissue without a good oxygen supply, which in the end would produce necrosis and reabsorption of most of the transfer (Coleman 2002, 2006; Coleman and Saboeiro 2007). More recently, basic science has evolved to the point where new immunohistochemical markers and immunostains have become available, so that some groups, such as the University of Tokyo research group led by Kotaro Yoshimura, gave us an insight into how aspirated fat behaved at the molecular level when it was transferred and the importance of adipose-derived stem cells (ADSC) in this whole process (Doi et al. 2015; Eto et al. 2009, 2012; Kato et al. 2014a, b; Mineda et al. 2014; Pu et al. 2015; Suga et al. 2010).

A.M.L. Caldeira, M.D., M.Sc., Ph.D., FACS, F.I.C.S (✉)
Global Plastic Surgery Department, Casa de Saúde Portugal, Instituto de Pós-Graduação Médica Carlos Chagas/Universidade Santa Úrsula, Rio de Janeiro, RJ, Brazil

Plastic and Reconstructive Surgery Department, Caldeira-Roth Institute, Rua Visconde de Pirajá, 414 – Suite 1012, Ipanema, Rio de Janeiro, RJ CEP 22410-002, Brazil
e-mail: lottcaldeira@gmail.com

W. Marrou Pautrat, M.D. • M. Bromley Cueva, M.D.
Plastic Surgery Resident Instituto Ivo Pitanguy, Rio de Janeiro, RJ, Brazil

Instituto de Pós-Graduação Médica Carlos Chagas, Rio de Janeiro, RJ, Brazil

J.M. Avelar (ed.), *Breast Surgery*, https://doi.org/10.1007/978-3-319-54115-0_48

48.2 What Do We Currently Know About Fat Transfer?

The first thing to realize nowadays is that adipose tissue is not primarily composed of adipocytes; they only make up 16% of the tissue. Instead, a much more complex arrangement of cells has been discovered to be part of it. A rough estimate of its components would be: ADSCs 30%, fibroblasts and smooth muscle cells 30%, adipocytes 16%, endothelial cells 15%, and blood-derived cells 9%. More interesting is the organization of these cells, which by means of whole mount staining, a well-organized network of large capillaries was revealed, measuring approximately 50 μm, running alongside adipocytes, giving them oxygen and exchanging the nutrients and endocrine molecules as needed (Eto et al. 2009).

48.2.1 Excised versus Aspirated Fat Transfer

The moment a free flap (deep inferior epigastric perforator, superficial inferior epigastric artery, superior gluteal artery perforator, anterolateral thigh) is transferred to the recipient site, the arterial and venous flow are reconstituted and the adipose tissue does not change its architecture or function; thus, the result will be very predictable, with very small reabsorption rates. Why doesn't this happen when aspirated fat transfer is used?

The answer is obvious: when aspirated fat transfer is used, the cellular architecture of the tissue is severely distorted. Some of the most relevant differences are related to the destruction of most of the 50-μm capillaries that were running along adipocytes. Now, the endothelial cells composing those capillaries are randomly distributed in the aspirated tissue rather than forming functional capillaries so the adipocytes will now need to survive by plasmatic imbibition until new vessels are formed (Fig. 48.1). Another important difference is related to the percentage of ADSCs. These cells are usually found attached to blood vessels in the subcutaneous layer; thus, as the tissue is aspirated and vessels are spared, not every ADSC is collected from the donor site. This results in 23% of ADSCs being in the aspirated tissue compared with 30% at the donor site or on excised fat transfer, thus giving a lower yield of new adipocytes when the fat is reinjected, as will be seen later in this chapter (Fig. 48.2). One last difference is the number of ruptured adipocytes, calculated using glycerol-3-phosphate dehydrogenase (GPDH) activity on the tissue, showing that aspirated fat has more GPDH, which means that there are more ruptured adipocytes compared with the donor site or an excised fat transfer (Eto et al. 2009).

Many of the future perspectives in fat transfer include finding ways to counterfeit the deleterious effects of aspiration, mainly by increasing the yield of ADSCs and decreasing the rupture of adipocytes in the transfer, which can be achieved with the use of certain aspiration techniques. Other procedures to increase the final yield that are under investigation are to use normobaric hyperoxygenation after the transfer, to use cell-assisted lipotransfer techniques, or even to add M2 macrophages to the aspirated tissue. To understand how these procedures could aid in increasing the final yield of the transfer, some facts from the behavior of adipose tissue in the recipient site need to be explained.

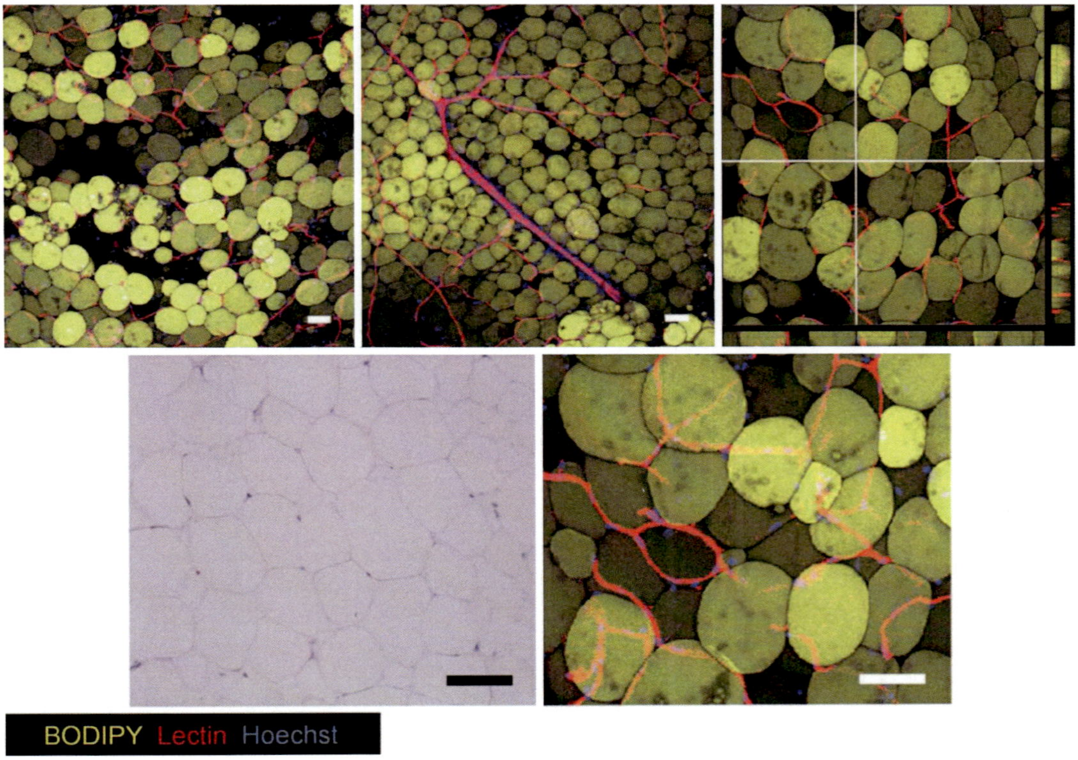

Fig. 48.1 Structure of living adipose tissue in whole-mount triple-stained images. Nonfixed aspirated and excised adipose tissues were stained with boron-dipyrromethene (adipocytes; *yellow*), lectin (endothelial cells; *red*), and Hoechst 33,342 (nuclei; *blue*) and investigated using a confocal microscope. There were many capillaries running alongside adipocytes in both aspirated and excised adipose tissue. Adipocytes, capillaries, and vessels were arranged in an organized manner in excised adipose tissue, whereas the disrupted tissue contained dead spaces, some adipocytes, and disrupted capillaries, with most of the large vessels lost in aspirated adipose tissue. Merged images of aspirated (*above, left*) and excised (*above, center*) adipose tissue respectively. Scale bars 100 μm. (*Above, right*) Dissected image example (excised adipose tissue). Images dissected horizontally and longitudinally at the levels of *white lines* are shown on the sides. Conventional histological image (*below, left*) and whole-mount triple-stained confocal image (*below, right*). Intact adipose tissue was processed with fixation, paraffin embedding, and sectioning (*below, left*). In the conventional histological examination, adipocytes appear hexagonal and there is little interstitial space between them. On the contrary, in whole-mount, triple-stained confocal micrographs of nonfixed, nonsectioned adipose tissue, adipocytes are spherical, with a substantial amount of interstitial space. Scale bars 100 μm. Reproduced with permission from Eto H, Suga H, Matsumoto D et al. (2009)Characterization of structure and cellular components of aspirated and excised adipose tissue, Plast Reconstr Surg; 124(4):1087-97. doi: 10.1097/PRS.0b013e3181b5a3f1)

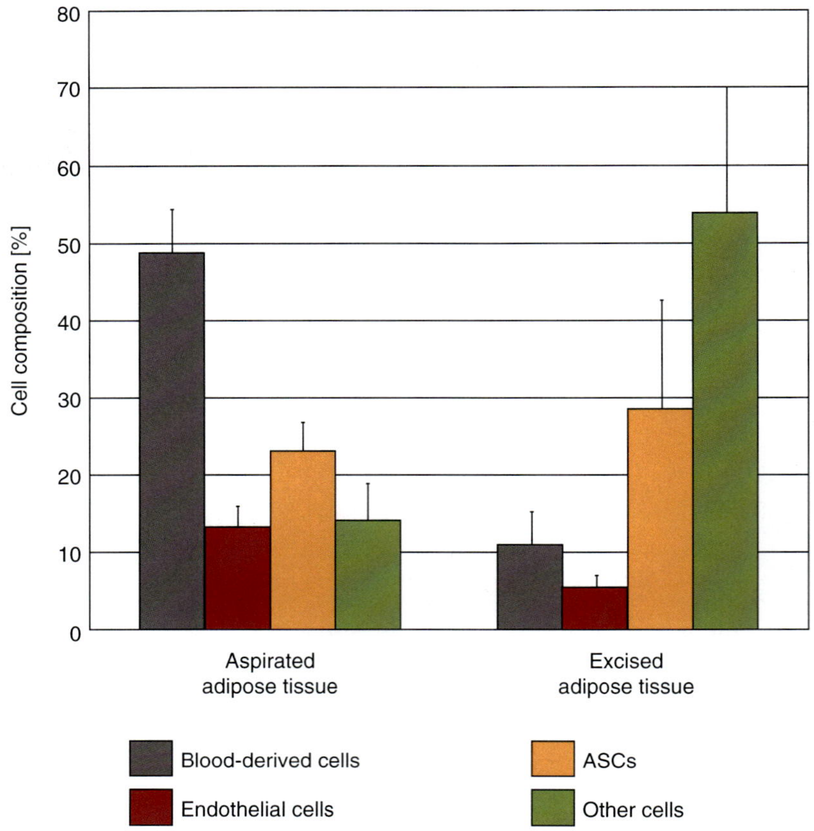

Fig. 48.2 Summarized data of cell composition obtained from stromal vascular fraction analyses (aspirated adipose tissue, $n = 9$; excised adipose tissue, $n = 3$). Values are mean ± SEM. *ASCs* adipose-derived stromal cells (Reproduced with permission from Eto H, Suga H, Matsumoto D et al. (2009) Characterization of structure and cellular components of aspirated and excised adipose tissue, Plast Reconstr Surg; 124(4):1087–97. doi: 10.1097/PRS.0b013e3181b5a3f1)

48.2.2 Degenerative Changes Induced by Ischemia

When aspired adipose tissue is transferred to a recipient site, it suffers moderate to severe ischemia because cells within the tissue are accustomed to a highly vascular environment at the donor site. Different cell types have a different resistance to ischemia. Blood-derived cells, vascular endothelial cells, and some adipocytes are the most susceptible cells and undergo apoptosis during the first 24 h. Most adipocytes resist longer and undergo a different process, known as necrosis during the third through seventh day (Fig. 48.3). This apoptotic/necrotic phenomenon starts when the oxygen threshold lies beneath 30–35 mmHg, but interestingly there is one type of cell that appears to be resistant to the effects of moderate and severe ischemia for more than 72 h. This is the ADSC, which survives long enough in an ischemic environment until vasculogenesis and angiogenesis take place to revascularize the tissue (Fig. 48.4). The function of the ADSC is to conduct the regenerative changes induced by ischemia, which takes place between the 4th day and the end of the 12th week after the fat transfer is performed (Suga et al. 2010).

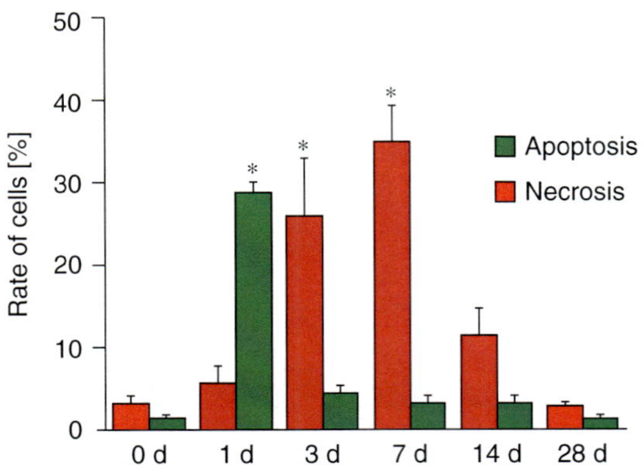

Fig. 48.3 Analysis of apoptotic and necrotic cells. Number of apoptotic (*green*) and necrotic (*red*) cells (n = 3). TUNEL-positive apoptotic cells and propidium iodide-positive necrotic cells were counted in histological sections. Apoptosis was most frequently observed on day 1, whereas necrosis was mostly observed on days 3 and 7. *p = 0.05 versus day 0 (Reproduced with permission from Suga H, Eto H, Aoi N et al. (2010) Adipose tissue remodeling under ischemia: death of adipocytes and activation of stem/progenitor cells, Plast Reconstr Surg; 126(6):1911-23. doi: 10.1097/PRS.0b013e3181f4468b)

But, why don't all these degenerative and further regenerative processes happen with free flaps, but do occur with aspirated fat transfers? Simply because what triggers the process is moderate to severe ischemia. Going into more detail, adipocyte death up-regulates two important proteins: HIF-1alpha and FGF-2. These two peptides are responsible for the activation of ADSCs and the beginning of the regenerative changes induced by ischemia (Fig. 48.5).

Moreover, it was discovered that dead adipocytes are reabsorbed much slower than the newly regenerated cells, thus serving as a scaffold for tissue remodeling, giving an imprint to the newly formed tissue (Kato et al. 2014b; Suga et al. 2010). Dead adipocytes cluster together to form oil droplets. The reabsorption of these droplets occurs by the macrophage lineage. It was not long ago that we thought indistinctly that macrophages were inflammatory cells scavenging the different tissues of the body. Now our knowledge indicates that there are two types of macrophages, M1 and M2. The former are the classic inflammatory cells that exist in the regenerating and necrotic zones whose job is to absorb the oil droplets by surrounding them in a single layer and eventually consuming the oil. The latter, in

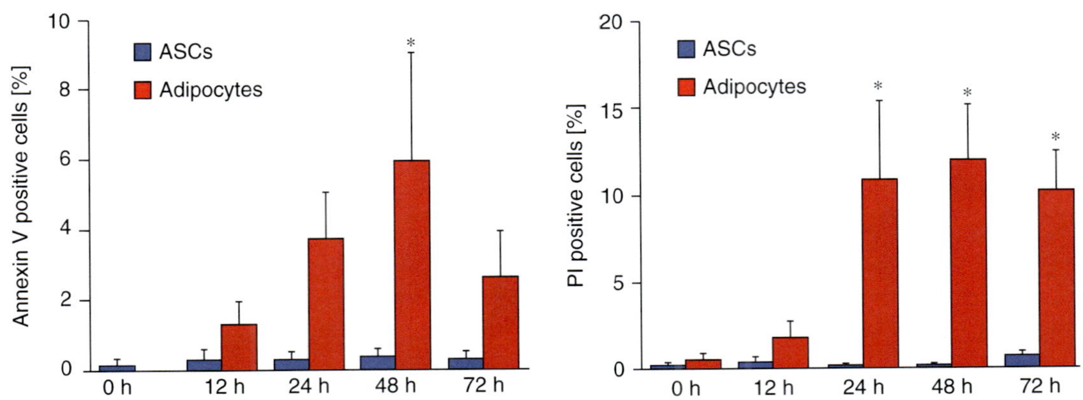

Fig. 48.4 Quantification of annexin V-positive apoptotic cells (*below, left*) and propidium iodide-positive necrotic cells (*below, right*; n = 4) is shown. *p = 0.05 versus 0 h (Reproduced with permission from Suga H, Eto H, Aoi N et al. (2010) Adipose tissue remodeling under ischemia: death of adipocytes and activation of stem/progenitor cells, Plast Reconstr Surg; 126(6):1911--23. doi: 10.1097/PRS.0b013e3181f4468b)

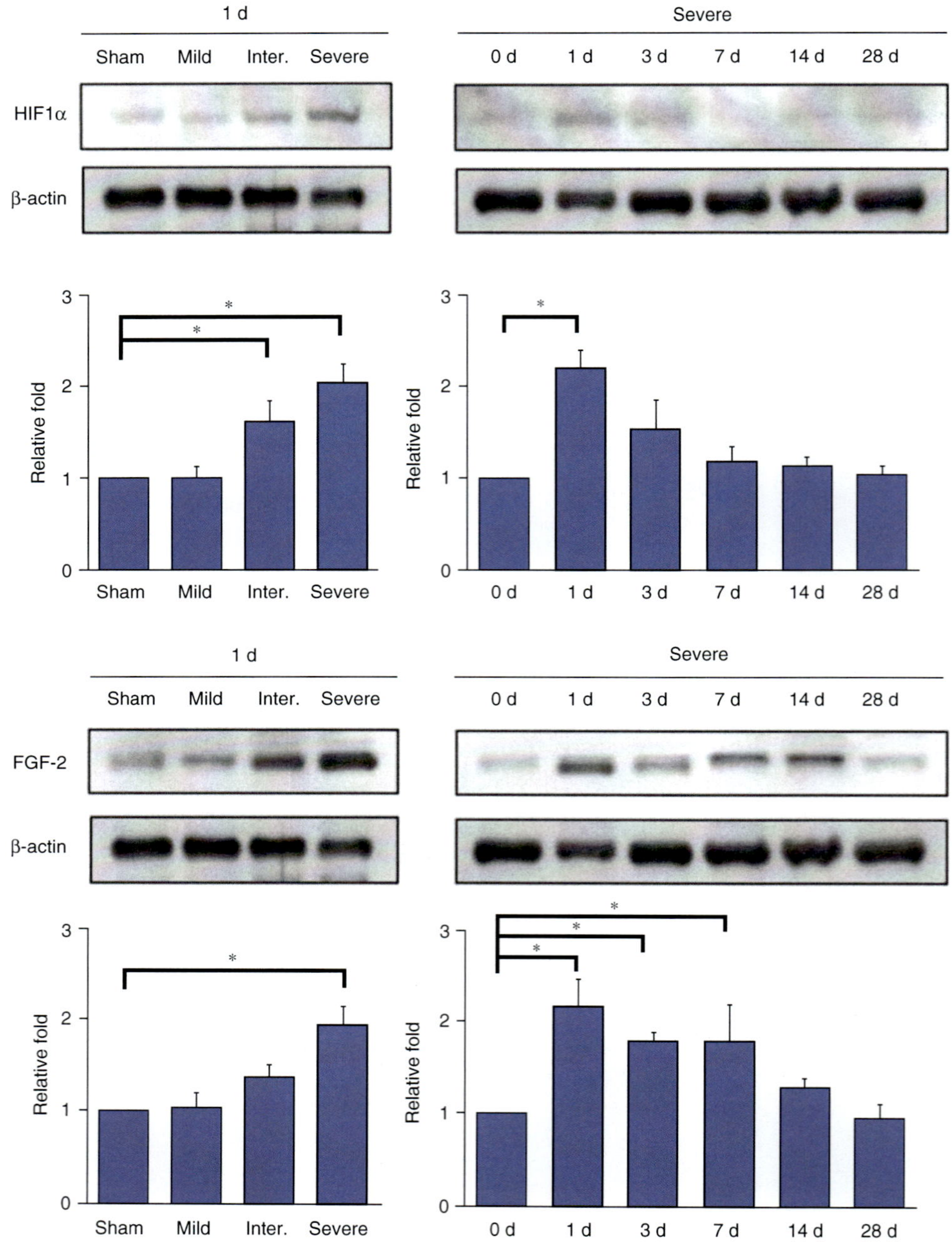

Fig. 48.5 Expression of HIF-1 and FGF-2 proteins in adipose tissue with hypoxia. (*Above*, *left*) Western blotting for HIF-1 was performed in each ischemia model on day 1. β-Actin was used as an internal control. HIF-1 protein was up-regulated in the intermediate and severe models. $*p = 0.05$ versus sham ($n = 3$). Sequential changes in HIF-1 protein expression were observed in adipose tissue exposed to severe ischemia (*above*, *right*). A significant elevation was observed on day 1. $*p = 0.05$ versus day 0 ($n = 3$). (*Below*, *left*) Images showing Western blotting for FGF-2 on day 1. FGF-2 protein was up-regulated in the intermediate and severe models. The β-actin signal served as an internal control. $*p = 0.05$ versus sham ($n = 3$). Sequential changes in FGF-2 protein expression in adipose tissue exposed to severe ischemia are shown (*below*, *right*). A significant elevation was observed on days 1, 3, and 7. $*p = 0.05$ versus day 0 ($n = 3$) (Reproduced with permission from Suga H, Eto H, Aoi N et al. (2010) Adipose tissue remodeling under ischemia: death of adipocytes and activation of stem/progenitor cells, Plast Reconstr Surg; 126(6):1911–-23. doi: 10.1097/PRS.0b013e3181f4468b)

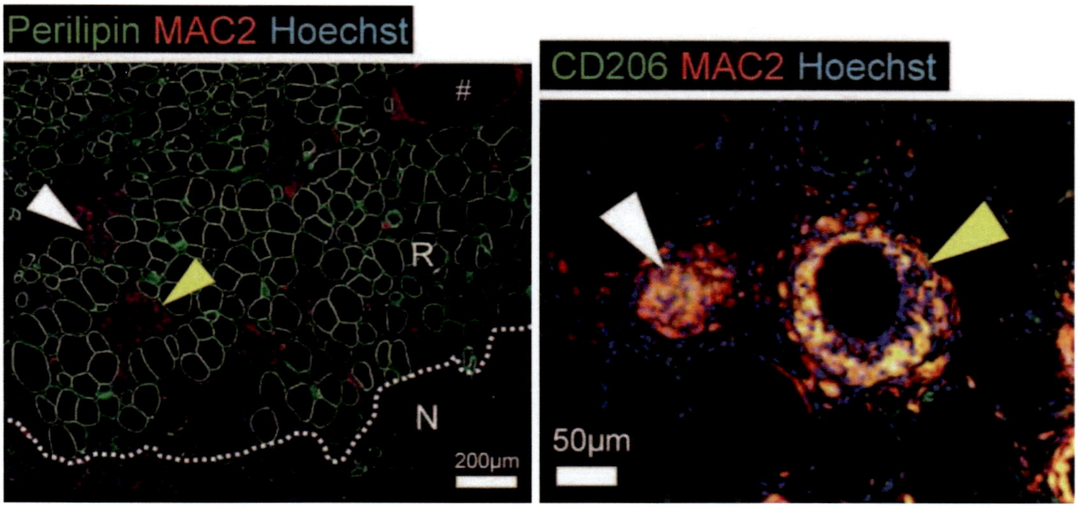

Fig. 48.6 At 12 weeks, in border areas between the regenerating (*R*) and necrotizing (*N*) zones, adipogenesis appeared to be complete, but oil absorption and fibrous replacement were still ongoing. In addition to large oil drops (#) surrounded by macrophages, adipocyte-sized macrophage clusters were observed with (*yellow arrowheads*) or without (*white arrowheads*) lipid droplets inside (*left*; scale bar = 200 μm). The lipid droplet-containing macrophage cluster was composed of an innermost single layer of M1 macrophages (MAC2 + CD206−) and outer multilayered M2 macrophages (MAC2 + CD206−; *right*; scale bar = 50 μm). It is suspected that M2 macrophages appeared in unfavorable conditions where adipocyte regeneration had failed and fibrous replacement of the space was needed. Reproduced with permission from KatoH, Mineda K, Eto H et al. (2014b) Degeneration, regeneration, and cicatrization after fat grafting: dynamic total tissue remodeling during the first 3 months, Plast Reconstr Surg; 133(3):303e-313e. doi: 10.1097/PRS.0000000000000066)

contrast to M1 macrophages, are a new type of cell that has been recently discovered and that has anti-inflammatory properties. When M1 macrophages are not able to reabsorb the oil droplet completely, M2 cells surround the M1 macrophages to form a crown-like structure with fibrous replacement properties causing fibrosis of the space occupied by the oil (Kato et al. 2014b; Suga et al. 2010). They only appear in unfavorable conditions, where adipocyte regeneration has failed, as in the necrotic zone, to help M1 macrophages (Fig. 48.6).

48.2.3 Regenerative Changes Caused by Ischemia

In the last section, the effects of ischemia on the fat transfer were determined and how it triggered a degenerative process of the tissue. Now it is time to see the other side of the coin: how the body responds and fights ischemia to preserve the tissue transfer in the best way possible. It is ambiguous, but ischemia not only destroys endothelial cells and adipocytes, but it also regenerates them. Going into a more detailed picture, we see that the HIF-alpha and FGF-2 molecules produced by dying adipocytes activate a more hypoxia-resistant cell lineage (Suga et al. 2010), the ADSC. As shown before (Fig. 48.4), these types of cells can adequately resist hypoxia for 72 h or more, the time needed for angiogenesis and vasculogenesis to rebuild the capillary network around the tissue transfer (Suga et al. 2010). More importantly, when activated, they are transformed into new adipocytes. This adipogenesis begins in the first week after the tissue transfer, peaks at 4 weeks and lasts for approximately for 12 weeks (Fig. 48.7) (Kato et al. 2014b).

What proof do I have that this is happening? Is it possible to discriminate dying adipocytes from newly formed ones under the microscope? Using modern immunohistochemistry, it has been noted that the small adipocytes shown on

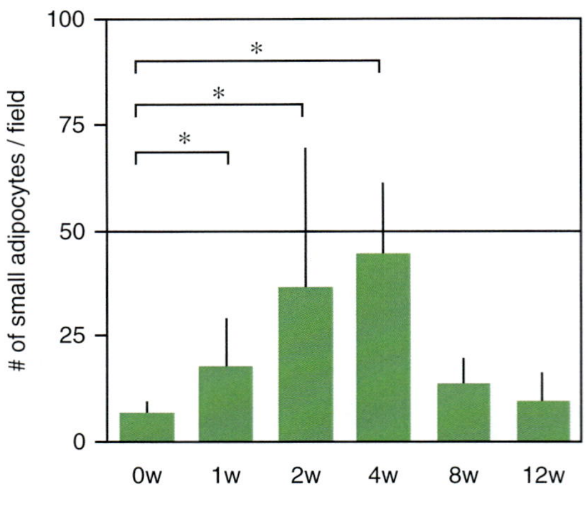

Fig. 48.7 Sequential changes in the number of new adipocytes. Newly born adipocytes (preadipocytes), which are small (<20 μm) and strongly positive for perilipin, were counted. Adipogenesis peaked at 4 weeks and returned to baseline level by 12 weeks (*$p < 0.05$) (Reproduced with permission from Kato H, Mineda K, Eto H et al. (2014b) Degeneration, regeneration, and cicatrization after fat grafting: dynamic total tissue remodeling during the first 3 months, Plast Reconstr Surg; 133(3):303e-313e. doi: 10.1097/PRS.0000000000000066)

days 7 and 14 were positive for perilipin, a membrane marker for viable adipocytes. They were also negative for propidium iodide, indicating newly formed adipocytes rather than necrotizing ones (Suga et al. 2010). Furthermore, the tissue was stained with CD34 (an ADSC marker) and Ki67 (a cell-proliferating marker) showing the small adipocytes located close to old dead adipocytes to be CD34 and Ki67 positive, meaning they were proliferating ADSCs, thus confirming our findings in a definitive manner (Fig. 48.8) (Suga et al. 2010).

Even more interesting are findings that show that ADSCs are cells that not only have the property to generate new adipocytes, but they also bear the capacity to hatch new endothelial cells (Suga et al. 2010). This closes a regeneration circle, by which activated ADSCs form new adipocytes that are nourished by newly generated capillaries formed by endothelial cells derived from the same activated ADSCs.

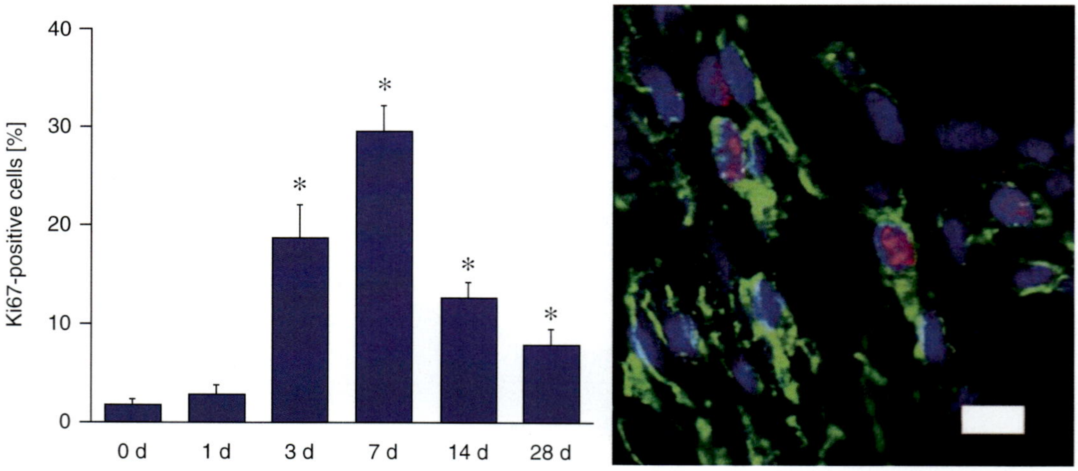

Fig. 48.8 Analysis of proliferating cells. (*Left*) Number of Ki67-positive proliferating cells ($n = 3$). Proliferative cells increased in number under ischemia, peaking on day 7. *$p = 0.05$ versus day 0. Immunohistochemistry for CD34 (*green*), Ki67 (*red*), and 4′ ,6-diamidino-2-phenylindole staining (nuclei, *blue*) on day 7 (*right*). Cells positive for both CD34 and Ki67 were observed. Scale bar 10 μm (Reproduced with permission from Suga H, Eto H, Aoi N et al. (2010) Adipose tissue remodeling under ischemia: death of adipocytes and activation of stem/progenitor cells, Plast Reconstr Surg; 126(6):1911–23. doi: 10.1097/PRS.0b013e3181f4468b)

48.2.4 Everything Has an Order

Compelling evidence has been presented in this chapter to support "compensatory proliferation," or the physiological turnover of adipocytes from fat transfer in response to ischemia (Eto et al. 2012). But how do these principles work throughout the tissue? Does all the transferred tissue behave the same? The research group from Tokyo University led by Yoshimura discovered that ischemia was the driving force behind the process. Moreover, it was observed that the fat transferred was not homogeneously hypoxic, but that the distance of plasmatic diffusion was strictly limited by a gradient of oxygen and nutrients. This meant that the tissue transferred further from recipient vessels would have higher rates of necrosis than the tissue located closer to them, because of the partial pressures of oxygen being smaller for the former tissue than for the latter (Eto et al. 2012).

This is how the "three-zone" model was created (Eto et al. 2012; Kato et al. 2014b). Here, the fat transfer is divided into three zones: a superficial surviving zone, an intermediate regenerative zone, and a deep necrotic zone (Figs. 48.9 and 48.10).

The surviving zone, which is the most superficial layer of the transfer, has an extent of 300 μm and is composed of one to several rows of mature adipocytes that remain intact over time. Neither degeneration nor regeneration of adipocytes is observed here. The reason is its proximity to receptor vessels; thus, oxygen and nutrients pass

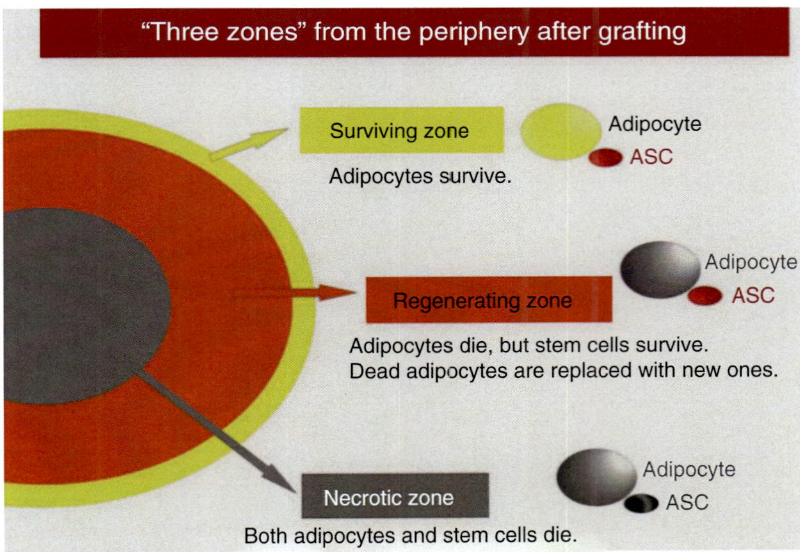

Fig. 48.9 Conclusive schema for three zones of the grafts. The most superficial zone is the "surviving zone," which is less than 300 μm thick. In the surviving zone, both adipocytes and adipose-derived stromal cells (*ASCs*) survive. The second zone is the "regenerating zone," the thickness of which varies depending on the microenvironmental conditions such as the vascularity of and attachment to the surrounding tissue. In this zone, adipocytes die as early as day 1, but adipose-derived stromal cells survive and provide new adipocytes to replace the dead ones. The most central zone is the "necrotic zone," where both adipocytes and adipose-derived stromal cells die, no regeneration is expected, and the dead space is absorbed or filled by scar formation (Reproduced with permission from Eto H, Kato H, Suga H et al. (2012) The fate of adipocytes after nonvascularized fat grafting: evidence of early death and replacement of adipocytes, Plast Reconstr Surg; 129(5):1081–-92.doi:10.1097/PRS.0b013e31824a2b19)

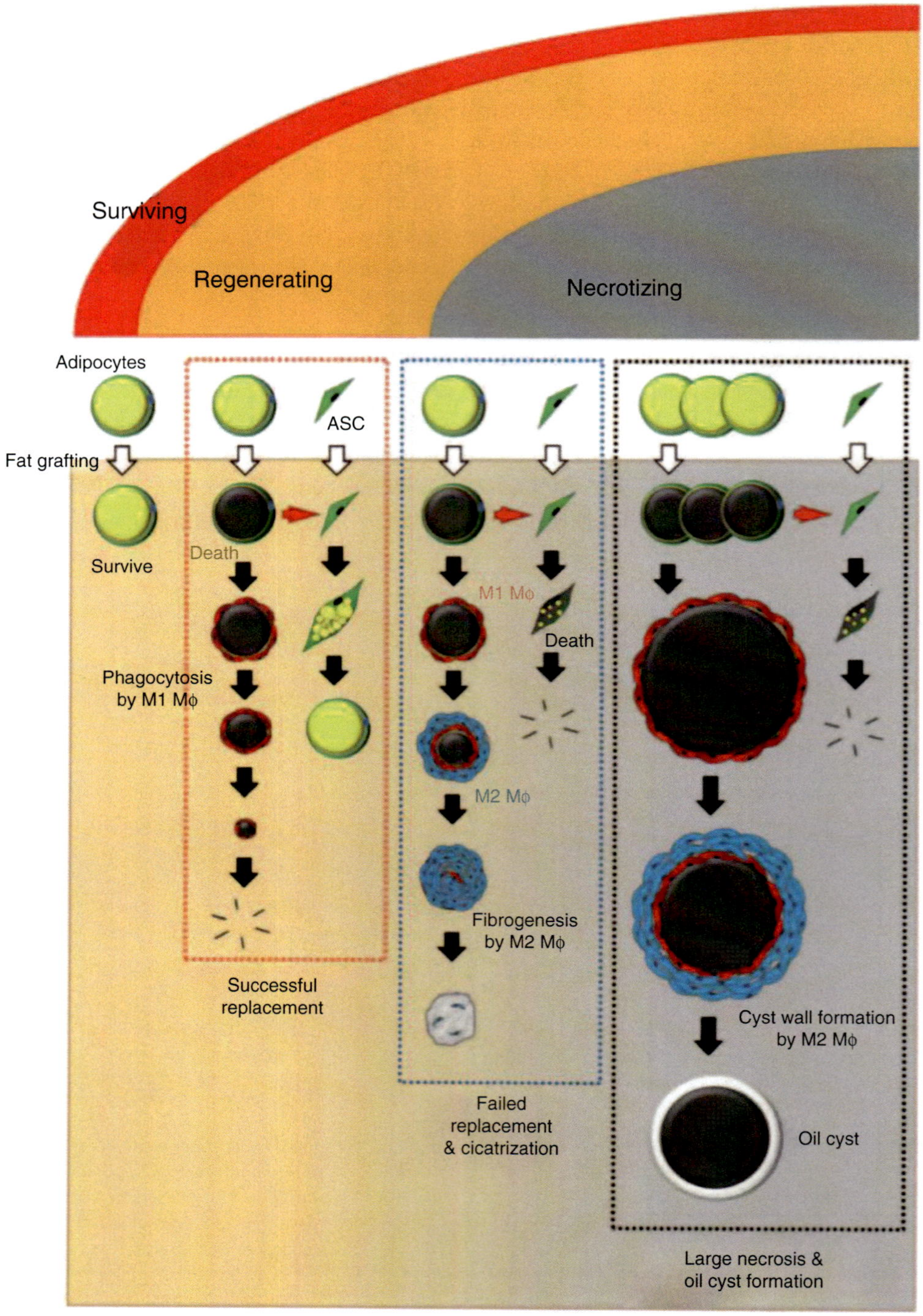

Fig. 48.10 Conclusive schema for the fate of adipocytes in grafted fat. During the first 3 months of adipose tissue remodeling, transplanted adipocytes have differential fates depending on their microenvironments. In this schema, complex cellular events are simplified and the adipocyte fate is categorized into four patterns: survival, successful regeneration, failed regeneration (cicatrization), and oil cyst formation. Cicatrization and oil cyst formation are often not complete at 3 months. *ASC* adipose stem/progenitor/stromal cells (Reproduced with permission from Kato H, Mineda K, Eto H et al. (2014b) Degeneration, regeneration, and cicatrization after fat grafting: dynamic total tissue remodeling during the first 3 months, Plast Reconstr Surg; 133(3):303e-313e. doi: 10.1097/PRS.0000000000000066)

freely to the transferred adipocytes, maintaining an O_2 partial pressure above 35 mmHg (Kato et al. 2014b).

The regenerative zone lays deeper within the tissue: from 300–1,200 μm. Here, the oxygen threshold is beneath 30 mmHg, and adipocytes, blood-derived cells, and endothelial cells die shortly after the procedure, but ADSCs survive. During the first 7 days, oil droplets are seen where the adipocytes have died. From the second week to the eighth week numerous growing pre-adipocytes emerge between oil droplets surrounded by M1 macrophages. At 12 weeks, the tissue is filled with matured adipocytes and appears intact, with all oil droplets successfully reabsorbed, thus confirming that the regeneration process has taken place (Kato et al. 2014b).

The necrotic zone accounts for the deepest areas of the transfer, those more than 1,200 μm from receptor vessels. An interesting concept arises within the necrotic zone: the deeper the tissue transfer is located, the further from nourishing capillaries it is. This limits the oxygen gradient to levels in which adipocytes and even ADSCs do not survive, thus increasing the size of the necrotic tissue, which translates into a greater fat reabsorption quotient. When put into practice, the best way to avoid placing fat deep into an avascular plane is to inject small amounts in a retrograde fashion, following Coleman's technique, being careful not to administer it as a bolus (Kato et al. 2014b).

Adipocytes placed in the necrotic zone travel through two different pathways depending on the amount of fat injected into this section of the transfer. If a small amount of fat is injected into the receptor area, then the necrotic area is small and oil droplets form, surrounded by crownlike structures of M1 and M2 macrophages unable to reabsorb the oil successfully, causing fibrosis of the tissue (Kato et al. 2014b; Suga et al. 2010). On the other hand, if large quantities of fat are placed in the necrotic zone, the oil droplets tend to cluster and form oil cysts, which contain M1 and M2 macrophages, degenerated fat, and fibrous tissue in their walls. This makes the microenvironment of the cyst inadequate for adipogenesis, favoring chronic inflammation that persists for years, associated with progressive fibrosis and calcifications, which are the worst outcomes possible for breast fat transfer procedures because of the potential to be confounded with malignant lesions (Mineda et al. 2014).

48.3 Future Perspectives in Fat Transfer

Everything tends to an equilibrium, especially in the human body where homeostasis is the ruling principle of human physiology. Thus, why it is surprising that when a tissue is transferred from one part of the body to another, it is not merely a mechanical transposition, but a dynamic remodeling of that tissue to comply with the specific functions of that organ or system? The fat transferred to the breast degenerates and activates some ADSCs to regenerate new adipocytes to function in the new organ. It can be seen as a balance of degeneration = regeneration. Up to this year, the variables hiding beneath the two processes could not be totally elucidated, consequently producing regeneration rates ranging from 20 to 70% of what was transferred in the first place. The aim for the years to come is to maximize this regeneration percentage to reach proportions of 80, 90, or 100% of the fat originally injected. This is clearly the future regarding fat transfer procedures. In the next paragraphs, some experimental proceedings that try to maximize regeneration rates are shown, to provide a clearer idea of the path that research is taking within this exciting branch of plastic surgery.

48.3.1 Supplementation of M2 Macrophages

It is now known that M2 macrophages are a new type of cell with anti-inflammatory properties, such as an increased expression of IL-10 and arginase-1 (Fig. 48.11). They also seem to produce pro-angiogenic factors such as vascular endothelial growth factor, basic fibroblast growth factor, and matrix metalloproteinases, thus promoting angiogenesis. Because of these data, a

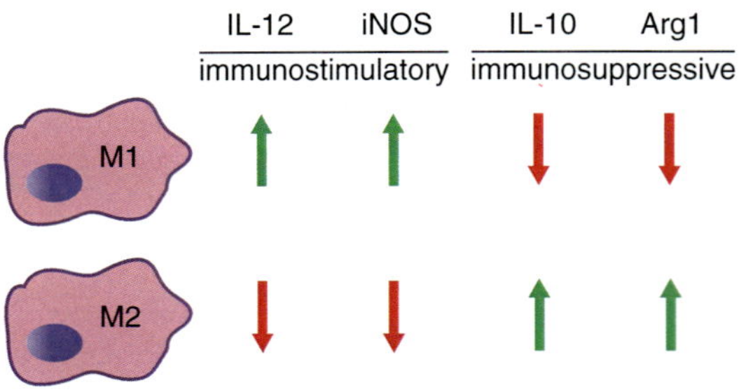

Fig. 48.11 Schematic representation of macrophage polarization. M1 macrophage polarization results in increased expression of interleukin-12 (*IL-12*) and inducible nitric oxide synthase (*iNOS*), and M2 macrophage polarization results in increased expression of arginase-1 (*Arg1*) and interleukin-10 (*IL-10*). Polarized M1 macrophages decrease the expression of interleukin-10 and arginase-1, and M2 macrophages decrease interleukin-12 and inducible nitric oxide synthase expression (Reproduced with permission from PhippsKD, Gebremeskel S, Gillis J et al. (2015) Alternatively activated M2 macrophages improve autologous Fat Graft survival in a mouse model through induction of angiogenesis, Plast Reconstr Surg; 135(1):140–9. doi: 10.1097/PRS.0000000000000793)

randomized clinical trial (RCT) comparing fat transfer supplemented with M2 macrophages vs fat transfer alone was performed, concluding that there was a significant difference ($p < 0.02$) between the groups. An increased number of blood vessels was observed in the M2 supplemented transfers, thus confirming the angiogenic effect of the M2 cell lineage (Fig. 48.12). This information is of utmost interest because increased angiogenesis means a reduction in the necrotic zone and an increase in regeneration rates (Phipps et al. 2015).

48.3.2 Effect of *N*-Acetylcysteine in Fat Transfer Survival

N-acetylcysteine is a widely known antioxidant that works by reducing oxygen free radicals using a sulfhydryl chemical group. It is established that during fat harvest, before the trans-

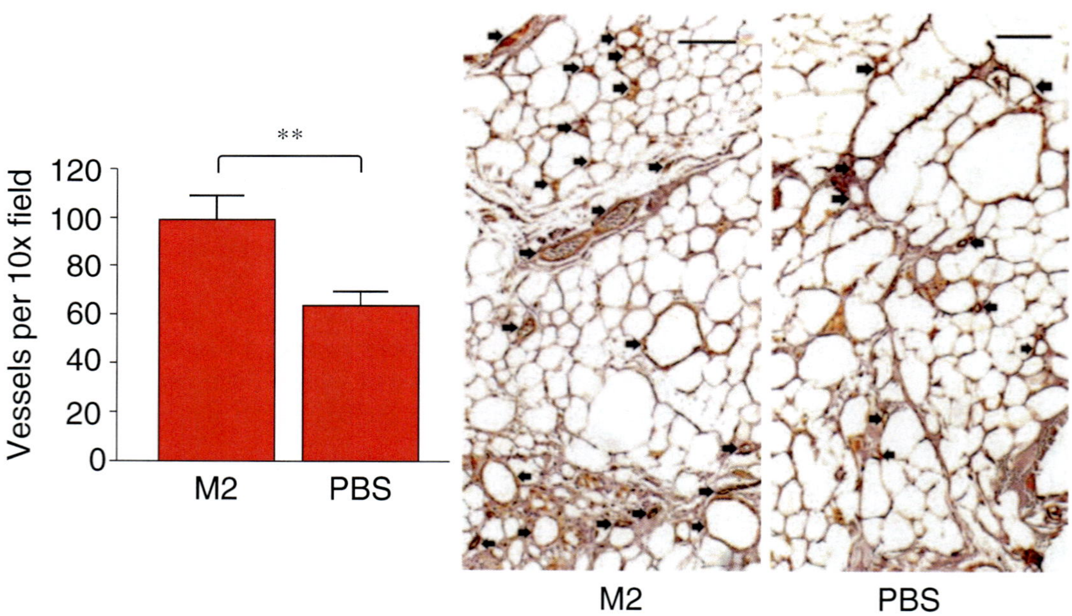

Fig. 48.12 CD31 immunostaining of fat grafts at 3 months after injection (scale bar = 100 µm). Increased numbers of CD31+ staining blood vessels (*arrows*) were observed in M2 macrophage-supplemented grafts (*center*) compared with phosphate-buffered saline (*PBS*) control (*right*) grafts. This difference in the number of blood vessels was significant (*left*) (**$p < 0.02$) (Reproduced with permission from Phipps KD, Gebremeskel S, Gillis J et al. (2015) Alternatively activated M2 macrophages improve autologous Fat Graft survival in a mouse model through induction of angiogenesis, Plast Reconstr Surg; 135(1):140–9. doi: 10.1097/PRS.0000000000000793)

fer, isolated cells are put under significant mechanical, ischemic, and oxidative stress, which results in cell injury and a reduced regeneration rate in the future. That is why in the last year, a research group was interested in determining whether *N*-acetylcysteine administered at the site of the harvest could improve long-term regeneration percentages. For this, an RCT was designed comparing the two groups, one adding *N*-acetylcysteine to the tumescent fluid of the lipoaspiration and the other using a normal tumescent fluid. Results at 3 months after injection of fat into mouse models showed a significant difference ($p < 0.01$) between the groups. Volumetric microcomputed tomographic data analysis exhibits a larger volume of the fat transferred in the *N*-acetylcysteine group compared with the control group (Fig. 48.13). This can be explained simply by the antioxidant mechanism of *N*-acetylcysteine limiting the damage done by reactive oxygen species in the necrotic zone, thus reducing the proportion of dead ADSCs and increasing the regeneration rate (Gillis et al. 2015).

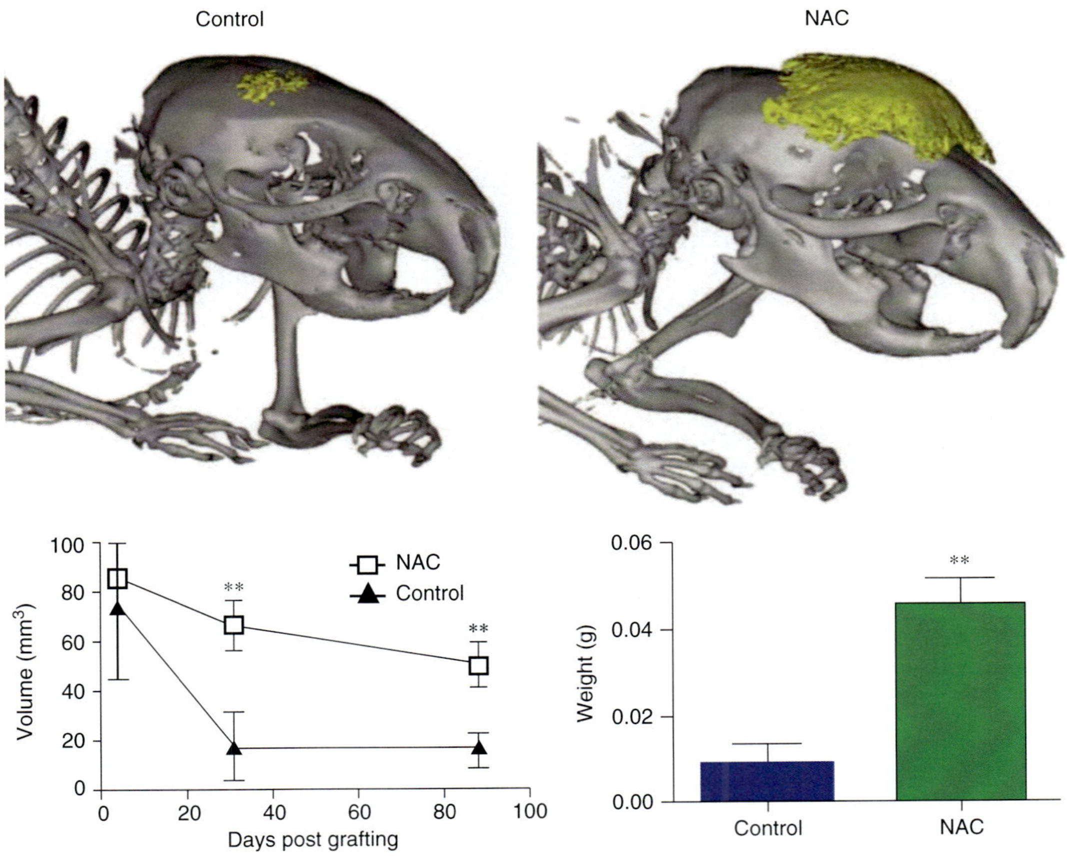

Fig. 48.13 Effects of *N*-acetylcysteine (*NAC*) on free fat grafting in vivo. Representative three-dimensional reconstructions of microcomputed tomographic data of control (no *N*-acetylcysteine) and *N*-acetylcysteine–treated fat grafts at 3 months after injection (*above*). (*Below, left*) Volumetric micro–computed tomographic data analysis of grafts at 4 days, 1 month, and 3 months after injection ($n = 15$ per group). (*Below, right*) Explanted fat graft weights at 3 months after injection ($n = 15$ per group). $^{**}p < 0.01$ (Reproduced with permission from Gillis J, Gebremeskel S, Phipps KD et al. (2015) Effect of N-Acetylcysteine on Adipose-Derived Stem Cell and Autologous Fat Graft Survival in a Mouse Model, Plast Reconstr Surg; 136(2):179e-188e. doi: 10.1097/PRS.0000000000001443)

48.3.3 The Role of Aging, Body Mass Index, and Harvest Site

During the last few years there has been discussion about what is the ideal age at which to harvest fat, and whether results differ regarding adipocyte viability when fat is harvested from young patients compared with older ones? Is the body mass index (BMI) a decisive factor with regard to adipocyte quality and regeneration rate? Finally, there was much controversy in relation to the site from which fat was harvested. Is abdominal fat better than fat from the inner thigh? Two years ago, a paper was published to address these issues with the use of a prospective, cross-sectional study of 24 healthy patients. It concerned the dry aspiration of fat from 24 female patients undergoing plastic surgery procedures. They were separated into different groups: younger (up to 45 years), older (more than 45 years), normal weight (BMI from 20.5 to 24), and overweight (BMI from 25 to 34.5). Fat samples of all patients were obtained from the following sites: flanks, lower abdomen, and inner thighs. The outcome was adipocyte viability, measured using propidium iodide. Results showed that adipocyte viability was similar (not statistically significant) in younger and older patients, between normal-weight and overweight patients, and finally among all three harvest sites. The only statistically significant results appear to be the interaction between age and harvest site (Fig. 48.14). Here, it is important to notice the difference in the younger group between the lower abdomen and flank harvest sites ($p = 0.014$), supporting adipocyte viability from the lower abdomen compared with the flanks in this age group. Similarly, it is observed that in young patients, fat is preferably harvested from the lower abdomen ($p = 0.0122$), whereas older patients benefit more from fat harvested from the flanks ($p = 0.0399$) (Geissler et al. 2014).

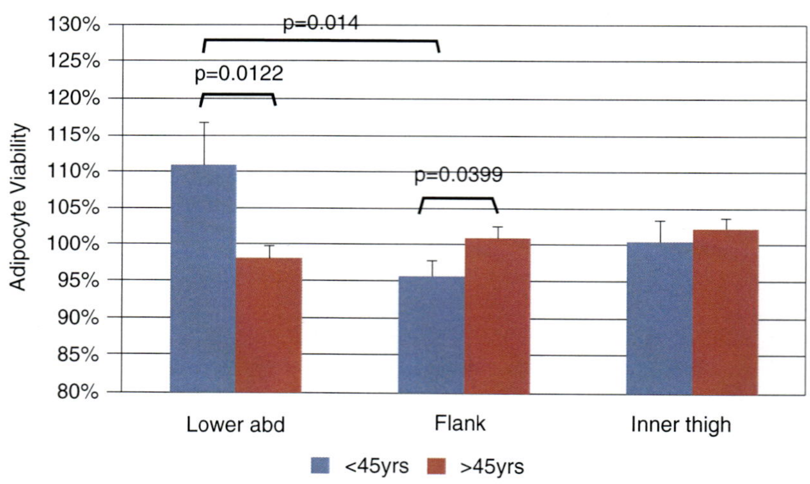

Fig. 48.14 Comparison of adipocyte viability calculated for adipocytes harvested from the lower abdomen, flank, and inner thigh depots of younger and older groups. A significant difference is observed in the younger group between the lower abdomen and the flank. No significant difference in adipocytes was observed among the three harvest sites in the older group. Adipocyte viability is reduced in the lower abdomen depot in the older group compared with the younger group. Adipocytes from the flank have greater viability in the older group compared with the younger group (Reproduced with permission from Geissler PJ, Davis K, Roostaeian J et al. (2014) Improving fat transfer viability: the role of aging, body mass index, and harvest site, Plast Reconstr Surg; 134(2):227–-32. doi: 10.1097/PRS.0000000000000398)

48.3.4 Impact of Local Anesthetics on Preadipocyte Viability

Until not long ago, no one thought that local anesthetics used in infiltration solutions used to harvest fat could affect preadipocyte viability. A few years ago, this paradigm suddenly changed with the publication of an article that tested different local anesthetics and their impact on preadipocyte survival, measured by propidium iodide. Results from this trial demonstrated that with the exception of bupivacaine, all local anesthetics significantly reduced cell viability, but to different extents (Fig. 48.15). Among the most common local anesthetics used, articaine and lidocaine were the most detrimental with regard to preadipocyte viability. These data are important in the context of choosing the right local anesthetic to maximize preadipocytes, and in the long run, adipocyte viability (Keck et al. 2010).

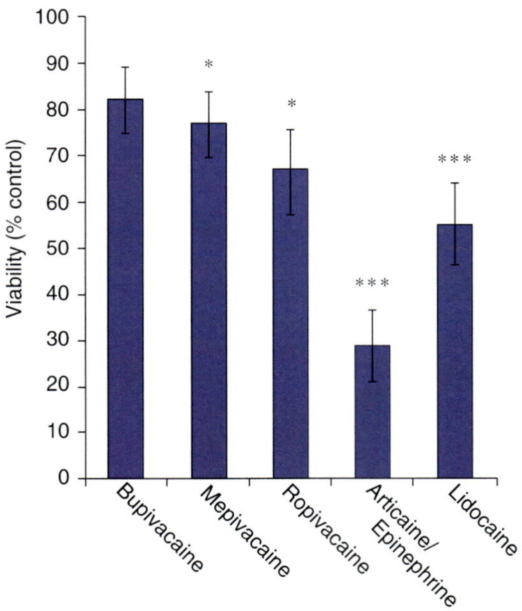

Fig. 48.15 Viability of preadipocytes after treatment with local anesthetics. Viability was assessed by flow cytometry immediately after treatment with the indicated local anesthetics. The diagram shows cell viability in mean SEM, with the saline control treatment taken as 100% (n = 15). Significant differences from controls are indicated by *asterisks*: *p = 0.05; ***p = 0.001 (Reproduced with permission from Keck M, Zeyda M, Gollinger K et al. (2010) Local anesthetics have a major impact on viability of preadipocytes and their differentiation into adipocytes, Plast Reconstr Surg; 126(5):1500–5. doi: 10.1097/PRS.0b013e3181ef8beb)

48.3.5 Effect of Normobaric Hyperoxygenation in Fat Transfer

This groundbreaking idea was published 2 years ago and consists in evaluating the effect of normobaric hyperoxygenation on the final retention rate of fat transfers. The theory states that recipient tissues are responsible for providing the tissue transferred with oxygen and nutrients through plasmatic diffusion until the ingrowing neovasculature develops. The driving force of this diffusion is the gradient of oxygen partial pressure, which is normally low in adipose tissue. An effective way of increasing oxygen partial pressure would be to increase the percentage of inhaled oxygen, thus forcing more oxygen to the recipient's adipose tissue, hosting an adequate environment for adipocyte regeneration. The experiment was performed using mouse models exposed to 60% normobaric hyperoxygenation therapy and a control group using 20% oxygen (room air) for the first 3 days after the tissue transfer. The results showed tree important findings:

1. The surviving zone was much thicker in normobaric hyperoxygenation samples than in control samples at 1 week (Fig. 48.16).
2. The preadipocyte number was significantly larger in normobaric hyperoxygenation grafts than in controls at 4 weeks ($p = 0.016$), showing an increase in the regeneration zone.
3. Postoperative hyperoxygenation reduces the de-necrotizing area of the tissue transfer at 12 weeks.

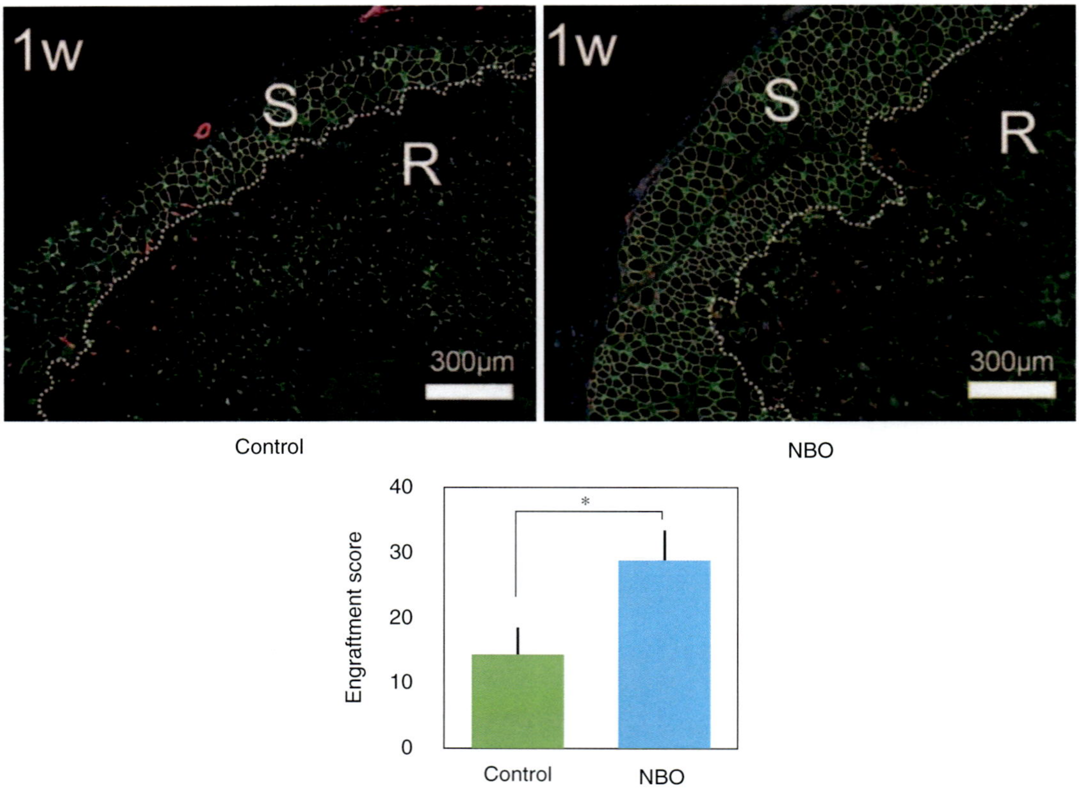

Fig. 48.16 Surviving zones in autologous fat grafts in controls and mice with normobaric hyperoxygenation. Adipocytes located in the most superficial layers (surviving zone) probably survived because of direct plasmatic diffusion of the required nutrients and oxygen from the surrounding intact recipient tissues. All adipocytes died within 1 week in the deeper zones (regenerating and necrotizing zones). (*Above*) Immunostained fat graft sections (*green*, perilipin for viable adipocytes; *red*, MAC-2 for macrophages; and *blue*, Hoechst 33,342 for nuclei) at 1 week after fat grafting. The surviving zone (area strongly positive for perilipin) was clearly demarcated by 1 week. *Dashed lines* indicate the border of the areas strongly and weakly positive for perilipin. The surviving zone was much thicker in normobaric hyperoxygenation samples than in control samples. Scale bars = 300 μm. *S* surviving zone, *R* regenerating zone. (*Below*) Mature adipocytes survived significantly longer in normobaric hyperoxygenation grafts than in controls. Engraftment scores (normalized sample weight/normalized initial sample weight × percentage of area of viable adipocytes) were calculated for comparison. (Reproduced with permission from Kato H, Araki J, Doi K et al. (2014) Normobaric hyperoxygenation enhances initial survival, regeneration, and final retention in fat grafting, Plast Reconstr Surg; 134(5):951–9. doi:10.1097/PRS.0000000000000600)

Normobaric hyperoxygenation is still under research, but possesses great potential for increasing the regeneration rate of the transfer (Kato et al. 2014a).

Conclusion

In this chapter, we have shifted paradigms from what was known about fat transfer procedures. The traditional "cell survival theory" was substituted for a "cell replacement theory," which explains much better the behavior of fat when injected into a recipient tissue. The balance between degeneration and regeneration is demonstrated, that is important for every system inside the body to maintain homeostasis.

After a thorough understanding of how a process works, we are capable of modifying parts of it to obtain different results. This is exactly what it is all about for the next few years, what can be done to increase the final retention rate of the tissue transfer. Some interesting techniques have been presented in the final section of the chapter, among which the normobaric hyperoxygenation concept is thought to have a bright future. There are other concepts currently being studied to increase the effectiveness of fat transfer procedures, one of which is estrogen modulation. It is known that estrogenic receptors are very important in adipose tissue; therefore, ongoing research is being carried out into increasing the final regeneration percentage of fat injected into a recipient site by altering the estrogen concentration gradient inside the tissue itself (Chung et al. 2014; Bills et al. 2015).

What does the future hold for fat transfer procedures? It is something that no one knows for sure. What is clear is only that the road is becoming much more interesting than before. We are lucky to live and work in the decade of the development of regenerative surgery.

References

Billings E Jr, May JW Jr (1989) Historical review and present status of free fat graft autotransplantation in plastic and reconstructive surgery. Plast Reconstr Surg 83(2):368–381

Bills JD, Derderian C, Barker J et al (2015) The role of estrogen in the modulation of autologous fat graft outcomes. Plast Reconstr Surg 135(1):103e–113e. doi:10.1097/PRS.0000000000000792

Chung MT, Paik KJ, Atashroo DA et al (2014) Studies in fat grafting. I. Effects of injection technique on in vitro fat viability and in vivo volume retention. Plast Reconstr Surg 134(1):29–38. doi:10.1097/PRS.0000000000000290

Coleman SR (2002) Hand rejuvenation with structural fat grafting. Plast Reconstr Surg 110(7):1731–1744

Coleman SR (2006) Structural fat grafting: more than a permanent filler. Plast Reconstr Surg 118(3 Suppl):108S–120S

Coleman SR, Saboeiro AP (2007) Fat grafting to the breast revisited: safety and efficacy. Plast Reconstr Surg 119(3):775–785

Doi K, Ogata F, Eto H et al (2015) Differential contributions of graft-derived and host-derived cells in tissue regeneration/remodeling after fat grafting. Plast Reconstr Surg 135(6):1607–1617. doi:10.1097/PRS.0000000000001292

Eto H, Suga H, Matsumoto D et al (2009) Characterization of structure and cellular components of aspirated and excised adipose tissue. Plast Reconstr Surg 124(4):1087–1097. doi:10.1097/PRS.0b013e3181b5a3f1

Eto H, Kato H, Suga H et al (2012) The fate of adipocytes after nonvascularized fat grafting: evidence of early death and replacement of adipocytes. Plast Reconstr Surg 129(5):1081–1092. doi:10.1097/PRS.0b013e31824a2b19

Geissler PJ, Davis K, Roostaeian J et al (2014) Improving fat transfer viability: the role of aging, body mass index, and harvest site. Plast Reconstr Surg 134(2):227–232. doi:10.1097/PRS.0000000000000398

Gillis J, Gebremeskel S, Phipps KD et al (2015) Effect of N-acetylcysteine on adipose-derived stem cell and autologous fat graft survival in a mouse model. Plast Reconstr Surg 136(2):179e–188e. doi:10.1097/PRS.0000000000001443

Kato H, Araki J, Doi K et al (2014a) Normobaric hyperoxygenation enhances initial survival, regeneration, and final retention in fat grafting. Plast Reconstr Surg 134(5):951–959. doi:10.1097/PRS.0000000000000600

Kato H, Mineda K, Eto H et al (2014b) Degeneration, regeneration, and cicatrization after fat grafting: dynamic total tissue remodeling during the first 3 months. Plast Reconstr Surg 133(3):303e–313e. doi:10.1097/PRS.0000000000000066

Keck M, Zeyda M, Gollinger K et al (2010) Local anesthetics have a major impact on viability of preadipocytes and their differentiation into adipocytes. Plast Reconstr Surg 126(5):1500–1505. doi:10.1097/PRS.0b013e3181ef8beb

Mineda K, Kuno S, Kato H et al (2014) Chronic inflammation and progressive calcification as a result of fat necrosis: the worst outcome in fat grafting. Plast Reconstr Surg 133(5):1064–1072. doi:10.1097/PRS.0000000000000097

Phipps KD, Gebremeskel S, Gillis J et al (2015) Alternatively activated M2 macrophages improve autologous Fat Graft survival in a mouse model through induction of angiogenesis. Plast Reconstr Surg 135(1):140–149. doi:10.1097/PRS.0000000000000793

Pu LL, Yoshimura K, Coleman SR (2015) Future perspectives of fat grafting. Clin Plast Surg 42(3):389–394. doi:10.1016/j.cps.2015.03.007

Suga H, Eto H, Aoi N et al (2010) Adipose tissue remodeling under ischemia: death of adipocytes and activation of stem/progenitor cells. Plast Reconstr Surg 126(6):1911–1923. doi:10.1097/PRS.0b013e3181f4468b

49 Importance of Regenerative Medicine in Breast Augmentation

Alberto M.L. Caldeira, Miluska Bromley Cueva, and Walter Marrou Pautrat

49.1 Introduction

Fat transfer to the breast is an interesting and popular procedure that can be used to fill soft-tissue and contour defects. The goal is to provide safe, long-lasting, and reproducible results. What began as a simple technique of suctioning fat and inserting it into the breast has developed into different surgical techniques, diverse technologies, and distinctive opinions around the world. These possibilities have created a confusing picture as to which technique is the best, which can only be achieved by updated knowledge of what is accepted and what is new in the field.

The first documented breast augmentation was performed by Czerny, when he transplanted a lipoma from the lumbar region to a breast defect (Czerny 1895). Others have described transplanting fat to the breast; however, none of the techniques had become neither standardized nor commonly used around the world until the beginning of the twentieth century. In the 1980s, liposuction was introduced, and became an impending foundation regarding fat transplantation. Because of this, different techniques were then created to inject autologous fat tissue into the breast (Bircoll 1987).

As with every novelty, the safety of fat transplantation was questioned. In 1987, the American Society of Plastic and Reconstructive Surgeons Ad-Hoc Committee on New Procedures declared the following: "The committee is unanimous in deploring the use of autologous fat injection in breast augmentation. Much of the injected fat will not survive, and the known physiological response to necrosis of this tissue is scarring and calcification. As a result, detection of early breast carcinoma through xerography and mammography will become difficult and the presence of disease may go undiscovered." (ASPRS Ad-Hoc Committee on New Procedures. Report on autologous fat transplantation, 30 September 1987). This statement was unfounded, as no studies had been carried out to support it. However, fat transfer became a very much discussed and feared topic among surgeons. This generated apathy for creating new research, made surgeons around the world become hesitant about using autologous fat, and a paradigm was created.

In 2013, The American Society of Plastic Surgery released a survey, in which 49% of respondents consider the lack of evidence supporting the

A.M.L. Caldeira, M.D., M.Sc., Ph.D., F.A.C.S. (✉)
Global Plastic Surgery Department, Casa de Saúde Portugal, Instituto de Pós-Graduação Médica Carlos Chagas/Universidade Santa Úrsula, Rio de Janeiro, RJ, Brazil

Plastic and Reconstructive Surgery Department, Caldeira-Roth Institute, Rua Visconde de Pirajá, 414 – Suite 1012, Ipanema, Rio de Janeiro, RJ CEP 22410–002, Brazil
e-mail: lottacaldeira@gmail.com

M. Bromley Cueva, M.D. • W. Marrou Pautrat, M.D.
Instituto Ivo Pitanguy, Rio de Janeiro, RJ, Brazil

Instituto de Pós-Graduação Médica Carlos Chagas, Rio de Janeiro, RJ, Brazil

J.M. Avelar (ed.), *Breast Surgery*, https://doi.org/10.1007/978-3-319-54115-0_49

oncological safety of lipofilling to be a significant obstacle to its use for breast reconstruction or cosmetic augmentation (Bircoll 1987). In 2007, Coleman and Saboeiro stated: "It is time to end the discrimination created by the 1987 position paper and judge fat grafting to the breast with the same caution and enthusiasm as any other useful breast procedure." Afterward, plastic surgeons around the world described their own reports and cases, supporting lipofilling (Coleman and Saboeiro 2007).

Although there are plenty of theories supporting the safety of fat transfer, there were no published studies with a control group regarding the oncological safety of lipofilling. Because of this, in 2016, Kronowitz et al., from the M.D. Anderson Cancer Center, created a match control study involving 1024 cases from 1981 to 2014, in which they analyzed the probability of locoregional recurrence in breast cancer patients, estimated using the Kaplan–Meier method. They concluded that there was no increase in locoregional recurrence, systemic recurrence, or a second breast cancer. Their findings support the oncological safety of lipofilling in breast reconstruction (Kronowitz et al. 2016).

Furthermore, there are plenty of studies stating that current radiologists have a better level of confidence in differentiating between fat necrosis calcification after breast surgery and that related to breast cancer (Rubin and Yoshimura 2010; Rubin 2011; Veber et al. 2011).

1 cubic centimeter of adipose tissue (Suga et al. 2010; Yoshimura et al. 2006; 2009) contains:

- One million adipocytes
- One million adipose-derived stem/progenitor cells
- One million endothelial cells
- One to two million other cells, such as blood-derived cells

To understand the cellular pathway of fat, we need to understand what we are transferring.

Because of experimental work led by Yoshimura et al., we now know that during transfer most of the adipocytes will die and are replaced with new adipocytes created by the adipose-derived stem/progenitor cells (Suga et al. 2009). Even under the severe ischemia induced by lipografting, adipose-derived stem/progenitor cells survive and play key roles in the repair process after ischemia–reperfusion injury to adipose tissue (Suga et al. 2008), contributing to adipogenesis and angiogenesis (Suga et al. 2009). Therefore, adipocyte death does not mean adipose tissue necrosis, but triggers a regeneration cascade; in contrast, death of both adipocytes and adipose-derived stromal cells results in adipose tissue necrosis (Eto et al. 2012).

49.2 Three Zones in Grafted Tissue: Surviving, Regenerating, and Necrotizing

Yoshimura et al. observed the three zones from the periphery to the center of the graft with immunohistochemistry (Kato et al. 2014):

- The surviving area (adipocytes survived)
- The regenerating area (adipocytes died, adipose-derived stromal cells survived, and dead adipocytes were replaced with new ones)
- The necrotic area (both adipocytes and adipose-derived stromal cells died) (Fig. 49.1)

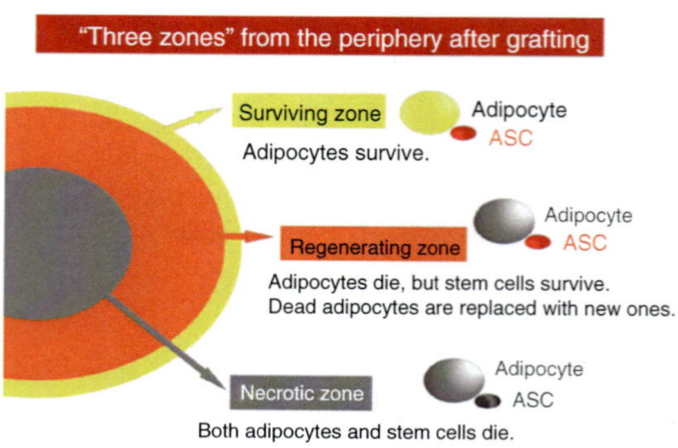

Fig. 49.1 The "three zones" from the periphery after grafting. Reproduced with Permission granted by Dr. Kotaro Yoshimura

Later, they described the histopathological timeline of the three zones.

1 week ***Surviving zone:*** Adipocytes remain intact. ***Regeneration zone:*** All adipocytes died and remain as adipocyte-sized oil droplets. ***Necrotic zone:*** All adipocytes died.	**2–4 weeks** ***Surviving zone:*** Adipocytes remain intact. ***Regeneration zone:*** Growing preadipocytes emerge. ***Necrotic zone:*** Dead adipocytes and inflammatory cells are observed, but no regenerative changes are seen.
8 weeks ***Surviving zone:*** Adipocytes remain intact. ***Regeneration zone:*** New adipocytes matured ***Necrotic zone:*** No adipogenesis is seen. Many small and large oil drops were seen along with numerous inflammatory cells.	**12 weeks** ***Surviving zone:*** Adipocytes remain intact. ***Regeneration zone:*** Matured adipocytes ***Necrotic zone:*** Number of small oil drops is reduced, but many large oil drops remain with surrounding inflammatory cells.

Interestingly, although most adipocytes had already died during the first week, the size of the grafted tissue did not change during the first 4 weeks. This indicates that the dead adipocytes generally maintained their size during this time, as the oil drops were slowly absorbed over a period of weeks or months, depending on their size. The size of the necrotizing zone depends on the size of the grafted tissue and the microenvironment into which it is placed. Necrotic zones are eventually absorbed, filled with fibrous tissue, or become problematic cysts. Stabilization of the grafted fat may not occur until many months after complete regeneration at 3 months, thereby emphasizing the importance of long-term follow-up to thoroughly evaluate the clinical results of micro-fat-grafting procedures.

49.3 How Much Fat Can We Transfer?

As previously mentioned, vascularization is the key point for fat survival. Moreover, fat plays the role of a tissue expander in the breast. This is not important when small volumes of fat are injected, as small amounts (with a good transfer technique) can still preserve an adequate recipient interface for oxygen and nutrient dispersal. However, when large amounts of fat are injected, there is great interstitial pressure, with large fat collections leading to inadequate nutrition, and most importantly, to fat necrosis and absorption (Zocchi and Zuliani 2008). Another important principle is the interstitial fluid pressure limit. There is a major limitation as to how much volume breast tissue can accept. As we inject more fat, the recipient site initially enlarges to accommodate the increased volume. However, beyond a certain injection volume, the compliance of tissue rapidly decreases and the interstitial fluid pressure suddenly increases (Gosset et al. 2008). As interstitial fluid pressure rises, capillary circulation drops precipitously (Mineda et al. 2014), inhibiting oxygen delivery, neovascularization, and subsequent graft survival. With small volume increases, the tissues are relatively compliant; however, as the volume transfer into a small recipient increases, the compliance drops rapidly, increasing interstitial fluid pressure, decreasing blood flow and oxygen delivery, and ultimately leading to graft necrosis and volume loss (Coleman 2001) (Fig. 49.2).

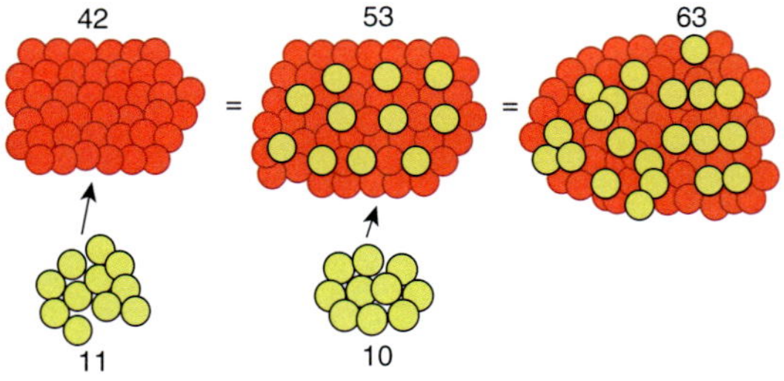

Fig. 49.2 Theoretical conceptual approximation of the overgrafting theory. Eleven 4-mm yellow droplets can be evenly spread inside a 42-droplet recipient bed without crowding, coalescence, or increased tightness of the recipient. However, squeezing another ten droplets results in confluence and inability of the recipient bed to expand enough to accommodate the additional size. Reproduced with permission from Coleman (2001)

49.4 Fat Necrosis and Calcification

Cysts are the worst consequence of fat transfer, as they show long-term inflammation and progressive calcification. Cysts and calcifications caused by fat necrosis have been reported frequently. Various studies have shown calcification in the breast of 3.9–25% after fat transfer (Veber et al. 2011; Peer and Walker 1951). Gosset et al. reported that mammograms detected microcalcifications in 19% and magnetic resonance imaging found cystic lesions in 47% (Carpaneda and Ribeiro 1994). Histopathology findings and clinical CT images revealed that oil cysts, which are formed by 6 months and are filled with necrotized materials, are continuously inflammatory and calcifications continue to develop – very slowly – over time for several years. Therefore, large fat necrosis-inducing oil cysts should be avoided, although small fat necrosis resulting in sand-like calcification may be within acceptable limits (Geissler et al. 2014). A bolus injection of fat must never be given as it always results in large central necrosis and a subsequent cyst. We can prevent this by distributing fat tissue evenly and diffusely as tiny aliquots or noodles.

There are three variables, which must be considered before starting a procedure: harvesting, processing, and transplanting. We will revise and describe some of the new trends affecting these three processes.

49.4.1 Harvesting

Liposuction is a low-cost, simple procedure with the advantage of giving its recipient autologous fat. However, because fat can be harvested from different body areas, survival rates have been reported to be highly variable from study to study, ranging from 30 to 95% (Cleveland et al. 2015; Guerrerosantos 1996; Salinas et al. 2014). The difference in fat survival as it relates to various patient characteristics is broadly lacking and may play a significant role. Criteria such as donor-site choice, patient age, and body mass index may all be significant in their effect on fat survival. According to R. Rohrich; age affects adipocyte viability differently across anatomical regions. The lower abdomen appears to be a preferred source of adipocytes in younger patients, whereas the flank showed higher adipocyte viability in the older ones (Coleman and Saboeiro 2015).

49.4.2 Processing

Fat transfer involves harvesting, isolating the adipocyte fraction, and subsequent injection. Many techniques exist to isolate the adipocyte fraction, including centrifugation, decantation, cotton gauze rolling, mesh filtering, the Telfa technique, and washing. The search for the best processing technique started in the early 2000s.

Since then, many theories have evolved; however, superiority has never been proven. In 2014, Austen et al. from the Massachusetts General Hospital proved that there are no differences in the number of stem cells isolated, comparing centrifugation with mesh filtering, and that the concentration efficacy of mesh/gauze is equivalent to centrifugation at 1200 × *g*, with equivalent in vivo outcomes (Khouri et al. 2000). In 2015, Cleveland et al. from New York University failed to find compelling evidence to advocate a single technique as the superior method for processing lipoaspirate in preparation for autologous fat grafting. Furthermore, they advocated that the lack of high-quality data limited the clinician's ability to determine the optimal method for purifying harvested adipose tissue (Khouri et al. 2012). Despite continued exploration in this field, further research is required to recognize the ideal methods of processing harvested adipose tissue.

49.4.3 Transplanting: Surgical Technique

- Liposuction is performed in the lower abdomen of young patients and in the flanks of older ones.
- Decantation of the fat is done using 60-mL syringes (Fig. 49.3).
- After decantation, transference of the fat to 10-mL syringes.
- The breast is marked into quadrants for easier fat distribution.
- 2-mm incisions are made in the center of the inframammary fold and at 12 o'clock on the areola (Fig. 49.4).
- Fat transfer is carried out using 1.7-to 1.9-mm blunt microcannulas.
- Layering the fat into different levels: subcutaneous, intraglandular, retroglandular, and intramuscular (Fig. 49.5).
- Injection of the fat, according to Coleman's tunneling technique, in a retrograde fashion

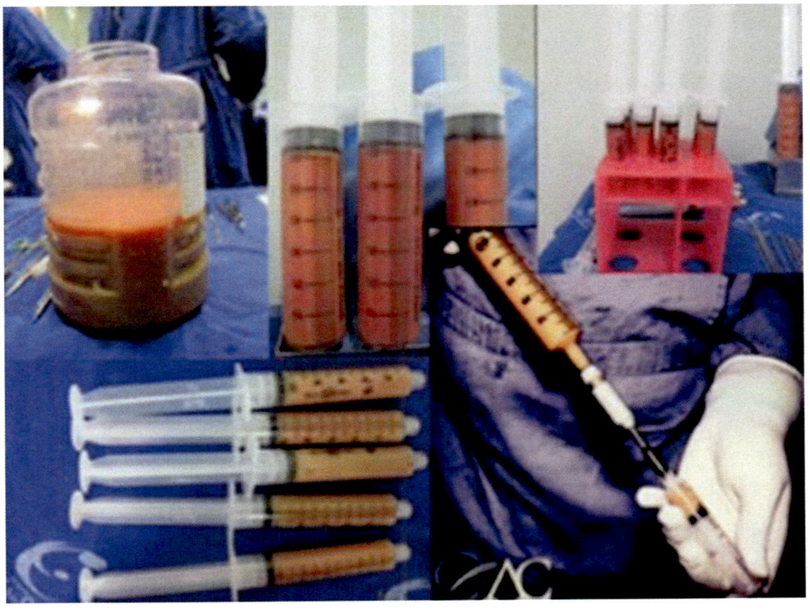

Fig. 49.3 Decantation of the fat and transfer to 10 mL syringes. Reproduced with permission from A. Caldeira's library

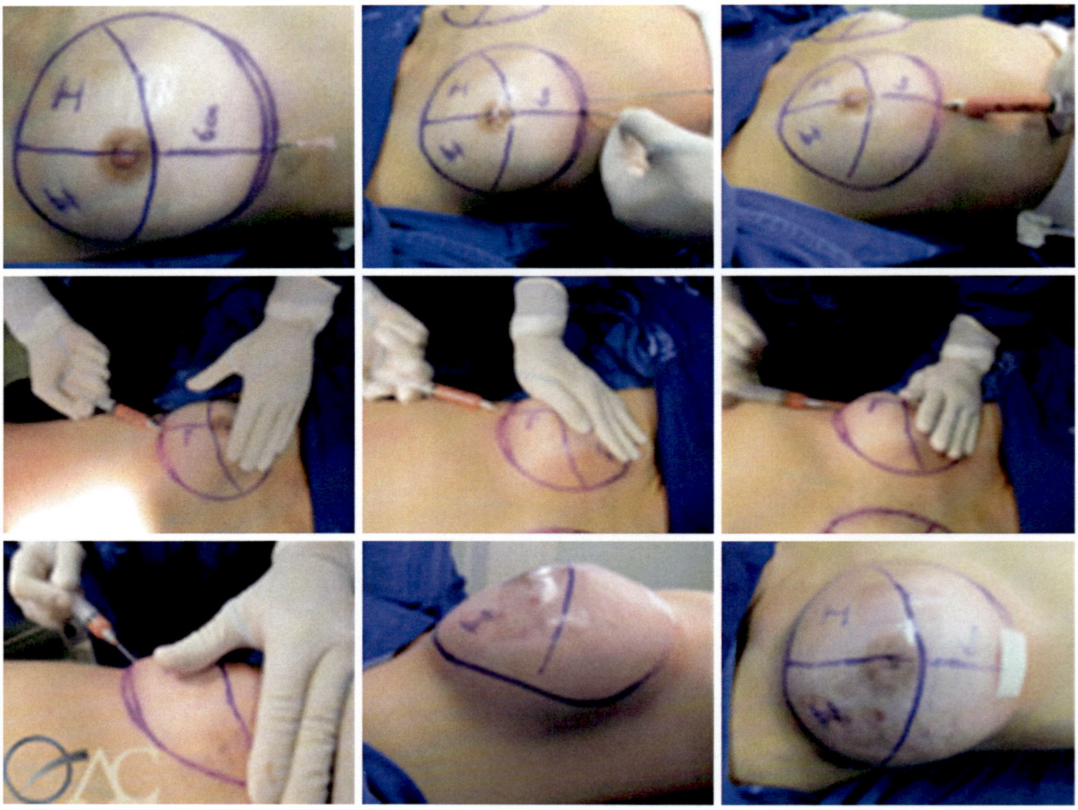

Fig. 49.4 Marking of the breast into quadrants and 2-mm incisions in the inframammary fold. Reproduced with permission from A. Caldeira's library

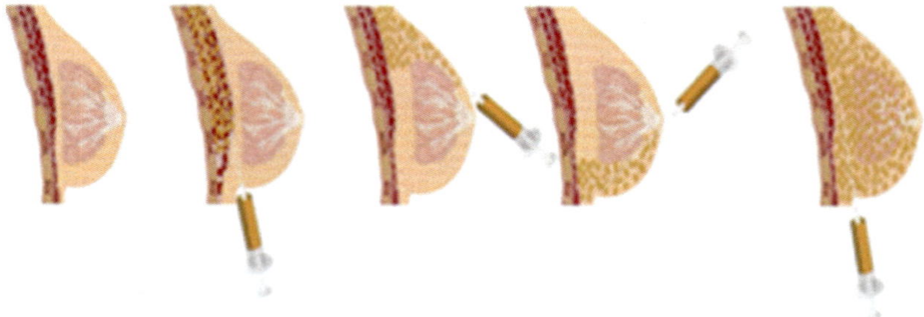

Fig. 49.5 Layering the fat into different levels. Reproduced with permission from A. Caldeira's library

Recommendations for a successful procedure:

- The outcome of breast augmentation through fat transfer is related to the surgeon's level of expertise and the technique used.
- The technique must include all precautions to ensure that the maximum amount of fat survives:
  - Reducing the possibility of trauma to the harvest site.
  - Demonstrating correct refinement to the tissue.
  - Minimal fat manipulation.
  - Delivering droplets of fat through thin cannulas, never exceeding the 2-mm limit (De Fillippo and Atala 2002).
  - Placement of small aliquots instead of large portions should be achieved.
  - Transferred fat should be placed in proximity to the patient's blood supply to increase fat survival rates and reduce both the implication of fat necrosis and calcification risk.
- A trained radiologist is necessary for reliable screening.

following fanning mode. Injecting 10 mL per tunnel, creating about 50 tunnels per breast depending on the amount of fat transfer.

- Dressing is applied.

Overgrafting is assessed by tissue turgor. Peau d'orange of subdermal tension should be avoided, keeping in mind that often less is best (Kato et al. 2010).

49.5 External Soft-Tissue Expander

Fifteen years ago Khouri introduced the BRAVA® external soft-tissue expander device to the market as an and has demonstrated modest augmentation after long-term use (Kato et al. 2010). According to Khouri, "Short-term use of BRAVA®, causes a marked temporary increase in breast size and generates a very large fibrovascular scaffold that would be an ideal recipient for fat grafts" (Moisidis et al. 2004).

According to Khouri, to successfully transfer a megavolume (more than 300 mL) of fat, we need compliant tissue that can be expanded and an abundant blood supply that can accept large fat volumes without significantly increasing interstitial fluid pressure. Khouri concludes that this can be achieved with the use of the BRAVA® external breast expander, which enables tissue compliance to be increased, the potential recipient space to be increased, and, equally as importantly, an abundant stromal/vascular platform to be created (Guyton 1965). Furthermore, he reported that successful rates depend directly on the use of BRAVA® wear; the more the patient uses it, the better the expansion, and the more pronounced the results will be. This gives the responsibility for a good outcome to the patient, making BRAVA® a predictable procedure.

For this to happen, Khouri describes the patient wearing the BRAVA® external breast

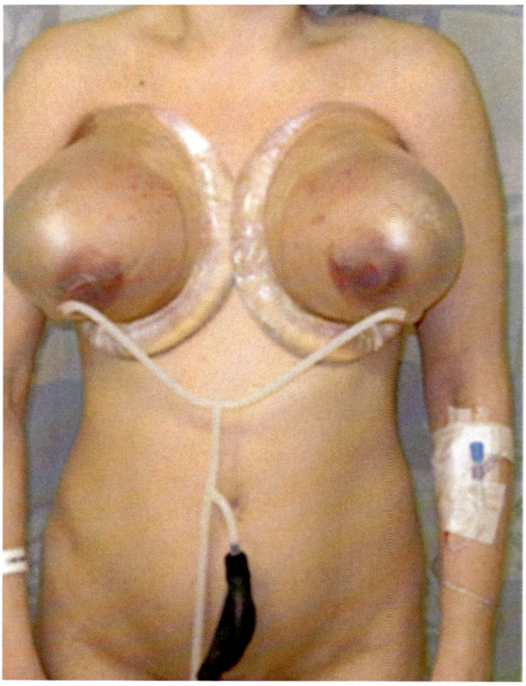

Fig. 49.6 BRAVA® device. Reproduced with permission from R. Khouri's library

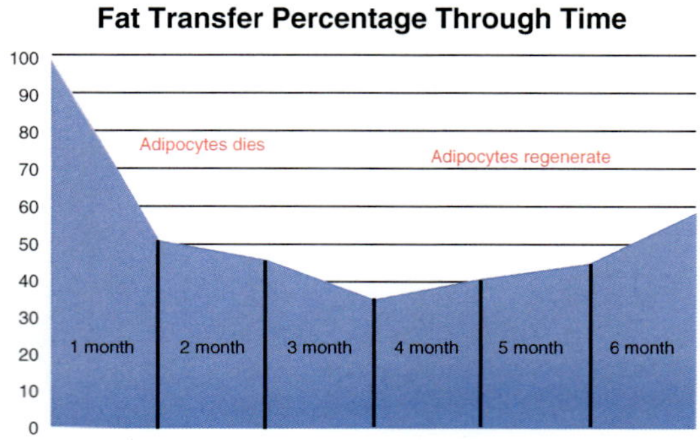

Fig. 49.7 Graph showing fat transfer over time. Notice how the fat volume decreases at months 1, 2, and 3 and then increases through months 4, 5, and 6. This result mimics the "cell replacement theory," where at the beginning, adipocytes die and they are later replaced by new adipocytes created by the adipose-derived stem cells. Reproduced with permission from Caldeira et al. (2016)

tissue expander for 10 h/day for 4 weeks (Fig. 49.6) (Khouri et al. 2014; Tufto and Rofstad 1999) before the surgery and for 48–72 h uninterrupted after the surgery.

49.6 Fat Behavior Over Time

In 2013, a quasi-experimental study was created to evaluate fat transfer over time, using a 3D simulation software named Crisalix® (Caldeira et al. 2016). This study was chosen and presented at the Aesthetic Meeting 2016, held in Las Vegas. In this study, patients were used as their own control group and compared with their own postoperative evaluation. The volume after fat transfer was evaluated after the first, second, third, fourth, fifth, and sixth months. The technique for fat transfer was previously explained in this chapter (without the use of any other device). The results showed how the fat transfer volume behaves over time and revealed a tendency, similar to that of cell replacement theory, proposed by Yoshimura (Fig. 49.7), where at the beginning, adipocytes die and they are later replaced by new adipocytes created by the adipose-derived stem cells (ADS). Furthermore, the mean fat volume percentage measured after 6 months was 58.9%. Last, a longer follow-up is needed, as by the end of the sixth month, there was still a tendency for it to rise.

This study confirms that with good harvesting, processing, and surgical techniques, fat transfer to the breast is a completely valid choice, and that no other device is needed to achieve success.

References

Bircoll M (1987) Cosmetic breast augmentation utilizing autologous fat and liposuction techniques. Plast Reconstr Surg 79(2):267–271

Caldeira A, Marrou W, Bromley M (2016) Fat transfer in augmentation mammography, a 3D volumetric evaluation. Oral presentation. ASAPS, Las Vegas

Carpaneda CA, Ribeiro MT (1994) Percentage of graft viability versus injected volume in adipose autotransplants. Aesthet Plast Surg 18(1):17–19

Cleveland E, Albano N, Hazen A (2015) Roll, spin, wash, or filter? Processing of lipoaspirate for autologous fat grafting: an updated, evidence-based review of the literature. Plast Reconstr Surg 136(4):706–713

Coleman SR (2001) Structural fat grafts: the ideal filler? Clin Plast Surg 28(1):111–119

Coleman SR, Saboeiro AP (2007) Fat grafting to the breast revisited: safety and efficacy. Plast Reconstr Surg 119(3):775–785

Coleman SR, Saboeiro AP (2015) Primary breast augmentation with fat grafting. Clin Plast Surg 42(3):301–306

Czerny V (1895) Plastischer Ersatz der Brustdrüse durch ein Lipom. Zentralbl Chir 22:72

De Fillippo RE, Atala A (2002) Stretch and growth: the molecular and physiological influences of tissue expansion. Plast Reconstr Surg 109(7):2450–2462

Eto H, Kato H, Suga H, Aoi N, Doi K, Kuno S, Yoshimura K (2012) The fate of adipocytes after nonvascularized fat grafting: evidence of early death and replacement of adipocytes. Plast Reconstr Surg 129(5):1081–1092

Geissler P, Davis K, Roostaeian J, Unger J, Huang J, Rohrich R (2014) Improving fat transfer viability: the role of aging, body mass index, and harvest site. Plast Reconstr Surg 134(2):227–232

Gosset J, Guerin N, Toussoun G, Delaporte T, Delay E (2008) Radiological evaluation after lipomodelling for correction of breast conservative treatment sequelae. Ann Chir Plast Esthet 53(2):178–189

Guerrerosantos J (1996) Autologous fat grafting for body contouring. Clin Plast Surg 23(4):619–631

Guyton AC (1965) Interstitial fluid pressure. II. Pressure-volume curves of interstitial space. Circ Res 16:452–460

Kato H, Suga H, Eto H (2010) Reversible adipose tissue enlargement induced by external tissue suspension: possible contribution of basic fibroblast growth factor in the preservation of enlarged tissue. Tissue Eng Part A 16(6):2029–2040

Kato H, Mineda K, Eto H, Doi K, Kuno S, Kinoshita K, Kanayama K, Yoshimura K (2014) Degeneration, regeneration, and cicatrization after fat grafting: dynamic total tissue remodeling during the first 3 months. Plast Reconstr Surg 133(3):303–13e

Khouri RK, Schlenz I, Murphy BJ, Baker TJ (2000) Nonsurgical breast enlargement using an external soft-tissue expansion system. Plast Reconstr Surg;105(7):2500–2512; discussion 2513–4

Khouri RK, Eisenmann-Klein M, Cardoso E, Cooley BC, Kacher D, Gombos E, Baker TJ (2012) Brava and autologous fat transfer is a safe and effective breast augmentation alternative: results of a 6-year, 81-patient, prospective multicenter study. Plast Reconstr Surg 129(5):1173–1187

Khouri RK, Rigotti G, Cardoso E, Khouri RK Jr, Biggs T (2014) Megavolume autologous fat transfer. I. Theory and principles. Plast Reconstr Surg 133(3):550–557

Kronowitz SJ, Mandujano CC, Liu J, Kuerer HM, Smith B, Garvey P, Jagsi R, Hsu L, Hanson S, Valero V (2016) Lipofilling of the breast does not increase the risk of recurrence of breast cancer: a matched controlled study. Plast Reconstr Surg 137(2):385–393. doi:10.1097/01.prs.0000475741.32563.50

Mineda K, Kuno S, Kato H, Kinoshita K, Doi K, Hashimoto I, Nakanishi H, Yoshimura K (2014) Chronic inflammation and progressive calcification as a result of fat necrosis: the worst outcome in fat grafting. Plast Reconstr Surg 133(5):1064–1072

Moisidis E, Heath T, Boorer C, Ho K, Deva AK (2004) A prospective, blinded, randomized, controlled clinical trial of topical negative pressure use in skin grafting. Plast Reconstr Surg 114(4):917–922

Peer LA, Walker JC (1951) The behavior of autogenous human tissue grafts. II. Plast Reconstr Surg 7(2):73–84

Rubin E (2011) Breast imaging considerations in fat grafting to the breast. Plast Reconstr Surg 128(5):570–51e

Rubin JP, Yoshimura K (2010) Mammographic changes after stem cell supplemented fat transfer compared with changes after breast reduction: a blinded study. Paper presented at International Federation of Adipose Therapeutics and Science Annual Meeting, October 2, 2010, Dallas, Texas; and at the 27th Annual Meeting of the Northeastern Society of Plastic Surgeons, October 30, Washington, DC.

Salinas HM, Broelsch GF, Fernandes JR, McCormack MC, Meppelink AM, Randolph MA, Colwell AS, Austen WG Jr (2014) Comparative analysis of processing methods in fat grafting. Plast Reconstr Surg 134(4):675–683

Suga H, Matsumoto D, Inoue K, Shigeura T, Eto H, Aoi N, Kato H, Abe H, Yoshimura K (2008) Numerical measurement of viable and nonviable adipocytes and other cellular components in aspirated fat tissue. Plast Reconstr Surg 122(1):103–114

Suga H, Eto H, Shigeura T et al (2009) IFATS collection: fibroblast growth factor-2-induced hepatocyte growth factor secretion by adipose-derived stromal cells inhibits postinjury fibrogenesis through a c-Jun N-terminal kinase-dependent mechanism. Stem Cells 27(1):238–249

Suga H, Eto H, Aoi N, Kato H, Araki J, Doi K, Higashino T, Yoshimura K (2010) Adipose tissue remodeling under ischemia: death of adipocytes and activation of stem/progenitor cells. Plast Reconstr Surg 126(6):1911–1923

Tufto I, Rofstad EK (1999) Interstitial fluid pressure and capillary diameter distribution in human melanoma xenografts. Microvasc Res 58(3):205–214

Veber M, Tourasse C, Toussoun G, Moutran M, Mojallal A, Delay E (2011) Radiographic findings after breast augmentation by autologous fat transfer. Plast Reconstr Surg 127(3):1289–1299

Yoshimura K, Shigeura T, Matsumoto D et al (2006) Characterization of freshly isolated and cultured cells derived from the fatty and fluid portions of liposuction aspirates. J Cell Physiol 208(1):64–76

Yoshimura K, Suga H, Eto H (2009) Adipose-derived stem/progenitor cells: roles in adipose tissue remodeling and potential use for soft tissue augmentation. Regen Med 4(2):265–273

Zocchi ML, Zuliani F (2008) Bicompartmental breast lipostructuring. Aesthet Plast Surg 32(2):313–328

Check for updates

Importance of Lipoinjection for Breast Augmentation

50

Marcelo Paulo Vaccari Mazzetti
and Ryane Schmidt Brock

50.1 Introduction

One of the first descriptions of improving breast size using lipografting was made by Czerny (1895). The lipoinjection provided from the liposuction of fat tissue was probably first used by Bircoll (1987) and was for cosmetic reasons.

There are many explanations for why the use of lipoinjection has not become popular in plastic surgery, such the unpredictable absorption of the fat tissue injected, inadvisable according to the American Society of Plastic Surgery at that time because of the risks of fat necrosis and the resultant scarring and calcification. This could make it difficult to correctly diagnose breast cancer. Since that time, several studies, e.g., Coleman (2001), Coleman and Saboeiro (2007, 2015), Cleveland et al. (2015), Caldeira et al. (2016), Khouri et al. (2000, 2012, 2014), Kronowitz et al. (2016), have been carried out and today give support to the use of this technique.

Breast augmentation is considered by the American Society of Plastic Surgeons to be one of the most common procedures in plastic surgery. The technique most frequently used is silicone implantation. However, autologous fat transplantation has attracted great interest in breast augmentation for cosmetic purposes. It is considered a technical alternative for increasing mammary volume without implants, using only lipoinjection (ASPS 2013; Li et al. 2014).

Silicone implantation is a very well established technique in breast augmentation; however, some patients refuse to have artificial materials in their body. Lipoinjection has the advantage of using autogenous tissue that is collected using a simple technique that is frequently done together with breast augmentation to achieve a better body shape than that associated with liposuction.

The clinical indications for the lipoinjection technique, in our practice, is the patient's desire to achieve a medium or small breast volume increase without implants.

Caldeira et al. (2016) have recently developed and established the regenerative surgery of breast augmentation using lipoinjection.

50.2 Surgical Procedure

All patients are photographed and marked beforehand. Areas for body liposuction and breast lipoinjection are marked with the patient in the upright position.

The surgical procedure is carried out under general or peridural endovenous anesthesia.

M.P.V. Mazzetti, M.D., M.Sc. (✉)
The Brazilian Society of Plastic Surgery, Face Defects Research and Study Center,
Av. Ceci, 475, São Paulo, SP, Brazil
e-mail: dr.marcelovaccari@gmail.com

R.S. Brock, M.D., M.Sc.
The Brazilian Society of Plastic Surgery,
São Paulo, SP, Brazil

J.M. Avelar (ed.), *Breast Surgery*, https://doi.org/10.1007/978-3-319-54115-0_50

The operating room is prepared to provide an increase in temperature. For the liposuction, we use a subcutaneous infiltration of a tumescent solution of lidocaine 2% (40 mL; only with general anesthesia), epinephrine (3 mL), and 1,000 mL of saline solution (1:333.333). The donor site is usually the abdomen or the flank, but other areas are also utilized as donor sites (knees, jowls, and arms), because we usually use lipoinjection in the gluteus in most of our cases and all available fat is required to supply all areas of lipoinjection (breast, gluteus and sometimes the face).

The liposuction is performed using a 3- or 4-mm Mercedes cannula with a closed system of collection.

After the liposuction, all the fat is decanted and the residual passed through a sieve and separated from the liquid part that consisted of tumescent fluid, blood, and destroyed fat. The fat tissue cannot stay out of the body for more than 30 min; thus, when the liposuction had been underway for 25 min we stopped it and proceeded to the lipoinjection. Then another 25 min of liposuction followed, before lipoinjection was carried out once again, and so on.

Only the fat is stored in 60-mL (submuscular injection) and 5 and 10-mL (subcutaneous injection) syringes.

A tiny (2- to 3-mm) incision is done in the central region of the inframammary fold, over the costal arch. Cannula number 5 is introduced, supported in the costal arch in the submuscular plane, under the pectoralis major muscle, and the fat graft is then introduced into a submuscular layer, under the pectoralis major muscle and over the pectoralis minor muscle. Intraoperative ultrasound could be used to determine the correct anatomical plan for the submuscular lipoinjection (Fig. 50.1). A large volume is introduced into this layer until the fat starts to overflow; we use 100–200 mL in each breast, usually in asymmetrical distribution for each breast (the larger volume in the small breast). In some cases, we performed lipoinjection in association with the inferior pedicle technique, under direct vision, using a lateral approach. After lipoinjection we closed the muscular approach to avoid fat extrusion (Fig. 50.2). It is possible to see the fat spreading under the pectoral muscle. After the submuscular injection, we performed a subcutaneous lipoinjection, under skin and over the gland, without intraglandular injection, with a cannula of 2.0 mm, in tunnels with retrograde injection, such as described by Coleman.

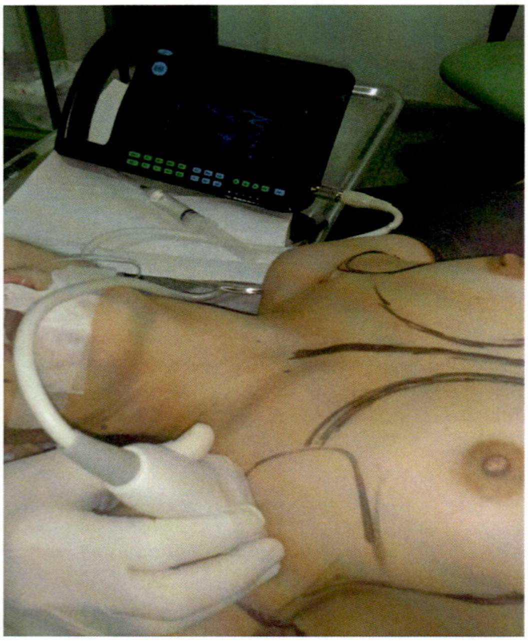

Fig. 50.1 Previous image study before lipoinjection under the pectoralis muscle, which can be guided by intraoperative ultrasound

Manual massage must be carried out to make all the lipografts uniform and a compressive dressing is applied after this procedure.

The incision used to introduce the cannula is sutured to avoid contamination of the fat graft. The superior pole is used, filled by submuscular injection, and subcutaneous lipoinjection is frequently used to fill the inferior breast pole (Figs. 50.3, 50.4, 50.5, and 50.6).

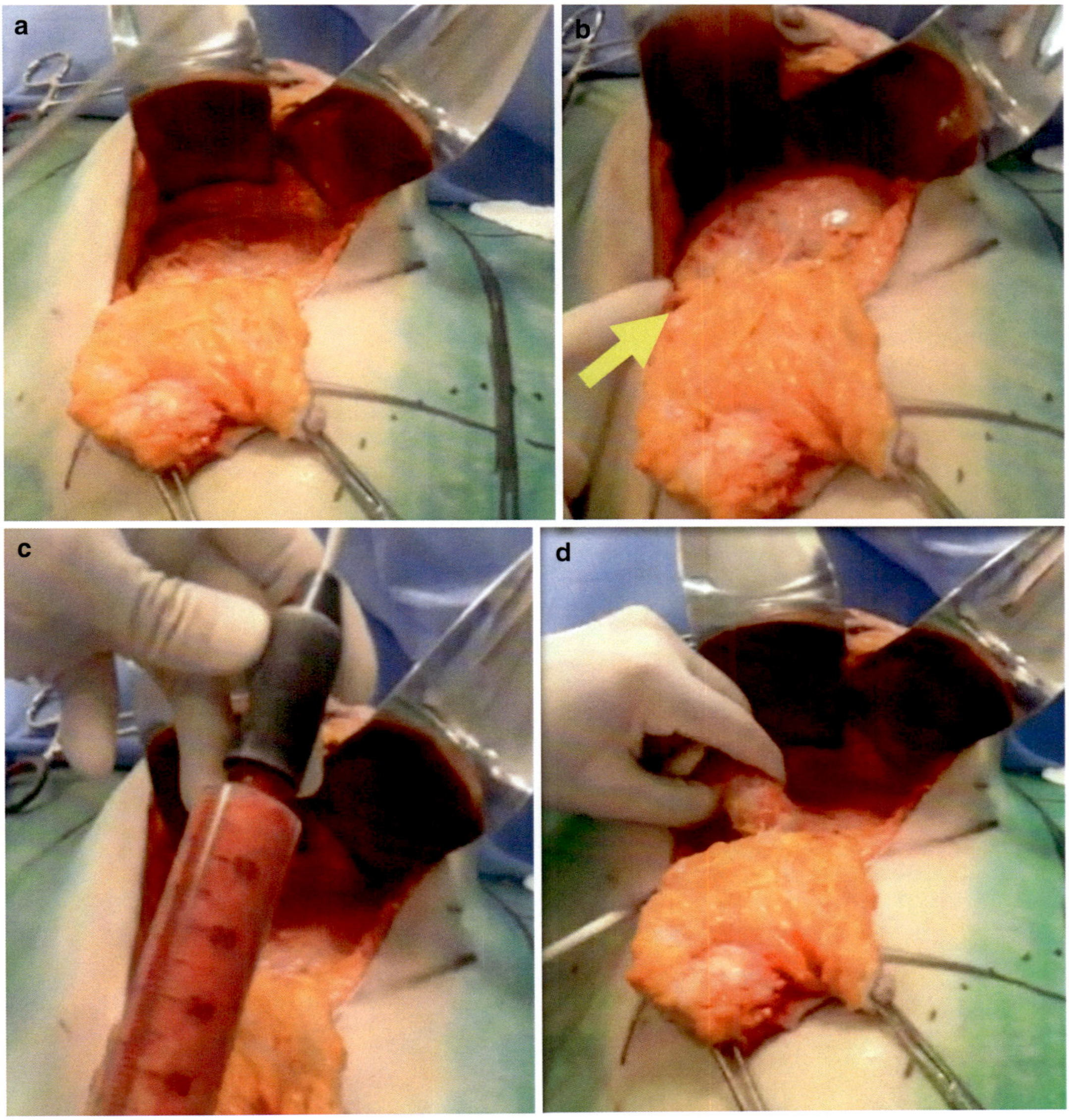

Fig. 50.2 Patient undergoing lipoinjection associated with inferior pedicle mastoplasty. (**a**) Displacement of the mammary gland with complete view of the pectoralis major muscle, which (**b**) received a 100-mL submuscular lipoinjection (*yellow arrow*) and more than70 mL subcutaneously. (**c**) The fat in a 60-cc syringe with a cannula number 5 for muscular lipoinjection. (**d**) The pectoralis major muscle is held with the fingers to perform lipoinjection

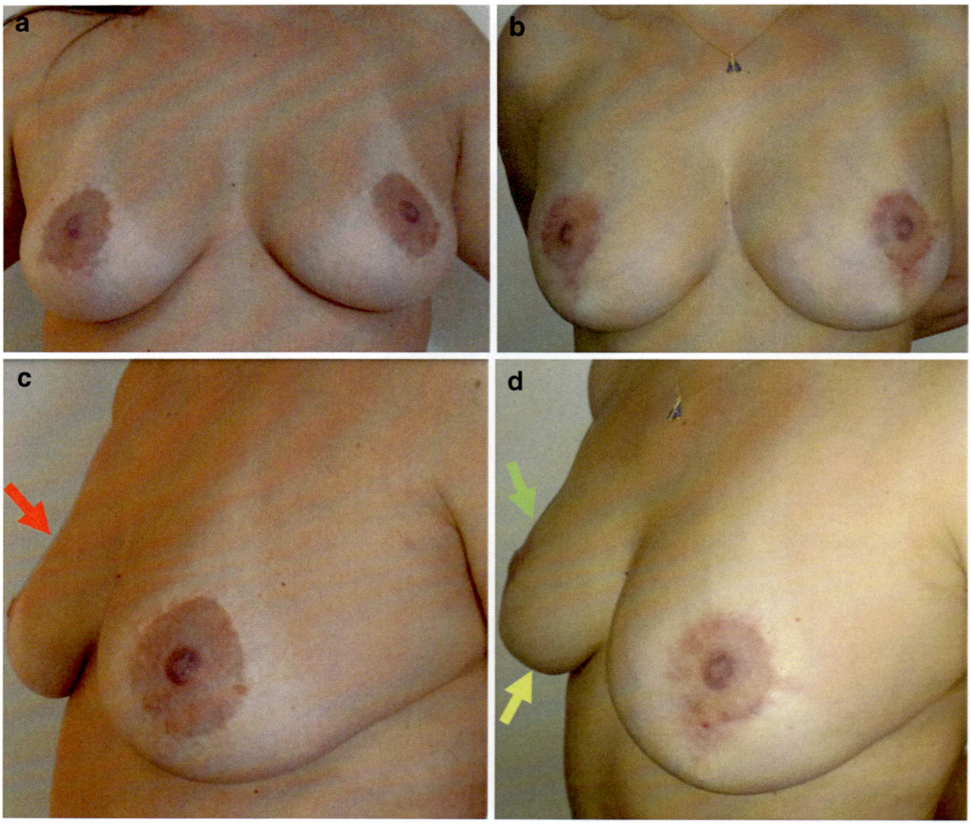

Fig. 50.3 Patient undergoing lipoinjection of 220 mL in the right side and 180 mL in the left side, under the pectoralis major muscle and subcutaneously. (**a**) Frontal preoperative view. (**b**) Frontal view 90 days postoperatively. (**c**) Preoperative oblique view: the patient's wish was to fill the superior pole (*red arrow*). (**d**) Postoperative oblique view with better projection of the superior pole (*green arrow*) and inferior pole (*yellow arrow*)

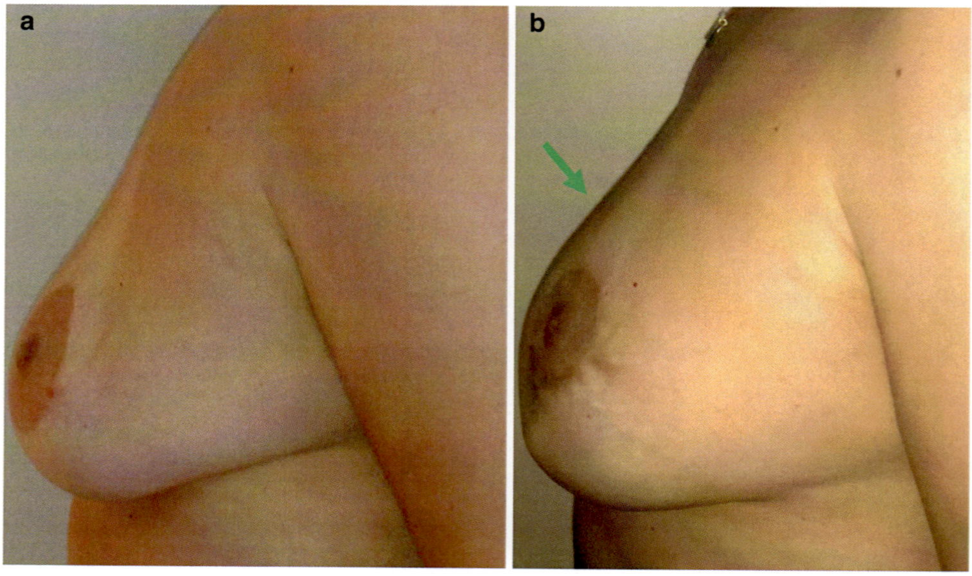

Fig. 50.4 Patient undergoing lipoinjection of 220 mL in the right side and 180 mL in the left side, under the pectoralis major muscle and subcutaneously. (**a**) Lateral preoperative view. (**b**) Lateral view 90 days postoperatively with better projection of the superior pole (*green arrow*). The nipple–areolar complex was also reduced

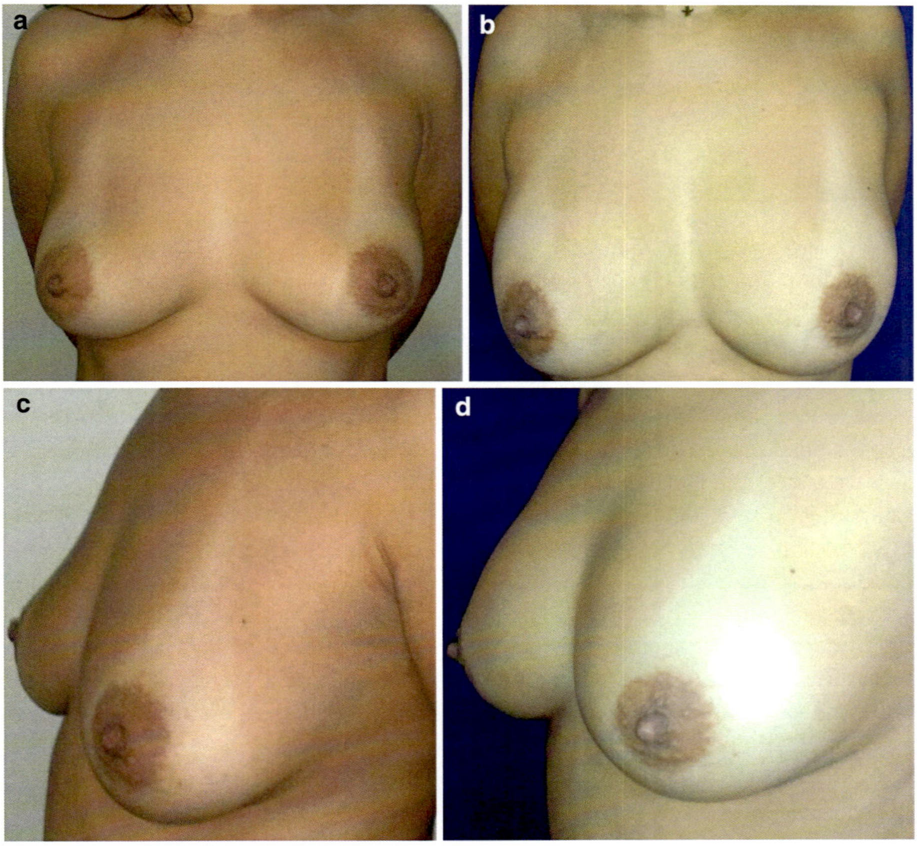

Fig. 50.5 Patient undergoing lipoinjection of 300 mL on both sides: 180 mL under the pectoralis major muscle and 120 mL subcutaneously. (**a**) Frontal preoperative view. (**b**) Frontal view 90 days postoperatively with filling of the superomedial poles (*yellow arrows*). (**c**) Preoperative oblique view. (**d**) Postoperative oblique view with better projection of the superior pole (*green arrow*)

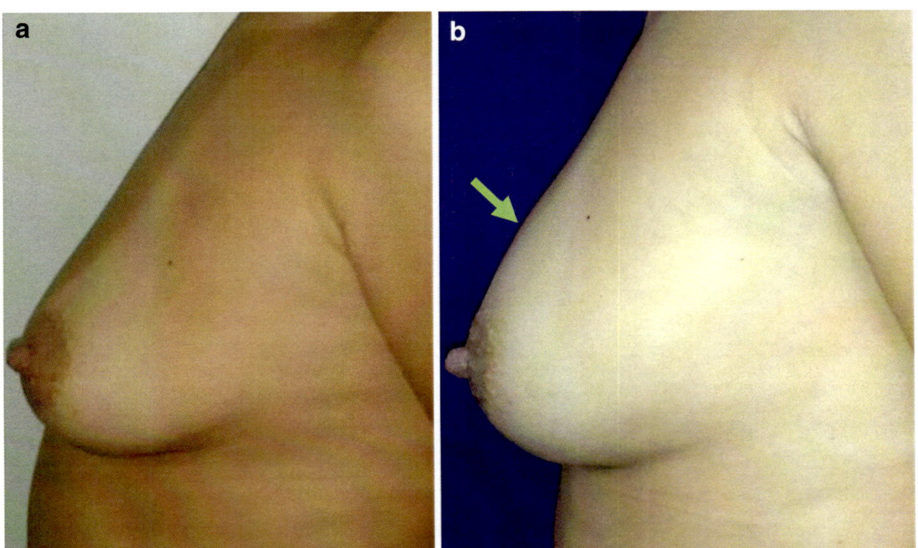

Fig. 50.6 Patient undergoing lipoinjection of 300 mL on both sides, 180 mL under the pectoralis major muscle and 120 mL subcutaneously. (**a**) Lateral preoperative view. (**b**) Lateral view 90 days postoperatively with better projection of the superior pole (*green arrow*). The nipple–areolar complex was also reduced

50.3 Complications

In our patients, we have one cyst related to lipoinjection. The necrosis cysts (fat necrosis and calcification) may be present and we suggested rigorous pre- and postoperative image control with MRI.

Infection is possible during lipoinjection and that of the lipografts should be prevented. Rigorous antiseptic care before, during, and after surgery, the period of the fat being out of the body not exceeding 30 min, a closed collection system, and prevention of hypothermia during the surgery are good practices.

Asymmetry is possible and a careful preoperative examination permits the observation that almost all breasts are asymmetrical; thus, different lipoinjection volumes must to be carried out in each breast to correct that.

If we consider absorption and loss of result to be complications, we believe that we have a loss of lipografts of 30% to 50%.

50.4 Discussion

Lipoinjection is an alternative to breast augmentation, it has the advantage of being autologous, which avoids rejection and capsular contracture, which happens with silicone implantation. It is biocompatible and in some cases abundantly available, can be easily harvested and processed, and can be injected in controlled amounts (Figs. 50.3, 50.4, 50.5, and 50.6). The fat can be harvested from a number of sites, including the abdomen, the medial, lateral or anterior thighs, the flank, the lower and upper back, and the knees (Cleveland et al. 2015).

For young patients, the inferior abdomen is the best donor area; for older patients the flank is better. For other areas, this difference is not well established.

Lipoinjection can be performed in association with liposuction, a very common surgical procedure in plastic surgery, that is used to achieve a better body contour. However, to achieve good results in breast augmentation with lipoinjection, at least 300 mL should be used in each breast.

Studies have demonstrated no cosmetic improvement in thin patients who had been injected with less than 150 mL of fat. For this reason, autologous fat transfer for breast augmentation is not suitable for thin women who have insufficient fat deposits (Li et al. 2014; Gabriel et al. 2015).

Our technique does not use intraglandular fat injection, as there are the potential drawbacks of autologous fat grafts, especially in reconstructed breasts, such as interference with breast cancer diagnosis using radiological studies (Gutowski and ASPS 2009; Kim et al. 2014).

Kronowitz et al. (2016) carried out research with safety in oncological patients over 33 years with lipoinjection for breast reconstruction, without loco regional and systemic recurrence.

The radiological studies permit differentiation between fat necrosis calcification and breast cancer (Rubin and Yoshimura 2010; Rubin 2011; Veber et al. 2011).

The biology of the fat injection was studied by Kato et al. (2014) in three zones of the lipografts: the surviving area, the regenerating area, and the necrotic area. In first two, the fat tissue is regenerated, but in the last one, all cells died and became necrotic cysts and calcification. The adipose-derived stem cells present in autogenous tissue had an important role to reconstitute the regenerating area and several factors are involved (see Chaps. 48 and 49).

An significant recipient is the pectoral muscle, with an important blood supply that avoids or minimizes the development of cysts and calcifications caused by fat necrosis. We use lipoinjection in a bolus under pectoral muscle and we observed that fat is spread; so far, we have not observed the presence of cysts or calcifications. Our only cyst was in a subcutaneous layer, caused by a non-observance of Coleman principles. It was excised with the help of a mastologist without major problems.

In male breasts lipoinjection can be performed for the correction of asymmetry (Fig. 50.7).

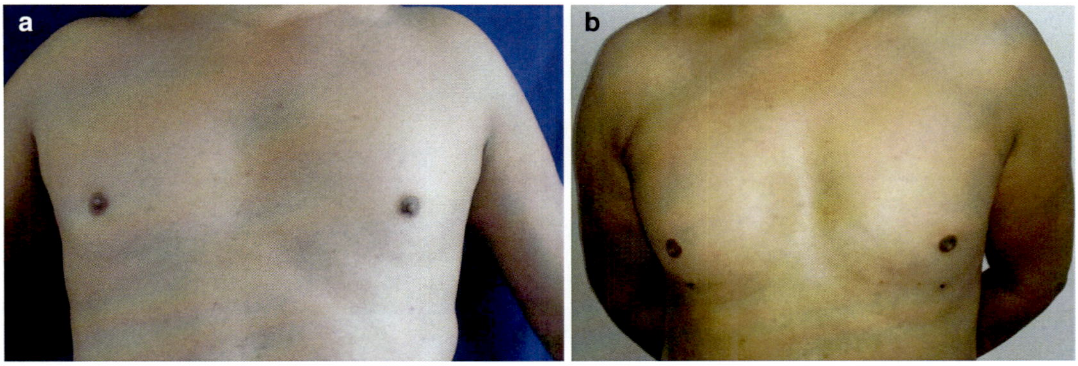

Fig. 50.7 Male patient with asymmetrical breasts with soft depression of the inferomedial pole in the left breast. (**a**) Preoperative view of liposuction with a lipoinjection only in the inferomedial pole of the left breast of 50 mL subcutaneously. (**b**) Frontal view of lipoinjection 40 days postoperatively

Conclusion

The lipoinjection technique represents a long-lasting and natural form of breast augmentation with improvement of size and shape. Volumes greater than 300 mL have not been used by us, but we have achieved good results with no major complications for patients searching for a small increase in the size of their breasts and who want to avoid having an implant in their bodies. Our technique avoids lipoinjection into the gland and uses the advantages of a rich vascular supply provided by the pectoral muscle for good maintenance of the lipografts.

Acknowledgment The authors have no conflicts of interest.

The study had no financial support.

References

American Society of Plastic Surgeons (ASPS) (2013) http://www.plasticsurgery.org/Documents/news-resources/statistics/2013-statistics/plastic-surgery-statistics-full-report-2013.pdf

Bicoll M, Novack BH (1987) Autologous fat transplantation employing liposuction techniques. Ann Plast Surg 18(4):327–329

Caldeira A, Marrou W, Bromley M (2016) Fat transfer in augmentation mammography, a 3D volumetric evaluation. Oral presentation. ASAPS, Las Vegas

Cleveland E, Albano N, Hazen A (2015) Roll, spin, wash, or filter? Processing of lipoaspirate for autologous fat grafting: an updated, evidence-based review of the literature. Plast Reconstr Surg 136(4):706–713

Coleman SR (2001) Structural fat grafts: the ideal filler? Clin Plast Surg 28(1):111–119

Coleman SR, Saboeiro AP (2007) Fat grafting to the breast revisited: safety and efficacy. Plast Reconstr Surg 119(3):775–785

Coleman SR, Saboeiro AP (2015) Primary breast augmentation with fat grafting. Clin Plast Surg 42(3):301–306

Czerny V (1895) Plastischer ersat der brustdruse durch ein lipom. Zentralbl Chir 27:72

Gabriel A, Champaneria MC, Maxwell GP (2015) Fat grafting and breast reconstruction: tips for ensuring predictability. Gland Surg 4(3):232–243

Gutowski KA, ASPS (2009) Fat graft task force. Current applications and safety of autologous fat grafts: a report of the ASPS fat graft task force. Plast Reconstr Surg 124(1):272–280

Kato H, Araki J, Doi K et al (2014) Normobaric hyperoxygenation enhances initial survival, regeneration, and final retention in fat grafting. Plast Reconstr Surg 134(5):951–959. doi:10.1097/PRS.0000000000000600

Khouri RK, Schlenz I, Murphy BJ, Baker TJ (2000) Nonsurgical breast enlargement using an external soft-tissue expansion system. Plast Reconstr Surg;105(7):2500–12; discussion 2513–4

Khouri RK, Eisenmann-Klein M, Cardoso E, Cooley BC, Kacher D, Gombos E, Baker TJ (2012) Brava and autologous fat transfer is a safe and effective breast augmentation alternative: results of a 6-year, 81-patient, prospective multicenter study. Plast Reconstr Surg 129(5):1173–1187

Khouri RK, Rigotti G, Cardoso E, Khouri RK Jr, Biggs T (2014) Megavolume autologous fat transfer.

I. Theory and principles. Plast Reconstr Surg 133(3): 550–557

Kim HY, Jung BK, Lew DH, Lee DW (2014) Autologous fat graft in the reconstructed breast: fat absorption rate and safety based on sonographic identification. Arch Plast Surg 41(6):740–747

Kronowitz SJ, Mandujano CC, Liu J, Kuerer HM, Smith B, Garvey P, Jagsi R, Hsu L, Hanson S, Valero V (2016) Lipofilling of the breast does not increase the risk of recurrence of breast cancer: a matched controlled study. Plast Reconstr Surg 137(2):385–393. doi:10.1097/01.prs.0000475741.32563.50

Li FC, Chen B, Cheng L (2014) Breast augmentation with autologous fat injection. A report of 105 cases. Ann Plast Surg 73(1):S37–S42

Rubin E (2011) Breast imaging considerations in fat grafting to the breast. Plast Reconstr Surg 128(5):570e–571e

Rubin JP, Yoshimura K (2010) Mammographic changes after stem cell supplemented fat transfer compared with changes after breast reduction: a blinded study. Paper presented at International Federation of Adipose Therapeutics and Science Annual Meeting, October 2, 2010, Dallas, Texas; and at the 27th Annual Meeting of the Northeastern Society of Plastic Surgeons, October 30, Washington, DC

Veber M, Tourasse C, Toussoun G, Moutran M, Mojallal A, Delay E (2011) Radiographic findings after breast augmentation by autologous fat transfer. Plast Reconstr Surg 127(3):1289–1299

A Critical Analysis of Breast Implants

51

Wanda Elizabeth Correa and Luis Bernardo Froes

51.1 Introduction

Silicone breast implants have been used for more than 50 years and are probably the most extensively studied device in the history of medicine.

Any critical analysis of implants necessarily focuses on the materials and history. Understanding the stages in the creation of products for augmenting or restoring the breast mound helps to explain why current implants are what they are, including their various characteristics, such as types of coating and filling, manufacturing processes, and safety criteria. (Reidel, 1994).

51.2 Raw Material

Silicone began to be used on a wide scale in the latter half of the twentieth century and is now present in countless products. In medicine as a whole, and in plastic surgery in particular, its use is extremely widespread, playing an outstanding role in breast implants.

W.E. Correa, M.D. (✉)
Department of Ivo Pitanguy Plastic Surgery, Pontifical Catholic University, Rio de Janeiro, RJ 22430-060, Brazil
e-mail: wandaelizabeth@fena.com.br

L.B. Froes, M.D.
Faculty of Medicine, University of Sao Paulo, Butantã, SP 03178-200, Brazil

Silicone is a family of polymeric organic silicon compounds. Silicon itself is a nonmetallic element highly abundant in nature, notably in quartz. Glass is the substance that most resembles silicone. Silicone emerged precisely through attempts to create a kind of pliant glass and can be obtained in various physical forms, such as oils, gels, elastomers, or solids such as resin. Silicone oil is formed by nonreactive short linear chains and silicone gel by reactive short-branched chains. The elastomer is formed by reactive short and long chains with high branch density, and the resin is a hard silicone, more like glass, formed by fully branched short and long chains. Silicone is a colorless, odorless, antioxidant, antifoaming, hydrophobic release agent (nothing adheres to it) that does not cause allergy or reactions in contact with the skin or mucosa. It is biocompatible when implanted in the human body.

The development of silicone dates to between 1863 and 1880, when two German scientists, Fridel and Crafts, made the first attempt to obtain an organic silane. Although unsuccessful, their studies were important for developing a methodology that later allowed Kipplin, a chemistry professor, to obtain a controlled polymeric organic silane in 1904, thus leading to the invention of silicone as we know it today (Brown et al. 1953; Correa n.d. 2011).

However, interest in the industrial use of silicone only emerged in World War II, sparking a huge demand for chemical products that were resistant to extreme conditions, withstanding

J.M. Avelar (ed.), *Breast Surgery*, https://doi.org/10.1007/978-3-319-54115-0_51

temperatures ranging from–50° to +350°, remaining stable, not conducting electricity, and with constant viscosity. Dow Corning, followed by GE, Bayer, and various Japanese and Chinese corporations, manufactured and marketed the first silicone-based products beginning in 1943.

The application of silicone to medicine came soon after its use in military products, with the development of artificial tubes. The first report dates to 1946, in a surgical intervention in which a silicone tube was used to replace the bile duct. Such silicone tubes were later used in shunts, urethras, and joints. (Brown et al. 1953) based on laboratory and clinical trials, described the tolerance and compatibility of silicone when used as a permanent subcutaneous implant. Marzoni was the first to describe the tissue reaction after subdermal implantation, although medical practice had already demonstrated that the material is well-tolerated at this level (Marzoni et al. 1959).

51.3 Use in Plastic Surgery

Czerny (1895) published one of the first reports of breast augmentation surgery. He transplanted a lipoma from the patient's flank to the mammary region in an attempt to correct a defect resulting from the removal of a fibroadenoma.

Attempts in this direction continued, and by the late nineteenth century various materials had been used in injected or implanted form, such as paraffin, ivory, glass balls, rubber, cartilage, glass wool, gutta-percha, or molded polyethylene. Each in its own way caused distortions in shape, with tissue and glandular involvement of the breasts, leading to consequences such as stiffening, necrosis, infection, or other breast deformities, with reports of death, in which infection was the most frequent cause.

In the 1950s and 1960s, other substances were tested to augment the breast mound, such as petroleum jelly, beeswax, epoxy resin, silicone oil, industrial silicone, and Ivalon sponge made of a polyvinyl polymer. These sponges were blocks that surgeons used to sculpt implants with the volume and model desired by each patient (Nahabedian 2007).

Both these and the previous materials resulted in misshapen, stiff, and painful breasts, often ending in bilateral mastectomy. In 1960, Arion developed and implanted for the first time a silicone shell filled with a predefined volume of saline solution, which can be considered the forerunner of subsequent implants.

In 1961, Thomaz Cronin created the first silicone implant. Assisted by Frank Gerow, in 1962, he performed the first surgery to introduce breast implants conceptually similar to those used today, a silicone shell that was also filled with silicone. (Cronin and Gerow, 1963).

These implants were developed jointly with Dow Corning and launched onto the market in 1963. The silicone shells had a smooth surface and were coated with a thick membrane, with a Dacron mesh on the posterior surface to promote suture fixation to the pectoral muscle and a teardrop shape, in an attempt to provide a natural look. They were filled with thick gel and had internal struts for support. The product was christened "natural feel" and can be considered the "first generation" of implants. (Moyer et al. 2012).

Despite the decrease in complications compared with previous products, these implants showed a high capsular contracture rate. Industry, in an attempt to avoid the "hardening" of the breasts, began to manufacture implants with thinner shells and more fluid gel, known as "second-generation" implants. The reduction in thickness increased the rupture rate, in parallel with manufacturing and quality control defects, leading to shell failures. The combination of a more fluid gel and thinner membrane led to the identification of filling gel leaks through the shell, a phenomenon known as "bleeding." (Brandon et al. 1999).

Complications or unfavorable outcomes, due in part to inherent implant factors such as capsular contracture, and in part to the need to improve implant manufacturing, the technique, and surgeons' training, did not stop the growing demand by patients. Drastic improvements compared with the results of previous attempts led to an exponential increase in the demand for breast augmentation, stimulating the gradual improvement of implants and the surgical technique in general (Handel et al. 1995).

51.4 Capsular Contracture and the Development of New Coating Surfaces for Implants

Inherent to implants, capsular contracture had always been by far the most significant problem to be solved or attenuated. The contracture rate in smooth implants, the only ones existing at the time, reached up to 50% in case series.

Implanting any foreign material leads the body to react immediately with local inflammation and cellular reaction against the invading substance. This natural reaction can have three consequences: the material can be rapidly degraded and replaced by scar tissue; the material can be degraded slowly and eventually replaced by scar tissue; or the material may not be degraded and absorbed by the body's defense mechanisms, and is isolated from the rest of the body by scar tissue. This membrane that interposes itself between the implanted material and the surrounding tissues is called a capsule and is formed around all implants, including silicone.

The body's defense against foreign bodies may then enter into two additional stages: contracture of the capsule, as if trying to reduce the implanted volume, and next, an attempt at expulsion from the body. The capsule and the object inside it are thus "pushed" against the outside milieu, and if the object has a sharp part, the resulting pressure slowly causes ischemia until a tiny point of necrosis occurs, leading the skin to rupture and giving rise to the object's systematic expulsion. The intensity and velocity of these reactions are directly proportional to the type of material. Silicone causes a slow reaction, whereas other materials are encapsulated and expelled more intensely and rapidly (Embrey et al. 1999).

Capsule formation always occurs in breast implants, but capsule contracture occurs at varying rates, depending on the type of implant surface, ranging from nearly 0 to almost 50%. Contracture can be unilateral or bilateral, or even recurrent, even after replacing the implants. Expulsion of the implant by the mechanism described above is extremely rare, because encapsulation tends to form a spherical volume without sharp angles that can rupture the skin and expel the implant. Although capsule formation is a natural and even desirable reaction by the body, isolating the material and preventing its contact with the body, capsule contracture can result in a breast mound that is stiff to the touch and unsightly.

Therefore, many of the modifications tested in implants have been aimed specifically at lowering the occurrence or minimizing the intensity of contractures. In 1968, Pangman launched a silicone gel implant coated with a 1-cm-thick layer of polyurethane foam with a Y-shaped polyurethane baffle or internal divider for support, marketed by the manufacturer under the name Natural Y. Ashley (1970) published the first study on this new type of implant, concluding that there was a relevant drop in the capsular contracture rate (Ashley 1972).

All patients develop capsular formation around breast implants. However, around smooth or textured implants, a fibrotic, avascular capsule with varying thickness is formed, containing some inflammatory cells. On polyurethane-coated implants, the capsule displays mild fibroplasia, more accentuated neovascularization, and chronic inflammatory reaction with multinucleated giant cells (Pitanguy et al. 1990). Such implants are believed to have bioactive properties, increasing the interaction between the material and the body, with random contraction vectors, providing lower capsular contracture rates, as reported by Pitanguy et al. (1991).

The greatly reduced capsular contracture rate in polyurethane-coated implants has been attributed (among other hypotheses) to the disruption or nonlinearity of the capsule's normally parallel collagen fibers. This nonlinearity inhibits the circumferential contractility of the fibers, similar to an antenna that is stretched: when crushed or folded, it loses its recoil capacity.

It has also been suggested that polyurethane-coated implants do not avoid capsular contracture, but rather delay its onset. This could be attributed to the progressive loss of the polyurethane layer, slowly degrading over the years, making the implant's coating similar to that of textured implants.

Other observations include an increase in the cell content and greater adherence to the implant. Although this protective layer continues to coat the implant, capsule formation can be up to twice as slow as in textured or smooth-coated implants. Some authors have observed very low short- and medium-term contracture rates in polyurethane-coated implants than in smooth or textured implants (when the latter have already reached the total number of contractures). However, they report that by extending the follow-up time, the contracture rate in polyurethane-coated implants continues to increase over the years, reaching 25% at 10 years.

In the 1980s, the polyurethane-coated implants known as "Meme implants" were widely marketed, especially in North America (Herman, 1984). In Brazil, Meme implants were introduced by Pitanguy in 1988 with highly positive results, decreasing capsular contracture in comparison with smooth surface implants, previously the only ones available on the market. Such implants were later manufactured by Silimed and obtained a significant market share, especially in Brazil (Hester et al. 1988).

The US Food and Drug Administration (FDA) changed the classification and regulations for breast implants in 1991, leading many manufacturers of this and other types of implants to lose interest in their marketing, development, and registration.

Nevertheless, the manufacturing process for these implants evolved, initially from polyurethane foam sheets adhering to the silicone surface to the polyurethane foam's vulcanization directly onto the shell's smooth surface. Among other improvements, this eliminated the potential reaction to the glue used in the process and improved the finishing of the implant's edges.

The satisfactory performance of the Meme implants in the mid-1980s led other manufacturers (who lacked the manufacturing technique) to question polyurethane itself and the possible risks of its byproducts. Later, attributing the low contracture rate to the rippled surface of polyurethane, they began to texture the smooth-coated silicone shells.

Initially, each manufacturer developed its own texturing method. One method used the polyurethane foam sheet itself to imprint its rippled effect onto the smooth silicone surface. Another method involved adhering rock salt to the silicone sheet and then washing it off to remove the residual salt by dilution. Other techniques included sandblasting and even laser printing.

Although the decrease in capsular contracture did not reach the same low rates as with polyurethane-coated implants, textured implants were widely accepted, leading to the gradual abandonment of smooth-surface implants by most surgeons worldwide.

51.5 Filling Gel Cohesivity and Barrier Processes

Improvements in implants were also aimed at decreasing the "bleeding" of filling gel. One solution was to use gel with greater cohesivity than that in the earlier implants (Fig. 51.1). Cohesivity is increased by modifications that provide greater attractive force between the silicone molecules. Another new feature was the development of barrier processes, which are membranes interspersed between the silicone sheets during manufacturing of the implant shell (Fig. 51.2). These features resulted in safer and more reliable implants in terms of the filling content's stability. Implants manufactured in this way were considered to be of the fourth and fifth generations. (Moyer et al. 2012.)

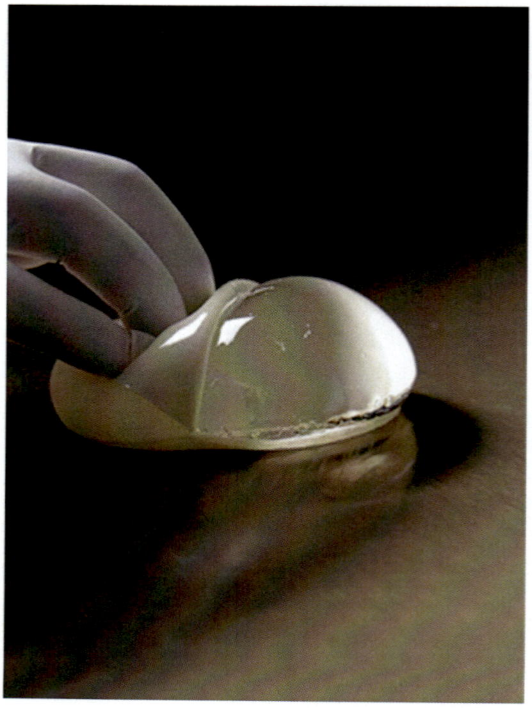

Fig. 51.1 Highly cohesive gel used in current implants

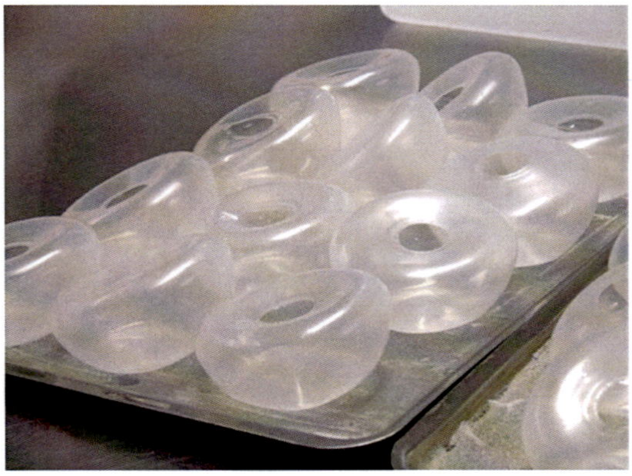

Fig. 51.2 Implant shell before the filling and texturizing process

51.6 1992: The American Moratorium on Silicone Gel Filling

A 30-year period witnessed the testing of numerous types of implants, varying in both surface and filling, and many of these were launched onto the market. Despite the huge number of patients with breast implants, the USA and other countries had previously had no regulation or standardized scientific studies that could certify the safety of using such devices, in the way that we understand safety certification today. There was much more of an empirical feeling by surgeons about the low or even nonexistent occurrence of health problems caused by silicone gel implants. This was widely accepted as sufficient to continue using the implants. However, in April 1992, for various reasons, especially the evolution in criteria for the use of products and substances in humans, with more scientifically rigorous criteria, and even pressure by lobbies and the media, the Food and Drug Administration (FDA) decided to suspend the use of silicone gel as a breast implant filler. The FDA required manufacturers to provide scientific proof that their implants did not cause harm to patients' health. Some European countries adopted similar attitudes to those of the FDA (Brody 2009).

Only in 2006, after one of the most extensive and rigorous tests ever performed in a medical product, was silicone gel filler released once again in the USA. However, most of the European countries had not found scientific evidence to maintain the suspension and had already authorized the use of silicone gel in the late 1980s, setting their own rules from then on. Agencies such as the European Committee for Quality Assurance, Medical Technologies and Devices in Plastic Surgery (EQUAM) were created or mandated to collect scientific documentation on which to base their recommendations and to continue monitoring the evolution of studies.

In the USA, 14 years of study and follow-up in patients with silicone gel implants have failed to prove any harm to their health. (Berry and Davies, 2010).

51.7 Implants Filled With Saline Solution

In addition to implants that are filled with highly cohesive gel, there are implants in which saline is used for filling. Like skin expanders, they are smooth- or textured-surface silicone shells that are filled after implantation. Used especially in the USA during suspension of silicone gel-filled implants, they were never widely accepted in Brazil. Even in the USA, they quickly lost popularity after the release of traditional implants. The hypothetical advantage of "choosing" the volume is negated, with distortions in shape as the filling limit is reached. There may even be problems when the injected volume is lower than the capacity of the implant, potentially folding when the implant is not completely full or a sloshing sound as the body moves, in addition to a more rigid texture to the touch. The implant also empties relatively quickly over the years, leading to a decrease in the volume and its consequences (Young and Watson, 2001).

51.8 Shape and Projection

Recent decades have seen a drop in the number of manufacturers, but also a considerable increase in uniformity of quality in most implants (Fig. 51.3). The reopening of the US market and the rapid increase in the demand for plastic surgeries in various countries have rekindled competition

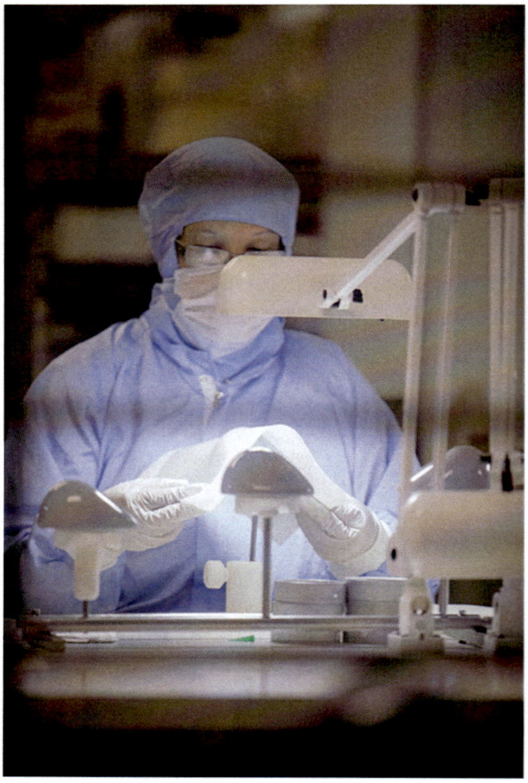

Fig. 51.3 First phase of an implant production process

between suppliers, in addition to demands by surgeons, leading manufacturers to increasingly diversify the shape, projection, and volume of implants. Although the wide range of market options greatly increases the surgeon's choices, the lack of precise equivalence among implants by different suppliers has required each surgeon to identify similarities among products made by various manufacturers.

51.9 How Current Implants are Manufactured

51.9.1 Textured Implants

The texturing process involves imprinting sodium chloride or ammonium carbonate grains on a sheet of silicone elastomer, which is used as the implant's last layer. While the implant is still empty and with the smooth membrane already vulcanized, it receives a layer of dispersed elastomer, over which is placed the last layer, already textured. The implant is then processed in a high-temperature furnace. The texture of the implant depends on the size of the salt grains used. Sodium chloride requires brush-washing the membrane to remove the residues. Even so, the salt leaves traces. With ammonium carbonate, when the implant is heated in the high-temperature furnace, the grains burst, forming a texture with open pores. The texture varies according to the size of the grains.

The implants are then filled with highly cohesive silicone, the open lower part of the implant is sealed with a silicone patch, generally round, and new vulcanization is applied (Fig. 51.4).

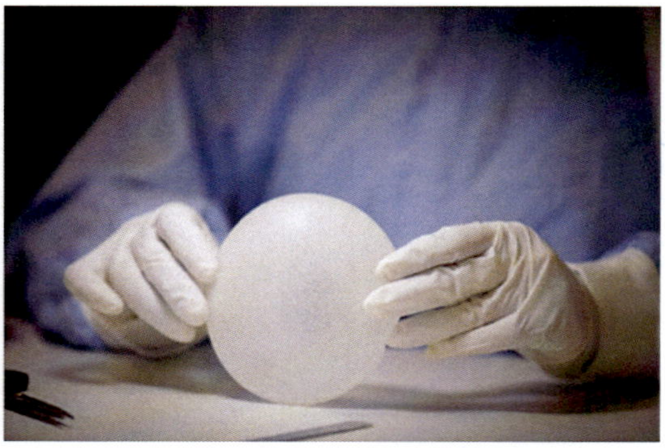

Fig. 51.4 Current texturized implant

51.9.2 Polyurethane-Covered Implants

The already vulcanized smooth shell is filled with highly cohesive gel, similar to a smooth implant. The sealing patch is placed on the posterior side, after which a last layer of elastomer is applied to the implant, and finally the

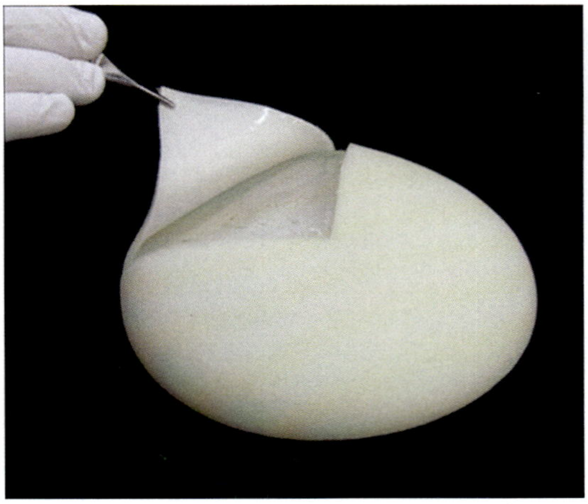

Fig. 51.5 Detail of a polyurethane-covered implant shell

polyurethane sheet covers the outside of the future implant (Fig. 51.5). The implant is then heated in the high-temperature furnace for another vulcanization process. Elastomer dispersion penetrates the polyurethane pores, drastically reducing the possibility of delamination of the polyurethane.

51.10 Quality Control

The implants, with their final shape, undergo individual inspection, in which they are discarded if there is any alteration in the shell, filling, or closing patch. Air bubbles that may occasionally remain inside the implant are removed by puncture with a needle developed for this purpose (Fig. 51.6), through the closing patch, which is then sealed with a drop of silicone gel (Fig. 51.7). The implant is then vulcanized.

Already complete, the implants are placed in blister packs and sterilized with either ethylene oxide (ETO) or dry heat. After this stage, implants that have been sterilized in ETO comply with the quarantine standard for the use of this process, for dispersion of the ETO.

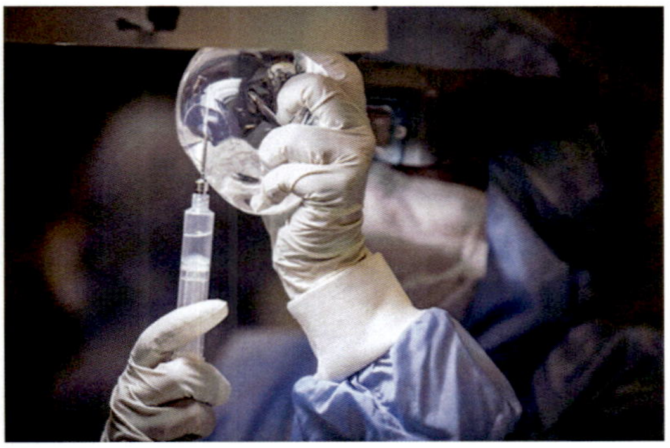

Fig. 51.6 Remaining air bubble being removed by puncture

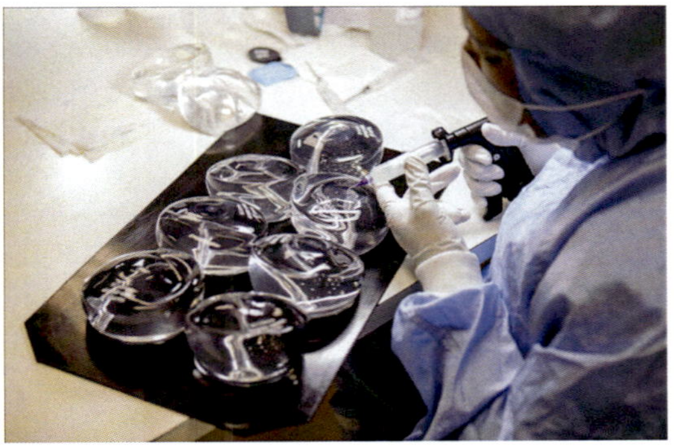

Fig. 51.7 Implant being sealed with a drop of silicone gel before vulcanization

51.11 Pregnancy and Breastfeeding

There is no scientific evidence for teratogenic or mutagenic effects, or interference with breastfeeding, or the presence of silicone in the breast milk of mothers with breast implants.

Conclusion

More than half a century has passed since the first use of breast implants as we know them today. Over the decades, various generations of plastic surgeons have accompanied and often actively participated in improvements to the manufacturing methods, the vast expansion of available implant models, the introduction of rigorous product quality control rules, the enforcement of the serious and systematic evaluation of implants and their risks to humans, and the elaboration of countless studies, many of which have focused on discrediting the materials and the implants themselves. Implants have also been highly visible in the lay media, which sometimes extols them, even presenting an unrealistic or misleading picture, as if they were magic solutions to different problems and types of patients, only to swing in the other direction by creating an atmosphere of fear, as if some malignant or destructive evidence had been discovered about them.

Implants have survived waves of pessimism about their use, present or future, not least the moratorium by the United States and other countries, having passed and resisted especially during the suspension, with tests and trials rarely seen in elsewhere in medicine in terms of number, quality, and intensity. Meanwhile, over the years, other materials such as soybean oil or fat in the form of autologous grafts have emerged with the aim of replacing silicone gel. All these other materials have come and gone, without demonstrating superiority or even equivalent results.

Today's implants obviously display inherent problems to be solved and improvements to be pursued, as with any other medical discovery. However, in the current scenario, to our knowledge, no trial or publication exists whose conclusions have achieved sufficient international scientific consensus to generate or even provide grounds for a universal recommendation to remove or replace implants based on the time since implantation, much less to generically condemn their use.

The first patient to receive breast implants, in 1963, still had her implants on the 50th anniversary of her surgery. This is probably the most striking image of one of the greatest milestones in medicine, and especially of plastic surgery, that has helped to reduce or overcome physical, psychological, and social losses and traumas for millions of patients worldwide.

References

Ashley FL (1970) A new type of breast prosthesis. Preliminary report. Plast Reconstr Surg 45(5):421–424

Ashley FL (1972) Further studies on the natural-Y breast prosthesis. Plast Reconstr Surg 49(4):414

Berry MG, Davies DM (2010) Breast augmentation. I. A review of the silicone prosthesis. J Plast Reconstr Aesthet Surg 63(11):1761–1768

Brandon HJ, Jerina KL, Wolf CJ et al (1999) Ultimate strength properties of control and explanted Silastic I and Silastic 0 silicone gel-filled breast implant shells. Aesth Surg J 19:381–387

Brody GS (2009) Breast implants, safety and efficacy of silicone. University of Southern California, California

Brown JB, Fryer MP, Randall P et al (1953) Silicones in plastic surgery: laboratory and clinical investigations, a preliminary report. Plast Reconstr Surg 12:374–376

Correa WEM (2011) Implantes Mamários de Silicone. Cirurgia Plástica - Para a Formação do Especialista. Ed. Carreirão S. Editora Atheneu, Rio de Janeiro.

Cronin TD, Gerow FJ (1963) Augmentation mammaplasty: a new "natural feel" prosthesis. Transactions of the 3rd international congress of plastic surgery. Excerpta Medica Foundation, Amsterdam, pp 41–49

Embrey M, Adams E, Cunningham B, Peters W, Young L, Carlo GL (1999) A review of the literature on the etiology of capsular contracture and a pilot study to determine the outcome of capsular contracture interventions. Aesth Plast Surg 23:197–206

Handel N et al (1995) The fate of breast implants: a critical analysis of complications and outcomes. Plast Reconstr Surg 96(7):1521–1533

Herman S (1984) The Meme implant. Plast Reconstr Surg 73(3):411–414

Hester TR Jr et al (1988) A 5-year experience with polyurethane-covered mammary prostheses for treatment of capsular contracture, primary augmentation mammoplasty, and breast reconstruction. Clin Plast Surg 15(4):569–585

Marzoni FA, Upchurch SE, Lambert CJ (1959) An experimental study of silicone as a soft tissue substitute. Plast Reconstr Surg 24:600–608

Moyer HR, Ghazi BH, Losken A (2012) The effect of silicone gel bleed on capsular contracture: a generational study. Plast Reconstr Surg 130(4):793–800

Nahabedian MY (2007) Explantation of 41-year-old implants following primary breast augmentation. Ann Plast Surg 58(1):91–94

Pitanguy I et al (1990) Implante de silicone gel com revestimento de poliuretano. Rev Bras Cir 80(2):119–130

Pitanguy I, Salgado FS, Radwanski HN, Stersa RM (1991) Estágio atual dos implantes mamários. Rev Bras Cir 81(6):291–299

Reidel, Bern (1994) História do silicone.

Young VL, Watson ME (2001) Breast implant research "where we have been, where we are, where we need to go". Clin Plast Surg 28(3):451–483

52 Augmentation Mastoplasty Using Polyurethane-Covered Prostheses

Arnaldo Miró

52.1 Introduction

Breast augmentation surgery using silicone implants is one of the most frequently performed aesthetical surgical procedures worldwide.

Silicone breast implants have undergone many developments since their introduction into plastic surgery by Cronin and Gerow (1964), minimizing any adverse effects and optimizing the results.

Evolution of the implant has encompassed variations in the gel density, barriers to reduce silicone transudation, and new shapes and volumes.

However, the most important new achievement was the introduction of a polyurethane coating over the surface of the implants, contributing substantially to reducing capsular contracture, widely considered to be the main adverse event in the use of silicone breast implants (Baker 1975; Baker et al. 1976, 1978).

In the literature an average of 1–2% capsular contracture is reported in patients using polyurethane coated implants (De la Pena-Salcedo et al. 2012; Gasperoni et al. 1992; Miró 2009; Vázquez 1999, 2005; Vázquez and Pellón 2007).

Since being described and released by Ashley (1970, 1972), the original polyurethane-coated implant has achieved many new advantages.

A. Miró
Clinica de Cirurgia Plastica e Reparadora Dr. Arnaldo Lobo Miró Ltda, Alameda Dom Pedro II, 80420-060 Curitiba, PR, Brazil
e-mail: arnaldomiro@clinicamiro.com.br

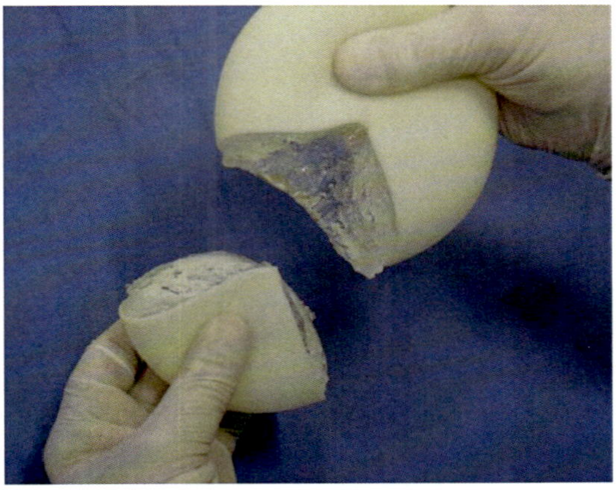

Fig. 52.1 Breast prosthesis with cohesive gel and polyurethane foam surface

By means of an innovative technology, the current implant has a highly cohesive filling with thinner additional polyurethane covering, via a new vulcanization process (Fig. 52.1).

The systematic use of polyurethane-coated implants has long been the subject of worldwide controversy among the scientific community owing to an article published by the National Cancer Institute (1979), reporting an increased risk for breast cancer in rats after the administration of large doses of 2,4-diaminotoluene (2,4-TDA). The FDA solicited extensive studies from the manufacturers regarding the safety and viability of using this substance in breast implants, and the manufacturers decided to temporarily suspend their trade while the research was being carried out (FDA 2004). Thereafter, the FDA

J.M. Avelar (ed.), *Breast Surgery*, https://doi.org/10.1007/978-3-319-54115-0_52

imposed a moratorium on silicone manufacture and trading in the USA. Since then, many manufacturers have ceased production.

Eventually, in 1995, supported by comprehensive studies, laboratory research, and the documented clinical experience of dozens of surgeons from around the world (Smahel 1978; Brand 1984, 1988; Hester et al. 1988, 1991; Kerrigan 1989; Sinclair et al. 1993), the FDA released a new update, in which they stated: "Based on the very small amounts of TDA found in urine, the potential cancer risk, if any, is likely to be negligible. FDA's estimate of excess cancer risk from exposure to TDA is about 1 in 1 million over a woman's lifetime." (Food and Drug Administration (FDA) 1995).

A retrospective review of scientific publications, by highly respected surgeons in the international scientific community, is favorable toward the use of polyurethane-covered implants, emphasizing a drastic reduction in the rates of capsular contracture (Brand 1984, 1988; Frame et al. 2015; Gasperoni et al. 1992; Hester et al. 1997; Kerrigan 1989; Melmed 1988; Pitanguy et al. 1990; Rebello 1993; Vázquez 1999, 2005; Vázquez and Pellón 2007).

52.2 Method

A personal sample of 563 medical records was retrospectively surveyed in which we could analyze each patient's characteristics, wishes, and surgical plan between 1995 and 2015. A total of 430 of these 563 patients were cases of primary breast augmentation and 120 were secondary cases with various presenting complaints.

52.3 Technical Highlights, Results, and Comments

52.3.1 Implant Volume Selection

To evaluate and select implant volume, oval-shaped plastic sizers with pre-established measurements are tested on the breasts. The sizers both simulate the implant volume during the initial consultation and help to visualize any asymmetries in shape and volume that should be addressed surgically (Fig. 52.2).

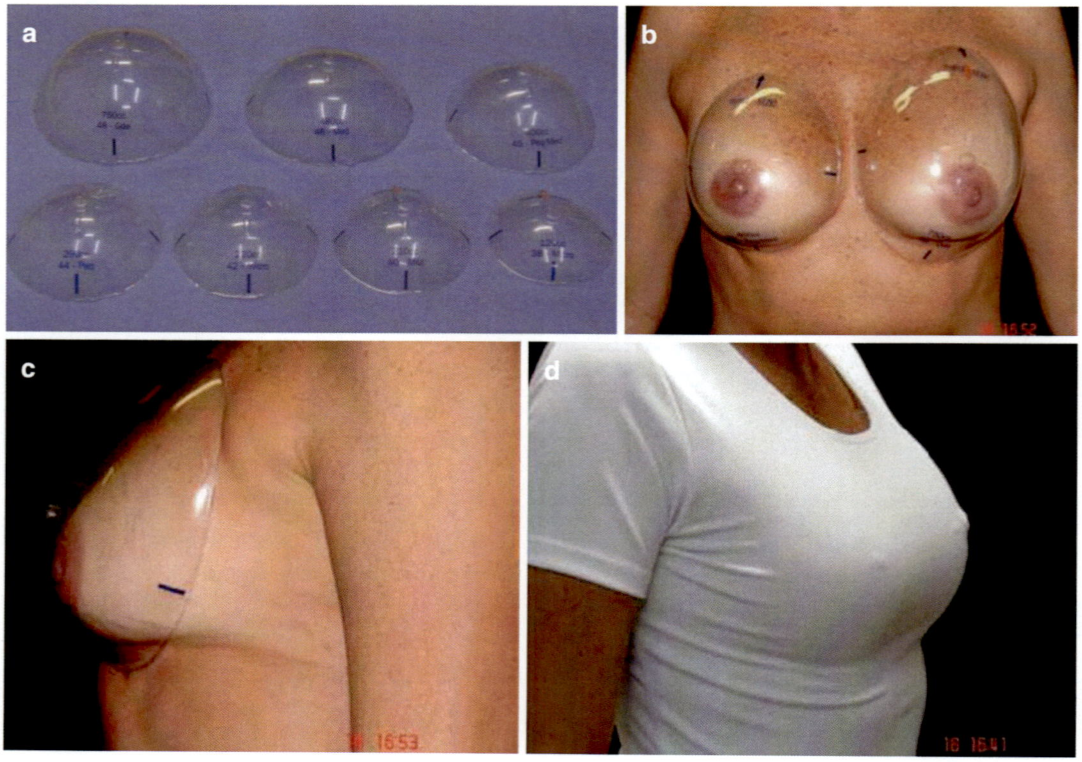

Fig. 52.2 (**a–c**) Transparent sizers used to evaluate the volume of breast augmentation. (**d**) A tight T-shirt aids in the evaluation of the desired implant volume

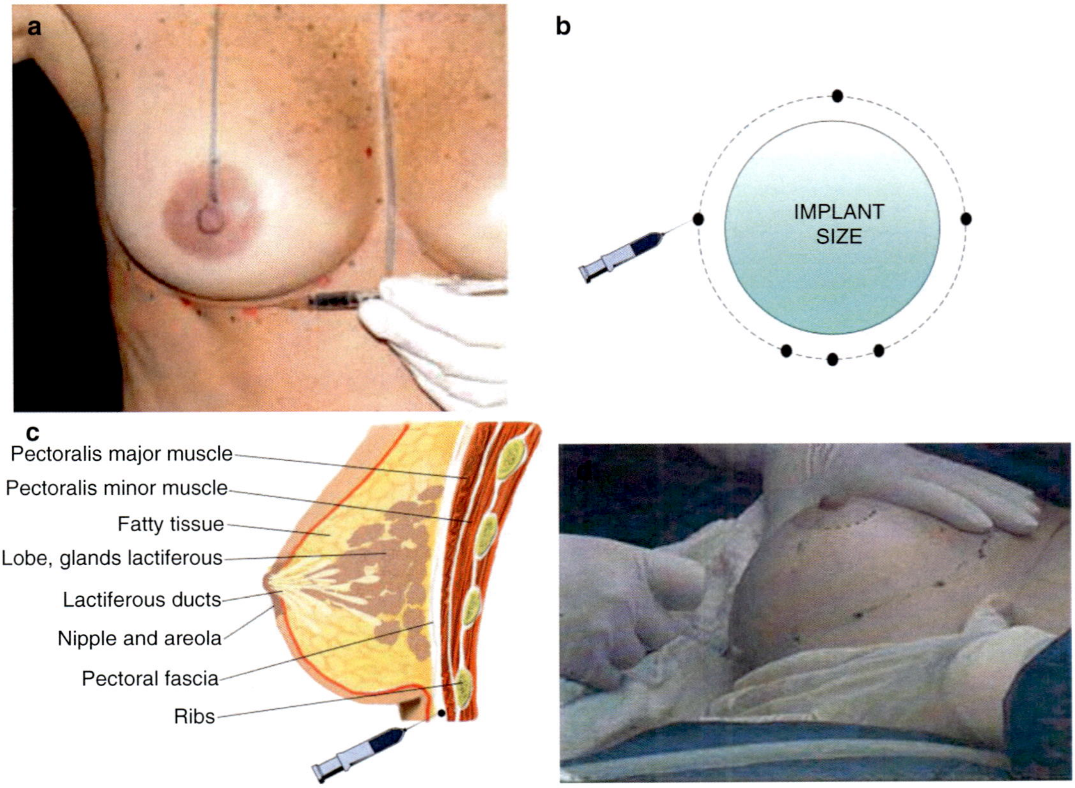

Fig. 52.3 (**a**) The implant position should be precisely set according to referential outlines: externally on the skin over the gland and internally in the underlying subcutaneous fat. The new mammary fold, a midsternal line, and a midclavicular-line locate the prosthesis in the new mammary shape. (**b**, **c**) Diagrammatic aspects of the cutaneous marking, with two concentric lines, the inner circle located at the edge of the prosthesis, and the outer circle located about 1–2 cm from the first; methylene *blue* injection outlines the subjacent adipose tissue, indicating the margins of the dissection. (**d**) Delimitation of the area to be manipulated

52.3.2 Anesthesia

Epidural block, with mild sedation is our usual choice for the procedure; however, general or local anesthesia with sedation may be used. Infiltration of saline solution and epinephrine (1:200,000) is employed in the retromammary space.

52.3.3 Marking

The position of the implants over the chest is noted with the patient in the upright position, marking the inframammary fold and two vertical, parallel lines: the first along the midsternal line and the second on the midclavicular line (Fig. 52.3a). The projection of the implant over the breast area is outlined according its diameter. The limit of the implant pocket dissection is marked with transcutaneous injection of methylene blue into the deep adipose tissue using an insulin syringe (Fig. 52.3b, c). The margin is always located 1–2 cm beyond the edge of the implant's diameter (Fig. 52.3d).

52.3.4 Incisions

In our approach, we consider the preference of the patient, the volume of the implants, and the diameter of the areola (Fig. 52.4). Whenever possible, the author's first choice is an infra-areolar incision and the second choice is the inframammary fold.

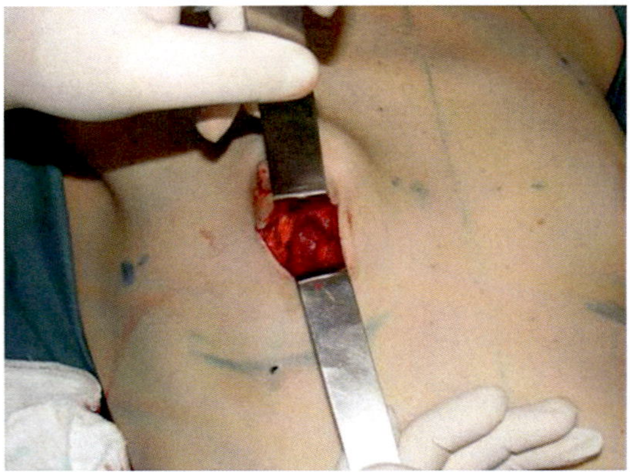

Fig. 52.4 Intraoperative detail of the inferior periareolar approach

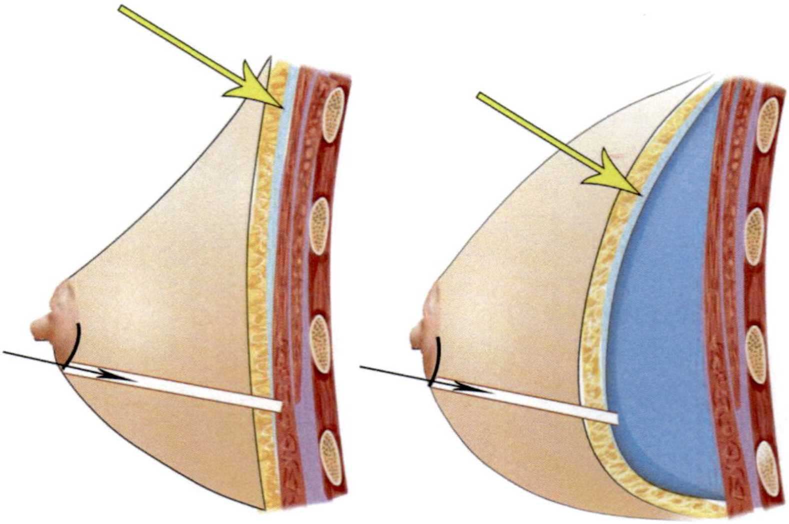

Fig. 52.5 Periareolar access approach and subfascial position of the implant

52.3.5 Dissection

The preference for undermining is the subfascial plane (De la Pena-Salcedo et al. 2012; Goes 2010; Hunstad and Webb 2010; Graf et al. 2003), whenever possible, and should be slightly larger than the diameter of the implant. The pectoral fascia is reached after the transfixation of the mammary gland (Fig. 52.5), and then, superior and lateral undermining is performed. The inferior portion is undermined in the retromammary space up to the margin of the new fold. The dissection limit is determined by the methylene blue, which was previously marked deeply subcutaneous into the breast fat (Fig. 52.6). At the end of dissection, only the upper pole is covered by the pectoral fascia.

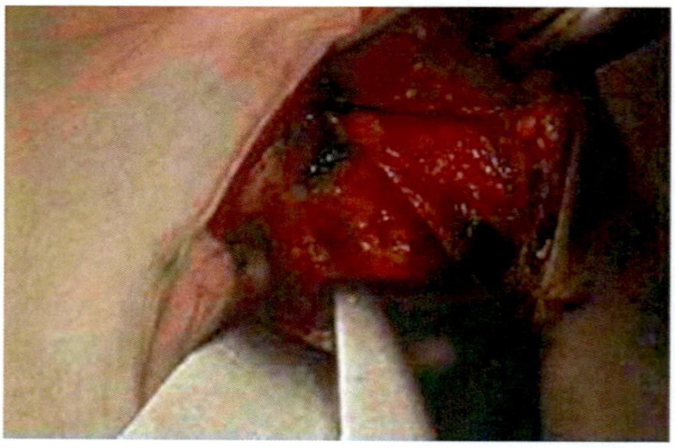

Fig. 52.6 The deep fat demarcation with methylene *blue* outlining the dissection limits

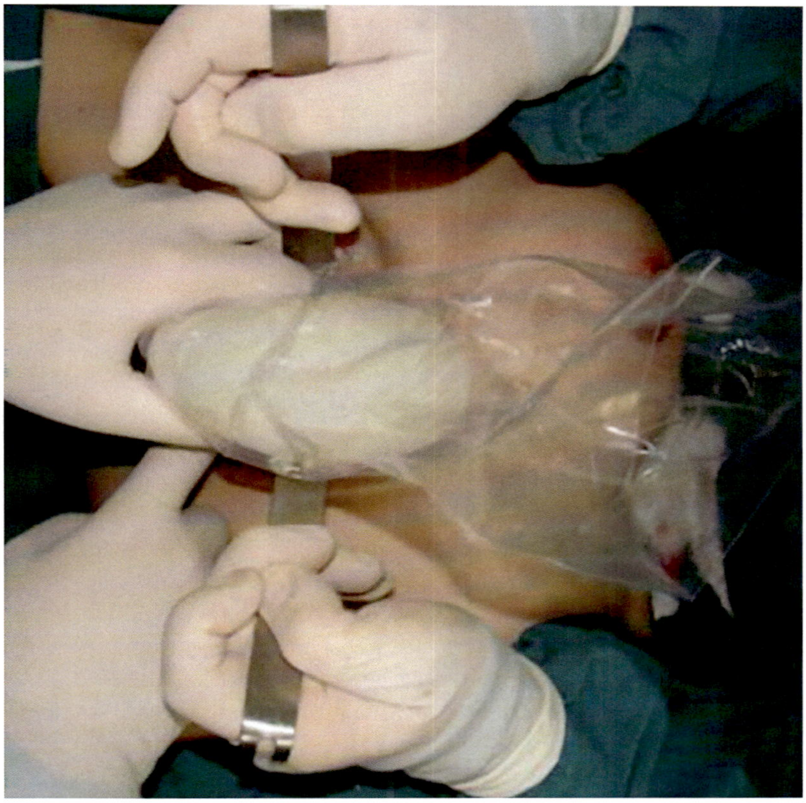

Fig. 52.7 Implant being inserted with the aid of the plastic sleeve

52.3.6 Insertion

Gloves should be changed and the pocket washed with antibiotics. The plastic sleeve that accompanies the implant facilitates its placement and avoids damage and contact with the edges of the incision (Fig. 52.7).

52.3.7 Stitches

Vicryl™ 3–0 is used to close glandular tissue, and vicryl™ 4–0 for subdermal closure. For the skin, intradermal sutures are made using 3–0 nylon. This is removed after 20–30 days. Suction drains are only used in secondary surgeries. Compression dressings, a support bra, and cotton gauze are worn.

52.3.8 Postoperative Care

Prophylactic use of 1 g intravenous cephalosporin-based antibiotics should be started at the time of sedation and is maintained intravenously for 24 h. Oral antibiotics are given for 5 more days.

Skin stretching, or the subjective feeling of the implant, is a common complaint in the first 30 days. An implant that is soft to the touch and that looks natural is expected 3–4 months after the procedure, as the final result. The use of a close-fitting (but not tight) support bra, adequate rest, and movement restriction of the upper limbs are also part of the postoperative protocol.

Massage of the breast area is not recommended or prescribed. Considering the adhesiveness of the implant to the surrounding tissue, massage could possibly be ineffective or harmful.

The patient may return to light activities 1 week after surgery. Sun exposure and sports activity are not allowed for 40 days.

Polyurethane-coated implants are slightly more difficult to handle owing to their "velvety" texture. Its introduction via small access incisions and its positioning in the dissected pocket require special care, and we stress the importance of a pocket that is larger than the diameter of the implant. The sliding and accommodation of the implants also require special attention to avoid the occurrence of folds, which could be particularly visible and/or palpable in very slim patients. The skin marks and the methylene blue marks in the fat, as a reference to a 1- or 2-cm larger pocket, is a safer guide to precise undermining. The adhesive characteristics of the implant in relation to the surrounding tissues does not permit later attempts to change the position of the implants. Therefore, suitable dimensions of the pocket that are adequate for the size of the implants are mandatory. A new inframammary fold must be precisely located too. Transoperative replacement of the implant can be more time-consuming and difficult compared with other types of implants.

52.4 Discussion

52.4.1 Considerations Regarding the Characteristics of the Polyurethane-Coated Implant

Differing from other implants in their process of accommodation of the pocket, polyurethane-coated prostheses present the following characteristics: (1) great adhesiveness to the adjacent tissues; (2) intense cellular response from the organism to their presence as foreign bodies; (3) a particular degradation process of the polyurethane; (4) singular capsule formation around the implant.

Their Velcro™-like adhesiveness to the tissue around the implant does not permit any rotation or displacement from its original position, offering particular benefit to patients with a natural profile or anatomically shaped prostheses, where any degree of malpositioning is markedly visible.

The reaction known as biodegradation of the polyurethane foam generates a range of known byproducts, including polyester and toluene diisocyanate, the latter breaking down further into MDA (methylenedianiline) and 2,4-TDA.

Following studies conducted in laboratory rats, 2,4-TDA was considered carcinogenic for several years. However, despite the FDA statement, in a monograph, Kerrigan (1989) asserted that, "...based on our study of breast prosthesis with polyurethane coating, we can state that we did not find any proof that would suggest that these prostheses are dangerous products for internal use in surgery. On the contrary, the data in the literature suggest that this implant markedly reduces morbidity and the necessity of secondary surgeries..." In 2013, the Brazilian Society of Plastic Surgery's Commission on Silicone, referring to the study by Sai Yi Pan et al. (2012, replied: "According to the analysis of this committee based on the material presented for evaluation, there is, up to this date, no new data that is known to this committee about the potential risks involving polyurethane coated breast implants and a possible association with breast cancer or neoplastic pathologies of any other nature." (Silicon Commission from Brazilian Plastic Surgeons Society 2013).

The most important feature of polyurethane-coated implants is the sharp reduction in rates of capsular contracture. According to numerous studies (Brand 1984; Hester et al. 1988; Rebello 1993), this has two main causes. The first is of a physical nature, in which the irregular surface of the implant favors the formation of a nonlinear pattern of fibrotic scarring around the implant, thus preventing the deforming spherical contracture. The second cause is of a biological nature, in which an intense inflammatory reaction to a foreign body occurs, characterized by the presence of giant cells and macrophages with active phagocytosis involving numerous polyurethane fragments, thus forming millions of microcapsules without coalescence, avoiding a synergic single capsular contracture around the implant (Fig. 52.8).

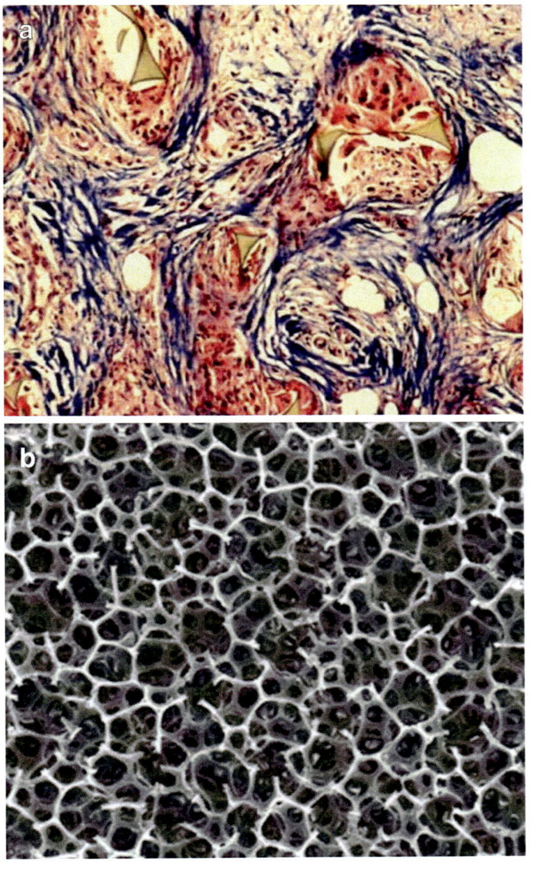

Fig. 52.8 (**a**) Polyurethane microscopic capsule. The stained blue collagen, surrounding single polyurethane structures, forming microcapsules. (**b**) Polyurethane foam surface view under the electron microscope. Imagens taken from Handel's paper (2006)

52.5 Intercurrences and Complications

The author's personal survey of 563 patients who underwent breast augmentation surgeries with polyurethane-coated implants, revealed the following complications.

Among the postoperative complications, there were three cases of unilateral infection, with *Staphylococcus epidermidis*. In these cases, the implant was removed, the infection successfully treated, and the patients were fully recovered in 6 months, at which point another breast augmentation was carried out. Four cases of seroma were detected 2 and 3 months postoperatively, as confirmed by breast ultrasound, and were treated with transcutaneous puncture using a thin, blunt cannula, with the aid of ultrasound. Three cases of medium-volume hematoma in the superior pole were treated with transincisional aspiration under sedation. Seven cases of cutaneous rash occurred during the first 15 days, but were resolved with the use of systemic corticosteroids. Last, we identified in our survey four cases of Baker grade III unilateral capsular contracture. These patients were reoperated with radical capsulotomy, pocket enlargement, and successfully received a new implant.

Conclusion

This systematic use of polyurethane-coated implants allowed us to minimize the intercurrences and/or postoperative complications, providing good results in most cases.

The natural look of the results, feeling soft to the touch, and the low rate of complications are important features of polyurethane-coated implants. A requirement for their use is more elaborate pocket preparation and more demanding implant accommodation, but the benefits and results achieved overcome these technical features, making this implant suitable for diversified aesthetic and reconstructive breast augmentation (Figs. 52.9, 52.10, 52.11, 52.12).

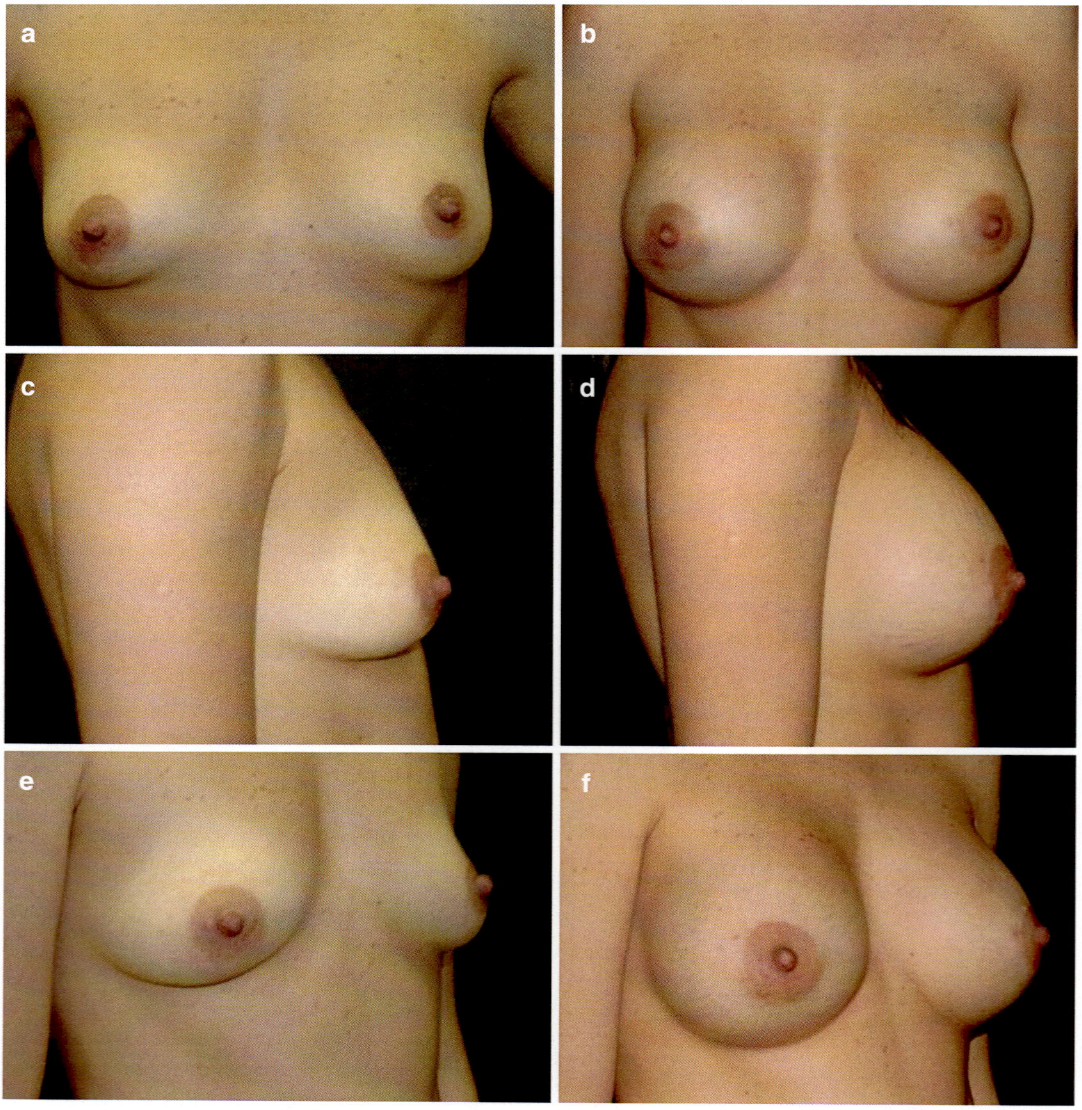

Fig. 52.9 A 29-year-old patient. (**a**, **c**, **e**) Frontal, profile, and lateral views: presenting moderate hypomastia without ptosis and slight asymmetry in shape and volume. (**b**, **d**, **f**) Five months after surgery, with high-profile prostheses of 285 cc on the right and 305 cc on the left

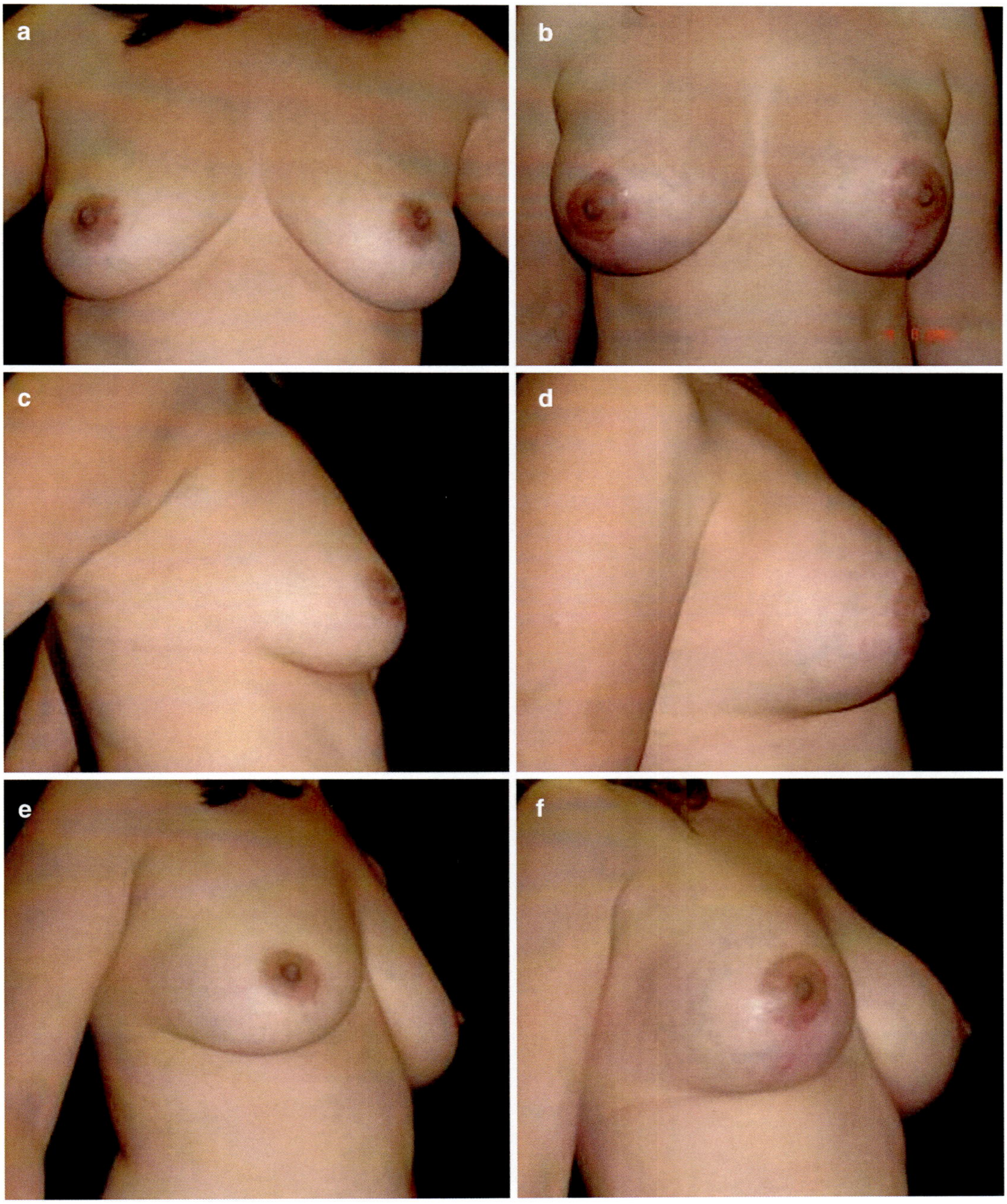

Fig. 52.10 A 46-year-old patient. (**a**, **c**, **e**) Frontal, profile, and lateral views: presenting mammary ptosis, asymmetry, and deficiency of the upper pole. (**b**, **d**, **f**) Four months postoperatively. Mastopexy with medial inferior incision and implants of 255 cc on the right and 235 cc on the left, with a high, round profile

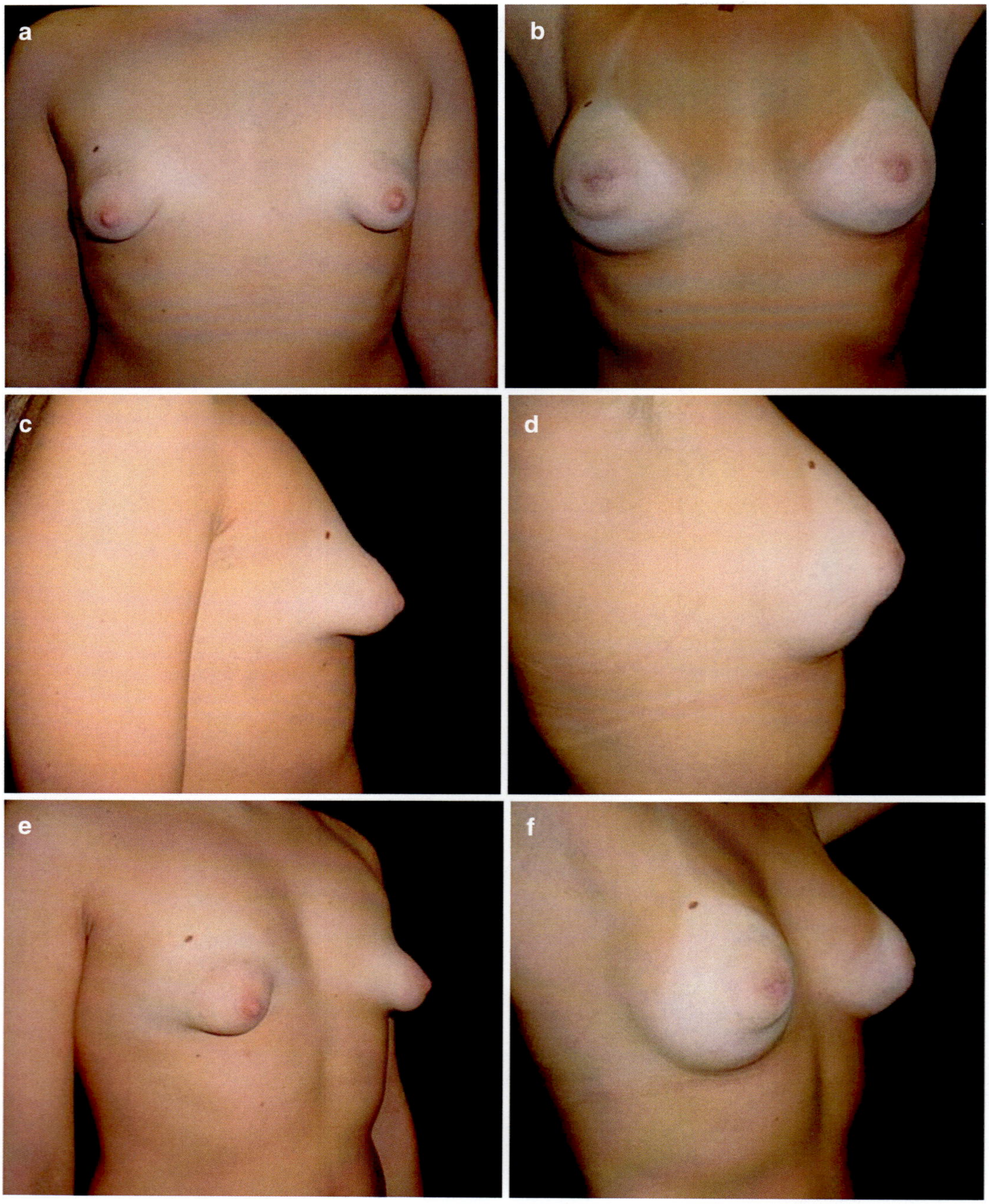

Fig. 52.11 A 21-year-old patient. (**a**, **c**, **e**) Frontal, profile, and lateral views: before surgery, presenting hypomastia and tuberous breasts. (**b**, **d**, **f**) Twelve months postoperatively, with high-profile 285-cc implants (no need for any specific treatment in the nipple–areola region)

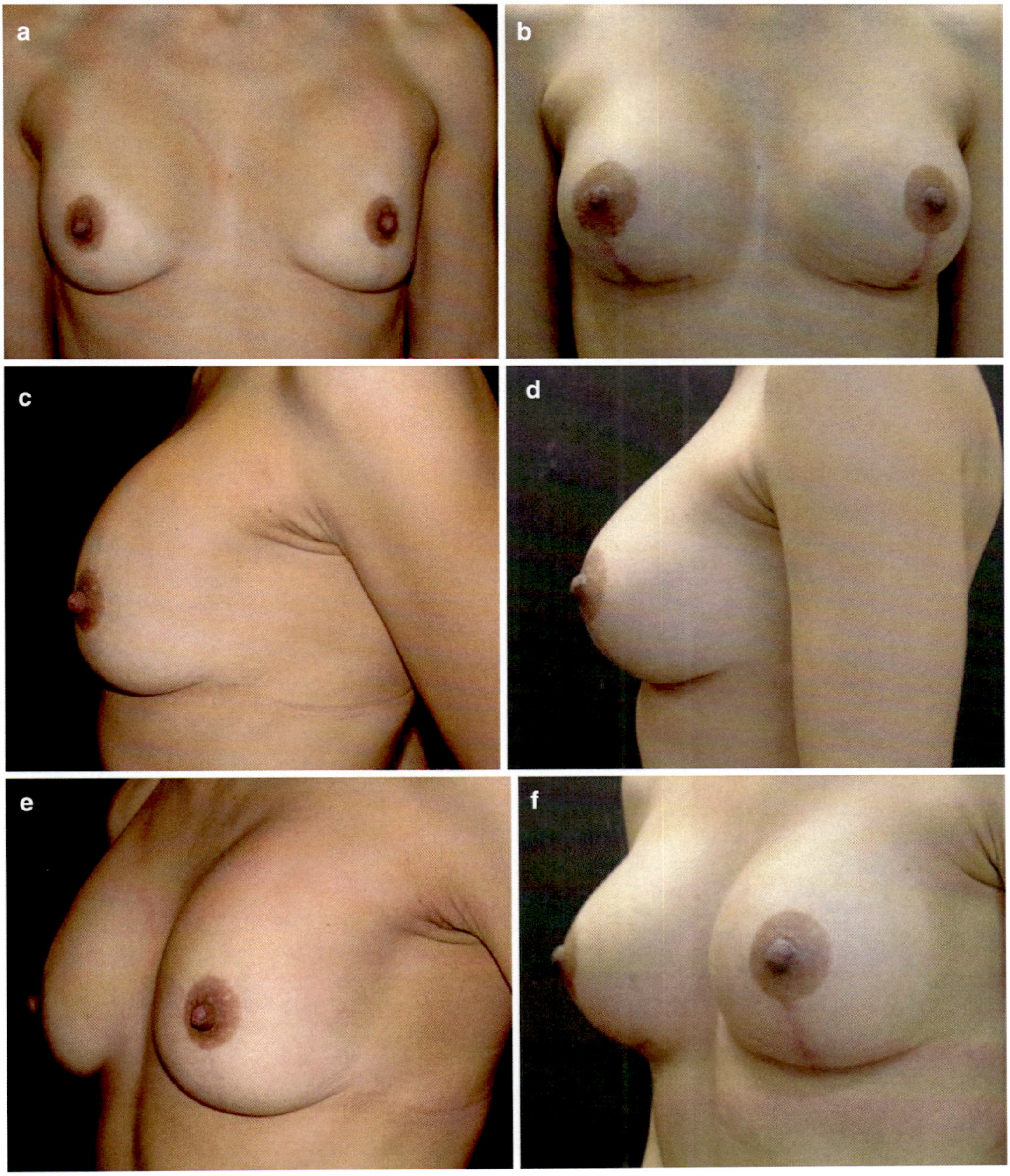

Fig. 52.12 A 43-year-old patient. (**a**, **c**, **e**) Frontal, profile, and lateral views before surgery. The patient had previously undergone a submuscular breast implant with Baker grade III contracture. (**b**, **d**, **f**) Four months postoperatively, after a change to the subfascial plane, capsulotomy, mastopexy, and 285-cc high-profile implants

References

Ashley FL (1970) A new type of breast prosthesis: preliminary report. Plast Reconstr Surg 45(5):421–424

Ashley FL (1972) Further studies on the natural-Y breast prosthesis. Plast Reconstr Surg 49(4):414–419

Baker JL Jr. (1975) Classification of spherical contractures. Presented at the Aesthetic Breast Symposium, Scottdale, Arizona

Baker JL Jr, Bartels RJ, Douglas WM (1976) Closed compression technique for rupturing a contracted capsule around a breast implant. Plast Recontr Surg 58(2):137–141

Baker DE, Retsky MI, Schultz S (1978) "Bleeding" of silicone from bag-gel breast implants, and clinical relation to fibrous capsule reaction. Plast Reconstr Surg 61(6):836–841

Brand KG (1984) Polyurethane-coated silicone implants and the question of capsular contracture. Plast Reconstr Surg 73(3):498

Brand KG (1988) Foam-covered mammary implants. Clin Plast Surg 15(4):533–539

Cronin TD, Gerow F. (1964) Augmentation mammoplasty: a new (natural feel) prosthesis. In: Transactions of the Third International Congress of Plastic Surgery, Amsterdam, Excerpta Medica, pp 41–9

De la Pena-Salcedo JA, Soto-Miranda MA, Lopez-Salguero JF (2012) Back to the future: a 15 years experience with polyurethane foam-covered breast implants using the partial subfascial technique. 36:331-338.

FDA (2004) Breast Implant Consumer Handbook. Timeline of breast implant activities

Food and Drug Administration (FDA) (1995) Update: Study of TDA released from polyurethane foam-covered breast implants

Frame J, Kamel D, Olivan M, Cintra H (2015) The in vivo pericapsular tissue response to modern polyurethane breast implants. Aesth Plast Surg 39:713–723

Gasperoni C, Salgarello M, Gargani G (1992) Polyurethane-covered mammary implants: a 12-year experience. Ann Plast Surg 29(4):303–308

Goes JCS (2010) Breast implant stability in the subfascial plane, and the new shaped silicone gel breast implants. Aesth Plast Surg 34:23–28

Graf RM, Bernanrdes A, Rippel R, Araujo LR, Damasio RC, Auerswald A (2003) Subfascial breast implant: a new procedure. Plast Reconstr Surg 111(2): 904–908

Handel N (2006) Long-term safety and efficacy of polyurethane foam-covered breast implants. Aesthetic Surg J 26:265–274

Hester TR Jr, Cukic J (1991) Use of stacked polyurethane-covered mammary implants in aesthetic and reconstructive breast surgery. Plast Reconstr Surg 88(3):503–509

Hester TR Jr, Nahai F, Bostwick J, Cukic J (1988) A 5-year experience with polyurethane-covered mammary prostheses for treatment of capsular contracture, primary augmentation mammoplasty, and breast reconstruction. Clin Plast Surg 15(4):569–585

Hester TR Jr, Ford NF, Gale PJ, Hammett JL, Raymond R, Turnbull D et al (1997) Measurement of 2,4-toluenediamine in urine and serum samples from women with meme or replicon breast implants. Plast Reconstr Surg 100(5):1291–1298

Hunstad J, Webb L (2010) Subfascial breast augmentation: comprehensive experience. Aesth Plast Surg 34:365–373

Kerrigan CA (1989) Report on the Meme breast implant. McGill University, Montreal

Melmed E (1988) Polyurethane implants: a 6-year review of 416 patients. Plast Reconstr Surg 82(2):285–290

Miró AL (2009) Polyurethane-coated silicone breast implants: evaluation of 14 years' experience. Rev Bras Cir Plast 24(3):296–303

National Cancer Institute (1979) Bioassay of 2.4 diaminotoluene for possible carcinogenicity. (DHEW/Pub. NIH-79-1718)

Pitanguy I, Brentano J, Castro RM (1990) Implante de silicone gel com revestimento de poliuretano [Silicone gel implant with polyurethane coating]. Rev Bras Cir 80:119

Rebello C (1993) Mamoplastia de aumento com próteses mamárias de silicone revestidas de poliuretano [Augmentation mammoplasty with polyurethane coated prostheses]. Rev Bras Cir Plast 8:58

Silicon Commission from Brazilian Plastic Surgeons Society (2013)—E-Plastiko's -official SBCP periodical magazine 19/2013 - News SBCP

Sinclair TM, Kerrigan CL, Buntic R (1993) Biodegradation of the polyurethane foam covering of breast implants. Plast Reconstr Surg. Nov;92(6):1003–13; discussion 1014.

Smahel J (1978) Tissue reactions to breast implants coated with polyurethane. Plast Reconstr Surg 61(1):80–85

Vázquez G (1999) A ten-year experience using polyurethane-covered breast implants. Aesthet Plast Surg 23(3):189–196

Vázquez G (2005) Modification of the anatomic silicone gel implant with polyurethane cover. Cir Plast Iberolatinamer 31:193–198

Vázquez G, Pellón A (2007) Polyurethane-coated silicone gel breast implants used for 18 years. Aesthet Plast Surg 31(4):330–336

53 Critical Analysis on Access to and Location of Breast Implants

Marcelo Paulo Vaccari Mazzetti
and Ryane Schmidt Brock

53.1 Introduction

For women, the breast is a particular and fundamental part of the human body. Although the gluteus has sexual significance, femininity is represented by breasts. In addition, they represent the important function of feeding a newborn.

Breast augmentation is the most popular form of cosmetic surgery in the USA and in Brazil. These two countries have the largest numbers of plastic surgeries in the world (American Society of Plastic Surgery 2016; Brazilian Society of Plastic Surgery 2004).

Throughout the decades, physiological changes were noticed in patients undergoing breast augmentation and these changes should be considered during the surgical planning. Breast surgery could be considered the most important form of plastic surgery for women (Headon et al. 2015).

The main technique involves an implant inserted into the breast to reshape and resize the breast. The options for implants include a variety of surface textures (smooth or textured), shapes (rounded or anatomically shaped), and the type of gel inside the implant (saline or silicone) (Lam et al. 2006).

The silicone implant is the most popular and accepted for breast augmentation,; the saline form is not authorized in many countries (Lam et al. 2006). However, there is a type of silicone implant that contains partly saline filling; this one is frequently used in reconstructive mammoplasty.

Several techniques have been presented for breast augmentation since the 1800s, such as fat transplant, local flaps or silicone injection, but have had unsatisfactory results. In 1964, the first clinical trial of silicone gel implants was carried out and after that it became the gold standard technique for breast augmentation (Zelken and Cheng 2015).

The choice of access, placement, and implant is very important and should be made by the surgeon together with the patient. The aim of this chapter is to present a wide and current review of all the options to achieve patient and surgeon satisfaction.

53.2 Breast Evaluation

Breast size can be classified in terms of hypotrophy, small, medium or large, and it is directly related to the chest size. They may be in a correct anatomical position or present several grades of ptosis.

M.P.V. Mazzetti, M.D., M.Sc (✉)
Face Defects Research and Study Center, Brazilian Society of Plastic Surgery, São Paulo, SP, Brazil
e-mail: dr.marcelovaccari@gmail.com

R.S. Brock, M.D., M.Sc
Brazilian Society of Plastic Surgery, São Paulo, SP, Brazil

J.M. Avelar (ed.), *Breast Surgery*, https://doi.org/10.1007/978-3-319-54115-0_53

53.3 Ptosis Classification

There are various classifications for mammary ptosis. The first was described by Binet and Binet (1951), Sim (2014), and Peters et al. (2014):

Grade I—the inferior breast margin up to 2 cm under the inferior mammary fold.

Grade II—the inferior breast margin over 2 cm under the inferior mammary fold, without trespassing over the costal margin.

Grade III—the inferior breast margin is between the costal margin and the umbilicus.

Grade IV—the inferior breast margin is under the umbilicus.

However, the most frequently used classification was described by Regnault (1976) and considered the position of the nipple and the inferior mammary fold (Sim 2014; Georgiade et al. 1979):

Grade I—the nipple is above the inferior mammary fold and above the inferior breast margin.

Grade II—the nipple is below the inferior mammary fold and above the inferior breast margin.

Grade III—the nipple is below the inferior mammary fold and below the inferior breast margin.

They can be symmetrical or asymmetrical; the most common prevalence of bilateral breasts for size, ptosis or mammary fold position is asymmetrical.

53.4 Surgical Technique

53.4.1 Implant Access

Access may be gained via the mammary fold, the nipple, the periareolar or the transaxillary approach. The umbilical approach is possible only with saline implants, which are unusual in Brazil, where silicone implants are preferred.

For all kinds of implant access, the patient is in a dorsal decubitus position with her arms open at a 90°extension. The anesthesia is general and a local infiltration with lidocaine solution 1:200,000 is also carried out at the beginning of the procedure.

The inframammary incision at the mammary fold is the most commonly performed in Western countries; however, in patients with hypertrophic healing (Takayanagi 2012), it leads to a visible scar and is not the first choice in these particular cases.

A 4-cm-long incision and dissection are performed in the subglandular, subfascial or submuscular anatomical plane. This allows good visualization of the pocket created and it is easier to carry out hemostasis.

The areolar approach includes perinipple, transareolar, and periareolar incisions. The periareolar one is most frequently used; however, it has restrictions on patients with a small areola, it may not enable adequate visualization of the pocket and it may make it difficult to include large implants without surrounding tissue injury (Johnson 2013).

The periareolar incision may cause contracture and abnormal pigmentation. A hypertrophic periareolar or transareolar scar may be disturbing to patients (Takayanagi 2012; Johnson 2013).

The postoperative precautions of these techniques include bandages and a surgical bra.

The transaxillary approach was first described by Hoehler in 1973. It is very popular in many countries because it does leave not any unaesthetic scars in the breast unit. The incision is made as a natural axillar deep line about 4 cm length (Fig. 53.1). The first dissection must be carried out in the subcutaneous rectangular area and after that the dissection under the pectoralis major muscle and above the pectoralis minor muscle. At this time, rigorous hemostasis is performed (Handel et al. 2006). After hemostasis, the major muscle dissection is performed in the lateral, inferior, and medial poles, and the prosthesis is introduced via transaxillary access (Figs. 53.2 and 53.3).

Antibiotic prophylaxis is recommended for every type of breast augmentation technique.

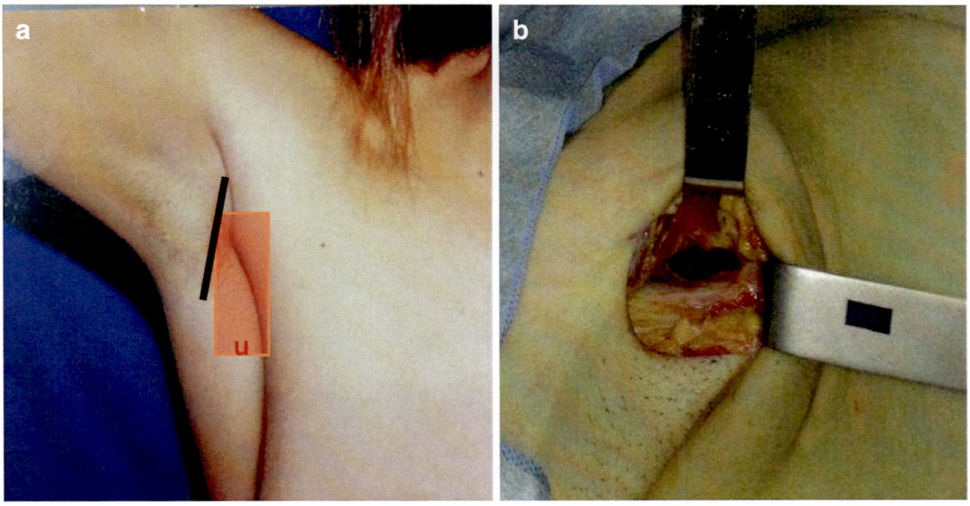

Fig. 53.1 Transaxillary approach to augmentation mastoplasty. (**a**) Peroperative photo shows the axillary region with marking of the incision, in *black*, and subcutaneous undermining (*u* + *red shadow*) of the area to facilitate the introduction of the implant. (**b**) Cutaneous incision was made in the axilla showing the dissected canal

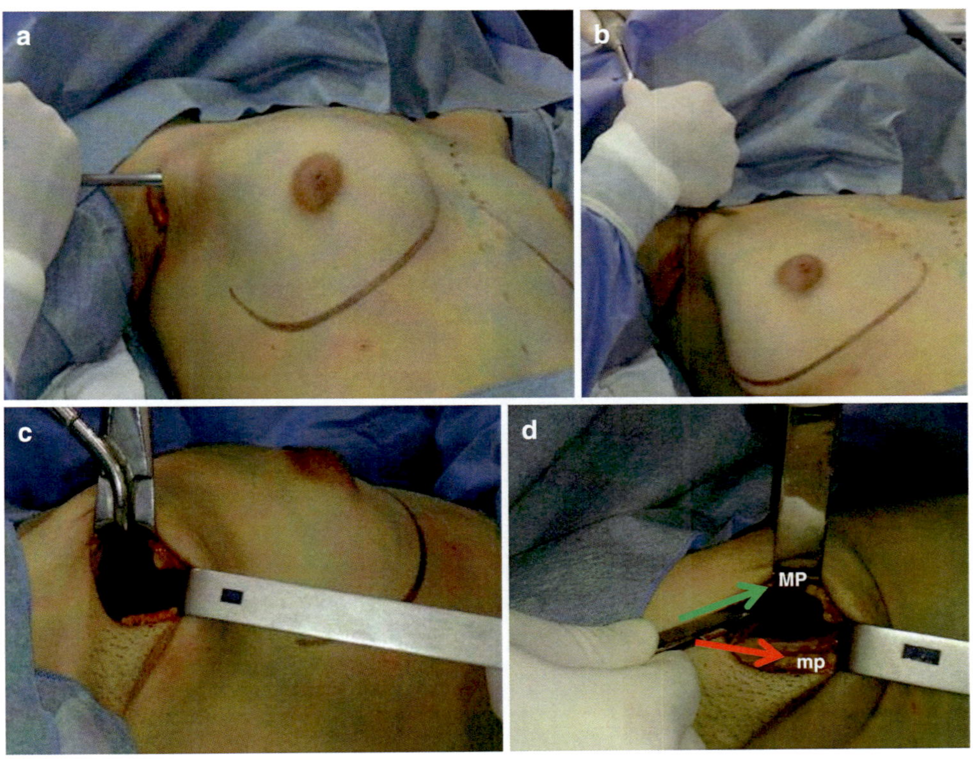

Fig. 53.2 (**a**) Dissection of the medial submuscular mammary area with a pectoral dissector that is introduced through the axillary incision. (**b**) Lateral dissection on an adequate level is performed with movements from one side to other. (**c**) Intraoperative view showing the cavity after dissection, with the pectoralis major muscle above the retractor and the subcutaneous undermined area. (**d**) The correct vector of dissection, parallel to the inferior border of the pectoralis major muscle, above the pectoralis minor muscle to avoid damage in the vascular and lymphatic structures (*green arrow*), because the use of the wrong vector under the pectoralis minor muscle (*red arrow*) damages these important structures. The pectoralis major muscle is retracted above to show the implant access

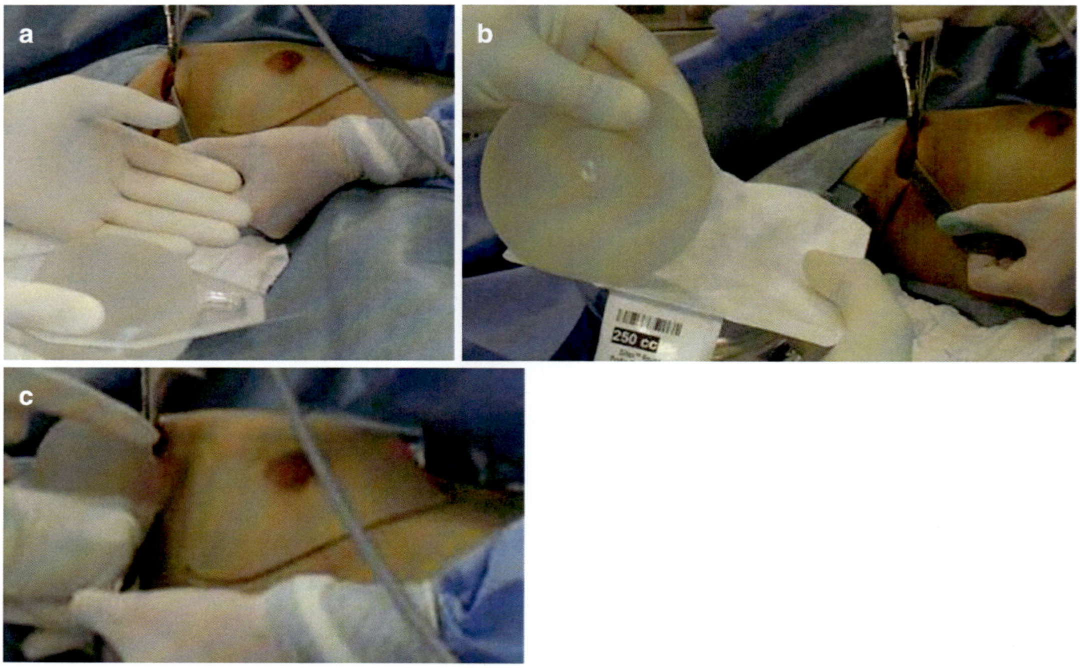

Fig. 53.3 Introduction of the silicone implant via the axillary approach. (**a**) Only the surgeon opens the envelope containing the implant and only he/she touches it. (**b**) The surgeon holds the prosthesis and checks that the size and serial number are correct. (**c**) The implant is carefully introduced via axillary access. The surgeon must use two pairs of gloves at this moment and the powdered gloves must be washed with saline solution, before he/she holds the implant

53.4.2 Implant Placement

Silicone implants can be placed above the muscle, under the fascia or under the muscle.

The subglandular pocket, above the muscle is indicated for small breasts with moderate glandular tissue and grade I ptosis. Patients with very little glandular tissue can develop an artificial result with use of a silicone implant, and the submuscular or subfascial location improves the final aspect.

The submuscular and subfascial placement results in a more natural shape, a breast augmentation with no evident implant shape seen under the skin. The muscle becomes a barrier between the prosthesis and the mammary glandular tissue, which diminishes the chance of glandular dysplasia and facilitates breast cancer control with mammography, ultrasound or magnetic resonance imaging. However, a negative characteristic of the submuscular placement is the pain caused by stretching the pectoralis major muscle fibers, which is more pronounced than in the other techniques. The patients must have a good analgesia in the postoperative period. It is very important to avoid the unfavorable occurrence of the postoperative period coinciding with the premenstrual period; the patient's pain in this case is almost intolerable.

Patients undergoing submuscular implants keep wearing the postoperative bra and an elastic strip over the implants for 2 until 3 months to avoid displacement of the implant because of the constant movement of the pectoral muscle constant. The difference between the subglandular and the submuscular approach is shown in Fig. 53.4.

ASPECT	SUBGLANDULAR LOCATION	SUBMUSCULAR LOCATION
NATURALITY	MINOR	MAJOR
TISSUE PROTECTION OVER PROSTHESIS	MINOR	MAJOR
MAMMARY CANCER DIAGNOSIS	SOME DIFFICULT	NO DIFFICULT
CAPSULAR CONTRACTURE	MORE CHANCE	VERY DIFFICULT
ELASTIC STRIP USE	DON´T NEED	NEED FOR 2-3 MONTHS
SOUTIEN	CAN USE	FORBIDEN FOR 2-3 MONTHS
POST OPERATIVE PAIN	NOT MUCH	HIGH
SURGERY COSTS	SMALLER	HIGHER
ANAESTHESIA	LOCAL (SEDATION) OR GENERAL	GENERAL

Fig. 53.4 Differences between implants located subglandularly or submuscularly

53.4.2.1 Type of Silicone Implants

The implants may be textured or smooth, round or anatomical, and they may have one of several different profiles. The choice of the ideal implant must be that of the plastic surgeon together with the patient.

53.5 Complications

Breast augmentation can present complications that are common in every surgical procedure, such as bleeding, infection, hematoma, seroma, and incision dehiscence, which are frequently diagnosed a few days after surgery.

Other complications such as unaesthetic scars, capsular contracture, and asymmetrical location could present later, after months, and in the case of capsular contracture, even years after the surgical procedure.

Georgiade et al., in 1979, first reported a late hematoma around a breast implant. It happened more than 2 years after breast augmentation with a saline-filled implant. It was suggested that these hematomas might have been caused by the intense, highly vascular inflammatory response that was induced by the polyurethane coating of the implant (Liu et al. 2015, Roça et al. 2014).

Late seroma may occur in textured silicone implants when the initial adherence of the capsule to the implant is separated, causing two rough surfaces. It has also been observed in polyurethane implants (Liu et al. 2015).

Regarding infections, the early ones are usually caused by endogenous bacteria from the skin or the milk ducts, and the later infections involve bacteremia from a distant site (Liu et al. 2015). However, some complications are specific to mammary augmentation with silicone implants. The most common complication is capsular contracture, followed by implant rupture and malpositioning. These complications lead to surgical revision (Lam et al. 2006; Binet and Binet 1951).

Capsular contracture can occur naturally as a biological response to a foreign body, but with the presence of hematoma, infection or leakage of silicone capsular contracture has become more frequent. Many specific techniques such as good hemostasis, use of perfectly sterile material, and a submuscular approach are reported to avoid capsular contracture. However, the etiology and pathogenesis are not yet clear, but seem to be multifactorial (Johnson 2013; Lam et al. 2006).

Capsular contracture is a local complication due to an excessive fibrotic foreign body reaction to the implant, an inflammatory reaction that produces collagen, and fibrosis that leads to excessively firm and painful breasts or contracture and asymmetry (Lam et al. 2006).

The classification of capsular contracture described by Baker is divided into four classes (Lam et al. 2006; Regnault 1976):

Class I—the breast looks completely natural.

Class II—the breast has minimal contracture, but there are no symptoms.

Class III—clinically significant, moderate contracture, some firmness felt by the patient.

Class IV—clinically significant, severe contracture, diagnosed by observation, and is symptomatic to the patient.

Research has demonstrated that smooth implants are more likely to cause capsular contracture, whereas the wrinkling of textured implants could prevent capsule formation, reducing the incidence of capsular contracture (Souza 2008).

The treatment is conservative for classes I and II; patients with capsular contractures class II or IV should undergo surgical revision with a capsulectomy with or without capsulotomy (Lam et al. 2006).

Some research suggests autologous fat transfer to treat capsular contracture as it increases the vascularity of the tissue around the implant. In a study with pigs, it was found that the fat injection caused the capsule to soften in the treatment group, potentially because of neovascularization in the adjacent tissue (Cheng and Huang 2009).

Leaking or rupture of the silicone implant may also occur because of closed capsulotomy, mammography or trauma, and aging of the implant and weakness of the shell can contribute to the rupture. In these cases, the patient should undergo surgical revision and the implant should be exchanged for a new one, which can be of a different type, texture, and size. The incision used is the same as the first one to avoid new scars, but the placement can be changed from subglandular to submuscular (Johnson 2013).

With so many options, newly qualified plastic surgeons frequently ask which one is the best. The proper answer is that the best choice is the technique and implant that the surgeon performs better and the one that will achieve patient satisfaction. However, knowledge and specific details of all techniques will provide all plastic surgeons with the possibility to choose, with the patient, the best choice for each specific woman.

53.6 Discussion

The important question to ask the patient is: "do you really need a breast implant?" The answer to this simple question is sometimes very difficult, because some patients have the wrong idea that the prosthesis could elevated the breast. They are not really interested in receiving a larger breast, but they are searching for better breast projection associated with a higher location. For these patients, we spend a lot of time explaining the real problem of their breasts and offer the option of undergoing a mastoplasty with inferior pedicle.

When the patient is sure that she wants a larger breast, it is important to explain to her about the presence or absence of ptosis and ask her if she wants to correct the breast ptosis. If she is satisfied with the breast location, the implant could be introduced via the mammary fold or transaxillary access.

There are two options for the treatment of breast ptosis: two operations, the first to correct the ptosis and the second to insert the prosthesis. This option is better for the surgeon. The second option is to treat ptosis and perform breast augmentation during the same operation, which is usually the patient's choice.

Treatment of breast ptosis associated with implant should be performed by a periareolar incision with excision of a semicircular area of skin and infra-areolar access (Fig. 53.5).

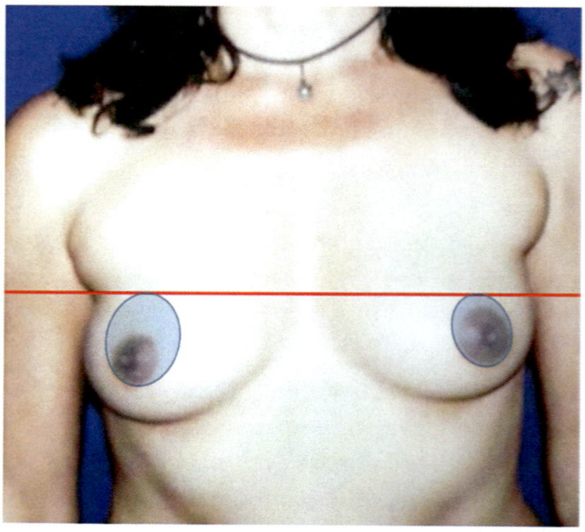

Fig. 53.5 Patient with the desire to increase the size of her breasts, asymmetry, and ptosis level I. the preoperative planning includes a periareolar incision, with skin resection above the nipple–areola complex in different proportions on each side and a submuscular location

The implant could be located in the subglandular or submuscular position.

This type of access usually results in an unfavorable scar (Rorich et al. 2006) and the patient must be informed about the real and predictive possibility of the surgical review of the scar. We suggest in these particular cases avoiding the large implants. The asymmetrical ptosis can be corrected at this time (Fig. 53.6).

When the surgeon has a patient without a breast ptosis, the decision regarding implant access could be via the inframammary fold or transaxillary access.

When the choice is transaxillary access, we recommend a submuscular location, because although a subglandular location is possible, the bleeding risks are high. Transaxillary access must be made in the correct anatomical plane to avoid

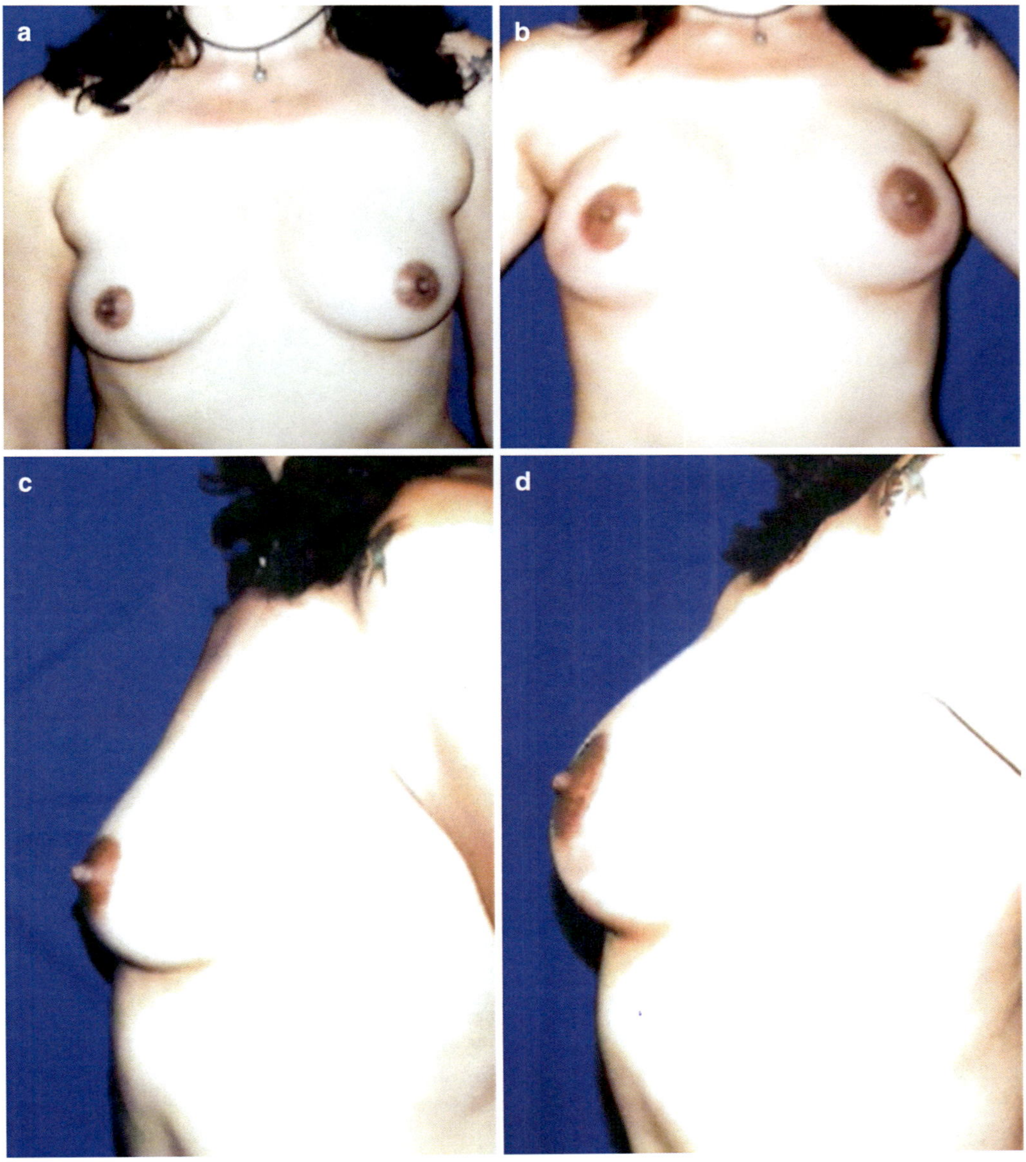

Fig. 53.6 Patient with a periareolar incision, with skin resection above the nipple–areola complex in different proportions on each side, to insert a submuscular implant of 300 ml, which was round and texturized. (**a**) Preoperative view with asymmetrical nipple–areola complex. (**b**) Postoperative frontal view. (**c**) Preoperative lateral view. (**d**) Postoperative lateral view

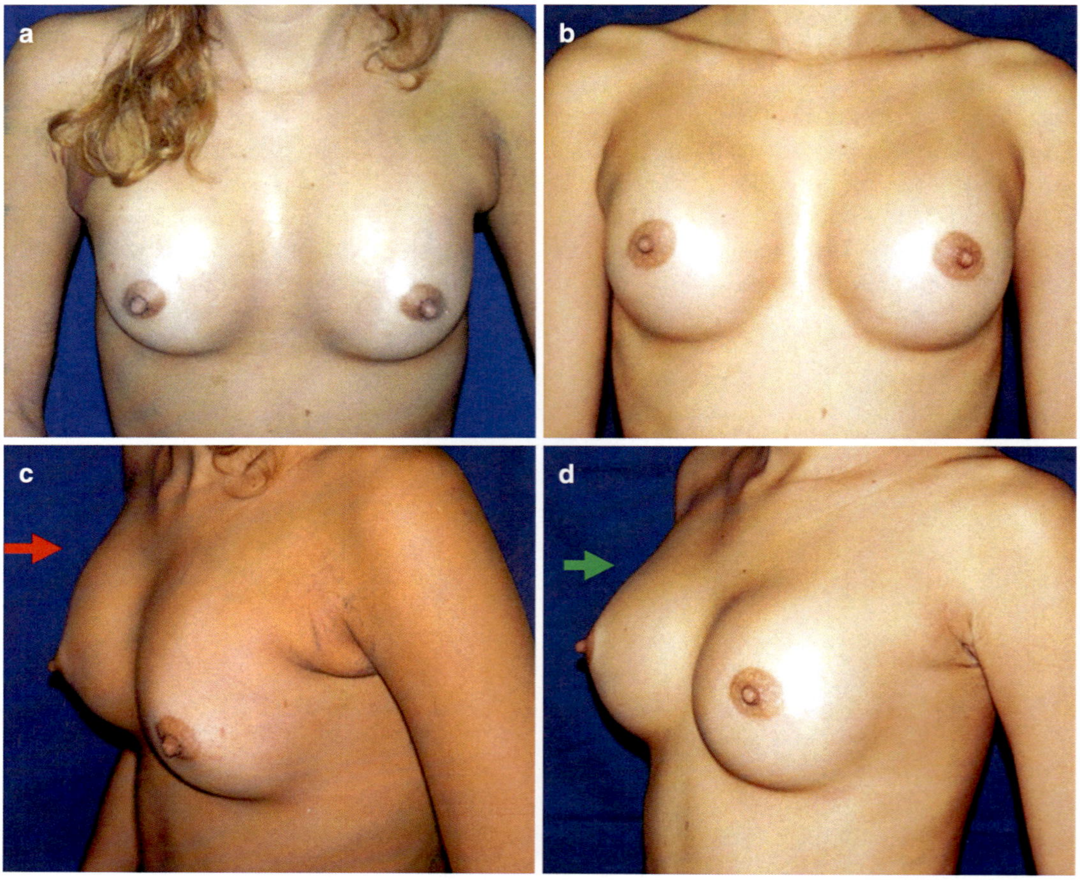

Fig. 53.7 Patient on (**a**, **c**) the 14th postoperative day and (**b**, **d**) 2nd postoperative month after application of a submuscular transaxillary 300-ml implant. (**a**) The frontal view showing the first days after an upper projection of the prosthesis with the nipple located at the inferior pole, and (**b**) after 2 months of elastic strip use, the implant moved to the correct position and the nipple was moved to a central position. (**c**) In the oblique view at 2 weeks, the wrong upper projection of the prosthesis (*red arrow*) moved down the nipple. After the use of the elastic strip, the upper pole was corrected (*green arrow*) and the nipple moved up

neurovascular and lymphatic damage. The use of elastic strip retention above the implant must be maintained for at least 60 days postoperatively to avoid upper dislocation of the implant (Fig. 53.7). After this time, the implant site is definitive.

For the patients who choose inframammary fold access, there are three possibilities of prosthesis location: subglandular, subfascial or submuscular. The surgeon may choose this according his/her experience. Some of the usual complications such as capsular contracture are uncommon in a submuscular location.

We prefer the transaxillary access with the implant in a submuscular location (Figs. 53.8 and 53.9). Asymmetry cannot be corrected via the trans-axillary approach (Fig. 53.10).

The final point of discussion concerns the size of the implant. This decision must be made according to three aspects: the anatomical size of the patient's chest, the distance between the inframammary fold and the nipple, and the desired breast projection of the patient. The size of the chest is important because the diameter of the implant should be sufficient to fill the lateral

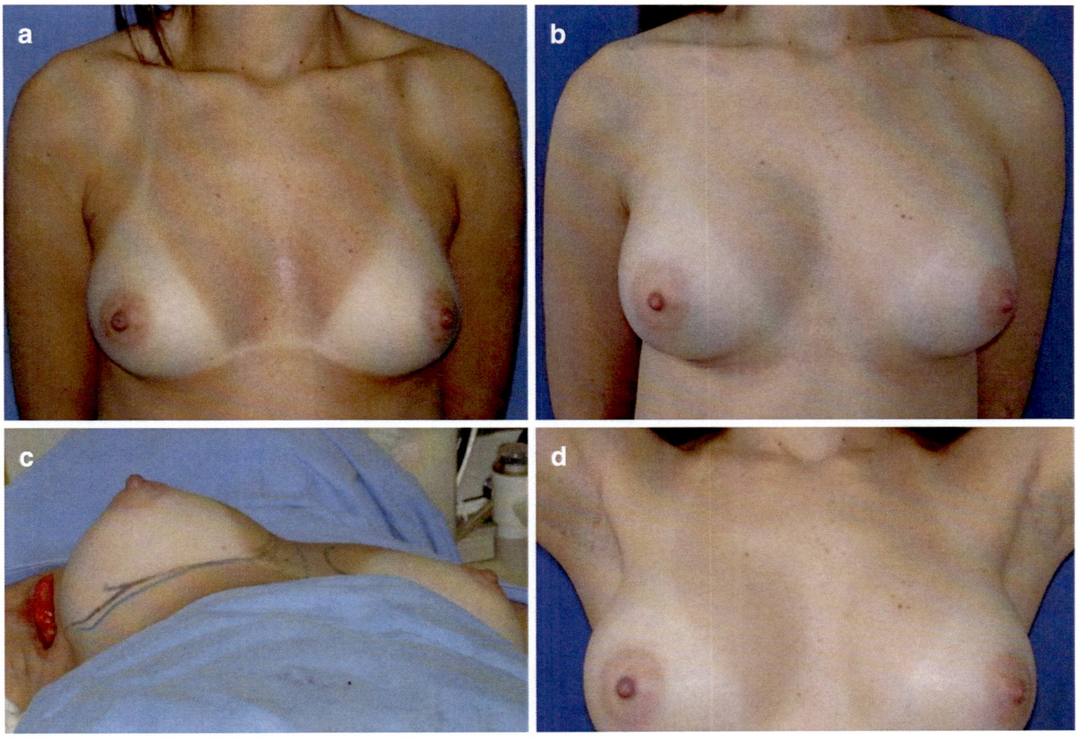

Fig. 53.8 Patient who received a 225-ml, round texturized subglandular transaxillary implant. (**a**) Frontal preoperative view. (**b**) Frontal postoperative view. (**c**) Transaxillary access intraoperative view, after the right side was performed. (**d**) Five months postoperative view of the axillary scar

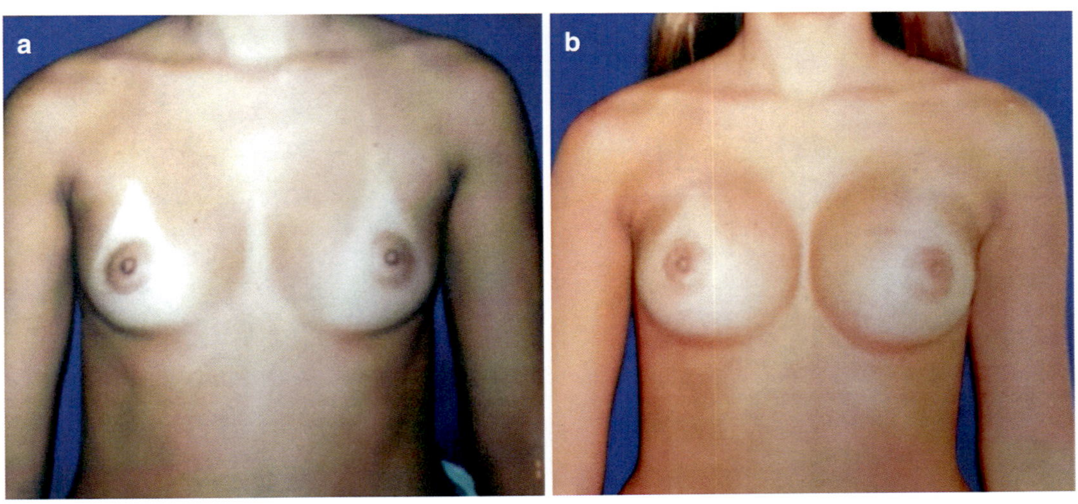

Fig. 53.9 Patient underwent the submuscular transaxillary approach to apply a 250-ml round texturized implant. (**a**) Frontal preoperative view. (**b**) Frontal postoperative view. (**c**) Lateral preoperative view. (**d**) Lateral view postoperatively with no breast scarring

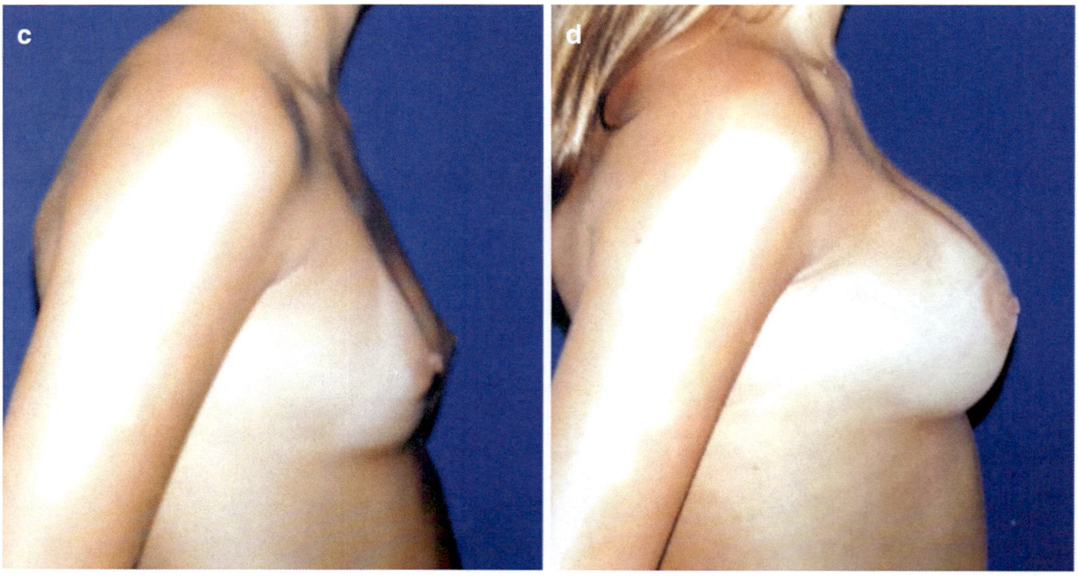

Fig. 53.9 (continued)

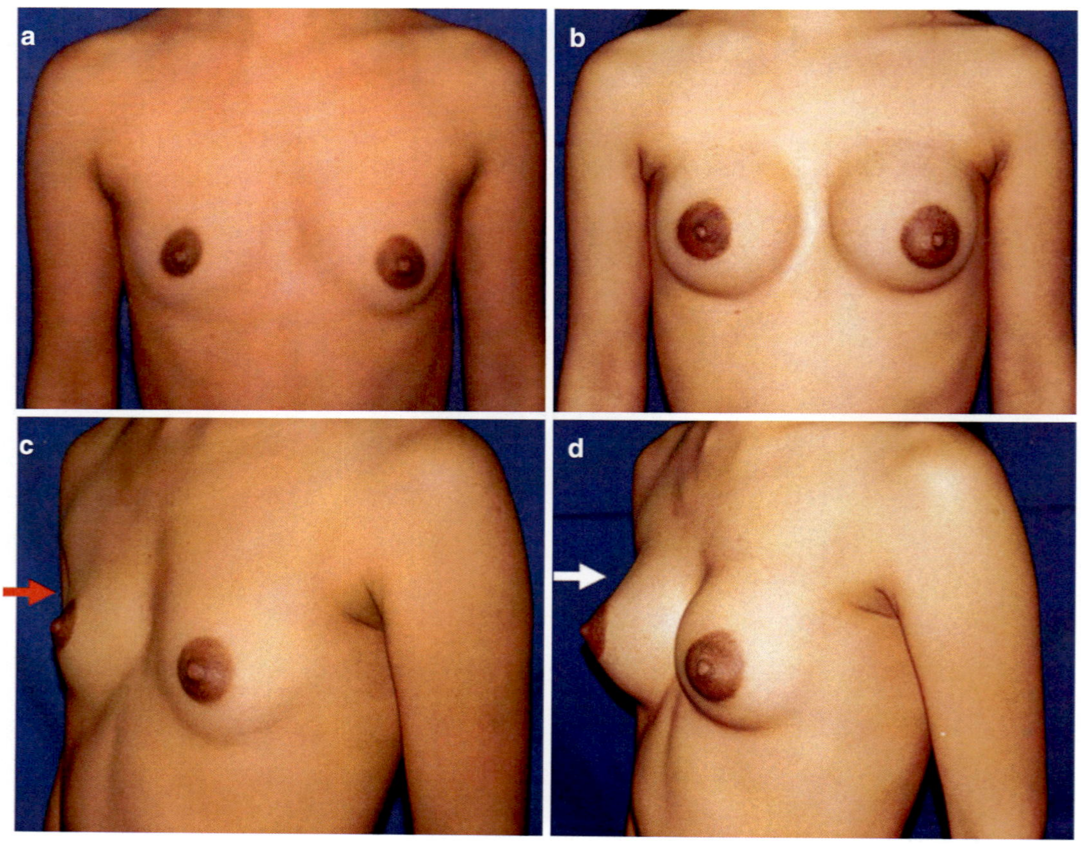

Fig. 53.10 Patient underwent a submuscular transaxillary approach to apply a 225-ml round texturized implant. (**a**) The frontal preoperative view shows asymmetrical nipple–areola complex and in (**b**) the postoperative view this had not been corrected because it is a limitation of transaxillary access. (**c**) In a preoperative oblique view a depression in the chest (*red arrow*) is shown; this depression matched the implant (*green arrow*), as was shown in (**d**) the postoperative oblique view

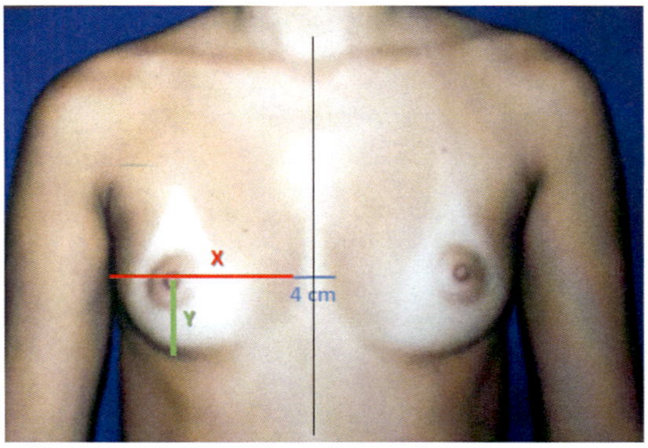

Fig. 53.11 Planning size of the prosthesis: after marking of a medium line (*black line*) we mark 2 cm on each side (*blue line*) to preserve the intermammary fold, and the mark the line of breast projection over the chest. This measurement will be "X" (*red*), after that the measurement from the nipple to the inframammary fold will be "Y" (*green*). The diameter of the implant will be "X," but "X"/2 must be equal to (ideal situation) or less than "Y." If "Y" is bigger, a smaller prosthesis or performing a surgical prolongation with a periareolar incision and upper semicircular skin resection should be considered

and medial portions of the chest, avoid lateral chest overcome, and maintain 2 cm distant on each side of the body's median line. The distance between the inframammary fold and the nipple must be the same (ideal situation) or longer than the beam of the prosthesis, but never smaller. According to these measurements, the ideal diameter of the implant is determined (Fig. 53.11). With the ideal diameter established, the surgeon will be able to offer to the patient different sizes according to the projection and will be able to better decide on the size. The surgeon will use his/her experience and professional sense to advise correctly the patient.

Conclusion

After discussing the different types of access and locations for the silicon prosthesis of the breast, we conclude with regard to the surgical access that for patients with breast ptosis, the best choice is a periareolar approach. For patients with scar hypertrophy, the better choice is the transaxillary approach with submuscular location. The regular patient could choose either inframammary fold or transaxillary access, with subglandular, submuscular or subfascial location. In the subglandular location, the pain is more acceptable, but the incidence of capsular contracture is greater. In the submuscular location, the pain and the care in the postoperative period are greater, but the incidence of capsular contracture is lower and the natural aspect is better. The size of the implant is determined by the chest size, the distance between the inframammary fold and the nipple, and the patient's desired breast projection.

Acknowledgment The authors have no conflicts of interest.

The study received no financial support.

References

American Society for Aesthetic Plastic Surgery (2016) Cosmetic Surgery National Data Bank Statistics. https://www.surgery.org/sites/default/files/ASAPS-Stats2016.pdf

Binet A, Binet M (1951) In: Les régions génitales de la femme: seins, ventre, bassin, vulve, vagin, formes normales et malformations (4):152

Conselho Federal de Medicina, 2004. https://www.portal.cfm.org.br/index.php

Lam T, Brennan M, French J (2006) Cosmetic and reconstructive breast surgery. Aust Fam Physician 35(6):423–428

Cheng MH, Huang JJ (2009) Augmentation mammaplasty in Asian women. Semin Plast Surg 23(1):48–54

Georgiade NG, Serafin D, Barwick W (1979) Late development of hematoma around a breast implant, necessitating removal. Plast Reconstr Surg 64:708–710

Handel N, Cordray T, Gutierrez J, Jensen JA (2006) A long-term study of outcomes, complications, and patient satisfaction with breast implants. Plast Reconstr Surg 117:757–767

Headon H, Kasem A, Mokbel K (2015) Capsular contracture after breast augmentation: an update for clinical practice. Arch Plast Surg 42(5):532–543

Johnson M (2013) Breast implants: history, safety, and imaging. Radiol Technol 84:439–515

Liu X, Zhou L, Pan F, Gao Y, Fan D (2015) Comparison of the postoperative incidence rate of capsular contracture among different breast implants: a cumulative meta-analysis. PLoS One 10(2):1–18

Peters W, Fornasier V, Howasth D (2014) Late unilateral hematoma after breast augmentation. Plast Surg 22(1):18–21

Regnault P (1976) Breast ptosis. Definition and treatment. Clin Plast Surg 3(2):193–203

Roça GB, Graf R, da Silva FR, Salles G Jr, Francisco JC, Noronha L, Maluf I Jr (2014) Autologous fat grafting for treatment of breast implant capsular contracture: a study in pigs. Aesthet Surg J 34:769–775

Rohrich RJ, Hartley W, Brown S (2006) Incidence of breast and chest wall asymmetry in breast augmentation: a retrospective analysis of 100 patients. Plast Reconstr Surg 111:1513–1519

Sim HB (2014) Transaxillary endoscopic breast augmentation. Arch Plast Surg 41(5):458–465

Souza SC (2008) Graduações de ptose mamária. Arquivos Catarinenses de Medicina 37(3):66–71

Takayanagi S (2012) Augmentation mammaplasty using implants: a review. Arch Plast Surg 39(5):448–451

Zelken J, Cheng MH (2015) Asian breast augmentation: a systematic review. Plast Reconstr Surg Glob Open 3:1–9

54 Mastopexy with Implant Inclusion

Ricardo Cavalcanti Ribeiro, Adrian Bermudez, and Marcelo Pastor

54.1 Introduction

In this chapter, we discuss breast ptosis, its classifications, different techniques, and complications. Breast ptosis or sagging is a natural consequence of aging. The key factors influencing breast ptosis are pregnancy, gravity, high BMI, breast size, smoking, and significant weight gain and/or loss.

Mastopexy with implant is considered one of the most complex surgeries because of the difficulty in achieving the right balance between two antagonist vectors: reduction and augmentation. Thus, variables such as implant volume, skin removal, and tension after surgery must be properly evaluated in this challenging procedure.

Many classifications for breast ptosis have been proposed; however, Regnault's classification is the most well-known and frequently used (Dufourmentel and Mouly 1959; Lalardrie and Jouglard 1974; Regnault 1976; Bostwick 1983; Kirwan 1999) (Fig. 54.1):

1. Mild ptosis: when the nipple–areola complex (NAC) is at the same level as the inframammary fold.

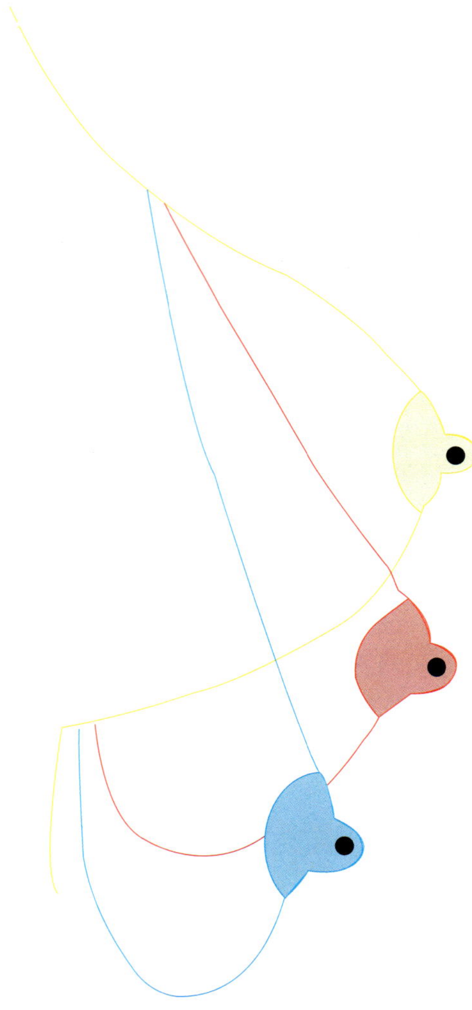

Fig. 54.1 *Yellow*: mild ptosis. *Red*: moderate ptosis. *Blue*: severe ptosis

Head of Division of Plastic and Reconstructive Surgery of Universidade Federal do Estado of the Rio de Janeiro (UNIRIO)

R.C. Ribeiro (✉) • A. Bermudez • M. Pastor
Condominio Peninsula, Avenida Das Acácias, NR 410–Apto 1.601–Bloco 2, 22.776-000 Rio de Janeiro, RJ, Brazil
e-mail: rribeiro@centroin.com.br

J.M. Avelar (ed.), *Breast Surgery*, https://doi.org/10.1007/978-3-319-54115-0_54

2. Moderate ptosis: when the NAC is lower than the inframammary fold, but above the lower edge of the breast.
3. Severe ptosis: when the NAC is below the inframammary fold and below the lower edge of the breast.
4. Pseudoptosis: when the NAC is above the inframammary fold, but the entire breast tissue is at the lower pole of breast (Bostwick 1983).

54.2 Discussion

54.2.1 Mild Ptosis

In many cases, the cause of mild ptosis is the short distance between the NAC and the inframammary fold (less than 4.5 cm) in patients with small breasts and a good volume in the upper pole. For small breasts, an implant is used to reduce the inframammary fold in relation to the size desired. Round, anatomical and conical implants can be used (Chekkoury et al 1991; Owaley 1979). Anatomical implants are preferred because they have the highest projection in the lower quadrants and are useful for expanding the lower pole, raising the NAC. Implants for this condition should be placed with 60% of the volume under the NAC and 40% above it Tebbetts (2001b). Following this maneuver, the NAC will rise 1.0–1.5 cm.

On the other hand, if the distance from the NAC to the inframammary fold is greater than 6 cm, it should be raised using the periareolar approach; in these cases, a round implant is preferred.

54.2.2 Moderate to Severe Ptosis

This type of ptosis is treated by raising the NAC using a periareolar approach with a vertical scar or an inverted T (Parsa and Parsa 2006). When more volume is desired, less skin is resected, resulting in a smaller scar.

54.2.3 Breast Implant Plane

One of the most important issues in this surgery is the plane in which the implant is placed. Depending on the surgical technique and the surgeons' preferences, the following anatomical sites for implant placement may be used:

- Subglandular: locates the implant below the glandular breast tissue.
- Subfascial: places the implant below the superficial fascia of the pectoralis major muscle. The fascia is thicker on its upper portion and becomes thinner on its lower portion.
- Submuscular: implant is inserted under the pectoralis major muscle. In this situation, the fibers of the muscle must be dislodged on the medial portion.
- Dual plane: implant is placed partially distributed among the submuscular and subglandular spaces Khan (2007).

54.2.4 Surgical Technique

In our experience, all patients are marked preoperatively in a standing position, and four anatomical reference points are needed: the inframammary fold, the midclavicular line, sternal notch, and the base of the mammary gland in its anatomical position. With these four points located, the necessary steps can be taken to perform practically any mastopexy technique. Once the four anatomical reference points are located, the following measurements are taken to mark the breast: the distance from the sternal notch to the NAC, the distance from the areola to the inframammary fold, the width of the base, and the height of the breast (Fig. 54.2).

The distance from the NAC to the inframammary fold and the distance from the NAC ascending to the desired position are key factors in selecting the proper surgical indication.

For cases in which the NAC is being migrated to a higher position, the breast implant is placed through the areola. On the other hand, if the inverted T technique is being used, the implant is placed through the inframammary fold.

The implant placement can be dual-plane, submuscular or subglandular. For tuberous breasts, the subglandular plane is the most appropriate.

All surgical techniques start by cutting the circumference of the areola to the desired size. The usual measurement is 4 cm, and the implant is placed by a 180° incision on the lower segment of the NAC, with a transglandular dissection reaching the fascia of the pectoral muscle. When repositioning of the NAC is required, a superior areolar incision is preferred instead of an inferior one. Once the new position of the NAC is confirmed with the patient in a semiseated position, a half-moon shape is bound and de-epithelialized (Fig. 54.3).

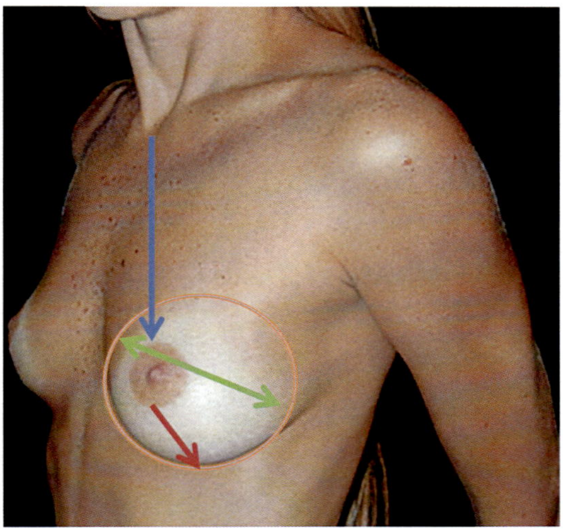

Fig. 54.2 *Blue*: the distance from the sternal notch to the nipple–areola complex. *Red*: distance from the areola to the inframammary fold. *Green*: width of the breast base. *Orange*: height of the breast base

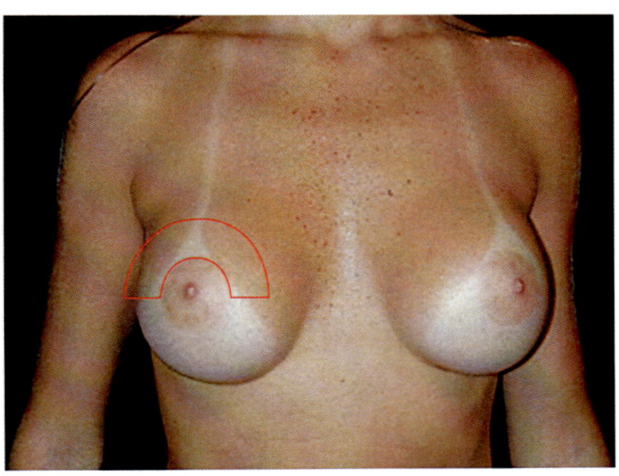

Fig. 54.3 Half-moon de-epithelialization

When the resected half-moon, which corresponds to the upper portion, does not exceed 1.5 cm, it can be closed directly using subdermal sutures with Monocryl® 4–0, and the skin is closed with a continuous intradermic suture with nylon 3–0. If the upper portion of skin of the half-moon exceeds 1.5 cm, or if the skin of the lower portion is resected to reduce the size of the areola, closure should be performed using a circumferential suture (round block), reducing the risk of periareolar scar enlargement Benelli (1990).

54.2.5 Periareolar Mastopexy Indications

A periareolar mastopexy is indicated when breast ptosis is less than 3 cm, or a greater distance than 5 cm from the NAC to the inframammary fold. This technique does not allow great elevation of the areola (a maximum of 4–5 cm); therefore, it is recommended only in patients who have mild or moderate ptosis de la Fuente and Martin del Yerro (1992). In these cases, we prefer the infra-areolar technique. This approach

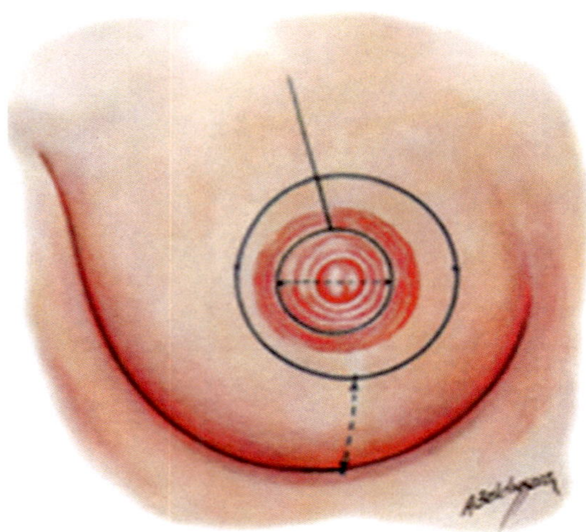

Fig. 54.4 Periareolar de-epithelialization

keeps the vascularization of the NAC and enough tissue in the lower pole to cover the implant Hoover et al. (2010).

The areola is marked with a cookie cutter, which must have a diameter greater than 3.5 cm, and then periareolar de-epithelialization is carried out (Fig. 54.4).

The dissection of the glandular tissue of the lower hemisphere is followed by the inclusion of the implant in the retromuscular or retroglandular plane, depending on the amount of tissue left to cover the implant.

Once the implant is placed, the dermal resection of the periareolar pexy is drawn; the upper and lower margins should be marked. These two points are placed on the midclavicular line marked previously. The top margin is marked 3 cm above this point. These 3 cm correspond to the 2-cm radius forming the new areola, plus 1 cm to compensate for the displacement of the skin when the periareolar dermal resection is closed.

Depending on the implant size, the distance from the inframammary fold to the bottom edge of the circumferential marking should be 5–7 cm. The larger the breast size, the greater the distance.

54.3 Indications for Inverted T Mastopexy

When breast ptosis is more severe with significant excess skin above and below the NAC, this technique should be used. In these cases, the distance for the NAC migration is greater than 3 cm, and the distance from the NAC to the inframammary fold is more than 5 cm.

Given these conditions, the implant is placed retromuscular or retroglandular through the inframammary fold. With the implant and drain in position, closing is performed with Monocryl 2–0 or 3–0 sutures, without skin closure. The first step is to choose a point on the midclavicular line, 8 cm below the center of the new NAC that had been marked preoperatively. These 8 cm correspond to 2 cm from the radius of the new areola plus 6 cm from the edge of the new NAC to the inframammary fold. The amount of skin to be resected is determined by bidigital pinching. This amount of tissue forms the bases of the two triangles, creating an ellipse with the apex of each triangle corresponding to the new NAC and the inframammary fold.

The diameter of the new areola is marked, and the tissue within the ellipse is resected. In the upper triangle, only the dermis is resected,

a

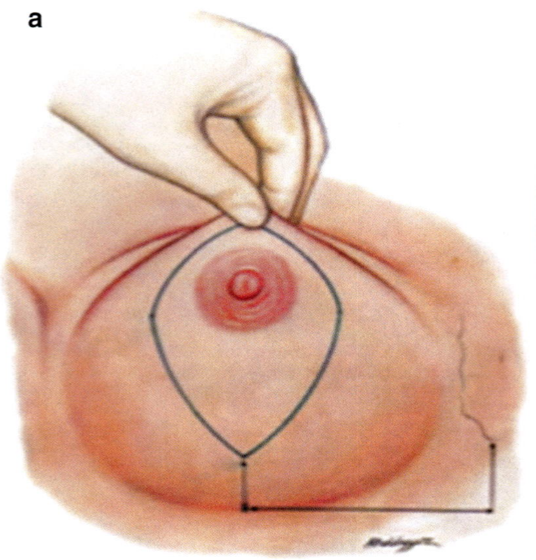

b

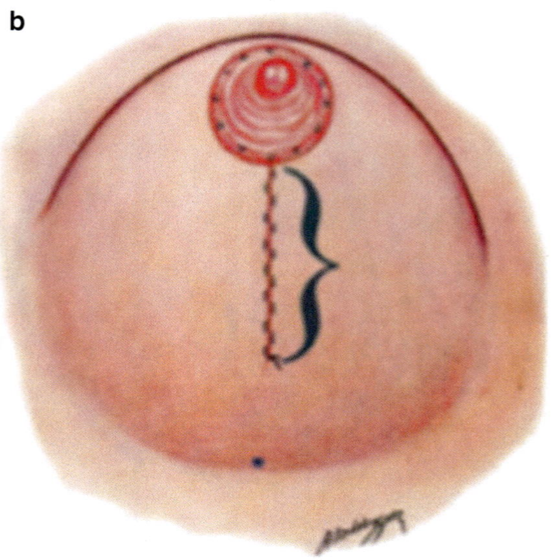

Fig. 54.5 (**a**) Losange marking. (**b**) Vertical scar, 4–7 cm

whereas the lower triangle is removed from the subcutaneous tissue to the pre-glandular fascia. This tissue is removed to allow the closure without tension (Fig. 54.5).

This removed tissue eliminates the lower pole of the breast, forming the two pillars that allow the mastopexy to take place by closing them with Monocryl 2–0 and 3–0.

The next step is the use of the Freeman areola marker to draw the new location of the NAC. Resection of the overlying skin in the areola is marked with a diameter of 3.5–4.5 cm, and the skin is removed. The areola is mobilized upward, and the vertical and horizontal incisions are closed according to the anatomical planes.

54.4 Secondary Mastopexy

Experience has shown that secondary mastopexy carries a high risk of potential complications, including fat necrosis, loss of skin flaps, and ischemia of the areola. Avoiding complications in such patients is an issue that does not receive the attention it deserves, but has become increasingly important over the years due to the return of a larger number of patients previously undergoing this procedure Handel (2006).

Over the years, the breast experiences changes in shape and volume. The mammary tissue is replaced by fat and the breast becomes progressively more ptotic Araco et al. (2007). Pregnancy, breastfeeding, and weight variations speed up these changes, increasing the risk of secondary mastopexy. Also, breast implants can cause thinning, atrophy, and stretching of the tissues, with the consequent acceleration of ptosis. Owing to gravity, the thinning of the tissue and atrophy occur at the lower pole of the breast. This can be demonstrated by physical examination and mammography.

In all cases, a capsule is formed around the implant, and many patients develop significant capsular contracture. The treatment for this complication is capsulotomy and capsulectomy that can compromise the blood supply, when breast tissue is thin. The surgical scars can further compromise the vascularization of the skin and nipple (Pitanguy 1961 and Spear et al. 2004).

Another fact is that few patients are willing to decrease their breast size, and indeed, larger sizes are requested. These cases are challenging for the plastic surgeon, on the grounds that a good aesthetic result is difficult to obtain, complications are relatively common, and disasters can happen. Some patients experience delayed healing, poor positioning of the papilla, and unaesthetic scarring. Some of the most serious complications are the extensive loss of the flaps, fat necrosis, infection, implant exposure, and partial or total loss of the papilla and areola.

Five surgical options are available for patients who need secondary mastopexy, whether presenting capsular contracture or not. The first is the removal of the implant without mastopexy and without repositioning the implant. The second is surgery of the capsule only, including repositioning of the implant without mastopexy. The third option is mastopexy only without manipulation of the implant. The fourth option is removal of the implant with mastopexy. The fifth and the riskiest option is removal of the implant, capsulotomy or capsulectomy, mastopexy, and new implant application.

54.5 Complications

Some of the most common complications are dehiscence, enlarged or hypertrophic scarring, bruising, patient dissatisfaction, infection, seroma, asymmetry, capsular contracture, double contour in the lower pole, and secondary ptosis (Lejour 1999; Araco et al. 2007; Pitanguy 1961; Rohrich et al. 2006).

Conclusion

There are several factors that can affect the outcome of the surgery. Every aspect of the patient should be evaluated, especially the patients' expectations.

The simultaneous implementation of mastopexy with implants is the rational solution to the problem of hypoplastic and ptotic breasts, as it provides results balancing the lower morbidity and cost with a high level of satisfaction and a low number of complications.

References

Araco A, Gravante G, Araco F et al (2007) A retrospective analysis of 3,000 primary aesthetic breast augmentations: postoperative complications and associated factors. Aesth Plast Surg 31(5):532–539. Epub 2007 July 20

Baran CN, Peker F, Ortak T et al (2001) Unsatisfactory results of periareolar mastopexy with or without augmentation and reduction mammaplasty: enlarged areola with flattened nipple. Aesth Plast Surg 25(4):286

Benelli L (1990) A new periareolar mammaplasty: the round block technique. Aesth Plast Surg 14:93–100

Bostwick J (1983) Correctin of the breast ptosis. In: Aesthetic and recent breast surgery. CV Mosby, St Louis, pp 209–249

Cárdenas-Camarena L, Ramírez-Macías R (2006) Augmentation/mastopexy: how to select and perform the proper technique. Aesth Plast Surg 30(1):21–33

Chekkoury IH, Rodier C, Keller P et al (1991) Our own experience in the treatment of hypotrophy and ptosis of the breast. Ann Chir Plast Esthetic 36(2):116–119

Daher C, Di Lamartini J (2012) Mastopexy associated with submuscular or subglandular silicone implants: indications and complications. Rev Bras Cir Plást. 27(2):294–300

De Benito J, Sánchez K (2010) Key points in mastopexy. Aesthet Plast Surg 34(6):711–715

Dufourmentel C, Mouly R (1959) Chirurgie plastique. Flammarion, Paris, pp 327–370

de la Fuente A, Martin del Yerro JL (1992) Periareolar mastopexy with mammary implants. Aesth Plast Surg 16(4):337–341

Gonzales-Ulloa M (1960) Correction of hypotrophy of the breast by means of exogenous material. Plast Reconstr Surg 25(1):15–40

Gruber R, Denkler K, Hvistendahl Y (2006) Extended crescent mastopexy with augmentation. Aesth Plast Surg 30(3):269–274. discussion 275-76

Handel N (2006) Secondary mastopexy in the augmented patient: a recipe for disaster. Plast Reconstr Surg 118(7 Suppl):152S–163S. discussion 164S-65S, 166S-67S

Hoover DJ, Paragi PR, Santoro E, Schafer S, Chamberlain RS (2010) Pro- phylactic mastectomy in high risk patients: a practice-based review of the indications. Do we follow guidelines? Breast Dis 31(1):19–27

Khan UD Lower pole enhancement in breast augmentation. In: 6th Croatian Congress of Plastic, Reconstructive and Aesthetic Surgery. Croatia: Opatja-Rijeka, 2006.

Khan UD (2007) Muscle splitting biplane breast augmentation. A new pocket in a different plane. Aesth Plast Surg 31:353–358

Kirwan L (1999) Augmentation of the ptotic breast: simultaneous periareolar mastopexy and breast augmentation. Aesth Surg 19:34

Lalardrie J, Jouglard JP (1974) La chirurgie plastique du sein. Masson, Paris, p 290

Lejour M (1999) Vertical mammaplasty: early complications after 250 personal consecutive cases. Plast Reconstr Surg 104(3):764

Owaley J Jr (1979) Simultaneous mastopexy and augmentation for correction of the small, ptotic breast. Ann Plastic Surg 2(3):195–200

Parsa FD, Parsa AA (2006) Breast ptosis: to augment, to lift, or to do both? Plast Reconstr Surg 117:2101–2102

Pesquisa Datafolha encomendada pela Sociedade Brasileira de Cirurgia Plástica. (n.d.) Disponível em http://www2.cirurgiaplastica.org.br. Accessed 22 August 2011

Pitanguy I (1961) Mammaplasty: study of 245 consecutive cases and presentation of a personal technique. Rev Bras Cir 42:201–220

Puckett CL (1985) Crescent mastopexy and augmentation. Plast Reconstr Surg 75(4):533

Regnault P (1976) Breast ptosis. Definition and treatment. Clin Plast Surg 3:193

Regnault P (1990) Breast reduction and mastopexy, an old love story: B technique update. Aesth Plast Surg 14(2):101

Rohrich RJ, Gosman AA, Brown SA et al (2006) Mastopexy preferences: a survey of board-certified plastic surgeons. Plast Reconstr Surg 118(7):1631–1638

Saldanha OR, Maloof RG, Dutra RT, Luz OAL, Saldanha Filho O, Saldanha CB (2010) Mamaplastia redutora com implante de silicone. Rev Bras Cir Plást. 25(2):317–324

Saleh KH, Letter A (2009) Incision periareolar mastopexy with breast implant augmentation. N Iraqi J Med 5(1)

Spear SL (2006) Augmentation/mastopexy: "surgeon, beware". Plast Reconstr Surg 118(7 Suppl):133S–135S

Spear SL, Low M, Ducic I (2003) Revision augmentation mastopexy: indications, operations and outcomes. Ann Plast Surg 51:540–546

Spear SL, Pelletiere CV, Menon N (2004) One-stage augmentation combined with mastopexy: aesthetic results and patient satisfaction. Aesth Plast Surg. 28(5):259–267

Stevens WG, Freeman ME, Stoker DA et al (2007) One-stage mastopexy with breast augmentation: a review of 321 patients. Plast Reconstr Surg 120(6):1674–1679

Tebbetts JB (2001a) Dual plane breast augmentation: optimizing implant-soft tissue relationship in a wide range of breast types. Plast Reconstr Surg 107:1255–1272

Tebbetts JB (2001b) Alternatives and trade-offs in breast augmentation. Clin Plast Surg 28(3):485–500

Breast Augmentation

55

Ricardo Cavalcanti Ribeiro, Renato Saltz,
Carlo Amaral, and Andrea Kocsis

55.1 Introduction

Through the ages, the female breast has always been a cause of interest. This is not surprising, as the woman's breast has been symbol of femininity, motherhood, and sexuality.

Interestingly, in South America small breasts were considered a standard of beauty and as a consequence of globalization, this concept has changed. With the influence of American and European fashion, the women in South America started to value larger breasts.

They have very high expectations and a strong demand for excellent results and minimal evidence of surgery. The second group is much older. They have complaints about low upper pole projection and early ptosis associated with postpartum involution. These patients have often been dissatisfied with the size of their breasts for many years and enjoyed the fullness and contours of the breast during pregnancy and lactation.

Recent advances are rather related to attempts at reducing the incidence of capsular contracture. In addition to preventive alternatives, such as subpectoral placement, the use of antibiotics and intraluminal steroids, and "bags" has come to the fore. Several implant types have been developed, and now we have textured, polyurethane, smooth, and saline implants.

55.2 Methods

55.2.1 Patient Selection

The best candidates for breast plastic surgery are physically healthy, psychologically stable patients who are realistic in their expectations, who want an improvement in their appearance with mammaplasty, and do not believe that surgery will change their life. An important issue for the selection of patients is related to the time of the procedure. It was suggested that postpartum patients should wait at least 6 months after cessation of lactation, and that patients must, likewise, pass through a period of 6 months between surgery and a new pregnancy. Any patient who wishes to become pregnant in the future should understand that changes may occur such as involution and/or ptosis after pregnancy and lactation. With the appropriate selection of

R.C. Ribeiro, M.D. (✉)
Head of the Plastic and Reconstructive Surgery Department, Federal University of the State of Rio de Janeiro (Unirio), Rio de Janeiro, RJ, Brazil

R. Saltz, M.D., F.A.C.S. • C. Amaral • A. Kocsis
Members of the Plastic and Reconstructive Surgery Department, Federal University of the State of Rio de Janeiro (Unirio), Rio de Janeiro, RJ, Brazil

Condominio Peninsula, Avenida Das Acácias, NR. 410–Apto 1.601–Bloco 2, 22776000 Rio de Janeiro, RJ, Brazil
e-mail: saltz@saltzplasticsurgery.com; tracee@saltzplasticsurgery.com

J.M. Avelar (ed.), *Breast Surgery*, https://doi.org/10.1007/978-3-319-54115-0_55

patients, combined with a thorough and open discussion and examination, excellent results and high rates of satisfaction of patients can be expected (Araco A, Gravante G, Araco F et al. 2007).

55.2.2 Types and Forms of Implant

–Various types of implants have been developed for breast enlargement, including saline solution (smooth) and silicone, which can be smooth, textured, and polyurethane-coated (Barone FE, Perry L, Keller T et al. 1992).

Breast implants are usually made with a silicone bag filled with silicone gel. The walls of the implant are silicone, but not in gel form. Silicone is biocompatible material with human tissues.

According to the profile, silicone implants can be low profile and have a wider base, which are indicated when greater projection of the pole and low anterior projection are desired. High profile implants have a smaller base, are higher, and, therefore, are better indicated when greater projection of the breast anteriorly is required, especially filling the upper pole (Becker H, Shaw KE, Kara M. 2005).

The anatomical profile implants, given this name because they have a "natural" or "drop" profile: low projection in its upper portion and larger dimensions above the inferior pole. They are indicated in situations where breast volume is increased to maintain its shape without modifying the upper part of the breast and are widely used in surgery for breast reconstruction.

There are also conical (available only in polyurethane) and round formats. The textured silicone implant has on its surface microroughness in an attempt to break capsular formation. It displays a smaller index of capsular contracture than the smooth silicone implants: 2–3%. Polyurethane-coated implants have the lowest rate of capsular contracture of breast implants (0.5%), being more sensitive to palpation and more likely to fold because of the difficulty of placing and sliding on the mammary tissue. It has a disadvantage when an implant exchange is needed, as it is extremely difficult to remove from the mammary pocket (Fig. 55.1) (Pennisi VR 1985).

55.2.3 Indications

The main indications for breast augmentation are:

Congenital absence or deformity of one or both breasts
Hypomastia
Dissatisfaction with the volume or breast form
Tuberous breasts
Desire to increase breast volume after losing previous volume (e.g., after pregnancy and breastfeeding)
Post-reducing mammoplasty
Breast reconstruction

55.3 Discussion

55.3.1 Ways of Access

Once the type and size of the implants have been determined, it is appropriate to choose the location of the incision with the patient.

We can mention pre-existing breast scars, inframammary, periareolar, tennis racket, transareolar–papillary, axillary, and umbilical (Fig. 55.2).

55.3.1.1 Inframammary

This is the incision most commonly used by most surgeons. It can be used when the nipple–areola complex (NAC) is too small for the size of the implant. It allows direct access to the retromammary or retropectoral space and development to the precise pocket with regard to the size.

The main criticism of this incision is the visibility of the scar and the small impact, but significant hypertrophy. Visibility can be minimized by making the incisions just above the inframammary crease. The length of the incision should only allow the passage of the implant to the pocket.

55.3.1.2 Periareolar

This is the incision that draws less attention between breast incisions.

The areola margin should be carefully and precisely followed. These incisions tend to be hypertrophied when extended to the surrounding skin and are hyperpigmented, if located within the areola. There is a higher risk of infection associated with transection of the ductus (colonized by

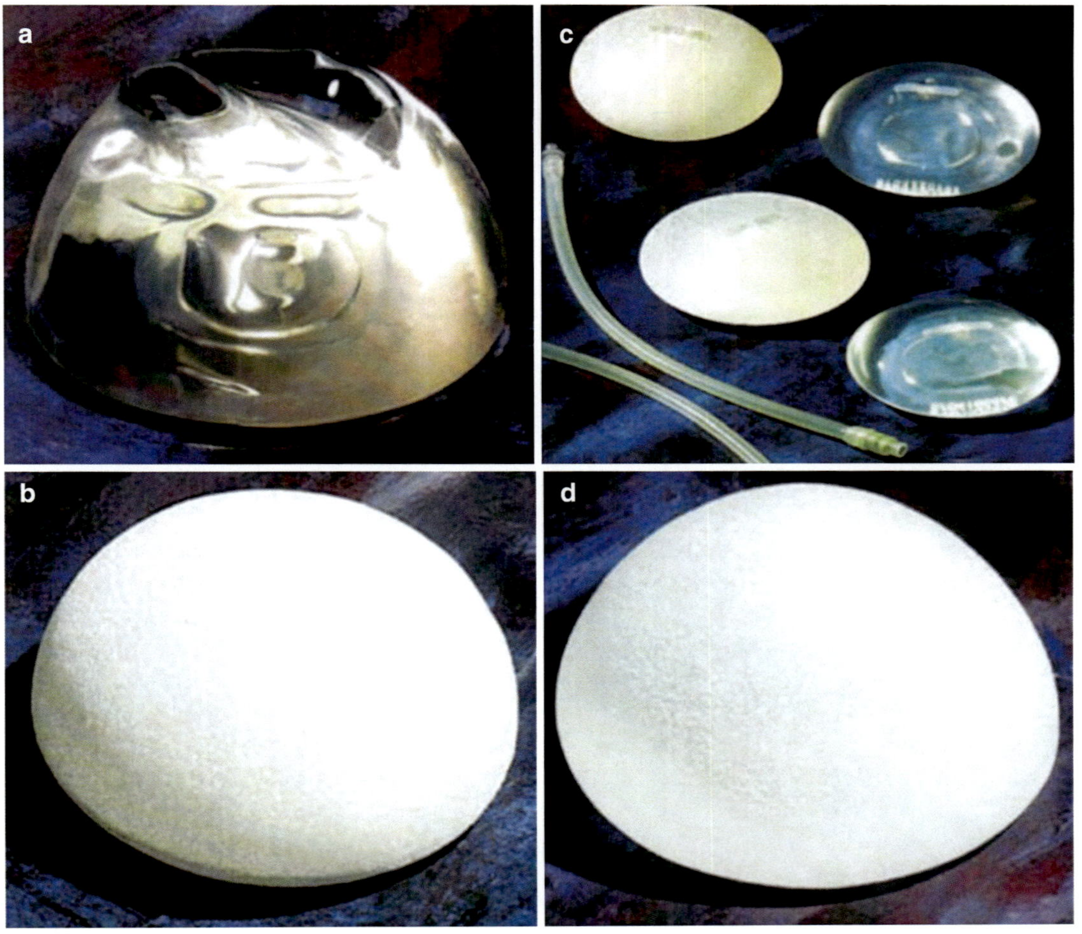

Fig. 55.1 Silicone implants. (**a**) Smooth. (**b**) Saline. (**c**) Textured. (**d**) Polyurethane

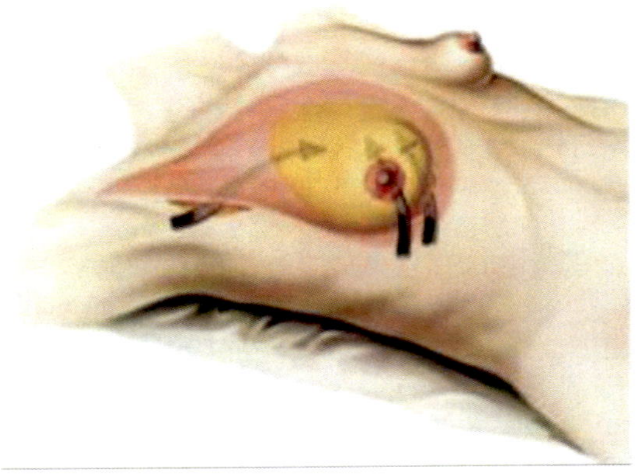

Fig. 55.2 The most frequent access route used for placement of breast implants

various species of bacteria). When using implants filled previously or texturized, access can be difficult in patients with an areolar diameter less than 35 mm. This is because the incision should comprise about half of the circumference to preserve irrigation, sensitivity, and lactation. What is most important in preserving the sensitivity of the papilla is not to extend to the lateral half (Hvilsom GB, Hölmich LR, Henriksen TF 2009).

55.3.1.3 Transareolar–Papillary

This approach is rarely used. The surgeon can opt for this access route in patients with papillary hypertrophy or inverted nipple, when those defects need to be corrected.

55.3.1.4 Tennis Racket

This is an excellent option in patients who have breast ptosis or require removal of excess skin.

55.3.1.5 Axillary

This is less common, but is sometimes requested by patients themselves. Implantation in this way is more difficult, requiring the use of endoscopy for better visualization of structures. Patients should clearly understand that there is a significant chance that subsequent surgery may be required to treat contracture or replace implants, an incision of an alternative type will then be used.

55.3.1.6 Umbilical

This approach requires specialized equipment, and inflatable implants are the only ones that can be used. Moreover, it has the same disadvantages as the axillary approach (Johnson et al. 1993).

55.3.2 Surgical Techniques

The technical changes turn around making the incisions and the desired location of the implant: submuscular or subglandular. In each case, the preoperative marks are similar.

All marks must be made with the patient standing with her arms beside her body. The pocket contour is then marked. The upper extent should be to approximately the second rib. Laterally, the pocket is limited to the extent of the breast proposal, usually in the mid-axillary line. Higher dissection can lead to uncomfortable lateral filling and a poor aesthetic result.

The inframammary fold should be marked with any changes that may be required to correct constrictions or asymmetries. The pocket is extended about 2 cm below the natural fold to prevent "high-position implants."

When deciding between subglandular and submuscular placement, various issues should be considered. The submuscular placement is preferred, in general, for several reasons. It allows better contouring, as the implant margins are located deep, and any undulations are obscured over the previous additional tissue. As previously observed, the deep placement of the implant also aids in the visualization of breast tissue on mammography. These reasons are particularly important in patients with minimal breast tissue. Likewise, the dissection plane is avascular and avoids possible contamination associated with the section of the ducts. It is thought that both these points, along with a massage, were proposed to be advantages of the implant by muscle movement, decreasing the incidence of capsular contracture. There may be a certain flattening of the upper pole and/or lateral displacement of the implant in very muscular patients when placed under the muscle. This may, however, be largely avoided by careful attention to release of the medial chest fibers. This plan is preferred in patients with micromastia, post-lactation involution, and congenital breast atrophy.

Subglandular placement also has its advantages (Fig. 55.3). As the tissue plane is further away from the pleural cavity, the injection of local anesthetic and subsequent removal of the capsule (if required) are simpler and safer. Additional advantages are significantly less postoperative pain and the possibility of correcting smaller degrees of ptosis. It is preferred in patients with first-degree hypoplasia.

With either method, some surgeons recommend a preoperative "prophylactic" dose of a first-generation cephalosporin. The patient is carefully positioned and secured with attention to the symmetry levels of the shoulders. The upper limbs should be kept at 90° and a protective belt should be placed so that the patient is securely secured and sufficient for intraoperative verification of the size and position of the implant, so it can be performed with the patient seated.

From an inframammary incision, the dissection is performed directly on the back of the subcutaneous Tissue in the pectoral fascia. For muscle subfield, parallel division is used to spread muscle fibers. This should be done directly on a rib to avoid entering the pleural space. the subpectoral space is entered and in the dissection fingers are used to develop the pocket according to the previously made marks. The muscle needs to be taken off medially from the third rib down, sideways below the anterior serratus and inferiorly from the costal cartilages. This can be aided by lifting the detached tissue to stretch the fibers and neurovascular bundles. Care should be taken to maintain a certain medial separation between the two pockets. If the finger length proves to be inadequate, a large urethral probe may be useful. Now, pressure a lot of attention to hemostasis in his pocket, which can be wrapped with a damp sponge, while continuing on the other side.

If subglandular placement is desired, dissection is continued down to the pectoral fascia, and then extended as previously outlined along the fascial plane, taking care to avoid letting the breast tissue deep into the pocket to improve cancer detection later.

If a periareolar approach is preferred (Figs. 55.4 and 55.5), the incision is made through the skin and subcutaneous tissue. Thereafter, the dissection takes an inferior direction to the deep subcutaneous tissue, going to the lower lateral pectoral fascia. This dissection needs to have a width of approximately two fingers to allow placement of the implant.

The axillary approach requires the placement of surgical fields on the arm plates to allow the surgeon to stand above them. The incision should be made under the arm and along a skin groove posterior to the lateral margin of the pectoralis. Dissection of the subcutaneous plane is

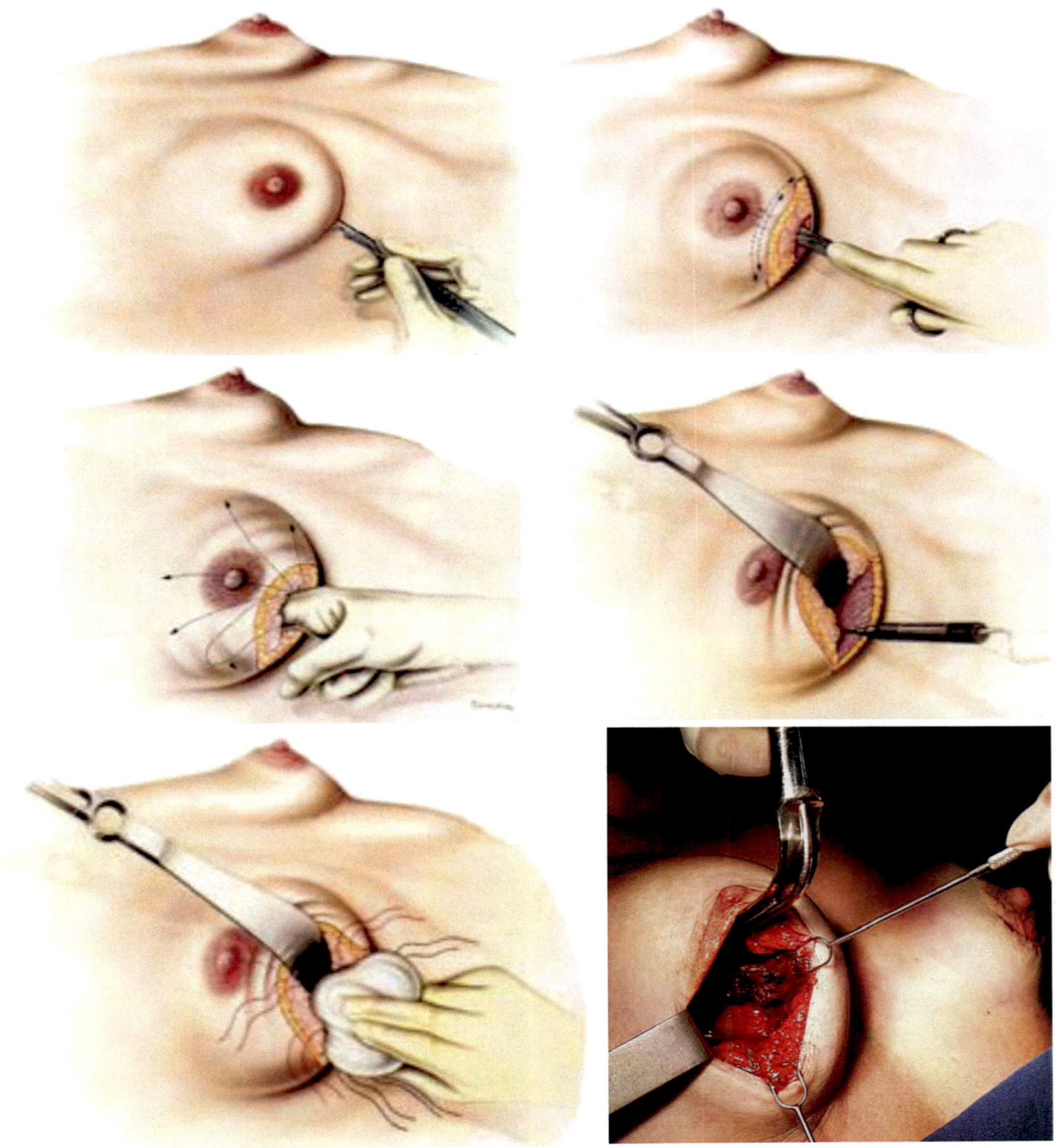

Fig. 55.3 Subglandular placement via periareolar access, submuscular placement

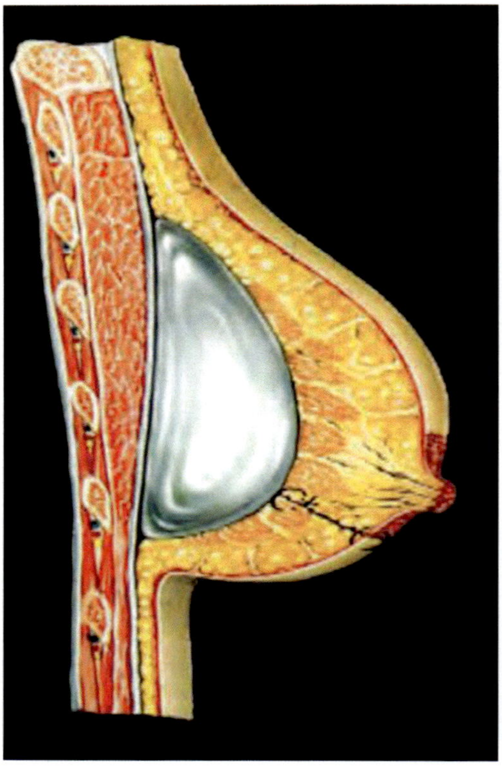

Fig. 55.3 (continued)

performed to achieve the lateral margin of the pectoralis. This tunnel should readily admit two fingers. If the implants are to be placed in the submuscular position, the fascia is sectioned at this point and the development of the pocket starts between the upper and lower pectorals. The dilatation is performed again using the fingers if possible and then a catheter can be used to complete the dissection. In this case, the side and bottom are superficial to the fascia.

Axillary access is best accomplished with the assistance of an endoscope to 30°, to allow direct visualization of the pocket.

The rest of the procedure is similar, independent of the choice of incision and placement of the implant. Hemostasis is carefully checked, and irrigation of the mammary pocket with saline solution or antibiotic solution of betadine should be carried out, according to the preference of the surgeon. The sizers can then be placed to confirm appropriateness, proportionality, and symmetry of the pockets or the surgeon can proceed with placement of the implant. In an effort to decrease the rate of capsular contracture, several steps are

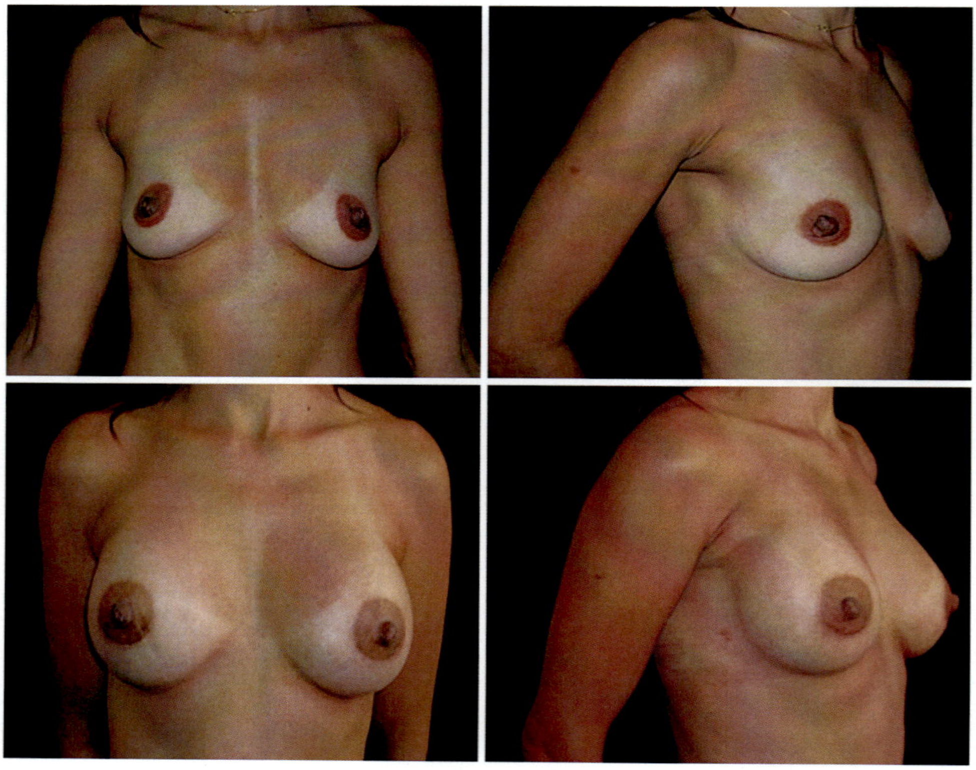

Fig. 55.4 Preoperatively and 6 months postoperatively, 280-mL silicone implant with subglandular placement

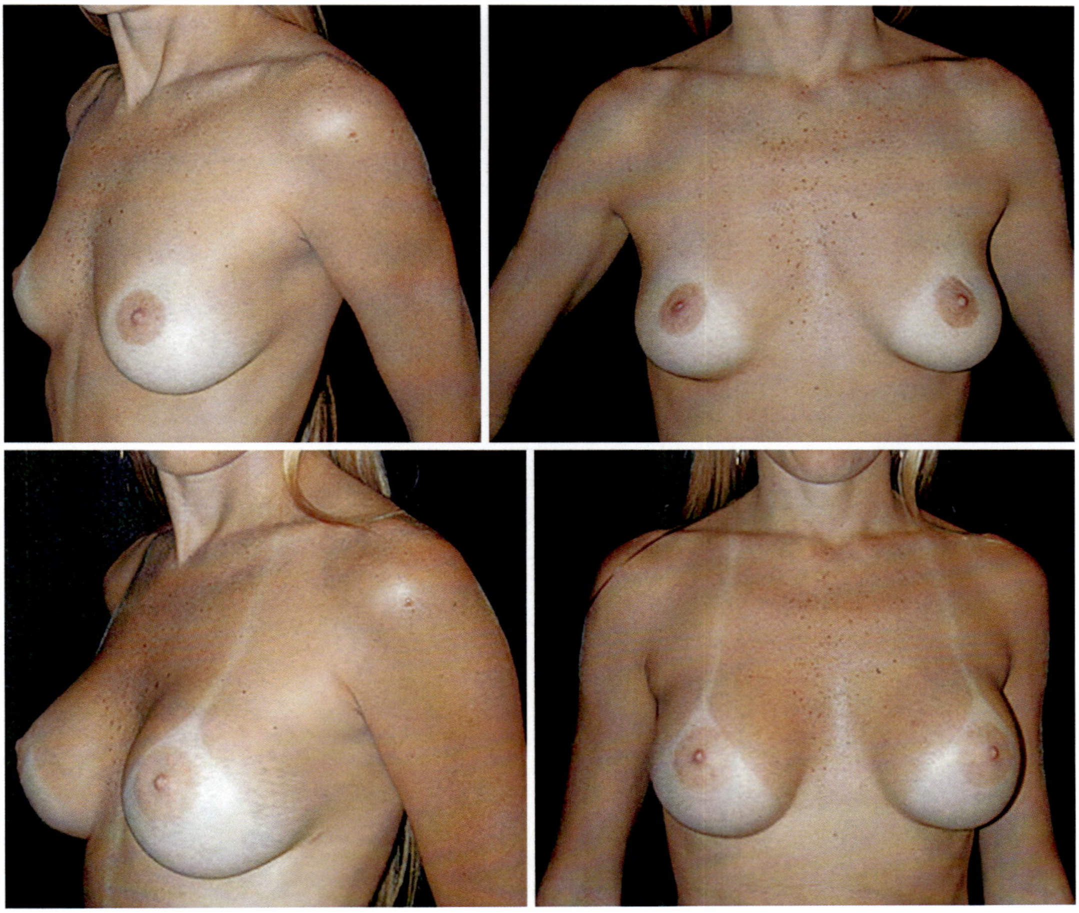

Fig. 55.5 Periareolar access, 245-mL silicone implant, subglandular placement

recommended to minimize contact of the implant with sleeve talc and the patient's skin. If saline implants are used, they are placed in the pocket with fixed tubes (after removal of all air). They must be carefully targeted (especially if they have an anatomical shape), and then inflated as much as desired, leaving the fixed tubes. Pre-filled implants are simply placed in the pocket and oriented (Ersek RA 1991).

At this point, it is desirable to raise the table to check the placement and size with the patient sitting. Any adjustments that need to be made to the extent and symmetry of the pocket, or the position or orientation of the implant, can usually be done at this point with a finger placed next to the implant to protect it. The amounts of saline solution may also be adjusted for symmetry. When the appearance is satisfactory, the table is lowered again. The incisions are closed in layers. Dressings consist of gauze over the incisions and a support bra or ace wrap over the top to increase pressure.

The use of steroids and antibiotics in a pocket or intraluminal is controversial, as is the use of drains and postoperative massage.

55.3.3 Postoperative Care

Postoperative care for breast implants is relatively simple. In the first 24 h, the food should be liquid or paste and the patient should have bed rest until the end of the second day, avoiding effort, with the head of the bed elevated at 45°. The prescribed medication must be interrupted after surgery. For 2 weeks, movements above the shoulders and behind the back should be avoided. Lifting weights, physical effort, driving, and public transport should be prohibited during this period.

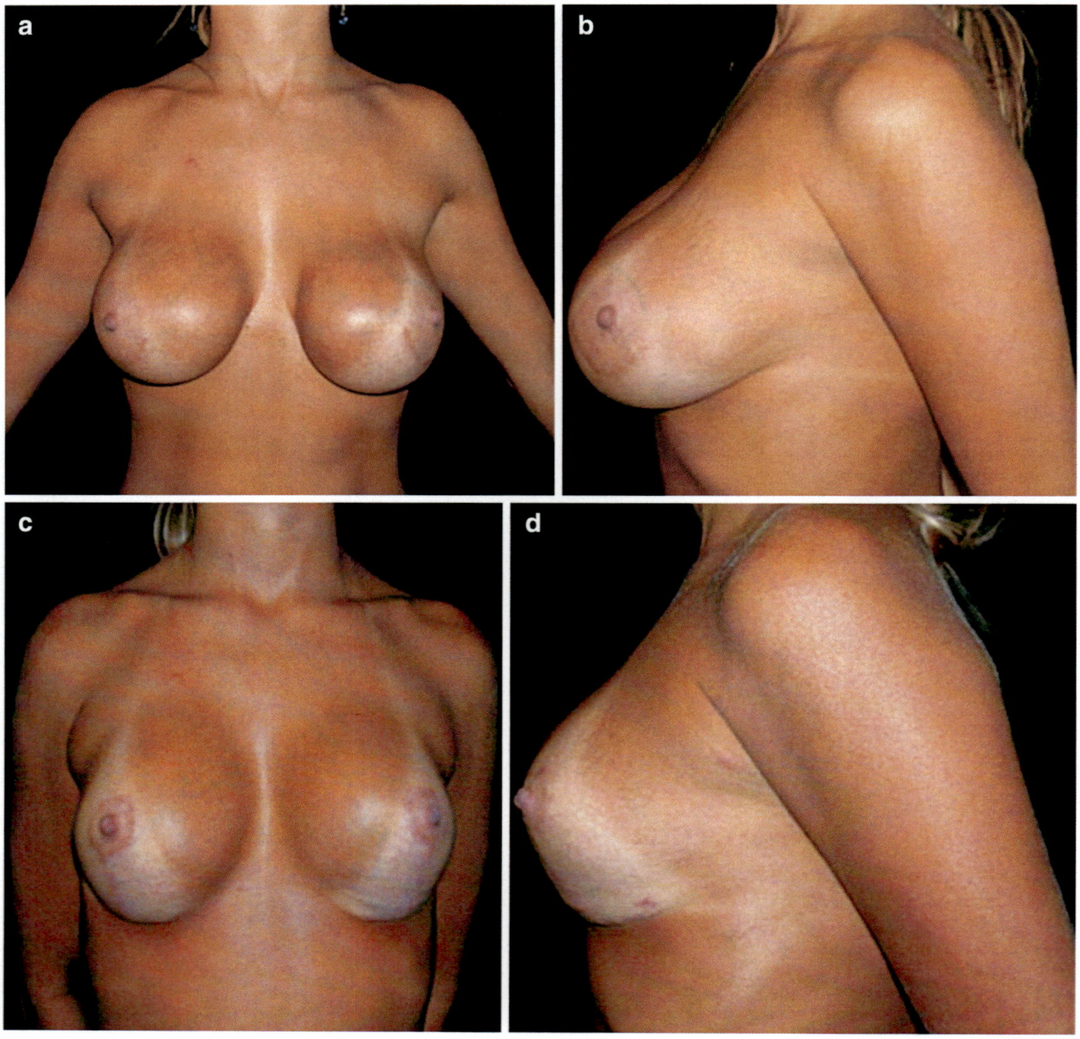

Fig. 55.6 (**a**, **b**) Inadequate subglandular and submuscular placement. (**c**, **d**) Correct repositioning with mastopexy

A special bra should be worn for 60 days and sunlight should be restricted for a minimum of 60 days.

The use of a drain is the surgeon's decision, and sutures should be removed after at least 15 days.

55.4 Complications

Under normal circumstances, breast augmentation is a safe and reliable operation. We must remember that every surgery carries a risk of complications and side effects (Haiavy J, Tobin H 2002).

According to the manifestation period, we can classify them as immediate (within the first 30 days) and late (Codner MA, Cohen AT, Hester TR 2001).

Hematoma, infections, seroma, extrusion, malposition, and hypertrophic scarring are the most common complications, in addition to pneumothorax and sensitivity changes (hypo- or hypersensitivity) (Rohrich RJ, Adams WP Jr, Beran SJ et al. 1998).

Although it is accepted that capsular contracture is the most common and persistent problem associated with breast augmentation, there may be other late complications such as displacement, a change of position (Figs. 55.6 and 55.7), incorrect indication for implants, glandular atrophy, apparent margin, folds (rip-

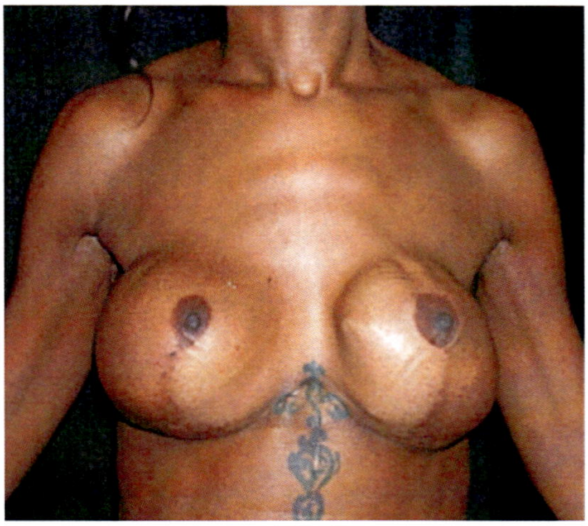

Fig. 55.7 Subglandular placement with capsular contracture

pling), unaesthetic scars, seroma, late infection, late erythema, and intracapsular and extracapsular rupture (Becker L, McCurdy LI, Taves DH 2001).

"Double bubble" is a contour irregularity that occurs when the implants are placed inadequately in a significantly ptotic breast (Shetty MK, Watson AB 2001). Finally, although MRI with spiral surface coils is very effective at predicting breakage, mammography should continue to be the initial study application for imaging complications relating to implants (Gabriel SE, Woods JE, O'Fallon WM et al. 1997).

Conclusions

Breast augmentation is a surgical procedure that aids in bringing back the patient's self-esteem and femininity.

Each implant type selection, surgical technique, and route of access has its indications, depending on the anatomical characteristics and desires of each patient and the surgeon's preferred technique.

There is no evidence that silicone implants are responsible for any major diseases of the whole body. Women are exposed to silicone constantly in their daily lives. There is no plausible evidence for a novel autoimmune disease caused by implants.

Implants do not last forever; risks accumulate over time, and many women should expect to have more than one implant.

References

Araco A, Gravante G, Araco F et al (2007) A retrospective analysis of 3,000 primary aesthetic breast augmentations: postoperative complications and associated factors. Aesth Plast Surg 31:532–539

Barone FE, Perry L, Keller T et al (1992) The biomechanical and histopathologic effects of surface texturing with silicone and polyurethane in tissue implantation and expansion. Plast Reconstr Surg 90:77

Becker L, McCurdy LI, Taves DH (2001) Superficial thrombophlebitis of the breast (Mondor's disease). Can Assoc Radiol J 52:193–195

Becker H, Shaw KE, Kara M (2005) Correction of synmastia using an adjustable implant. Plast Reconstr Surg 115:2124

Codner MA, Cohen AT, Hester TR (2001) Complications of breast surgery. Clin Plast Surg 28:587

Ersek RA (1991) Rate and incidence of capsular contracture: a comparison of smooth and textured silicone double-lumen breast prostheses. Plast Reconstr Surg 87:879

Gabriel SE, Woods JE, O'Fallon WM et al (1997) Complications leading to surgery after breast implantation. N Engl J Med 336:677–682

Haiavy J, Tobin H (2002) Mycobacterium fortuitum infection in prosthetic breast implants. Plast Reconstr Surg 109:2124–2128

Hvilsom GB, Hölmich LR, Henriksen TF (2009) Local complications after cosmetic breast augmentation: results from the Danish registry for plastic surgery of the breast. Plast Reconstr Surg 124(3):919–925

Johnson GW, Christ JE (1993) The endoscopic breast augmentation: the transumbilical insertion of saline-filled breast implants. Plast Reconstr Surg 92:801

Pennisi VR (1985) Polyurethane-covered silicone gel mammary prosthesis for successful breast reconstruction. Aesth Plast Surg 9:73

Rohrich RJ, Adams WP Jr, Beran SJ et al (1998) An analysis of silicone gel-filled breast implants: diagnosis and failure rates. Plast Reconstr Surg 102:2304. discussion 2309

Shetty MK, Watson AB (2001) Mondor's disease of the breast: sonographic and mammographic findings. AJR Am J Roentgenol 177:893–896

56 Approach to Ptotic Breasts: Surgical Options for Solving the Problems

Sérgio Levy Silva

56.1 Introduction

The correction of breast ptosis has been addressed in different techniques over several decades. However, even today, despite various types of surgical options that have been offered (Fig. 56.1), it is difficult to choose which technique or tactic to select. This is because there are several factors that contribute to this pathological condition. For this to be done properly, you need to know about skin aging, changes that lead to sagging skin, such as body weight changes, hormonal issues of each patient, benign or malignant diseases that can reach the breasts, etc. With this knowledge in our hands, we can choose the correct treatment to fulfill those requirements. In some cases, after surgery, the fall of the breasts may recur, which leads to a second surgical procedure. Patients must be alerted to this possibility so that doctors do not have surprises and unnecessary charges in the postoperative period.

The aim of this chapter is to demonstrate what should we know about anatomy and pathophysiology (aging, loss of skin volume, breasts, etc.), and also to know about the classification of ptosis, the history of the pathological condition and its technical and surgical descriptions.

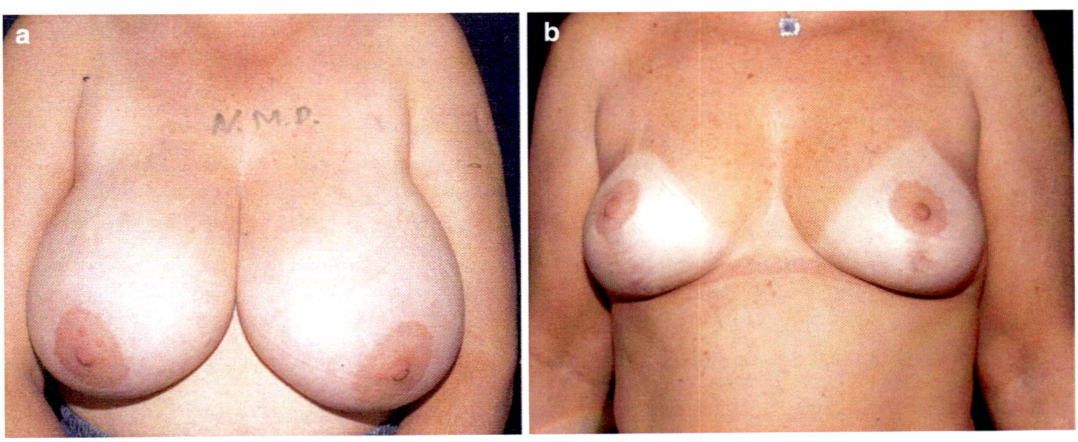

Fig. 56.1 Brazilian authors who described tactics to improve the final results. The Pitanguy's technique is of universal use, it can be used in any breast dysmorphy. (**a**) Preoperative photo (**b**) postoperative photo

S.L. Silva
Rua Real Grandeza, 108–sala 313, 22281034
Botafogo, RJ, Brazil
e-mail: slevy@br.inter.net

J.M. Avelar (ed.), *Breast Surgery*, https://doi.org/10.1007/978-3-319-54115-0_56

56.2 Anatomy

Located in the mammary region, which occupies part of the thoracic region on each side of the sternum, in front of the pectoral muscles, between the third and the seventh rib, are the presternal line and the anterior axillary line. The surface boundaries are not clear. At the bottom, there is the submammary fold, the result of greater adherence to the dermal deep plane, which is accentuated in ptosis and hypertrophy.

The breasts are glandular pairs, organs that are susceptible to neuroendocrine stimulation, and are primarily destined for milk secretion to nourish the new born. Therefore, it is an accessory to the reproductive system. It is also considered an attachment of the skin and an element of beauty, libido, and female differentiation. The mammary gland secretes exocrine and contains a mixture of proteins, lactose, fat, and minerals. It consists in 15–20 blister glands composed of lobes, each with a separate lactiferous duct and opening in the breast papilla. The whole mammary gland is surrounded by Cooper's ligament and is separated from the pectoral muscle by the Chassaignac space. Arterial blood supply is venous and lymphatic and served by the internal thoracic artery (internal mammary), lateral thoracic artery, and the anterior lateral branches of the posterior intercostal arteries.

Venous drainage is provided by a superficial system and another deeper one.

Lymph is provided by the deep cervical axillary lymph nodes, thoracic lymph nodes, and internal deltoid pectorals on both sides.

Innervation is done by the intercostal nerves (second to sixth), brachial plexus, and nerves for the thoracic axial and brachialis muscles.

56.3 Physiopathology

Depending on the volume, loss of elasticity, loss of weight and the hormonal changes of each woman, the breasts may drop or show ptosis to many different degrees. Anamnesis will lead to an accurate diagnosis of what happened and how we can reverse this pathological condition.

56.4 Classification

56.4.1 Regnell Classification

According to Regnell, the ptosis can be classified as:

Bilateral breasts hypertrophy (with or without ptosis)

Normal sized breasts with ptosis

Bilateral breast hypertrophy (with or without ptosis)

Mammary asymmetry with or without hypertrophy or with or without ptosis

56.4.2 Binet Classification

According to Binet, the ptosis is classified as:

Ptosis by atrophy (senile, post-puerperal involution, etc.)

Ptosis by hypertrophy or pseudohypertrophy (increase in weight)

Pendulous breasts, distance from the submammary fold to the bottom edge of the breast of less than 2 cm

Ptotic breast distance from the submammary fold to the bottom edge of the breast of more than 2 cm

Level I—Breast lower edge not exceeding the costal edge

Level II—The lower edge is between the costal edge and the navel.

Level III—The lower edge is below the horizontal umbilical plane.

56.5 History

We describe below a brief report on the evolution of breast ptosis correction.

The correction of ptosis corresponds to a form of surgery named mastopexy (masto = mammary and pexy = fixing); thus, several techniques were presented with this purpose.

In 1922, Torek advocated the amputation technique of the lower pole and a free graft. In 1988, Biesenberger described the displacement with recession of the entire gland and remaining skin rotation of 180° and transposition of the nipple–areola complex (NAC). Authors such as Maliniac (1950) and Gillies and McIndoe (1939), added to their techniques Schwarzmann's concept (1930).

Aufricht (1949) and Barnes (1950), reported the plot points of the breasts to help the recession, modeling, and symmetrization of the breasts. Penn (1955) reported the point in the external region that forms an equilateral triangle with a distance of 18–21 cm from the NAC. Wise et al. (1963) described fixed mammoplasties. Strombeck (1971), uses the molds designed by Wise. Regnault (1967) described the classification of breast ptosis. Goulian (1971), and Pitanguy (1967) described the recession technique in the lower pole, transposition of the NAC combined with the Schwarzmann maneuver, with the final suture ending in the submammary fold or in an inverted T (Lexer and Kraske 1923).

National authors who embraced Prof Ivo Pitanguy's technique have described several tactics with the goal of improving and promoting greater durability of results.

56.6 Technique

As we said earlier, to choose which surgical technique to pick for the resolution of breast ptosis, the surgeon should consider not only the experience and knowledge of various surgical techniques and tactics, but also the knowledge of the various elements that strike the breasts. With this in mind, we correct this pathological condition with precision.

With the experience gained over 25 years, we gradually selected the best technique to obtain in the end, breasts with volume, shape, symmetry, and a good postoperative time (Figs. 56.2, 56.3, 56.4, 56.5, 56.6, 56.7, 56.8, and 56.9).We chose Professor's Ivo Pitanguy's technique (Fig. 56.10), combined with other tactics, such as retail superior pedicle, dermal belt, inverted

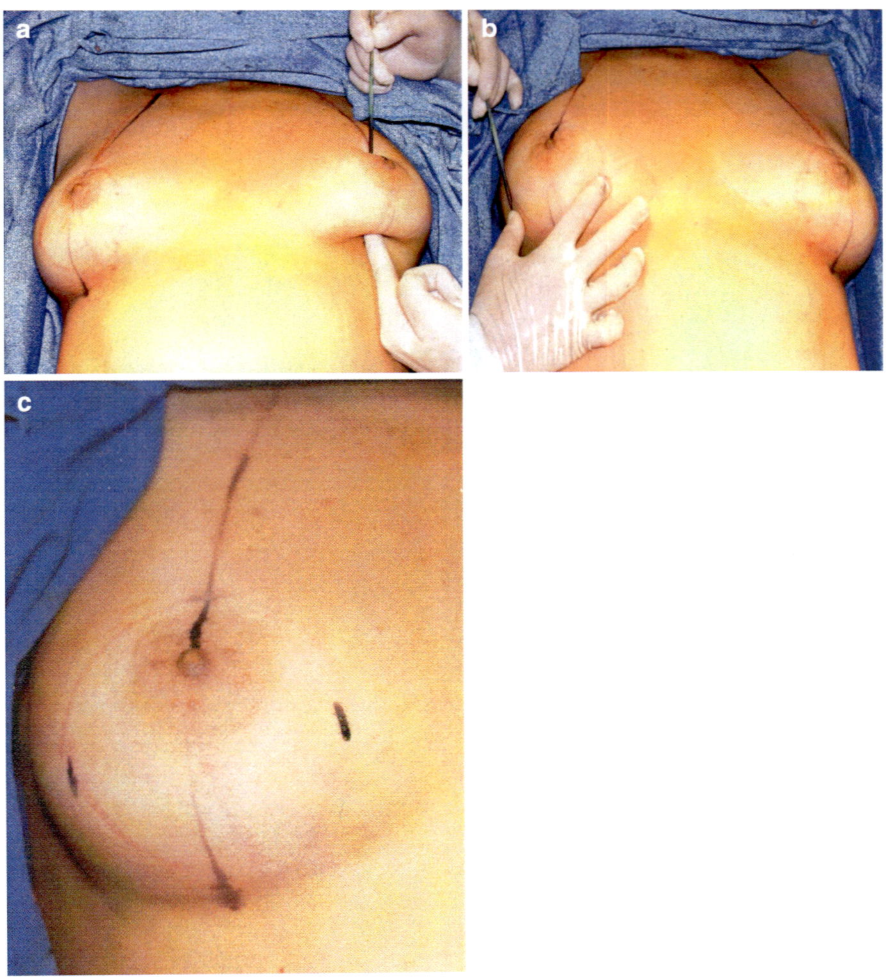

Fig. 56.2 Postoperative results between 1 and 10 years. (**a**, **b** and **c**) The Pitanguy's technique aggregate to tactical changes, enables us to achieve better and more lasting results

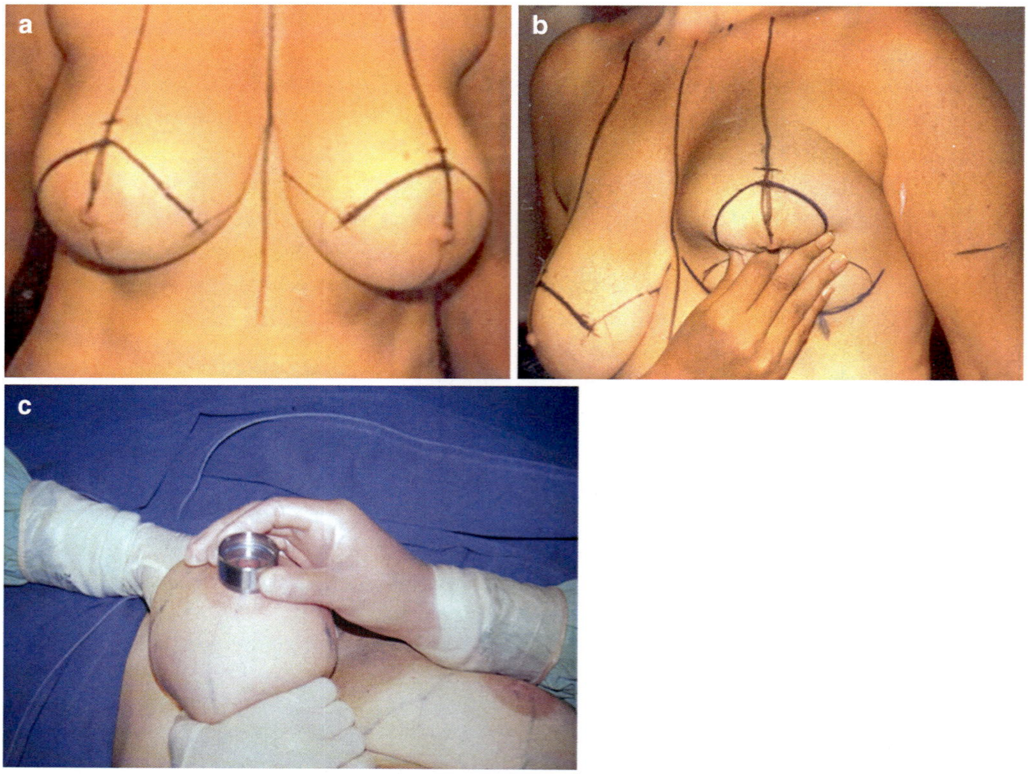

Fig. 56.3 Point marks. (**a**) (projection of the submammary fold in breast middle region), points (**b**) and (**c**) (by digital pressure)

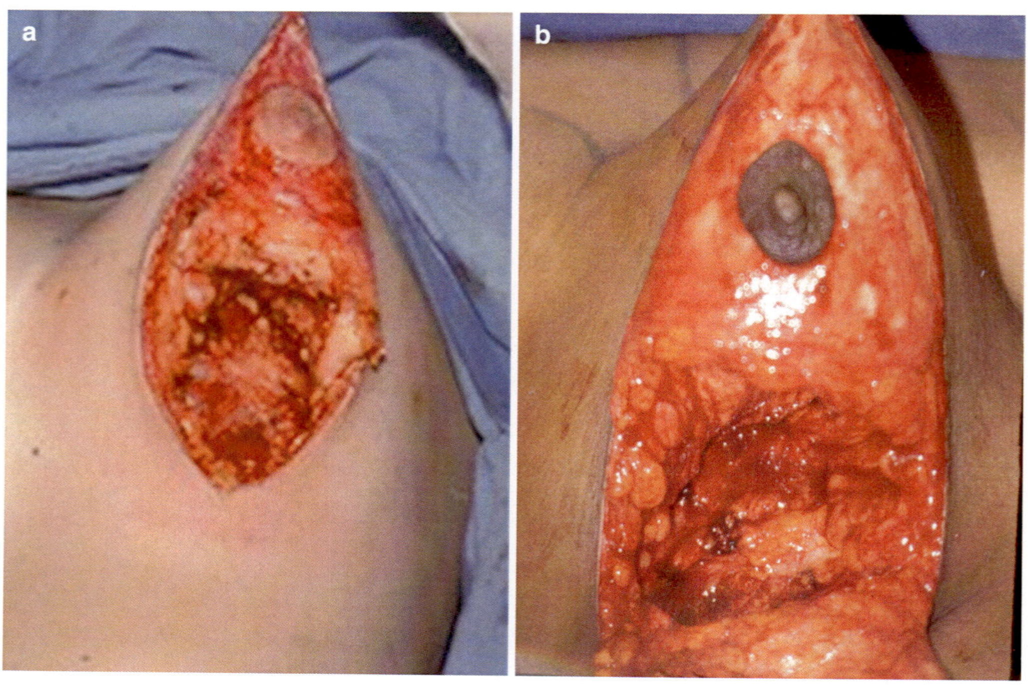

RESECTION IN KEEL

RESECTION FLAT

Fig. 56.4 (**a**) and (**b**) Confirmation of pre-defined points and marking of the CAM

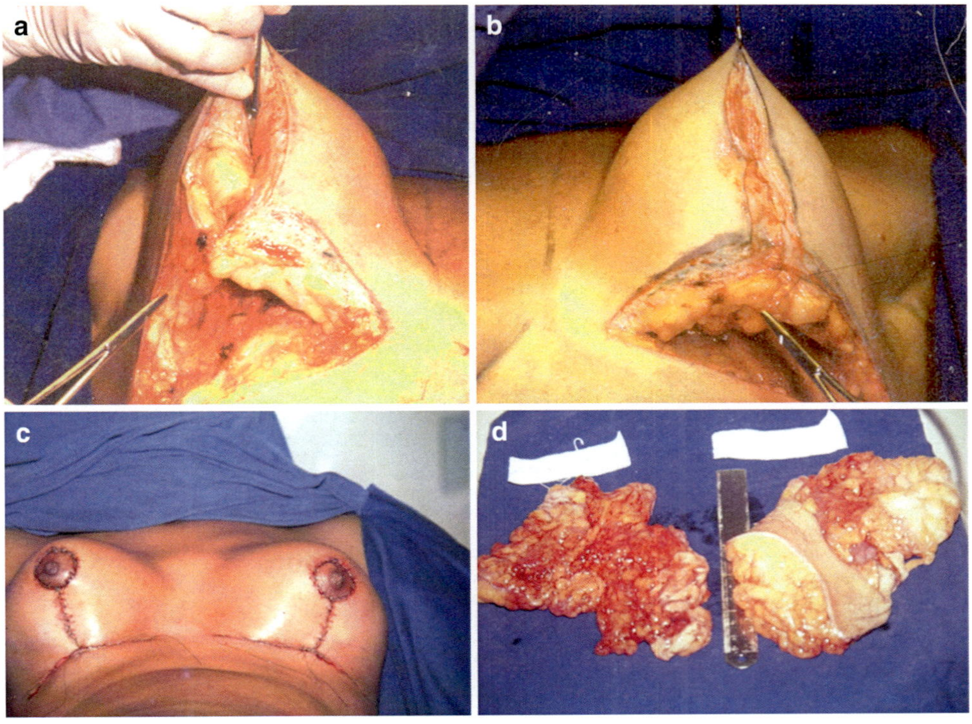

Fig. 56.5 (**a**, **b**, **c** and **d**) Marking of the CAM and resection maneuver in keel or Gothic cathedral (in glandular tissue or mixed)

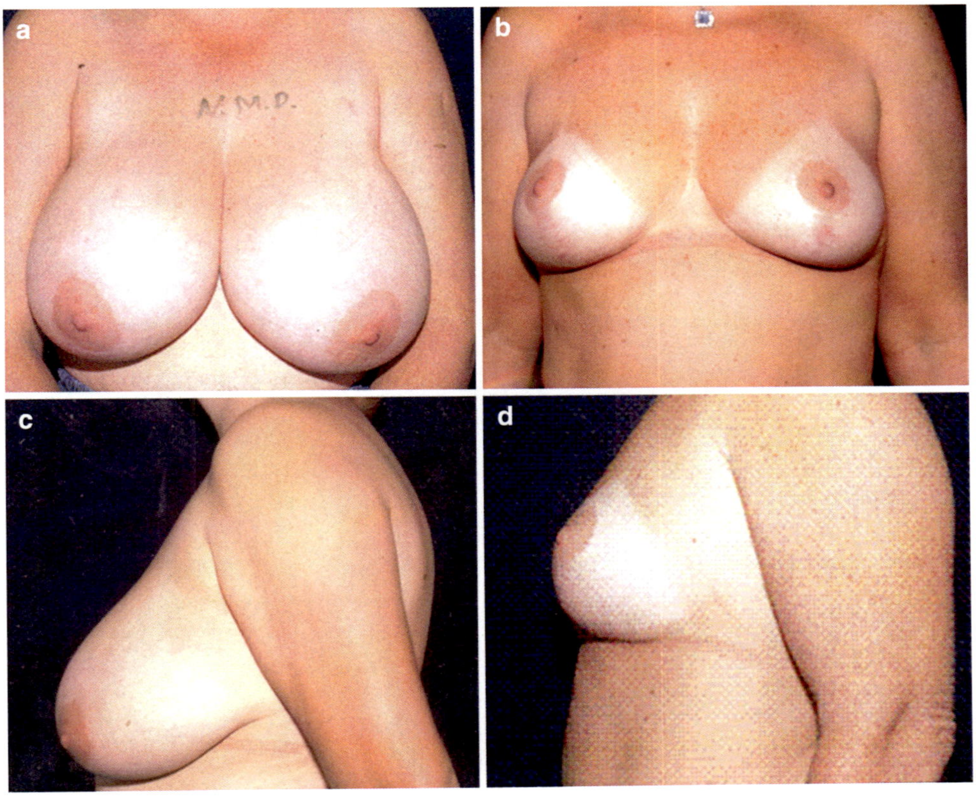

Fig. 56.6 confection of a dermal belt will result in less stress and better shape of the breasts. In this technique, we can remove (as showed in this case), 3 kg of tissue on each side. (**a**, **c**) Preoperative photos (**b**, **d**) postoperative photos

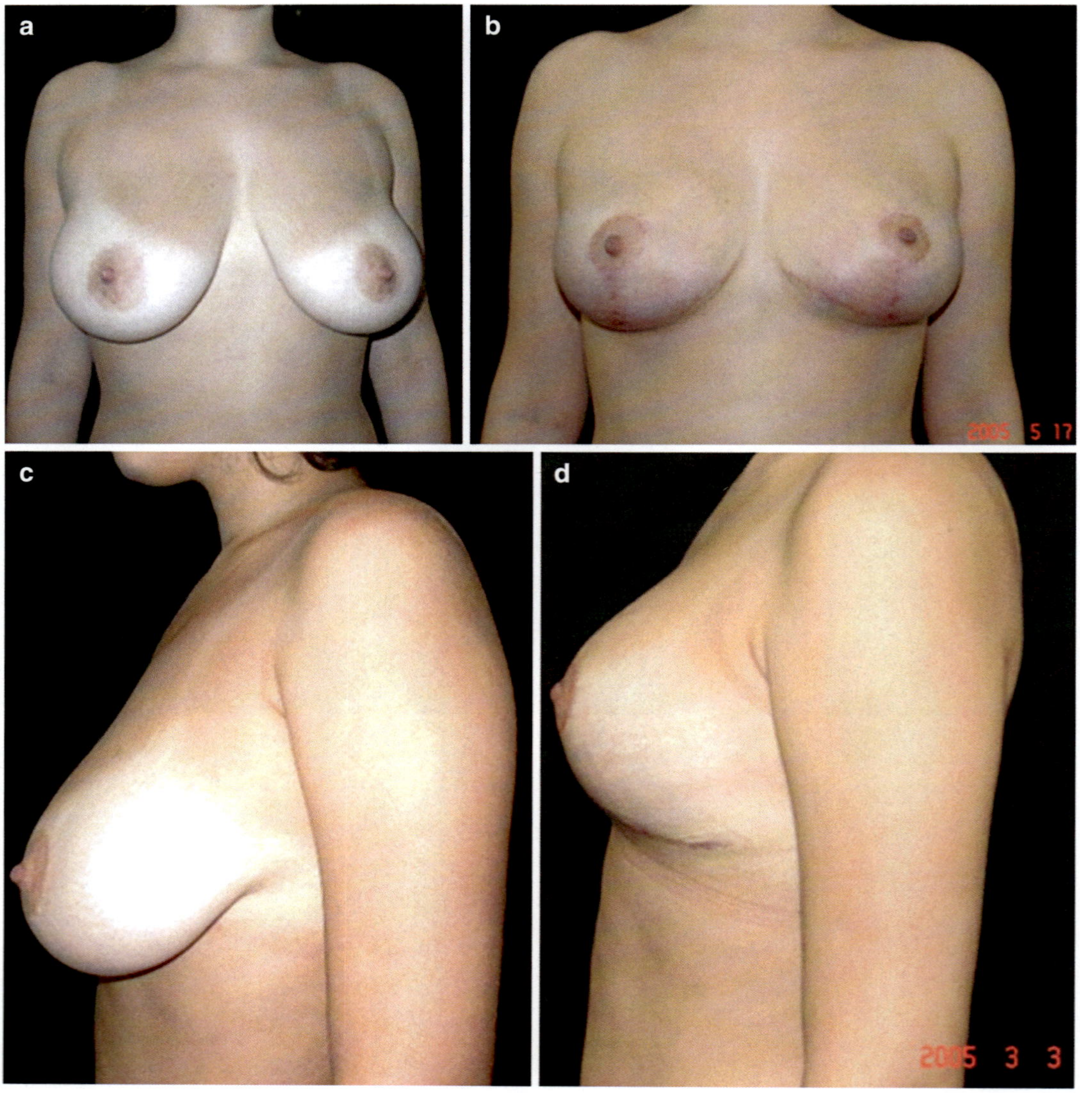

Fig. 56.7 Post-operative results between 1 to 10 years. (**a**, **c**) Preoperative photos (**b**, **d**) postoperative photos

suture, liposuction, and breast implants (Figs. 56.11, 56.1, 56.12, 56.13 and 56.14). These elements are the subject of this chapter.

For patients with large or medium breast hypertrophy with ptosis and/or asymmetry to various degrees (Fig. 56.15), we always choose Professor Pitanguy's usual technique. When possible, we always try to reduce the scar on the submammary fold and always use the dermal belt (CHDID). In patients with moderate or small hypertrophy with ptosis and asymmetry, we normally use a superior pedicle (Ribeiro), and a dermal belt (CHIDID). In some cases, we use textured breast implants (between 250 and 350 ml; Figs. 56.11, 56.16, 56.17, 56.18).

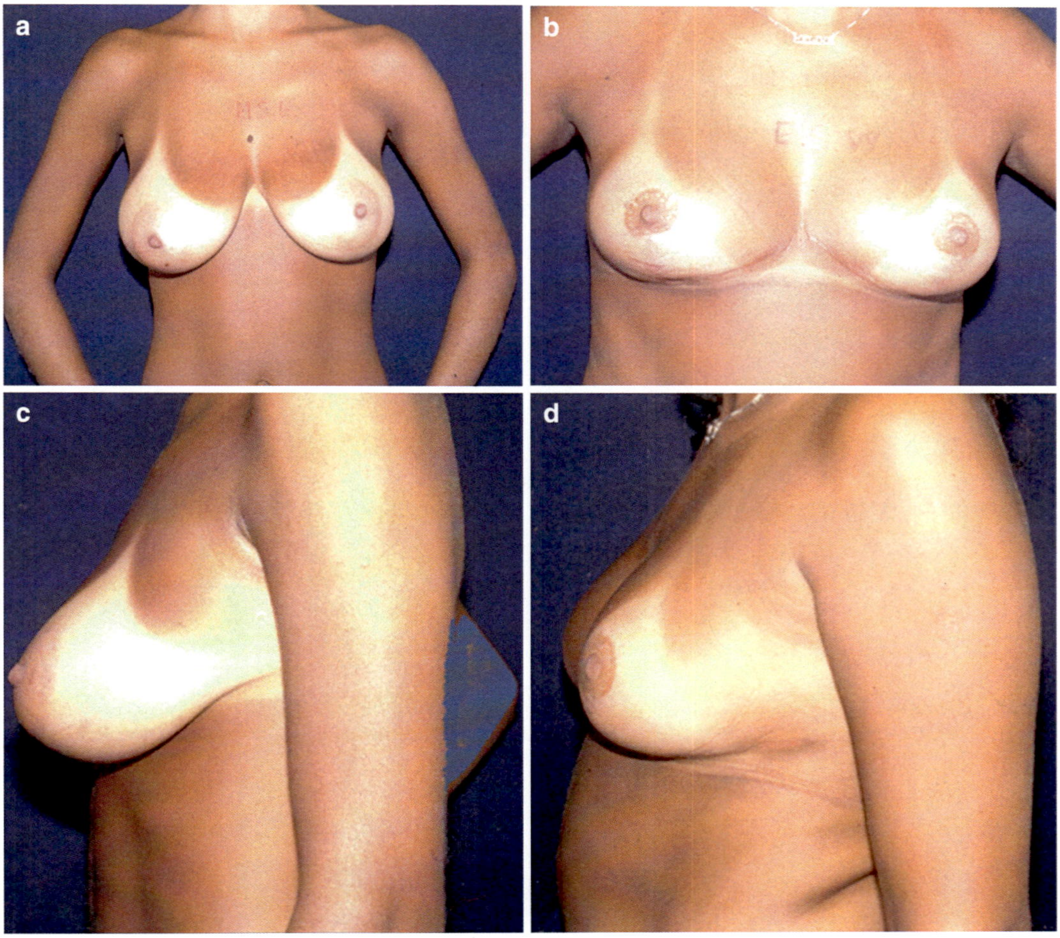

Fig. 56.8 Final results (**a**) (**b**): Post-operative results between 1 to 10 years. (**a**) Preoperative photos (**b**) postoperative photos (**c**) (**d**) Same patient ilustrated on Fig. 56.8 on profile view. (**a**) before surgery, (**b**) post operative result

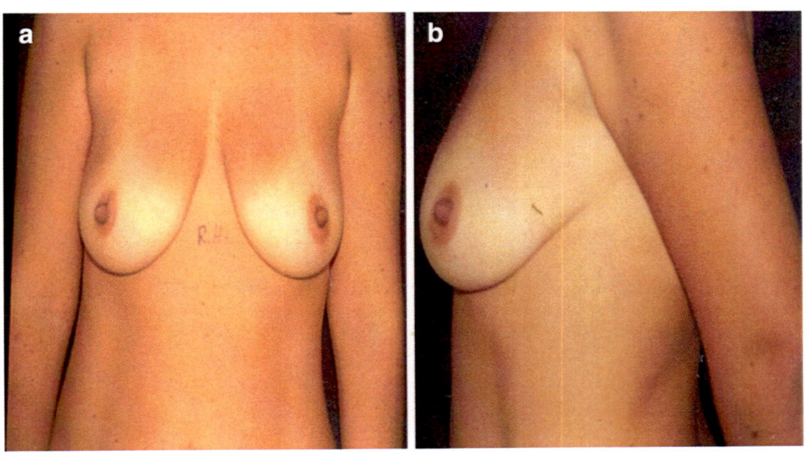

Fig. 56.9 Final results (**a**) and (**b**) severe ptosis of the breast with moderate hypertrophy with asymmetry. Those deformities may be treated through techniques described by brazilian authors who described personal approches to improve the final results. From 1961 to 1992: Pitanguy, Peixoto, Bozzola, Sinder, Ribeiro, Bolivar, Pontes, Hakme, Jurado, Lima, Sepulveda, Chidid

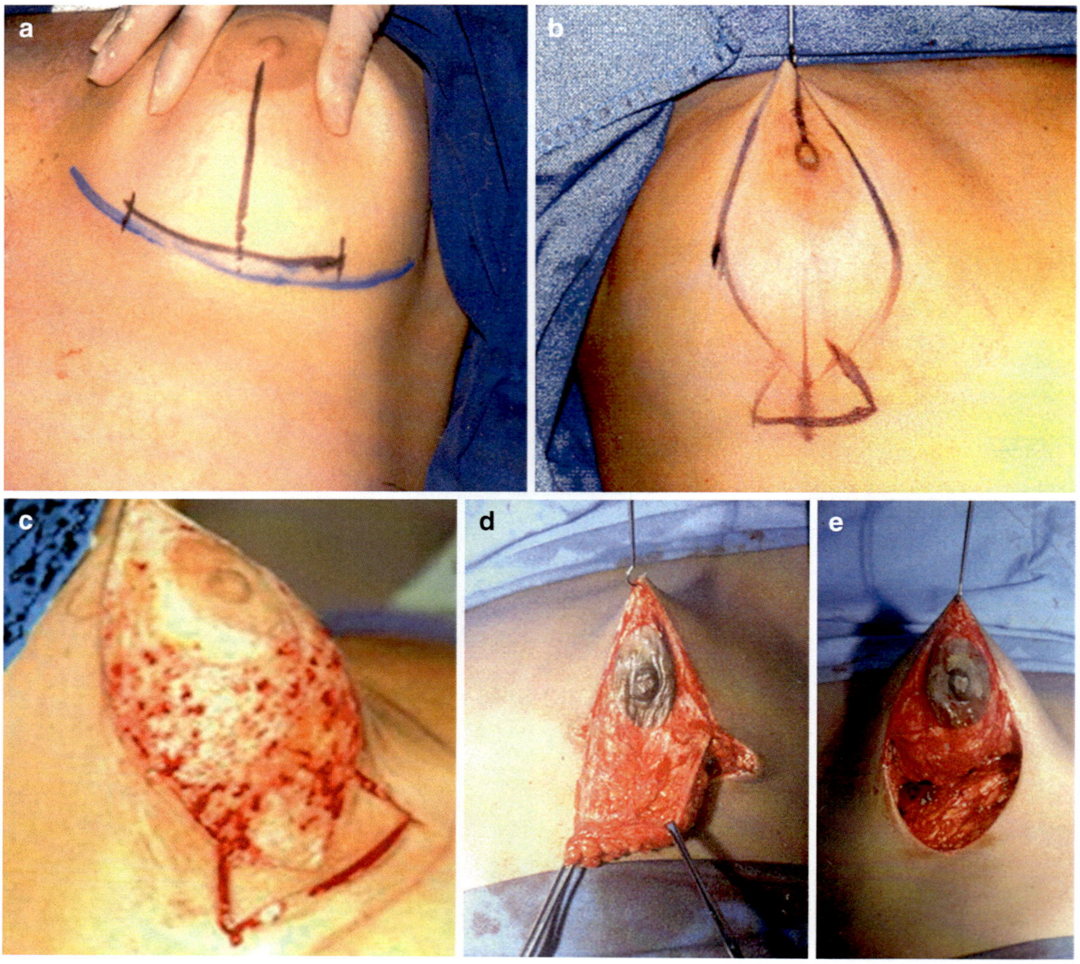

Fig. 56.10 Pitanguy's technique combined with tactical changes enables us to achieve better and more lasting results. (**a**, **b**, **c** and **d**) Inverted suture (from the bottom up, in order to decrease the medial scar aspect), liposuction (internal and external) and marking the new CAM; (**e**) photo shows after inverted suture

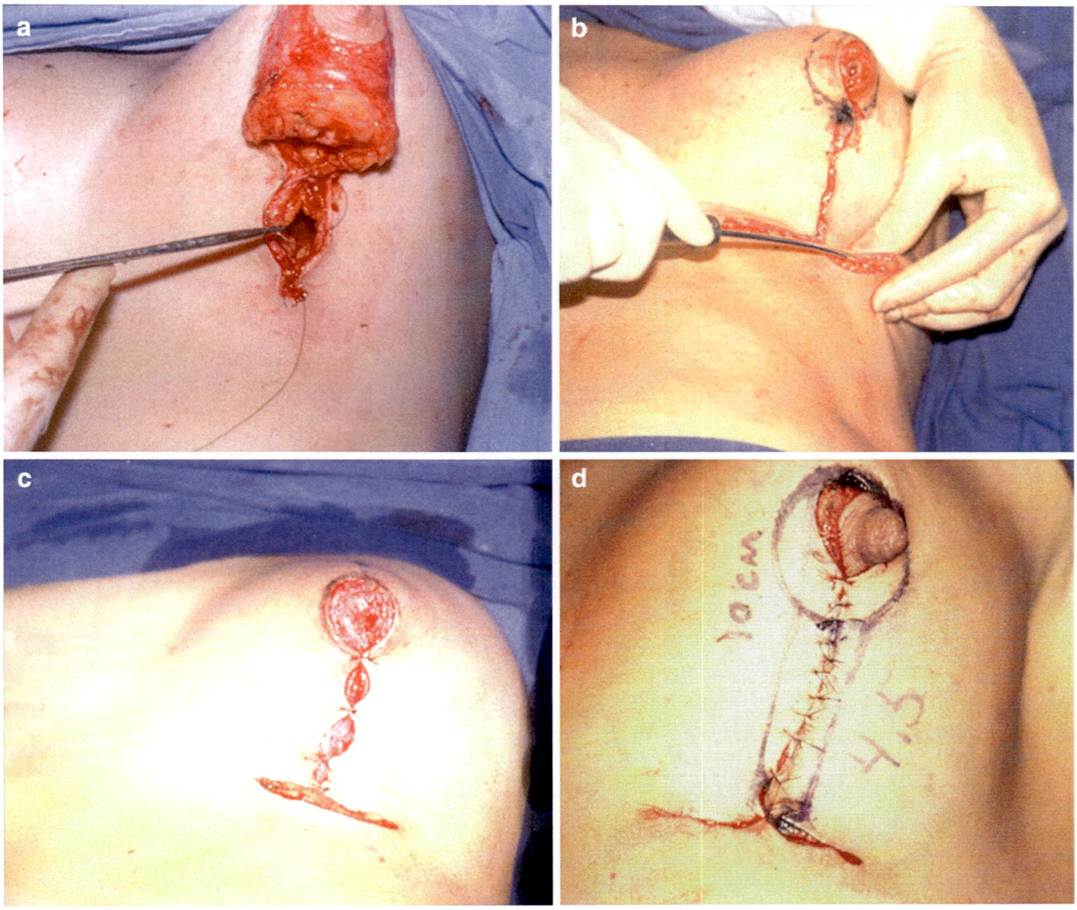

Fig. 56.11 Creation of a dermal belt results in less stress and a better shape of the breasts. In this technique, we can remove (as shown in this case) 3 kg of tissue from each side. (**a**, **b**, **c** and **d**) Inverted suture (from the bottom up, in order to decrease the medial scar aspect), liposuction (internal and external) and marking the new CAM

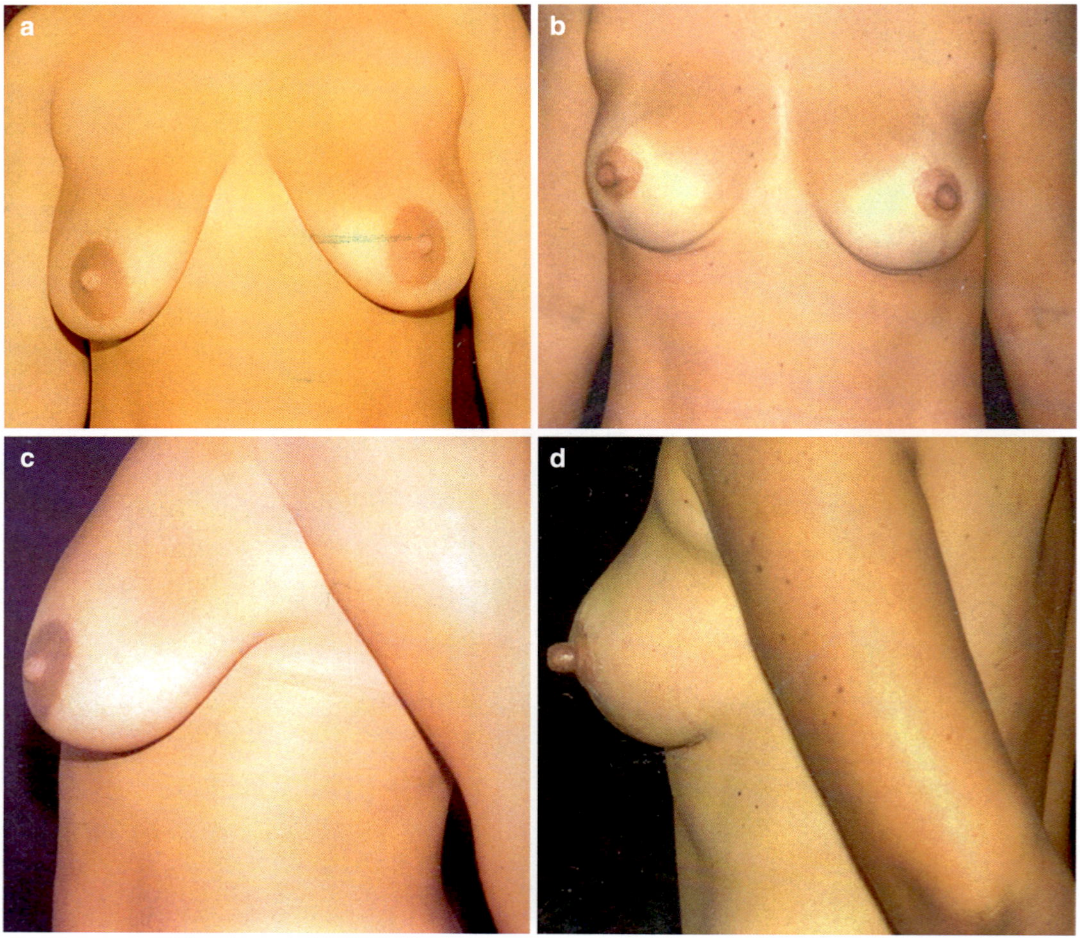

Fig. 56.12 Patient with arms elevated to check the possibility of reducing the scar in the submammary fold. Marking and preparation of retail as a superior pedicle and final mounting without the use of breast implants. (**a**, **c**) Preoperative photos (**b**, **d**) postoperative results

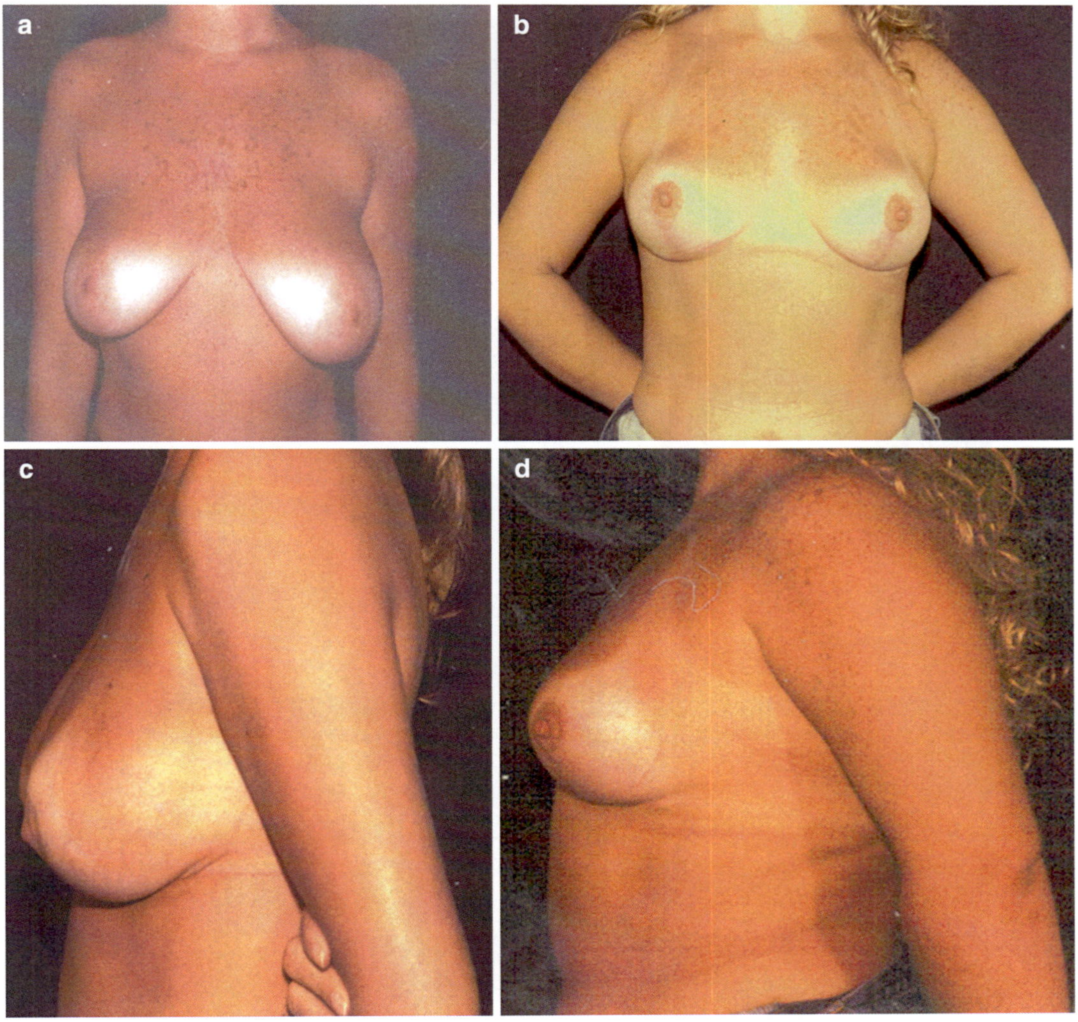

Fig. 56.13 Inverted suture (from the bottom up, to decrease the medial scar), liposuction (internal and external), and marking of the new nipple–areolar complex (NAC): (**a**, **c**) Preoperative photos (**b**, **d**) postoperative results

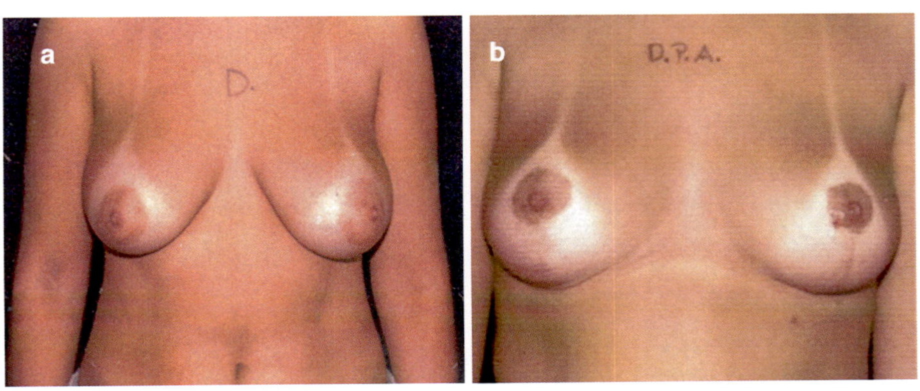

Fig. 56.14 (**a**, **d**) Preoperative photos (**b**, **e**) postoperative photos results (**c**, **f**) ten year later

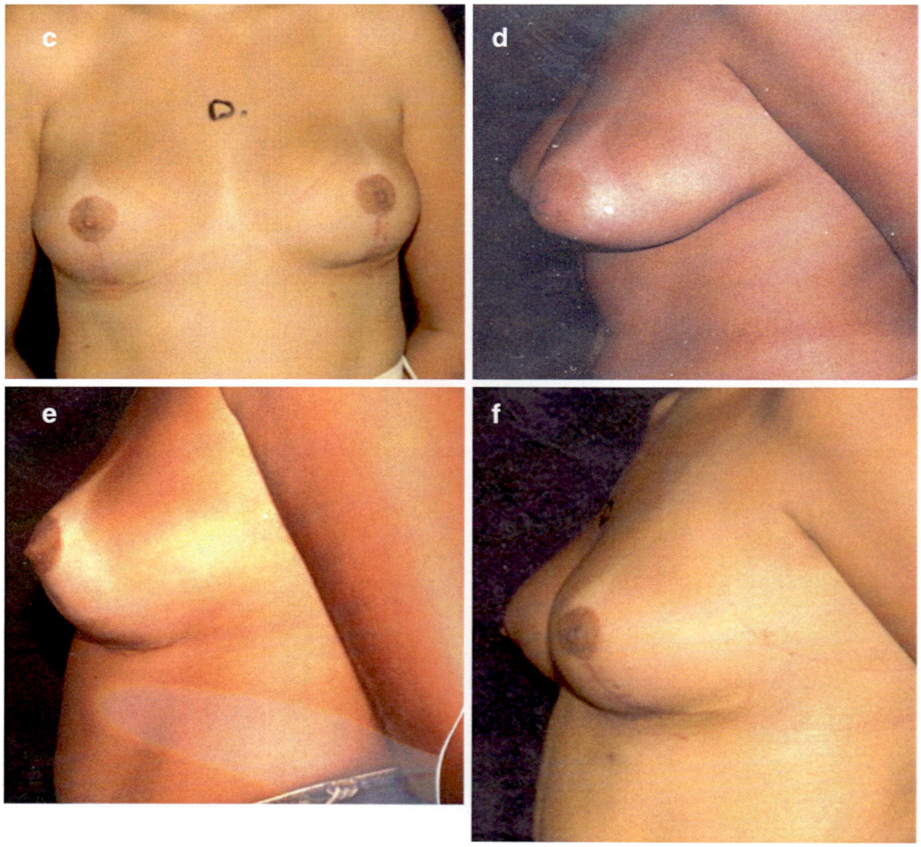

Fig. 56.14 (continued)

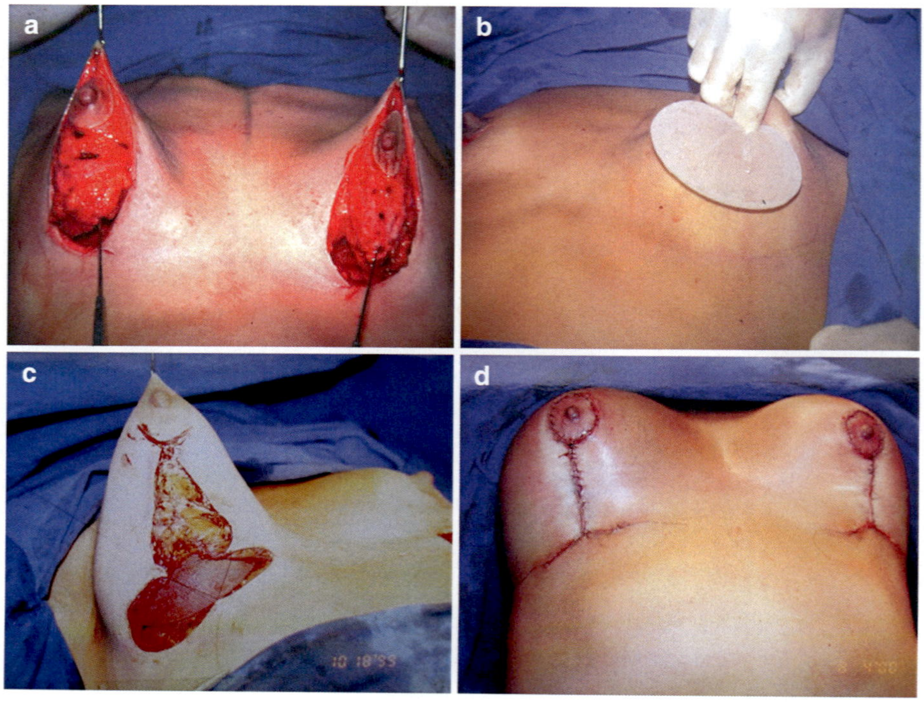

Fig. 56.15 (**a**, **b**, **c** and **d**) Retail finished and inclusion of the implant to increase the volume, shape and final suture

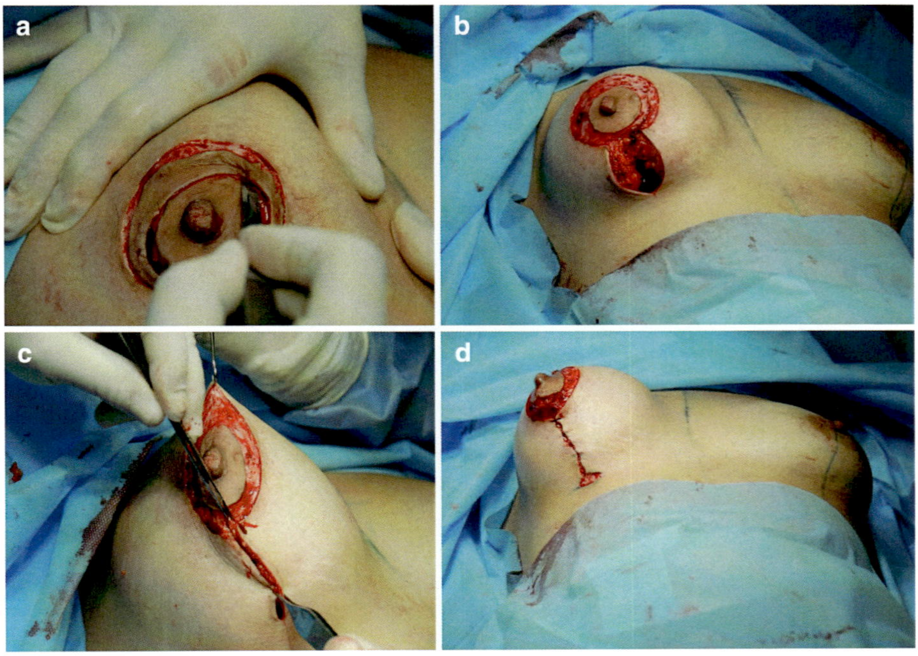

Fig. 56.16 (**a**, **b**, **c** and **d**) Tactic made without previous resection, placement of the implant, removal of the skin, modeling and final suture

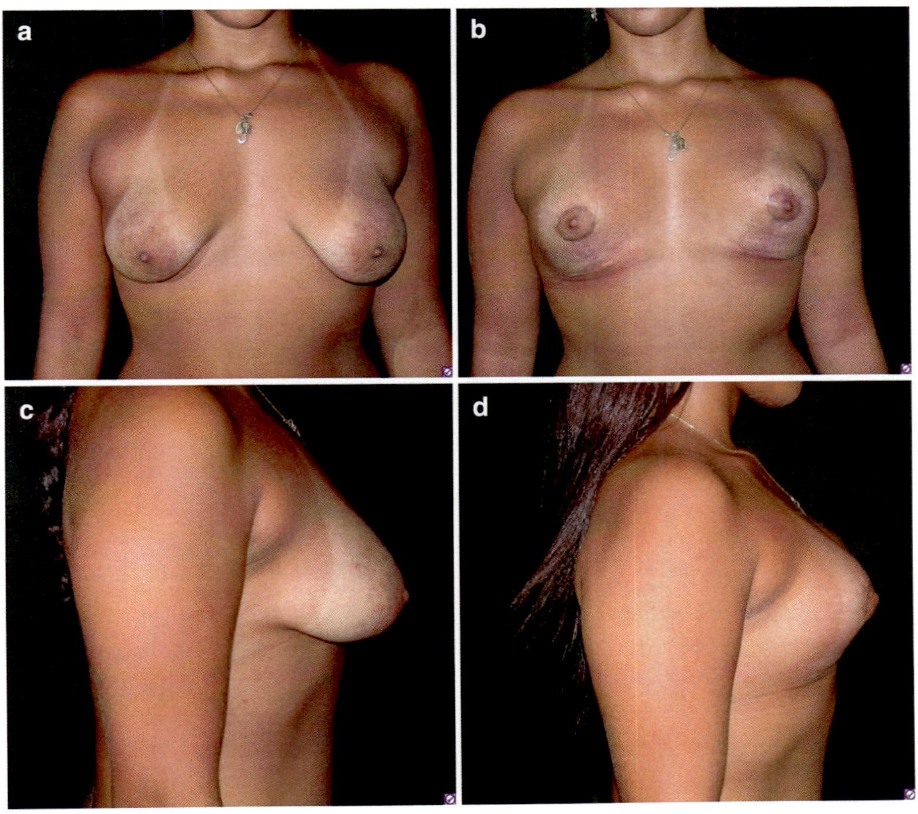

Fig. 56.17 Final Results. (**a**, **c**) Preoperative photos (**b**, **d**) postoperative photos results

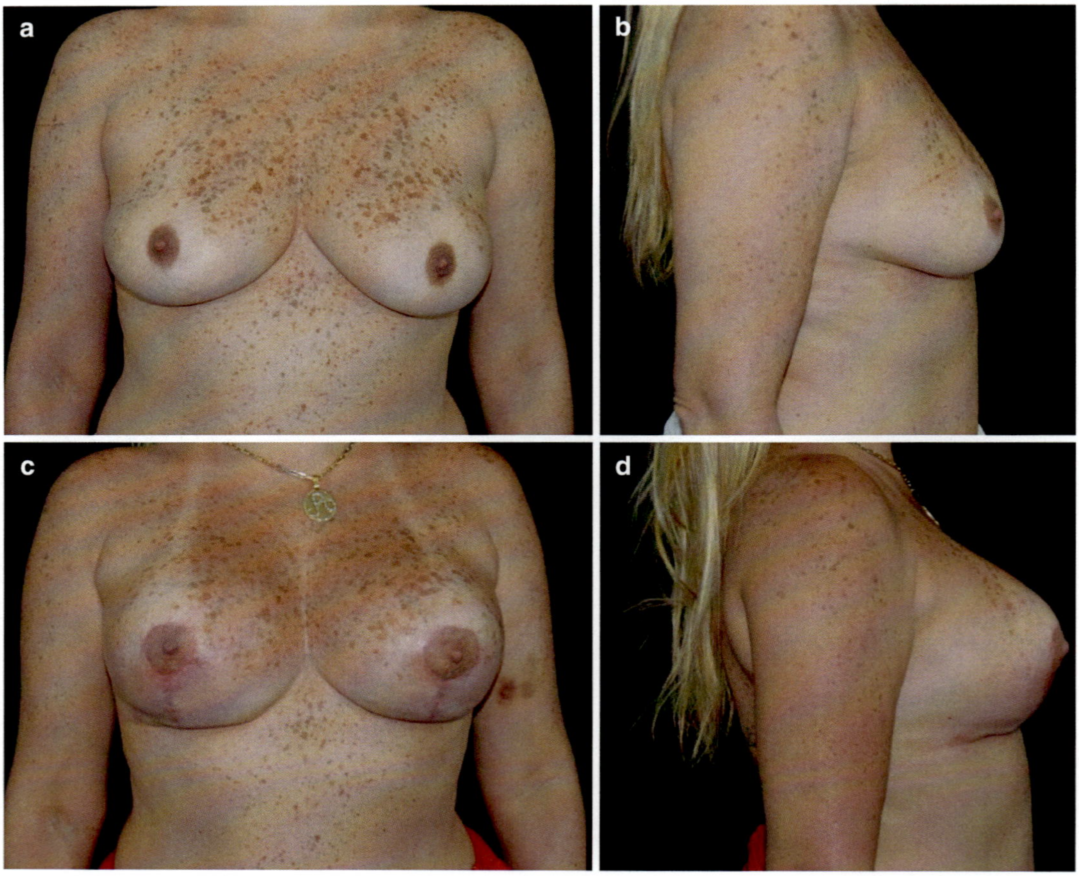

Fig. 56.18 Marking of the NAC and resection maneuver in a keel or Gothic cathedral shape (in glandular tissue or mixed. Final Results. (**a**, **c**) Preoperative photos (**b**, **d**) postoperative photos results

56.7 Technical Description

The marking of points A, B, and C is carried out according to parameters described by the Professor Pitanguy's usual technique. Point A is located in the projection of the submammary fold in the mammary medial line, approximately 18–22 cm away from the upper segment the sternal bone.

Points B and C are marked by digital pressure, evaluating the amount of skin to be resected. These lines shall not be located above the projection of the NAC (Fig. 56.16). After these markings (8–10 cm long) have been made, we follow them to achieve the lateral and medial portions of those points to reach the previously marked inframammary fold (Fig. 56.17).

We start the surgery by marking the NAC; after that, we use Schwarzmann's maneuver. The resection of the gland is flat (when greasy) or keel-shaped (when glandular or mixed), depending on the content (Fig. 56.18). After this, we set up the skin and gland by making a skin belt (Fig. 56.11). Finally, we mark the new location of the NAC, remove the skin, and perform the final suture (Figs 56.2, 56.3, 56.4). In cases of moderate breasts or small hypertrophy, we use all breast tissue and the dermis to model and fill the breasts. By doing so, points A, B, and C are marked according to Professor Pitanguy's original technique and remain in the form of an ellipse (according to Arié), until the submammary fold is found (Figs. 56.12 and 56.16).

With the patient raising her arms, we copy the site before breast ptosis; at this point, we try to make two triangles (medial and lateral), to try to reduce the scar on the submammary fold (Fig. 56.12). We mark with an Areolotomos the size of the NAC, taking Schwarzmann's maneuver throughout the area of the ellipse, we unstick the gland up to the third or fourth intercostal space, using the flap as a superior pedicle to fill, enhance, and give shape to the breast. To do so, this flap is fixed in the pectoralis major muscle at the level of the fourth intercostal space (Figs. 56.18, 56.12 and 56.13). After this, we use the inverted suture (from top to bottom, from the submammary fold). In some cases, we carry out a lateral and medial liposuction of the breasts. We finish with suturing of the dermal belt (Fig. 56.13), the mounting of the breasts (Fig. 56.13), and the final suture (Figs. 56.5, 56.6, 56.7).

In cases of hypomastia with severe ptosis, we use breast implants to give greater volume and shape to the breasts. Retail as a superior pedicle is used to cover and protect the implant. We prefer to use implants of textured types, of between 250 and 350 ml (Fig. 56.14). We can also use the technique recommended by Hakme and others. We mark Pitanguy's point A with a Mamilotoma, set the size of the NAC and then perform Schwarzmann's maneuver(Fig. 56.5). We incise the skin, unstick the gland, and put in the mold of the implant. The removal of the skin is progressive clamping, until we get to the point where such withdrawal is without tension. Finally, we remove the mold, put in the implant, carry out modeling, and the final suture (Figs. 56.8, 56.9, 56.19, 56.20).

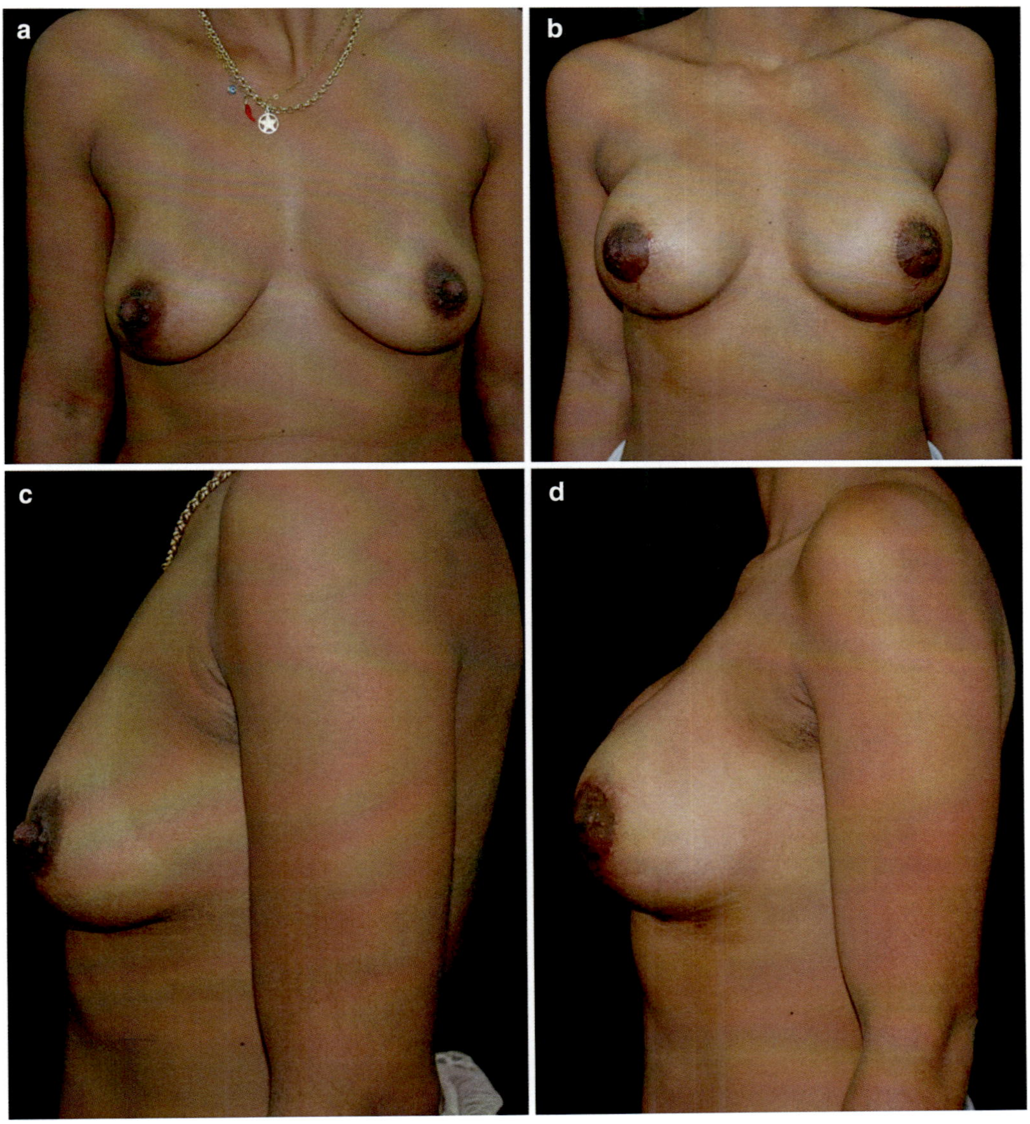

Fig. 56.19 Tactic carried out without previous resection, placement of the implant, removal of the skin, modeling, and final suture. Final Results. (**a**, **c**) Preoperative photos (**b**, **d**) postoperative photos results

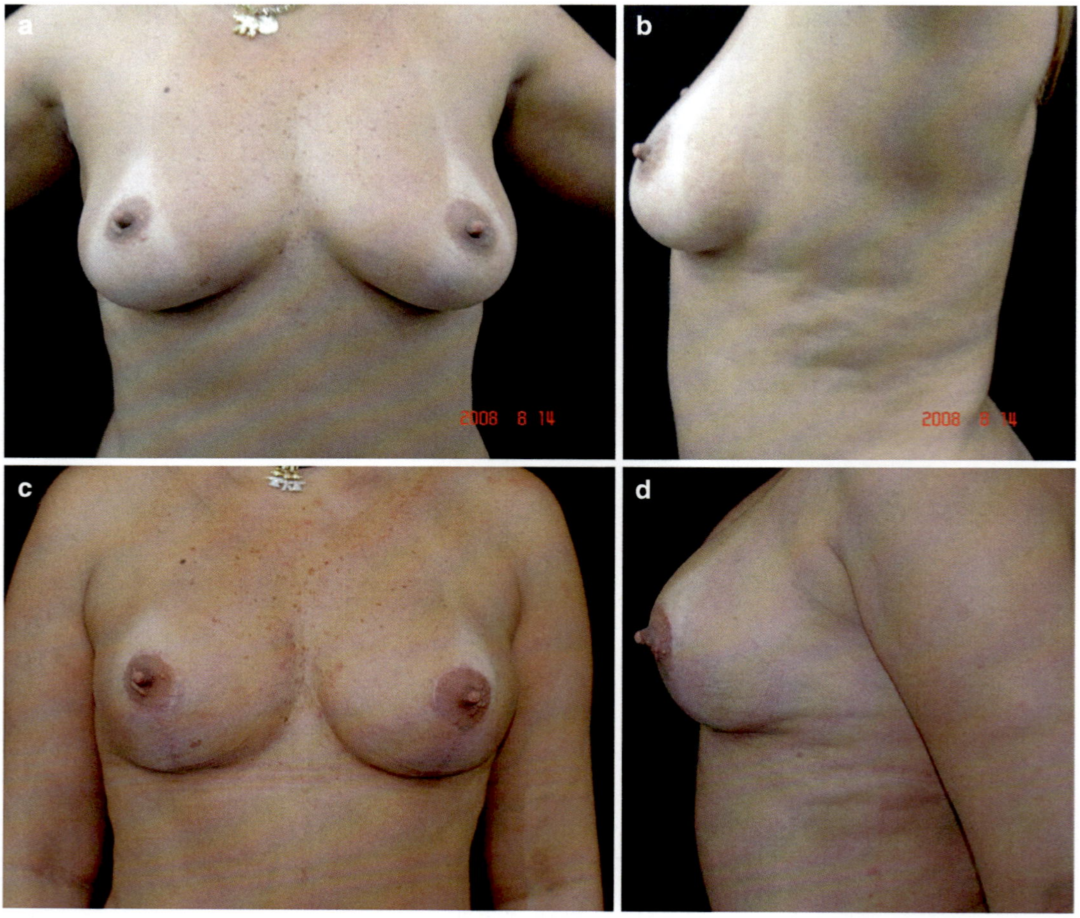

Fig. 56.20 Final Results. (**a**, **c**) Preoperative photos (**b**, **d**) postoperative photos results

Acknowledgments This work is the result of the teachings and publications that have been granted by Ivo Pitanguy and Ramil Sinder, teachers who taught us how to solve the issues of breast dysmorphia, showing that behind every case, there is a woman with distress, anxiety, and a perspective on the final results. Finally, we should point out that the patient's expectations may not always can be fulfilled by the professional as they wish. To the teachers Ivo Pitanguy and Ramil Sinder, our eternal gratitude.

References

Arié G (1957) Nova técnica em mamaplastia. Ver LatAmer Cir Plást 3:28

Ashley DL (1970) A new type of breast prosthesis preliminary report. Plast Rec. Surg. 45:421

Aufricht G (1949) Mamaplasty for pendulous breast. Empiric and geometry planning. Plast Rec Surg 4:13

Barnes HO (1950) Breast malformations and a new approach to the problem of the small breast. Plast Rcconstr Surg 5:499–506

Biesenberger H. (1931) Deformitäten und kosmetische Operationen der weiblichen Brust. Ed. W. Maudrich. Wein

Bozzona AR, Oliveira HC, Sanchez WH, Miura O, DDandréia S (1982) Momoplastia em L contribuição pessoal R. Amrggs, Porto Alegre 26(3), 207

De Castro CC (1983) De castro redução mamária pela técnica do retalho dermoadiposo de pediculo inferior. Rev Bras De Cir 73:47

Dufourmentel L (1925) La mastopexie par déplacement sous-cutané avec transposition du mamelon. Bull Mem Soc Chir Paris, 20 Mars 1925

Franco T (1976) Incisão EM fechadura no tratamento cirurgico das pequenas ptoses mamárias. Rev Bras De Cir 66(1/2):43

Franco T (1980) Axial flap from the inferior pole of the breast. Ann Plast Surg 5(4):260–265

Gillies M, McIndoe AH (1939) The technique of mammaplasty in conditions of hypertrophy of the breast. Surg Gynecol Obstet 68:658

Goulian D Jr (1971) Dermal mastopexy. Plast Reconstr Surg 47(2):105

Lima JC (1979) Breast reduction: new methods and refinements. Trans Intern SAO Paulo Congress of Plastic. Rec. Cartgraf. Surg

Maliniac JW (1950) Breast deformities and their repair. Grune & Stratton, New York

Marino H (1964) Nuevos conceptos en el tratamiento quirurgico de la hipertrofia Y de la ptosis mammaria. Bol Soc Sirug B Aires 48:122

Marino HE, Uriburuj V (1957) La mama buenos aires editorial científico arg

Peixoto G (1980) Reduction mammaplasty: a personal techique. Plast Rec Surg 65:217

Peixoto G (1984) Reduction mammaplasty. Aesth Plast Surg 8:231–236

Pitanguy I (1961) Mamaplastias: estudo de 245 casos consecuticos e apresentação de tecnica pessoal. Rev Bras Cir 42:201

Penn J (1955) Breast reduction. Br J Plast Surg 7:357

Pitanguy I (1967) Surgical treatment of the breast hypertrophy. Plast Surg 20:78

Pitanguy I (1978) Mamaplastia Guanabatra Koogan Rio de Janeiro

Pontes R (1981) Reduction mammaplasty—variations I and II. Ann Plast Surg 6(6):437

Regnault P (1967) Indications for breast augmentations. Plast Rec Surg 40:524

Ribeiro L (1973) Mastoplastia moditicotion personal de Técnica prensa med. Argentina 60:944

Ribeiro L (1975) A new technique for reduction mammaplasty. Plast Rec Surg 55(3):330

Ribeiro L (1989) Cirurgia plastica da mama medsi, vol. 1, 2, 3, 6 E 8

Ribeiro L (2005) Pediculos em mamaplastia atlas E texto. medsi gaunabara koogan. Pag 19 Á 113

Ribeiro L, Baker E (1983) Technical consideration (Chapter 22). In: Georgiade NG (ed) Aesthetic breast surgery. William Wilkins, Baltimore, p 260

Schwarzmann E (1930) Die technik der mammaplastik. Chirurg 2(1930):932–943

Sinder R (1970) Tese apresentada á faculdade nac. De med. para concorrer á livre docência

Strombeck JO (1971) Reduction mammaplasty. Surg Clin Amer 51:453

Talita F, Rebello C (1977) Cirurgia Plastica Estética. R.J. Atheneu

Wise RJ, Gannon JP, Hill JR (1963) Further experience with reduction mammaplasty. Plast Reconstr Surg 32(1):12

57

Augmentation Mastoplasty with Silicone Implant Associated with Mastopexy via an Initial Periareolar Approach (*Safety Pocket*)

Ataliba Ronan Horta de Almeida,
André Villani Correa Mafra,
and Leandro Ramalho Chaves Isobe

57.1 Introduction

The correction of different degrees of breast ptosis includes resection of excess skin in addition to repositioning of the nipple–areola complex (NAC) at the apex of the breast cone.

The most widely adopted classification of breast ptosis was described by Regnault in 1976. This classification has three distinct degrees based on NAC height in relation to the inframammary fold. Two intermediate forms, namely, partial ptosis and pseudoptosis, were also described (Table 57.1).

A.R.H. de Almeida, M.D. (✉)
Sociedade Brasileira de Cirurgia Plástica (Brazilian Society of Plastic Surgery–SBCP), Plastic Surgery Training Center, Hospital Mater Dei (Mater Dei Hospital), Belo Horizonte, MG, Brazil

Plastic Surgery Medical Center, Hospital Mater Dei (Mater Dei Hospital), Belo Horizonte, MG, Brazil
e-mail: ronan838@gmail.com

A.V.C. Mafra • L.R.C. Isobe
SBCP, Plastic Surgery Medical Team, Hospital Mater Dei (Mater Dei Hospital),
Belo Horizonte, MG, Brazil

Sociedade Brasileira de Cirurgia Plástica (Brazilian Society of Plastic Surgery–SBCP), Plastic Surgery Training Center, Hospital Mater Dei (Mater Dei Hospital), Belo Horizonte, MG, Brazil

In Brazil, there is growing interest in the association of silicone prosthesis implant surgery with the correction of pre-existing breast ptosis because of the inability of augmentation mastoplasty to correct sagging skin and the patients' demand for a larger breast volume. Moreover, the use of surgical correction of ptosis simply repositions the pre-existing tissues and cannot restore the texture of a young breast.

Several authors have reported the presence of breast ptosis in patients who wish to undergo prosthesis implantation in combination with breast pexy techniques because augmentation mastoplasty for the correction of breast ptosis tends to increase the degree of ptosis.

Table 57.1 Regnault's classification of breast ptosis

Complete or true ptosis	Grade I	Areola at the height of the inframammary fold and above the breast
	Grade II	Areola below the inframammary fold and above the breast contour
	Grade III	Areola below the inframammary fold and the contour of the breast
Partial ptosis	Areola above the mammary fold and gland ptosis	
Pseudoptosis	Areola above the mammary fold; loose, hypoplastic skin (e.g., marked weight loss after pregnancy)	

J.M. Avelar (ed.), *Breast Surgery*, https://doi.org/10.1007/978-3-319-54115-0_57

This text proposes a surgical maneuver that provides greater safety for breast implants and lower visibility and palpation of the edges of breast implants in the lower pole of the breast. The prosthesis remains protected because of the breast tissue (glands and subcutaneous tissue) integrity within the lower pole of the breast, where only skin is removed.

57.2 Methods

Marking of the breast skin was performed with the patient in an orthostatic position. The points of the sternal notch and acromion were tagged, and the midpoint between these two points and the midclavicular line was set.

The median of the breast was drawn and Pitanguy's point A, the apex of the future NAC, was marked. The excess skin was marked so that it could be removed in the perioperative period after insertion of the mammary prosthesis. The patient was then positioned on the operating table in the supine position with the arms parallel and juxtaposed to the body.

Under sedation assisted by the anesthesiologist, strict asepsis with 4% chlorhexidine digluconate solution and 2% alcoholic chlorhexidine was performed, followed by placement of sterile surgical fields. These fields allow visualization of the shoulders and cervical region as reference anatomical elements determined by the breasts.

The breast boundaries and incision sites in the periareolar regions were marked with methylene blue. The areolae were marked with an areola cutter measuring 4.5 cm in diameter. The breast was infiltrated with saline solution comprising 0.9% sodium chloride combined with 1% lidocaine and epinephrine (1:500,000 IU).

A semicircular skin incision was made in the lower portion of the areola, and access to the mammary pocket was accomplished through the lower portion of this incision (Webster incision). Skin, subcutaneous tissue, and breast glandular tissue were incised in this sequence in a 90° inclination to reach the fascia of the pectoralis major muscle (Fig. 57.1).

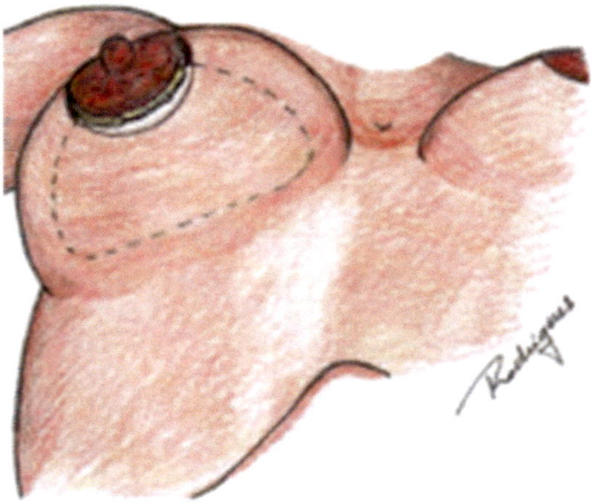

Fig. 57.1 Periareolar incision and inclusion of the prosthesis

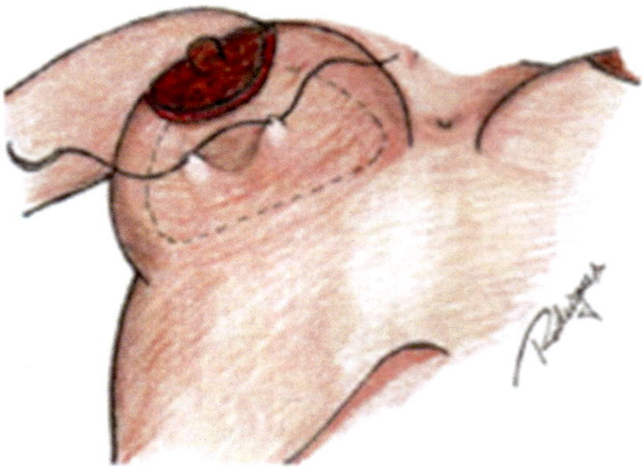

Fig. 57.2 Vertical suture of the skin to adjust for excess skin in the area between the areola and the inframammary fold

The retromammary pocket was constructed in the upper and lower poles of the breast. The breast implant was included after hemostasis and cavity review. There is no break in the vertical and horizontal incisions, thus characterizing the surgical maneuver as a "safety pocket." During pocket construction, emergence of the neurovascular pedicle in the fourth intercostal space was observed in the outer lower quadrant. This pedicle should not be damaged because it is responsible for innervation of the NAC. Suturing was performed using poliglecaprone 3–0 in the anatomical planes.

A vertical suture of the skin was completed to adjust the excess skin in the area between the nipple

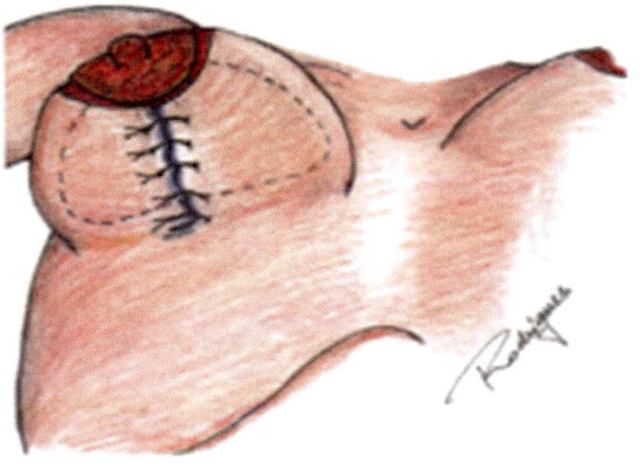

Fig. 57.3 Marking with methylene blue after the vertical skin suture

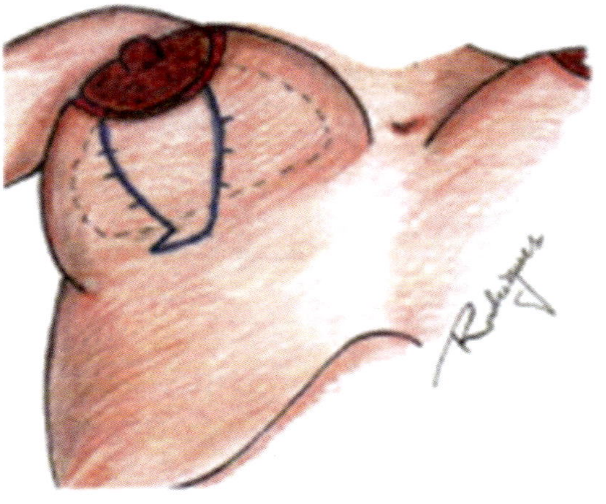

Fig. 57.4 Skin marking with methylene blue after suture removal

and the inframammary fold using a 3–0 nylon monofilament suture (Fig. 57.2). After the necessary tension was checked, the stitches were removed and methylene blue was used to mark the excess skin to be removed (Figs. 57.3 and 57.4). Thus, the excess skin observed after inclusion of the breast implant can be safely removed (Fig. 57.5). Whenever possible, longitudinal markings were preferred. We also used "L" or "T" markings when there were greater amounts of excess skin.

The neoareola was marked to maintain a distance of 4.5–6.5 cm between the lower portion of the NAC and the inframammary fold. The areola cutter was used to correct possible sagging periareolar skin. The NAC was repositioned with simple poliglecaprone 5–0 sutures in the

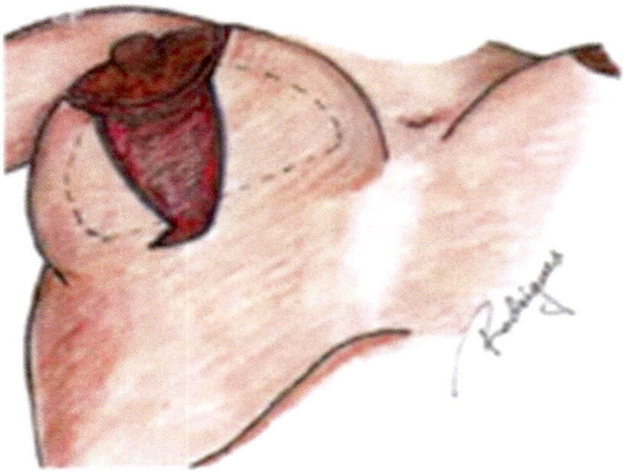

Fig. 57.5 Surgical appearance after skin decortication

subdermal plane and 4–0 polypropylene sutures in the intradermal plane.

57.3 Discussion

Augmentation mastoplasty associated with mastopexy, which has always been a controversial issue, has been discussed by several authors since its initial description in 1960 by Gonzalez-Ulloa.

In 2003, Carramashi and Tanaka found that the combination of pexy and prosthesis provided adequate volume and shape for the treatment of the sequelae of reductive mastoplasty.

In 2008, Sanchez et al. suggested the use of an inferior pedicle to protect breast implants. Soares et al. proposed the construction of a dual space consisting of an upper subglandular space and a lower submuscular space for placing the implant. In 2008, Gomes described a mastopexy technique with breast augmentation that used a superior pedicle flap surrounding the implant.

In 2009, Mansur and Bozola reported the use of an inferior breast pedicle to protect and support the breast implant and prevent it from sliding down the mammary fold and emptying the breast. Spear (2003) also observed alleviation in patient discomfort on palpation of the implants in the lower pole.

In 2003, Graf et al. described a new approach to breast augmentation in which the prosthesis was positioned in the subfascial plane. These authors observed lower visibility of the prosthesis with greater protection because the new structure was added among the skin, subcutaneous tissue, and the implant. In these operations, the anatomical planes of the inferior pedicle are sectioned; this may expose the prosthesis in the case of dehiscence.

Preservation of the tissue integrity of the lower pole was a relevant factor in this study because the only communication between the breast pocket and the skin lies in the lower periareolar region. The implants are protected from the external environment and are not supported by flaps or surgical incisions.

A decrease in palpation of the prosthesis and external evidence for its edges occurred because of the placement of the implants in the retrofascial plane only in the inferior pole of the breast. Preservation of the neurovascular pedicle of the fourth intercostal space maintains NAC sensitivity and vascularization. The choice not to use flaps to cover the lower breast implant was considered positive because it avoids glandular lesions that predispose the breast to infection and the prosthesis to extrusion or exposure.

In the patient who presented with aseptic steatonecrosis, protection of the prosthesis by the unexposed glandular tissues was crucial for a favorable prognosis. We believe that there was no dehiscence increase or implant compromise in this case because we preserved the tissues intact without breaking the skin in the lower breast pole.

57.4 Results

Figures 57.6 and 57.7 illustrate some of the cases in this series.

57.5 Complications

The principal complications observed in this group of patients: hematoma, scar retraction, ecchymosis, steatonecrosis, and dehiscence.

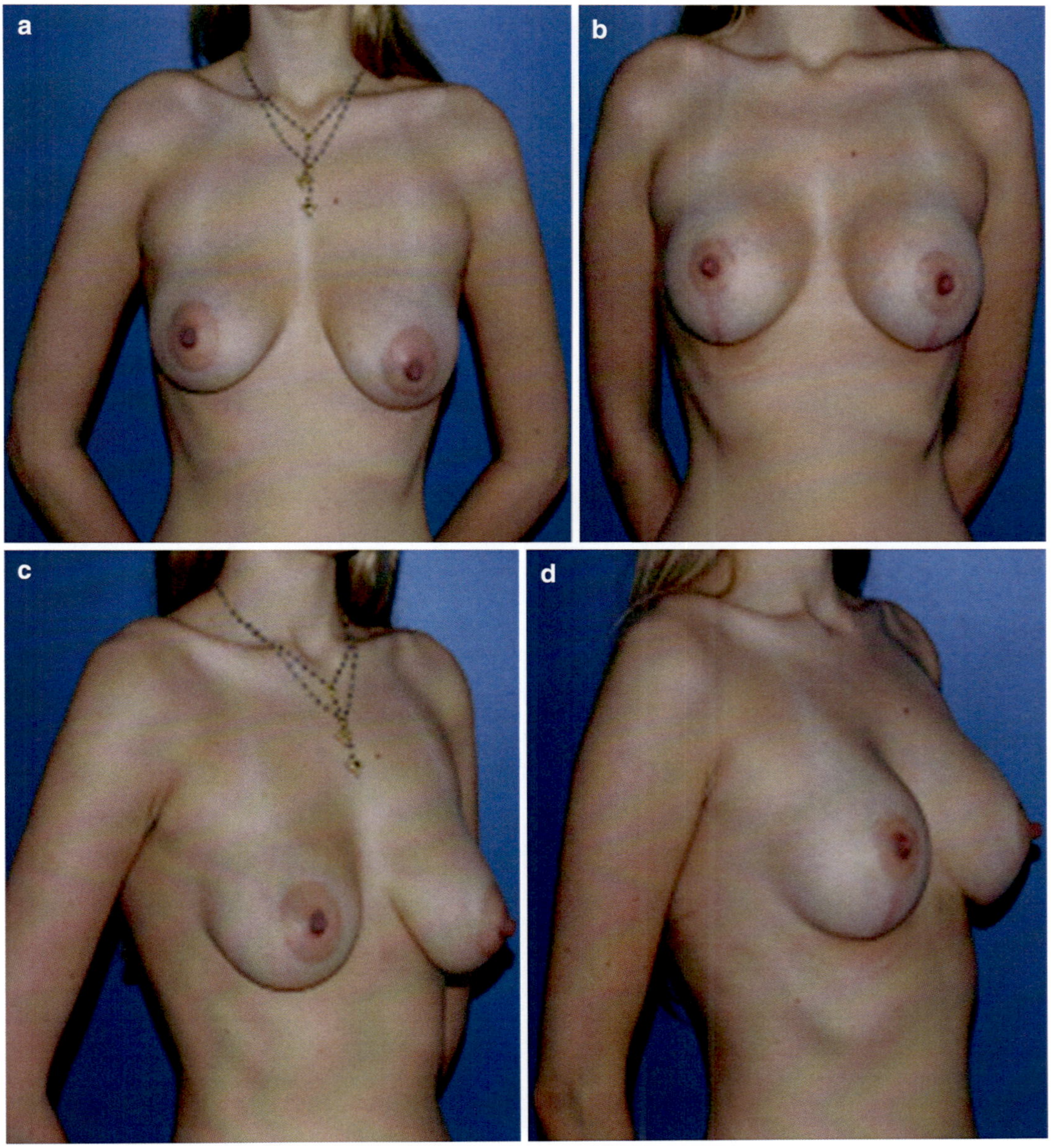

Fig. 57.6 Patient who underwent augmentation mastoplasty with the inclusion of silicone implants associated with the initial periareolar approach mastopexy. (**a**, **c**) Preoperative appearance. (**b**, **d**) Appearance 1 year postoperatively

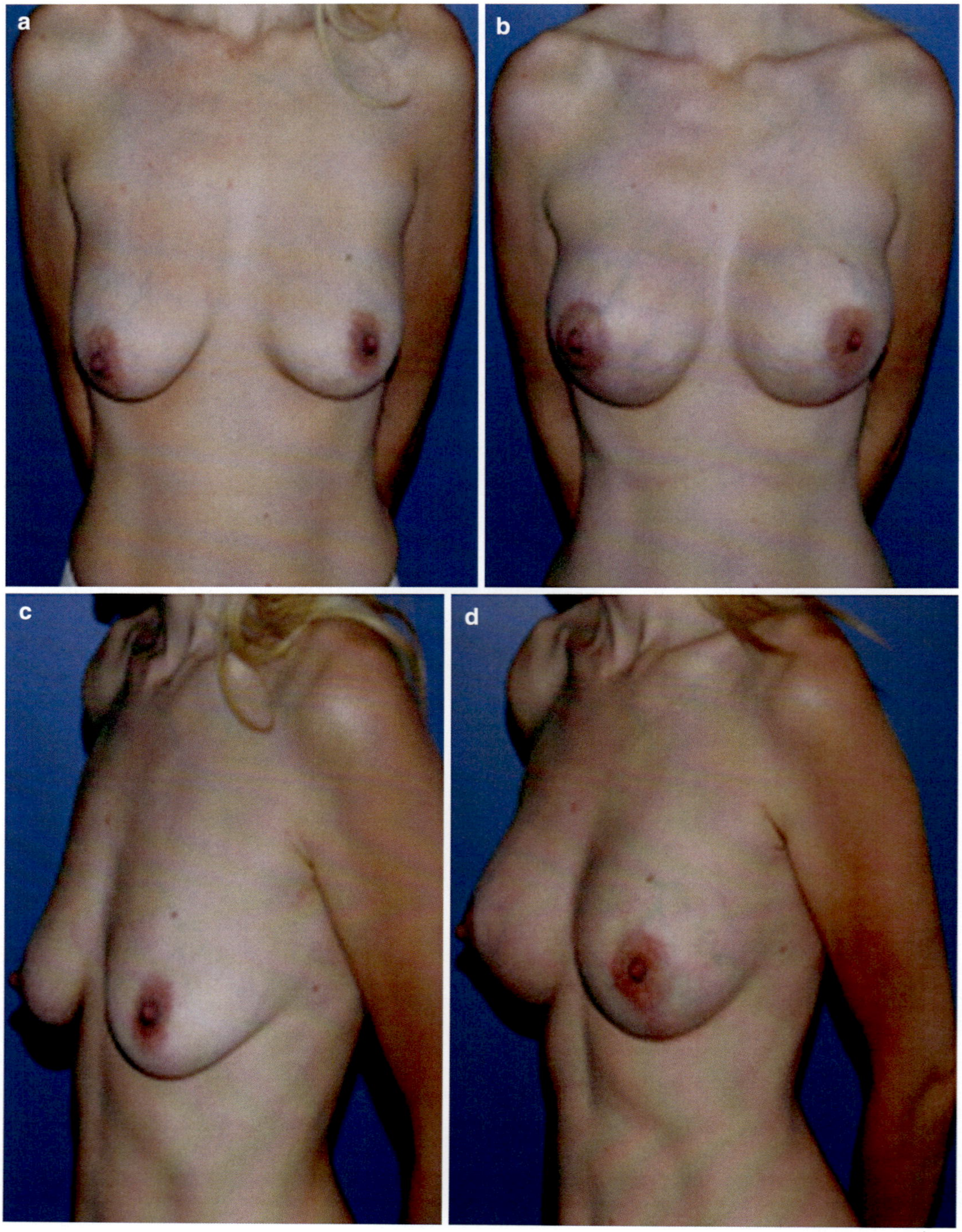

Fig. 57.7 Patient who underwent augmentation mastoplasty with the inclusion of silicone implants associated with the initial periareolar approach mastopexy. (**a**, **c**) Preoperative appearance. (**b**, **d**) Appearance 1 year postoperatively

Conclusions

The inclusion of silicone implants followed by mastopexy using the initial periareolar approach (safety pocket) is a good option in cases of augmentation mastoplasty associated with the correction of pre-existing ptosis.

The conservative skin removal approach after implantation of the prosthesis, the vertical periareolar access, and the use of a subfascial plane are the differential and relevant points that characterize this technique.

Suggested Reading

Carramaschi FR, Tanaka MP (2003) Mastopexia associada à inclusão de prótese mamária. Rev Soc Bras Cir Plást 18(1):25–36

Chem RC (1991) Plástica mamária estética de aumento com a utilização de próteses. Rev Soc Bras Cir Plást. 6(1/2):28–32

Gomes RS (2008) Mastopexia com retalho de pedículo superior e implante de silicone. Rev Bras Cir Plást 23(4):241–247

Gonzalez-Ulloa M (1960) Correction of hypotrophy of the breast by means of exogenous material 25(1):15–40

Graf RM, Bernardes A, Rippel R, Araujo LR, Damasio RC, Auersvald A (2003) Subfascial breast implant: a new procedure 111(2):904–908

Mansur JRB, Bozola AR (2009) Mastopexia e aumento das mamas com proteção e suporte inferior da prótese com retalho de pedículo inferior. Rev Bras Cir Plást 24(3):304–309

Pitanguy I, Carreirão S, Mazzarone F, Fróes LB, Cló TT (1991) Mastopexia associada à inclusão de prótese. Rev Soc Bras Cir Plást 81(2):101–111

Regnault P (1966) The hypoplastic and ptotic breast: a combined operation with prosthetic augmentation 37(1):31–37

Regnault P (1976) Breast ptosis. Definition and treatment. Clin Plast Surg 3(2):193–203

Sanchéz J, Carvalho AC, Erazo P (2008) Mastopexia com prótese: técnica em "D" espelhado. Rev Bras Cir Plást 23(3):200–206

Soares AB, Franco FF, Rosim ET, Renó BA, Hachmann JOPA, Guidi MC et al (2011) Mastopexia com uso de implantes associados a retalho de músculo peitoral maior: técnica utilizada na disciplina de cirurgia plástica da unicamp. Rev Bras Cir Plást 26(4):659–663

Spear S (2003) Augmentation/mastopexy: "surgeon, beware" 112(3):905–906

Spear SL, Pelletiere CV, Menon N (2004) One-stage augmentation combined with mastopexy: aesthetic results and patient satisfaction. Aesthetic Plast Surg 28(5):259–267

Mastopexy With and Without Prostheses

58

João Erfon, Claudio Mauricio M. Rodrigues, and Guilherme Teles

58.1 Introduction

Breast ptosis essentially results from the synergism of two factors: the involution of mammary parenchyma with decreased volume and looseness of the skin envelope, which reduces elasticity (Kim et al. 2010). Mastopexy, one of the most common procedures in plastic surgery, can correct this issue. Several approaches described in the literature use dermoglandular pedicles with the nipple-areola complex (NAC) (Bonomi et al. 2012).

This chapter describes an approach for mastopexy and mastopexy supplemented with the use of silicone implants, using a single central block of lipoglandular tissue and the NAC, which is separated from the skin flaps and includes the superior base vascular pedicle (Erfon et al. 1996). A new concept for modeling the breast parenchyma is presented that maintains its central part. Tissue is taken from external quadrants in cases of mastopexy. The lateral and medial flaps are sutured together to improve the central block, providing greater protection and support to the silicone implant. The incisions can be designed as an inverted T or vertical, according to the skin resection required in each case. The simplicity of marking and technical implementation, the favorable aesthetic results, and the preservation of the breast's functions are guaranteed to satisfy both surgeons and patients.

This approach aims to create a good breast shape with reduced scarring and less tension on the sutures by properly redistributing the lipoglandular tissue with surrounding skin (Lima 1979; McKissock 1972). Silicone implants are used, when properly indicated, to achieve the desired breast volume. The optimal arrangement of the skin flaps and breast cone promotes more satisfactory results. A reduction in the size of scars, which has been advocated by many authors (Arié 1957; Bozola et al. 1987; Franco and Rebello 1977; Peixoto 1980, 1984; Sepúlveda 1981; Souza Pinto 1983; Wise et al. 1963) is respected within reasonable limits, with possible accommodation and contraction of the skin. These results vary from one patient to another.

In the last 30 years, mastopexy has been carried out both alone and with silicone implants by the senior author under the principles that are

Work performed at ArtClinic.

J. Erfon (✉)
Department of Surgery, Walter Cantídio Hospital of the Federal University of Ceará, Rua Atilano de Moura, Fortaleza, CE 60810-180, Brazil
e-mail: erfon@artclinic.com.br

C.M.M. Rodrigues, M.D.
Unichristus University, Rua Atilano de Moura, Fortaleza, CE 60810-180, Brazil

G. Teles
Defeitos da Face Hospital and Santa Cruz Hospital, Rua Atilano de Moura, Fortaleza, CE 60810-180, Brazil

J.M. Avelar (ed.), *Breast Surgery*, https://doi.org/10.1007/978-3-319-54115-0_58

described in this chapter. Five principles are observed: (a) modeling the breast parenchyma in a single central block, separate from the skin flaps, without disconnecting the NAC and including a silicone implant when necessary; (b) using the superior vascular pedicle, as described by Weiner (1973) and modified by the senior author (Erfon et al. 1992); (c) reducing scars by retraction of the skin, the markings with incisions of the same size, and the mounting of the parenchyma separated from the skin (Erfon et al. 1996; McKissock 1972); (d) using lipoglandular tissue from the external quadrants, which is folded medially to increase the single central block; and (e) creating medial and lateral skin flaps that contain lipoglandular tissue, which are superimposed onto the central block of tissue to provide greater protection and support for silicone implants, when used.

58.2 Method

This retrospective study included female patients who underwent mastopexy with and without silicone implants using a single central block technique from July 1985 to December 2015. The patients were classified into two groups: (a) patients with breast ptosis and sufficient lipoglandular tissue to fill the volume of the new breast and (b) patients with breast ptosis associated with atrophy, requiring silicone implants to obtain adequate volume in the new breast. These two procedures were adapted for all operations performed by the senior author.

The following basic principles were observed: (1) modeling the breast parenchyma in a single central block, separate from the skin flaps, without disconnecting the NAC; (2) using the superior vascular pedicle flap, as described by Weiner (1973) and modified by the senior author (Erfon et al. 1992, 1996); (3) reducing scars by retraction of the skin, the markings with incisions of the same size, and the mounting of the parenchyma separated from the skin flaps; (4) using lipoglandular tissue from the external quadrants, which is folded medially to increase the single central block; and (5) dissecting and superimposing two lipoglandular, medial, and lateral flaps onto the single central block in cases of mastopexy with silicone implants (Fig. 58.2d, e).

58.3 Technique

Marking begins with the patient in an upright position, after frontal, semi-profile (oblique), and profile photos have been taken. A dotted line is drawn from the sternal notch to the xiphoid (mean anterior body line), which will be used to check the symmetry between the breasts (Figs. 58.1a and 58.2a–c). The inframammary fold and point A are marked. Point A is marked 2 cm above the projection of the inframammary fold (Fig. 58.1a). Starting from point A, with the patient on the operating table, points B and C are drawn; they are always around the NAC and can be within 5–9 cm from point A, forming a triangle (Fig. 58.1b). This marking defines the vascular superior pedicle of the flap. A semicircular line connecting points A, B, and C is marked, improving the width of the vascular pedicle (Fig. 58.2c). When the NAC is very lateralized, the distance between A and C may be greater than the distance between A and B, allowing greater medial rotation of the same (Fig. 58.2c, g, h).

Starting from points B and C downward, two straight 5-cm segments are marked; the angle between them varies based on the amount of skin to be resected (Fig. 58.1b). The marking is concluded by joining the distal ends of these two segments to the submammary fold (Fig. 58.1c, d). The symmetry of the marking in the contralateral breast is made using the above midline of the body, keeping equal distances between them and drawing a medial incision in each breast. According to the distance between the end of these two segments and the submammary fold, the marking can be concluded in inverted T or V incisions (Fig. 58.1c, d).

Sedation plus local anesthesia is routinely used. The retromammary area and the perimeter of the breast are infiltrated with a solution of epinephrine (1:1000) with saline (1:160 mL) plus 40 mL of 2% xylocaine.

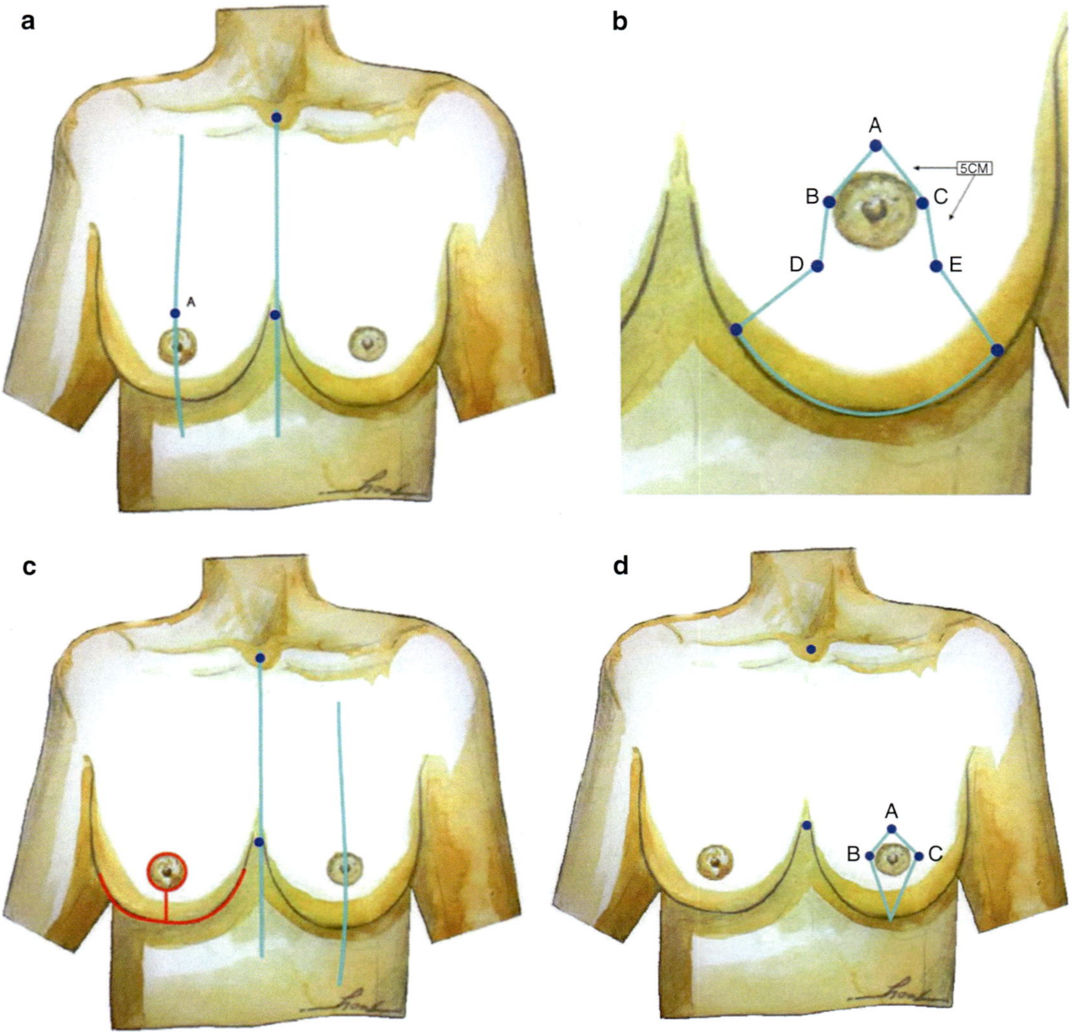

Fig. 58.1 Planning and marking the incisions. (**a**) Marking the breasts while standing, starting with the average previous line of the body and points A, B, and C. (**b**). Marking the other incisions (see text). (**c**) Marking an inverted T. (**d**) Marking V for periareolar and vertical scars

The surgery begins with the de-epithelization of the area around the NAC, extending 2 cm below it. Then, a total skin excision is carried out in the previously marked area in the lower pole of the breast (Fig. 58.2d). In cases of mastopexy without implants, the medial and lateral skin flaps are dissected to be approximately 2 cm thick, extending to 1 or 2 cm above points B and C, then continuing to the muscle fascia (Fig. 58.2d). Dissection of the retromammary space is performed by completely freeing the breast from the thoracic plate, resulting in a single central block comprising the breast parenchyma and the NAC that is maintained by the superior vascular pedicle.

The external quadrants are folded medially and sutured to the medial quadrants with 3-0 colorless mononylon stitches, forming a single central block that maintains the NAC on ttop. This block is pulled to the chest using two 3-0 colorless mononylon stitches: one stitch is in the posterior projection of the NAC, in its new position; the other stitch is at the distal end of the flap, fixing it to the center of the submammary fold.

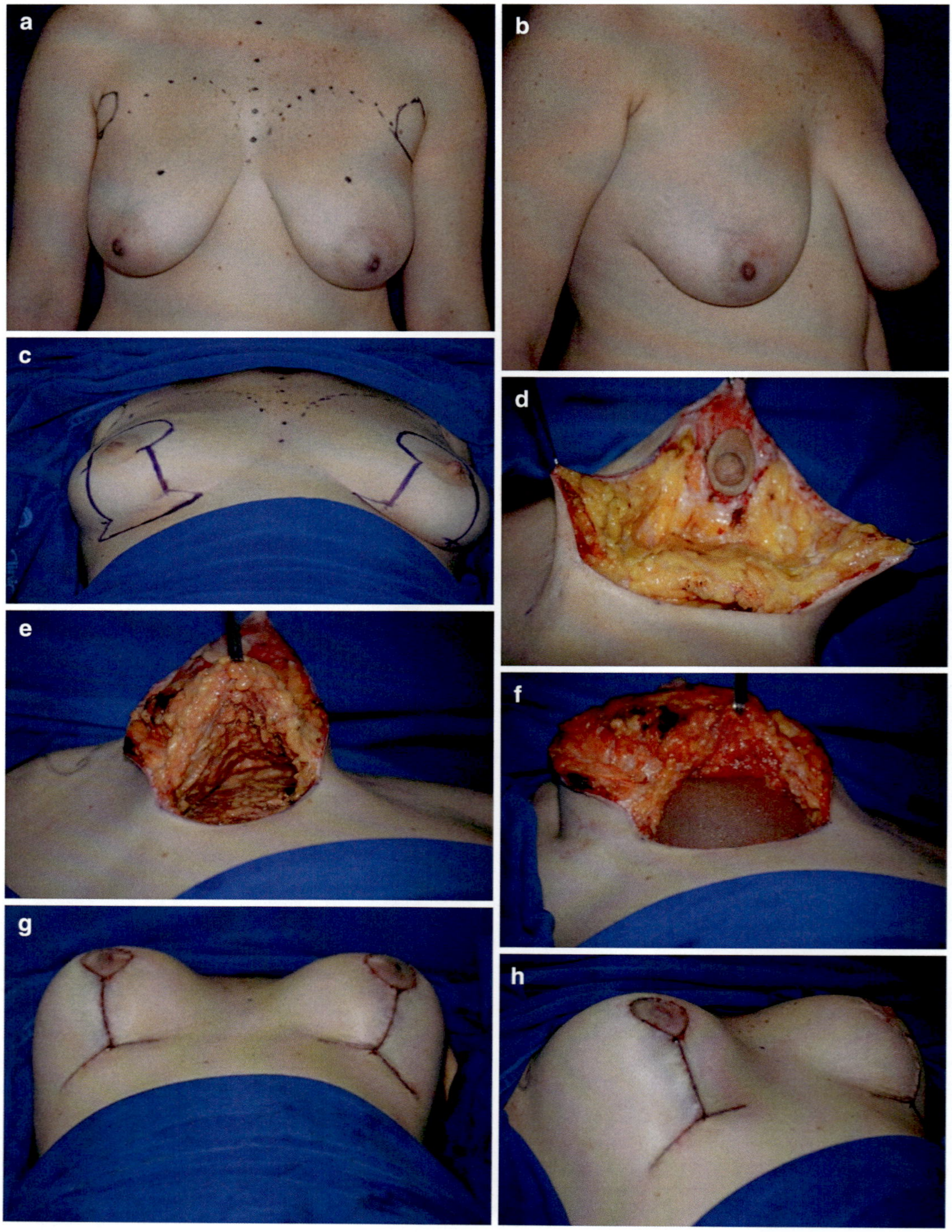

Fig. 58.2 Preoperative, intraoperative, and immediate postoperative mastopexy combined with silicone implants. (**a–c**) Preoperative breast ptosis and planning of mastopexy with silicone implants. (**d–f**) Intraoperative dissection of the breast for a breast lift with implants (see text) and placement of the prostheses. (**g**, **h**) Early postoperative results

Skin suturing begins with 3-0 colorless mononylon stitches, uniting the medial and lateral skin flaps from the inframammary fold to points B and C, which will form the vertical scar. At this time, the symmetry of the breasts is checked and adjustments are made if necessary. The NAC is positioned in its entirety (Fig. 58.2g, h). The suture is concluded with 4-0 colorless mononylon stitches in the skin flaps and 5-0 clear sutures in the NAC. All stitches are internal.

In cases of breast ptosis with hypotrophy, silicone implants are used to add volume to the breast. In such cases, a modified technique reduces the dissection of the skin flap to 3 or 4 cm medially and laterally, allowing it to slide on the single central block of breast tissue; sutures without tension (Fig. 58.2d, g, h) provide the central block of tissue with greater protection and support the implant (Fig. 58.2f). The retroglandular space is dissected in proportion to the prosthesis for each case (Fig. 58.2e).

The bandage is simple: dry gauze and a special bra that should be worn for 2 months.

58.4 Results

We performed 474 mastopexies using this technique from July 1985 to December 2015: 132 (27.85%) simple mastopexies and 342 (72.15%) mastopexies with silicone implants. The female patients ranged in age from 17 years to 75 years. The incidence of mastopexy with silicone implants has greatly increased, especially over the last 15 years.

The results of this technique have been better than those obtained with other techniques used previously by the senior author (Peixoto 1980; Pitanguy 1976; Strombeck 1960). We found the following advantages: (a) ease of shaping the breast into a cone, as if it were a simple placement of implants; (b) ease of lifting the NAC; (c) good maintenance of NAC vascularization and the skin flaps; (d) preservation of sensitivity; (e) preservation of the primary function of the breasts (i.e., the possibility of breastfeeding); (f) good-quality scars from the reduction of tension on the skin flaps and natural elevation of the NAC, which is pushed into its new position by the breast tissue of the central block. When the central block of tissue is not enough to form a new breast mound, a silicone implant is used (Fig. 58.2d-h).

Patients are free to return to activities within a week. Driving and exercise can be resumed with 1 month.

58.5 Discussion

We believe that this technique is easy to plan and execute, even for young surgeons. It allows for a final result that is within the preoperative expectations. Even with a well-defined plan, the position of the NAC (in addition to the other incisions) can be easily changed during the procedure, if the surgeon so desires, due to the versatility of the marking. Maintaining a single central block that includes the mammary parenchyma and NAC facilitates the modeling of the new breast and the elevation of the NAC, which is naturally pushed into its new position without the need for traction (as in other techniques). However, it is necessary to leave enough tissue volume below the NAC, as the skin flaps are thin (about 2 cm thick) and are not part of the new breast volume. If adequate volume is obtained, the NAC will be on top of the single central block without tension (Fig. 58.2g, h). The single central block of tissue also facilitates symmetry between the breasts because it is very easy to identify specific differences in these flaps. As the elevation necessary for the NAC increases, the parenchymal flap should become longer, narrower, and thicker.

The vascularization and sensitivity of the NAC are preserved and can be identified by simple sensitivity tests using touch. No severe ischemia to the areola was noted in our cases. Furthermore, the lactiferous ducts are preserved in addition to the muscles of the NAC; along with the preservation of vascularization and sensitivity, this helps to maintain the primary functions of breastfeeding and sensitivity, which are both important for reproductive-age women.

After it is fixed to the chest in its new position, the single central block of parenchymal tissue (with the NAC on top) maintains a firm and well-shaped breast that does not depend on the skin flaps to shape it. The skin flaps are sutured without tension, which leads to good-quality scar tissue.

Working with a single central block of tissue, it is easy to check for symmetry and set the volume when the first three sutures are completed. It is extremely easy to check which quadrant needs correction.

The preoperative evaluation of the patient should take into account the degree of ptosis, the quality of the supporting tissue (skin elasticity and thickness of the subcutaneous layer), and the breast tissue volume (Erfon et al. 1996; Parsa et al. 2010). This analysis allows the best approach to be determined, with or without the use of implants.

When there is a need to use implants, the subglandular pocket has demonstrated effective and lasting results. The detachment in the double plane, as described by Tebbetts (2001), can be reserved for exceptional cases.

When planning the new NAC positioning and cutaneous resections, the surgeon should ensure that the width of the breast base, breast height, and relationship between the submammary fold and areola are taken into account (Tebbetts 2013). This approach allows for a tension-free skin envelope without compromising the breast projection.

Creating a single centralized block allows greater projection of the breasts with upper pole filling, which maintains itself in the long term. As noted by Swanson (2011), such results have been limited when using other techniques.

Mastopexy can be a challenging procedure for the plastic surgeon. It is necessary to obtain a three-dimensionally harmonious result with contralateral symmetry while dealing with several other factors, such as breast enlargement, skin elasticity, liposubstitution, atrophy, and implants. Gonzalez-Ulloa first described mastopexy associated with implants in 1960 and established some important principles, including inserting the implant without being aggressive to the skin, protecting the tissue, and making the space for the implant large enough so that the region can be closed without tension (Gonzalez-Ulloa 1960).

Spear et al. (2003) observed that the main reasons for surgical revisions are capsular contracture and the recurrence of ptosis (Spear et al. 2003). In the senior author's experience, secondary ptosis is more common than capsular contracture, especially in patients who have undergone previous bariatric surgery. Spear et al. (2003) described mastopexy with implants as being more complex than either one of the procedures performed individually, with an increased risk of revision in the future. However, Stevens et al. (2007) reported that the complication rates for mastopexy with implants were comparable with those for mastopexy or breast lift performed separately (Stevens et al. 2007). Although proceeding in two stages provides more predictable results, many patients choose to undergo breast augmentation with mastopexy in one procedure because of the inconvenience of undergoing additional surgery and anesthesia (Stevens et al. 2014).

Khavanin et al. (2014) conducted a meta-analysis with 4856 cases of mastopexy with implants and showed a total complication rate of 13.12%, with the most common complications being the recurrence of ptosis (5.2%) and areola asymmetry (2.94%). The reoperation rates with this approach were lower than those observed for other techniques (Khavanin et al. 2014). Therefore, a discussion of the possibility of a future reintervention should be part of the preoperative consultation.

Kelemen et al. (2013) stated that the success of mastopexy is related to the distribution of the breast parenchyma, particularly with the completion of the upper pole of the breast, rather than to the amount of skin removed (Kelemen et al. 2013). Using a single central block of lipoglandular tissue has been very helpful in completing and maintaining the upper pole with long-lasting results.

58.6 Complications

The most common complication in cases of simple mastopexy was steatonecrosis at the distal end of the lipoglandular flap in 22 (4.64%) patients. In 2 (0.42%) of these cases, there was spontaneous drainage of fat without infection, which resolved with conservative treatment and required revision surgery after 6 months. There were no cases of NAC necrosis. Bruising occurred in 2 (0.42%) patients and seroma in 4 (0.84%) patients. Dehiscence in the inverted T was not very frequent because there is not as much skin tension as in techniques that shape the breasts using strong tension on the skin flaps; this complication occurred in 28 (5.90%) cases. Reoperations were performed in 19 (4.00%) patients for skin or implant placement adjustment after 6 months. In most cases, the reoperation was performed through the vertical scars of the breasts.

Conclusion

The mastopexy technique using a single central block and mastopexy with silicone implants, as described in this chapter, resulted in improved aesthetic and functional outcomes compared with other techniques used before by the senior author. The complications associated with mastopexies were reduced substantially with this technique.

Both patients and surgeons reported satisfaction with this technique, which is important. With this technique, it is easy to obtain similar results whether or not silicone implants are used (Figs. 58.3 and 58.4).

In summary, the advantages of this technique are as follows: (a) maintenance of function; (b) maintenance of good vascularization of the NAC and skin flaps; (c) preservation of sensitivity; (d) good-quality scars; (e) ease in obtaining a conical shape by working with a single central block of tissue; (f) ease of NAC elevation; and (g) greater protection of the

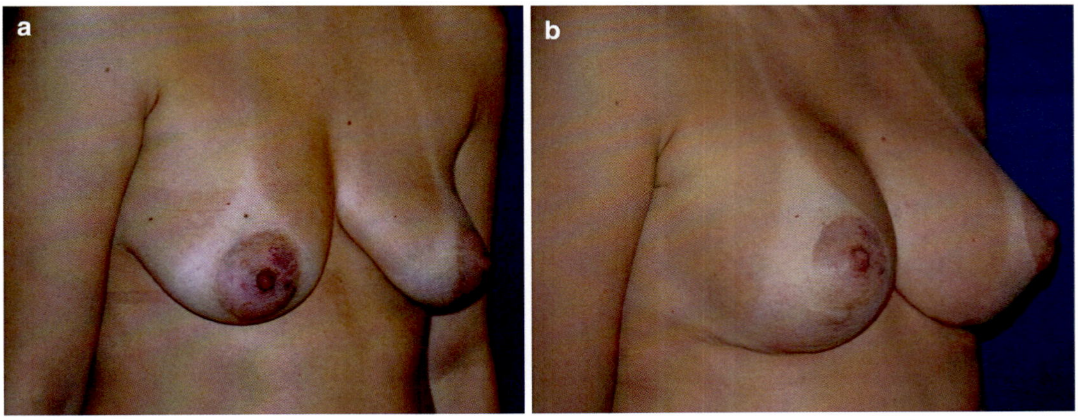

Fig. 58.3 Preoperative and late postoperative mastopexy with silicone implants. (**a**) Preoperative atrophy and breast ptosis. (**b**) Six months postoperative

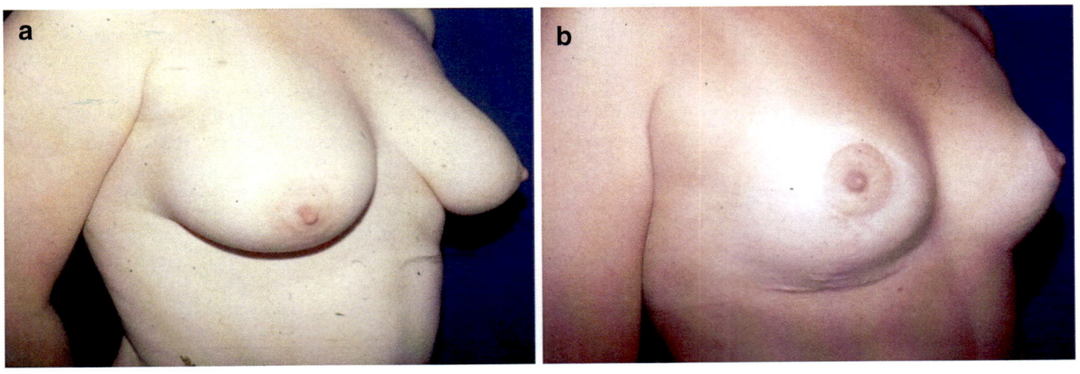

Fig. 58.4 Preoperative and late postoperative mastopexy. (**a**) Preoperative breast ptosis. (**b**) Mastopexy without silicone implants at 6 months postoperative

silicone implant by increasing the thickness of the central block of lipoglandular breast tissue. These advantages have encouraged the use of and indications for this technique, which is easy to learn and perform and has few complications.

References

Arié G (1957) Una nueva técnica de mastoplastica. Ver Lat Americana Cir Plástica III 23:8

Bonomi S, Salval A, Settembrini F, Gregorelli C, Musumarra G, Rapisarda V (2012) Inferiorly based parenchymal flap mammaplasty: a safe, reliable, and versatile technique for breast reduction and mastopexy. Plast Reconstr Surg 130(1):116e–125e

Bozola AR et al (1987) Sistematização de mamaplastia em "L". Rev Bras Cir Plást 2(1):13–33

Erfon J, Barbosa V, Brasil Jr A (1992) Reduction mammaplasty in a single block. In Hinderer UT (ed) Plastic surgery, vol 2. Madrid, p 629–634

Erfon J, Hochberg J, Ardenghy M, et al. (1996) Central block reduction mammaplasty and mastopexy. In: Proceedings of the 65th Annual Scientific Meeting of the American Society of Plastic and Reconstructive Surgeons, vol 14. Dallas, p 176–178

Franco T, Rebello C (1977) Cirurgia Estética, 1ª Edição edn. Liv. Atheneu, Rio de Janeiro, p 211

Gonzalez-Ulloa M (1960) Correction of hypotrophy of the breast by means of exogenous material. Plast Reconstr Surg 25(1):15–40

Kelemen N, Kannan RY, Offer GJ (2013) A stacked technique of mastopexy: volume redistribution mastopexy with inferior flap and superomedially based pedicle. Aesthet Plast Surg 37:349–353

Khavanin N, Jordan SW, Rambachan A, Kim JYS (2014) A systematic review of single-stage augmentation-mastopexy. Plast Reconstr Surg 134(5):922–931

Kim P, Kim KK, Casas LA (2010) Superior pedicle autoaugmentation mastopexy: a review of 34 consecutive patients. Aesthet Surg J 30(2):201–210

Lima JC (1979) Breast reduction: new method and refinements. In: Ely JF (ed) Transaction of the seventh international congress of plastic reconstructive surgery. Cartigraf, Rio de Janeiro, p 508

McKissock PK (1972) Reduction mammaplasty with a vertical dermal flap. Plast Reconstr Surg 49(3):245–252

Parsa AA, Jackowe DJ, Parsa FD (2010) A new algorithim for breast mastopexy/aumengtation. Plast Reconstr Surg 125(2):75–77

Peixoto G (1980) Reduction mammaplasty: a personal technique. Plast Reconstr Surg 65(2):217–225

Peixoto G (1984) Reduction mammoplasty. Aesthet Plast Surg 8:231–236

Pitanguy I (1976) Personal preferences for reduction mammaplasty. In: Goldwyn R (ed) Plastic and reconstructive surgery of the breast. Little Brown, Boston, p 167

Sepúlveda A (1981) Tratamento das assimetrias mamárias. Ver Bras Cir 71:11–18

Souza Pinto EB et al (1983) Dermoadipose and adenoadipose flaps in mammaplasty. Aesthet Plast Surg 7(7):101–108

Spear SL, Low M, Ducic I (2003) Revision augmentation mastopexy: indications, operations, and outcomes. Ann Plast Surg 51(6):540–546

Stevens WG, Stoker DA, Freeman ME, Quardt SM, Hirsch EM (2007) Mastopexy revisited: a review of 150 consecutive cases for complication and revision rates. Aesthet Surg J 27(2):150–154. https://doi.org/10.1016/j.asj.2006.12.014

Stevens WG, Macias LH, Spring M, Stoker DA, Chacón CO, Eberlin SA (2014) One-stage augmentation mastopexy: a review of 1192 simultaneous breast augmentation and mastopexy procedures in 615 consecutive patients. Aesthet Surg J 34(5):723–732. https://doi.org/10.1177/1090820X14531434

Strombeck JD (1960) Mammaplasty: report of a new technique based on the two pedicle procedure. Br J Plast Surg 13:79–83

Swanson E (2011) A retrospective photometric study of 82 published reports of mastopexy and breast reduction. Plast Reconstr Surg 128(6):1282–1301

Tebbetts JB (2001) Dual plane breast augmentation: optimizing implant–soft-tissue relationships in a wide range of breast types. Plast Reconstr Surg 107:1255–1272

Tebbetts JB (2013) A process for quantifying aesthetic and functional breast surgery. I. Quantifying optimal nipple position and vertical and horizontal skin excess for mastopexy and breast reduction. Plast Reconstr Surg 132(1):65–73

Weiner PL, Aiache AE, Silver L, Ttitanonda TA (1973) Single dermal pedicle for nipple transposition in subcutaneous mastectomy, reduction mammaplasty or mastopexy. Plast Reconstr Surg;510(2):1115–1120.

Wise RJ, Gannon JP, Hill JR (1963) Further experience with reduction mammaplasty. Plast Reconstr Surg;32(1):12.

59 Breast Augmentation

Farid Hakme, Célio Coelho Neto Leão, Barbara de Castro Fonseca, Bruna Jacobowski, and Christiane Vigné Alvarez de Abreu

59.1 Introduction

Through the ages the breast has been the center of femininity, being an important element in the psychosocial balance of women. Because of the speed of the media and, consequently, globalization, the concept of beauty has become manipulable and uniform in South America, where traditionally small breasts have been considered to be the standard concept of beauty. This has changed with the influence of American and European fashion, and South American women now want larger breasts, which has become possible thanks to breast augmentation surgery. For some years this has been improving and making possible the dreams of thousands of women whose breast volume is smaller than their expectations.

To restore body harmony in patients with hypoplasia or an absence of breast tissue, constitutional or acquired deformities, inert materials such as paraffins, ivory, oils, body fat, autograft, sponges of different compositions, silicone fluid or gel, and in recent years textured or polyurethane material with a thicker consistency, have been sought.

F. Hakme (✉) • C.C.N. Leão, M.D.
B. de Castro Fonseca, M.D. • B. Jacobowski, M.D.
C.V.A. de Abreu, M.D.
Hospital of Plastics, Rio de Janeiro, RJ, Brazil
e-mail: faridhakme@uol.com.br

59.2 Types and Sizes

Currently, there is a trend toward using textured implants in our service, totaling almost 90% of cases.

We have found that the preference has been for increasing the volume of implants. Between 1979 and 1981, the most frequently used volume was 120 cc, from 1988 to 1998 this increased to 160 cc; in 1999, it was 175 cc; from 2005 to 2012, implants of 235 cc predominated, and in recent years they have reached a volume of 260 cc, the high profile implants that used in most cases.

59.3 Indications

Surgical indications were mammoplasty sequelae, unilateral and bilateral amastia, hypomastia and breast ptosis, and age range between 18 and 45 years.

59.3.1 Access

The various routes of access are shown in Table 59.1.

Table 59.1 Routes of access for breast augmentation

Transareolopapillary	0%
Axillary	5%
Pre-existing scars	5%
Tennis racket incision	20%
Periareolar	30%
Inframammary	40%

J.M. Avelar (ed.), *Breast Surgery*, https://doi.org/10.1007/978-3-319-54115-0_59

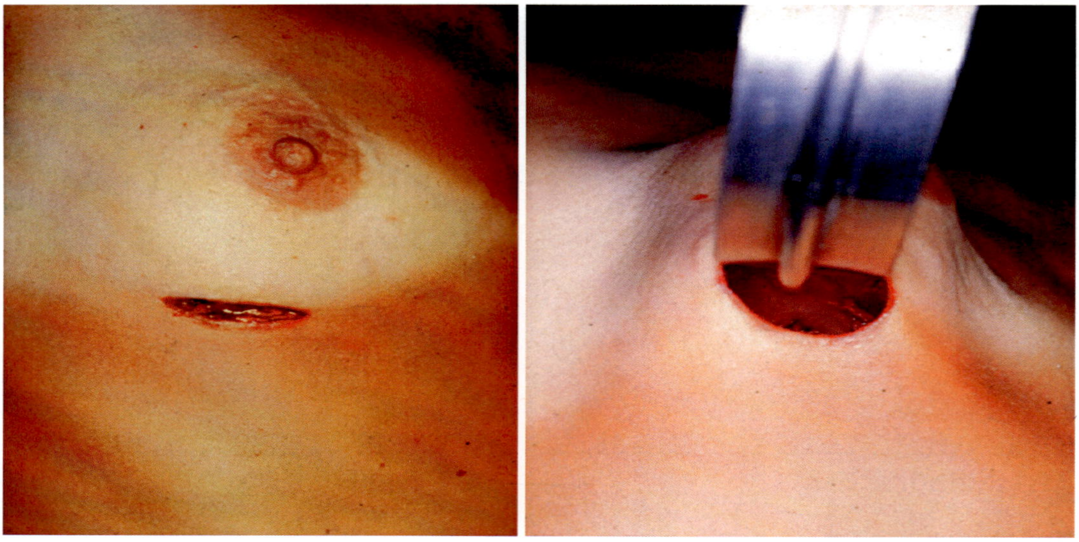

Fig. 59.1 Inframammary incision

- *Pre-existing mammary scars*: in patients who had already undergone breast reduction or insertion of previous implants, taking advantage of the existing incision in 5% of cases.
- *Axillary*: the axilla was used in those patients who did not want scars on the breast, complemented by endoscopy, which helped to dissection area "pocket" for implants placement could to be under direct vision, and enable adequate hemostasis of 4%.
- *Inframammary*: the incision was used in 40% of cases, when the patient had a very small nipple–areola complex (NAC), and the indication was for placement of a large volume implant (Fig. 59.1).
- *Transareolopapillary*: currently not used because of major trauma/damage to the milk ducts interfering with possible future breast-feeding. This route was only used in patients with an inverted nipple or nipple hypertrophy, when we attempted to reduce the nipple (Fig. 59.2).
- *Tennis racket incision*: in cases of breast ptosis, when there is need for excess skin removal, the preferred access route was the tennis racket incision in 20% of our cases (Fig. 59.3).

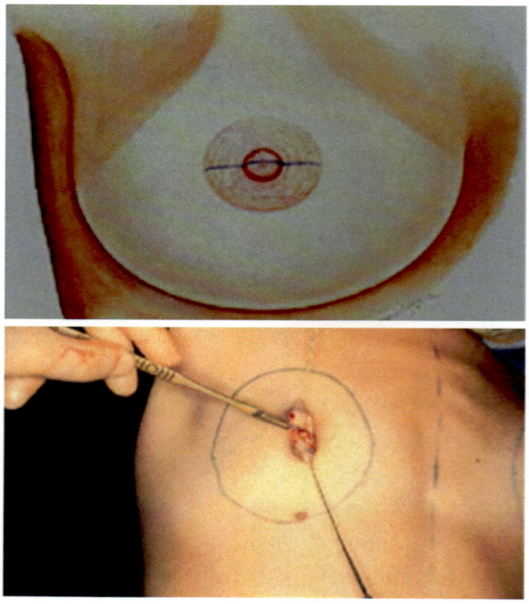

Fig. 59.2 Transareolopapillary incision

- *Periareolar* (lower half): used by 30% of our cases, in patients with a NAC of normal size (Fig. 59.4).

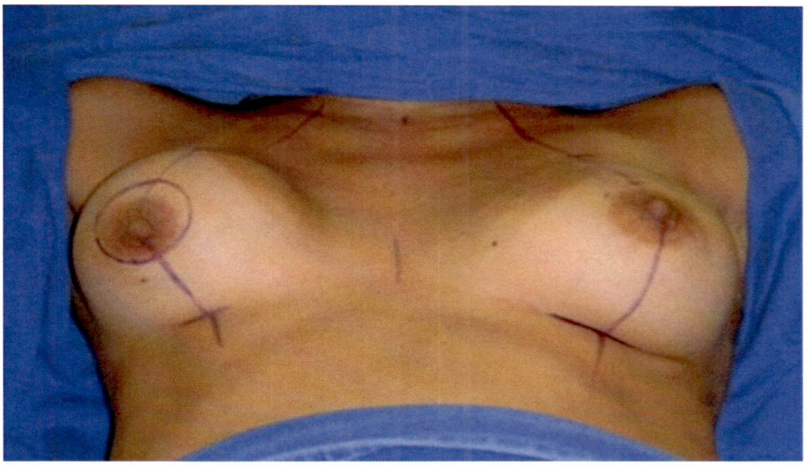

Fig. 59.3 Tennis racket incision

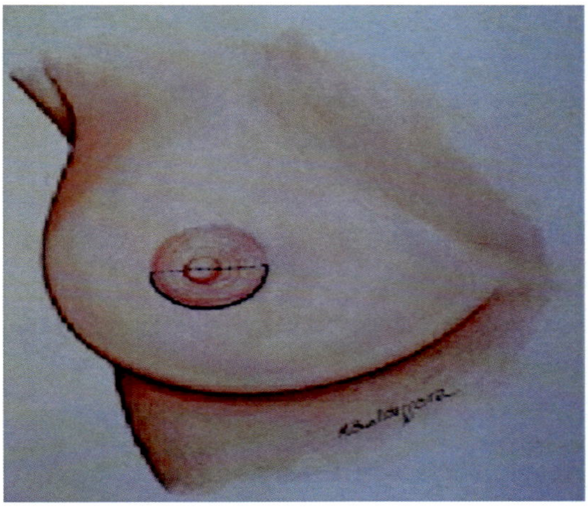

Fig. 59.4 Periareolar incision

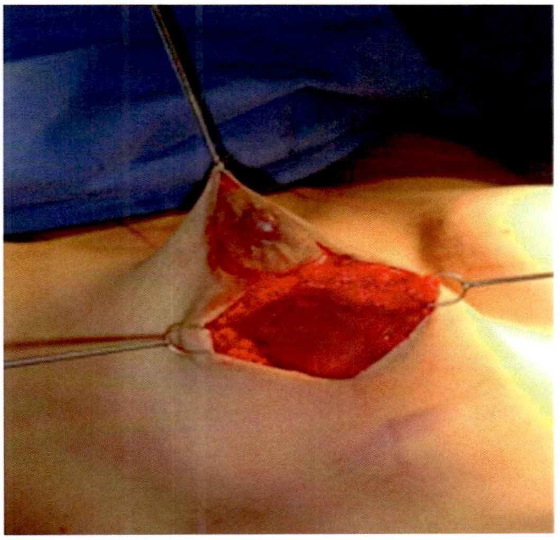

Fig. 59.5 Detachment

59.3.2 Store Creation

Large, conventional detachment was carried out in the ante-pectoral region below the muscle fascia with direct manipulation, exceeding 1 cm below the inframammary crease and symmetrically to the contralateral side, centering on the NAC. In the sternal region, detachment and partial incision of the pectoralis major were performed, leaving an adherent muscle layer of subcutaneous tissue and skin (Fig. 59.5).

59.3.3 Implant Placement and Templates

We position the implants inside the (pectoral muscle implant pocket) through direct manipulation, making sure that the edges of the implant do not become bent, which could cause its projection onto the skin. In the sternal region, the implant is placed below or on the hip muscle flap, and the flap is folded down to the subcutaneous tissue and skin over the implant, for protection (Fig. 59.6).

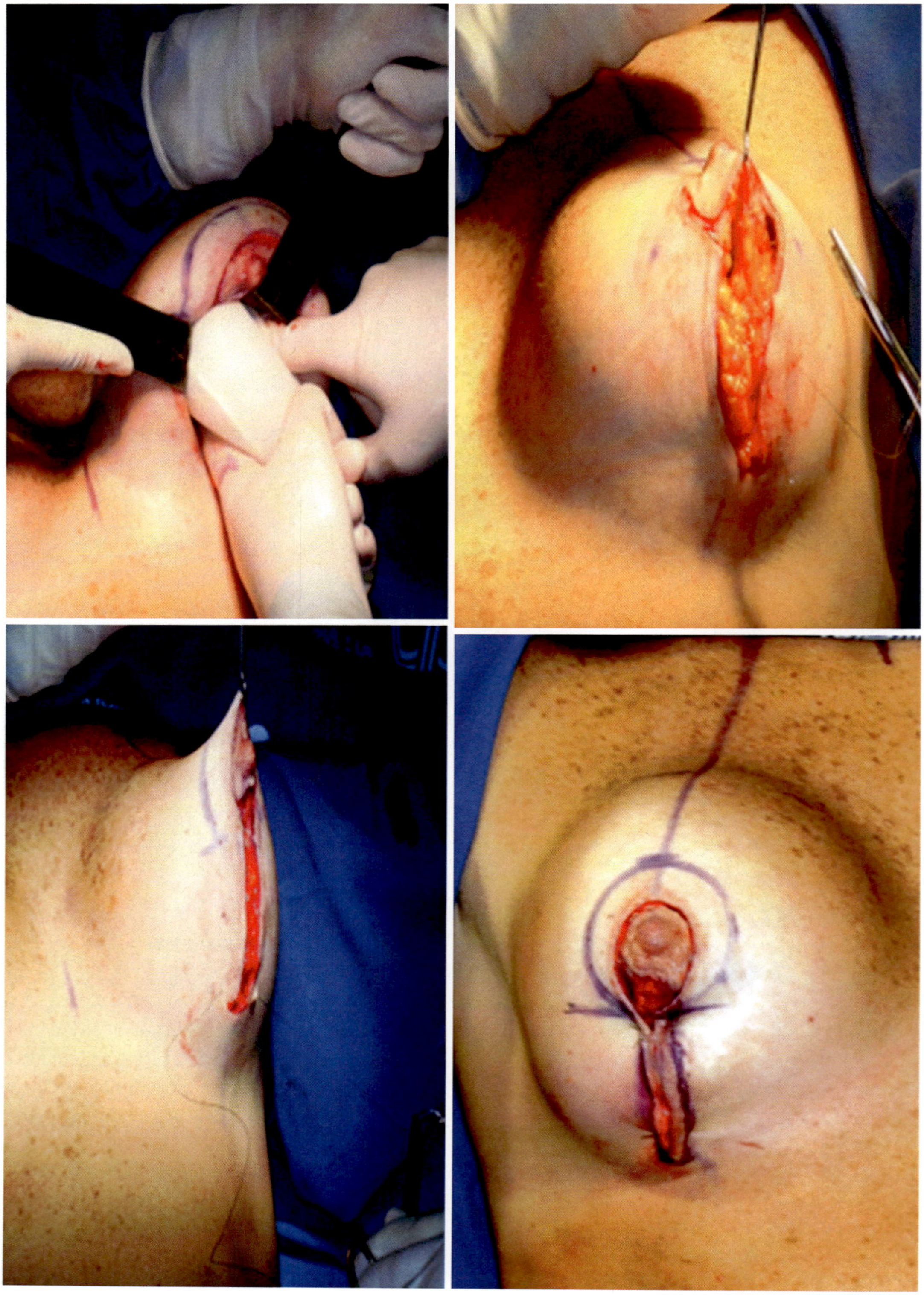

Fig. 59.6 Implant placement

The choice of route of placement varies among subglandular, submuscular or subfascial. The subglandular route stands out because of its lower morbidity and ease of implant placement. The submuscular route, despite the greater technical difficulty, has become more high profile in recent years, and is mainly indicated in very thin patients.

Implants placed in the submuscular plane, whether total or partial, also have some drawbacks. Although the plane achieves better coverage, the possibility of displacement of the upper implants or laterally, in addition to deformities in the lower pole described as the "double bubble signal. Tebbetts described a new possibility for plan the placement of the implant, which is called "dual plane." The implant must be located behind the breast parenchyma and the pectoralis major (in two planes simultaneously). The breast parenchyma is peeled from the pectoral muscle to a greater or lesser extent, depending on the type of breast, allowing a dynamic change between the implant and the gland. The pectoralis major is completely divided into specific portions of the insertion, thus changing the relationship with the breast implant and the breast parenchyma. This technique is aimed at bringing together the advantages of each type of plane that is possible for the implant, in addition, to reducing the limitations of each technique, its necessary to be molded for each type of treated breast.

The use of molds is not part of the routine in our service, based on the advisory of ANVISA (National Sanitary Surveillance Agency in Brazil) prohibiting sterilization of the mold in an autoclave. This fact is explained by the reporting of numerous cases in which molds were contaminated with the residual liquid of sterilization, resulting in an increased risk of infection, especially with mycobacteria.

59.3.4 Removal of Skin

Skin is removed in the shape of an ellipse in the lower pole of the breast, as indicated by an incision below the breast. In specific cases, periareolar skin can be removed.

In cases of breast ptosis, when we perform the tennis racket incision, we proceed to removal of excess skin after implant placement when we can make a proper assessment of the excess skin to be resected.

59.3.5 Synthesis

We closed the wound in the anatomical planes and we do not use drains (Fig. 59.7).

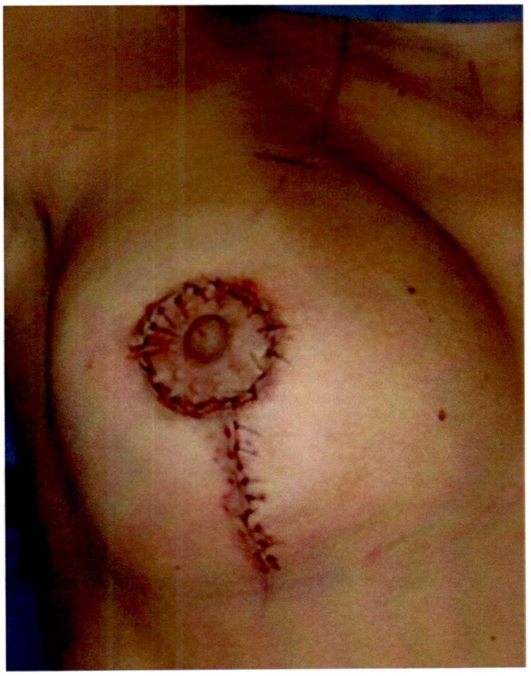

Fig. 59.7 Tennis racket incision

59.3.6 Complications

Infection and bruising are the main immediate complications of breast implants. When they occur, conservative treatment may be attempted by drainage in aseptic conditions and antibiotic therapy supported by culture and sensitivity. In the event of no regression of signs and symptoms after 7 days, the implant is removed.

In the case of infection, the implant should be removed and thorough washing of the cavity promoted, and the implant should not be replaced until after a period of 6 months, when the tissues have completely recovered.

In cases of hematoma, the implant is removed and the cavity washed, with the removal of clots and hemostasis reviewed. The implant can be reattached during surgery.

Changes in sensitivity of the skin of the breast and areola may occur transiently or definitively. We carry out the detachment of the implant store cautiously, avoiding major displacements in the lateral chest to minimize this complication.

Mondor's syndrome, which occurs in 2% of cases presented with a fibrous cord that goes to the breast and is painful on palpation. This is a self-limited thrombophlebitis of the upper abdominal vein that lasts a few weeks. Management is conservative, consisting only in the use of symptomatic and local heat.

In cases of capsular contracture after MRI examination proving incarceration of the implant by a fibrous capsule, the treatment depends on each case. In patients with thin and little glandular integument, it is preferable to keep the cap for added protection of the implant to be placed during the same surgery; thus, only capsulotomy should be performed.

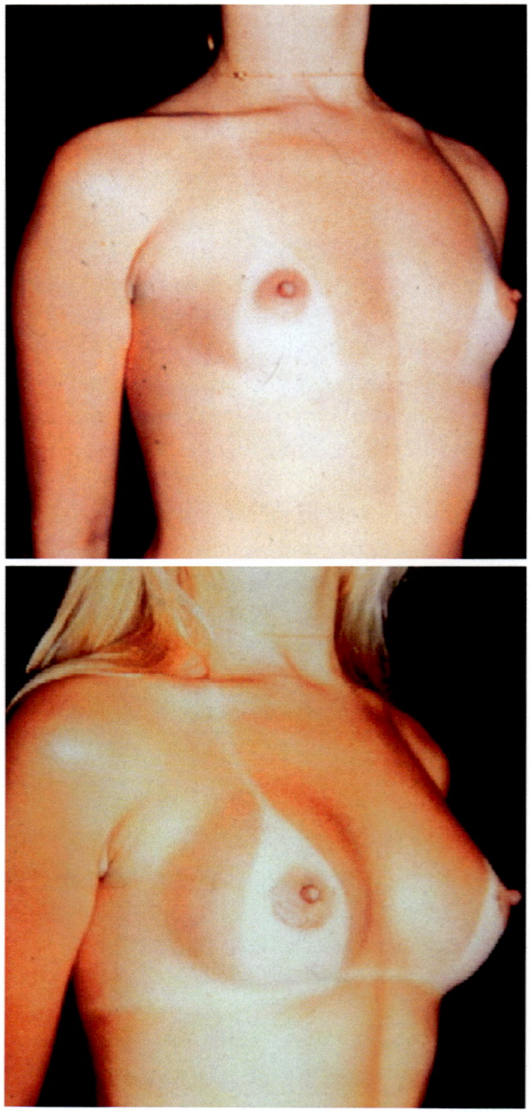

Fig. 59.8 Case 1: implant via the periareolar route. Pre- and postoperatively

59.4 Preoperative and Postoperative Results

The results of each case are presented:

Case 1: implant insertion via a periareolar route (Fig. 59.8).

Case 2: periareolar 220 mL, pre- and postoperatively (Fig. 59.9).

Case 3: tennis racket incision: 1 month postoperatively, implant 280 mL (Fig. 59.10).

Case 4: tennis racket incision: 1 month postoperatively, implant 280 mL (Fig. 59.11).

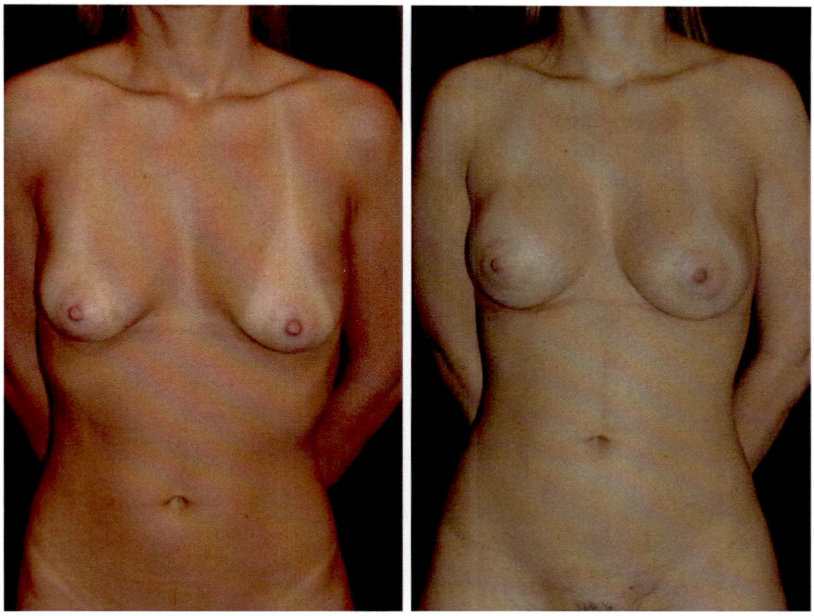

Fig. 59.9 Case 2: periareolar incision, 220 mL, pre- and post-operative

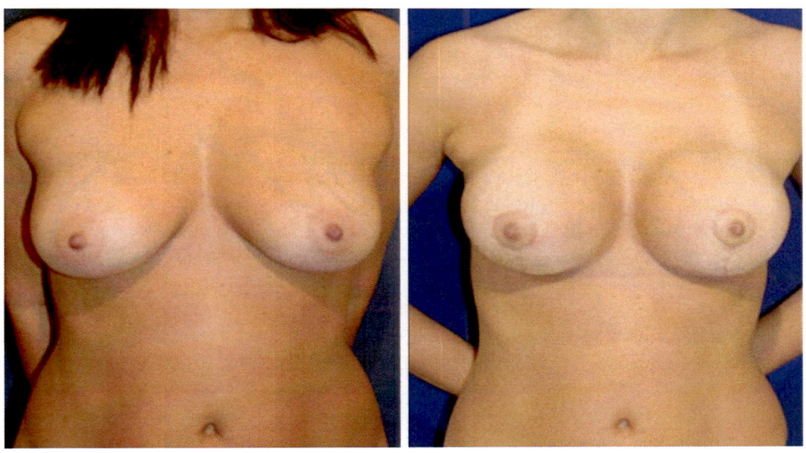

Fig. 59.10 Case 3: tennis racket incision, 1 month postoperatively, implant 280 mL

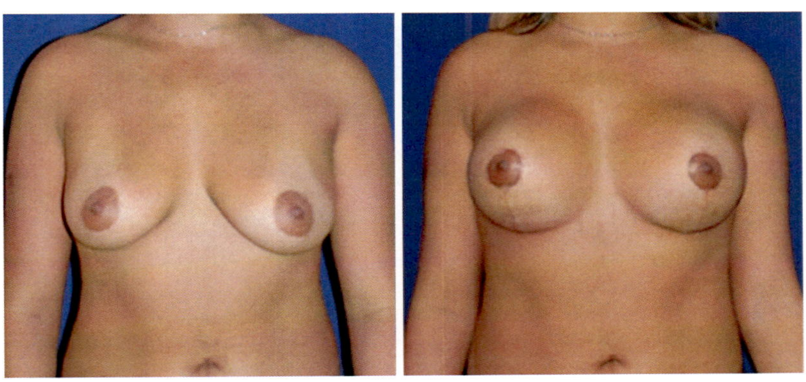

Fig. 59.11 Case 4: tennis racket incision, 1 month postoperatively, implant 280 mL

59.5 Final Considerations

Regarding the type of implants used, such as anatomical, round or conical, in addition to a high or super-high profile, Frank List in the year 2016, the US Congress showed no difference in the long-term results between the different types, when after demonstrating a series of photographs of patients with different types of implants, most of the surgeons present did not recognize significant differences between them. In our experience, we also observed low rates of complications and good results, both in the use of textured implants such as polyurethane, high or super-high profile, round or anatomical implants. That is, the size, profile, access route, and texture of implants are selected according to the surgeon's personal preference.

References

Adams GA, Santerre JP (1992) The polyurethane foam covering the meme breast prosthesis: biomedical breakthrough or a biomaterial baby? Ann Plast Surg 29(5):477

Artz JS, Dinner MI, Fogliettl DO, Samplier J (1991) Breast reconstruction utilizing subcutaneous tissue expansion followed by polyurethane-covered silicone implants: a 6 year experience. Plast Reconstr Surg 88(4):635–641

Ashley FL (1970) A new type of breast prothesis. Plast Reconstr Surg 45(5):421–424

Ashley FL (1972) Further studies on the natural-Y breast prothesis. Plast Reconstr Surg 49(4):414–419

Barone FE, Perry RNL, Keller T, Maxwell GP (1992) The biomechanical and histopathologic effects of surface texturing with silicone and polyurethane in tissue implantation and expansion. Plast Reconstr Surg 90(1):77–86

Berrino P, Galli A, Rainero ML, Santi PL (1986) Long-lasting complication with the use of polyurethane-covered breast implants. Br J Plast Surg 39(4):549–553

Bondurant S, Ernster V, Herdman R (1999) Safety of silicone breast implants. National Academy Press, Washington, DC

Brand KG (1984) Poliurethane-coated silicone implants and the question of capsular contracture. Plast Reconstr Surg 73:498

Brand MG (1988) Foam-covered mammary implants. Clin Plast Surg 15(4):533

Bruck MG (1990) Long term results of polyurethane-covered prostheses. Aesthet Plast Surg 14:85–86

Bucky LP, Ehrlich HP, Sohoni S, May JW Jr (1994) The capsule quality of saline filled smooth-silicone texturized, and polyurethane implants in rabbits; a long term study. Plast Reconstr Surg 93(6):1123–1131

Caftee HH, Hathaway C (1990) Polyurethane foam-covered implants, and capsular contracure a laboratory investigation. Plast Reconstr Surg 86(4):708–712

Caleel R (2000) Transumbilical endoscopic breast augmentation: submammary and subpectoral. Plast Reconstr Surg 106:1177–1182

Camirand A, Doucet J (2000) Breast augmentation: teaching our patient how compression can help prevent capsular contracture. Aesthet Plast Surg 24:221–226

Capozzi A (1981) Clinical experience with polyurethane-covered gel-filled mammary prostheses. Plast Reconstr Surg 68(4):512–520

Capozzi A (1982) Polyurethane-covered gel mammary implants. Plast Reconstr Surg 69:904

Capozzi A (1991) Long-term complication of polyurethane-covered breast implants. Plast Reconstr Surg 88(3):458–481

Chajchir A et al (1994) Endoscopic augmentation mastoplasty. Aesthet Plast Surg 18:377–382

Cocke WM, Leathers HK, Lynch JB (1975) Foreign body reaction to polyurethane covers of some breast prostheses. Plast Reconstr Surg 56:527–530

Cohen S, Rohrich RJ (1994) Evaluation of the patient with silicone gel breast implants and rheumatic complaints. Plast Reconstr Surg 94:120–125

Cohney BC (1991) Nineteen years experience with polyurethane foam-covered mammary prostheses: a preliminary report. Ann Plast Surg 27(1):27–30

Collis N, Shape DT (2000) Recurrence of subglandular breast implant capsular contracture: anterior versus total capsulectomy. Plast Reconstr Surg 106:792–797

Collis N, Sharpe DT (2000) Silicone gel-filled breast implant integrity: a retrospective review of 478 consecutively explanted implants. Plast Reconstr Surg 105:1979–1985

Cronin TD, Gerow FJ (1963) Augmentation mammaplasty: a new "natural feel" prosthesis. Excerpta Medica International Congress Series, number 66

Czerny V (1985) Plastischer Ersatz der Brustdruse durch ein Lipom. Zentralbl Chir 27:72

Dolsky RL (1984) Inserting the Meme prosthesis. Plast Reconstr Surg 73(3):466–468

Doslky RL (1985) Polyurethane-coated implants. Plast Reconstr Surg 76(6):974–975

Eyssen JE, Von Werssowetz AJ, Middlethon GD (1984) Reconstruction of the breast using polyurethane-coated prostheses. Plast Reconstr Surg 73(3):415–421

Food and Drug Administration (FDA) (1995) Department of Health & Human services update: study of TDA released from polyurethane foam-covered breast implants, p 36

Fryzer JP et al (2000) Characteristics of women with comestic breast augmentation surgery compared with reduction surgery patients and women in the general population of Sweden. Ann Plast Surg 45:349–356

Gasperoni C, Salgarello M, Gargani G (1992) Polyurethane-covered mammary implants: a 12-years experience. Ann Plast Surg 29(4):303–308

Graf RM, Bernardes A, Auersvald A, Damasio RCC (2000) Subfascial endoscopic transaxillary augmentation mammaplasty. Aesthet Plast Surg 24:216–220

Handel N, Silvertein MJ, Jensen A, Collins A (1991) Comparative experience with smooth and polyurethane breast implants using the Kaplan-Meier method of survival analysis. Plast Reconstr Surg 88(3):475–481

Handel N, Jensen JA, Black Q, Waisman JR, Silvertein MJ (1995) The fate of breast implant: a critical analysis of complication and outcomes. Plast Reconstr Surg 96:1521

Heinstein JB, Mangino JE, Ruberg RL, Bergese JJ (2000) A prosthetic breast implant infected with Mycobacterium fortuitum. Ann Plast Surg 44:330–333

Herman S (1984) The meme implant. Plast Reconstr Surg 73(3):411–414

Hester TR Jr, Cukic J (1991) Use of stacked polyurethane-covered mammary implants in aesthetic and reconstructive breast surgery. Plast Reconstr Surg 88(3):503–509

Hester TR Jr, Nahai F, Bostiwick J, Cukic J (1988) A 5-year experience with polyurethane-covered mammary prostheses of treatment of capsular contracture, primary augmentation mammoplasty and breast reconstruction. Clin Plast Surg 15(4):569–585

Hoefflin SM (1990a) Extensive experience with polyurethane breast implants. Plast Reconstr Surg 86(1):166–167

Hoefflin SM (1990b) Polyurethane implants and closed capsulotomies. Plast Reconstr Surg 87(4):811

Hoefflin SM (1991) Stacked polyurethane implants and mammographic misinterpretation. Plast Reconstr Surg 84:998

Hoffman S (1991) Treatment of breast contractures with open capsulotomy and replacement of gel prostheses with polyurethane-covered implants. Plast Reconstr Surg 87:808

Independent Review Group (1998) Silicone gel breast implants: the report of the independent review group. Jill Rogers, Cambridge

Jabaley ME, Das SK (1986) Late breast pain following reconstruction with polyurethane-covered implants. Plast Reconstr Surg 78(3):390–395

Karnes J et al (2000) Simultaneous breast augmentation and lift. Aesthet Plast Surg 24:148–154

Kerrigan CA (1995) Report on the Meme breast implant. McGill University, Montreal

PJ LV, Kellerher JC (1986) "Saline float" positioning of the polyurethane-covered breast prosthesis. Plast Reconstr Surg 78:845–846

Melmed EP (1988) Polyurethane implants: a 6-year review of 416 patients. Plast Reconstr Surg 82(2):285–290

Melmed EP (1990) Treatment of breast contractures with open capsulotomy and replacement of gel prostheses with polyurethane-covered implants. Plast Reconstr Surg 86(2):270–274

Niazi ZMN, Salzberg CA, Montcalvo M (1996) Infection of bilateral polyurethane coated silicone gel breast implants. Ann Plast Surg 37:91–93

O'Connell JB (1992) Removal of stacked polyurethane-covered mammary implants. Plast Reconstr Surg 90(5):930

Okunski WJ, Chowdary RP (1987) Infected Meme implants: salvage reconstruction with latissumus dorsi myocutaneous flaps and silicone implants. Aesthet Plast Surg 11:49–51

Pennisi VR (1985) Polyurethane-covered silicone gel mammary: prosthesis for successful breast reconstruction. Aesthet Plast Surg 9:73–77

Pennisi VR (1990) Long-term use of polyurethane breast prostheses: a 14-years experience. Plast Reconstr Surg 86(2):368–371

Picha GJ, Goldstein JA, Sthor E (1990) Natural-Y Meme polyurethane versus smooth silicone analysis of the soft-tissue interaction from 3 days to 1 year in the rat animal model. Plast Reconstr Surg 85(6):903–916

Pitanguy I, Brentano J, Ramalho MC, Porto MJ (1990) Implante de silicone com revestimento de poliuretano. Rev Bras Cir 80(2):119–130

Pitanguy I, Salgado F, Radwanski HN, Stersa RM (1991) Estagio atual dos implantes mamários. Rev Bras Cir 81(6):291–299

Pollock H (1984) Polyurethane-covered breast implant. Plast Reconstr Surg 74(5):729

Rebello C (1993) Mamoplastia de aumento com proteses mamarias de silicone revestidas de poliuretano. Rev Bras Cir Plast 8(1–3):58

Rees TD (1964) Plastic surgery of the breast. In: Converse JM (ed) Reconstructive plastic surgery. Saunders, Philadelphia, pp 1903–1938

Ribeiro RC, Saltz R (2001) Cirurgia de mama estetica e reconstrutiva. Revinter, Rio de Janeiro, pp 351–386

Rohrich RJ et al (1999) Factors predictive of quality of life after silicone implant explanation. Plast Reconstr Surg 104:1334–1337

Russel MB (1984) Polyurethane-covered breast implant. Plast Reconstr Surg 74(5):728–729

Schatten WE (1984) Reconstruction of breasts following mastectomy with polyurethane-covered, gel-filled prostheses. Ann Plast Surg 12(2):147–156

Sinclair TM (1995) Biodegradation of the polyurethane foam, revisited in the rat model. Plast Reconstr Surg 96:1326

Sinclair TM, Kerrigan CL, Buntic R (1993) Biodegradation of the polyurethane foam covering of breast implants. Plast Reconstr Surg 92(6):1003–1013

Slade CL, Peterson HD (1982) Disappearance of the polyurethane cover of the Ashley Natural-Y prosthesis. Plast Reconstr Surg 70(3):379–382

Smahel J (1978) Tissue reaction to breast implants coated with polyurethane. Plast Reconstr Surg 61(1):80–85

Spear SL, Elmaraghy M, Hess C (2000) Textured-surface saline-filled silicone breast implants for augmentation mammaplasty. Plast Reconstr Surg 105:1542–1552

Umansky C (1985) Infection with polyurethane-coated implants. Plast Reconstr Surg 75(6):925
Villafane O, Garcia-Tutor E, Taggart I (2000) Endoscopic transaxillary subglandular breast augmentation using silicone gel textured implants. Aesthet Plast Surg 24:212–215
Wilkinson TS (1985) Polyurethane-coated implants. Plast Reconstr Surg 76(6):925–926

60 Removal of Breast Implants Followed by Mastopexy

Juarez M. Avelar

60.1 Introduction

Augmentation mastoplasty is an important field concerning aesthetic breast procedures. Before Cronin and Gerow (1963) introduced silicone implants, several other materials were employed but used to present a very high rate of complications. In fact, the new implant solved several problems and surgeons all around the world were soon employing them. Nevertheless, the criteria for indication and selection of patients are very important topics before surgery, which quite often are not well considered. The own patients usually indicate as much as the breasts may be augmented, which should not be accepted for surgeons. Nowadays, the size of the implant is much larger than a few decades ago owing to the great demands of patients caused by lay information on television, magazines, and in the cinema. This is a risk, as the patient's taste before surgery may change afterward. Such a misunderstanding between patients and surgeons is the main reason for performing breast augmentation, with undesirable consequences (Broadbent and Woolf 1978).

In addition to the unaesthetic appearance of the breast with a very large implant, several other circumstances may motivate patients to feel disappointed with the surgical results. Excessive weight of the breasts and ptosis after augmentation are the most frequent patient complaints are caused by too large a implant inserted during primary surgery.

For this reason, before operation the surgeon must talk peacefully with patients and listen to their complaints and afterward a careful physical evaluation is carried out, to avoid misunderstanding, as reported by Maliniac (1959), related to severe consequences after surgery. Each patient has the chance to choose her surgeon; nevertheless, each surgeon may also select his or her patients (Avelar 1986, 1988). During consultation, it is the right moment for both surgeon and patient to evaluate before taking the decision. If a patient has been disappointed with a previous of breast augmentation surgery result, her anxiety must be well-evaluated, as sometimes she wants to get rid of the implant and may decide without confidence to have them removed .

60.2 Method

60.2.1 Surgical Planning

Before any operation, surgical planning is an important step that must be done after careful examination of the breasts. Mammography or ultrasound may be performed to evaluate the implant, the capsule around it, and the mammary

J.M. Avelar
Brazilian Institute of Surgery Plastic and Reconstructive, Alameda Gabriel Monteiro da Silva, São Paulo, SP CEP 01442000, Brazil
e-mail: juarezavelar@bol.com.br

J.M. Avelar (ed.), *Breast Surgery*, https://doi.org/10.1007/978-3-319-54115-0_60

gland. The surgeon must evaluate the relationship between the thickness of the mammary tissue and the implant. If the patient wants to have them removed, it is mandatory to analyze whether or not it is possible to remodel a new breast afterward. The patient's wish is not enough for a surgeon to remove the implant, as reshaping the breasts may be a difficult task during the operation. In fact, surgical planning is similar to reduction mastoplasty. The remaining mammary tissue is incised to create glandular flaps that can be rotated to reshape the breasts.

60.2.2 Surgical Marking: Pre-marking

It is my routine to carry out pre-marking 1 day before surgery, as there is one more chance to examine the patient.

Similar to reduction mastoplasty, the operation is demarcated with the patient in a standing position in front of two vertical mirrors in the examination room at my clinic (Fig. 60.1). The basic reference is to determine Pitanguy's point A, which is the result of some lines drawn on the patient's chest (Pitanguy 1959; Pitanguy and Garcia 1972). First, the center of the sternal notch is marked following other points on the midclavicular line, 7 cm away from it (Fig. 60.2). A vertical line is drawn until it reaches the nipple on each side. The inframammary fold is also marked by elevating the breast. Afterward, I follow Pitanguy's description, such as placing my index finger under the submammary crease and behind the breast with the implant inside (Fig. 60.2). With my opposite index finger the future position of the nipple area is then estimated where point A is marked. From this point, the rest of the markings are done in the operating room. These reference points are marked and it is recommended that the patient preserves them until the next day. At that moment, the patient signs the informed consent.

Usually, I perform surgery with the patient under local anesthesia combined with intravenous sedation under the care of an anesthesiologist (Fig. 60.3). With the patient placed in the supine position, the operating table is bent about 30° with elevation of the chest so that the breasts show the ptotic position than the inframammary creases are marked. As long as Pitanguy's point A is marked, all demarcations of the surgery must be made, including the submammary folds (Fig. 60.3).

60.2.2.1 Anesthesia

This type of operation may be performed under general anesthesia. My preference is to employ

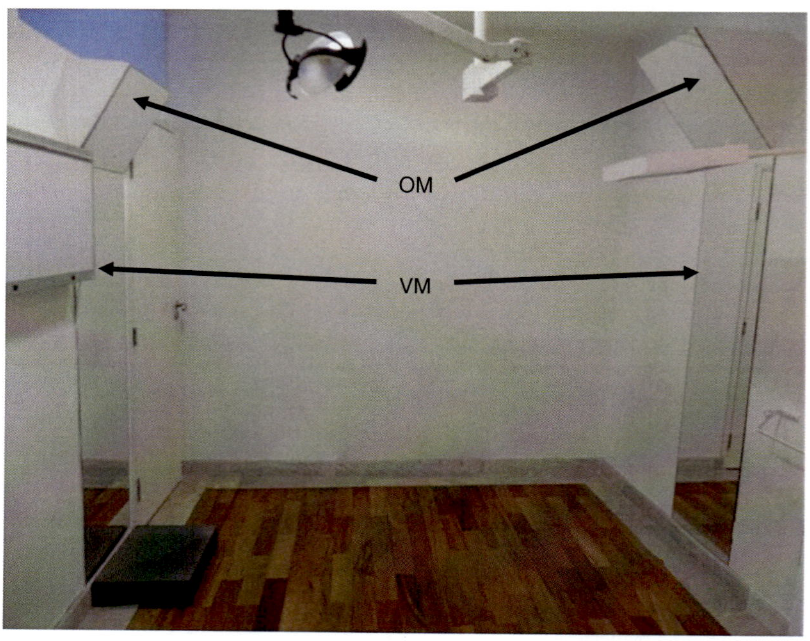

Fig. 60.1 Photo of the examination room at my clinic. Two vertical mirrors (VM) are placed one in front of the other, combined with two oblique mirrors (OM) are strategically located on top of the vertical ones making 45° inclination from the others. When a patient is in a standing position in front of one vertical mirror she sees herself from the frontal and back views at the same time

local anesthesia combined with intravenous sedation under the care of an anesthesiologist, even for large breasts.

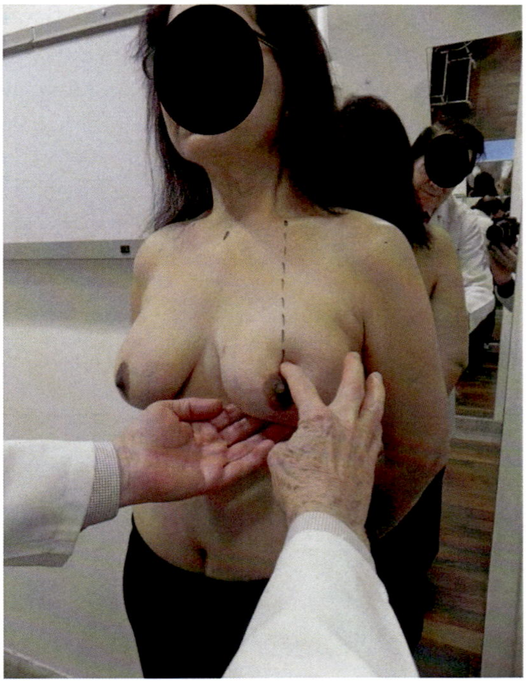

Fig. 60.2 A patient is being examined by a surgeon in the examining room in a standing position in front of a vertical mirror and she follows the examination. Pitanguy's point A is being marked during pre-demarcation 1 day before the operation for removal of the silicone implant followed by mastopexy

60.2.3 Anesthetic Infiltration

The anesthetic solution is: lidocaine (2%) 40 mL, plus distilled water 160 mL, plus epinephrine (1/1000) 1 mL. The total solution is 201 mL, which is enough to infiltrate both breasts.

It is important to emphasize that the local infiltration must be performed very carefully because of the presence of implants inside the breasts. I start the infiltration of one breast at the segment of the inframammary crease, followed by the subcutaneous layer of the external border of the breast (Fig. 60.3) to infiltrate the ending of the intercostobrachial nerve and ends of the intercostal nerves in the subcutaneous plane. The base of the breast is then infiltrated, which means below the mammary implant and above the pectoralis muscle. I clamp the breast with one hand and a long microcannula is employed passing underneath the implant (Fig. 60.3a, b). As a final step, the subcutaneous plane corresponding to the technical markings, even those below the areola, is infiltrated (Fig. 60.3c).

60.2.4 Removing the Mammary Implant

I employ an elastic rubber band all around the breast or the surgeon's assistant holds the breast with two hands to expose the nipple–areola complex (NAC). Then, a careful incision circumscribing the areola is made followed by

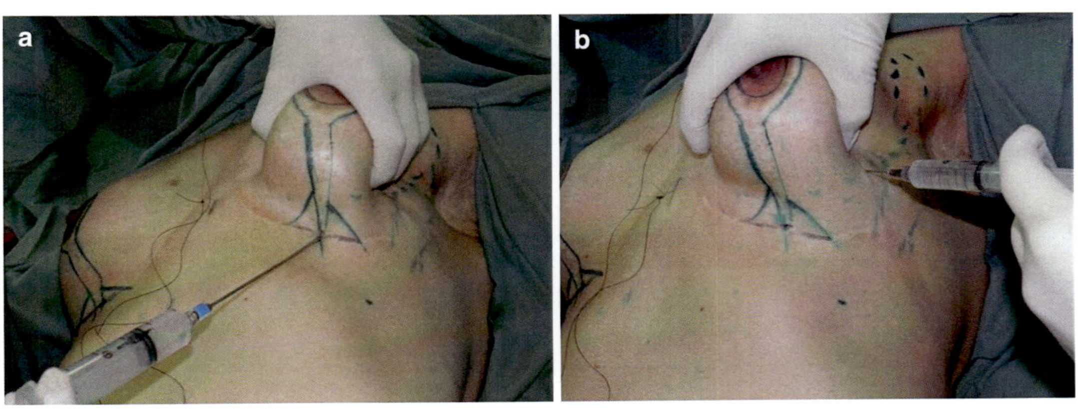

Fig. 60.3 Local anesthesia combined with intravenous sedation under the care of anesthesiologist for removal of a silicone implant followed by mastopexy. (**a**, **b**) Photos show the surgeon holding the left breast with one hand and with the other one he uses a long needle to infiltrate below the implant and above the pectoralis muscle. (**c**) Using a regular needle, subcutaneous infiltration is being performed to block the fiber ends of the intercostobrachial nerve

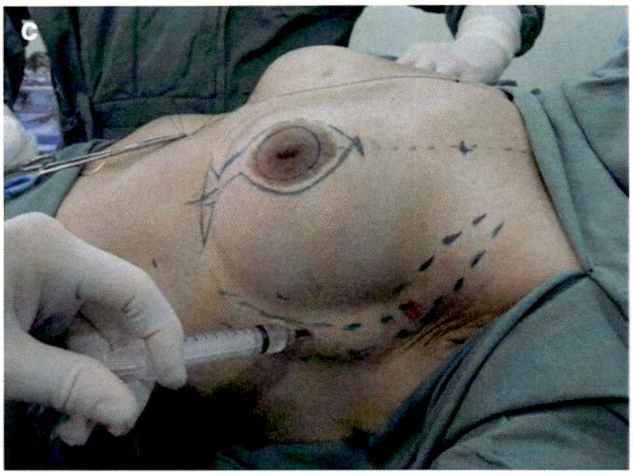

Fig. 60.3 (continued)

Schwarzmann's maneuver (Schwarzmann 1930) all around, for maintenance of the blood supply to the nipple.

Afterward, a cutaneous incision is made following the surgical markings to de-epithelialize the area of excess skin. My dermal–adipose–glandular flap with superior pedicle is outlined on the raw area (Fig. 60.4a) (Avelar 1980, 1993). The breast is suspended by the assistant through its top corner using a strong hulk, which is kept in the ideal position for performing glandular incisions (Fig. 60.4b). Two parallel incisions are made following previous marking until the capsule of the mammary implant is reached to create

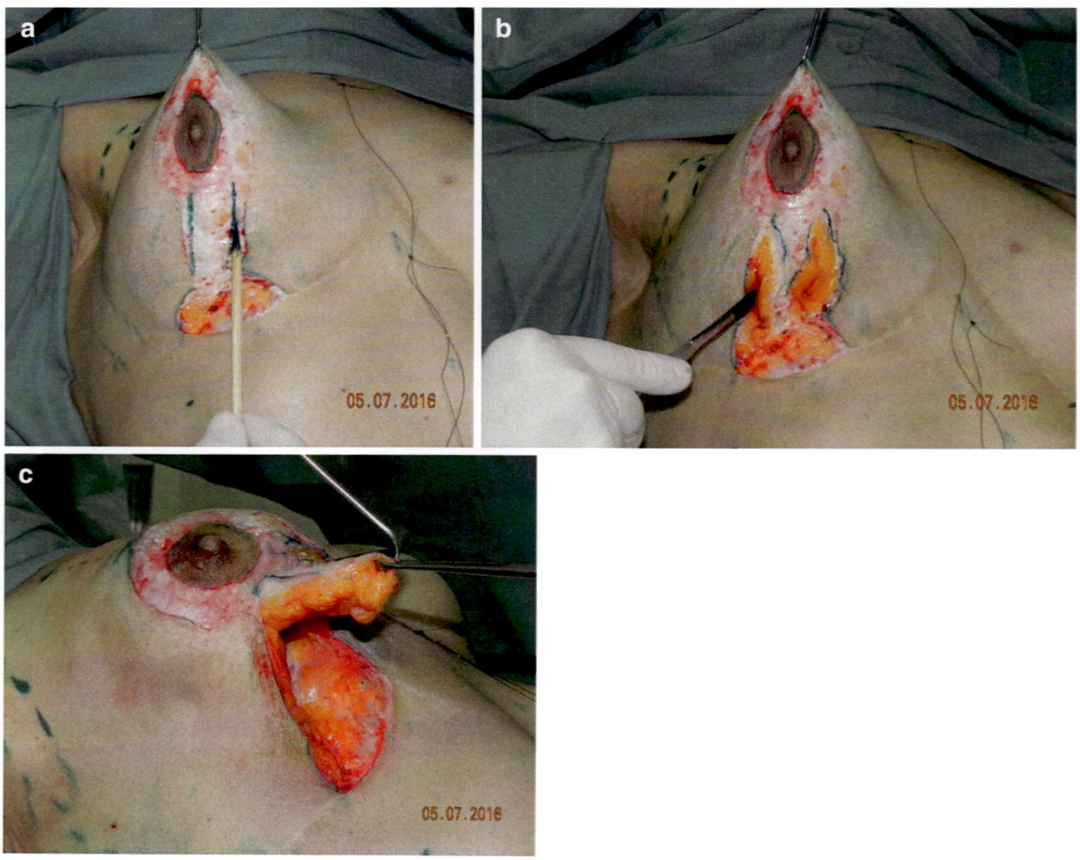

Fig. 60.4 Creation of a medial adipose–glandular flap with a superior pedicle. (**a**) Peroperative photo showing marking of the flap with two lines. (**b**) Two incisions are made following demarcation lines. (**c**) The flap is already created and pulled forward by a gentle hulk. (**d**) Drawing demonstrates that the flap is marked and incised. (**e**) The flap is created and pulled forward

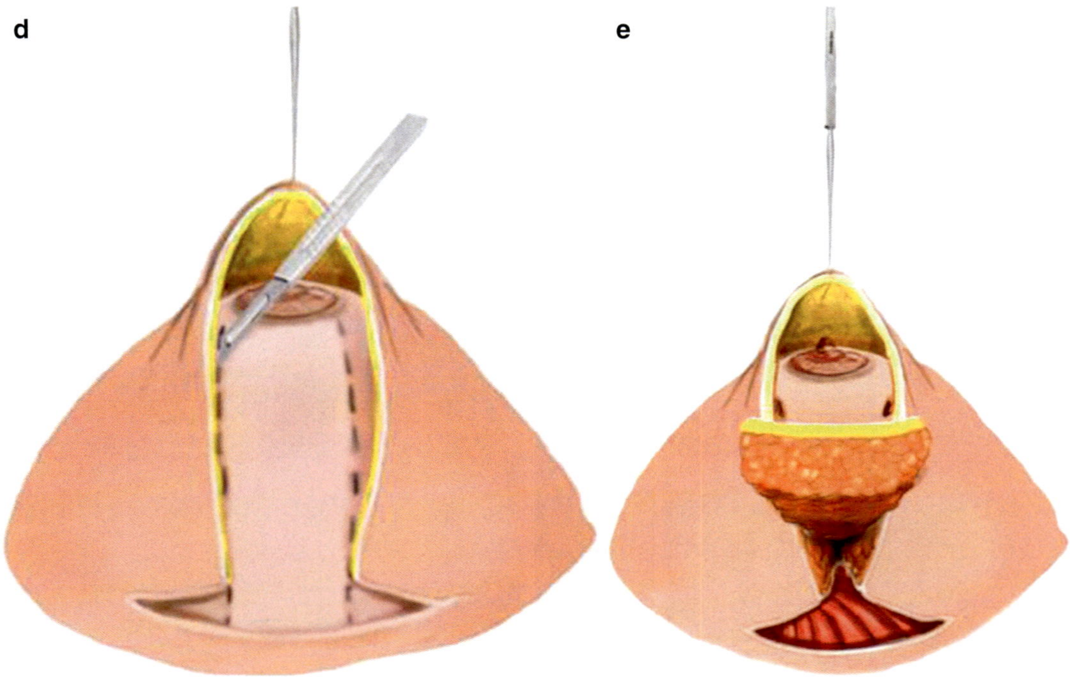

Fig. 60.4 (contiuned)

the main glandular flap. The width of the flap is established according to the dimensions of the mammary parenchyma (Fig. 60.4b). A gentle hulk is placed on the tip of the dermal–adipose–glandular flap to pull it forward and to elevate it to expose the capsule of the implant (Fig. 60.4c–e). An incision is made and the implant is then removed (Fig. 60.5). It is not necessary to resect the capsule. Some incisions are made in the internal surface of the capsule, just to create some raw areas for adequate healing (Fig. 60.6).

After removing the implant from one breast the anesthetic infiltration is performed on the opposite one according to the above description. Although there is little bleeding during such a procedure, hemostasis should be carefully carried out.

To facilitate the internal suture, my Z instrument is introduced inside the cavity created after removing the implant under the remaining glandular tissue between the two columns (Fig. 60.7). The tip of the dermal–adipose–glandular flap is then stitched to the deep concavity of the capsule and the lateral borders are sutured laterally, as I have previously described (Fig. 60.7) (Avelar 1980, 1993). Afterward, the medial and external walls of the remaining mammary parenchyma are sutured over the dermal–adipose–glandular flap similar to the two glandular columns described by Pitanguy (1959), Pitanguy and Garcia (1972).

The surgeon's assistant maintains pulling up the Z instrument to suture both columns to the aponeurosis of the pectoralis muscle (Fig. 60.7). Afterward, a cutaneous temporary stitch is inserted to approximate the points B and C on the midline of the submammary crease. Thus, it is possible to evaluate the size and shape of the future breast (Fig. 60.8).

Next, I move to the other side of the operating table to perform the same procedure on the opposite breast, as it has already been infiltrated.

After temporary stitching on the second breast, it is the exact moment to evaluate the two breasts with regard to the size, shape, and the position (Fig. 60.8).

60.2.5 Repositioning the New Nipple–Areola Complex

After a temporary suture, the new nipple–areolar area is demarcated and the superficial layer of the

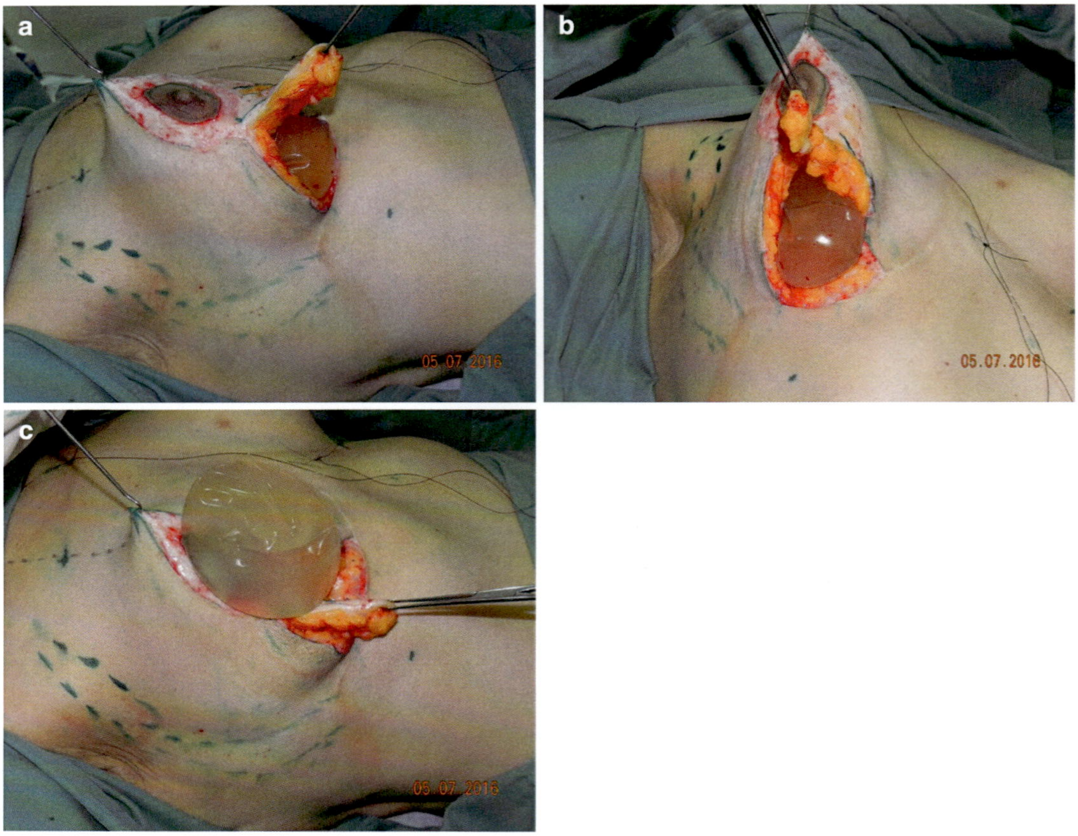

Fig. 60.5 Sequential peroperative photos showing removal of the silicone implant after creation of the medial adipose–glandular flap. The implant is still inside the breast on the right side of the patient. (**a**) Lateral view. (**b**) Frontal view. (**c**) The implant is already out of the breast

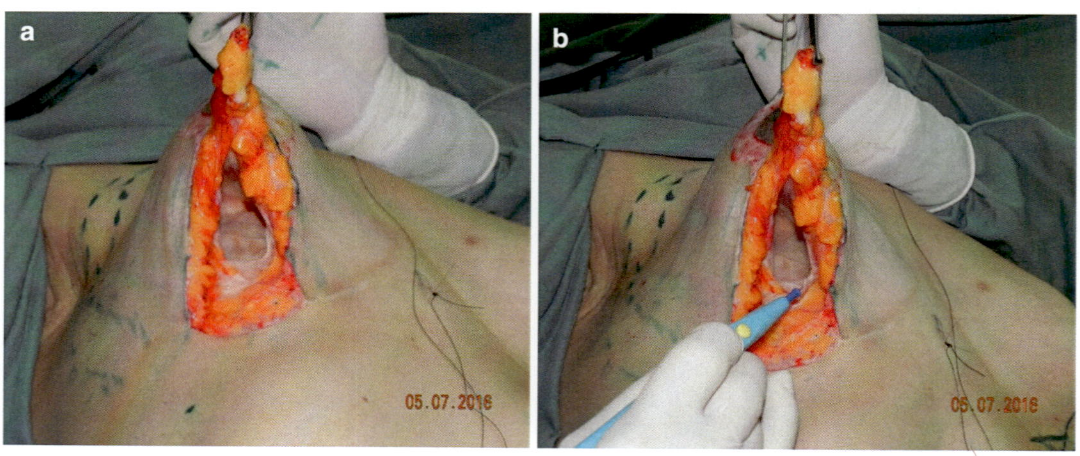

Fig. 60.6 After removal of the silicone implant, the fibrotic capsule is inside the breast and the adipose–glandular flap is pulled forward in the frontal view. (**a**) Internal view. (**b**) Cauterization is performed on the capsule just to cut it. (**c**) Internal view of the cavity showing the two columns of breast tissue

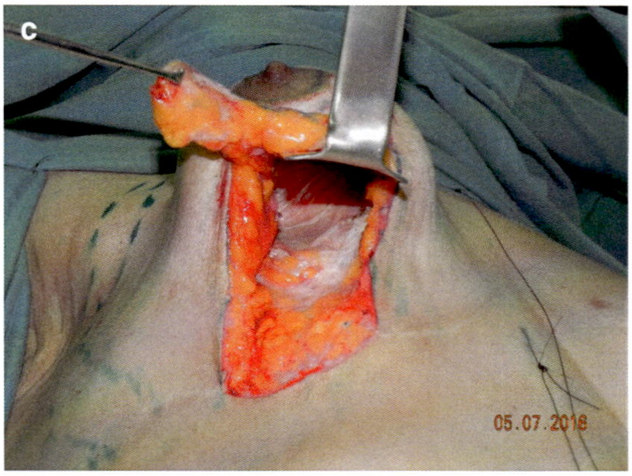

Fig. 60.6 (continued)

dermis is removed. Also, I perform dissection of the dermis on the vertical border of the wound to create two dermal flaps on each side. The dermal flaps are sutured with isolated stitches, creating a dermal structure that works as a reinforcement of the vertical suture to adjust content and container (Avelar 1980, 1993). The dermal structure works as a plane to support the weight of the breast as a new dermal brassiere. Afterward, using special forceps, the skin is pulled forward to evaluate the exact amount of cutaneous excess to be resected (Fig. 60.8). Running intradermal suture is applied to close the wound. The nipple–areola region is drawn on the vertices of the new breast using a

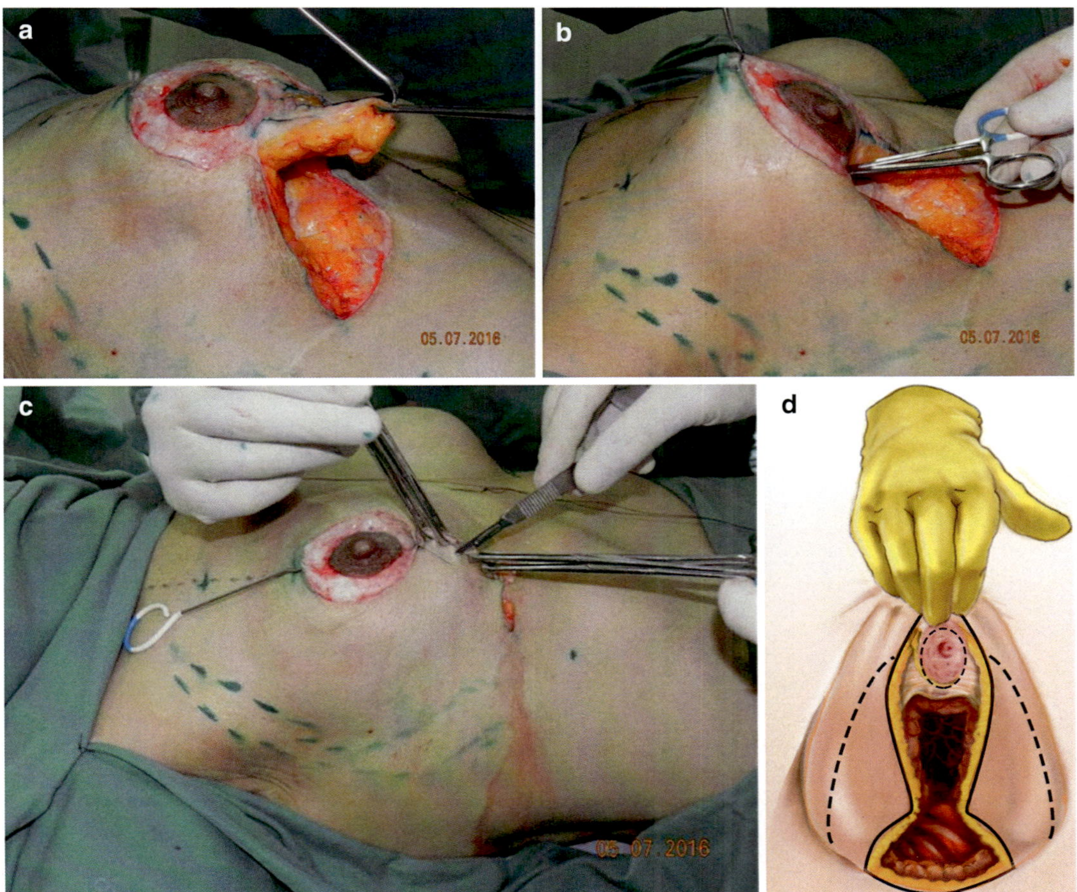

Fig. 60.7 Rotation and suture of the adipose–glandular flap. (**a**) The flap is pulled forward. (**b**) The flap is rotated backward to the inside of the cavity to be sutured to the mammary gland. (**c**) The two glandular columns were sutured together. (**d**) Drawing shows in a frontal view that the flap was sutured, but the two columns had not yet been sutured. The *dotted lines* show Pitanguy's marking, indicating that a smaller area of skin is resected

special round marker. The new areolar area is de-epithelialized and the nipple–areola segment is then pulled from deep to outside so that it can be sutured (Fig. 60.8).

60.2.6 Bandaging after Surgery

Adhesive tapes are placed, covering the wound after internal suturing. Elastic tapes are applied, covering both breasts, similar to a brassiere and a garment is placed over it all. No drainage is used as there is no cutaneous undermining, bleeding during surgery, and "dead space" as well. Patients usually go home the next day with all the postoperative instructions to avoid any strain on the upper limbs for at least 2 weeks. They return to my clinic 1 week after surgery when the first bandaging is removed and replaced by another one. The new bandaging is changed every 1 or 2 weeks for 2 months. There are no stitches to be removed, as only an internal suture is performed.

The final result may be achieved 6 months to 1 year after the operation, showing a good balance between the breast and the chest (Figs. 60.9 and 60.10).

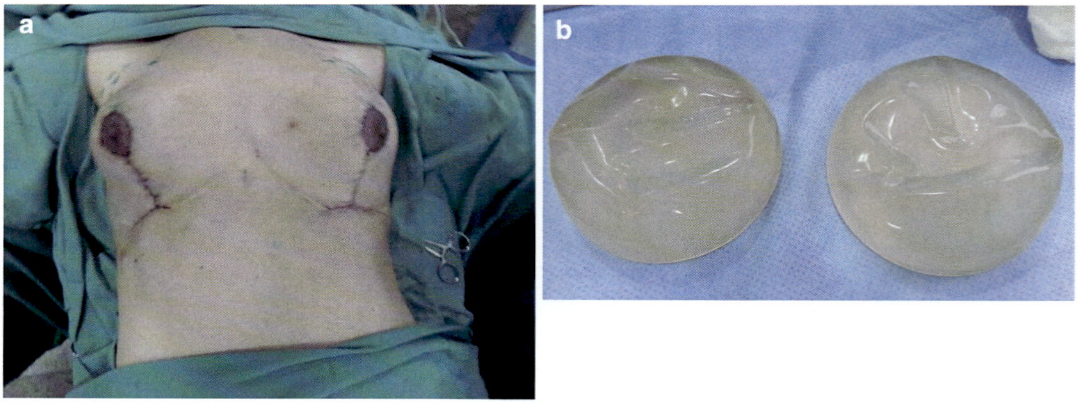

Fig. 60.8 Final of the surgery. (**a**) After intradermal suture, the nipple–areola region is repositioned and sutured. (**b**) Photo of both silicone implants removed

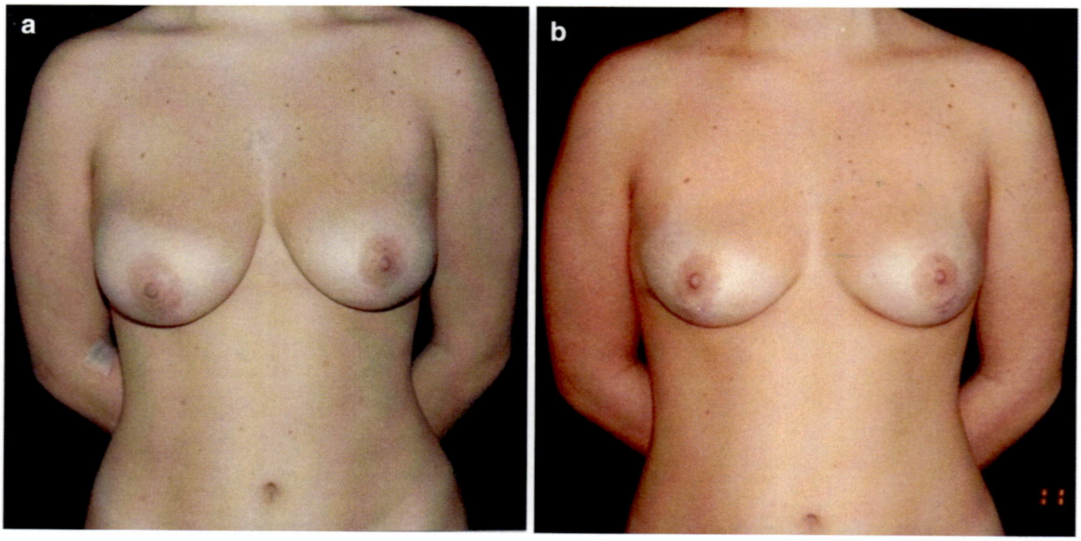

Fig. 60.9 A 32-year-old patient with silicone implants in her breasts presenting ptosis with physical discomfort. (**a**, **c**, **e**, **g**) preoperative view, (**b**, **d**, **f**, **h**) after removal of the implant followed by mastopexy

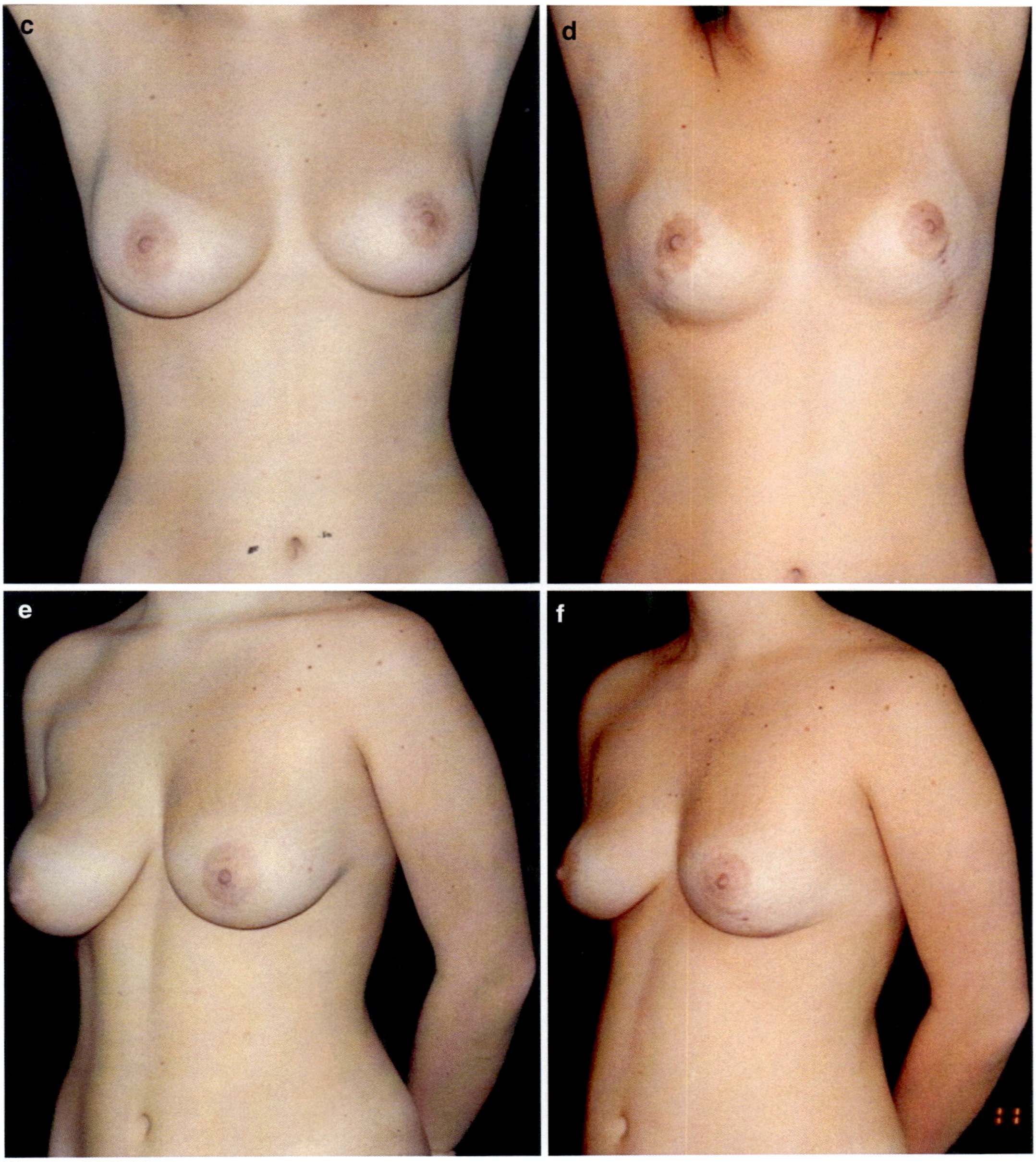

Fig. 60.9 (continued)

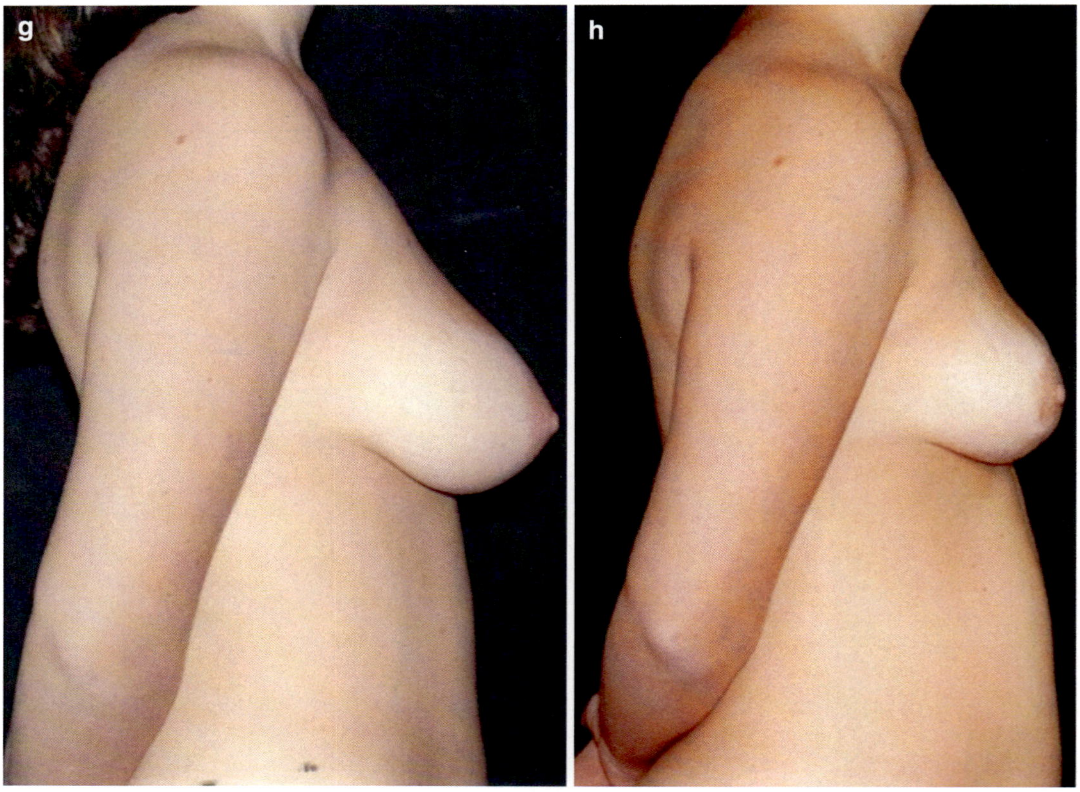

Fig. 60.9 (continued)

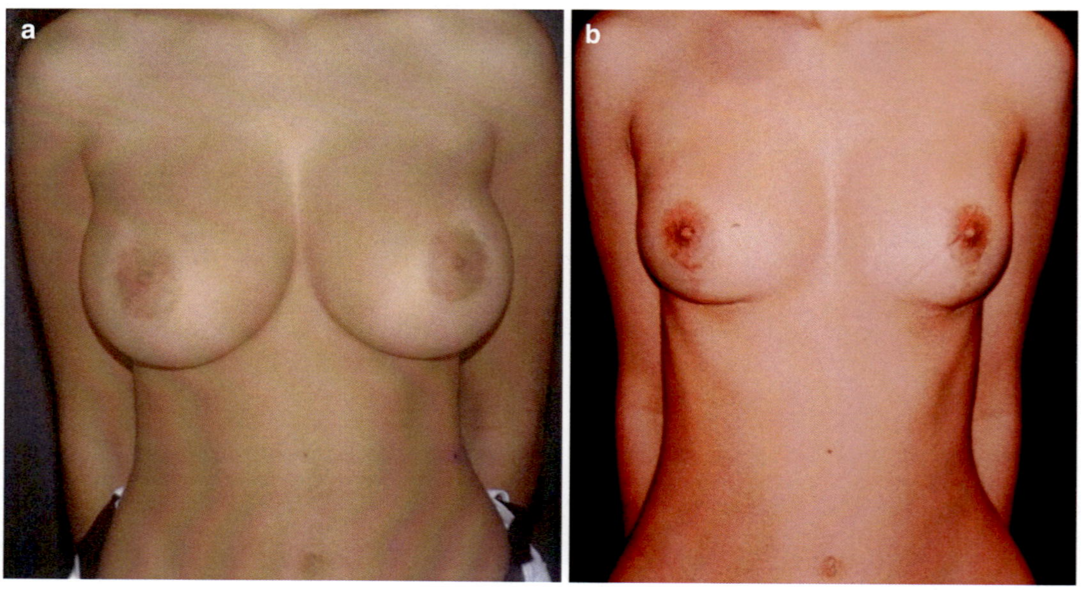

Fig. 60.10 A 36-year-old patient with large breasts due to previous augmentation mastoplasty performed elsewhere presenting ptosis with physical discomfort caused by the implant. (**a**, **c**, **e**) Pre-operative view, (**b**, **d**, **f**), after removal of the implant followed by mastopexy with an adipose–glandular flap with a superior pedicle sutured to the aponeurosis of the pectoralis major muscle

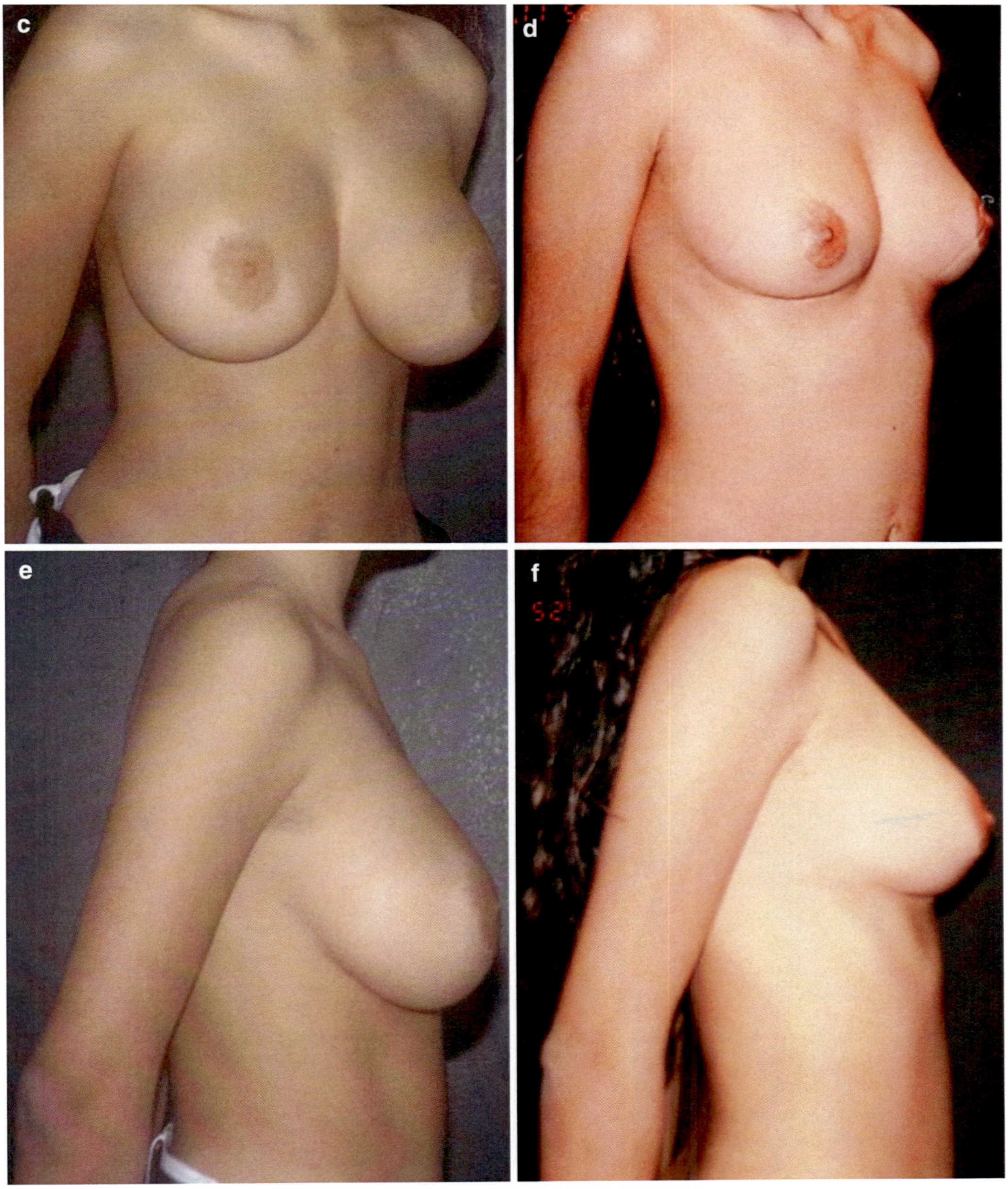

Fig. 60.10 (continued)

If the breast presents a large amount of mammary tissue, my adipose–glandular flap with superior pedicle is quite long; thus, it is possible to be sutured onto the aponeurosis of the pectoralis major muscle (Fig. 60.11). So far, in all cases, the two columns created after removal of the implant are sutured in a similar way to Pitanguy's mastoplasty technique, with good surgical results (Figs. 60.12 and 60.13).

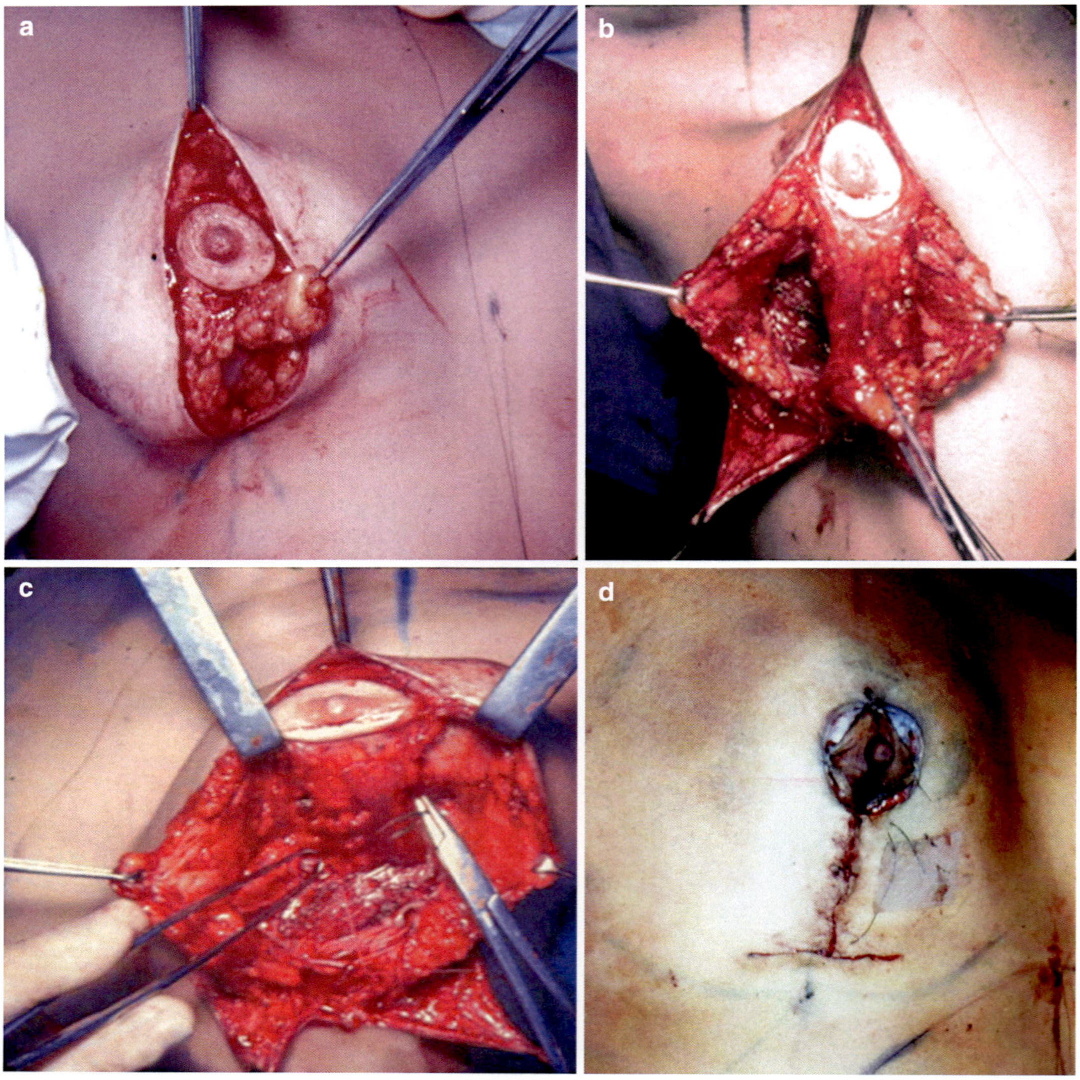

Fig. 60.11 Sequential peroperative photos in frontal view showing removal of the silicone implant and creation of a long dermal–adipose–glandular flap with a superior pedicle to be sutured onto the pectoralis muscle. (**a**) The implant is still inside the right breast and the flap is pulled forward. (**b**) The adipose–glandular flap is raised. (**c**) The flap is being sutured onto the pectoralis muscle. (**d**) final result after suturing of the flap to the pectoralis muscle and the skin as well

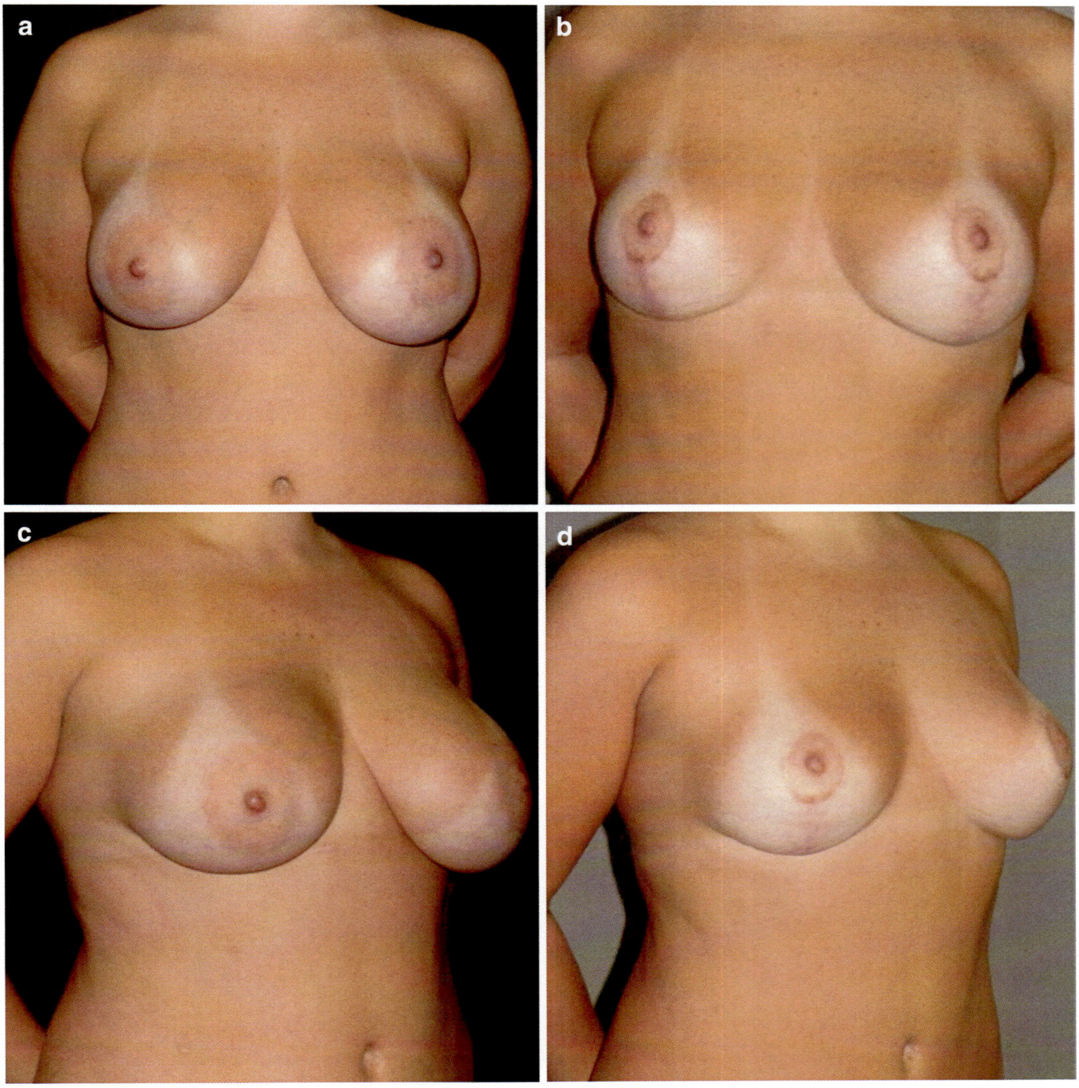

Fig. 60.12 A 38-year-old patient complained about large breasts due to previous augmentation mastoplasty performed elsewhere, presenting ptosis with asymmetry (the left breast was larger than the right). Photos (**a**, **c**, **e**) preoperative view, (**b**, **d**, **f**) after surgery. The implants removed were the same size with a volume of 280 mL. She had enough mammary gland that a long adipose–glandular flap was created on each side and sutured to the aponeurosis of the pectoralis major muscle. 110 g of breast tissue was resected on the left side to achieve a good balance between the two breasts

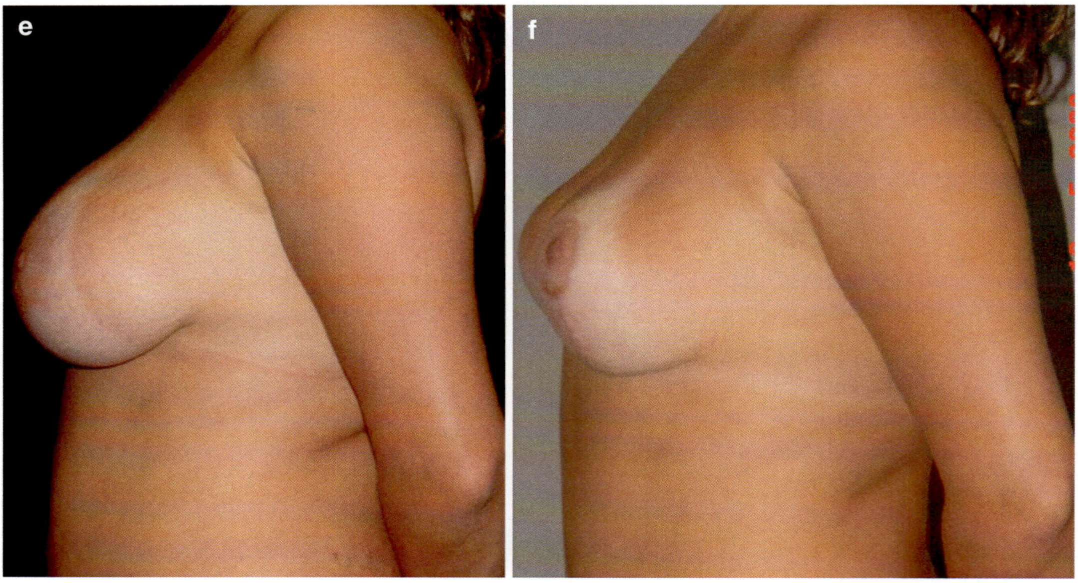

Fig. 60.12 (continued)

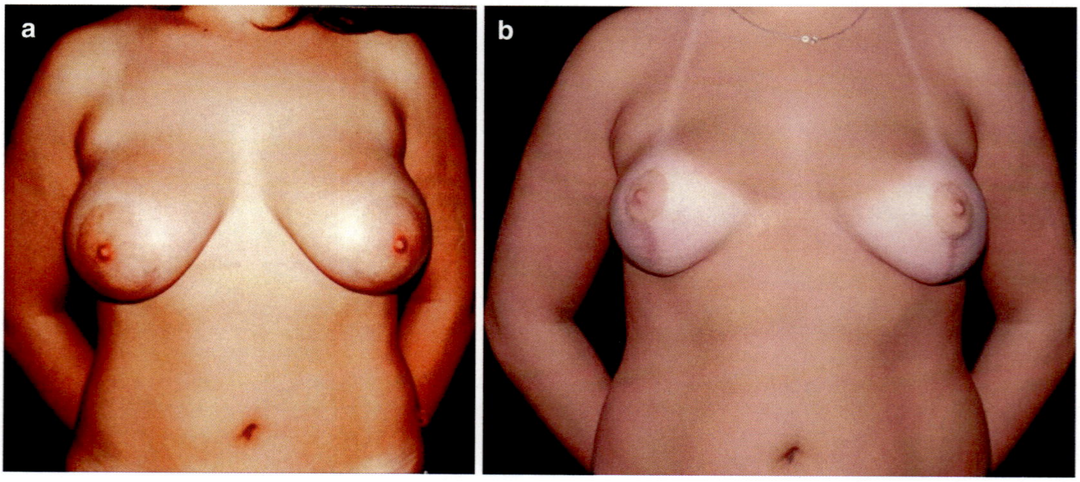

Fig. 60.13 A 27-year-old patient complained about large breasts because of previous augmentation mastoplasty performed elsewhere. The first operation was done against her desire, as she wanted to undergo mastopexy. (**a**, **c**, **e**) Pre-operative view showing ptotic breasts. (**b**, **d**, **f**) After removal of an implant weighing 295 mL from each side, mastopexy was performed according to the technique described

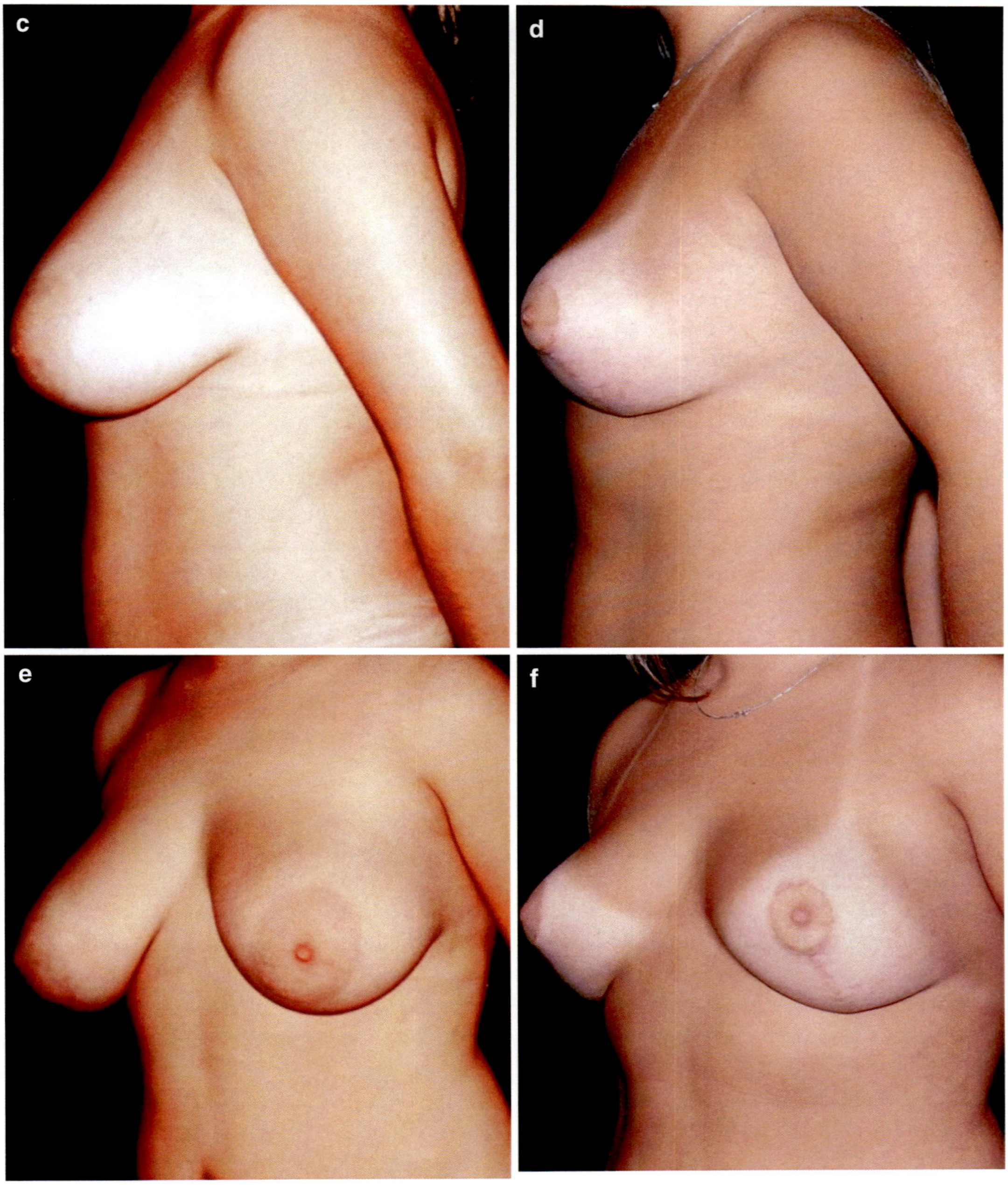

Fig. 60.13 (continued)

60.3 Discussion

Breast implant removal after augmentation mastoplasty is a quite common procedure in my practice because of breast abnormalities. The patients feel uncomfortable concerning the shape, size, and weight of them. It is a bad result due to the misunderstanding between surgeon and patient, as she had previously been looking for a better appearance to her breasts. For this reason, it is mandatory to have a good relationship between the patient and surgeon so that they to choose an adequate size of implant during the first operation. Even in an accurate evaluation of whether she really needs implants, as in all patients, I have removed them and it was possible to create new breasts with a normal size that balances well with body contouring.

The patient wants the best for her, but sometimes the final decision concerning the size of the implant was not well understood before operation, that is, the main reason why a patient feels uncomfortable about the surgical result of the augmentation mastoplasty. Each surgeon may inform the patient about content and container before performing the operation, as mentioned by Noel (1933) and later May (1943), concerning the relationship between the volume of the breast and the skin covering. An imbalanced result is the most frequent complaint after previous operation.

Because of this unexpected situation some patients want to have the implant removed, as the large volume makes it too heavy and gives similar symptoms as for hypertrophic breasts. Patients complain about the sulcus on the shoulders and they feel like they have two large balls on their chests.

Therefore, the decision to remove the implant is a mandatory procedure as long as the breasts are ptotic, heavy, and have an unaesthetic appearance.

Augmentation mastoplasty is a useful procedure for achieving a good balance and harmony with a patient's chest. However, when such situations are not well-accepted, the patient usually begs for the implant to be removed. The operation is similar to the mastopexy procedure, through which it is necessary to remove the implant and to perform rotation of the glandular.

Usually, the size and shape of the breast after surgery must be in a good balance with the whole body. Even the final scars must be well planned before operation. Often, the scars may present with an inverted T to adjust the cutaneous flaps (Figs. 60.14 and 60.15).

I have removed the silicone implant in 53 patients operated elsewhere owing to unsatisfactory results such as the exaggerated volume of the implants causing similar symptoms of mammary hypertrophy. Thus, very heavy breasts with ptosis, physical discomfort, back pain, some with asymmetry are patients' most frequent complaints. After careful surgical planning, removal of the implant was carried out followed by mastopexy. In my publication, (Avelar 1980), I described an adipose–glandular flap with a superior pedicle during my regular mastopexy. This flap has been created in all patients with a good surgical solution as it is rotated up and backward and sutured on the posterior aspect of Pitanguy's "third pedicle of the breast" (Figs. 60.12, 60.13, 60.14, and 60.15; Pitanguy and Garcia 1972). In fact, my adipose–glandular flap replaces the space on the upper pole of the breast due to removal of the implant.

60.4 Complications

There are some points that may occur when the surgeon has planned to remove the implant. For this reason, he or she must be cautious about planning such an operation. The most feared situation is to remove implant and the patient does not have enough glandular tissue to recreate the new breasts. For this reason, it is mandatory to carry out an accurate examination before the operation, or even mammography or magnetic resonance imaging for adequate evaluation. The surgeon must be sure that the patient has enough glandular tissue to create flaps so as to remodel the new breasts. The new nipple–areola region must be well placed, as they may be in an ectopic location, which is an unaesthetic situation. Asymmetry of the breasts must be very well resolved during the operation, as if the patient had presented it previously for the augmentation mastoplasty.

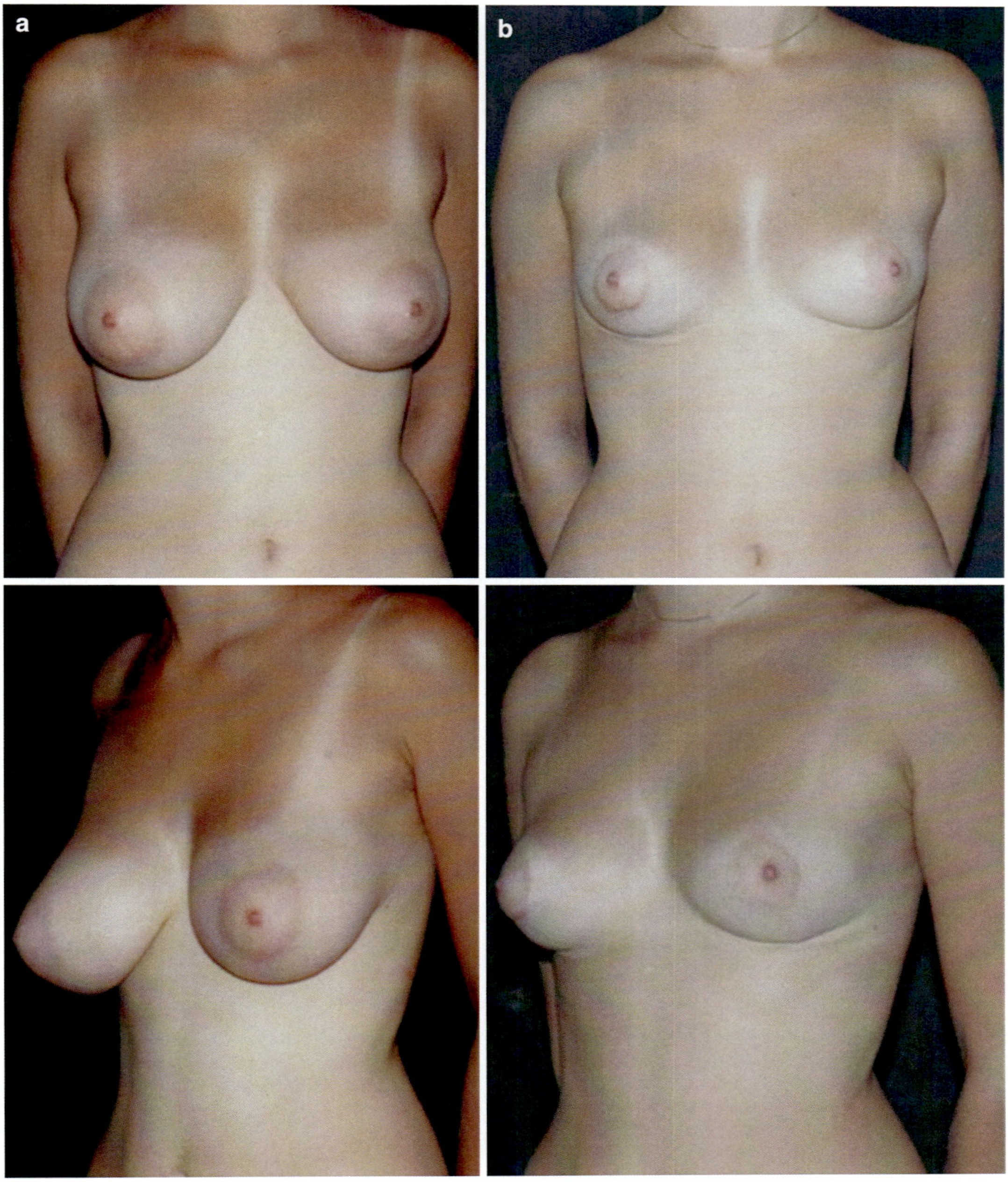

Fig. 60.14 A 24-year-old girl complained about the large volume of her breasts caused by previous silicone implantation done elsewhere. Her first operation had been performed 3 years ago against her decision, as she had wanted to undergo mastopexy. (**a**, **c**) Preoperative view showing large, ptotic breasts. (**b**, **d**) After removal of a 285-mL implant from each side, mastopexy was performed following the technique described

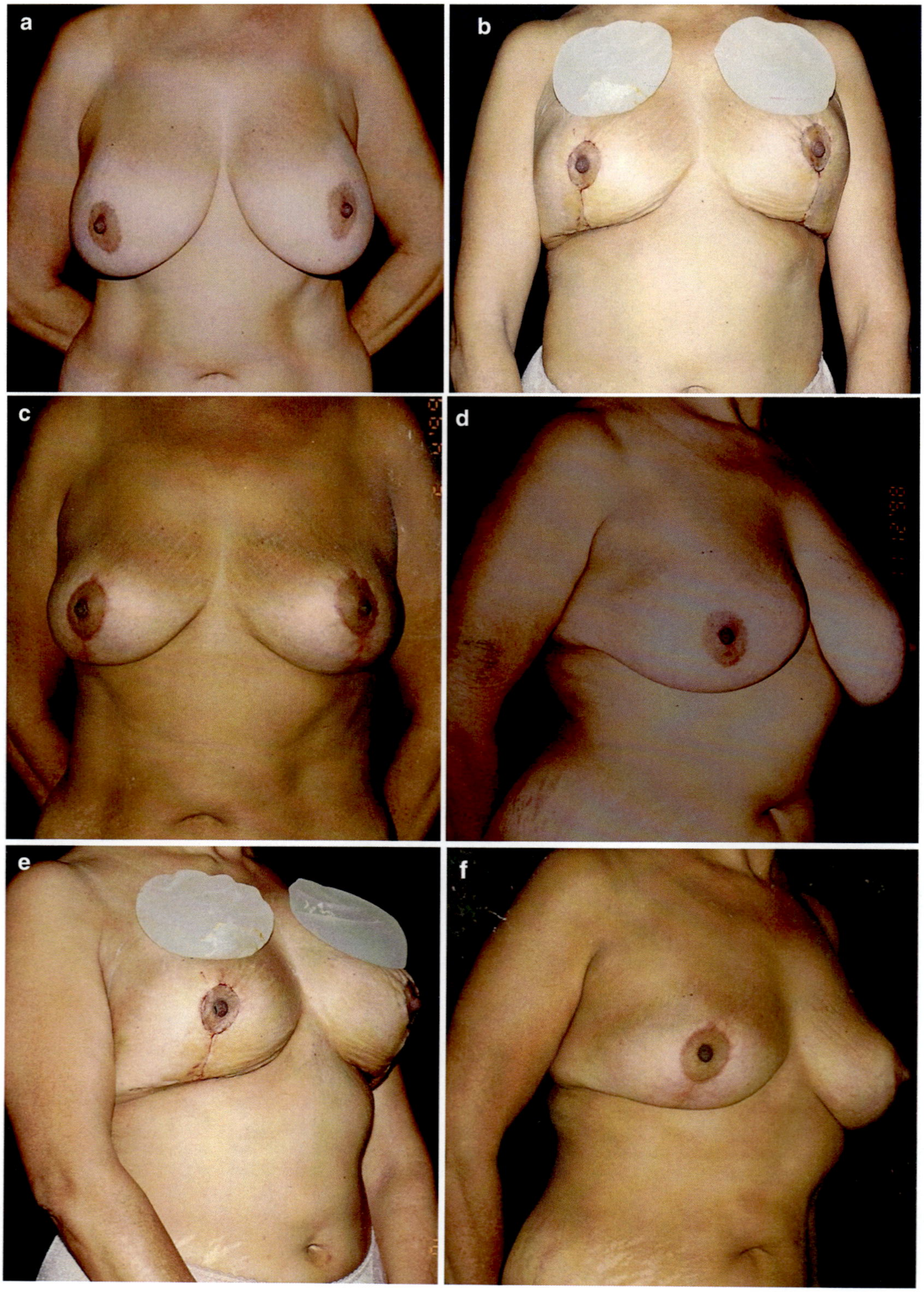

Fig. 60.15 A 59-year-old female presented large and ptotic breasts caused by silicone implant application done elsewhere about 20 years ago. (**a**, **d**) Preoperative views showing large and ptotic breasts. (**b**, **d**) Same patient 3 months after the operation for the removal of an implant followed by mastopexy. The removed implant of 300 mL on each side can be seen. (**c**, **f**) Same patient 1 year after mastopexy

Conclusions

Removal of breast implants is not a single procedure, as the rotation of the glandular flaps requires meticulous planning and an efficient operation. The final decision must include a good understanding between surgeon and patient. The operation is aesthetic one, but with components of reconstruction owing to the reorganization of the mammary gland after suture. The patient's problem is due to an imbalance between the size of the implant and the size of the breast. For this reason, it is necessary to have a good relationship between content and container.

References

Avelar JM (1980) Retalho dermo-adiposo-glandular superior nas ptoses mamárias. In: Simpósio Brasileiro de Cirurgia da Mama, São Paulo

Avelar JM (1986) Psychological profile of the patient—introducing to the subject (Perfil psicológico do paciente—introdução ao estudo). In: Avelar JM, Illouz YG (eds) Lipoaspiração (liposuction), vol 2. Hipócrates, São Paulo, pp 8–18

Avelar JM (1988) Abdominoplasty—reflections and biopsychological perspectives (abdominoplastia reflexões e perspectiva biopsicológicas). Rev Soc Bras Cir Plast 3(2):152–154

Avelar JM (1993) Augmentation mastoplasty—mastopexy versus silicone inclusion (mastoplastia de aumento—mastopexia X Inclusão de silicone). In: Avelar JM (ed) Loco-regional anesthesia on aesthetic surgery (anestesia loco-regional em cirurgia estética), vol 33. Hipócrates, São Paulo, pp 284–300

Broadbent TR, Woolf RM (1978) Unsatisfactory results in augmentation mammaplasty—chest and breast asymmetry. Aesthet Plast Surg 2(3):251–269

Cronin TD, Gerow FJ (1963) Augmentation mammaplasty: a new "natural feel" prosthesis. In: 3rd International Congress Plastic Surgery, vol 20. Excerpta Medica, Amsterdam, pp 41–49

Maliniac J (1959) Harmful fallacies in mammaplasty. Abstract, International Congress of Plastic Surgery, London

May H (1943) Reconstruction of breast deformities. Surg Gynecol Obstet 77:523

Noel A (1933) Refection plastique du mamelon apres necrose survenue a la suite d'une operation esthétique des seins. Le Bull Méd

Pitanguy I (1959) Breast hypertrophy. In: Wallace AB (ed) Transaction International Society of Plastic Surgeons, Second Congress. E&S Livingstone, Edinburgh and London, pp 509–517

Pitanguy I, Garcia LC (1972) Important aspects of the personal technique of mammaplasty (aspectos importantes da tecnica pessoal em mammaplastia). Bol Soc Cir Plast Reconstr 4:7

Schwarzmann E (1930) Die Technik der Mammaplastik. Chirurg 2:932–943

Index

J.M. Avelar (ed.), *Breast Surgery*, https://doi.org/10.1007/978-3-319-54115-0

FSC
www.fsc.org
MIX
Papier | Fördert gute Waldnutzung
FSC® C083411

Kolibri 360 GmbH
Ferdinand-Jühlke-Straße 7
99095 Erfurt, Deutschland
produktsicherheit@kolibri360.de